LOW
BACK
PAIN

MEDICAL DIAGNOSIS AND
COMPREHENSIVE
MANAGEMENT

LOW BACK PAIN

MEDICAL DIAGNOSIS AND COMPREHENSIVE MANAGEMENT

DAVID G. BORENSTEIN, M.D.

Professor of Medicine
Medical Director
The Spine Center
Associate Director for Education and Research
Division of Rheumatology
The George Washington University Medical Center
Washington, D.C.

SAM W. WIESEL, M.D.

Professor and Chairman
Department of Orthopaedic Surgery
Georgetown University School of Medicine
Washington, D.C.

SCOTT D. BODEN, M.D.

Assistant Professor of Orthopaedics
Director, The Emory Spine Center
Emory University School of Medicine
Atlanta, Georgia

W.B. SAUNDERS COMPANY
A Division of Harcourt Brace & Company
Philadelphia, London, Toronto, Montreal, Sydney, Tokyo

W.B. SAUNDERS COMPANY

A Division of
Harcourt Brace & Company

The Curtis Center
Independence Square West
Philadelphia, Pennsylvania 19106

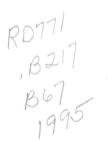

Library of Congress Cataloging-in-Publication Data

Borenstein, David G.

Low back pain : medical diagnosis and comprehensive management / David G. Borenstein, Sam W. Wiesel,
Scott D. Boden.—2nd ed.

p.   cm.

Includes bibliographical references and index.

ISBN 0–7216–5411–8

1. Backache.   2. Lumbar vertebrae—Diseases.   3. Sacrum—Diseases.   I. Wiesel, Sam W.
  II. Boden, Scott D.   III. Title.   [DNLM: 1. Low Back Pain—diagnosis.   2. Low Back Pain—
  therapy.   3. Spinal Diseases.   4. Lumbar Vertebrae.   WE 755 B731L 1995]

RD771.B217B67 1995   617.5′64—dc20

DNLM/DLC   93–41601

LOW BACK PAIN: Medical Diagnosis and   ISBN   0–7216–5411–8
               Comprehensive Management

Printed in the United States of America.

Last digit is the print number: 9   8   7   6   5   4   3   2   1

For the sacrifice of effort and resources of my parents so that I could attend medical school

and

For the inspiration of my brother to become a physician

This book is dedicated to Murray and Mollie Borenstein, and Alan Borenstein, M.D.

For a good man and one who will help a good friend in need at any time, my brother, Bert H. Wiesel, Jr.

To my family, especially my parents, without whose support and encouragement, I could not have become a physician, I dedicate this book to Herbert and Claire Boden

ACKNOWLEDGMENTS

The authors would like to recognize all those individuals who have supplied support, encouragement, constructive criticism, and expertise.

Members of the George Washington University medical community have been essential for the development and completion of this book. They have included the professional and support staff of the Division of Rheumatology: Arnold M. Schwartz, M.D., Associate Professor of Pathology; William M. Steinberg, M.D., Professor of Medicine; Joseph M. Giordano, M.D., Professor of Surgery; David O. Davis, M.D., Professor of Radiology; Edward M. Druy, M.D., Professor of Radiology; Michael C. Hill, M.D., Professor of Radiology; Stanley C. Marinoff, M.D., Clinical Professor of Obstetrics and Gynecology; Arnold M. Kwart, M.D., Clinical Professor of Urology; Randall J. Lewis, M.D., Associate Clinical Professor of Orthopaedic Surgery; Patience H. White, M.D., Professor of Medicine; Werner Barth, M.D., Professor of Medicine; Ace Lipson, M.D., Associate Clinical Professor of Medicine; Rhea Jett, Word Processing Specialist; Robert Irving, Photographer; and Judith Guenther, Medical Illustrationist; and Thomas Welsh, Chief Physical Therapist, Georgetown University Hospital.

Individuals at other institutions have also been willing to share their expertise, patient histories, or radiographs when requested, and their kindness is greatly appreciated: Anne Brower, M.D., Professor and Chairperson of Radiology, Eastern Virginia Medical School (Author of *Arthritis in Black and White*); David Caldwell, M.D., Associate Professor of Medicine, Duke University Medical Center; Peter M. Levitin, M.D., Private Rheumatologist, Tannenbaum Medical Associates, Greensboro, North Carolina; Eric Gall, M.D., Professor of Medicine, University of Arizona Health Science Center; Alan Borenstein, M.D., Private Neurologist, Florida Medical Center, Ft. Lauderdale, Florida; and Theodor Schifter, M.D., Rheumatologist, Ramat-Gan, Israel.

For the second edition, we wish to thank Thomas S. Dina, M.D., Associate Professor of Radiology and William O. Bank, M.D. Professor of Radiology, The George Washington University Medical Center.

We wish to acknowledge the constructive criticism of the editorial and production staff of W. B. Saunders Company including Kimberly Kist, Lorraine Kilmer, Frank Polizzano, Agnes Byrne, and Nancy Matthews.

FOREWORD

Drs. Borenstein, Wiesel and Boden are to be highly commended for both conceiving and then organizing and writing this important book on the diagnosis and management of low back pain. The text fills a great need in providing detailed information for physicians on how to evaluate thoroughly patients presenting, in many different ways, with low back pain.

Low back pain is a major national problem. At some point in our lives, four of five Americans are affected with the painful and disabling disorder of low back pain. It involves people of all ages. According to national health surveys, back pain is the leading cause of limitation of activity in young persons between 17 and 44 years of age in the United States.

Low back pain, we now know today, is neither a single disorder nor simply due to a straightforward mechanical derangement as it was often previously held to be. Rather, it is a complex topic involving many structures in this region of the body and caused by a very large number of diverse diseases and conditions. These have been magnificently catalogued and thoroughly described as the largest component of this textbook. Each of these diseases causing low pain is systematically discussed in full with appropriate sections such as Clinical History, Laboratory Data, and Therapy. A more than adequate list of references appears at the end of each disease section. As a result, the book serves as a highly valuable reference text for physicians, as the authors had intended. A special feature for the busy practitioner (are there other kinds?) is a capable summary placed strategically at the very front of each disease description. Another inventive special feature for the even busier practitioner is an appendix that tabulates the special features of each disease/condition that is described in the body of the text.

The "expert" (specialized) care, referred or primary, in the past has been assumed by the surgeon, orthopaedic or neurologic; osteopathic or chiropractic physician; or physical therapist. There is now a new cadre of medical specialists (such as internists, rheumatologists) who are developing expertise in the diagnosis and care of patients with low back pain. This excellent and much needed volume reflects this new expertise. The volume is appropriately subtitled "Medical Diagnosis and Comprehensive Management"; these are the essential characteristics of the authors' contributions to professional education and clinical guidance for this important health problem. The various surgical approaches to the management of back pain are concisely described; and the book concludes with a fitting description of the multidisciplinary approach to the management of chronic back pain.

We are grateful to Drs. Borenstein, Wiesel and Boden for providing physicians and other health professionals with a highly informative, eminently readable, and well-organized textbook on the important topic of low back pain, a major health problem in the Nation.

LAWRENCE E. SHULMAN, M.D., PH.D.
Director, National Institute of Arthritis and Musculoskeletal and Skin Diseases,
National Institutes of Health,
Bethesda, Maryland

PREFACE

Since the publication of the first edition of *Low Back Pain: Medical Diagnosis and Comprehensive Management*, significant progress has been made in the evaluation and treatment of low back pain patients. Advances in radiographic technology have allowed for anatomic identification of abnormalities in the lumbar spine that previously required invasive techniques. While technology has changed, the appropriate place of diagnostic tests in the evaluation of low back pain patients has not. Diagnostic tests remain confirmatory for the impressions developed during the evaluation of a patient's history and physical examination. In a time of diminishing financial resources, the appropriate selection of diagnostic tests and therapeutic interventions is essential. Expensive tests should be limited to those individuals in whom the results of the tests will necessitate specific therapeutic interventions. Surgery must be reserved for those individuals who have failed appropriate nonoperative therapy and have a disorder that is correctable with an invasive procedure. We believe that the revised algorithm in this volume offers practicing physicians guidance in obtaining appropriate diagnostic tests in a timely manner and selecting patients who are good surgical candidates.

The dual role of this book remains the same. *Low Back Pain: Medical Diagnosis and Comprehensive Management* is a practical guide to the diagnosis and management of low back pain patients. This text is also a reference book for the 70 or more disorders associated with the symptom of low back pain. We hope that practicing physicians will find its guidance useful in both roles.

The publication of a book is like the birth and development of a child. The idea for a book is conceived and nurtured for a number of months before it is presented to the public. One never knows how an offspring will be judged by the public. Will your offspring be deemed worthy so that a second effort is warranted? We would like to thank those individuals who read our first edition and complimented us on our effort. Your good wishes and constructive criticism resulted in our producing an updated version. Dr. Scott Boden has joined us in revising this new edition. Dr. Boden has published a number of articles in the area of low back pain and brings another perspective to the diagnosis and management of low back pain patients. We hope that this second edition also will be helpful to those physicians who found the first edition useful in the care of their patients with low back pain.

DAVID BORENSTEIN, M.D.
SAM W. WIESEL, M.D.
SCOTT D. BODEN, M.D.

CONTENTS

11
Rheumatologic Disorders of the Lumbosacral Spine

12
Infections of the Lumbosacral Spine

13
Tumors and Infiltrative Lesions of the Lumbosacral Spine

14
Endocrinologic and Metabolic Disorders of the Lumbosacral Spine

ANATOMY AND PHYSIOLOGY OF BACK PAIN

Anatomy and Biomechanics
of the Lumbosacral Spine

The structure of the lumbosacral spine is complex. To diagnose and treat this area effectively, one must have a clear knowledge of the normal anatomy. The purpose of this chapter is to present a working description of the anatomy and biomechanics of the lumbosacral spine. This information will provide a keystone from which to build as the various pathologic entities affecting the lumbosacral spine are discussed.

LUMBAR VERTEBRAE

The lumbar spine is composed of five vertebrae. Each vertebra consists of a body anteriorly and a neural arch posteriorly that encloses the vertebral canal (Fig. 1–1). The spinal cord and cauda equina pass through and are protected by the structures surrounding the vertebral canal.[1] The neural arch has two pedicles on its sides and a lamina posteriorly (Fig. 1–1). A spinous process projects posteriorly from the lamina in the midline and is usually palpable through the skin. A transverse process projects laterally from each side at the junction of the pedicle and lamina (Figs. 1–2 and 1–3).

The body of each vertebra has a dense bony cortex surrounding spongy medullary bone. The cortices of the inferior and superior aspects of the body are called the vertebral endplates. The endplate which is thicker in its center is covered by a cartilaginous plate. The periphery of the endplate is thickened to form a distinct rim that is derived from the epiphys-

eal plate and becomes fused to the body at 15 years of age. The trabecular pattern of the spongy bone in the interior of the vertebral body follows the lines of force placed on the bone. In the frontal plane, vertical lines link the superior and inferior surfaces; horizontal lines, the lateral surfaces; and oblique lines, the inferior surface with the lateral surfaces. In the sagittal plane, the trabeculae follow a fan-like arrangement. The first arrangement transfers force from the superior surface to the two pedicles, superior articular surfaces, and spinous process. The second transfers force from the inferior surface to the inferior articular surfaces and spinous process. The overlapping trabecular pattern leaves an area in the anterior portion of the vertebral body with a lesser number of trabeculae. This area of the vertebral body fractures at 75% of the force needed to fracture the posterior portion of the vertebral body (Fig. 1–4).

The facet joints are composed of articular processes arising from adjacent vertebrae. The articular processes project superiorly and inferiorly from the junction of the pedicles and the laminae. They form true synovial joints with synovial fluid (one superior process from below with one inferior process from above), and their purpose is to stabilize the motion between two vertebrae with respect to both translation and torsion while allowing sagittal plane flexion and extension. Each joint is enclosed in a fibrous capsule. The zygapophyseal or facet joints contain menisci that are rudimentary invaginations of the joint capsule that project into the joint space.[2] The menisci function as fillers that provide stability and distribute loads over greater articular areas. The me-

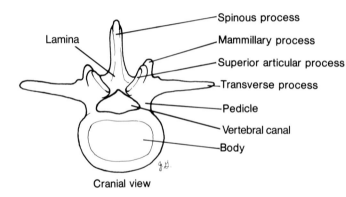

Lamina

Spinous process

Mammillary process

Superior articular process

Transverse process

Pedicle

Vertebral canal

Body

Cranial view

Figure 1–1. Cranial view of a typical lumbar vertebra.

Figure 1–2. Posterior view of a typical lumbar vertebra.

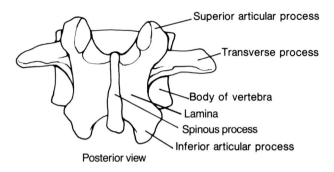

Superior articular process

Transverse process

Body of vertebra

Lamina

Spinous process

Inferior articular process

Posterior view

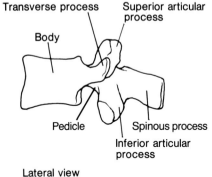

Transverse process

Superior articular process

Body

Pedicle

Spinous process

Inferior articular process

Lateral view

Figure 1–3. Lateral view of a typical lumbar vertebra.

Figure 1–4. Lines of force in the interior of a vertebral body. *A,* Lines attaching vertebral endplates. *B,* Lines attaching the superior endplate with the pedicles, superior articular surface, and spinous process. *C,* Lines attaching the inferior endplate with inferior articular surface and spinous process. *D, Arrow* points to the weakest area of a vertebral body, a common location for vertebral fractures.

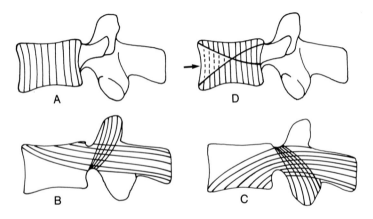

A

D

B

C

nisci are rarely entrapped between the articular cartilage.

Nerve roots exit from the spinal canal through the intervertebral foramina. Each foramen is bordered by pedicles inferiorly and superiorly. Anteriorly, the foramen is bordered by the intervertebral disc and vertebral body, and posteriorly by the lamina as well as the anterior aspect of the facet joint and its capsule. The intervertebral foramina are longer in their vertical dimension than in their horizontal with the largest cross-sectional area at the L1-L2 foramen and the smallest at the L5-S1 foramen.

Since the spinal cord ends at the L1 level, the course of the exiting nerve roots becomes longer and more obliquely directed as they approach the lower segments (Fig. 1–5). Therefore, in the lumbar region, the nerve roots are located in the superior aspect of the foramen. The exiting nerve roots cross the disc immediately above the foramen from which they exit (Fig. 1–6). For example, the L4 nerve root crosses the L3-L4 foramen and then exits the foramen formed by the L4 and L5 vertebral bodies. The nerve leaves the foramen in a

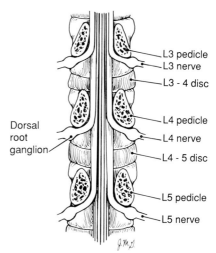

Figure 1–6. A coronal schematic view of the exiting lumbar spinal nerve roots. Note the exiting root takes the name of the vertebral body pedicle under which it travels into the neural foramen. It is also evident why L4-L5 disc pathology generally affects the L5 root rather than the L4 root which has already exited.

downward, anterolateral direction. At the lateral extent of the foramen, the dorsal root ganglion and anterior ramus have not yet joined to form the spinal nerve. The spinal nerve forms just lateral to the foramen. The dorsal (sensory) root is twice the thickness of the anterior (motor) root. The motor root is located anteriorly and inferiorly in the foramen. The nerve roots are covered by both arachnoid and dura. The arachnoid covers the nerve roots to the level of the dorsal root ganglion. The outer dura covers the roots through the foramen and continues along the spinal nerves as the perineurium. Within the foramen, the nerve and its sheath occupy 35% to 40% of the area. The largest of the lumbar spinal nerves is L5 which is housed in the smallest lumbar foramen. Consequently, the L5 spinal nerve is most vulnerable to compression by foraminal structures. Connective tissue, ligamentum flavum, arteries, veins, lymphatics, and the sinuvertebral nerve fill the remaining space (Fig. 1–7).[3]

The spinal canal in cross-section is surrounded by the neural arch posteriorly and the posterior surface of the vertebral body anteriorly. The canal itself is triangular in shape with an anterior base. It progressively widens from L1 to the sacrum. However, the lateral angles of the triangle are smaller in the fourth and fifth lumbar vertebral bodies. These are locations of potential nerve impingement. The lumbosacral area of the spinal canal contains the cauda equina. The true spinal cord termi-

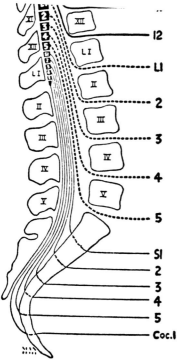

Figure 1–5. A lateral schematic of the spine showing the relationship of the conus medullaris to L1 and L2, and the relationship of the individual spinal nerves to each of the vertebral bodies at skeletal maturity. (From Haymaker W, Woodhall B: Peripheral Nerve Injuries. 2nd ed. Philadelphia: W B Saunders Co, 1953.)

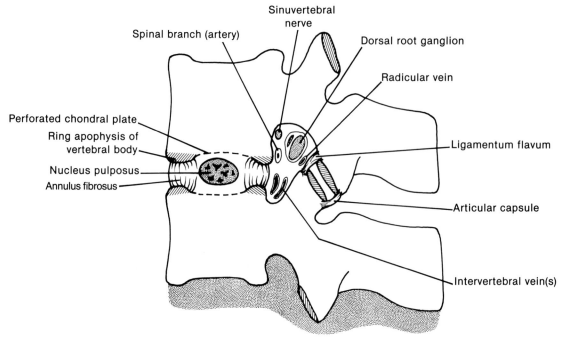

Figure 1-7. Schematic of a sagittal section of the spine showing contents of an intervertebral foramen in relation to a disc. The two vertebral bodies and intervertebral disc along with supporting structures constitute a motor unit, which includes all components of a somite present in an embryo.

nates with the conus medullaris approximately at the level of the inferior margin of the first lumbar vertebra.

SACRUM AND COCCYX

The sacrum is a large triangular bone (Figs. 1–8 and 1–9). It is composed of five fused vertebrae and is inserted like a wedge between the two pelvic bones. The sacral and iliac sides of the sacroiliac amphiarthrodial joint are covered with thicker hyaline cartilage (1–3 mm) and thinner fibrocartilage (1 mm), respectively (Fig. 1–10).[2] The ventral, or anterior, portion of the joint is lined by synovial membrane, which produces a small amount of synovial fluid. The dorsal, or posterior, portion of the joint does not contain synovial tissue and is joined by fibrous attachments (Fig. 1–11). The most common segments articulating

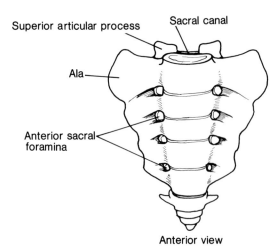

Anterior view
Figure 1-8. Anterior view of the sacrum and coccyx.

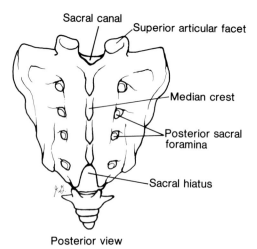

Posterior view
Figure 1-9. Posterior view of the sacrum and coccyx.

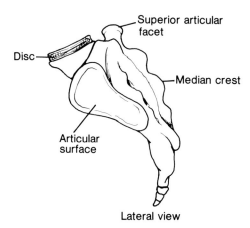

Figure 1–10. Lateral view showing the articular surface of the sacrum.

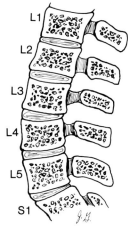

Figure 1–12. Lateral view of the lumbar spine including the lumbosacral articulation at the L5-S1 interspace.

with the ilium include S1, S2, and S3. Occasionally, L5 may be an articulating segment, while S4 and L4 are rarely involved. Usually fewer sacral segments are involved in the female pelvis than in the male pelvis. There is a wedge-shaped intervertebral disc interposed between the base of the sacrum and the last lumbar vertebrae (lumbosacral disc) (Fig. 1–12). The spinal canal continues into the sacrum and the sacral nerves exit through bony foramina situated both anteriorly and posteriorly.

The coccyx, which is often referred to as the tail bone, is made up of four tiny fused vertebrae. It is connected to the inferior end of the sacrum and is solid. There is no spinal canal in the coccyx.

INTERVERTEBRAL DISCS

The intervertebral discs (Fig. 1–13) are the major structural link between adjacent vertebrae. Together they make up 33% of the

height of the lumbar spine.[3] They function as universal joints, permitting far greater motion between vertebral bodies than if the vertebral bones were in direct contact with each other.

Each intervertebral disc is made up of a gelatinous nucleus pulposus surrounded by a laminated, fibrous annulus fibrosus. Each disc is situated between the cartilaginous endplates of vertebrae above and below.

The nucleus pulposus is posterocentrally situated within the disc and consists of collagen fibrils enmeshed in a mucoprotein gel (see Fig. 1–13). The nucleus pulposus occupies about 40% of the disc's cross-sectional area. It has a high water content at birth (88%), which mechanically lets it absorb quite a bit of stress.[4–5] However, with age the percentage of water decreases reflecting both an absolute decrease in available proteoglycans and a change in the ratio of the different proteoglycans present. This desiccation (loss of water) reduces the ability of the nucleus pulposus to function as a gel and withstand stress.

The annulus fibrosus forms the outer boundary of the disc.[6] It is composed of fibrocartilaginous tissue and fibrous protein arranged in concentric layers or lamellae that run obliquely from one vertebra to another. Successive layers of these fibers slant in alternate directions so that they cross each other at different angles which vary with the intradiscal pressure of the nucleus pulposus. Thus, the annulus fibrosus can absorb stress by expanding and contracting like a Japanese finger trap. Its peripheral fibers pass over the edge of the cartilaginous endplate to unite with the bone of each vertebral body. The most superficial fibers blend with the anterior and posterior

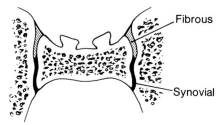

Figure 1–11. Transverse view of the sacroiliac joint. The anterior portion of the joint is lined by synovial tissue. The posterior portion is joined by fibrous tissue.

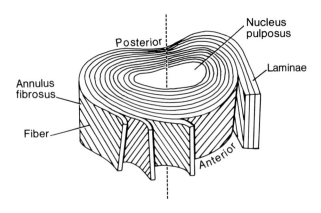

Figure 1–13. The intervertebral disc. The outer portion, the annulus fibrosus, is composed of 90 sheets of laminated collagen fibers which are oriented vertically in the peripheral layers and more obliquely in the central layers. Successive laminae run at angles to each other.

longitudinal ligaments. With age, the annulus fibrosus fibers deteriorate, become fissured, and lose their capacity to contain the nucleus pulposus. If there is sufficient internal stress, the nucleus pulposus material can penetrate through the annulus, and the resulting injury is termed a herniated disc.

LIGAMENTS OF THE LUMBAR VERTEBRAL COLUMN

The vertebral bodies are bordered front and back by two major ligaments.[7] The anterior longitudinal ligament is a broad, strong band of fibers extending along the front and sides of the vertebral bodies (Fig. 1–14). Its deepest fibers blend with the intervertebral discs and are firmly bound to each successive vertebral body. The ligament increases in thickness to fill the concavities formed by the configuration of the vertebral body.

The posterior longitudinal ligament extends along the posterior surface of the vertebral bodies (Fig. 1–15). It forms the anterior boundary of the spinal canal. In the lumbar canal, it becomes narrow as it passes over each vertebral body and then expands laterally as it passes over each disc. It thus takes on the configuration of a series of hourglasses, with the attenuated lateral expansions over the intervertebral discs being the weakest and most vulnerable to disc herniation. The posterior longitudinal ligament starts to narrow at the first lumbar level (L1) and becomes one half its original width at the fifth lumbar (L5)–first sacral (S1) interspace. A third ligament, the lateral vertebral ligament, lies between the anterior and posterior ligaments and passes from one vertebral body to the next, firmly adhering to the intervertebral disc.

The ligamenta flava run posteriorly between adjacent laminae (Fig. 1–16). These yellow, elastic ligaments extend from the base of the articular processes on one side to those on the opposite side, as well as laterally into the intervertebral foramina. They are attached inferiorly to the superior edges and posterosuperior surfaces of the laminae and superiorly to the inferior and anteroinferior surfaces of the laminae. This unique arrangement, combined

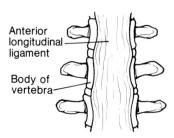

Figure 1–14. Anterior view of the lumbar spine. The anterior longitudinal ligament covers the anterior surface of the vertebral bodies and meshes with the anterior fibers of the annulus fibrosus.

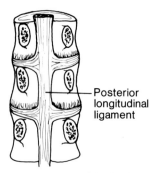

Figure 1–15. Posterior view of the lumbar vertebrae. The posterior longitudinal ligament expands laterally to cover the intervertebral discs. The posterior longitudinal ligament is weakest in this location.

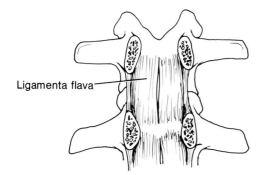

Figure 1–16. The ligamenta flava attach to the anterior surface of the lamina above and extend to the posterior surface of the upper margin of the lamina below.

with the anterior tilt of the laminae and elastic properties of the ligament that resist buckling, has the effect of creating an extremely smooth posteroinferior wall that remains smooth and protects the neural elements in spite of whatever position into which the spine is bent or twisted.

In the posterior portion of the vertebrae, the intervertebral joints are strengthened by a series of ligaments that lie between adjacent transverse spinous processes (intertransverse ligaments) and spinous processes (interspinous and supraspinous ligaments) (Fig. 1–17). In the lumbar region, the supraspinous ligament is indistinct as it merges with the insertion of the lumbodorsal muscles. These ligaments help reduce the anterior force (shear) placed on the lumbar spine because of the lordotic curve and the lumbosacral angle. Iliolumbar ligaments that attach to the transverse processes connect the lower two lumbar vertebrae to the iliac crest, limiting the movement of the sacroiliac joint. During lateral flexion, the contralateral iliolumbar ligaments become taut, allowing on average only 8° of movement

of L4 relative to the sacrum. Flexion and extension of the lumbar spine is also limited but to a lesser degree than lateral flexion.

The stability of the sacroiliac joint is dependent not only on the interdigitation of the articular surfaces of the ilium and sacrum but also on the several large accessory ligaments surrounding the joint. Ligaments attach the sacrum and ilium (anterior sacroiliac, posterior sacroiliac, and interosseous sacroiliac) and the sacrum and ischium (sacrotuberous and sacrospinous) (Fig. 1–18). The relative strength of the ligaments is different between the sexes. After puberty, in contrast to the increasing strength of the ligaments in the male, the strength of the ligaments is sacrificed in the female for increased mobility, particularly during pregnancy and labor.

BLOOD SUPPLY OF THE LUMBAR SPINE

The lumbar spine's blood supply arises directly from the aorta.[7] There are four paired lumbar arteries that arise directly from the posterior aspect of the aorta in front of the bodies of the first four lumbar vertebrae. In front of L5, a fifth pair may come off the middle sacral artery. These vessels (Fig. 1–19) curve posteriorly around the bodies of the vertebrae and give off posterior rami as they pass between the transverse processes. These posterior rami, in turn, furnish the vertebral or spinal branches, which supply the bodies of the vertebrae and their ligaments. The sacrum is supplied by medial branches of the superior gluteal or hypogastric arteries. The arteries follow the contour of the sacrum and send branches to each anterior sacral foramen. The arteries supply the sacral canal and exit the

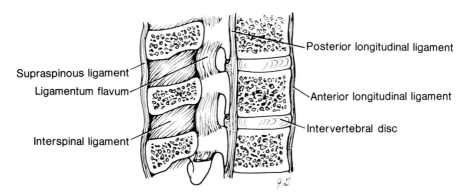

Figure 1–17. Lateral view of the lumbar spine demonstrating the ligaments that support the anterior (anterior longitudinal, posterior longitudinal) and the posterior (supraspinous, intraspinous) elements of the vertebrae. Note the position of the ligamentum flavum forming a smooth posterior wall of the neural foramen.

Anterior view   Posterior view

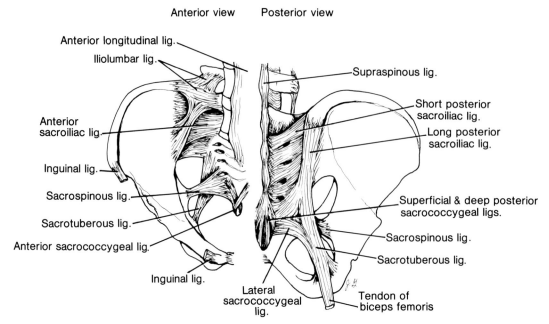

Figure 1–18. Anterior and posterior views of the sacroiliac joint ligaments. The anterior and posterior ligamentous attachments are very strong. Disruption of these attachments usually occurs only with severe trauma to the pelvis.

posterior sacral foramen to supply the lower back muscles.

The venous supply to the lumbar spine mirrors the arterial supply. The venous system is valveless, draining the internal and external venous systems into the inferior vena cava. The venous system is arranged in an anterior and posterior ladder-like configuration with multiple cross-connections (Fig. 1–20). The functional result of this extensively anastomotic, valveless system is the constant shifting of blood from larger to smaller vessels and vice versa depending on the degree of intra-abdominal pressure. Batson described retrograde venous flow from the lower pelvic organs to the lumbosacral spine.[8] He claimed that these venous connections provide the route for metastases to spread from pelvic neoplasms (prostate) to the spine.

During the adult phase of life, there is no active blood supply to the intervertebral discs. Although up to 8 years of age, there are small vessels supplying the discs, which are gradually obliterated during the first three decades of life. By the time growth has stopped, the nucleus pulposus and annulus fibrosus no longer have an active blood supply and receive only marginal sustenance from the transfer of tissue fluid across the cartilaginous endplates.

MUSCLES AND FASCIA OF THE LUMBOSACRAL SPINE

The most superficial layer of tissue below the subcutaneous tissue contains the lumbodorsal fascia (Fig. 1–21). Medially it attaches to the dorsal spinous processes, inferiorly it attaches to the iliac crest and lateral crest of the sacrum, laterally it serves as the origin of the latissimus dorsi and transversus abdominis muscle, and superiorly it attaches to the angles of the ribs in the thoracic region. It also surrounds the sacrospinalis muscles. Below the fascia lie superficial multisegmental muscles, collectively named the erector spinae muscle. Its origin is a thick tendon attached to the posterior aspect of the sacrum, iliac crest, lumbar spinous processes, and supraspinous ligament. The muscle fibers split into three columns at the level of the lumbar spine: the lateral iliocostalis (insertion—angles of ribs), the intermediate longissimus (insertion—transverse processes of the lumbar and thoracic vertebrae), and the more medial spinalis (insertion—posterior spines) (Fig. 1–22). The muscle also is divided into distinct thoracic and lumbar portions.[11] The thoracic portions consist of tiny muscles with segmental origins from the thorax and the erector spinae apo-

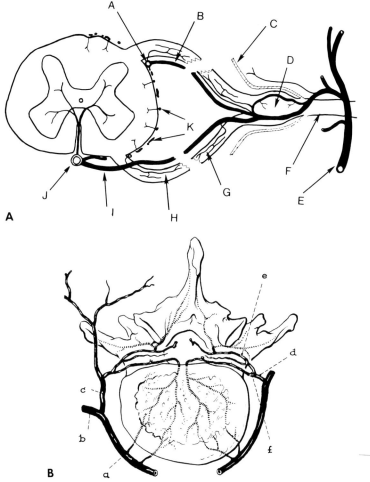

Figure 1–19. Arterial system of the lumbosacral spine. *A,* A schema illustrating all of the possible vascular relations of the spinal roots in which both medullary and radicular arteries are present. The break in the roots indicates that the schema applies to either the short cervical roots or the long lumbosacral elements of the cauda equina. The dorsolateral spinal artery (A) receives the dorsal medullary artery (B) and directly supplies the dorsal proximal radicular artery. The anterior spinal artery (J) receives the ventral medullary artery (I) and supplies the ventral proximal radicular artery (H) through the vasa corona (K). The segmental artery (E) gives a spinal branch that accompanies the spinal nerve (F) through the intervertebral foramen to supply the plexus of the dorsal root ganglion (D), which gives origin to the proximal radicular arteries (G) and (when present) the medullary vessels. The dura (C) receives fine meningeal branches. Note that medullary arteries usually do not supply roots in mid-course. (From Parke W, Gammell K, Rothman R: Arterial vascularization of the cauda equina. J Bone Joint Surg 63A:53, 1981.) *B,* Diagram of the blood supply to a vertebra as seen from below and from behind with the laminae removed: (a) is a segmental (in this case a lumbar) artery; (b) is its ventral continuation; (c) is its dorsal branch; (d) is the spinal branch; and (e) and (f) are the spinal branch's dorsal and ventral twigs to tissue of the epidural space and to the vertebral column; the unlabeled middle twig is to the nerve roots, and at some levels, to the spinal cord. (From Hollinshead WH: Anatomy for Surgeons, Vol. 3. 3rd ed. Philadelphia: (Harper Medical) Lippincott, 1982.)

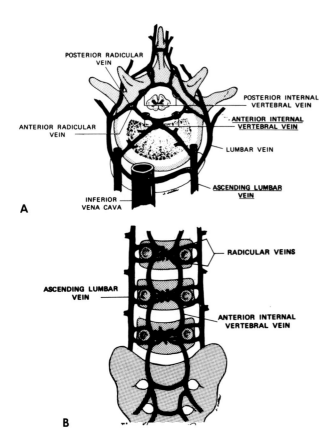

Figure 1–20. Venous system of the lumbosacral spine. (From Wiesel SW, Bernini P, Rothman RH: The Aging Lumbar Spine. Philadelphia: WB Saunders Co, 1982.)

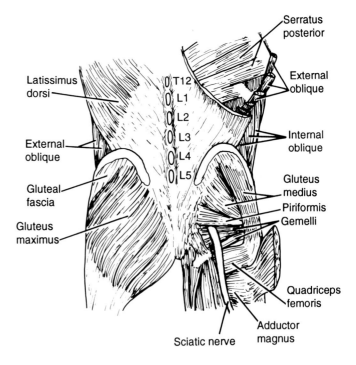

Figure 1–21. Posterior view of the superficial fascia and muscles of the lumbar spine and buttocks (left) and deeper posterior muscles of the lumbar spine and buttocks (right).

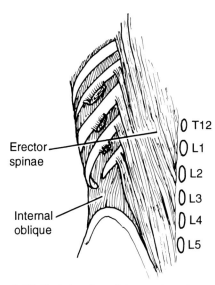

Figure 1–22. Posterior view of the erector spinae muscle, primary extensor muscle of the lumbar spine.

neurosis. The lumbar portions insert into the ilium and arise from the accessory processes of the vertebrae. The action of this group of muscles is to extend the spine and with unilateral action bend the spinal column to one side.

Deep to the erector spinae lie the transversospinal muscles including the multifidus and rotators. The multifidus originates from the posterior surface of the sacrum, aponeurosis of the sacrospinalis, posterior superior iliac spine, and posterior sacroiliac ligament and inserts two to four segments above their origin into spinous processes. The multifidus extends the spine and rotates it toward the opposite side. The rotators have similar attachments and action but ascend only one or two segments. Additional deep muscles include the interspinalis, connecting pairs of adjacent lumbar spinous processes, and the intertransversarii (medial, dorsal lateral, and ventral lateral groups), which connect pairs of adjacent transverse processes. They extend and bend the column to the same side, respectively.

The forward and lateral flexor muscles of the lumbar spine are located anterior and lateral to the vertebral bodies and transverse processes (Fig. 1–23). The iliopsoas consists of two separate muscular heads, the iliacus and psoas major. The origins of the psoas major arise from the intervertebral discs by five slips, each of which starts from adjacent upper and lower margins of two vertebrae, the transverse processes of the lumbar vertebrae, and membranous arches emanating from the bodies of the four upper lumbar vertebrae, permitting

the lumbar arteries and veins and sympathetic rami communicantes to pass beneath them. The iliacus arises from the iliac fossa and joins the psoas under the inguinal ligament, crosses the hip joint capsule, and inserts into the lesser trochanter of the femur. These muscles flex the lumbar spine and bend it toward the same side. The quadratus lumborum lies lateral to the vertebral column arising from the posterior part of the iliac crest and iliolumbar ligament and inserts into the twelfth rib and the tips of the transverse processes of the upper four lumbar vertebrae. This muscle fixes the twelfth rib down against traction exerted by the diaphragm during inspiration and bends the trunk toward the same side when acting alone.

Although not anatomically part of the low back, anterior abdominal muscles, such as the rectus abdominis, external abdominal oblique, internal abdominal oblique, transversalis (flexors of the lumbar spine), gluteal muscles (extensors of the hip and trunk), hamstrings (flexors of the knee), quadriceps (extensors of the knee), gastrocnemius, and soleus (plantar flexors of the foot), are important support structures of the lumbosacral spine. Abnormalities in these muscles (shortening, increased muscle tone) may result in abnormal kinetics of the lumbosacral spine and low back pain. The location and function of the lumbosacral and abdominal muscles that affect spinal motion are illustrated in Figure 1–24.

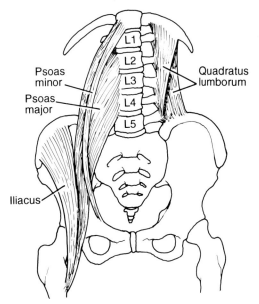

Figure 1–23. Anterior view of the intrinsic flexors of the lumbar spine. The quadratus lumborum contains two layers. The psoas major and iliacus muscles have a conjoined attachment on and around the lesser femoral trochanter.

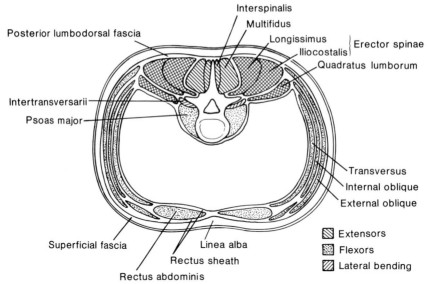

Figure 1–24. Cross-section of body musculature and fascia through the third lumbar vertebra. The primary motions of the lumbar spine are flexion, extension, and lateral bending. (Only a small proportion of rotation occurs in the lumbar spine.) Flexors are anterior to the spine and extensors are posterior. The muscles that cause lateral bending are contiguous to the vertebral bodies in a lateral position.

NERVE SUPPLY OF THE LUMBOSACRAL SPINE

A familiarity with the neuroanatomy of the lumbosacral spine is essential in understanding the pain patterns that are associated with disease processes affecting individual anatomic components of the low back.[7, 9–11] The sinuvertebral nerve is felt to be the major sensory nerve supplying the structures of the lumbar spine. It arises from its corresponding spinal nerve before it divides into posterior and anterior primary divisions. It is joined by a sympathetic branch from the ramus communicans and enters the spinal canal by way of the intervertebral foramen, curving upward around the base of the pedicle and proceeding toward the midline on the posterior longitudinal ligament (Fig. 1–25). The nerve divides into ascending, descending, and transverse branches, which anastomose with the contralateral side and sinuvertebral nerves at adjacent levels from above and below (Fig. 1–26). The sinuvertebral nerve innervates the posterior longitudinal ligament, the superficial layers of the annulus fibrosus, the blood vessels of the epidural space, the anterior but not the posterior dura mater (posterior dura is devoid of nerve endings), the dural sleeve surrounding the spinal nerve roots, and the posterior vertebral periosteum. The posterior longitudinal ligament is most heavily innervated while the anterior, sacroiliac, and interspinous ligaments

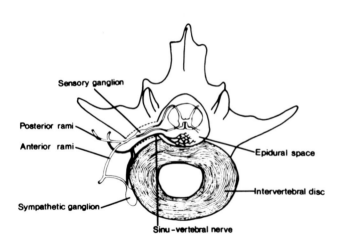

Figure 1–25. An axial view of the spine showing the sinuvertebral nerve. The nerve reenters the neural foramen from the spinal nerve to innervate the posterior longitudinal ligament. (From Wiesel SW, Bernini P, Rothman RH: The Aging Lumbar Spine. Philadelphia: WB Saunders Co, 1982.)

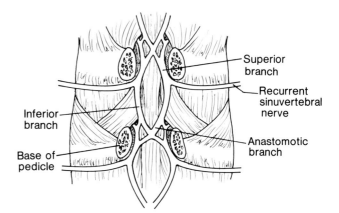

Figure 1–26. Branches of the recurrent sinuvertebral nerve anastomosing with nerve branches from above and below.

receive nociceptive (pain) nerve endings to a lesser degree.[12] The lumbar intervertebral discs are innervated posteriorly by the sinuvertebral nerves and laterally by branches of the ventral rami and grey rami cummunicantes.[13] Afferent sympathetic nerves may also supply the annulus fibrosus in the anterior portion of the intervertebral disc.[14]

The posterior primary rami arise from each corresponding spinal nerve and divide into medial and lateral branches. The medial (posterior) branch descends posteriorly at the back of the transverse and superior articular processes to supply sensory fibers to two facet joint levels. The sensory fibers supply the inferior portion of a posterior joint facet and the superior part of the joint capsule at the next lower level. Therefore, each facet joint is supplied by sensory nerves from spinal nerves from two different segments (Fig. 1–27). The medial branch continues caudally to supply innervation of dorsal muscles including the multifidus, intertransversarii mediales, interspinales, fascia, interspinous ligaments, blood vessels, and periosteum and anastomoses with sensory nerves from adjacent levels. The spinous processes and laminae are supplied by branches of the posterior primary rami (Fig. 1–28). The surface layer of the ligamentum flavum may receive sensory fibers from the posterior primary rami. The substance of the ligamentum flavum is not innervated. The interspinous and supraspinous ligaments are supplied by branches arising from nerves that innervate surrounding muscles. The lumbodorsal fascia receives sensory innervation from cutaneous nerves of the posterior primary rami that originate at one level cephalad to the lumbar level.

The lateral (anterior) branches of the posterior primary rami supply small branches to the sacrospinalis muscle and continue to innervate cutaneous structures in the lumbar area (Fig. 1–28). In the lumbar spine, only the posterior primary rami from the upper three lumbar levels supply cutaneous sensory nerves to the lumbar area. The cutaneous innervation may supply areas of skin as distal as the greater trochanter.

The nucleus pulposus of the intervertebral discs is devoid of any nerve endings. The posterior portion of the annulus fibrosus shares free nerve endings with the fibrous tissue that binds it to the posterior longitudinal ligament.

Figure 1–27. Lateral view of the posterior primary rami supplying facet joints at two vertebral levels.

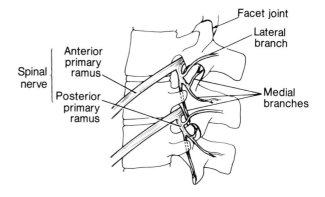

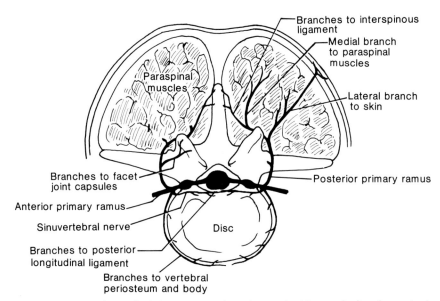

Figure 1–28. Cross-sectional view depicting nerve supply to the anterior (sinuvertebral) and posterior (posterior ramus) portions of the lumbar spine.

Lesions of the nucleus pulposus cause no pain. Only when the nerve fibers near the annulus are stimulated are nociceptive impulses transmitted to the spinal cord.

RETROPERITONEAL ABDOMINAL STRUCTURES NEIGHBORING THE LUMBOSACRAL SPINE AND SURFACE ANATOMY

Anterior to the lumbosacral spine are a number of organs that are retroperitoneal in location. These structures may be enveloped in their own fascia or may be partially covered by peritoneum. During the embryonic development of the abdominal cavity, some organs come to lie relatively immobile against one another or against the retroperitoneal organs of the posterior body wall. The abdominal organs that are located posteriorly include the middle portion of the duodenum and the ascending and descending colon. Other retroperitoneal structures include the kidneys, ureters, aorta, inferior vena cava, bile duct, pancreas, and periaortic lymph nodes. Inferior to the abdominal cavity is the pelvic cavity. The rectum is directly anterior to the sacrum and coccyx. The anatomic relationships of the retroperitoneal structures and lumbosacral spine are depicted in Figure 1–29. The pancreas and duodenum lie anterior to the L1 vertebral body. The kidneys are at the same level in a paraspinous location. They extend to the L3 level.

The ureters are also paraspinous in location, anterior to the aorta, running caudad to the bladder in the pelvis. The moveable portion of the sigmoid colon may reach the L1 vertebral level. The sigmoid colon enters the pelvis and is attached to the sacrum at the S2 level. The renal arteries take off from the aorta at the L1 level. The aorta branches into the common iliac arteries at the L4 vertebral body.

Superficial landmarks help localize portions of the lumbosacral spine. The L4 vertebral body is in the same plane as a line connecting the superior portions of the iliac crests. The junction of the lumbar spine with the sacrum is localized by the sacroiliac "dimples." On the anterior surface, in a patient without a panniculus, the umbilicus is situated anterior to the L5 vertebral body.

BIOMECHANICS OF THE LUMBOSACRAL SPINE

Familiarity with the anatomy of the lumbosacral spine helps identify those structures that are at risk of developing pain but is not adequate to explain all the mechanisms by which back pain develops. The normal function of the lumbosacral spine requires both great flexibility and strength. Recognition of deviations from normal function, such as hyperlordosis, helps explain the source of pain in those individuals who may not have specific anatomic abnormalities.

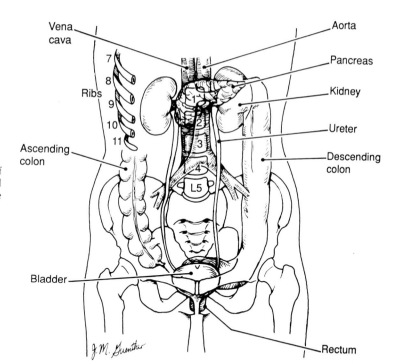

Figure 1–29. Diagrammatic view of the anatomic relationships of visceral organs in the retroperitoneum and the lumbosacral spine.

Better understanding of the biomechanics of back disorders has been garnered from laboratory studies of cadaveric spine segments. The whole vertebral column, cervical, thoracic, and lumbosacral components, supports man in a balanced, upright position while allowing locomotion. The mobility of the spine is correlated with its organization whereby multiple components (functional units) are superimposed on one another interlocked by ligaments and muscles that allow flexion and extension. Flexor and extensor muscles also play a role in maintaining the rigidity of the spine.

The function of the spine is divided between the anterior (static) and posterior (dynamic) portion of each functional unit. Each functional unit is composed of two vertebral bodies, an intervertebral disc anteriorly, and facet joints posteriorly. The anterior portion is a weight-bearing, shock-absorbing, flexible structure. The posterior portion protects the neural elements, acts as a fulcrum, and guides movement for the functional unit.

The intervertebral disc in the anterior portion of the functional unit gives the spine its flexibility. The disc is attached closely to the vertebral endplates. Between these endplates and the annulus fibrosus, the matrix (nucleus pulposus) of the disc is enclosed in a circle of unyielding tissues. Compressive pressure placed on the disc is dissipated circumferentially in a passive manner. In response to the greater axial forces exerted on the lumbar spine in comparison to the cervical and thoracic spines, the nucleus pulposus has its greatest surface area in the lumbar spine. The intervertebral disc is not the only structure that helps dissipate stresses placed on the spine. With flexion, extension, rotation, or shear stress, the load distribution on the functional unit is shared by the intervertebral disc, anterior and posterior longitudinal ligaments, the facet joints and capsules, and other ligamentous structures such as the ligamentum flavum and the interspinous and supraspinous ligaments that attach to the posterior elements of the functional unit. In addition, muscle attachments both intrinsic and extrinsic to the spine interact to accommodate the load-bearing requirements of the spine. The lower lumbar discs may need to bear a load of 1000 kilograms when stressed with pure compressive forces.[15] This degree of pressure generated by these compressive loads when progressively applied would fracture the vertebral endplates before herniating the nucleus pulposus. These fractures do not occur. The intrinsic muscles that help dissipate these compressive loads are the posterior segment muscles, which actively contract in response to load stresses. In addition, the excessive force is also borne by the abdominal muscles, which contract to increase intraabdominal pressure.

The degree of pressure on the intervertebral

disc varies depending on the position of the lumbar spine. Nachemson has recorded in vivo intradiscal pressures of volunteers in various positions, while exercising, and when wearing external supports (Fig. 1–30).[16] The load on a lumbar disc may vary from as little as 25 kilograms in the supine position to over 250 kilograms in the seated, forward flexed position.

The nucleus pulposus is spherical and acts like a ball between the two vertebral endplates. The nucleus acts like a "joint" from the standpoint of motion, allowing movement in many directions: flexion, extension, lateral flexion, rotation right and left, and gliding in the sagittal and frontal planes. The nucleus pulposus may be thought of as a flattened tennis ball, constantly placing tension on the surrounding annular fibers. Examination of the disc under tension reveals that it is strongest in its anterior and posterior regions and weakest in its center.

While the nucleus pulposus affords shock absorbency to the disc, the annulus fibrosus allows for flexibility of the functional unit. With compressive forces, the nucleus pulposus stretches the annular fibers. Flexion or extension of the functional unit occurs in part because of the horizontal shift of fluid within the disc, resulting in the expansion of the annular fibers posteriorly or anteriorly, respectively. The annular fibers tend to oppose the movement of the nucleus pulposus, thereby tending to restore the functional unit to its resting state. As the disc ages, the annular fibers are replaced with fibrous elements with less elastic

properties. The capability of the disc to recoil from compressive forces diminishes.

Resistance to stress by the vertebral column is further augmented by the vertebral ligaments. The ligaments run longitudinally along the anterior and posterior portion of the functional unit. The ligaments resist excessive movement in any direction and prevent any significant translational (shearing) action. Although the ligaments prevent excessive movement and support the annulus, they do not limit the normal motion and elasticity of the functional unit. Of pathologic importance is the narrowing of the posterior longitudinal ligament to half its original width at the lumbosacral interspace. The L5-S1 interspace undergoes the greatest static stress on the spine in general and the greatest movement of the lumbar spine, yet is also the segment with the least posterior ligamentous support.

The posterior portion of the functional unit is composed of the two vertebral arches, two transverse processes, a spinous process, and paired superior and inferior facet joints. The posterior elements share some of the compressive loads and influence the pattern of spine motion. In cadaveric lumbar spines, Adams and Hutton determined the mechanical function of the facet, or apophyseal, joints to be resistance to intervertebral shear forces and compression. Furthermore, the facet joints serve to prevent excessive motion from damaging the discs. In particular, the posterior annulus is protected in torsion by the lumbar facet surfaces and in flexion by the capsular ligaments of the facet joints.[13]

In the lumbar spine the facet joint planes of motion are vertical, permitting flexion and extension of the spine. In the neutral lordotic position, lateral or rotational movements are prevented owing to the apposition of the joint surfaces. In a slightly forward flexed position (decreased lordosis) the facet surfaces separate, allowing some lateral and rotatory movement. With extension, the facet surfaces approximate, preventing any lateral or oblique movement.

The surface area of the posterior elements plays an important physiologic role as the site of muscular attachments. The pattern of muscular origins and insertions provides balance for the segments of the lumbar spine while allowing wide ranges of motion. The maintenance of erect posture is in part achieved by the support derived from the ligamentous structures of the lumbar spine as well as the sustained, nonvoluntary tone generated by the surrounding lumbosacral muscles.

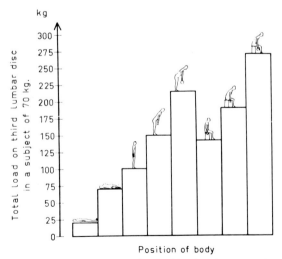

Figure 1–30. Total load on the third lumbar disc in a subject weighing 70 kg in a variety of positions. (From Nachemson AL: In vivo discometry in lumbar discs with irregular nucleograms. Acta Orthop Scand 36:426, 1965.)

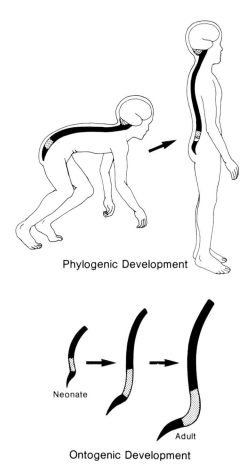

Phylogenic Development

Neonate

Adult

Ontogenic Development

Figure 1–31. The phylogenic development of the lumbar lordosis (walking on all fours to upright position) is recreated in the development of the neonate to an adult (ontogenic development).

To understand the function of the lumbosacral spine, it must be viewed in its relationship to the other components of the vertebral column. In the sagittal plane, the vertebral column shows four curvatures: cervical (concave posterior), thoracic (convex posterior), lumbar (concave posterior), and sacral (fixed and nonmobile). These curves developed during phylogeny (evolution) with the transition from the quadruped to the biped state. Initially, the spine was concave anteriorly. The lumbar spine first became straight, then inverted. The same changes are observed during ontogeny (development of the individual). On the first day of life, the lumbar spine is concave anteriorly. At 5 months of age, the lumbar spine is slightly concave anteriorly, and at 13 months the concavity disappears. From the age of 3 years onward, the lumbar lordosis begins to appear, assuming its definitive adult state at age 10 (Fig. 1–31). The curvature of the ver-

tebral column increases its resistance to axial compressive forces in comparison to the forces that could be sustained if the spine had remained with a completely straight orientation.

The entire spine with its three physiologic curves is balanced on the sacrum. The sacrum is part of the pelvis, which also includes the two iliac bones, the pubis and ischium. The two sacroiliac joints and symphysis pubis and the attached bones form a closed ring that transmits forces from the vertical column to the lower extremities. The weight supported by L5 is distributed equally into the pelvic wing, ischium, and acetabulum on both sides. Back pressure from the weight of the body against the ground is transmitted to the acetabulum by the head and neck of the femur. Stress placed on both pubic bones is counterbalanced across the symphysis pubis.

The sacrum and iliac bones move as one unit. The pelvis is balanced on a transverse axis between the hip joints, which allow rotatory motion in an anterior-posterior plane. The anterior portion of the pelvis can rotate upward, lowering the sacrum with a decrease in the lumbosacral angle. A downward movement of the front portion of the pelvis elevates the rear portion of the pelvis and sacrum and increases the lumbosacral angle. The lumbosacral angle is determined as the line drawn parallel to the superior border of the sacrum measured in relationship to a horizontal line (average 30°).

The balance of the spine is related to the reciprocal physiologic curves in the three areas of the vertebral column. The balance in curvature results in an individual's posture. The lumbosacral angle plays a significant role in determining posture and the degree of spinal curvature. With a decrease in the lumbosacral angle, the angle between the lumbar spine and sacrum is decreased (decreased or flattened lordosis). An increase in the lumbosacral angle results in an increased lumbar lordosis (Fig. 1–32). The change in angle will result in compensatory alterations in thoracic and cervical curves to maintain the head over the center of gravity. The shape of the lumbar lordosis is also influenced by the shape of the intervertebral discs, the supraspinous ligaments, the facet joints, the posterior erector muscles, and the traction of the hip flexors on the lumbar vertebral bodies.

An individual's posture is good if it can be maintained for extended periods of time in an effortless, nonfatiguing fashion. Maintenance of normal posture is essentially a ligamentous function relieved by intermittent small muscu-

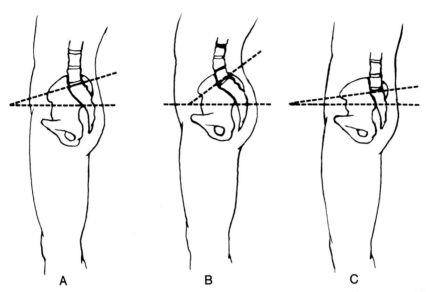

Figure 1–32. Lumbosacral angle: *A,* normal angle—normal lordosis; *B,* increased angle—increased lordosis; *C,* decreased angle—flattened lordosis.

lar contractions that are triggered by mechanoreceptors in the joints and ligaments.[14] Deviations from physiologic static spinal curves necessitate increased voluntary muscular action, which may result in fatigue, discomfort, and disability.

The proper alignment of posture requires the function of a number of structures in the lumbar spine, pelvis, and lower leg. Pelvic position is held in ligamentous balance by the anterior hip joint capsule and the iliopectineal ligament, which prevent hyperextension of the hip. The tensor fasciae latae also support the pelvis by limiting lateral shift. The tendency to increase the lumbosacral angle and increase the lumbar lordosis is also counterbalanced by the hamstrings and gluteus maximus, which decrease the lumbar lordosis.

The curvature of the lumbar spine tenses the anterior longitudinal ligament, which limits the degree of lordosis. Increased abdominal pressure generated by contracted abdominal muscles (rectus abdominis) also decreases the lumbar lordosis.

The knee joint is extended and locked during normal posture. The locking of the knee eliminates the need for muscular effort. The ankle cannot be locked in any position. Therefore, continued muscular effort from the gastrocnemius and soleus is needed to stabilize the foot.

In the resting static position, ligamentous, nonmuscular structures maintain posture. Rotation of the pelvis will uncouple the balance of the ligaments and joints and will necessitate the initiation of muscular effort.

The movements of the lumbar spine are flexion, extension, lateral bending, and rotation. The extent of motion in these planes is limited by the extensibility of the longitudinal ligaments, articular surface and capsule, fluidity of the disc, and pliability of the muscles. Extension of the lumbar spine has a range of 30° and is limited by the anterior longitudinal ligaments. Forward flexion has a lumbar range of 40°, which occurs to the greatest degree (75%) at the intervertebral space between L5 and S1. The remaining range of forward flexion is apportioned between the remainder of the lumbar vertebral interspaces. Lateral flexion is limited to 20 to 30°. The segmental range is maximal between L3 and L4 and is minimal between L5 and S1. The degree of lumbar rotation exclusive of thoracic rotation is difficult to determine. For the lumbar column as a whole, the range of rotation is estimated to be only 10°. Rotation is sharply limited by the orientation of the articular facet surfaces.

The movement of the lumbar spine is done in conjunction with other components of the spine and pelvis. The lumbar-pelvic rhythm is the simultaneous reversal of the lumbar lordosis and change in position of the pelvis. The lumbar component of the rhythm takes the lumbosacral spine from a concave, to flat, to convex configuration. During the progressional change, the pelvic component of the rhythm is rotating the pelvis around the transverse axis connecting the two hip joints, increasing the lumbar angle. In the normal individual, the rhythm is a smooth progression with equal alteration in lumbar reversal and pelvic rotation.

In forward flexion, the lumbar joints flex as the extensor muscles lower the torso. After 45° of flexion, the tension in the ligaments has increased and contraction in the paraspinal muscles has decreased.[17] As flexion continues, the pelvis rotates further by the relaxation of the hamstring and gluteus muscles. As the trunk is returned to the upright position, the order of muscle recruitment is reversed with initial contraction of the hamstrings, then the glutei, which rotate the pelvis to 45° of flexion, at which point the erector spinae muscles become active and return the torso to its fully upright position.

The flexion and extension of the lumbosacral spine is an unimpeded process when the various components of the spine and surrounding muscles are normal. The integrity of the discs must be intact to allow the migration of the nucleus pulposus in the annulus. Symmetric facet joints permit smooth flexion and extension. The supporting ligaments must not be too long or too short. The paraspinous and hip girdle muscles must have matching elasticity, strength, and flexibility. Normal motion also requires good hip joint function. In addition, lower leg function must be normal.

Abnormalities in any of these component parts will result in static and/or kinetic dysfunction. Understanding of normal function will pinpoint those factors that impede normal motion and identify those structures that cause low back pain.

References

1. Louis R: Surgery of the Spine. New York: Springer-Verlag, 1983, pp 32–42.
2. Bellamy N, Park W, Rooney PJ: What do we know about the sacroiliac joint? Semin Arthritis Rheum 12:282, 1983.
3. Bradford FK, Spurling RG: The Intervertebral Disc. Springfield, Illinois: Charles C Thomas, 1945.
4. Compere EL: Origin, anatomy, physiology, and pathology of the intervertebral disc. Instruc Lect Amer Acad Orthop Surg 18:15, 1961.
5. Coventry MB, Ghormley RK, Kernohan JW: The intertebral disc: Its microscopic anatomy and pathology. Part I: Anatomy, development and physiology. J Bone Joint Surg 27A:105, 1945.
6. Galante JO: Tensile properties of the human lumbar annulus fibrosis. Acta Orthop Scand (Suppl) 100:1, 1967.
7. Hollinshead WH: Anatomy for Surgeons, Vol 3. The Back and Limbs. 3rd ed. Philadelphia: (Harper Medical) JB Lippincott, 1982.
8. Batson OV: The function of the vertebral veins and their role in the spread of metastasis. Ann Surg 112:138, 1940.
9. Edgar MA, Ghadially JA: Innervation of the lumbar spine. Clin Orthop 115:35, 1976.
10. Hirsch C, Ingelmark B, Miller M: The anatomical basis for low back pain. Acta Orthop Scand 1:33, 1963.
11. Pedersen HE, Blunck CFJ, Gardner E: The anatomy of lumbosacral posterior rami and meningeal branches of spinal nerves (sinu-vertebral nerves). J Bone Joint Surg 38A:377, 1956.
12. Jackson HC, Winkelman KK, Bichel WH: Nerve endings in the human lumbar spinal column and related structures. J Bone Joint Surg 48A:1272, 1966.
13. Adams MA, Hutton WC: The mechanical function of the lumbar apophyseal joints. Spine 8:327, 1983.
14. Cailliet R: Low Back Pain Syndrome. Philadelphia: FA Davis Co, 1983.
15. Perey O: Fracture of vertebral endplates in the lumbar spine. An experimental biomechanical investigation. Acta Orthop Scand (Suppl) 25:10, 1957.
16. Nachemson A, Morris J: In vivo measurements of intradiscal pressure. J Bone Joint Surg 46A:1077, 1964.
17. Farfan HF: Muscular mechanism of the lumbar spine and the position of power and efficiency. Orthop Clin North Am 6:135, 1975.

2

Epidemiology of Low Back Pain and Sciatica

Epidemiology, the study of the incidence, prevalence, and control of disease in a population, can provide important insights to the physician caring for patients with back problems. Through epidemiology, the linkage between pain and individual or external factors can be determined, which allows risk factors to be identified and minimized. More importantly, it provides an understanding of the natural history of the condition, which is relevant to patient counseling about prognosis, and provides a standard to which the efficacy of various treatments may be verified.

No discussion of epidemiology can begin without reviewing the two most basic concepts: incidence and prevalence. *Incidence* is the rate at which healthy people develop a new symptom or disease over a specified period of time. It is dependent solely on the rate at which the disease occurs. In contrast, *prevalence* is a measure of the number of people in a population who have a symptom or disease at a particular point in time. The 1-year prevalence of back pain, for example, is a measure of all those with back pain identified over a 1-year period, regardless of whether the problem began during or before the survey period. Therefore, prevalence depends both on incidence and duration of disease.

Information on the prevalence and incidence of back pain is available from multiple sources including insurance and hospital data, interviews or questionnaires, and clinical studies. The quality of the data bases is variable, especially if their primary purpose is financial rather than scientific. Another problem which alters the measured prevalence is the lack of a uniform definition of the problem. For example, a study that defines low back pain as an episode lasting at least a week will report a much higher prevalence than one defining it as an episode lasting more than 2 weeks.

PREVALENCE OF LOW BACK PAIN

Back pain is the second leading cause of work absenteeism (after upper respiratory tract complaints) and results in more lost productivity than any other medical condition.[1-3] Spine or back impairments result in an annual average of 175.8 million restricted activity days.[4] The lifetime prevalence of back pain exceeds 70% in most industrialized countries.[5] National statistics from the United States indicate a 1-year prevalence rate of 15% to 20% (Fig. 2–1).[6, 7]

Using the definition of low back pain of the National Health and Nutrition Examination Survey II (NHANES II)—an episode lasting 2 weeks, the prevalence of back pain among both men and women is 16% for persons 25 to 74 years of age (Table 2–1).[4] The highest prevalence was in the 45 to 64 age group. Rates were also higher for whites (16.5%) than for either blacks (13.2%) or other racial groups (11.3%). The primary site of pain was lower back (85.1%) with middle back pain reported in 7.9% and upper back pain in 7.0%.

Data from the National Center for Health Statistics (NCHS) show that 14.3% of new patient visits to physicians are for low back pain, and each year there are nearly 13 million physician visits for chronic low back pain.[8] The mean days of restricted activity due to back

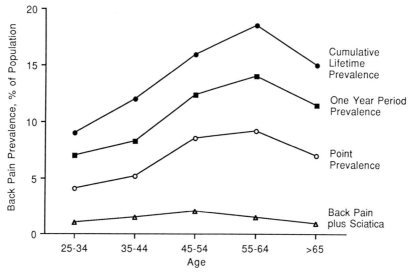

Figure 2–1. Prevalence of low back pain. Only episodes lasting for at least 2 weeks are included. Sciatica is defined as pain radiating to the legs, increasing with cough, sneeze, or deep breathing. (From Deyo RA, Tsui-Wu Y-J: Descriptive epidemiology of low-back pain and its related medical care in the United States. Spine 12:264, 1987.)

problems was 23.5. Eight days were completely lost from work. Chronic disability resulting from low back pain was reported to affect 2.4 million Americans permanently with an additional 2.4 million temporarily disabled.

Data from NHANES II has been analyzed for the use of health professionals by subjects with back pain (Table 2–2). Overall, 84% of those with low back pain (> 2 weeks) had seen a health care professional, 30.9% had been admitted to a hospital, and 11.6% had undergone surgery.[7] It is worth noting that 75% to 85% of subjects reported success with the standard nonoperative treatments (excluding traction and cold application).

A prospective Swedish study analyzed all patients of Gothenburg with low back pain. Of 49,000 residents aged 20 to 65 years, a total of 7,526 absence episodes were reported due to low back pain in an 18-month period.[9] This study also provided important natural history data for this condition: 57% of patients recovered in 1 week, 90% in 6 weeks, 95% after 12 weeks. At the end of 1 year, 1.2% remained disabled and out from work. Recurrent pain and disability were common and occurred in 12% over the 18-month observation period.

The impact of back pain on society is staggering. Back pain is the most frequent cause of activity limitation in people below age 45, the second most frequent reason for physician visits, the fifth most frequent for hospitalization, and the third ranking reason for surgical procedures.[10–14] About 1% of the United States population is chronically disabled because of back pain and an additional 1% is temporarily disabled, representing a total of 400,000 compensable back injuries each year.

PREVALENCE OF SCIATICA AND DISC HERNIATIONS

The definitions of sciatica used in epidemiologic surveys vary. In general, sciatica is considered to be pain radiating along the course of the sciatic nerve to one or both legs to below the knee. A herniated nucleus pulposus (HNP) is one cause, but not the only explanation, for sciatica. Sciatica is present in about 25% of those with back problems. The average absence of patients with sciatica exceeds that of patients with back pain alone.

In the United Kingdom, the estimated prevalence of herniated disc is from 1% to 3%—3.1% of men and 1.3% of women.[15] In men age 55 to 64, the prevalence was 9.6%; in women the maximum prevalence of 5% occurred after the age of 64. Similarly, in Sweden the lifetime prevalence of sciatica was found to be 3.6% in those younger than 25 and 22.4% among those aged 45 to 54.[16]

Sciatica usually resolves with nonoperative treatment, but a minority of patients may need hospitalization and surgery. Operation rates for herniated lumbar discs vary. It is estimated that the rate per 100,000 is 100 in Great

TABLE 2–1. PREVALENCE OF JOINT PAIN BY SITE OF JOINT AND SELECTED DEMOGRAPHIC CHARACTERISTICS

		(RATE PER 100 PERSONS)			
		Back, Neck or Other Joint Pain	Back Pain[1]	Neck Pain[2]	Other Joint Pain[3]
Total ages	25–74 years	21.0	16.0	8.2	19.0
Male		19.6	16.0	7.0	16.6
Female		22.4	16.0	9.4	21.3
Age	25–44 years	15.8	12.3	6.6	12.3
	45–64 years	38.4	20.3	10.1	25.1
	65–74 years	40.1	18.2	9.3	28.1
Race	White	21.9	16.5	8.6	19.4
	Black	15.5	13.2	5.6	16.8
	Other	13.7	11.3	7.2	12.5

[1]Have you ever had pain in your back on most days for at least 2 weeks?
[2]Have you ever had pain in your neck on most days for at least 2 weeks?
[3]Have you had pain or aching in any joint other than the back or neck on most days for at least 6 weeks?
From Praemer A, Furner S, Rice DP: Musculoskeletal conditions in the United States. Illinois: American Academy of Orthopaedic Surgeons, 1992, pp 23–33.

Britain,[17, 18] 350 in Finland,[19] 200 in Sweden,[20] and over 450 in the United States.[21, 22] Over 95% of operations are at the L4 and L5 levels.[23] The mean age at surgery is 40 to 45 years, with males being operated on twice as often as females.

GENERAL RISK FACTORS

Back pain is a multifactorial disorder with many possible etiologies; consequently, determining risk factors for low back pain is difficult. In addition, many of the proposed risk factors have a high prevalence in the general (asymptomatic) population and require large data base studies to make statistically valid statements about risk factors. Thus, the literature is filled with a myriad of studies with con-

TABLE 2–2. THE USE OF HEALTH PROFESSIONALS BY NHANES II SUBJECTS WITH LBP (N = 1516)*

HEALTH PROFESSIONAL	PERCENTAGE
General practitioner	58.6
Orthopedist	36.9
Chiropractor	30.8
Osteopath	13.8
Internist	7.6
Rheumatologist	2.5
Any	84.6

*From Deyo RA, Tsui-Wu Y-J: Descriptive epidemiology of low-back pain and its related medical care in the United States. Spine 12:264, 1987.

flicting conclusions. The following discussion is intended to summarize the consensus of studies concerning risk factors.

The maximal frequency of low back pain symptoms appears to be in the age range of 35 to 55, while absences and duration of symptoms increase with increasing age.[24] While gender seems to be of little importance with respect to low back symptoms,[25–29] surgery for disc herniations is performed about 1.5 to 3 times more often in males.[23, 30–35] Postural deformities such as scoliosis, kyphosis, and leg length discrepancy do not predispose to low back pain in general.[36–47] Studies of scoliosis have shown that there is no increased association with back pain unless the curve is severe (> 80°).[48–55] Anthropometric data are contradictory with no strong relationship between height, weight, body build, and low back pain.[56–59] Physical fitness is not a predictor of acute low back pain, but the physically fit have a lesser risk of chronic low back pain and a more rapid recovery after a pain episode.[60–62] Several investigators have found an association between smoking, herniated discs, and low back pain.[63–66]

OCCUPATIONAL RISK FACTORS

The relationship between occupational factors and low back pain is difficult to study because exposure is usually difficult or impossible to quantify. The problem is further complicated by several factors: (1) workers may be exposed to multiple risk factors in the same job; (2) workers in the same industry or occupation may have substantially different exposure, and (3) workers with back pain may shift to less strenuous jobs leaving a preponderance of healthy workers on the heavy tasks and shifting the apparent prevalence of back pain. In addition, the recall of occupational exposures is notoriously poor and often influenced by financial manipulation of the insurance system.[65]

Physical factors found to be associated with increased risk of low back pain include heavy work, lifting, static work postures (prolonged sitting or standing), bending and twisting, and vibration.[24, 64, 67–72] Psychologic and psychosocial work factors including monotony at work, job dissatisfaction, and poor relationship with coworkers have been found to increase complaints about low back pain.[73–76] Prospective studies have concluded that these psychologic risk factors were more predictive than any of the physical risk factors.[48, 77]

SUMMARY

The epidemiology of low back pain and sciatica is both a critical and confusing topic. All data must be carefully analyzed in light of the data base from which it was extracted as well as the potential motivation for secondary gain on the part of the patients or physicians who provide the input information. Nevertheless, a working knowledge of the prevalence, incidence, and natural history of this problem is essential to evaluate and counsel patients with the proper perspective. Most episodes of low back pain or sciatica resolve spontaneously within the first 2 weeks, and a relative minority take 6 to 12 weeks. Only 1% to 2% of cases should require evaluation for operative management. Knowledge of the physical and psychosocial risk factors can help prevent and minimize the severity of recurrences.

References

1. Deyo RA, Bass JE: Lifestyle and low back pain. Spine 14:501, 1989.
2. Rowe ML: Low back pain in industry. A position paper. J Occup Med 11:161, 1969.
3. Salkever DS: Morbidity costs: National estmates and economic determinants. NCHSR Research Summary Series, October 1985, Department of Health and Human Services Publication No. (PHS) 86-3393, 1986.
4. Praemer A, Furner S, Rice DP: Musculoskeletal conditions in the United States. Illinois: American Academy of Orthopaedic Surgeons, 1992, pp 23–33.
5. Damkot DK, Pope MH, Lord J, Frymoyer JW: The relationship between work history, work environment and low-back pain in men. Spine 9:395, 1984.
6. Cunningham LS, Kelsey JL: Epidemiology of musculoskeletal impairments and associated disability. Am J Public Health 74:574, 1984.
7. Deyo RA, Tsui-Wu Y-J: Descriptive epidemiology of low-back pain and its related medical care in the United States. Spine 12:264, 1987.
8. Anderson GBJ: The epidemiology of spinal disorders. In Frymoyer JW (ed): The Adult Spine: Principles and Practice. New York: Raven Press, 1991, pp 107–146.
9. Choler U, Larsson R, Nachemson A, Peterson LE: Back Pain. Spri Report 188, 1985 (in Swedish).
10. National Center for Health Statistics: Physician visits, volume and interval since last visit, United States, 1971. Series 10, Number 97, 1975.
11. National Center for Health Statistics: Inpatient utilization of short stay hospitals by diagnosis, United States, 1973. Series 13, Number 25, 1976.
12. National Center for Health Statistics: Surgical operations in short stay hospitals, United States, 1973. Series 13, Number 24, 1976.
13. National Center for Health Statistics: Limitation of activity due to chronic conditions, United States, 1974. Series 10, No. 111, 1977.
14. National Center for Health Statistics: Prevalence of selected impairments, United States, 1977. Series 10, No. 134, 1981.
15. Lawrence JS: Rheumatism in populations. London: Heinemann, 1977.
16. Hirsh C, Jonsson B, Lewin T: Low back symptoms in a Swedish female population. Clin Orthop 63:171, 1969.
17. Benn RT, Wood PH: Pain in the back: An attempt to estimate the size of the problem. Rheumatol Rehabil 14:121–128, 1975.
18. Wood PHN, Badley EM: Epidemiology of back pain. In Jayson M (ed): The Lumbar Spine and Back Pain. London: Churchill Livingstone, 1987, pp 1–15.
19. Heliövaara M: Epidemiology of sciatica and herniated lumbar intervertebral disc. Helsinki: The Research Institute for Social Security, 1988, pp. 1–47.
20. Nachemson A, Eck C, Lindstrom IL, et al.: Chronic low back disability can largely be prevented: A prospective randomized trial in industry. AAOS 56th Annual Meeting, Las Vegas, 1989.
21. Frymoyer JW: Back pain and sciatica. N Engl J Med 318:291, 1988.
22. Kelsey JL, White AA III: Epidemiology and impact on low back pain. Spine 5:133, 1980.
23. Spangfort EV: The lumbar disc herniation. Acta Orthop Scand (Suppl) 142:1, 1972.
24. Andersson GBJ: Epidemiologic aspects on low back pain in industry. Spine 6:53, 1981.
25. Battié MC, Bigos SJ, Fisher LD, et al.: Isometric lifting strength as a predictor of industrial back pain reports. Spine 14:851, 1989.
26. Horal J: The clinical appearance of low back disorders in the city of Gothenburg, Sweden. Acta Orthop Scand (Suppl) 118:1, 1969.
27. Svensson HO, Andersson GBJ: Low back pain in forty to forty-seven year old men. I. Frequency of occurrence and impact on medical services. Scand J Rehab Med 14:47, 1982.
28. Svensson HO, Andersson GBJ, Johansson S, et al.: A retrospective study of low back pain in 38- to 64-year-old women. Frequency and occurrence and impact on medical services. Spine 13:548, 1988.
29. Valkenburg HA, Haanen HCM: The epidemiology of

low back pain. In White AA, Gordon SL (eds): Symposium on Idiopathic Low Back Pain. St. Louis: Mosby Yearbook, 1982, pp 9–22.

30. Braun W: Ursachen des lumbalen Bandscheibervefalls. Die Wirbelsaule in Forschung und Praxis 43, 1969.

31. Brown JR: Factors contributing to the development of low back pain in industrial workers. Am Industr Hyg Assoc J 36:26, 1975.

32. Heliövaara M, Knekt P, Aromaa A: Incidence and risk factors of herniated lumbar intervertebral disc or sciatica leading to hospitalization. J Chronic Dis 40:251, 1987.

33. Kelsey JL, Ostfeld AM: Demographic characteristics of persons with acute herniated lumbar intervertebral disc. J Chronic Dis 28:37–50, 1975.

34. Lawrence JS, Graft R, deLaine VAI: Degenerative joint diseases in random samples and occupational groups. In Kellgren JH, Jeffrey MR, Bull J (eds): The Epidemiology of Chronic Rheumatism, Vol. I. Oxford: Blackwell Scientific Publications, 1983, pp 98–119.

35. Weber H: Lumbar disc herniation. A controlled, prospective study with ten years of observation. Spine 8:131, 1983.

36. Battié MC, Bigos SJ, Fisher LD, et al.: A prospective study of the role of cardiovascular risk factors and fitness in industrial back pain complaints. Spine 14:141, 1989.

37. Biering-Sorensen F: The prognostic value of the low back history and physical measurements. Unpublished doctoral dissertation, University of Copenhagen, 1983.

38. Biering-Sorensen F: A prospective study of low back pain in a general population. I. Occurrence, recurrence and aetiology. Scand J Rehabil Med 15:71, 1983.

39. Biering-Sorensen F: A prospective study of low back pain in a general population. III. Medical service—work consequence. Scand J Rehabil Med 15:89, 1983.

40. Hansson T, Bigos S, Beecher P, et al.: The lumbar lordosis in acute and chronic low back pain. Spine 10:154, 1985.

41. Hodgson S, Shannon HS, Troup JDG: The prevention of spinal disorders in dock workers. Report to National Dock Labour Board, London, 1974.

42. Kostuik JP, Bentivoglio J: The incidence of low back pain in adult scoliosis. Spine 6:268, 1981.

43. Hult L: Cervical, dorsal, and lumbar spinal syndromes. Acta Orthop Scand (Suppl) 17:1, 1954.

44. Magora A: Investigation of the relation between low back pain and occupation. 7. Neurologic and orthopedic condition. Scand J Rehab Med 7:146, 1975.

45. Pope MH, Bevins T, Wilder DG, Frymoyer JW: The relationship between anthropometric, postural, muscular, and mobility characteristics of males, ages 18–55. Spine 10:644, 1985.

46. Rowe ML: Low back pain in industry. A position paper. J Occup Med 11:161, 1969.

47. Sorensen KH: Scheuermann's juvenile kyphosis. Doctoral dissertation, Copenhagen, Munksgaard, 1964.

48. Battié MC, Bigos SJ, Fisher LD, et al.: Anthropometric and clinical measurements as predictors of industrial back pain complaints: A prospective study. J Spinal Disorders 3:195, 1990.

49. Battié MC, Bigos SJ, Fisher LD, et al.: The role of spinal flexibility in back pain complaints within industry: A prospective study. Spine 15:768, 1990.

50. Bradford DS, Moe JH, Winter RB: Scoliosis and kyphosis. Operative management of idiopathic scoliosis.

In Rothman RH, Simeone FA (eds): The Spine, 2nd ed. Philadelphia: WB Saunders Co, 1982, pp 316–349.

51. Collis DK, Ponseti IV: Long term follow-up of patients with idiopathic scoliosis not treated surgically. J Bone Joint Surg [AM] 51:425, 1969.

52. Kostuik JP, Bentivoglio J: The incidence of low back pain in adult scoliosis. Spine 6:268, 1981.

53. Kostuik JP, Israel J, Hall JE: Scoliosis surgery in adults. Clin Orthop 93:225, 1973.

54. Nachemson AL: Back problems in childhood and adolescence. Lakartidningen 65:2831, 1968 (in Swedish).

55. Nilsonne U, Lundgren KD: Long-term prognosis in idiopathic scoliosis. Acta Orthop Scand 39:456, 1968.

56. Battie MC: The reliability of physical factors as predictors of the occurrence of back pain reports. A prospective study within industry. Thesis, University of Goteborg, Goteborg, Sweden, 1989.

57. Kelsey JL, Githens PB, Walter SD, et al.: An epidemiologic study of acute prolapsed cervical intervertebral disc. J Bone Joint Surg [AM] 66:907, 1984.

58. Riihimaki H, Wickstrom G, Hanninen K, Luopajarvi T: Predictors of sciatic pain among concrete reinforcement workers and house painters. A five year follow-up. Scand J Work Environ Health 15:415, 1989.

59. Westrin C-G: Low back sick-listing. A nosological and medical insurance investigation. Scand J Soc Med (Suppl) 7:1, 1973.

60. Cady LD, Bischoff DP, O'Connell ER, et al.: Strength and fitness and subsequent back injuries in fire fighters. J Occup Med 21:269, 1979.

61. Cady LD Jr, Thomas PC, Karwasky RJ: Program for increasing health and physical fitness of firefighters. J Occup Med 27:110, 1985.

62. Nachemson AL: Report to the Swedish Department of Economy 1989 (in Swedish).

63. Frymoyer JW, Pope MH, Clements JH, et al.: Risk factors in low back pain. An epidemiological survey. J Bone Joint Surg [Am] 65:213, 1983.

64. Frymoyer JW, Pope MH, Costanza MC, et al.: Epidemiologic studies of low-back pain. Spine 5:419, 1980.

65. Kelsey JL: An epidemiological study of the relationship between occupations and acute herniated lumbar intervertebral discs. Int J Epidemiol 4:197, 1975.

66. Kelsey JL, Githens PB, O'Connor T, et al.: Acute prolapsed lumbar intervertebral disc. An epidemiologic study with special reference to driving automobiles and cigarette smoking. Spine 9:608, 1984.

67. Chaffin DB, Park KS: A longitudinal study of low-back pain as associated with occupational weight lifting factors. Am Ind Hyg Assoc J 34:513, 1973.

68. Kelsey JL, Hardy RJ: Driving of motor vehicles as a risk factor for acute herniated lumbar intervertebral disc. Am J Epidemiol 102:63, 1975.

69. Magora A: Investigation of the relation between low back pain and occupation. 3. Physical requirements: sitting, standing and weight lifting. Industr Med Surg 41:5, 1972.

70. Magora A: Investigation of the relation between low back pain and occupation. 4. Physical requirements: bending, rotation, reaching and sudden maximal effort. Scand J Rehab Med 5:186, 1973.

71. Snook SH: Low back pain in industry. In White AA, Gordon SL (eds): Symposium on Idiopathic Low Back Pain. St. Louis: Mosby-Year Book, 1982, pp 23–28.

72. Troup JDG, Roantree WB, Archibald RM: Survey of cases of lumbar spinal disability. A methological

study. Med Officers' Broadsheet. National Coal Board, 1970.

73. Bergenudd H, Nilsson B: Back pain in middle age: occupational workload and psychologic factors: An epidemiologic survey. Spine 13:58, 1988.

74. Magora A: Investigation of the relation between low back pain and occupation. 5. Psychological aspects. Scand J Rehab Med 5:191, 1973.

75. Svensson HO, Andersson GBJ: Low back pain in forty to forty-seven year old men: Work history and work environment factors. Spine 8:272, 1983.

76. Westrin C-G: Low back sick-listing. A nosological and medical insurance investigation. Acta Soc Med Scand 2:127, 1970.

77. Bigos SJ, Spengler DM, Martin NA, et al.: Back injuries in industry: A retrospective study. III. Employee-related factors. Spine 11:252, 1986.

3

Sources of Low Back Pain

The patient with low back pain presents a challenge to the family practitioner, internist, rheumatologist, orthopedist, neurosurgeon, psychiatrist, osteopath, and physical therapist. The patient's complaint is a symptom, not a diagnosis. The number of anatomic parts of the lumbosacral spine that have the potential to cause pain is substantial. In addition, the spectrum of disease processes that may affect back structures is broad. Compounding the problem is the patient who presents with back pain associated with a work-related injury. The extent and intensity of symptoms may be exaggerated by nonphysiologic factors. The physician's task in caring for patients with low back pain is to identify the likely source of pain and its pathologic process. Only then may the treating physician feel reasonably confident in instituting what he or she believes to be appropriate therapy.

Unfortunately, in many circumstances a physician may not fully examine a patient with low back pain. There are many factors that contribute to this incomplete examination, which include the number of patients with the symptom of low back pain, the natural history of the disease, the effect of nonphysiologic factors on severity and duration of symptoms, and the extent of the physician's knowledge of functional anatomy of that part of the body.

Second to the common cold, back pain is the most prevalent affliction of man. Physicians with busy practices see many patients with this symptom. The natural course of back pain is one of rapid improvement. Eighty to 90% of patients are better within a 2-month period, with or without intervention on the part of the physician. Making a specific diagnosis at the initial visit is not important from a practical standpoint. Most patients are going to improve over time irrespective of the physi-

cian's therapeutic intervention. Most patients have a mechanical cause for their back pain (muscle strain, annular tear) and do not have an underlying serious, systemic medical illness. Identifying the source of a patient's pain as ligamentous, muscular, or articular in origin in the acute circumstance does not significantly alter therapy or hasten response to it.

Some physicians may be skeptical about the severity of the patient's back pain symptoms. This skepticism arises from interaction with patients who are involved in accidents or have work-related injuries. Some physicians see so many of these patients that they have stopped "evaluating" them. Some patients have an ulterior motive for continuing to have pain—for example, to increase their monetary reward or to get a light-duty job at work. Physicians are taught to believe that patients will be honest about the severity of their symptoms because it is in their own best interest to do so. When that honesty is brought into question, the physician believes there is a breach of trust. This distrust is destructive to the doctor-patient relationship, with the result that patients who might be helped are denied appropriate care. The manipulation of worker's compensation or insurance systems by a few individuals should not color the way physicians view patients with back pain in general.

It is not uncommon for a practicing physician to be more familiar with the functional anatomy of organs of the chest and abdomen than with those of the lumbosacral spine. It is left to the orthopedists and neurosurgeons to be concerned with anatomic relationships and sensory innervation of the structures of the low back. Unfortunately, this is a short-sighted view of a very complicated problem. Only with familiarity with anatomic sources of pain in the lumbosacral spine and the mechanism of pain transmission and inhibition is it possible to adequately evaluate patients who have low back pain. With greater knowledge of the functional anatomy and pathophysiology of the structures of the lumbosacral spine, physicians are better able to distinguish those individuals with a potentially more ominous cause of low back pain from those with mechanical abnormalities. Also, they may be better able to differentiate the various causes of mechanical low back pain. The significant differences between acute and chronic pain take on greater importance with regard to therapy goals. Not only does understanding the sources of pain help in the differential diagnosis of diseases of the lumbosacral spine, but also it explains the rationale for a variety of therapeutic modalities used for patients with low back pain. The purpose of this chapter is to review pain physiology, and discuss the sources and character of pain associated with abnormalities involving the anatomic structures of the lumbosacral spine.

PAIN PRODUCTION AND TRANSMISSION

Pain is defined by pain specialists (algologists) as an unpleasant sensory and emotional experience associated with actual or potential tissue damage or described in terms of such damage. Pain is a subjective, individual perception related to mechanical and chemical alterations of body tissues. This means that pain is perceived in the cortical portions of the cen-

tral nervous system and is not dependent on the precise nature or absolute amount of tissue destruction peripherally. This potential separation of tissue destruction from the perception of pain emphasizes the fact that pain messages can be modified at many levels of the nervous system.

The peripheral nervous system contains a wide range of nerve fibers. Myelinated somatic nerves are called A fibers and are subdivided into four groups according to decreasing size: alpha, beta, gamma, and delta. The largest are the alpha fibers, which conduct impulses that serve motor function, proprioception, and reflex activity. Beta fibers also innervate muscle and convey touch and pressure sensations. Gamma fibers control muscle spindle tone. The delta fiber mechanoreceptors subserve reflex withdrawal while thermal receptors subserve pain and temperature functions. The thinly myelinated B fibers are preganglionic autonomic axons that innervate smooth muscle. The unmyelinated C fibers transmit nociceptive impulses (Table 3–1).

Bare nerve endings and specialized corpuscular receptors are the two kinds of receptor organs serving body sensory function.[1] They differ in their capacity to transform mechanical, thermal, and chemical energy into electrical impulses. The corpuscular receptors (mechanoreceptors) are most sensitive to mechanical and vibratory energy. They are larger myelinated fibers (A-alpha and A-beta) that rapidly transmit information about innocuous mechanical stimuli to the cerebral cortex.

TABLE 3–1. PERIPHERAL NERVE FIBER CHARACTERISTICS

	MYELINATION	RECEPTOR TYPE	TRANSMISSION (m/sec)	THRESHOLD	DISTRIBUTION	MODALITY
A-alpha	+	Mechanoreceptor	Rapid (70–120)	Low	Local	Vibration (proprioception) Pain (prick)
A-beta	+	Mechanoreceptor	Rapid (40–70)	Low	Local	Vibration (proprioception) Reflex withdrawal
A-gamma	+	Mechanoreceptor	Rapid (20–40)	Low	Local	Muscle spindle
A-delta	+	Mechanonociceptor	Slow (5–15)	High	Local	Damaging pressure
A-delta	+	Thermal mechanonociceptor	Slow (5–15)	High	Local	Noxious Temperature (sharp)
B	+	Autonomic	Slow (10–15)	High	Diffuse	Preganglionic fibers
C	−	Mechanonociceptor	Slow (0.2–1.5)	High	Diffuse	Noxious
C	−	Polymodal nociceptor	Slow (0.2–1.5)	High	Diffuse	Pressure (sharp) Any noxious stimulus (dull)

Another set of fibers that respond only to stimuli associated with actual tissue damage are called nociceptors. Mechanoreceptors and polymodal nociceptors are two primary forms of these nerve fibers. Mechanoreceptors transmit information about mechanical forces that cause tissue injury. Bare nerve endings, in contrast, are sensitive to all physical modalities (e.g., heat, chemical injury) but differ in their individual sensitivity and threshold to different stimuli.

Nociceptive impulses are carried by two sizes of bare nerve endings. The largest of the two types of pain fiber is the A-delta, 6 to 8 μm in diameter, which is thinly myelinated and conducts impulses relatively quickly (12 or greater m/sec). Some A-delta fibers respond mainly to mechanical energy and accurately locate a site of injury. Others respond to chemical or thermal stimulation proportionately with the degree of injury. More frequent nerve firings are associated with greater tissue damage.[2] Some A-delta fibers may be polymodal responders, which will fire after a high threshold has been reached and actual tissue damage has occurred. These fibers have the property of lowering their active thresholds once they have been exposed to other noxious stimuli.[3] In the sensitized state, innocuous mechanical stimuli that previously evoked no response produce nociceptive impulses, which continue following cessation of the stimulus. Sensitization plays a role in the prolongation of acute pain and the development of chronic pain. Complete destruction of a receptor does not block the sensitized transmission of impulses from undamaged receptors of the same axon.[4] Focal areas of demyelination due to chronic irritation may give rise to spontaneous action potentials that travel in an anterograde or retrograde direction. In these injured nerves, normal stimulation may evoke sustained afterdischarges.

The smaller, unmyelinated C fibers, 0.3 to 1.0 μm in diameter, conduct impulses slowly (0.4 to 1.0 m/sec), are polymodal responders (mechanical, chemical, heat), and are activated only by tissue destruction. These receptors show continued or delayed firing after the physical stimulus has been discontinued. After repeated or prolonged stimulation, their threshold for activation can diminish to levels of intensity that are usually innocuous.[5] Humoral mediators and chemical substances released during acute inflammation and tissue destruction may temporally play a role in C fiber transmission. Peptides, such as bradykinin, are released after a latency of 15 to 30 seconds and reach a peak 15 seconds after the latency period, which may contribute to the delayed and continued firing of high-threshold receptors. Other factors that may play similar roles in nociceptive potentiation are potassium, histamine, substance P, serotonin, and prostaglandins.[6, 7] In combination, these nociceptive A-delta and C fibers detect noxious stimuli damaging body structures. For example, muscle pain is mediated by both A-delta and C fibers. The A-delta fibers are activated by release of histamine, serotonin, and bradykinin during intense exercise. The C fibers respond to rapid contractions of muscle but not to byproducts of muscle metabolism.

The interaction of the mediators of inflammation and neuropeptides that mediate nociceptive stimulation is complex.[8] The products of inflammation released during tissue destruction sensitize and stimulate peripheral nociceptors. The nociceptors produce neurotransmitters that stimulate the C fiber (Table 3–2). The excitation of the primary afferent receptors also produces an axon reflex that results in the peripheral release of neuropeptides such as substance P, neurokinin A, and calcitonin gene-related peptide. These neuropeptides are the same mediators that stimulate second order neurons in the spinal cord. The tissue damage caused by the direct stimulation of peripheral nociceptive fibers is referred to as neurogenic inflammation.[9]

The two groups of pain fibers are associated with two dissociable types of sensory input. The pinprick sensation, which is quick in onset and well localized, is carried in the larger, myelinated A fibers. These fibers are phylogenetically part of a newer sensory system that ascends to the sensory cortex with few interposed relays. This type of pain results in rapid movement, quick protection and reflex withdrawal from a potentially damaging stimulus. The later dull, aching, less localized sensation is carried by the unmyelinated C fibers. These smaller fibers belong to a phylogenetically older sensory system with multiple relays in the

TABLE 3–2. MEDIATORS OF PERIPHERAL NOCICEPTIVE TRANSMISSION

Chemical Mediators	Neurotransmitters
Bradykinin	Substance P
Prostaglandins	Norepinephrine
Leukotrienes	Neurokinin A
Histamine	Calcitonin gene-related peptide
Serotonin	

PAIN RELATED FIBERS IN THE DORSAL HORN OF THE SPINAL CORD

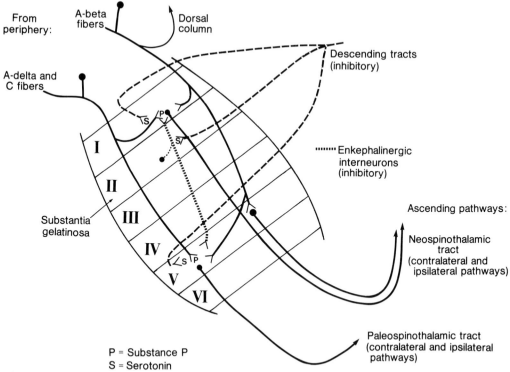

Figure 3–1. Organization of the pain-related fibers in the dorsal horn. Nociceptive A-delta and C fibers carry pain messages from the periphery to laminae I and V. These nerves release substance P. These neurons synapse with second-order relay neurons, which ascend in the rapid pathway (neospinothalamic tract) and/or the slow pathway (paleospinothalamic tract). The nociceptive messages of these neurons are modified presynaptically by collateral branches of the large low-threshold cutaneous mechanoreceptors (A-beta fibers) whose main branches ascend in the ipsilateral dorsal columns. The nociceptive fibers are also inhibited by enkephalinergic interneurons whose cell bodies are situated in lamina II. The enkephalinergic cells are driven by the large peripheral A afferents or the serotoninergic fibers descending in the dorsolateral white funiculus of the spinal cord. Descending tracts also attach presynaptically to nociceptors in laminae I and V to inhibit pain transmission.

medulla and thalamus.[10] The pain associated with C fiber stimulation produces tonic contraction, serving the function of guarding and protecting the injured part.

The Dorsal Horn

Dorsal horn neurons are classified according to their response to primary afferent input. Low-threshold neurons respond only to nonnoxious stimuli such as hair movement or touch. High-threshold neurons are nociceptive specific responding to excessive joint movement. Dorsal horn neurons stimulated by noxious and non-noxious stimuli are classified as wide dynamic range neurons. These neurons have graded responses that increase with increasing intensities of stimulation. Wide dy-

namic range neurons respond to hair movement, pressure, pinch, or pinprick.

The nociceptive A-delta and C fibers with nerve endings in the periphery and their cell bodies in the dorsal root ganglion have destination points in the dorsal horn of the spinal cord.[11] Of the six specialized layers of nerve endings that are laminated in the dorsal horn, I, II, and V receive nociceptive fibers (Fig. 3–1). Laminae III and IV receive primary afferent input from large fiber, low-threshold neurons involved with spinal cord processing of proprioception. Lamina VI has low-threshold and wide dynamic range neurons that may share some function with lamina V in transmission of nociceptive information to supraspinal sites. This organization of the dorsal horn has physiologic importance. Small-caliber myelinated fibers ascend or descend in Lissauer's tract for one or two segments before entering the dorsal gray matter. They terminate in lamina I and the bottom of lamina II. Lamina I receives A-delta mechanoreceptors and some polymodal C afferents. The sensory input is from the skin and muscle nociceptors that have a small peripheral receptive field. These neurons are important in signaling the presence of pain but are unlikely to transmit information concerning the intensity or nature of the painful stimulus.[12] In contrast, cells in lamina V receive more specific information because of the convergent input of rapidly conducting A-beta fibers along with more slowly conducting A-delta and C nociceptive fibers (wide dynamic range neurons). These fibers respond to mechanical or thermal stimuli, steadily increasing their discharge frequency with the intensity of the noxious stimulus. This layer conveys the information concerning the location, intensity, and form of harmful stimuli. These axons contain substance P, a neurotransmitter, which is most highly concentrated in the superficial layers of the dorsal horn.[13] Substance P plays an important role in dorsal horn transmission of nociception. Dorsal horn nociceptors are substantially stimulated by substance P. Depletion of substance P in the spinal cord with capsaicin is associated with decreased transmission of nociceptive impulses.[14]

Substance P is only one of an ever increasing number of neuropeptides associated with modulation of sensory input in the spinal cord (Table 3–3).[8] Many fibers produce more than one neuropeptide. For example, substance P and calcitonin gene-related peptide are released simultaneously by neurons in the spinal cord.[15] Excitatory amino acids, such as aspartate and glutamate, are also neurotransmitters in the spinal cord. One hypothesis has suggested that excitatory amino acids are the mediators of fast nociceptive transmission while the neuropeptides are the mediators of slow transmission.[16] The repertoire of neuropeptides and excitatory amino acids associated with a specific noxious stimulus has not been determined.

The unmyelinated fibers from lamina V supply not only the skin and muscles but also other somatic structures, such as joints and ligaments. In addition, visceral afferents converge on the wide dynamic range neurons in lamina V that supply sensory innervation for somatic structures, including skin. It is important to remember that on entering the spinal cord the visceral fibers travel caudally or cranially for several segments in the posterior horn of gray matter before synapsing with neurons in the dorsal horn. The "referred pain" associated with visceral disease processes occurs secondary to "cross-talk" between visceral sensory afferents and the wide dynamic range neurons that supply sensation to cutaneous structures. This convergence of afferent nerves allows for the summation of nociceptive input on a spatial and temporal basis. Stimulation of the visceral afferents results in a wide field of cutaneous nerve stimulation that activates secondary neurons ascending to the midbrain. This diffuse stimulation results in the perception that the skin has been stimulated when in fact the actual source of the sensory input is the visceral afferents.[17]

Lamina II (substantia gelatinosa) receives the majority of the slow, unmyelinated C afferents. Although a small number of cells in this lamina have projections that reach the cortex, most cells in the substantia gelatinosa have local connections with other neurons in other laminae at the same segmental level and with the substantia gelatinosa on the opposite side of the spinal cord. This connection is accomplished through commissural fibers that cross the spinal cord. These nerves have inhibitory effects on pain transmission. Most of the C fibers interconnect with descending inhibitory neurons.[18]

Spinothalamic Tract

The majority of second-order neurons connect with incoming afferent neurons in laminae I and V of the dorsal horn, then cross to the contralateral side at the same spinal cord level to ascend rostrally in the anterolateral spinothalamic tract (neospinothalamic tract) (Fig. 3–2). Phylogenetically, the spinothalamic

TABLE 3–3. NEUROPEPTIDES MODULATING NOCICEPTIVE INPUT IN THE SPINAL CORD

Stimulatory	Inhibitory
Substance P	Serotonin
Neurokinin A	Somatostatin
Glutamate	Cholecystokinin
Aspartate	Norepinephrine
Vasoactive intestinal polypeptide	Gamma-aminobutyric acid
Calcitonin gene-related peptide	Glycine
	Endogenous opioid peptides
	β-endorphin
	Enkephalin
	Dynorphin

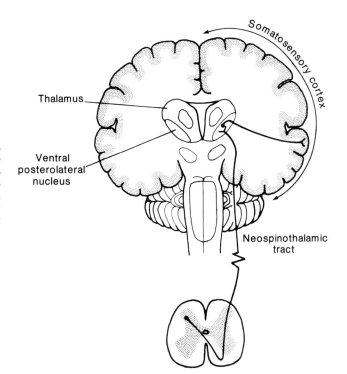

Figure 3–2. The neospinothalamic tract consists of a rapid three-neuron relay system from the dorsal horn to the ventral posterolateral nucleus of the thalamus to the somatosensory cortex. This rapid system, with its somatotopic organization, allows for analysis of the site, intensity, and nature of pain but provides no means to activate evasive motor action.

tract is the newer nociceptive sensory tract in the human nervous system. The neospinothalamic tract courses upward in the spinal cord with new fibers, at each spinal level, joining medially pushing axons from more caudal segments laterally. This organization preserves the somatotopic organization of the tract in the spinal cord. These fibers terminate in the posterior nuclear group of the thalamus, particularly the ventral posterolateral nucleus. Third-order neurons carry impulses from the thalamus to the posterior central gyrus of the parietal cortex. This rapid system with it somatotopic organization allows for analysis of the site, intensity, and nature of pain (pricking, pressing, throbbing, stabbing, or burning). However, this rapid transit system provides no means to mediate reflexes to activate the motor system for evasive action, or to alter cortical function to increase alertness. The neospinothalamic tract also has a polysynaptic portion with fibers branching with collaterals that enter the reticular system of the brainstem. Some of these collaterals synapse on cells that provide nociceptive information to the descending inhibitory system.[19]

The phylogenetically older anterior division, the paleospinothalamic tract, supplies the connections for the cortical response to pain (Fig. 3–3). These include suffering, which is a negative affective response to pain, fear, and depression. The second-order neurons of this tract send multiple connections to the reticular formation of the brainstem while traveling to the midline and intralaminar nuclei of the thalamus. The higher-order neurons that emerge from the reticular formation and thalamic nuclei connect with other thalamic nuclei, hypothalamus, the basal ganglia, and the midbrain central gray area. From these structures, a multitude of higher-order neurons synapse with a number of cortical areas, including the frontal lobe (pain perception), temporal lobe (recent and long-term memory), and hypothalamus (autonomic sympathetic and parasympathetic reflexes).[20] These cortical functions work independent of each other; that is, the intensity of nociceptive input does not necessarily result in a specific emotional response or autonomic reflexes such as increased heart rate or blood pressure or increased gastrointestinal secretion and motility.

The connections of the nociceptors with a number of different areas of cerebral cortex underscore the definition of pain as a subjective response that is a summation of total sensory input. Pain has sensory-discriminative, motivational-affective, and cognitive-evaluative dimensions.[21] The neospinothalamic tract contributes to the sensory-discriminative dimension of pain. The cortical projection of this system transmits information that characterizes the spatial, temporal, and magnitude properties of a noxious stimulus. The brain-

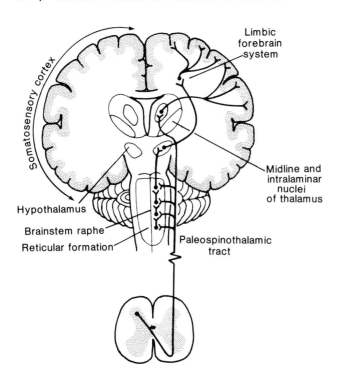

Figure 3–3. The paleospinothalamic tract consists of a slow multi-neuron relay system from the dorsal horn to the brainstem, hypothalamus, thalamus, and limbic forebrain system. This tract mediates reflexes and integrated responses (fear, memory, suffering) related to nociceptive impulses.

stem reticular formation and the limbic system play a significant role in the motivational-affective dimension of pain. The paleospinothalamic tract supplies the nerves with multiple synapses in the reticular system. These nerves do not carry spatial or temporal information, since target cells in the brainstem and cortex have wide receptive fields covering half or more of the body surface. Effects of sight and sound on pain perception occur through connections in the reticular system. Escape and protective behaviors are mediated through the reticular-limbic system. This system acts as an intensity monitor and contributes to the quality of unpleasantness, mobilizes internal defenses, and elicits behavior geared to avoiding or stopping the distress.

Cognitive functions—memory, cultural values, and anxiety—also play a significant role in the perception of pain. A new pain with little associated damage may be perceived as severe because of the fear of the unknown, while a pain associated with greater tissue damage may not elicit the same degree of discomfort because its cause is familiar. This central cognitive system evaluates and analyzes input in terms of past experience, probability of outcome, and symbolic importance. This system facilitates or inhibits activities in the sensory and motivational systems by modulating activity of inhibitory neurons in the substantia gelatinosa.

Another important connection between nerves at the level of the dorsal horn is the synapse between dorsal horn sensory fibers and anterior horn motor fibers. Through direct synapse with internuncial nerves, input from sensory nerves stimulates motor neurons at the same or neighboring segmental levels. This stimulation may result in reflex action that causes an instantaneous contraction of a muscle or a more tonic contraction (spasm) with repeated stimulation of nociceptive fibers.

Descending Analgesic Pathways

In addition to the two distinct sensory pathways that transmit nociceptive signals to brainstem and cortical structures, the cortex and midbrain have descending pathways that modulate pain input at the level of the dorsal horn (Fig. 3–4).[22] Neurons surrounding the cerebral aqueduct of the midbrain and the brainstem raphe in the medullopontine reticular formation terminate on interneurons present in lamina II (substantia gelatinosa).[23] The neurotransmitter for this descending pathway is serotonin (5-hydroxytryptamine). Serotoninergic cells activate enkephalinergic interneurons, which exert presynaptic inhibition of the small unmyelinated nociceptors that produce substance P.

Enkephalins are pentapeptides that are secreted by neurons where there are opiate receptors.[24] Substance P is an 11-amino-acid pep-

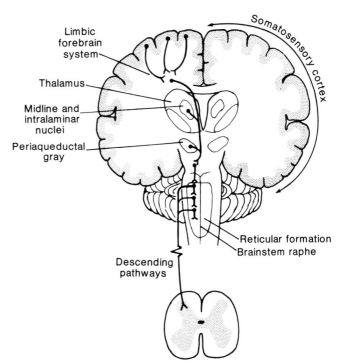

Figure 3–4. Descending pathways carry signals from higher brain centers through the periaqueductal gray and the brainstem raphe back to the dorsal horn. Neurons that compose the inhibitory descending pathways release serotonin and inhibit pain transmission through nociceptive fibers.

tide produced by unmyelinated nociceptive fibers.[25] The release of enkephalin inhibits substance P–sensitive nociceptors, decreasing ascending signals. This inhibitory process relies on opiate receptors for its action. Naloxone, an opiate antagonist, temporarily reverses the analgesic effects of activation of the periaqueductal gray and raphe neurons. Two other descending analgesic fiber systems include neurons from the locus ceruleus (neurotransmitter—norepinephrine) and Edinger-Westphal nucleus (neurotransmitter—cholecystokinin). The exact location for the interaction of these systems and neurons in the dorsal horn is unknown.

In addition to the descending analgesic pathways, segmental input from myelinated mechanoreceptors that synapse with small-diameter nociceptive afferents inhibits pain transmission. The modulation of nociceptive input by massage, compression, or vibration of tissues is the cornerstone of the "gate theory of pain."[26] A limited amount of sensory information can activate ascending fibers terminating in the brainstem and cortical portions of the nervous system. A gate at the level of the spinal cord can swing open to allow nociceptive impulses or proprioceptive impulses to pass through. Stimulation of myelinated A-beta (mechanoreceptor) fibers inhibits (closes the gate to) transmission of A-delta and C nociceptive fibers. The substantia gelatinosa

(lamina II) is the location for this interaction. This inhibition is not related to opioid receptors, since this effect is independent of naloxone (narcotic antagonist).[27] The enkephalinergic interneurons and the descending inhibitory neurons also serve to close the gate to pain transmission.

The clinical correlation of pain moderation by proprioceptive stimulation is the practice of rubbing the area after it has been injured. This maneuver activates large low-threshold fibers, reducing the effects of small fiber input to a level where pain is less severe. The benefit of transcutaneous electrical nerve stimulation (TENS) in diminishing pain is based on this principle. On the other hand, disease processes that diminish large fiber input may magnify painful stimuli. Herpes zoster viral infection, which preferentially damages large-fiber vibratory, dorsal ganglion cells, may result in hyperesthesia in the sensory field of the affected nerve secondary to the loss of large-fiber, proprioceptive input.

Visceral Sensory System

The sensory nerves for the abdominal and pelvic viscera have cell bodies in the dorsal root ganglia but do not use the spinal nerves to reach the target organ. Instead these nerves pass through the pathways of the sympathetic and parasympathetic nervous systems. The sympathetic nerve trunks extend from the skull to the coccyx. There are four paired lumbar ganglia, four paired sacral ganglia, and one single coccygeal ganglion. The sympathetic trunks are anterolateral to the spinal column, pass medially in the sacrum, and join centrally at the ganglion impar at the coccyx (Fig. 3–5). Arising from the thoracic and first two lumbar spinal nerves are white rami communicantes that pass to the trunk or ganglia. These rami allow the passage of peripheral processes of the visceral dorsal root ganglion cells to the sympathetic chain. These visceral sensory nerves do not synapse in the sympathetic ganglia, but pass directly through them, each on its way to its visceral destination by way of the associated artery. The peripheral

processes may ascend or descend through the sympathetic chain, eventually exiting through splanchnic nerves arising from the sympathetic trunk, which contain autonomic nerves with various functions. Thoracic segments on both sides form the greater, lesser, and least splanchnic nerves, which run from the thorax through the diaphragm to the abdomen, reaching the aortic plexus. The preaortic plexus is a large, elongated, dense network of nerve fibers and ganglion cells located on the anterior aspect of the aorta and its branches. Increased densities of cells on the aorta as it travels to its bifurcation are arbitrarily designated celiac, superior mesenteric, and inferior mesenteric ganglia. Below the level of the bifurcation of the aorta at the fourth lumbar vertebra, the hypogastric plexus runs over the

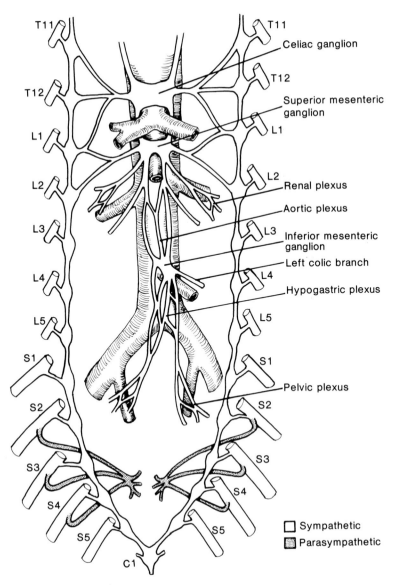

Figure 3–5. Sympathetic nerve trunks with bilateral ganglia at each spinal level are located lateral to the spinal column. The sympathetic nerves pass from the bilateral nerve chains to the aortic plexus, which consists of the celiac, superior mesenteric, and inferior mesenteric ganglia. The hypogastric and pelvic plexuses are located at the level of the aortic bifurcation and below. The parasympathetic nerves travel through the second, third, and fourth sacral nerves to supply organs in the pelvis.

Labels in figure:
T11
T12
L1
L2
L3
L4
L5
S1
S2
S3
S4
S5
C1

Celiac ganglion
Superior mesenteric ganglion
Renal plexus
Aortic plexus
Inferior mesenteric ganglion
Left colic branch
Hypogastric plexus
Pelvic plexus

☐ Sympathetic
▦ Parasympathetic

sacral promontory and passes into the pelvis, where it divides into bilateral pelvic plexuses which supply the rectum and genitourinary organs (Fig. 3–5).

The parasympathetic autonomic nervous system also supplies sensory innervation to the pelvic organs. The cell bodies for the sensory parasympathetic nerves are, like the sympathetic system, found in the dorsal root ganglia of the corresponding segment. However, in contrast to passing through the sympathetic chain of splanchnic nerves, the parasympathetic nerves pass through the splanchnic branches of the third, fourth, and fifth sacral nerves (nervi erigentes). These nerves pass to the pelvic plexus and inferior mesenteric plexus (Fig. 3–5).

It is important to remember that the segmental innervation of a visceral organ is not dependent on its location in fully developed humans but rather on its embryologic segment of origin, since sensory nerves grow into the viscera early in their development before they migrate to their final anatomic destinations. In addition, the organization of visceral afferents in the dorsal horn also plays an important role in the distribution of visceral pain. Visceral afferents synapse in lamina V with wide dynamic range neurons. These visceral neurons have a wide field of innervation. A single visceral fiber may synapse with a number of cutaneous afferents. Stimulation of a visceral afferent will activate a wide field of cutaneous nociceptors whose activity will be perceived as "referred pain." The field of activated nociceptors may be transmitted to several segmental levels, whereas somatic pain is transmitted to a single level.

The visceral afferents are also closely associated with activation of sympathetic and parasympathetic nerves. Stimulation of visceral afferents, in the appropriate circumstances, will activate autonomic nerve fibers, leading to responses such as vasoconstriction, vasodilatation, flushing, or tachycardia.

Segmental Innervation

A brief review of the embryologic origin of the axial skeleton and the peripheral nervous system provides the anatomic background for understanding the clinical symptoms associated with disorders of the lumbosacral spine. By the end of the second week, the notochord forms on the dorsum of the embryonic disc between the endoderm and ectoderm. The notochord is the central framework of the spine which is eventually absorbed into the vertebral column, where its remnants form the nucleus pulposus of the intervertebral disc. By the third week, mesodermal cells that parallel the notochord start to segment into individual somites. The somites subsequently differentiate into three primary parts—skin (dermatome); muscle, tendon, and ligaments (myotome); and bone (sclerotome). Simultaneously, the corresponding spinal nerve for each somite develops from the neural tube, supplying innervation for the three components of the somite. As the skin, muscle, and bone develop and migrate to their final location in the body, each segment's cells take along its corresponding nerve supply. Structures from one somite, for example parts of the buttock, posterior thigh, leg, and lumbosacral spine, may all become painful if one component is damaged.

The embryologic organization of segmental structures is evident in the innervation of skin, muscle, and bones of the lumbosacral spine and lower extremities. The sensory nervous system is segmentally organized. Each dorsal root ganglion supplies a particular segment. Topographically, on the surface of the body, the segments are ordered into cutaneous dermatomes. The same dermatomes cover areas both in the lumbar spine and in the lower extremity. While this organization may seem confusing when the body is viewed in an upright position, the organization of the dermatomes becomes clearer when the body is placed in a quadruped orientation (Fig. 3–6). Dermatomes stretch from areas in the lumbar spine to contiguous areas in the lower extremity. The L4 and L5 segments have no cutaneous branches supplying the lumbar spine. These nerve segments innervate cutaneous structures in the lower leg situated below the L3 and S1 segments.

It is important to remember that the distribution of these dermatomes is not absolute and may vary from individual to individual. The dermatomes overlap with each other and extend slightly past the midline (Figs. 3–7 and 3–8). For deeper somatic structures (muscles, joint capsule, tendons), the sensory fibers correspond to the same spinal cord segment that supplies motor nerves to those muscles. On the other hand, as previously mentioned, the segmental innervation of the viscera that are supplied with visceral afferents corresponds to the level of embryologic origin rather than to the actual anatomic location. Table 3–4 lists the cutaneous, somatic, and visceral innervation for lumbosacral and abdominal structures. Figures 3–9 through 3–16 list the der-

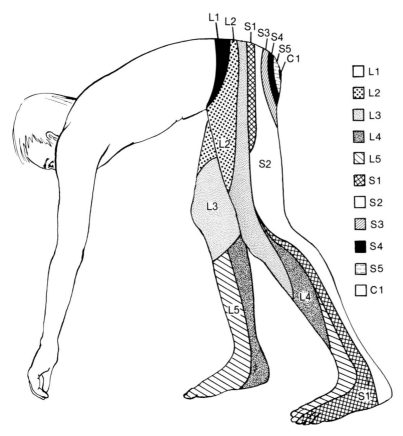

Figure 3–6. Organization of the lumbosacral dermatomes in the quadruped orientation.

matome, myotome, and sclerotome for the lumbar and sacral nerves. Review of these figures reveals the extent of the innervation of structures from individual spinal cord levels and marked overlap among the levels. The complexity of innervation of the lumbosacral spine and surrounding organs occurs not only because of structural duplication but also on the basis of individual variation. It is important for physicians evaluating patients with low back pain to keep the overlap and variation of innervation from individual to individual in mind when evaluating referred pain.

CLINICAL INTERPRETATION OF LOW BACK PAIN

The challenge for the clinician is to interpret the patient's description of his or her pain into anatomic and physiologic correlates that will identify the structure that has been "injured" and the pathologic process that has resulted in pain. Anatomically, structures of the lumbosacral spine receive specific types of sensory innervation that are associated with distinct qualities of pain (e.g., sharp, dull, aching,

throbbing, burning). An understanding of the quality of pain associated with pathologic processes in specific structures helps identify the source of the pain. In addition to the qualitative aspect of pain, pain may be categorized by its location, intensity, onset and duration, aggravating and alleviating factors, and behavioral response (Table 3–5).[28, 29] The sources of low back pain include superficial somatic, deep somatic (spondylogenic), radicular, visceral-referred, neurogenic, and psychogenic (Table 3–5).

Superficial Somatic Pain

The skin and subcutaneous fibers of the back are innervated by nociceptive nerve fibers that cover very small areas. Pathologic processes in the skin result in localized lesions whose intensity correlates with the extent of tissue distention and damage. The involvement of superficial tissues of the back from trauma (laceration, burns, compression), ulceration, superficial neoplasms, or infections (cellulitis) is usually rapidly recognized because of location and is not of great diagnostic

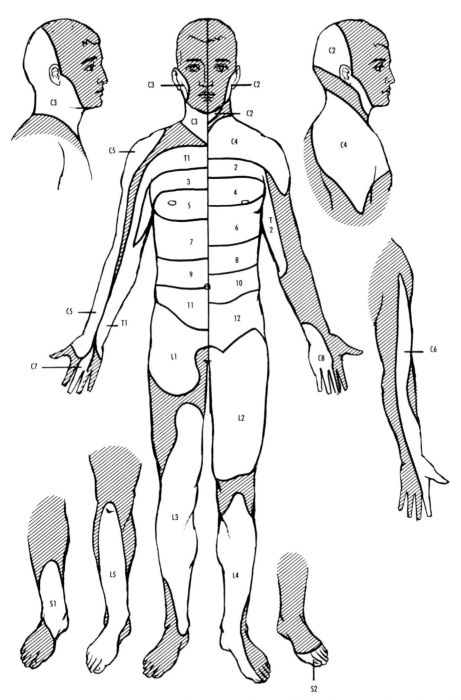

Figure 3–7. Dermatomal distribution (frontal view). The right and left halves show the total distribution of the alternating dermatomes, illustrating the overlap which may involve two or more dermatomes. The insets demonstrate the broad distribution of certain dermatomes (From Gardner E, Gray DJ, O'Rahilly R: Anatomy. 4th ed. Philadelphia: WB Saunders Co, 1975.)

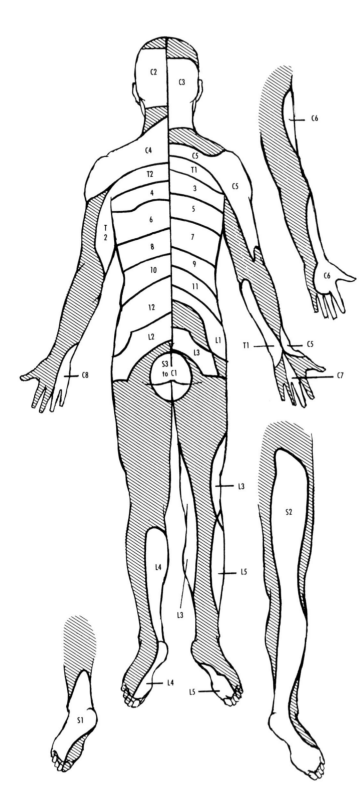

Figure 3–8. Dermatomal distribution (posterior view). (From Gardner E, Gray DJ, O'Rahilly R: Anatomy. 4th ed. Philadelphia, WB Saunders Co, 1975.)

TABLE 3–4. INNERVATION OF CUTANEOUS, SOMATIC, AND VISCERAL STRUCTURES OF THE LUMBOSACRAL SPINE, ABDOMEN, AND PELVIS

	DERMATOME	MOTOR	SEROSAL SURFACE	VISCERAL
Lumbar 1	Groin Level of L1 vertebral body descending to flanks	Iliopsoas	Anterior and lateral abdominal wall Posterior abdominal wall	Kidney Ureter Body of uterus Abdominal aorta Small intestine
Lumbar 2	Anterior thigh Level of L2–L3 vertebral body to lateral thigh (L5 dura—posterior longitudinal ligament)	Iliopsoas Sartorius Adductors	Posterior abdominal wall	Vault of bladder Abdominal aorta Ascending colon
Lumbar 3	Lower anterior thigh to anterior knee Level of L4–L5 vertebral body	Iliopsoas Quadriceps femoris Sartorius Adductors	Posterior abdominal wall	Abdominal aorta
Lumbar 4	Inner calf to medial portion of foot (first 2 toes)	Tibialis posterior Quadriceps femoris Gluteus medius Gluteus minimus Tensor fasciae latae	Posterior abdominal wall	Abdominal aorta
Lumbar 5	Dorsum of foot and big toe (lateral side of lower leg)	Tibialis anterior Extensor hallucis longus Gluteus maximus Hamstring Extensor digitorum longus	—	—
Sacral 1	Sole, heel, and lateral edge of foot	Gastrocnemius Gluteus maximus Hamstring Foot muscles Peroneus longus Peroneus brevis	Pelvic walls	—
Sacral 2	Posterior medial lower and upper leg	Flexor digitorum longus Hallucis longus Foot muscle	Pelvic walls	—
Sacral 3	Medial portions of buttocks	—	Pelvic walls	Rectum Upper anus Base of bladder Cervix Upper vagina Prostate
Sacral 4	Perirectal	—	Pelvic walls	Rectum Upper anus Base of bladder Cervix Upper vagina Prostate
Sacral 5	Perirectal	—	Pelvic walls	
Coccyx 1	Tip of coccyx	—		

L1

L1

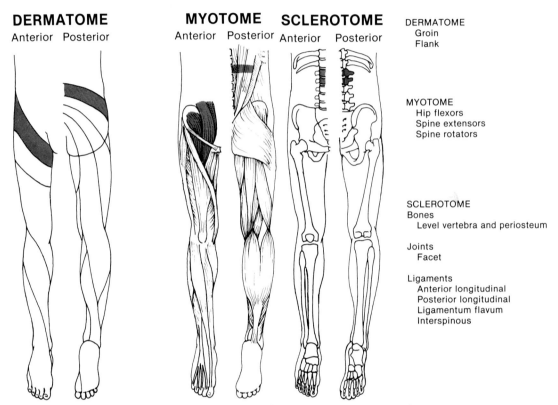

DERMATOME
Anterior Posterior

MYOTOME
Anterior Posterior

SCLEROTOME
Anterior Posterior

DERMATOME
   Groin
   Flank

MYOTOME
   Hip flexors
   Spine extensors
   Spine rotators

SCLEROTOME
Bones
   Level vertebra and periosteum

Joints
   Facet

Ligaments
   Anterior longitudinal
   Posterior longitudinal
   Ligamentum flavum
   Interspinous

Figure 3–9. Dermatome, myotome, and sclerotome distribution for L1.

difficulty. The exception may be patients who present with the burning pain of herpes zoster infection prior to the appearance of vesicles. The acute onset and distribution in a dermatomal pattern should alert the clinician to this possibility.

Deep Somatic (Spondylogenic) Pain

The sources of deep somatic pain in the dnlumbosacral spine are the vertebral column, the surrounding muscles, and the attaching tendons, ligaments, and fascia. Processes that mechanically disrupt these structures will result in back pain. In addition, inflammatory processes that destroy tissue or increase tissue tension and increased vascular pressure that results in distended vessels may cause pain.

In general, with the exception of inflammatory and neoplastic processes, spondylogenic pain is characterized by a deep, dull ache that is maximal over the involved site. The pain is exacerbated by specific motions and relieved with recumbency. The most common cause of spondylogenic pain is the production of high tensions in the muscles of the lower back (lifting a heavy object in a rotated position), which leads to avulsion of tendinous attachments of muscles to bony structures or rupture of muscle fibers or tearing of muscle sheaths (sudden recruitment of muscle bundles when muscles are flexed and relaxed).[30] Pain associated with tendinous lesions is more severe than that associated with direct muscle injury. Either injury is associated with a sharp stab of pain at the moment of injury followed by a dull ache that may persist for weeks and may be associated with tenderness on palpation and reflex muscle spasm. The initial pain originates in the unmyelinated nerve fibers that are stimulated by the mechanical disruption of the tendons, fascial sheaths of muscles, or surrounding intramuscular blood vessels. The prolonged aching pain is a result of the same nerve endings being stimulated by chemical mediators associated with the healing inflammatory response.[20]

L2

L2

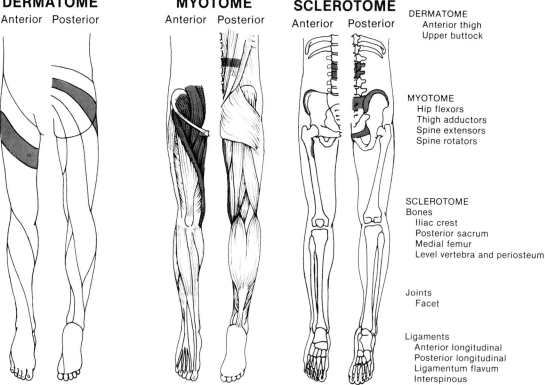

Figure 3–10. Dermatome, myotome, and sclerotome distribution for L2.

Muscle pain may occur in the absence of true muscle injury. Persistent utilization of muscle groups results in muscle pain and, potentially, tonic contraction (spasm). The chronic use of muscle, which occurs more commonly in untrained than in trained muscle, results in increase metabolic activity and the production of chemical byproducts that may stimulate unmyelinated nerve fibers. These factors may include lactic acid and potassium. Physical factors (ambient temperature) and muscle training (sedentary versus athletic) may explain the reason for spondylogenic pain in the individual whose abnormal posture results in persistent contraction of erector spinae muscles, as often occurs in pregnancy. Muscle fatigue may predispose to muscle injury in the workplace.[31] Repetitive trunk motions associated with lifting, bending, and twisting increase the risk for back injuries. With increasing fatigue, primary muscles are unable to complete physical tasks requiring the recruitment of secondary muscle groups at greater risk of injury. The endurance of mus-

cles may be more important as a predictor of pain than absolute strength of muscles.

Muscle hyperactivity may also develop secondary to nociceptive input from nonmuscular sources. Pathologic processes resulting in inflammatory or degenerative processes in facet joints, periosteum, skeleton, or visceral organs may cause muscle pain. The differentiation of reflex spasm secondary to mechanical, structural abnormalities from inflammatory lesions of the lumbosacral spine or viscera is difficult to make. Careful history and physical examination may help in suggesting the primary source of tissue injury. Of great importance is a history of partial injury in separating traumatic muscle spasm from reflex spasm. However, an episode of trauma is not always remembered by the patient. In other circumstances, patients ascribe their symptoms of muscle pain to an insignificant episode of trauma, when in fact their symptoms are secondary to a more serious illness (multiple myeloma).

Other sources of spondylogenic nociceptive

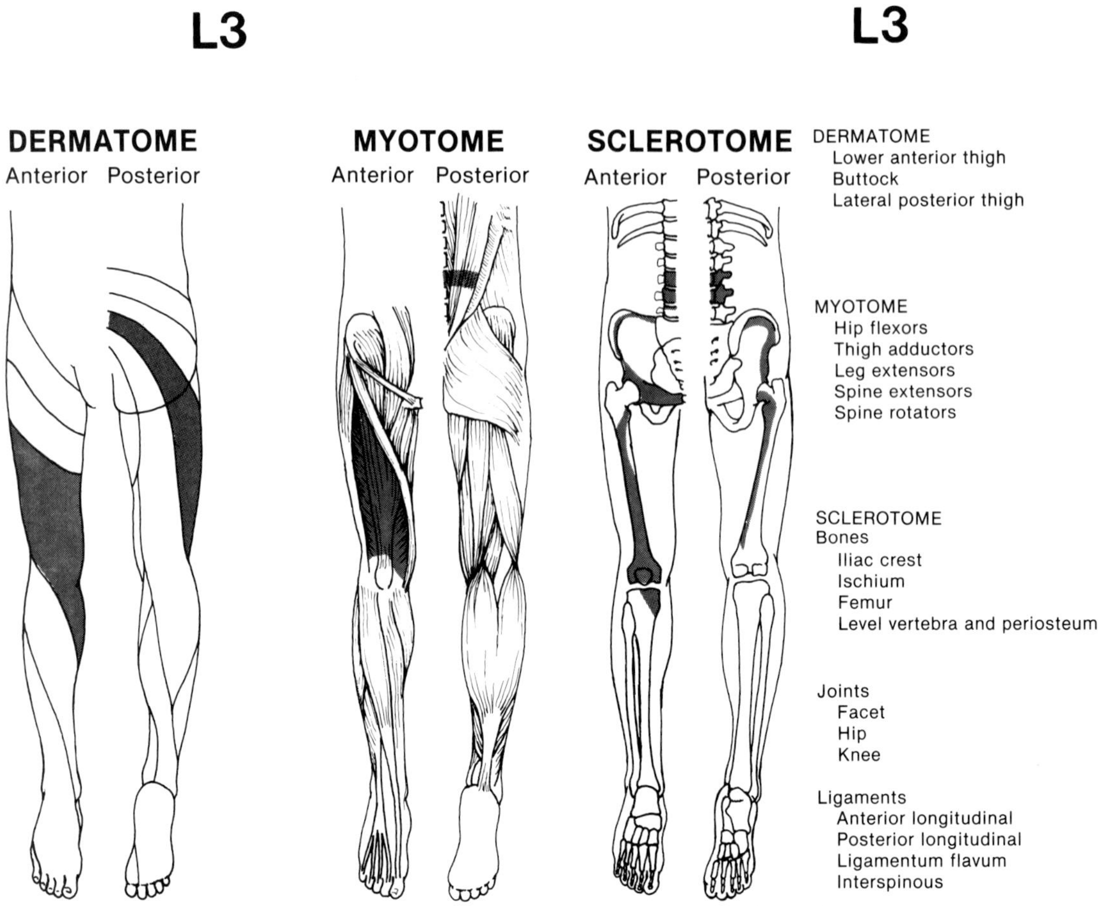

L3

DERMATOME
Anterior Posterior

MYOTOME
Anterior Posterior

SCLEROTOME
Anterior Posterior

DERMATOME
  Lower anterior thigh
  Buttock
  Lateral posterior thigh

MYOTOME
  Hip flexors
  Thigh adductors
  Leg extensors
  Spine extensors
  Spine rotators

SCLEROTOME
Bones
  Iliac crest
  Ischium
  Femur
  Level vertebra and periosteum

Joints
  Facet
  Hip
  Knee

Ligaments
  Anterior longitudinal
  Posterior longitudinal
  Ligamentum flavum
  Interspinous

Figure 3–11. Dermatome, myotome, and sclerotome distribution for L3.

input are the anatomic components of the vertebral column including joints, ligaments, bone, vessels, and the dural and epidural structures. Mechanical injury and resultant inflammation of the apophyseal and sacroiliac joint capsule and ligamentous structures of the lumbosacral spine may cause pain. Nerves that supply joints with sensory innervation frequently also supply surrounding muscle, bones, and skin. There is usually an overlap of nerve innervation with several nerves supplying a single joint (see Fig. 1–27). Terminal branches of unmyelinated and myelinated fibers are distributed through the synovium and periosteum. The joint capsule is richly supplied with sensory innervation. Sensory innervation to the joints includes mechanoreceptors in the joint capsule and nociceptors surrounding blood vessels and near the surface of synovial cells. The most painful stimuli to a joint are twisting, tearing, and stretching of the joint capsule or surrounding ligaments. The unmyelinated C nerve fibers of the posterior primary rami of multiple segments supply

these structures. Therefore, the patient has difficulty identifying the exact location of sources of pain. Usually patients point to the midline or the sacroiliac joint area. Percussion tenderness does not cause as much discomfort in the joints as percussion over muscles in spasm. However, because of the distribution of the sensory and motor nerves, patients with articular and ligamentous disease may develop reflex spasm on both sides of the lumbosacral spine and cutaneous hyperesthesia over the same areas.

Mechanical or inflammatory processes may cause joint pain. Mechanical stresses that stimulate nociceptors in the joint capsule may occur secondary to prolonged sitting or standing in inappropriate postures (hyperlordosis with high-heel shoes, soft chair, sagging mattress), atrophy of back muscles, excess joint motion secondary to decreased disc or vertebral body height, or malformations. Inflammatory diseases of the axial skeleton joints may cause the production of joint swelling along with release of inflammatory mediators that are irritating

L4

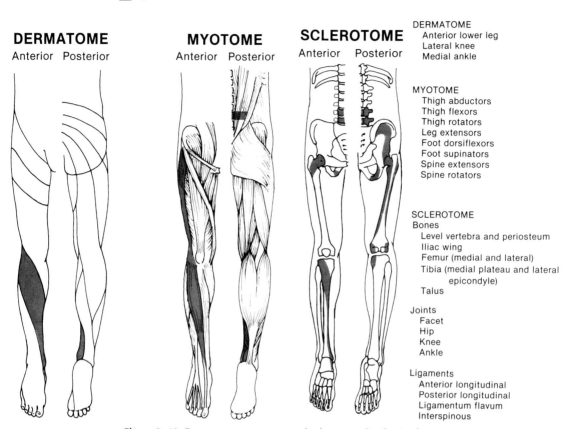

DERMATOME
Anterior Posterior

MYOTOME
Anterior Posterior

SCLEROTOME
Anterior Posterior

L4

DERMATOME
Anterior lower leg
Lateral knee
Medial ankle

MYOTOME
Thigh abductors
Thigh flexors
Thigh rotators
Leg extensors
Foot dorsiflexors
Foot supinators
Spine extensors
Spine rotators

SCLEROTOME
Bones
Level vertebra and periosteum
Iliac wing
Femur (medial and lateral)
Tibia (medial plateau and lateral
epicondyle)
Talus

Joints
Facet
Hip
Knee
Ankle

Ligaments
Anterior longitudinal
Posterior longitudinal
Ligamentum flavum
Interspinous

Figure 3–12. Dermatome, myotome, and sclerotome distribution for L4.

to nociceptors in the fibrous capsule. Structural changes affecting articular cartilage and synovium without inflammation may not be associated with pain since these tissues contain no free nerve endings. The clinical correlate of this fact is the lack of relationship between the extent of structural joint changes associated with aging on radiographic evaluation of the back and the severity of pain.[32]

Another source of spondylogenic pain is ligaments surrounding the vertebral column and fascia that attach muscles to each other and to bone. Although noncontractile tissue, the ligaments of the lumbosacral spine play an essential role in the static postural support of the low back in the upright, sitting, and flexed positions. When the lower back is in its normal configuration (normal lordosis), the ligaments stretch to a natural length that supports the lower back without muscular contraction other than what is generated by autonomic muscle tone. Pain is generated by nociceptors in the ligaments if they are placed under mechanical stress by poor posture, chronic contraction, ex-

cessive force (lifting heavy objects), or a loss of elasticity associated with aging. The same inflammatory diseases that affect joints may also engulf ligamentous structures, resulting in pain that may spread beyond the margins of articular structures. The exact segmental distribution of pain arising from ligamentous structures is hard to define. Experimental injection of hypertonic saline into ligamentous structures has defined locations of pain, but it is unclear whether the tension caused by the injection or the chemical irritation was the source of pain.[33] Whether pain generated in this fashion is the same as that generated by a mechanical injury is conjecture, since pain is related not only to the location of injury but also to the form of the noxious stimulus.

Bone pain is particularly intense when the periosteum is disrupted. Mechanical trauma, crush fractures, neoplasms, or infections may be causes of pain. For example, lumbar spine extension may cause pain by impaction of contiguous spinous processes or an inferior articular process on the lamina below.[34] Pain from

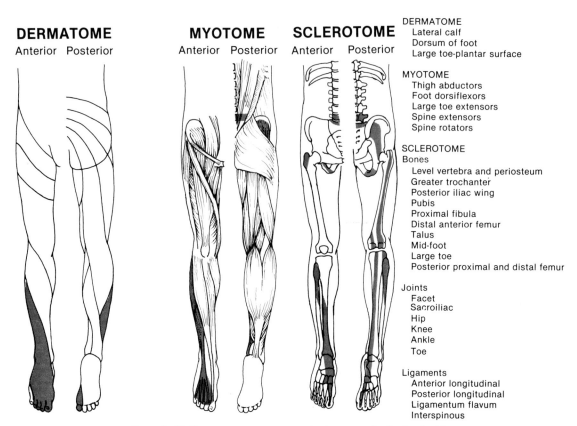

L5   L5

DERMATOME
Anterior Posterior

MYOTOME
Anterior Posterior

SCLEROTOME
Anterior Posterior

DERMATOME
 Lateral calf
 Dorsum of foot
 Large toe-plantar surface

MYOTOME
 Thigh abductors
 Foot dorsiflexors
 Large toe extensors
 Spine extensors
 Spine rotators

SCLEROTOME
Bones
 Level vertebra and periosteum
 Greater trochanter
 Posterior iliac wing
 Pubis
 Proximal fibula
 Distal anterior femur
 Talus
 Mid-foot
 Large toe
 Posterior proximal and distal femur

Joints
 Facet
 Sacroiliac
 Hip
 Knee
 Ankle
 Toe

Ligaments
 Anterior longitudinal
 Posterior longitudinal
 Ligamentum flavum
 Interspinous

Figure 3–13. Dermatome, myotome, and sclerotome distribution for L5.

a vertebral body may be insignificant, despite destruction and replacement of trabecular bone, if the process is slowly progressive and does not cause fractures or irritation of the periosteum. Once bone has been replaced to a significant degree, minor trauma may result in a pathologic fracture and intense pain.

Another potential cause of somatic back pain is the distention of veins of the vertebral plexus.[20] Nociceptive fibers supply the venous plexus. When sufficiently stretched with prolonged coughing, vomiting, parturition, or obstructed micturition, these fibers produce a dull, deep pain that may be associated with headache. In patients with herniated nucleus pulposus or intraspinal tumor, a moderate degree of increased pressure may provoke or exacerbate existing pain. These are patients who described increased back pain secondary to coughing or straining with a bowel movement.

The nociceptive innervation of the dura explains the association of pain with pathologic processes affecting the anterior dural membrane. The posterior dura has no nociceptive

innervation. The anterior dura, along with the dural sleeves which extend into the neural foramina, are densely innervated. Pain associated with dural lesions is of a deep, aching quality, located near the midline.

The annulus fibrosus receives nociceptive innervation, which is limited to the outer fibers of the annulus. Tears of the annulus fibrosus produce somatic pain predominantly located in the low back. Abnormalities of the nucleus pulposus unassociated with disruption of annular fibers are devoid of pain. The nucleus pulposus does not receive any sensory innervation.

Radicular Pain

The source of radicular pain is not peripheral sensory nerves but the proximal spinal nerves that form from the ventral and dorsal roots. Processes that decrease blood flow to the spinal nerve (ischemia) cause radicular pain. The large mechanoreceptor fibers, be-

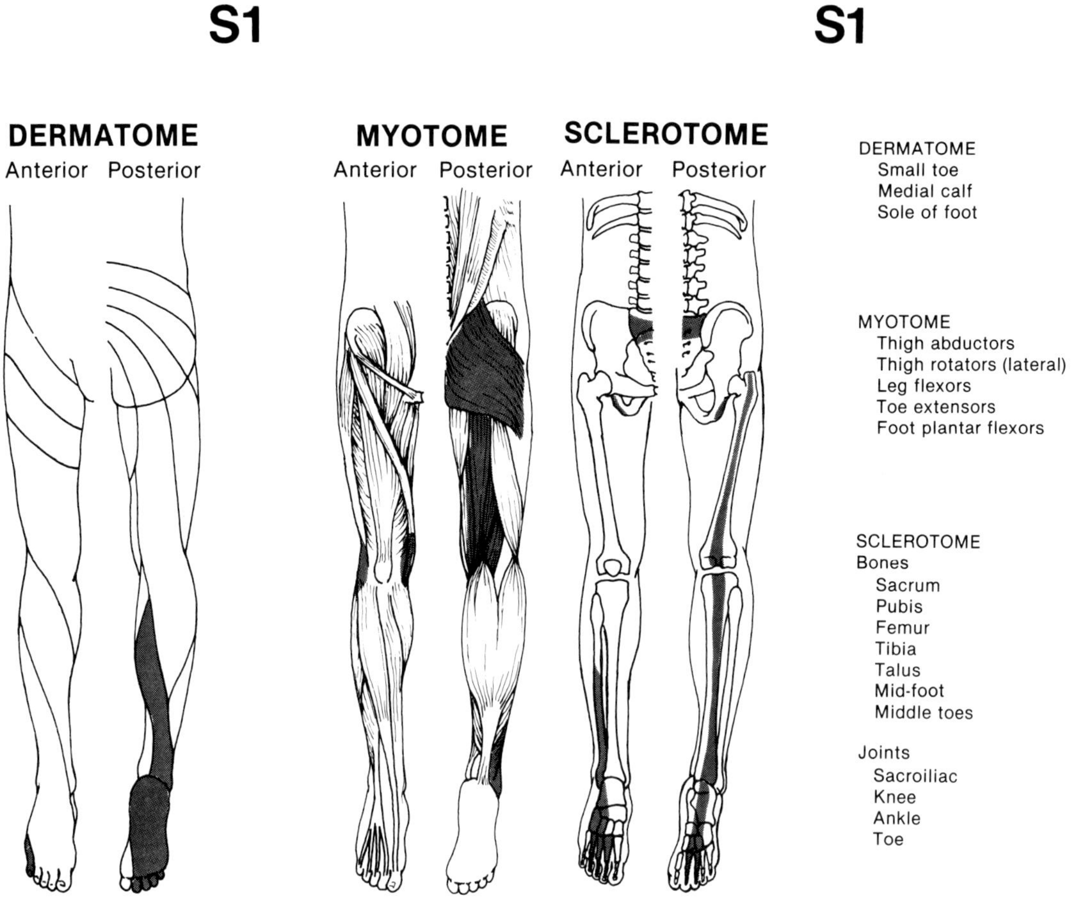

S1

S1

DERMATOME
Anterior Posterior

MYOTOME
Anterior Posterior

SCLEROTOME
Anterior Posterior

DERMATOME
Small toe
Medial calf
Sole of foot

MYOTOME
Thigh abductors
Thigh rotators (lateral)
Leg flexors
Toe extensors
Foot plantar flexors

SCLEROTOME
Bones
Sacrum
Pubis
Femur
Tibia
Talus
Mid-foot
Middle toes

Joints
Sacroiliac
Knee
Ankle
Toe

Figure 3–14. Dermatome, myotome, and sclerotome distribution for S1.

cause of their large diameters, have greater metabolic activity and are more sensitive to disturbances of blood flow. This results in the loss of inhibitory pain impulses, allowing for preferential nociceptive input into the dorsal horn. Another mechanism of pain production is inflammatory chemical irritation. Traction on a normal, noninflamed nerve root does not produce pain. However, slight tension on an inflamed root is associated with production of radicular pain.

Radicular pain has a lancinating, shooting, burning, sharp, tender quality, which may radiate from the back to the lower extremity and foot, in the distribution of the compromised spinal nerve. This pain radiating from the back to the leg is commonly called sciatica. In addition to sciatic pain, achiness and spasm may be experienced in thigh and calf muscles. The pain is exacerbated by any motion that increases tension on the involved nerve root, while bed rest relieves pain.

A frequent cause of compressive lesions that result in radicular pain are lesions of the lumbar vertebral discs (most commonly L4-L5 and L5-S1). Factors that cause disruption of normal disc architecture facilitate degeneration of discs and increase the potential of rupture and the production of radicular pain. A great deal of research involving the lumbar spine has taken place over the past decade and much of the work has been focused on the behavior of healthy and degenerated discs. The research effort has been multidisciplinary, focusing on biomechanical, biochemical, nutritional, immunologic, and nociceptive (pain) factors. A review of these factors helps in recognizing individuals who are at risk of developing this problem.

DISC BIOMECHANICAL FACTORS

Most of what is known about the pathomechanics of low back disorders has been gleaned by studying the mechanical behavior of cadaveric spinal motor segments. A motor segment is composed of two adjacent vertebral bodies, the interposed disc, and surrounding

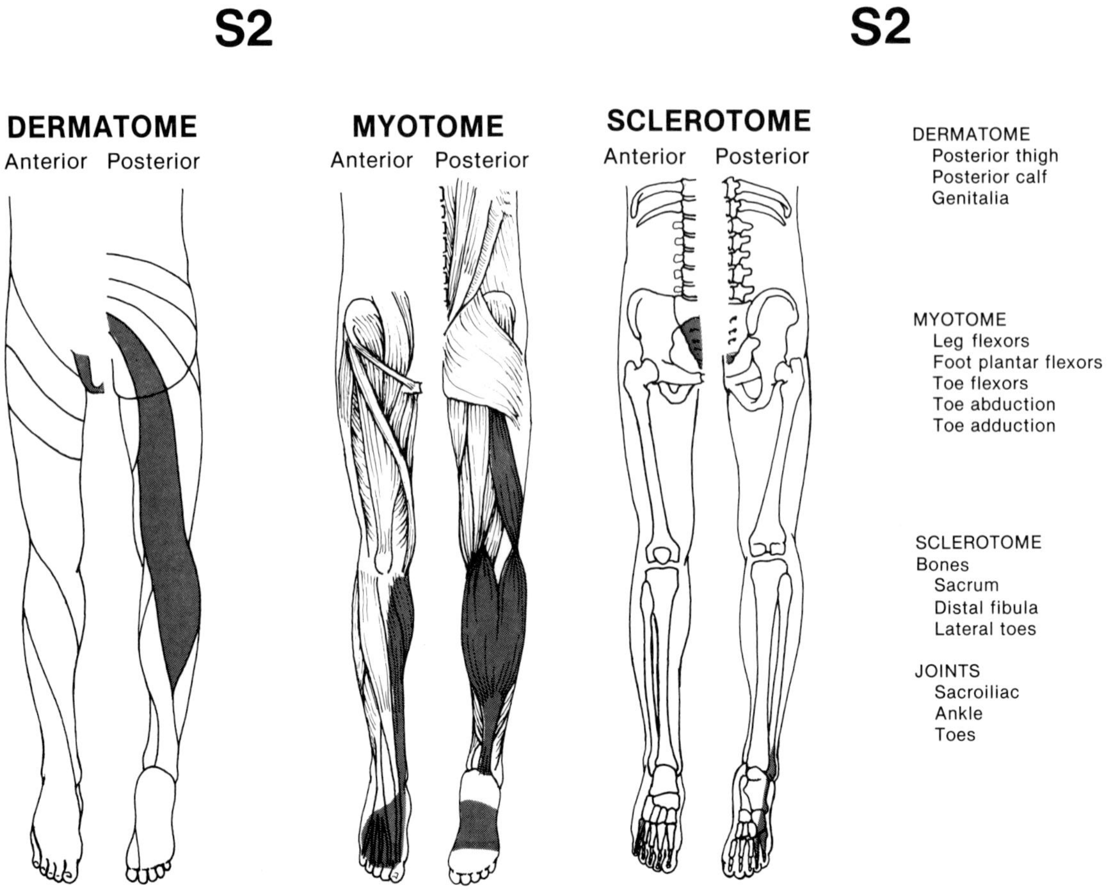

S2

S2

DERMATOME
Anterior Posterior

MYOTOME
Anterior Posterior

SCLEROTOME
Anterior Posterior

DERMATOME
  Posterior thigh
  Posterior calf
  Genitalia

MYOTOME
  Leg flexors
  Foot plantar flexors
  Toe flexors
  Toe abduction
  Toe adduction

SCLEROTOME
Bones
  Sacrum
  Distal fibula
  Lateral toes

JOINTS
  Sacroiliac
  Ankle
  Toes

Figure 3–15. Dermatome, myotome, and sclerotome distribution for S2.

structures. It seems clear that under flexion, extension, rotation, and shear stress, the load distribution in the motor segment is not confined to the intervertebral disc alone but is shared between the strong anterior and posterior longitudinal ligaments, the facet joints and capsules, and the other ligamentous structures, such as the ligamentum flavum and the interspinous and supraspinous ligaments (see Fig. 1–17). In vivo, these same structures, as well as the muscle and fascial attachments, intrinsic and extrinsic to the vertebral column, interact to accommodate the load-bearing requirements of the lumbar spine. For pure compression loads, it has been calculated that the lower lumbar disc may have to bear a load of up to 1000 kilograms of force, which may well exceed the compressive strength of the vertebral endplates. This excess is probably largely absorbed by other mechanisms, such as the hydraulic effect of intra-abdominal pressure produced by contraction of the abdominal wall musculature.

When pure compressive loads are progressively applied to an intervertebral disc, the vertebral endplate will give way before the nucleus pulposus will herniate. The disc itself behaves like a viscoelastic structure and protrudes circumferentially. It should be appreciated that there is no difference in the failure pattern between normal and degenerated intervertebral discs.

It has been suggested that abnormal torsional stresses, applied particularly to the lordotic motion segments, may be the mechanism by which radial and circumferential fissures are produced within the annulus fibrosus. Furthermore, these fissures tend to occur in the posterolateral segments of the annulus because of the eccentric geometry of the intervertebral disc. The effects of this torsional stress concentration are also intensified in the presence of asymmetry of the facet joints as well as in advanced degeneration of the disc. In these situations the disc tends to fail after a few degrees of torsion. When torsion and compression loads are applied simultaneously to the lumbar discs, a component of shear loading is created. The two lowest lumbar discs are affected to a greater degree than those above.

S3-C1

DERMATOME
Anterior   Posterior

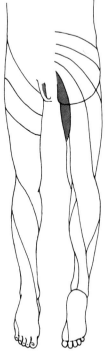

DERMATOME
Perirectal
Tip of coccyx

MYOTOME
Pelvic floor

SCLEROTOME
—

Figure 3–16. Dermatome, myotome, and sclerotome distribution for S3-C1.

It has been shown in vitro that extremely high loads must be applied in a direct horizontal plane to the disc to produce failure into the shear mode. An example of shear failure of the disc can be seen in cases of high-velocity motor vehicle collisions when the patient has been wearing a lap seat belt.

Under tension, the disc is strongest in the anterior and posterior regions and weakest in the center. It is somewhat paradoxical to note that the tensile strength of the annulus has been found to be greatest in its posterolateral segment, which is usually the location where the nucleus pulposus will herniate.

Most of the biomechanical knowledge of the lumbar spine deals with the normal and abnormal function of the intervertebral disc. The bony elements have only recently been evaluated. It appears that the anterior elements provide the major support for the lumbar column and absorb various impacts. The posterior structures share some of the loads, but they mainly influence the potential patterns of mo-

tion. The facet joints resist most of the intervertebral shear force and in lordotic postures share in resisting intervertebral compression. The facet joints also serve to prevent excessive motion from damaging the discs. In particular, the posterior annulus is protected in torsion by the facet surfaces and in flexion by the capsular ligaments of the facet joints. Rotation of a lumbar motion segment is normally limited to 3°. Motion beyond this range occurs secondary to facet joint failure or rotation around a new axis located in the impacted facet joint. The vertebral body slides laterally and posteriorly applying shear forces to the associated disc. Beyond 3° of motion, the annular fibers in the innervated outer portion of the disc are disrupted. This injury is a potential source of low back pain.[34, 35]

DISC BIOCHEMICAL FACTORS

On a microscopic level, the intervertebral disc consists of two adjacent hyaline cartilage endplates, an annulus fibrosus composed of sheets of collagen fibers obliquely aligned in layered sheets at angles varying between 40° and 80°, and a nucleus pulposus consisting of a loosely arranged network of collagen fibers and cells in an extracellular matrix. The annular fibers are attached to the endplates and for a short distance into the vertebral bodies. The annulus is thicker anteriorly than posteriorly and gradually thins out as it approaches the nucleus pulposus internally.

To function efficiently, the disc largely depends on the physical properties of the nucleus pulposus, which in turn are closely related to its water binding capacity. The higher the hydration content, the more effectively the disc functions. Unfortunately, the hydration of the disc drops progressively from early life, when the water content is 88%, to a level of 69% in the eighth decade of life.[36] Ultrastructurally, 99% of the tissue mass of the disc is formed by its matrix, which contains glycoproteins, proteoglycans, collagen, and other proteins. It is presently felt that structural insufficiency of the disc is guided by an alteration in this biochemical composition.

The bulk of the connective tissue matrix in an intervertebral disc is collagen. There are seven major subtypes of collagen identified in intervertebral discs. The annulus fibrosus contains types I, II, III, V, VI, IX, and XI and the nucleus pulposus types II, VI, IX and XI.[37] Type I, found predominantly in tendons, skin, bones, and ligaments, accounts for about 90% of the collagen in the body. Type II is absent

TABLE 3–5. CLASSIFICATION OF LOW BACK PAIN*

CATEGORY	SENSORY NERVES	PATHOLOGIC ENTITY	QUALITY
Superficial somatic (skin with subcutaneous tissue)	Cutaneous A fibers, small field	Cellulitis	Sharp
		Herpes zoster	Burning
Deep somatic (spondylogenic) (muscles, fascia, periosteum, ligaments, joints, vessels, dura)	Sinuvertebral	Muscular strain	Sharp (acutes)
	Posterior primary ramus unmyelinated	Arthritis	Dull ache (chronic)
		Fracture Increased venous pressure	Boring
Radicular (spinal nerves)	—	Herniated vertebral disc	Segmental
		Spinal stenosis	Radiating
			Shooting
Visceral referred (abdominal and pelvic viscera, aorta)	Autonomic sensory, unmyelinated C fibers, large field	Pancreatitis	Deep
		Intestinal diseases	Boring
		Prostatitis Endometriosis Abdominal aneurysm	Colicky Tearing
Neurogenic	Mixed motor sensory nerves	Herpes zoster Femoral nerve neuropathy	Burning
Psychogenic	—	Depression Conversion reaction Malingering	Variable

*Modified from Engel GL: Pain. In Blacklow R (ed): Signs and Symptoms: Applied Pathologic Physiology and Clinical Interpretation. Philadelphia: JB Lippincott, 1983, pp 41–60 and Macnab I: Backache. Baltimore: Williams and Wilkins, 1983, pp 16–18.

from these tissues but is found in high concentrations in hyaline cartilage. In the human, approximately 65% of the collagen in the annulus fibrosus is type II, with the remainder being type I. More than 95% of the collagen in the nucleus pulposus is type II. The significance is that type I collagen has a restricted water content and is thus better able to handle tensile stress; conversely, type II, with its hydrophilic physical properties, is ideally suited to absorb compressive forces. Type II, V, and XI are fibril forming collagens. Type III is found in both the nucleus and the inner annulus fibrosus. Type V is distributed in noncartilagi-nous tissues in combination with type I collagen. Type V collagen forms a scaffold for type I and these are copolymerized within the same fibril network in the annulus. Type XI copolymerizes with type II to control fibril diameter and may also serve as the site of binding of cartilage proteoglycans, heparin, and chondroitin sulfate. Type VI collagen is located in the nucleus pulposus and encircles interstitial collagen fibers forming an independent network for organization of extracellular components including proteoglycans. Type IX is found primarily in the nucleus pulposus and cross-links type II to bridge collagen fibrils covalently. In

TABLE 3–5. CLASSIFICATION OF LOW BACK PAIN *Continued*

LOCATION	INTENSITY	ONSET AND DURATION	AGGRAVATING AND ALLEVIATING FACTORS	BEHAVIOR
Well localized	Correlates with intensity of nerve stimulation (mild to moderate)	Acute	Intensified by direct contact	Mild concern
		Correlates with status of lesions	Diminished by light touch in adjacent areas	Able to see lesion
Diffuse	Correlates with intensity of nerve stimulation (mild to severe)	Acute or chronic	Intensified with movement	Avoidance of movement
Multiple segments affected			Diminished with rest	Abnormal posture secondary to protective spasm
Low back	Mild to severe	Acute	Intensified with standing, sitting	Avoidance of movement
Afferent distribution of affected nerve root (superficial and deep)	Correlates with intensity of nerve impingement		Diminished with bed rest	Abnormal gait
Segmental with radiation inside body	Mild to severe	Acute or chronic	Related to factors affecting each organ system	Movement to find comfortable position
	Correlates with intensity of nerve stimulation			
Peripheral nerve	Severe	Chronic Persistent	Intensified with palpation	Apprehension
Nondermatomal	Variable	Persistent	No consistent correlation	Emphasis on suffering

addition, collagens VI, IX, and XI form a porous capsule around chondrocytes that provide a compliant but inelastic barrier during compression. The interactions of the component collagens result in a three-dimensional meshwork of fibrils that influence the biologic properties of the disc.[37]

After collagen, the proteoglycans make up the major component of the extracellular matrix of the disc. These molecules consists of noncollagenous protein cores along with the attached sulfated glucose aminoglycans of chondroitin-4-sulfate, chondroitin-6-sulfate, and keratan sulfate. The proteoglycans are, in turn, attached to long chains of hyaluronic acid by small glycoprotein links. These molecules are found in great abundance within the nucleus pulposus but form only a small proportion of the dry weight of the annulus fibrosus. They are hydrophilic and, therefore, regulate the fluid content of the nucleus.

Proteoglycans are synthesized in chondrocytes. After the protein core is manufactured, up to 100 chondroitin sulfate and 50 keratan sulfate chains are added during post-translational processing in the chondrocyte.[37] The proteoglycan monomers aggregate as they encounter hyaluronate. The process of aggregation immobilizes the proteoglycans within the extracellular matrix. A link protein cements the proteoglycan to hyaluronate. Approximately 100 to 200 proteoglycan monomers are bound to a single hyaluronate chain.

Many age-related changes have been noted in disc proteoglycans. With time, these molecules lose their ability to associate with collagen, have a lower molecular weight, have a reduced aggregation potential, and develop an increased keratan sulfate content. These changes adversely affect the ability of the disc to imbibe water, which in turn decreases its capacity to dissipate energy when loaded. The changes in disc composition may also be related to topographic variations in the synthesis of disc proteoglycans.[38] Proteoglycan synthesis rates for annulus fibrosus in fetal discs is five times greater than for similar locations in adult discs. Synthesis rates are highest in the inner annulus for fetal discs and the mid-annulus for adult discs. The clinical correlate is that injuries to certain portions of an intervertebral disc may not heal secondary to inadequate production of proteoglycan. Injuries to the annulus fibrosus may have a limited potential for healing.[39] A greater understanding of the mechanisms by which chondrocytes synthesize and degrade extracellular matrix and collagen may help in differentiating between normal aging and pathologic degeneration of intervertebral discs.

DISC NUTRITIONAL FACTORS

The intervertebral disc is a relatively avascular structure and beyond 15 to 20 years of age has no direct blood vessels. Diffusion is the main transport mechanism for disc nutrition in the adult. Small uncharged solutes such as glucose and oxygen mainly gain access to the metabolizing cells through the vertebral endplates. The diffusion of negatively charged solutes such as sulfates, which are important for proteoglycan production, occurs mainly through the annulus fibrosus. Since the area available for diffusion of these negatively charged solutes is smaller in the posterior region of the annulus, turnover of both collagen and proteoglycan is slower in this critical zone. It is felt that this nutritional inadequacy in conjunction with the concentration of mechanical stress in the posterolateral annulus accounts for the high incidence of intervertebral disc ruptures in this area. Also, it is most likely that when fissures and cracks do occur in this area, even prior to the stage of rupture, the propensity for healing is liable to below or inadequate at best.

Decreased oxygen concentrations through-out intervertebral discs result in increased lactate concentrations. The increased lactate levels result in decreased pH. The acid milieu causes a decrease in matrix synthesis and increased degradative enzyme activity. The eventual consequence of inadequate nutrients is degeneration and poor healing of disc constituents.[40]

DISC IMMUNOLOGIC FACTORS

In its normal state, the intervertebral disc, owing to its avascular structure, seems to be an immunologically privileged site. However, as the disc degenerates, its chemical constituent parts are exposed to the host's normal immune defense mechanism, causing an autoimmune reaction to some degree. The phenomenon was first demonstrated in rabbits when it was found that their nucleus pulposus can induce the production of autoantibodies. This autoimmune reaction has been confirmed in the human, and there is particularly strong evidence that this sequestration within the spinal canal elicits a strong cell-mediated immune response to the autogenous disc material.

These findings can help explain, in part, the etiology of the acute sciatic pain associated with disc ruptures. It seems clear that mechanical compression on the nerve root that is being irritated by the herniated disc material is an important factor in the production of pain. As far as the inflammation that occurs around the nerve root, no one is certain whether it is related to an autoimmune phenomenon, ischemic neuropathy from alteration in blood flow patterns, or defects in the neuronal transport mechanism of the nerve root itself. Regardless, it has been shown that inflammation is a necessary ingredient in the production of root pain from disc herniations. This was demonstrated by the use of thin silk threads that were passed around lumbar nerve root sheaths at times of surgery for the removal of herniated discs. The threads were brought out through the skin during wound closure. Postoperatively, when pressure was applied to the roots that had not been compressed by the disc herniation, the patient experienced only paresthesias in the dermatomal distribution of the nerve. There was no pain. When tension was applied to the inflamed root that had previously been compressed by the disc herniation, radicular pain was perceived. This perhaps explains the reason why many patients with sciatica can be effectively treated with anti-inflammatory medications.

DISC NOCICEPTIVE FACTORS

In the lumbosacral region, free nerve endings supplied by the sinuvertebral nerves and posterior primary ramus provide sensory innervation to the anterior and posterior longitudinal ligaments, the facet joint capsules, the superficial lamellae of the annulus fibrosus, the dural envelope, the periosteum of the vertebrae, and the blood vessels. A review of the anatomy of the neural foramina elucidates the structures at risk from compression by a herniated disc.

As the nerve roots descend from the L1 level where the true spinal cord terminates, they cross the disc immediately above the foramen they exit. They enter the foramen below the pedicle and leave the foramen in a downward and forward fashion. By virtue of this configuration, the nerve is located in the superior portion of the foramen. The nerve carries along with it the arachnoid, until the confluence of the ventral and dorsal roots, and the dura, which invaginates in the foramen. The dura continues along the distal nerve forming the outer sheath, the perineurium. Debate exists whether the dural sleeves are firmly or loosely attached to the walls of the foramen.[20, 41]

Flexion of the spine allows motion of these elements in the foramina. When tension is placed on the structures, the nerve will elongate, while the dura increases in tension. In the foramen, 50% of the space is occupied by the nerve and its sheath. Connective tissue, adipose tissue, vessels, lymphatics, and the sinuvertebral nerves fill the remainder. The sinuvertebral nerve winds back into the foramen supplying the posterior longitudinal ligament, fibrous tissue near the annulus, and the anterior but not the posterior dural sheath. The posterior dura has no nociceptive innervation.

In the initial stage of protrusion, the sinuvertebral nerve on the posterior longitudinal ligament is irritated, which gives rise to pain in the lower back without sciatica. As the impingement increases, the dural sleeves and nerve root are involved. As a result, back pain becomes more severe and widely distributed. With greater pressure, pain in the sciatic distribution is elicited along with paresthesias and numbness, and the motor fibers in the inferior portion of the spinal nerve are compressed, resulting in reflex muscle spasm. With greater duration and extent of nerve pressure, numbness replaces pain as a symptom and muscle weakness replaces spasm. Additional clinical features of herniated vertebral discs are discussed in Chapter 10.

It is known that not all radicular-like pain is related to disc herniation. Distention of degenerated intervertebral discs or facet joints with injections of saline or contrast material can produce pain in the low back that radiates down the leg.[42, 43] This is not true radicular pain. It is referred pain that appears in mesenchymal structures of the same embryonic sclerotome as the injured tissue. When this type of pain is referred into the buttocks and legs, it has a dull, aching quality unlike the sharp, lancinating pain of true sciatica.

Herniated vertebral discs are not the only cause of radicular pain. Overgrowth of bone from the facet joints intrudes into the spinal canal, decreasing the room for the neural elements. This entity is referred to as lumbar spinal stenosis. Affected patients experience back and radicular pain in body positions that decrease room in the spinal canal or with walking (positions of extension).

Back pain and radicular pain may also occur secondary to obstruction of veins in the intervertebral foramen.[44] Direct compression of the nerve root may not be necessary to develop radicular pain. Intraforaminal venous dilatation secondary to venous compression from a disc or osteophyte may result in adjacent neural fibrosis. Nerve root fibrosis may be a source of pain in patients with degenerative disc disease without herniation.

Nerve root compression is also seen with fracture-dislocation of the spine, infections, and neoplasms. Neoplasms that cause radicular pain are usually extradural (metastatic) or intradural (neurofibroma). Intramedullary tumors of the spinal cord are unassociated with radicular pain.

Neurogenic Pain

Neurogenic pain arises from abnormalities of the peripheral or central nervous systems. The structures associated with neurogenic pain include the peripheral nerves, the dorsal root ganglia, spinal cord, thalamus, and sensory area of the cerebral cortex. Damage to the sensory portion of the nervous system results in pain produced spontaneously or with otherwise nonpainful sensory stimulation (light touch). The pain follows a distribution that corresponds to the damaged neural structure. The response to simple light touch can be excruciating pain similar to that experienced with causalgia or reflex sympathetic dystrophy.[45] The pain may have a delayed onset or occur in paroxysms. It may be sustained for some time after cessation of the provoking stimulus (hyperpathia). Particularly with injuries of the central nervous system, pain may begin abruptly without evident peripheral stimulation. Neurogenic pain is described as burning, tingling, crushing, gnawing, or skin crawling. In many circumstances, it is a unique pain that the patient has not experienced previously.[46] As opposed to radicular pain, increases in intraspinal pressure produced by coughing or sneezing rarely exacerbate nerve pain. Instead, pain is intensified by sensory stimulation of the damaged nerve. Because of this fact, patients actively protect the limb from contact and develop behavior that protects it from the environment.

The abnormality causing neurogenic pain is the loss of the pain inhibitory system in the peripheral nerves and/or central nervous system. Those processes that diminish the large, myelinated fiber input to the dorsal horn allow for increased transmission of nociceptive information. Also, nociceptive transmission is increased by diminished input from the nerves originating in the periaqueductal gray area of the midbrain.

An example of neurogenic pain is diabetic mononeuropathy of the femoral or sciatic nerve. The neuropathy presents with sudden onset of burning pain in the peripheral distribution of the nerve associated with loss of sensory and motor function. Another example of neurogenic pain is postherpetic neuralgia. Herpes zoster preferentially affects dorsal root ganglion cells of mechanoreceptors and causes neurogenic pain distributed in a dermatomal pattern.

Viscerogenic Referred Pain

Viscerogenic referred back pain arises from abnormalities in organs that share segmental innervation with structures in the lumbosacral spine. These organs include the pancreas, part of the duodenum, the ascending and descending colon, rectum, kidney, ureter, bladder, and pelvic organs including uterus, cervix, and prostate. Visceral afferents that supply these organs transmit impulses to the dorsal horn, where somatic and visceral pain fibers share second-order neurons.[47] Impulses from visceral nerve endings arrive at the same reception point among the posterior horn cells as do impulses of somatic origin. Visceral pain will be noted in the same somatic segment with which it shares neurons in lamina V of the dorsal horn.

The precise localization of somatic pain differs from the wider distribution of visceral pain since the latter is transmitted to multiple segments. In addition to superficial cutaneous pain, reflex muscle spasm and vasomotor changes may also occur. The back pain may have a gripping, cramping, aching, squeezing, crushing, tearing, stabbing, or burning quality, depending on the affected organ. The degree of tissue injury is correlated with the intensity of the pain and is associated with recruitment of additional segmental levels above and below, as well as neighboring segments that have transmitted past or concurrent nociceptive impulses. A clinical correlate of this recruitment of segments is the radiating quality of visceral pain.

The duration and sequence of viscerogenic referred back pain is helpful in identifying its organ of origin. Back pain caused by referred impulses will follow the periodicity associated with the diseased organ. Rhythmic peristaltic waves of a hollow viscus attempting to expel its contents against resistance produce pain that rises quickly to its greatest intensity in 20 to 30 seconds, lasts 1 to 2 minutes, and quickly subsides, only to recur again in minutes. Lesions in the ureter, uterus, or colon are associated with this quality of pain. Throbbing pain is associated with vascular lesions. Lesions that result in inflammation and the release of chemical mediators that facilitate pain are associated with pain that increases in intensity and lasts for extended periods of time.[6]

Back pain is rarely the sole symptom of visceral disease. Changes in gastrointestinal or urinary function may be clues to the potential source of pain. Viscerogenic pain may be differentiated from deep somatic pain by the response to activity and rest. Somatic pain is frequently exacerbated by activity and improved by rest. Patients with viscerogenic pain get no relief from bed rest. In fact, they may feel more comfortable moving about trying to achieve a comfortable position.

Psychogenic Pain

Psychogenic pain arises not from structures located in the lumbosacral spine but at levels of the cortex. Patients with psychogenic pain experience discomfort, but it is not based upon tissue damage. Patients with psychogenic pain may suffer from depression, hysteria, or conversion reaction. They respond to their environment with symptoms that help control their situation.[48]

The pain is poorly defined and does not

follow dermatomal patterns. It is superficial or deep, sharp or dull, radiating or nonradiating, constant or intermittent, excruciating or mild. Pain may be associated with specific social activities, such as work or sexual intercourse, while other activities requiring similar physical effort elicit little pain.

The time course of pain defies physiologic time sequences. Pain may last for seconds or for years and may be unrelenting and unmoved by therapy during this extended time. The language used to describe the pain may reflect the patient's thoughts of suffering or punishment, such as, "a knife sticking you," "being hit," "burned with a red hot poker," or "having your skin peeled off."[49]

Psychogenic pain is resistant to most conventional therapies that are effective in treating somatic causes of back pain. Therapy must be directed not at the pain but at the reasons causing an agitated depression, conversion reaction, or reluctance to return to work. These patients experience pain that is just as incapacitating as that felt by those suffering from muscle strain. These patients will not improve unless the source of pain is recognized.

Duration of Pain

The function of pain as it affects the whole body is closely related to its duration. Acute pain frequently has an understandable cause (trauma), normally has a characteristic time course, and resolves once healing has occurred. The purpose of acute pain is to inform the host that tissue damage has occurred and to prevent further injury. The rapidly conducting systems (neospinothalamic, dorsal column tracts, for example) are suited to the speedy relay of both nociceptive and light touch sensations necessary to determine the initial phase of tissue injury. The overlap between systems allows one to be responsive to proprioceptive stimuli while another is primed to receive nociceptive stimulation. The organization of multiple ascending systems allows the individual to be constantly primed for nociceptive impulses, which are important to prevent injury, while the central nervous system is flooded with non-nociceptive inputs.[50] This rapid system activates appropriate motor responses that attempt to minimize damage to the affected part.

The slowly conducting system, including the paleospinothalamic tract, carries information about the state of the injury and its susceptibility to further damage. This tonic stimulation

determines the general behavioral state of the individual to prevent further damage and foster rest and care of the damaged area to promote healing. Tonic pain also resolves with healing of the injury. The functions of the rapid and slow conducting systems may be controlled by different neurochemical mechanisms. This may have therapeutic implications, since the phasic and tonic components of pain may respond to different drugs.[50]

Chronic pain may persist long after the injury has healed. Chronic pain, which is continuous over several months, results from habituation of the sensory system to nociceptive stimuli. Constant stimulation results in an activation of the cerebral cortical function of memory. The central nervous system becomes habituated to the sensory input to the point where pain is perceived in the absence of a detectable lesion. As the duration of pain continues, the area affected may spread to adjacent or distal body areas. Chronic pain also results in autonomic responses that are depressive (vegetative) in quality: poor sleep, decreased appetite, irritability, withdrawal of interests, strained interpersonal relationships, and increased somatic preoccupation.[51] Chronic pain is associated with significant depression.[52] In addition, resolution or reduction of pain reverses the reactive depression caused by the pain.[53] The marked psychologic effects, including depression and anxiety associated with chronic pain, do not serve a useful purpose.

The changes associated with chronic pain that occur in the central nervous system (CNS) are related to alterations in molecular control of neuropeptide synthesis and neuroreceptor production.[54] Immediate early genes (IEG) are oncogenes that are activated by a variety of stimuli to nerve cells. IEG, such as c-fos and c-jun, act as transcription messengers that control the transcription mechanisms of a cell. Repetitive noxious stimulation is a potent promotor of IEG activation.[55] Noxious stimulation of C fibers results in alterations in postsynaptic receptors for excitatory amino acids, such as N-methyl-D-aspartate (NMDA). The ensuing increase in sensory nerve cell excitability is related to the emergence of NMDA receptors at the afferent synapses of dorsal horn neurons.[56] Increased excitability may persist for weeks following a transient peripheral injury. The development of chronic pain results in the modification of the transmission of stimuli in the nervous system. The persistence of chronic pain may become independent of ongoing nociceptive stimulation if neural cells have been modified to have a lower threshold for stimulation. The nervous system is malleable and will change in accordance with environmental stimuli. In the future, the therapy for chronic pain may be directed at control of cellular gene products that normalize receptor distribution on cell membranes or neurotransmitter production.

SUMMARY

Pain is a complex, subjective experience that is mediated through multiple components of the peripheral and central nervous systems. Factors at all levels of the neuraxis modulate pain perception. The summation of these inputs results in a perception that can be described in terms of its intensity, location, onset and duration, aggravating and alleviating factors, and elicited emotional responses. In acute circumstances, pain marks the onset and location of damage. It serves the purpose of protection. With chronic pain, the pain itself becomes the disease, since the injury that initiated the nociceptive response has healed. The therapy goals for patients experiencing back pain must take into account these anatomic, physiologic, and psychologic factors. The choice of specific forms of therapy for patients with low back pain should be made in light of these factors. The potential for individual patients to respond to a wide variety of therapeutic interventions is great, in view of the multitude of factors that result in pain.

References

1. Iggo A: Activation of cutaneous nociceptors and their actions on dorsal horn neurons. In Bonica JJ (ed): International Symposium on Pain. Adv Neurol 4:1, 1974.
2. Collins WF, Nulsen FE, Randt CT: Relation of peripheral fiber size and sensation in man. Arch Neurol 3:381, 1960.
3. Fitzgerald M, Lynn B: The sensitization of high threshold mechanoreceptors with myelinated axons by repeated heating. J Physiol (London) 365:549, 1977.
4. Thalhammer JG, LaMotte RH: Spatial properties of nociceptor sensitization. Brain Res 231:257, 1982.
5. Bessou P, Perl ER: Response of cutaneous sensory units with unmyelinated fibers to noxious stimuli. J Neurophysiol 32:1025, 1969.
6. Keele CA: Chemical causes of pain and itch. Ann Rev Med 21:67, 1970.
7. Ferreira SH: Prostaglandins, aspirin-like drugs and analgesia. Nature 240:200, 1972.
8. Aimone LD: Neurochemistry and modulation of pain. In Sinatra RS, Hord AH, Ginsberg B, Preble LM (eds): Acute Pain: Mechanisms and Management. St Louis: Mosby Year Book, 1992, pp 29–43.
9. Lynn B: Neurogenic inflammation. Skin Pharmacol 1:217, 1988.
10. Bishop GH: The relation between nerve fiber size and sensory modality: phylogenetic implications of the afferent innervation of the cortex. J Nerv Ment Dis 128:89, 1959.
11. Maciewicz R, Landrew BB: Physiology of pain. In Aronoff GM (ed): Evaluation and Treatment of Chronic Pain. Baltimore: Urban and Schwarzenberg, 1985, pp 17–38.
12. Christensen BN, Perl ER: Spinal neurons specifically excited by noxious or thermal stimuli. Marginal zones of the dorsal horn. J Neurophysiol 33:293, 1970.
13. LaMotte CC, de Lanerolle N: Substance P, enkephalin and serotonin. Ultrastructural basis of pain transmission in primate spinal cord. In Bonica JJ, Lindblom V, Iggo A (eds): Advances in Pain Research and Therapy, Vol 5. New York: Raven Press, 1983, pp 247–256.
14. Yaksh TL, Farb D, Leeman S, Jessell T: Intrathecal capsaicin depletes substance P in the rat spinal cord and produces prolonged thermal analgesia. Science 206:481, 1979.
15. Morton CR, Hutchison WD: Release of sensory neuropeptides in the spinal cord: studies with calcitonin gene-related peptide and galanin. Neuroscience 31:807, 1989.
16. Schneider SP, Perl EF: Selective excitation of neurons in the mammalian spinal cord by aspartate and glutamate in vitro: correlation with location and excitatory input. Brain Res 360:339, 1985.
17. Procacci P, Zopp M: Pathophysiology and clinical aspects of visceral and referred pain. In Bonica JJ, Lindblom V, Iggo A (eds): Advances in Pain Research and Therapy, Vol 5. New York: Raven Press, 1983, pp 643–660.
18. Cervero F, Iggo A: The substantia gelatinosa of the spinal cord. A critical review. Brain 103:717, 1980.
19. Willis WD, Maunz RA, Foreman RD, Coulter JD: Static and dynamic responses of spinothalamic tract neurons to mechanical stimuli. J Neurophysiol 38:587, 1975.
20. Wyke B: Neurological aspects of low back pain. In Jayson MIV (ed): The Lumbar Spine and Back Pain. New York: Grune & Stratton, 1976, pp 189–256.
21. Melzack R: Neurophysiological foundation of pain. In Sternbach RA (ed): The Psychology of Pain. New York: Raven Press, 1986, pp 1–24.
22. Reynolds DV: Surgery in the rat during electrical analgesic induced by focal brain stimulation. Science 164:444, 1969.
23. Fields HL, Basbaum AI: Brainstem control of spinal pain-transmission neurons. Ann Rev Physiol 40:217, 1978.
24. Aronin N, DiFiglia M, Liotta AS, Martin JB: Ultrastructural localization and biochemical features of immunoreactive leu-enkephalin in monkey dorsal horn. J Neurosci 1:561, 1981.
25. Hökfelt T, Kellerth JO, Nilsson G, Pernow B: Substance P: localization in the central nervous system and in some primary sensory neurons. Science 190:889, 1975.
26. Melzack R, Wall PD: Pain mechanisms: a new theory. Science 150:971, 1965.
27. Sjolund BH, Eriksson MBE: The influence of naloxone on analgesia produced by peripheral conditioning stimulation. Brain Res 173:295, 1979.
28. Engel GL: Pain. In Blacklow R (ed): Signs and Symptoms: Applied Pathologic Physiology and Clinical Interpretation. Philadelphia: JB Lippincott Co, 1983, pp 41–60.

29. Macnab I: Backache. Baltimore: Williams and Wilkins, 1983, pp 16–18.
30. Floyd WF, Silver PHS: Function of erectores spinae and flexion of the trunk. Lancet 1:133, 1951.
31. Parnianpour M, Nordin MA, Kahanovitz N, Frankel V: The triaxial coupling of torque generation of trunk muscles during isometric exertions and the effect of fatiguing isoinertial movements on the motor output and movement. Spine 13:982, 1988.
32. Lawrence JS, Bremner JM, Bier F: Osteoarthrosis: prevalence in the population and relationship between symptoms and x-ray changes. Ann Rheum Dis 25:1, 1966.
33. Kellgren JH: On the distribution of pain arising from deep somatic structures with charts of segmental pain areas. Clin Sci 41:46, 1939.
34. Bogduk N: The sources of low back pain. In Jayson MIV (ed): The Lumbar Spine and Back Pain. Edinburgh: Churchill Livingstone, 1992, pp 61–88.
35. Bogduk N, Twomey LT: Clinical Anatomy of the Lumbar Spine. Melbourne: Churchill Livingstone, 1987, pp 139–147.
36. Eyre DE: Biochemistry of the intervertebral disc. Connect Tissue Res 8:227, 1979.
37. Bayliss MT, Johnstone: Biochemistry of the intervertebral disc. In Jayson MIV (ed): The Lumbar Spine and Back Pain. Edinburgh: Churchill Livingstone, 1992, pp 111–131.
38. Bayliss MT, Johnstone B, O'Brien JP: Proteoglycan synthesis in the human intervertebral disc: variation with age, region, and pathology. Spine 13:972, 1988.
39. Hampton D, Laros G, McCarron, Franks D: Healing potential of the anulus fibrosus. Spine 14:398, 1989.
40. Eyre D, Benya P, Buckwalter J, et al.: The intervertebral disc: Basic science perspectives. In Frymoyer JW, Gordon SL (eds): New Perspectives on Low Back Pain. Park Ridge: American Academy Orthopaedic Surgeons, 1988, pp 147–207.
41. Cailliet R: Low Back Pain Syndrome. Philadelphia: FA Davis Co, 1983, p 31.
42. Hirsch C, Inglemark BE, Miller M: The anatomical basis for low back pain: studies on the presence of sensory nerve endings in ligamentous, capsular, and intervertebral disc structures in the human lumbar spine. Acta Orthop Scand 33:1, 1963.
43. Mooney V, Robertson J: The facet syndrome. Clin Orthop 115:149, 1976.
44. Hoyland JA, Freemont AJ, Jayson MIV: Intervertebral foramen venous obstruction: a cause of periradicular fibrosis? Spine 14:558, 1989.
45. Melzack R, Loeser JD: Phantom body pain in paraplegics: evidence for a central "pattern generating mechanism" for pain. Pain 4:195, 1978.
46. Denny-Brown D: The release of deep pain by nerve injury. Brain 88:725, 1965.
47. Selzer M, Spencer WA: Convergence of visceral and cutaneous afferent pathways in the lumbar spinal cord. Brain Res 14:331, 1969.
48. Devine R, Merskey H: The description of pain in psychiatric and general medical patients. J Psychosomat Res 9:311, 1965.
49. Klein RF, Brown W: Pain descriptions in medical settings. J Psychosom Res 10:367, 1967.
50. Dennis SG, Melzack R: Pain-signaling systems in the dorsal and ventral spinal cord. Pain 4:97, 1977.
51. Sternbach RA: Clinical aspects of pain. In Sternbach RA (ed): The Psychology of Pain. New York: Raven Press, 1986, pp 223–239.
52. Krishnan KR, France RD, Pelton S, et al.: Chronic pain and depression. I. Classification of depression in chronic low back pain patients. Pain 22:279, 1985.
53. Sternbach RA, Timmermans G: Personality changes associated with reduction of pain. Pain 1:177, 1975.
54. Zimmermann M: Basic neurophysiological mechanisms of pain and pain therapy. In Jayson MIV (ed): The Lumbar Spine and Back Pain. Edinburgh: Churchill Livingstone, 1992, pp 43–59.
55. Sheng M, Greenberg E: The regulation and function of c-fos and other immediate early genes in the nervous system. Neuron 4:477, 1990.
56. Davies SN, Lodge D: Evidence for involvement of N-methylaspartate receptors in "wind-up" of class 2 neurones in the dorsal horn of the rat. Brain Res 424:402, 1987.

CLINICAL EVALUATION OF LOW BACK PAIN

Low back pain is a ubiquitous problem.[1] Most individuals reading this book have personally experienced this disorder. It is also fair to say that a physician with a busy general practice will evaluate patients with low back pain on a daily basis.

Between 70% and 80% of the world's population experience low back pain sometime during their lives. The incidence of low back pain has been reported to range from a high of 20% of Western industrialized society in any given 2-week period to a "low" of 10% of adults in a 2-year period.[2, 3] Obviously to determine the occurrence of back pain in any group, complete survey information must be obtained from the entire population at risk. The definition of back pain plays a great role in determining who will in fact have it. The definition of the investigator and patient may not coincide. In any case, we can agree that low back pain is a very common clinical problem that affects most of a physician's population whether it consists of heavy laborers or sedentary office workers.[4–6] Back pain is second only to the common cold as the most common reason for visiting a physician.[7]

Even though most of the population is affected by this clinical problem, many individuals will not seek the advice of a physician in the diagnosis and treatment of this malady. Most low back pain is a self-limited illness. Of those individuals who are evaluated by their physician, 40% to 50% are better in 1 week, 51% to 86% in 1 month, and 92% within 2 months.[4] A similar pattern is also seen in work-related low back pain, with 70% to 90% of affected individuals being better within 2 months. Another study suggests that only about 14% of adults who do develop back pain have an episode that has a duration greater than 2 weeks.[8] Most individuals believe that their back pain is related to bad posture or a strain that will be transient in duration and is not of such a significant degree of discomfort as to warrant a visit to a physician's office. Those with more severe degrees of pain may choose to do nothing or to treat themselves with limited activity, over-the-counter medications, or temperature modalities (ice, hot packs). Others will bypass the family physician and go to the chiropractor, "the practitioner with an interest in spine problems." All of these interventions seem to work, since the natural history of the symptom is resolution over a short period of time. Some patients place too much confidence in their own understanding of the source of their pain and their initial response to therapy. The 50- or 60-year-old patient who develops persistent back pain after a minor trauma may ascribe all subsequent symptoms to the injury. Such patients may overlook the symptoms of fatigue, anorexia, and weakness, which have more ominous significance. They optimistically believe that the increasing doses of analgesics will eventually be effective and that their pain will subside.

In contradistinction to patients who belittle their symptoms, other patients may amplify their symptoms and express great anxiety in regard to the presence of back pain. These patients have unreasonably high expectations. They believe that 100% pain relief should be the end result of therapy even though their pain has been present for months. They want to undergo simultaneous therapies without forethought to a progression of modalities that offer a range of benefits and risks. These are the patients who undergo many of the 200,000 back operations done each year in the United States.[7] The vast majority of these operations are done for appropriate indications and result in good outcomes. However, many patients with persistent back pain of unknown etiology undergo exploratory back surgery, usually with poor results.

The clinician is faced with a constant dilemma. Back pain is common and affects any group of patients. Most episodes of back pain are related to mechanical regional abnormalities. Up to 95% of patients who have mechanical, self-limited back pain will improve. In 85% of patients, no specific diagnosis can be determined despite a thorough history, physical examination, and radiographic evaluation.[9] Some researchers have suggested that the absence of pathoanatomic abnormalities implicates psychosomatic mechanisms for the source of back pain.[10, 11] Although psychosomatic disorders may play a role in the perpetuation of pain, the initiating factor is usually physical in origin. Spinal pathology must be excluded before psychologic disorders are considered the source of a patient's pain. Therefore, an appropriate medical evaluation, including history and physical examination, are essential in the initial investigation of every patient with low back pain. The therapy chosen for this common problem should relieve symptoms, with toxicities limited to a minimum, while natural healing occurs. Intermixed in this large population of patients are individuals (2% to 10%) with potentially more serious causes of their pain.[8] Overlooking the correct diagnosis in these patients can have dire consequences.

Through careful review of the history, physical examination, and appropriate laboratory and radiographic tests, it should be possible for the clinician evaluating the patient's symptoms of back pain to formulate a logical diagnosis and implement an appropriate treatment plan.

References

1. Horal T: The clinical appearance of low back disorders in the city of Gothenburg, Sweden: comparisons of incapacitated probands with matched controls. Acta Orthop Scand (Suppl)118:1, 1969.
2. Nervell RLM, Turner JG: Orthopaedic Disorders in General Practice. Boston: Butterworths, 1985, pp 35–49.
3. Frymoyer JW, Pope MH, Costanza MC, et al: Epidemiologic studies of low-back pain. Spine 5:419, 1980.
4. Dillane JB, Fry J, Kaiton G: Acute back syndrome: A study from general practice. Br Med J 3:82, 1966.
5. White AWM: Low back pain in men receiving workmen's compensation. Can Med Assoc J 95:50, 1966.
6. Troup JDG, Martin JW, Lloyd DCEF: Back pain in industry: a prospective study. Spine 6:61, 1981.
7. Cypress BK: Characteristics of physician visits for back symptoms: a national perspective. Am J Public Health 73:389, 1983.
8. Deyo RA, Rainville J, Kent DL: What can the history and physical examination tell us about low back pain? JAMA 268:760, 1992.
9. White AA, Gordon SL: Synopsis: workshop on idiopathic low-back pain. Spine 7:141, 1982.
10. Sarno JE: Etiology of neck and back pain: an autonomic myoneuraliga? J Nerv Mental Dis 169:55, 1981.
11. Waddell G: Understanding the patient with backache. In Jayson MI (ed): The Lumbar Spine and Back Pain. Edinburgh: Churchill Livingstone, 1992, pp 469–485.
12. Bonica JJ: The nature of the problem. In Canon H, McLaughlin R(eds): Management of Low Back Pain. Littleton, Massachusetts: John Wright-PSG, Inc., 1982, pp 1–16.
13. Scott JHS: Backache. J Roy Col Surg (Edin) 25:477, 1980.

History

4

The history is the essential initial step in evaluating the patient with the symptom of low back pain. The history should include the patient's chief complaint, family history, past history, social history, review of systems, and present illness. Some physicians may concentrate only on the present illness, leaving out parts of the review of systems or social history. Others will utilize reproduced forms that list a succession of questions that are complete in evaluating the patient's pain but do not integrate the back symptoms with other medical, social, or psychologic problems. In circumstances involving patients with cauda equina symptoms (saddle anesthesia, progressive muscular weakness, incontinence), the necessity to do a complete history is reduced in face of the need to evaluate the patient for emergency surgical decompression. In others with chronic low back pain, a thorough review of all the components of the patient's history is essential to understanding the patient's difficulties.

Common sense is an essential component of this process. The astute clinician allows the patient to tell his story in his own words, but also steers him in directions that elicit the essential information needed for the diagnostic process. The clinician knows when the history must be abbreviated in order to administer essential therapy or prolonged to gather all the facts that may pertain to the patient's problem.

The expenditure of time in obtaining a complete history reaps the clinician great dividends in understanding the patient's disease. If not all the information is obtained during the initial evaluation, it is worthwhile to review the history on subsequent visits. The patient may have forgotten an essential piece of history. Repeated questions about the back pain

may jar the patient's memory. It also allows the patient to monitor his response to therapy.

CHIEF COMPLAINT

The recording of the chief complaint should include the patient's age, sex, and duration of low back pain. It is at this point that the possibility of a life-threatening cause of back pain needs to be considered. A leaking or ruptured abdominal aneurysm is one of the few catastrophic causes of acute low back pain that requires emergency intervention. Patients with an expanding aneurysm develop abdominal pain, distention, and circulatory collapse. This pattern of symptoms and signs should be recognizable by the emergency room physician or general practitioner. In such cases only essential history needs to be obtained. This might include history of prior vascular surgery, anticoagulant therapy, or severe hypertension.

Another potentially life-threatening emergency associated with low back pain is abrupt paraplegia. Acute paraplegia occurs secondary to a major insult to the spinal cord. In addition to muscle weakness, bladder, bowel and sexual function need to be assessed. Disorders associated with acute paraplegia include spinal cord tumors, epidural hemorrhage, epidural abscess, embolus, spinal artery thrombosis, and central herniation of a nucleus pulposus (cauda equina syndrome).[1] These disorders are associated with a history of progressive muscle weakness, anticoagulant therapy, fever, or cardiac disease (atrial fibrillation or atherosclerosis). Physical examination will help establish the potential causes of the paraplegia. Neurologic dysfunction, although not life-

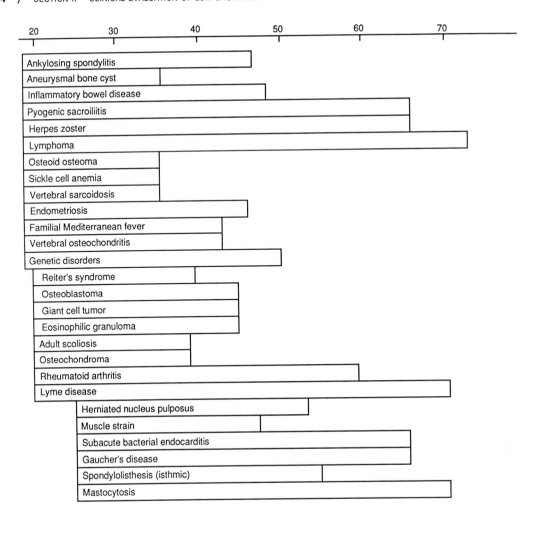

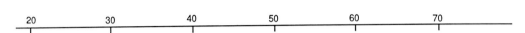

Figure 4–1. Age at peak incidence of back pain associated with mechanical and nonmechanical disorders.

threatening, results from a spinal cord insult and requires immediate evaluation. After the life-threatening causes of back pain have been eliminated as potential diagnoses, a complete history is obtained.

Age

Figure 4–1 lists causes of low back pain by the age range at which they occur. Spondylo-arthropathies, including ankylosing spondylitis, Reiter's syndrome, spondylitis associated with inflammatory bowel disease, and benign tumors of the spine (aneurysmal bone cyst, osteoid osteoma, osteoblastoma, and giant cell tumor), occur between the third and fourth decades. Diseases of middle age include diffuse idiopathic skeletal hyperostosis (D.I.S.H.), gout, Paget's disease, and osteomyelitis. A dif-

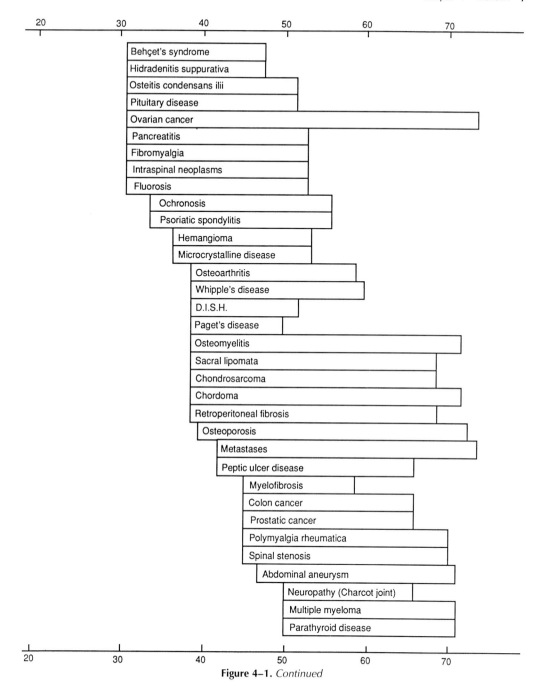

Figure 4–1. *Continued*

ferent set of diseases occurs more commonly during and following the sixth decade, which includes malignant (metastases, colon cancer, prostatic cancer), metabolic (osteoporosis), and degenerative diseases (expanding abdominal aortic aneurysm). Approximately, 80% of patients with malignant disease affecting the lumbar spine are over 50 years of age.[2]

Sex

Back pain occurs predominantly in men. Occupational exposure to heavy-duty labor explains some of the increased prevalence of this symptom. Many illnesses, including the spondyloarthropathies, infections, and malignant and benign tumors, also occur more commonly in men. Endocrinologic disorders, including osteoporosis and parathyroid disorders, and muscle disease (polymyalgia rheumatica and fibromyalgia) are more likely to appear in women. Psoriatic spondylitis, spondylitis associated with inflammatory bowel disease, hemangioma, Gaucher's disease, pituitary disease, and subacute bacterial endocarditis occur with equal frequency in both sexes. Table 4–1 lists illnesses associated with low back pain according to sexual predominance.

FAMILY HISTORY

Familial predisposition does occur in certain medical illnesses that are associated with back pain. A prime example is the spondyloarthropathies. In the presence of a particular histocompatibility locus antigen (HLA-B27), members of a family are at risk of developing ankylosing spondylitis, Reiter's syndrome, pso-

riatic spondylitis, and spondylitis associated with inflammatory bowel disease. Other spondyloarthropathies, such as those occurring in familial Mediterranean fever and Whipple's disease, occur more commonly in family members without any specifically associated genetic factor. The ethnic background of the family may predispose members to specific illnesses. Caucasian women of Northern European extraction are at greater risk of developing osteoporosis. Ashkenazic Jews develop Gaucher's disease. Many of the other illnesses that cause back pain have no specific familial predilection. However, it is always prudent for the examining physician to inquire about other family members with similar symptoms and the diagnoses associated with their complaints. This information can help direct the clinician in formulating the diagnostic evaluation of the patient.

OCCUPATIONAL/SOCIAL HISTORY

The occupational history is essential for evaluating the patient's risk of developing mechanical low back pain. Workers doing heavy lifting at their job are at risk of developing mechanical low back pain. However, this symptom also occurs in sedentary workers. Lifting a light object from a rotated position or stretching far overhead to reach an object on a shelf may be associated with the onset of low back pain. The relationship of work and onset of pain is important in evaluating the patient in regard to compensation. Whether the symptoms of back pain are work-related or not, it is important to discuss their association from the patient's viewpoint.

Ankylosing spondylitis is not caused by heavy lifting at work. The patient may have difficulty accepting the fact that his work has no correlation with the onset of his illness. A positive therapeutic outcome has a better chance of occurring when the patient realizes the source of his difficulties and does not have false expectations in regard to compensation for his symptoms.

It is appropriate to inquire about any pending litigation in regard to the patient's back pain. It is incumbent on the physician not to assume, because workmen's compensation is involved or litigation is pending, that the patient's symptoms are factitious or exaggerated. The patient should be given the benefit of the doubt. Patients who are hurt on the job or in an accident develop low back pain secondary to mechanical or medical causes. An inciden-

TABLE 4–1. SEX PREVALENCE FOR ILLNESSES ASSOCIATED WITH LOW BACK PAIN

Male Predominant	
Ankylosing spondylitis	Multiple myeloma
Reiter's syndrome	Chondrosarcoma
Familial Mediterranean fever	Chordoma
	Lymphoma
Behçet's syndrome	Ochronosis
Whipple's disease	Gout
Diffuse idiopathic skeletal hyperostosis	Abdominal aneurysm
	Prostatic cancer
Osteomyelitis	Vertebral sarcoidosis
Discitis	Retroperitoneal fibrosis
Pyogenic sacroiliitis	Peptic ulcer disease
Paget's disease	Osteochondroma
Osteoblastoma	Vertebral osteochondritis
Eosinophilic granuloma	
Osteoid osteoma	
Female Predominant	
Rheumatoid arthritis	Osteoporosis
Osteitis condensans ilii	Parathyroid disease
Polymyalgia rheumatica	Calcium pyrophosphate deposition disease
Fibromyalgia	
Giant cell tumor	Endometriosis
Aneurysmal bone cyst	Pregnancy
Sacroiliac lipomata	Ovarian cancer
	Adult scoliosis
Equal Frequency	
Psoriatic spondylitis	Mastocytosis
Enteropathic arthritis	Mechanical disorders
Hemangioma	Muscle strain
Gaucher's disease	Herniated disc
Pituitary disease	Osteoarthritis/spinal stenosis
Subacute bacterial endocarditis	
	Spondylolysis
Herpes zoster	
Skeletal metastases	

tal trauma may be assumed to be the source of pain while its actual cause, such as a pathologic fracture secondary to a tumor, goes unrecognized. Only a thorough physical examination can uncover the true cause of a patient's back pain.

Pressures to return to work may be different for the salaried employee versus the self-employed business person. The self-employed individual may push the physician into cutting corners in evaluation and therapy to obtain the "quick fix" needed to allow him to return to his normal activities. On the other hand, the salaried employee may delay the return to his usual activities because of fear of re-injury. The treating physician must keep these concerns of patients in mind when developing an appropriate diagnostic and therapeutic program.

Social history also includes quantification of consumption of alcohol, coffee, and recreational drugs and cigarette smoking. Increased consumption of alcohol or coffee and cigarettes smoking are associated with osteoporosis, while illicit drug use results in immunosuppression and predisposition to infection. Smoking may also be associated with increased risk for herniated intervertebral disc and low back pain.[3]

Review of leisure-time activities is another important way to measure level of function prior to the onset of back pain. Are recreational activities limited to the same degree as work-related tasks? Response to therapy can be measured by the patient's resumption of recreational activities.

PAST MEDICAL HISTORY

Past medical history should list in chronologic order all hospitalizations, operations, and previous severe injuries that affected the lumbosacral spine. Childhood back injuries, remembered by the patient, are usually significant in the amount of damage sustained by anatomic structures. A history of slipping on the ice and "cracking" the back resulting in bed rest for a few days may be the initial episode in the development of disc disease in adulthood. All general medical problems should be reviewed. Certain diseases, including diabetes, other endocrinopathies, malignancies, and metabolic bone disease, may have a direct effect on structures in the lumbosacral spine. A past history of cancer has high specificity as the cause of back pain but has low

sensitivity with only one third of patients with an underlying malignancy having this history.[4] Other disorders may not have a direct effect on the low back per se but may be associated with physical disorders (congestive heart failure, angina) or require specific medications (anticoagulants) that limit the therapeutic options for the treating physician. In addition, allergies to medications are listed.

REVIEW OF SYSTEMS

Although frequently thought to be redundant or superfluous, review of systems is an essential part of the low back pain history. A completely negative review is added evidence for the regional (mechanical) nature of the pain. Positive responses help organize symptoms into patterns associated with systemic illness that cause back pain. The presence of constitutional symptoms is a worrisome finding and requiries a more thorough evaluation. Fever in the setting of new-onset back pain may be associated with the "flu," pyogenic sacroiliitis, or osteomyelitis. The sensitivity of fever as a marker of spinal infection runs the gamut from 27% for tuberculous osteomyelitis to 83% for spinal epidural abscess.[2]

Review of the integumentary system may reveal a history of scaling patches over the elbows that respond to topical agents (psoriasis) or nail opacification that never responded to antifungal therapy (Reiter's syndrome). History of conjunctivitis, iritis, or oral ulcers should raise the possibility of a spondyloarthropathy as the cause of back pain. Decreased cardiopulmonary function may be a manifestation of a spondyloarthropathy or endocrinopathy. Visceral causes of back pain should be considered in the patient with a positive gastrointestinal or genitourinary history. History of anemia may be related to a systemic illness, gastrointestinal blood loss of an iatrogenic nature (drugs), or a primary hematologic disorder (sickle cell disease).

Neuropsychiatric history should not be skipped. Descriptions of local versus generalized sensory and motor abnormalities help categorize low back symptoms as a component of a systemic neurologic disease or as a regional disturbance associated with local nerve dysfunction. Review of any psychiatric disturbance is essential. During this part of the examination, it is helpful to have the patient describe his personality. Is he obsessive, compulsive, or driven? Is he passive? Is he depressed about his physical condition? Is he overly anxious or unconcerned about the potential cause of his back pain (anxiety neurosis, hysteria)? Answers to these questions alert the physician to those individuals who may have psychogenic back pain.

PRESENT ILLNESS

The history of the present illness should include the chronologic development of low back pain and its character, results of previous diagnostic tests, and response to therapy.

Onset

Mechanical causes of back pain (muscle strain, herniated nucleus pulposus) have an acute, sudden onset. The onset of pain is frequently associated with a specific task done in a mechanically disadvantaged position. Muscle bundles may be torn, fascia stretched, and facet joints irritated. Pain starts instantaneously or within a few hours.

Medical causes of low back pain have a more gradual onset of pain. Pain from tumors starts insidiously except for episodes of acute pain associated with pathologic fractures of skeletal structures. Patients with the early constitutional symptoms of Lyme disease may describe onset of disease during the summer months when the risk for tick bites is greatest.

Duration and Frequency

Mechanical low back pain generally has a duration of a few days to a few months. Most muscle strains are relieved within a week. Disc herniations may require 8 weeks for resolution. Disc degeneration may cause a low-grade chronic discomfort that is exacerbated during acute attacks, which last for 2 to 4 weeks. Most mechanical pain is intermittent. Frequency of episodes depends to a certain degree on exposure of an individual to mechanical stresses that worsen their condition.

Medical conditions cause chronic pain that is persistent rather than episodic. Patients with spondyloarthropathies develop chronic aching low back pain that has a long duration measured in months. Tumors of the spine cause persistent pain that builds in intensity over months.

Psychogenic pains are constant and unrelenting. Histories of years of constant, excruciating pain are not uncommon.

Location and Radiation

Most mechanical and medical causes of back pain are localized to the lumbosacral spine. Damage to musculoskeletal structures (discs, posterior apophyseal joints) may cause referred pain in surrounding areas of the lumbosacral spine. These structures include adjacent paraspinous, buttock, and thigh muscles. Abnormalities in facet joints, annular disc fibers, and supporting ligaments also will result in lumbosacral pain. Pain may be localized to a specific midline structure such as a spinous or transverse process. The identification of the point of maximum tenderness helps differentiate bone lesions from soft tissue lesions. Bilateral lower back pain is common in patients with sacroiliac joint disease associated with a spondyloarthropathy.

Pain radiating to the lower leg from the lumbar spine or exclusively in the lower limb is more suggestive of nerve root irritation. Discs that disrupt annular fibers will cause pain in the low back. As the disc impinges the nerve root, pain is referred down the leg. Once the disc is extruded and the pressure on the annulus from disc protrusion is relieved, leg pain continues while back pain resolves. Spinal stenosis also causes radiation of pain into the lower extremity. Disc herniation causes radiating pain at rest, while with spinal stenosis radiating pain occurs in positions that extend the spine and decrease room in the spinal canal for the neural elements.

Radiating pain to the lower extremity is not limited to mechanical abnormalities. The piriformis syndrome includes leg pain associated with back pain but without persistent abnormal neurologic signs. The sciatic nerve is compressed by the piriformis muscle. The muscle undergoes sustained contraction because of its attachment to an inflamed sacroiliac joint. Therapy that decreases joint inflammation reduces muscle contraction, resulting in diminished radicular symptoms. This syndrome is easily confused with a herniated disc. If the existence of pseudosciatica is not recognized unnecessary diagnostic tests are done.

In contrast to pain from nerve root irritation, psychogenic pain is not well localized. Large nondermatomal areas are affected. Radiation of pain follows no consistent pattern.

Aggravating and Alleviating Factors

Characteristically, mechanical lesions of the lumbosacral spine improve with rest and worsen with increased activity. Increased activity includes prolonged sitting with forward flexion if the patient has a herniated disc or prolonged standing in an extended position if the patient has spinal stenosis. Patients with muscle strain improve with bed rest. Not all lumbosacral spine movements exacerbate muscle strain pain. A careful history will define those motions that are painless and those that irritate the injured muscle resulting in reflex spasm.

Increases in cerebrospinal fluid pressure increase nerve root irritation caused by disc herniation. Coughing, sneezing, and the Valsalva maneuver increase pressure and exacerbate radicular pain. It is important to remember that the sudden, reflex motions associated with coughing or sneezing may increase muscle strain as well. However, pain due to muscle strain remains localized and does not radiate into the lower extremities.

Some patients with medical low back pain feel worse with bed rest. Patients with spondyloarthropathy have exacerbation of pain after a few hours of bed rest. Frequently they wake up during the night because of pain associated with rolling over in bed. Early morning is the worst time of the day for these patients.

The pain of tumors involving bone, muscle, or spinal cord is increased with recumbency. Patients with such tumors seek relief by sleeping in a chair or pacing the floor.

Other medical patients find relief only with absolute immobility. This is a sign of acute infection, compression fracture related to metabolic bone disease, or pathologic fracture secondary to a tumor or infiltrative disease.

Patients with viscerogenic referred pain rarely describe any association of their discomfort with position. Bed rest has little effect on their pain. Patients with colic are constantly moving, trying to find a comfortable position. Interventions that are effective at reducing genitourinary symptoms (antibiotics) or gastrointestinal symptoms (antacids) control back pain in these individuals.

Patients with psychogenic pain have difficulty describing factors that relieve or worsen their pain. The pain is present all the time. No position is comfortable. Activities involving little physical effort have an exaggerated effect on their pain.

Time of Day

Mechanical disorders (muscle strain, degenerative disc disease, spinal stenosis, osteoarthritis) cause pain that is increased with activity. The most pain occurs at the end of the day after the patient has been up and around. Diurnal changes in spinal mechanics may also explain maximal stresses on structures in the lumbar spine that correlate with patient symptoms.[5] The risk of disc herniation is greatest in the morning when the disc is extended to its greatest degree. At the end of the day, when the disc is less tense, symptoms related to joint compression are more likely.

Medical disorders are most problematic in the morning or after the patient has gone to sleep. Classically, inflammatory arthropathies cause morning stiffness. Patients have great difficulty getting out of bed in the morning because of stiffness and pain. As the patient ambulates, the stiffness and pain lessen.

Tumors of the spine and spinal cord cause pain that increases with recumbency. Therefore, most individuals with lumbar spine tumors have maximal pain during the night. This characteristic of tumors is not solely reserved to malignant processes. Benign tumors, such as an osteoid osteoma, cause severe nocturnal pain. Patients with spinal tumors may get up and walk in order to diminish their discomfort.

Quality and Intensity

Description of the quality of pain can be very helpful in identifying its source. The adjectives used to describe back pain are numerous. Initially the patient should describe the quality of pain in his own words without suggestions from the examining physician. Some patients are unable to describe their pain in their own words. At this point it is helpful to supply a list of choices. An example of such a list is the McGill Pain Questionnaire[6] (Fig. 4–2). The questionnaire divides words into three major groups: those that describe the sensory quality of pain: temporal, spatial, pressure, thermal, and other properties; those that describe the affective qualities of pain in terms of tension, fear, and autonomic properties; and those that describe the subjective, overall intensity of pain. In each category the words are listed with increasing intensity. In addition, a line drawing of the body is included demarcating the location of pain. A pain rating index (PRI) is determined by adding together the

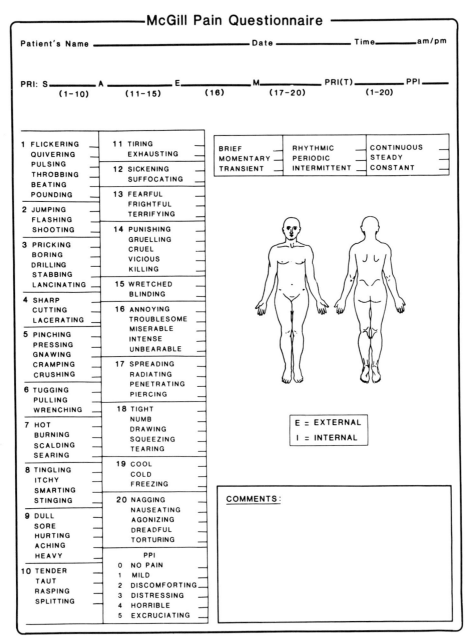

Figure 4–2. The McGill Pain Questionnaire. (From Melzack R [ed]: Pain Measurement and Assessment. New York: Raven Press, 1983.)

rank values of the words in each subclass. The number of words chosen is quantified. The scale can be administered on successive visits to help quantify response to therapy. If the McGill Pain Questionnaire is not used, the patient's history should include a line drawing of the body. The pictorial representation of the patient's pain helps delineate its extent. A patient's response to therapy may also be monitored by review of the extent of painful areas on serial line drawings.

The intensity of pain may be measured not only by verbal means but also by visual means.[7] The visual analogue scale is a visual way to quantify pain.[8] A visual analogue scale is a line, 10 cm in length, where one end represents no pain and the other severe, incapacitating pain (Fig. 4–3). A patient marks a point on the line corresponding to the severity of his pain. The distance of the point to the end of the line represents pain severity. The visual analogue scale has greater sensitivity to quantify pain than verbal descriptors. It is a continuum. Verbal descriptors correspond to points along the line. There are not enough words to describe all the possible points on the line. The visual analogue scale is quick and easy to do, understood by the patient, and accurately scored by measuring the line. The scale has its limitations in that certain patient categories clump responses to one or the other end of the spectrum. In addition, each patient's score must be regarded in light of his or her own response range. One patient's 4 value may be another's 8.

Another differentiation is between organic and psychogenic pain. A standardized way to differentiate psychogenic from organic pain is to use the Minnesota Multiphasic Personality Inventory (MMPI). The MMPI is a 566 question, self-administered true-false test formulated to identify psychologic traits, for example, hypochondriasis, depression, hysteria, or psychopathic deviance, associated with elevated scale scores in patients with chronic pain.[9] Although MMPI may help differentiate organic from functional pain, the test does not correlate well with patient physical findings. A test that validates the presence of pain is the Mensana Clinic Back Pain Test (MPT).[10] MPT is a 15 item questionnaire that takes about 10 minutes to complete (Table 4–2). Patients are classified as objective-pain patients, exaggerating-pain patients, and affective-pain patients corresponding to increasing test scores.[11] The MPT is more successful than MMPI in differentiating organic from functional low back pain and is useful for patients with chronic low back pain.[11] It also predicts the presence or absence of physical abnormalities better than MMPI. Other tests developed to measure the validity of the presence of pain rather than the patient's personality profile include the Oswestry Disability Questionnaire, Sickness Impact Profile, and Waddell Disability Index.[12]

Another means of testing the severity of pain is to measure the degree of disability an individual experiences with the discomfort. Roland and Morris developed a questionnaire consisting of 24 items (Table 4–3).[13] The test not only measures disability resulting from back pain but also measures response to therapy.

Superficial somatic, deep somatic, neurogenic, viscerogenic referred, and psychogenic pain have qualities that differentiate them.

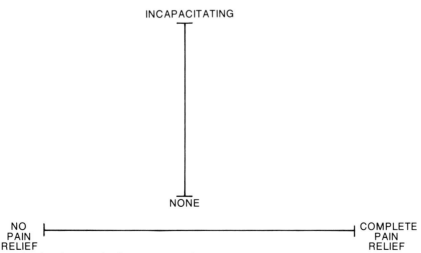

Figure 4–3. Visual analogue scales for pain *(top)* and pain relief *(bottom)*. The physical orientation of the scales may be vertical or horizontal.

TABLE 4–2. MENSANA CLINIC BACK PAIN TEST*

	POINTS		POINTS
1 How did the pain that you now experience occur?		(b) The pain is always worse with damp weather or with cold weather.	1
(a) Sudden onset with accident or definable event.	0	(c) The pain is occasionally worse with cold or damp weather.	2
(b) Slow, progressive onset without acute exacerbation.	1	(d) The weather has no effect on the pain.	3
(c) Slow, progressive onset with acute exacerbation without accident or event.	2	**5 How would you describe the type of pain that you have?**	
(d) Sudden onset without an accident or definable event.	3	(a) Burning; or sharp, shooting pain; or pins and needles; or coldness; or numbness.	0
2 Where do you experience the pain?		(b) Dull, aching pain, with occasional sharp, shooting pains not helped by heat; or the patient is experiencing hyperesthesia.	1
(a) One site, specific, well-defined consistent with anatomic distribution.	0	(c) Spasm-type pain, tension-type pain, or numbness over the area, relieved by massage or heat.	2
(b) More than one site, each well-defined and consistent with anatomic distribution	1	(d) Nagging or bothersome pain.	3
(c) One site, inconsistent with anatomic considerations, or not well-defined.	2	(e) Excruciating, overwhelming, or unbearable pain, relieved by massage or heat.	4
(d) Vague description, more than one site, of which one is inconsistent with anatomic considerations, or not well-defined or anatomically explainable.	3	**6 How frequently do you have your pain?**	
3 Do you ever have trouble falling asleep at night, or are you ever awakened from sleep?		(a) The pain is constant.	0
If the answer is "no," score 3 points and go to question 4. If the answer is "yes," proceed.		(b) The pain is nearly constant, occurring 50–80% of the time.	1
		(c) The pain is intermittent, occurring 25–50% of the time.	2
3a What keeps you from falling asleep?		(d) The pain is only occasionally present, occurring less than 25% of the time.	3
(a) Trouble falling asleep every night due to pain.	0	**7 Does movement or position have any effect on the pain?**	
(b) Trouble falling asleep due to pain more than three times a week.	1	(a) The pain is unrelieved by position change or rest, and there have been previous operations for the pain.	0
(c) Trouble falling asleep due to pain less than three times a week.	2	(b) The pain is worsened by use, standing, or walking, and is relieved by lying down or resting the part.	1
(d) No trouble falling asleep due to pain.	3	(c) Position change and use have variable effects on the pain.	2
(e) Trouble falling asleep which is not related to pain.	4	(d) The pain is not altered by use or position change, and there have been no previous operations for the pain.	3
3b What awakens you from sleep?		**8 What medications have you used in the past month?**	
(a) Awakened by pain every night.	0	(a) No medications at all.	0
(b) Awakened from sleep by pain more than three times a week.	1	(b) Use of nonnarcotic pain relievers, nonbenzodiazepine tranquilizers, or antidepressants.	1
(c) Not awakened from sleep by pain more than twice a week.	2	(c) Use of a narcotic, hypnotic, or benzodiazepine less than three times a week.	2
(d) Not awakened from sleep by pain.	3	(d) Use of a narcotic, hypnotic, or benzodiazepine more than four times a week.	3
(e) Restless sleep, or early morning awakening with or without being able to return to sleep, both unrelated to pain.	4		
4 Does weather have any effect on your pain?			
(a) The pain is always worse in both cold and damp weather.	0		

*Modified from Hender N, Vierstein M, Gucer P, Long D: A preoperative screening test for chronic back pain patients. Psychosomatics 20:801, 1979.

Each test question is asked by an examiner, who assigns the appropriate points for each response.

Score 17 or less: Patient is in the objective-pain category and reporting a normal response to chronic pain and is willing to participate in all modalities of therapy, including exercise and psychotherapy. This individual is a good surgical candidate. The patient with conversion reaction or post-traumatic neurosis may score less than 18 points. The person scoring 14 or less usually is considered more of an objective-pain patient than one scoring between 14 to 18.

TABLE 4–2. MENSANA CLINIC BACK PAIN TEST *Continued*

		POINTS				POINTS
9	**What hobbies do you have, and can you still participate in them?**			(b)	Experiencing financial difficulty with family income only 50–75% of the prepain income.	1
(a)	Unable to participate in any hobbies that were formerly enjoyed.	0		(c)	Patient unable to work, and receives some compensation so that the family income is at least 75% of the prepain income.	2
(b)	Reduced number of hobbies or activities relating to a hobby.	1		(d)	Patient unable to work and receives no compensation, but the spouse works and family income is still 75% of the prepain income.	3
(c)	Still able to participate in hobbies but with some discomfort.	2		(e)	Patient doesn't work, yet the income from disability or other compensation sources is 80% or more of gross pay before the pain; the spouse does not work.	4
(d)	Participates in hobbies as before.	3				
10	**How frequently did you have sex and orgasms before the pain, and how frequently do you have sex and orgasms now?**			**13**	**Are you suing anyone, or is anyone suing you, or do you have an attorney helping you with compensation or disability payments?**	
(a¹)	Sexual contact, prior to pain, three to four times a week, with no difficulty with orgasm; now sexual contact is 50% or less than previously, and coitus is interrupted by pain.	0		(a)	No suit pending, and does not have an attorney.	0
(a²)	(For people over 45) Sexual contact twice a week, with a 50% reduction in frequency since the onset of pain.	0		(b)	Litigation is pending, but is not related to the pain.	1
(a³)	(For people over 60) Sexual contact once a week, with a 50% reduction in frequency since the onset of pain.	0		(c)	The patient is being sued as the result of an accident.	2
(b)	Prepain adjustment as defined above (a¹-a³), with no difficulty with orgasm; now loss of interest in sex and/or difficulty with orgasm or erection.	1		(d)	Litigation is pending or workmen's compensation case with a lawyer involved.	3
(c)	No change in sexual activity now as opposed to before the onset of pain.	2		**14**	**If you had three wishes for anything in the world, what would you wish for?**	
(d)	Unable to have sexual contact since the onset of pain, and dificulty with orgasm or erection prior to the pain.	3		(a)	"Get rid of the pain" is the only wish.	0
(e)	No sexual contact prior to the pain, or absence of orgasm prior to the pain.	4		(b)	"Get rid of the pain" is one of the three wishes.	1
11	**Are you still working or doing your household chores?**			(c)	Doesn't mention getting rid of the pain, but has specific wishes usually of a personal nature such as for more money, a better relationship with spouse or children, etc.	2
(a)	Works every day at the same prepain job or same level of household duties.	0		(d)	Does not mention pain, but offers general, nonpersonal wishes such as for world peace.	3
(b)	Works every day but the job is not the same as prepain job, with reduced responsibility or physical activity.	1		**15**	**Have you ever been depressed or thought of suicide?**	0
(c)	Works sporadically or does a reduced amount of household chores.	2		(a)	Admits to depression, or has a history of depression secondary to pain and associated with crying spells and thoughts of suicide.	1
(d)	Not at work, or all household chores are now performed by others.	3		(b)	Admits to depression, guilt, and anger secondary to the pain.	2
12	**What is your income now compared with before your injury or the onset of pain, and what are your sources of income?**	0		(c)	Prior history of depression before the pain or a financial or personal loss prior to the pain; now admits to some depression.	3
(a)	Any one of the following answers scores 1. Experiencing financial difficulty with family income 50% or less than previously. 2. Was retired and is still retired. 3. Patient is still working and is not having financial difficulties.			(d)	Denies depression, crying spells, or feeling blue.	4
				(e)	History of a suicide attempt prior to the onset of pain.	

Score 18 to 20: This group has features of the objective-pain and the exaggerating-pain patient and personality difficulties. Organic lesions result in a more extreme response because of a premorbid condition.

Score 21 to 31: Patient is in the exaggerating-pain category. This type of patient has a prepain personality that may increase the likelihood of obtaining secondary gain from the complaint of pain. This patient responds to therapy that alters his attitude toward chronic pain. Surgery should be undertaken with caution.

Score above 32: Patient is the affective-pain category and has considerable difficulty in coping with chronic pain. This individual may need psychiatric consultation.

TABLE 4–3. ROLAND DISABILITY QUESTIONNAIRE*

1. I stay at home more of the time because of my back.
2. I change position frequently to try and get my back comfortable.
3. I walk more slowly than usual because of my back.
4. Because of my back I am not doing any of the jobs that I usually do around the house.
5. Because of my back, I use a handrail to get upstairs.
6. Because of my back, I lie down to rest more often.
7. Because of my back, I have to hold on to something to get out of an easy chair.
8. Because of my back, I try to get other people to do things for me.
9. I get dressed more slowly than usual because of my back.
10. I only stand up for short periods of time because of my back.
11. Because of my back, I try not to bend or kneel down.
12. I find it difficult to get out of a chair because of my back.
13. My back is painful almost all the time.
14. I find it difficult to turn over in bed because of my back.
15. My appetite is not very good because of my back pain.
16. I have trouble putting on my socks (or stockings) because of the pain in my back.
17. I only walk short distances because of my back pain.
18. I sleep less well because of my back.
19. Because of my back pain, I get dressed with help from someone else.
20. I sit down for most of the day because of my back.
21. I avoid heavy jobs around the house because of my back.
22. Because of my back pain, I am more irritable and bad tempered with people than usual.
23. Because of my back, I go upstairs more slowly than usual.
24. I stay in bed most of the time because of my back.

*The questions should be answered as your back feels today.

From Roland M, Morris R: A study of the natural history of back pain: Part 1: Development of a reliable and sensitive measure of disability in low-back pain. Spine 8:141, 1983.

These qualities have been described in Chapter 3 as well as the characteristics associated with the pain categories.

The patient should list all physicians consulted in regard to his back pain. In addition, information about the diagnostic tests used for evaluation of back pain and treatment should be obtained from the patient.

SUMMARY

The history is the foundation on which the rest of the diagnostic process is built. By listening carefully to the patient's description of the chief complaint, the clinician should be able to generate a list of potential diagnoses that could be causing the difficulties. The next step in the process is a complete and appropriate physical examination. With the myriad of tests that can be done during the physical and laboratory evaluations, the history allows the clinician to select those parts of the examination that will help in making the correct diagnosis from the possibilities included in the differential diagnosis list.

References

1. Kostuik JP, Harrington I, Alexander D, et al.: Cauda equina syndrome and lumbar disc herniation. J Bone Joint Surg 68A:386, 1986.
2. Deyo RA, Rainville J, Kent DL: What can the history and physical examination tell us about low back pain? JAMA 268:760, 1992.
3. Deyo RA, Bass JE: Lifestyle and low back pain: the influence of smoking and obesity. Spine 14:501, 1989.
4. Deyo RA, Diehl AK: Cancer as a cause of back pain: frequency, clinical presentation, and diagnostic strategies. J Gen Intern Med 3:230, 1988.
5. Adams MA, Dolan P, Hutton WC, Porter RW: Diurnal changes in spinal mechanics and their clinical significance. J Bone Joint Surg 72B:266, 1990.
6. Melzack R: The McGill Pain Questionnaire. In Melzack R (ed): Pain Measurement and Assessment. New York: Raven Press, 1983, pp 41–47.
7. Lipman JJ: Pain measurement. In Parris WCV (ed): Contemporary Issues in Chronic Pain Management. Boston: Kluwer Academic Publishers, 1991, pp 123–146.
8. Huskisson EC: Visual analogue scales. In Melzack R (ed): Pain Measurement and Assessment. New York: Raven Press, 1983, pp 33–40.
9. Sternbach RA, Wolff SR, Murphy RW, Akeson WH: Traits of pain patients: the low-back "loser." Psychosomatics 14:226, 1973.
10. Hendler N, Vierstein M, Gucer P, Long D: A preoperative screening test for chronic back pain patients. Psychosomatics 20:801, 1979.
11. Hendler N, Mollett A, Talo S, Levin S: A comparison between the Minnesota Multiphasic Personality Inventory and the Mensana Clinic Back Pain Test for validating the complaint of chronic back pain. J Occup Med 30:98, 1988.
12. Deyo RA: Measuring the functional status of patients with low back pain. Arch Phys Med Rehabil 69:1044, 1988.
13. Roland M, Morris R: A study of the natural history of back pain: Part 1: development of a reliable and sensitive measure of disability in low-back pain. Spine 8:141, 1983.

Physical Examination

5

After completion of the medical history, the physical examination is the next step in the diagnostic process. The history has alerted the physician to those individuals who have medical emergencies that require the initiation of therapy after only an abbreviated examination. These include patients with ruptured abdominal aneurysm or acute cauda equina syndrome. The history of severe, tearing pain and dizziness associated with an abdominal pulsatile mass alerts the physician to the problem of an expanding aneurysm. Patients with the cauda equina syndrome present with acute paraplegia, saddle anesthesia, and rectal or urinary incontinence. These patients are evaluated expeditiously for abnormalities of the aorta and spinal cord so that therapy may be instituted before a life-threatening bleed or permanent neurologic damage occurs. Fortunately, the number of patients who present in this manner is extremely small.

GENERAL MEDICAL EXAMINATION

Examination of the lumbosacral spine is done after the completion of the general medical physical examination for a number of reasons. Examining the painful part of the body is best left for the last portion of the evaluation. Putting the patient through the various maneuvers required to evaluate lumbosacral spine function may leave him in a condition that limits cooperation in completing the general medical examination. It also allows the physician an opportunity to observe the patient's motions and posture. The patient may be unaware that observation is the initial portion of the physical examination. In fact, unbeknownst to the patient, the chief complaint is being evaluated as soon as the physician introduces himself to the patient.

Clues to the "systemic" character of back pain are discovered during the general physical examination. Vital signs can document the presence of fever associated with an infection or neoplasm. Tachycardia may be a sympathetic nervous system response to the patient's pain. Normotension in a patient with a history of hypertension suggests acute blood loss.

The skin examination is particularly helpful in alerting the physician to the presence of systemic illness. A number of the spondyloarthropathies cause dermatologic abnormalities. Keratodermia blennorrhagica is a rash over the palms and soles characterized by hyperkeratotic, yellowish, confluent plaques. Psoriasis causes erythematous, raised plaques with overlying scales that occur on extensor surfaces (elbows, knees) and on the scalp, umbilicus, and perianal area. Erythema nodosum (erythematous, raised nodules, particularly noted on the lower extremities) is associated with inflammatory bowel disease and sarcoidosis. Dermal plaques are also associated with sarcoidosis. Chronic hidradenitis suppurativa, sometimes accompanied by acne conglobata and cystic acne, on the face and torso can lead to the development of spondyloarthropathy. Painful vesicles distributed in a dermatomal pattern are a telltale sign of herpes zoster. Petechiae raise the possibility of thrombocytopenia associated with a primary hematologic disorder (multiple myeloma) or secondary to metastatic tumor or subacute bacterial endocarditis. The presence of small skin ulcers or needle marks raises the possibility of intravenous drug use, though the patient may deny substance abuse. Erythema chronicum migrans, a large raised annular erythematous skin lesion, is the cutaneous hallmark of Lyme disease.

The eye examination may reveal the presence of conjunctivitis (Reiter's syndrome) or iritis (ankylosing spondylitis). In a rare circumstance, pingueculae, yellowish deposits in the sclerae extending from the cornea to the inner canthus may be noted, which are associated with Gaucher's disease. Examination of the oropharynx may demonstrate painless (Reiter's syndrome) or painful (Behçet's syndrome) oral ulcers. Examination of the neck may reveal thyromegaly, indicative of thyroid gland dysfunction. Lymphadenopathy may be associated with neoplastic processes (lymphoma), infectious processes (tuberculosis, subacute bacterial endocarditis), or idiopathic processes (sarcoidosis).

Excursion of the chest wall is important to measure. Arthritis of the costovertebral joints associated with a spondyloarthropathy will limit motion, decreasing chest excursion, and lung capacity. Chest excursion should be measured with the patient's arms held straight up over the head. The tape measure is placed at the fourth intercostal space in men and just below the breasts in women and is pulled tight. The patient is instructed to take in a deep breath. (Normal excursion is 2.5 cm or greater.) Auscultation of the lung fields may result in discovery of abnormal breath sounds indicative of fibrosis. Pulmonary fibrosis is found in patients with spondyloarthropathies, sickle cell anemia, and sarcoidosis. Cardiac examination may demonstrate cardiomegaly, gallops, and murmurs. These abnormal findings may be associated with cardiac disease related to ankylosing spondylitis (aortic insufficiency), sickle cell disease (cardiomyopathy), and subacute bacterial endocarditis (valve insufficiency).

Abdominal examination is necessary to identify pathologic processes associated with back pain. These processes include gallbladder, pancreatic, and ulcer disease. A pulsatile mass, particularly in the horizontal plane, should make the examiner suspicious of an expanding abdominal aneurysm. Abnormalities of bowel sounds should be noted. Organomegaly or masses are of diagnostic importance and need to be evaluated in greater detail. The inguinal area is examined for the presence of a direct or indirect hernia. Palpation of the costovertebral angles will elicit pain in patients with kidney abnormalities. Rectal and/or gynecologic examination is done after the completion of the lumbosacral spine evaluation.

Musculoskeletal examination is helpful in identifying peripheral joint arthritis, which is often associated with lumbosacral spine disease. For example, distal interphalangeal (DIP) joint arthritis is characteristic of psoriatic arthritis. Proximal interphalangeal (PIP) joint disease in conjunction with DIP joint arthritis is commonly found in patients with osteoarthritis. Reiter's syndrome causes lower extremity arthritis in addition to sacroiliitis and spondylitis. Ankle arthritis associated with erythema nodosum is frequently associated with sarcoidosis. During the musculoskeletal examination, it is appropriate to check for peripheral pulses, particularly in the lower extremities.

EXAMINATION OF THE LUMBOSACRAL SPINE

Common sense needs to be used in the conduct of the physical examination. Some patients who are in extreme pain will not tolerate an extensive general medical examination prior to evaluation of the lumbosacral spine. In these patients, an examination that concentrates on the lumbosacral spine is appropriate. The remainder of the examination may be completed after evaluation of the lumbosacral spine or at a subsequent visit.

The objective of the physical examination of the lumbosacral spine is to demonstrate those physical abnormalities that sort out the possible disease entities causing pain that were elicited during the medical history. Abnormalities of the lumbosacral spine may be discovered while the spine is static or during motion. Unless the tests are done in an orderly fashion, important observations may be missed. Therefore, it is helpful to evaluate the patient in a series of positions that test the function of musculoskeletal and neurologic structures of the lumbosacral spine.[1]

The patient is examined initially *standing*. The patient should be undressed. The spine is viewed from behind, as well as laterally and anteriorly, to see if the alignment is normal. From behind, the levels of the shoulders and any lateral spinal curves (scoliosis) should be noted. The patient stands with the head centered over the feet and the eyes level. Therefore, any deviation of the spine from the vertical is compensated by an opposite deviation elsewhere in the spine. The spine is compensated if the first thoracic vertebra is centered over the sacrum. A list occurs if the first thoracic vertebra is not over the center of the sacrum. The degree of list may be measured by dropping a perpendicular line from the first thoracic vertebra and measuring how far to the right or left of the gluteal cleft it falls. In one study, 52% of patients had a detectable lumbar scoliosis.[2] The posterior superior iliac spines should be of equal height. Any prominence of bones in the thorax or pelvis should be listed. Infection, fracture, or congenital abnormalities cause bony prominences. The gluteal folds and knee joints should be at an equal height. The feet should be in normal alignment without any limitation of movement from the Achilles tendons. The patient with lumbar muscle spasm may demonstrate a list to one side, with loss of normal spinal contours. Movement of the sacroiliac joint may be examined with the patient standing. The examiner places one thumb on the posterior superior iliac spine and the other on the sacral spine. The patient flexes the ipsilateral hip. Normally, the iliac spine moves downward. Upward motion is indicative of a fixed sacroiliac joint (Fig. 5–1).

Laterally, any exaggeration or decrease of normal spinal curvatures is noted. Does the patient have a hyperlordosis (increased lumbosacral angle) or flattened lumbosacral curve (decreased lumbosacral angle)? Is a kyphosis present with drooped shoulders as seen in Scheuermann's disease? In the lower extremity, are the legs straight or bent with flexion or extension deformities of the knees? Abnormalities in the lower extremity will be mirrored with similar abnormalities in the lumbosacral spine (flexion or extension deformity, respectively).

Anteriorly, the head should be straight, with level shoulders. The highest points on the flanks or the iliac wings should be of equal height. There should be no tilt to the pelvis. Anatomic structures in the lower extremities (patellae, malleoli) should be of equal height and aligned appropriately.

Abnormalities of any superficial structures are noted. These abnormalities include a tuft of hair over the spine, which may indicate a congenital abnormality, such as diastematomyelia or spina bifida occulta. Vesicles in a dermatomal pattern are suggestive of herpes zoster. Café-au-lait spots are associated with neurofibromatosis.

The patient should squat in place. This maneuver tests not only general muscle strength but also the integrity of function of the joints from the hips to the feet in the lower extremity. Specific areas of decreased function must be identified if the patient is unable to complete this maneuver.

With the patient in the standing position, the range of motion of the lumbosacral spine in forward flexion, extension, lateral bending (side flexion), and rotation is observed. The normal range of motion for forward flexion is 40° to 60°, for extension 20° to 35°, for lateral bending 15° to 20°, and for rotation 3° to 18°.

Spinal motion is important in terms of symmetry and rhythm. The absolute range of motion is not of major diagnostic significance because of wide individual variance. The statement is frequently made that the patient bends forward and reaches to within 6 inches of the floor or 12 inches of the floor or places his palms to the floor. The important part of the observation of the patient as he bends toward the floor is the quality of spinal flexion in terms of the smooth reversal of the normal lumbar lordosis as the spine flexes forward. This is termed lumbosacral rhythm, and when abnormal (patient keeps his lumbar lordosis and bends from the hips) signifies local back disease. Although limitation of spine flexion is of limited diagnostic value, the improvement of spine flexion is a means to monitor response to therapy of an individual patient.[3]

Forward flexion of the spine is a segmental motion, with bending occurring at each functional unit (a functional unit comprising two adjacent vertebrae along with their interposed disc). These units also contain the ligaments, nerves, and facet joints of the two adjacent vertebrae. The most movement occurs at the lumbosacral L5-S1 and L4-5 levels. As a result, most of the damage and most symptoms relate to these two functional units. In forward bending, each unit flexes about 8° to 10°. This means that the entire lumbar spine has only 45° of excursion, and as a person reaches to touch the ground the rest of the motion comes from the pelvis rotating through the hip joints.

When a person with an injury to one of the functional units attempts to bend forward, his flexion will frequently be inhibited by protective muscle spasm. The lumbar spine will not have the normal curve in the erect position nor is there any reversal of the sway of the back on attempting to bend forward. As the patient attempts to touch the floor, all of the motion occurs at the hip joints.

Although this inability to flex the lumbar spine can be due to injury, it also may be voluntary in that the patient either is afraid or does not wish to bend forward. Consequently, this restriction is not necessarily indicative of an injury. A good examiner can generally differentiate between actual spasm and just a reflex, protective response. Flexion from an up-

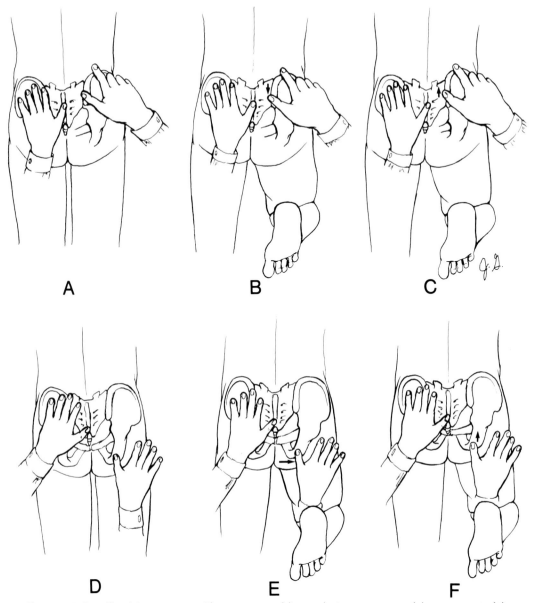

Figure 5–1. Sacroiliac joint movement. The upper row of figures depicts movement of the upper part of the joint. The lower row depicts movement of the lower part of the joint. *A,* The examiner places one thumb on the posterior superior iliac spine and the other thumb over one of the sacral spinous processes. *B,* Normal movement is associated with downward movement of the iliac spine with flexion of the ipsilateral hip. *C,* Abnormal movement associated with a fixed joint results in an upward motion of the iliac spine with flexion of the ipsilateral hip. *D,* The examiner places one thumb over the ischial tuberosity and the other thumb over the apex of the sacrum. *E,* Normal movement is associated with lateral movement of the ischial tuberosity with hip flexion. *F,* Abnormal movement associated with a fixed joint results in an upward movement of the ischial tuberosity with flexion of the hip.

right position should be compared with similar movement while kneeling. In the kneeling position, the sciatic nerve is not under tension and the hamstring muscles are relaxed; thus the back can move untethered.

It also should be appreciated that flexion is relative and its limitation may be only an indication of poor conditioning. The patient's perceived stiffness may actually represent very little loss of flexibility in respect to a preinjury state.

If the protective spasm is unilateral owing to injury of the tissues on one side of the spine, a scoliosis develops. The spine is tilted to one side because of one-sided muscle spasm. Scoliosis is difficult to mimic and may go unnoticed by the patient with back pain. It frequently will increase with forward flexion. Disc herniation can also cause a scoliosis by irritating nerves on one side of the spine (Fig. 5–2). This usually occurs at the L4-5 level. This diagnostic finding must be supplemented by other signs and symptoms to justify a diagnosis of a disc herniation. Scoliosis may be classified as structural or nonstructural. With structural scoliosis, anatomic changes in the vertebral column and thoracic ribs cause an asymmetry of structures, which appears with forward flexion. The high side (shoulder elevated) is on the convex side of the scoliotic curve. Nonstructural scoliosis is related to pain, has no associated anatomic change, and has no asymmetry with forward flexion. The scoliosis is of a lumbar variety if the apex of the curve is situated at the lumbar level.

Measurement of the distance from the floor to the patient's fingertips is an inexact measurement of lumbar flexion. However, the measurement is a useful way to follow the response of patients to therapy. Improvement in forward flexion will be manifested as a decrease in finger-to-floor distance whether the improvement is from decreased muscle spasm, increased hip motion, or decreased hamstring tightness.

After the patient has fully flexed, it is helpful to observe how he regains the erect posture. How this maneuver is performed reflects past habits as well as the constraints of any tissue injury. Normally a return to erect position is accomplished by a derotation of the pelvis without alteration of the kyphosis of the spine until the person has raised up to 45°. During the remaining 45° of re-extension, the low back resumes its lordosis. Patients with legitimate back pain tend to resume the erect position with a fixed lordosis and without any spine movement. It is all done by the pelvis with the help of knee and hip flexion.

The ability to bend sideways in lateral flex-

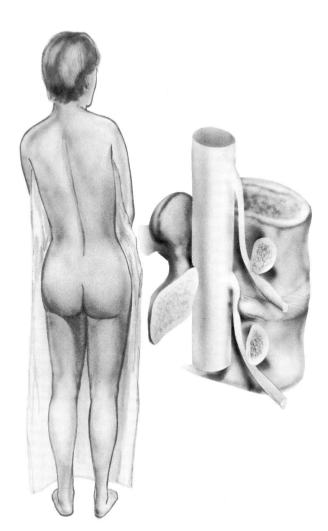

Figure 5–2. Herniation of a nucleus pulposus *lateral* to the corresponding nerve root. The sciatic list is away from the side of the irritated nerve root. (From Rothman RH, Simeone FA: The Spine. 2nd ed. Philadelphia, WB Saunders Co, 1982.)

ion has no major diagnostic significance as long as the patient is not simultaneously flexing or extending. The patient is asked to run a hand down the side of the leg and not to bend forward or backward while performing the movement. Lateral bending simply causes ligamentous or muscular stretching and can be free or restricted without diagnostic significance. However, pain that increases with flexion to the ipsilateral side may be related to an articular disease or a disc protrusion lateral to the nerve root. If pain is increased with flexion to the contralateral side, the lesion may be articular, muscular (muscles are stretched), or a disc protrusion medial to the nerve root (Fig. 5–3). Quantification of right and left lateral flexion can be measured by noting the distraction of two points, 20 cm apart in the midaxillary line on contralateral flexion.[4]

Hyperextension can cause pain by changing several anatomic relationships. Arching the back and increasing the lordosis forces the facet joints together, narrows the foramen through which the nerves exit the spine, and compresses the disc posteriorly. A combination of these three factors can create pressure on the nerves as they leave the spine and cause back pain, leg pain, or both.

Rotation may be examined in the standing position but care must be given to stabilize the pelvis to eliminate accessory motion of the hips. Rotation may be examined more accurately in the seated position. The hips and pelvis are stabilized with seating, limiting rotating motion of the spine.

The strength and stamina of the back and leg muscles can be tested by repeated active movement, especially flexion and extension of the lumbosacral spine. The patient should perform 10 toe raises on both feet and 10 more on each foot separately. Repeated testing causes fatigue, which accentuates differences in strength in the lower extremities. The strength of the examiner's arms may be less

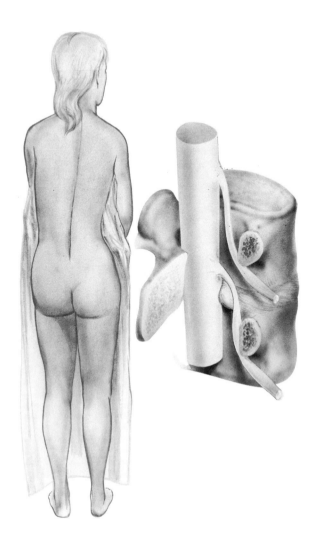

Figure 5–3. Herniation of a nucleus pulposus *medial* to the corresponding nerve root. The sciatic list is toward the side of the irritated nerve root. (From Rothman RH, Simeone FA: The Spine. 2nd ed. Philadelphia: WB Saunders Co, 1982.)

than that of the patient's legs. By using the patient's own weight, instead of the examiner's strength, differences of strength between the legs are discovered.

The patient may also be asked to walk on his heels to test for strength of the dorsiflexors of the foot. These muscles are more appropriately tested with the patient in the seated position.

The Trendelenburg sign may be elicited at this point. The patient is asked to stand on one leg. With a positive test, the buttock away from the affected muscle will fall when the patient is asked to stand on one leg. This may be related to an S1 nerve root lesion or hip disease (Fig. 5–4).

The physician should palpate the lumbosacral spine when the patient is standing, sitting, and during testing of motions. It is helpful to palpate both groups of paraspinous muscles simultaneously to discern differences of firmness or tenderness in the muscle bodies. Muscles become more prominent as they contract with spasm. Observation may demonstrate this muscle prominence on one side of the midline of the spine. Very localized areas of muscle tenderness, which may be trigger points for referred pain to other areas of the lumbosacral spine, should be identified. In the lumbosacral region, trigger points are located on both sides of the lumbosacral junction and in the superior portion of the buttocks near the iliac wings. Posterior thighs should also be palpated.

In addition to the soft tissue, bony structures should be palpated. The spinous processes are covered by ligamentous structures, not muscle, and are easily palpated. Localized tenderness suggests the presence of an isolated process, such as an infection, tumor, or fracture affecting that vertebral body. Pressure on the lateral surface of the vertebral body will elicit pain if an abnormality has involved the transverse process of the vertebra.

Palpation of the lumbar spine in the midline usually elicits pain at the level of a symptomatic degenerative disc. Moving laterally from the midline 1 to 3 cm, palpation of the facet joints may generate pain in the patient with degenerative joint disease. Palpation should

Trendelenburg test

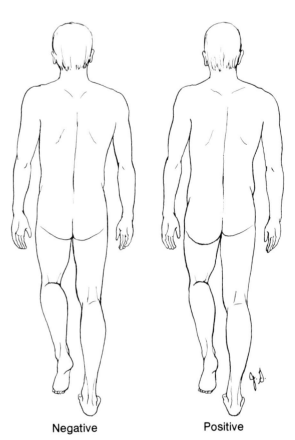

Negative   Positive

Figure 5–4. Trendelenburg test measuring integrity of the S1 nerve root and ipsilateral hip joint. A positive test is associated with a fall of the buttock contralateral to the affected nerve root or hip joint. In this figure, the right side is affected.

also be performed in the sciatic notch along the course of the sciatic nerve. Hyperesthesia along the irritated nerve is often found, and in addition, local tumors of the nerve may be discovered in this manner.

Vertebral tenderness may be a sensitive sign of spine pathology but is not discriminating in differentiating mechanical from medical disorders. Spinal pain with palpation may be from degenerative joint disease, spondyloarthropathy, or a vertebral infection.[5] Additional physical signs, such as fever and decreased chest expansion, will help differentiate mechanical from medical causes of vertebral tenderness.

The patient should next be examined *kneeling*. The patient should kneel on a chair facing the back rest. The ankle reflex corresponding to the S1 level is more easily tested in this position. Reinforcement of the reflex is obtained by having the patient grab the back of the chair or having the examiner dorsiflex the foot.

Persistence of limited motion and muscle spasm may be evaluated in this position. Some patients voluntarily guard their back muscles and are unwilling to flex forward in the standing position. In the kneeling position, their muscles may relax and soften remarkably. The spine may become more mobile, allowing the patient to bend forward.

The patient is examined in the *seated* position with feet on the floor. The strength of the dorsiflexors of the foot is measured by the examiner maintaining steady downward pressure on the dorsum of the foot. The maneuver should be continued for a minute to allow for detection of weakness in the muscles supplied by the L5 nerve roots. The patient generates uniform resistance to pressure that is overcome in a smooth fashion. Patients who fein weakness may either resist pressure for a few seconds and then suddenly release the muscle or demonstrate a stepwise release of the muscle resulting in a cogwheel effect.[1]

The patient is asked to *bend forward* over the examining table, allowing his weight to rest on his abdomen. This position flattens the lumbar lordosis and tilts the sacrum, allowing examination of the inferior portion of the sacroiliac joint, ischial tuberosities, and sciatic notch. Palpation over these anatomic structures may elicit pain. Patients with inflammatory processes of the sacroiliac joints (ankylosing spondylitis) are among those who experience increased pain with percussion over the sacroiliac joints. The gait of the patient should be examined as the patient walks from the

chair to the examining table. Back pain usually decreases the mobility of the lumbar spine and produces restriction of normal spinal movement. The back is stiff, as if frozen in one position. The patient walks in a stiff, guarded fashion depending mainly on hip movement and lateral spine flexion rather than using a normal gait involving a more complete range of active spinal movements.

The positions of *sitting* with legs dangling, *lying supine, lying on one side* and *lying prone* are used for the neurologic examination. Assessment of the neurologic status of the patient is very important in the overall back evaluation. A positive neurologic finding will give objectivity to the patient's subjective complaints. Each nerve root must be examined. Abnormalities of motor, sensory, and reflex function are tested. It is worthwhile to review the anatomy of the nerve roots in order to better understand abnormalities discovered on neurologic examination.

Each nerve root, as it leaves the spinal canal through the neural foramen, is enclosed within a sleeve that contains spinal fluid and very small blood vessels about and within the nerve. This sac, referred to as the dural sleeve, provides nourishment to a particular nerve root. Any compression and/or traction on the dura will compress its contents and encroach upon the nerve and its blood supply. Secondary to compression, pain is produced along the course of the peripheral nerve and is accompanied by dysesthesias, motor weakness, and decreased reflex function associated with the affected nerve root. The goal of many of the maneuvers done during this phase of the examination is to increase nerve compression to uncover neurologic dysfunction. Of the possible neurologic abnormalities, true muscle weakness is the most reliable indicator of persistent nerve compression with loss of nerve conduction.[6] Sensory changes are subjective and are easily affected by the emotional and energy state of the patient. As the patient fatigues, consistent sensory findings are difficult to reproduce. In addition, reflex changes may be lost in a previous episode of nerve root compression. Reflexes may not return even with recovery of sensory and motor function.[7] With age, reflexes are more difficult to elicit even without any prior history of nerve compression. However, the loss of reflexes is symmetric. Patients who lose reflexes in both lower extremities on the basis of compression have a central herniation of a disc.

In addition to nerve root lesions, upper motor neuron and peripheral nerve disease cause abnormalities that may be discovered during neurologic examination. With upper motor neuron lesions, the fine control of muscles is lost while the trophic effects of the peripheral nerves remain intact. Muscle strength is maintained initially, but patients develop spasticity of muscles (tonic contractions) and hyperreflexia. Patients will also develop a positive Babinski reflex (extension of the large toe and spreading of the other toes with stroking of the sole of the foot). Ankle clonus, an involuntary rhythmic plantarflexion motion after rapid dorsiflexion of the ankle, may also indicate upper motor neuron compression.

Peripheral nerve injuries may cause sensory and/or motor abnormalities, depending on the damaged nerve. Peripheral nerves receive nerve fibers from a number of nerve root levels. The locations of nerve root and peripheral nerve lesions affecting cutaneous structures in the lower extremity are depicted in Figures 5–5 and 5–6. A lesion at one nerve root level may cause a minor change in function if a structure is supplied by multiple spinal cord levels (hip flexion—psoas) (Fig. 5–7). However, if a peripheral nerve is injured, innervation to specific muscles and cutaneous areas is interrupted. In this circumstance, specific muscles may become paralyzed or areflexic (obturator nerve—thigh adduction) or specific cutaneous areas anesthetized (lateral femoral cutaneous nerve—lateral thigh) (Fig. 5–8). The differentiation of upper motor neuron, nerve root, and peripheral nerve lesions is an important one. The locations of the abnormalities causing these neurologic manifestations are different. Also, the category of pathologic process causing upper motor neuron, nerve root, and peripheral nerve abnormalities may be different (multiple sclerosis, disc herniation, and diabetes, respectively).

Sitting with legs dangling is the preferred position for testing knee reflexes (L4 nerve root). Minor differences in reflexes are usually caused by incomplete relaxation of the quadriceps or hamstrings by the patient. Reinforcing the reflex by having the patient attempt to pull apart his locked hands will distract him,

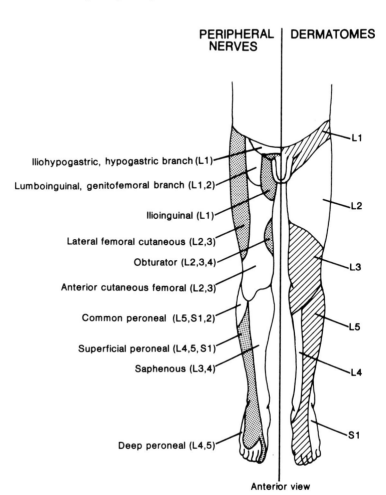

Figure 5–5. Anterior view of the lower extremities depicting skin areas innervated by nerve roots *(right)* and peripheral nerves *(left).*

PERIPHERAL NERVES | DERMATOMES

Iliohypogastric, hypogastric branch (L1)
Lumboinguinal, genitofemoral branch (L1,2)
Ilioinguinal (L1)
Lateral femoral cutaneous (L2,3)
Obturator (L2,3,4)
Anterior cutaneous femoral (L2,3)
Common peroneal (L5,S1,2)
Superficial peroneal (L4,5,S1)
Saphenous (L3,4)
Deep peroneal (L4,5)

L1
L2
L3
L5
L4
S1

Anterior view

DERMATOMES | PERIPHERAL NERVES

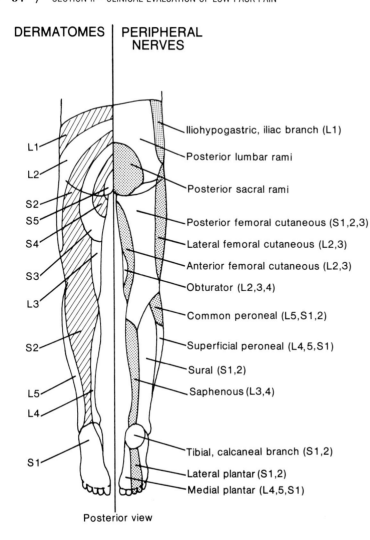

Iliohypogastric, iliac branch (L1)

Posterior lumbar rami

Posterior sacral rami

Posterior femoral cutaneous (S1,2,3)

Lateral femoral cutaneous (L2,3)

Anterior femoral cutaneous (L2,3)

Obturator (L2,3,4)

Common peroneal (L5,S1,2)

Superficial peroneal (L4,5,S1)

Sural (S1,2)

Saphenous (L3,4)

Tibial, calcaneal branch (S1,2)

Lateral plantar (S1,2)

Medial plantar (L4,5,S1)

Posterior view

Figure 5–6. Posterior view of the nerve root *(left)* and peripheral nerve *(right)* areas of the lower extremities.

allowing for relaxation of muscles. True asymmetry of reflex action should be present on repeated testing. The Babinski reflex may be tested in this position. This is done by lifting the leg to stroke the sole of the foot. By raising the foot, the examiner has performed a modified straight leg raising test. Since the thigh is already flexed to 90° in this position, straightening the knees to the horizontal places stretching forces on the nerve roots. The results of this sitting tension sign should correspond to those of the test done in the lying position.[8] This is a useful test in those situations where there is a suspicion of malingering. The patient with hamstring tightness may also experience leg pain. With extension of the knee, the patient will extend the trunk to relieve pressure (positive tripod sign). The patient with nerve root irritation will have a similar response. The localization of pain to the thigh or lower leg helps differentiate these patients.

Lying supine on the examining table is an excellent position for testing the status of the nerve roots and peripheral nerves. The classic test of sciatic nerve (L4, L5, S1) irritation is the straight leg raising test. Its purpose is to stretch the dura. The more useful straight leg raising test is done by raising the leg with the knee extended; first described by J. J. Forst, a contemporary of Lasègue, in the late 1800s.[9] When the sciatic nerve is stretched and its nerve roots and corresponding dural attachments are inflamed, the patient will experience pain along its anatomic course to the lower leg, ankle, and foot. Symptoms should not be produced in the lower leg until the leg is raised to 30° to 35°. Until that elevation, these is no dural movement. Between 30° and 60° to 70°, tension is applied to the dura and nerve roots (Fig. 5–9). The rate of deformation of the roots diminishes as the angle increases. Symptoms produced at elevations above 70° may represent nerve root irritation but may also be related to mechanical low back pain secondary to muscle strain or to joint disease.[10] The test is considered positive when the patient's radicular symptomatology is reproduced; the production of back pain does not indicate a positive test. Some patients will experience limitation of motion and posterior thigh pain secondary to hamstring muscle tightness. The degree of tightness is determined by raising the nonpainful side first, quantifying the degrees of painless motion.

In the Lasègue test, which is frequently mistaken as a straight leg test, the patient is supine with the hip flexed to 90° and the knee is slowly extended until sciatic pain is elicited (Fig. 5–10). This test is less valuable than the straight leg raising test since both hip and knee joints are moved, resulting in greater difficulty interpreting the test.

The patient with a positive straight leg raising test will have pain that radiates to the lower leg. To confirm the presence of nerve irritability, the raised leg should be lowered until the pain is relieved. At that position, the foot is dorsiflexed, which will cause a recurrence of pain as a result of stretching of the posterior tibial branch of the sciatic nerve (Fig. 5–11). Although this is not the test described by Lasègue, pain with dorsiflexion of the foot is commonly referred to as a positive Lasègue sign. This test is also known as Bragard's test.

A bilateral straight leg raising test may also detect sciatic nerve irritation (Fig. 5–12). The test is performed in the supine position by raising both legs by the ankles with knees extended. Raising both legs simultaneously tilts the pelvis upward, diminishing some of the tethering of the sciatic nerve. Therefore, the legs may be raised to a greater angle before radicular pain appears. Pain that occurs before 70° of motion is caused by stress on the sacroiliac joints. Above 70°, pain is related to a lesion in the lumbar spine. When the examination reveals a psychogenic cause of pain, a bilateral straight leg raising test is routinely painful at a lower elevation than a unilateral test.

The presence of a positive straight leg raising test at 60° is a sensitive test but a nonspecific test for disc herniation.[11] Radicular pain at a lower angle of elevation is associated with a larger disc protrusion documented at the time of surgery.[10] A positive crossed straight leg raising test is less sensitive but more specific for disc herniation.[12]

Measurements of the lower extremity are made with the patient in the supine position. Leg lengths are measured using the bony land-

marks of the anterior superior iliac spine and medial or lateral malleolus (Fig. 5–13). In addition, measurements of the thigh and calf at equivalent points above and below the patellae should be recorded.

Examination of the hip and sacroiliac joints is an essential part of the evaluation of the lumbosacral spine. Although hip pain may rarely be referred to the low back it is more characteristically felt in the groin and down the anteromedial thigh to the top of the knee. Flexion of the hip is measured first. Normal flexion has a range to 120°. As the examiner flexes the hip, a Thomas test detects the presence of hip flexion contracture. As the hip is flexed, the lumbar lordosis is flattened. With flattening of the lordosis, a flexion contracture of the contralateral hip will appear with raising of that leg. The number of degrees the contralateral hip is above the horizontal is the extent of the flexion contracture. To evaluate abduction of the hip, the examiner places one hand on the iliac crest, grasps the ankle with the other, and moves the leg away from the midline, noting the angle at which the pelvis moves. Hip abduction is maximum at 45°. Abduction may also be measured by quantifying the distance between the medial malleoli when both legs are maximally abducted. Adduction is measured with the examiner's hands in the same position, with note taken of when the pelvis moves after the leg is brought across the neutral position. Normal adduction ranges to 30°.

Examination of the hip for internal and external rotation is particularly sensitive for detecting early abnormalities of the hip. Flexion and extension of the hip may be normal while first internal rotation and then external rotation become painful. The range of motion is 45° for external rotation and 35° for internal rotation. Rotation is measured with the hip and knee in 90° flexion. Internal rotation is measured by rotation of the lower leg away from the midline of the trunk, and external rotation by rotating the lower leg toward the midline of the trunk.

Another test that stresses both the hip and sacroiliac joint is the Patrick or ''faber'' (flexion, abduction, external rotation) test (Fig. 5–14). The test is done by positioning the lateral malleolus of the tested leg on the patella of the opposite leg. Downward pressure is then placed on the medial aspect of the knee. Pain associated with a quick pulse of downward pressure is usually localized to the lateral aspect of the lumbar spine and originates in the sacroiliac joint. Slow pressure may elicit groin

SEGMENTAL MOTOR INNERVATION

Muscle	L1	L2	L3	L4	L5	S1	S2	S3	S4	S5
Erector spinae	X	X	X	X	X	X	X	X	X	X
Multifidus	X	X	X	X	X	X	X	X		
Interspinales	X	X	X	X	X					
Intertransversarii	X	X	X	X	X					
Quadratus lumborum	X	X	X	X						
Iliacus	X	X	X	X						
Psoas major	X	X	X	X						
Psoas minor	X	X								
Pectineus		X	X	X						
Sartorius		X	X	X						
Quadriceps femoris		X	X	X						
Gracilis		X	X	X						
Adductor brevis		X	X	X						
Adductor longus		X	X	X						
Quadratus femoris				X	X	X				
Adductor magnus			X	X	X					
Obturator externus			X	X						
Gluteus medius				X	X	X				
Gluteus minimus				X	X	X				
Tensor fasciae latae				X	X	X				
Gemellus inferior				X	X	X				
Extensor digitorum brevis				X	X	X				
Plantaris				X	X	X				
Popliteus				X	X	X				
Tibialis anterior				X	X	X				
Tibialis posterior				X	X					
Gluteus maximus					X	X	X			
Piriformis					X	X	X			
Gemellus superior					X	X	X			
Obturator internus					X	X	X			
Biceps femoris					X	X	X			

SEGMENTAL MOTOR INNERVATION (Continued)

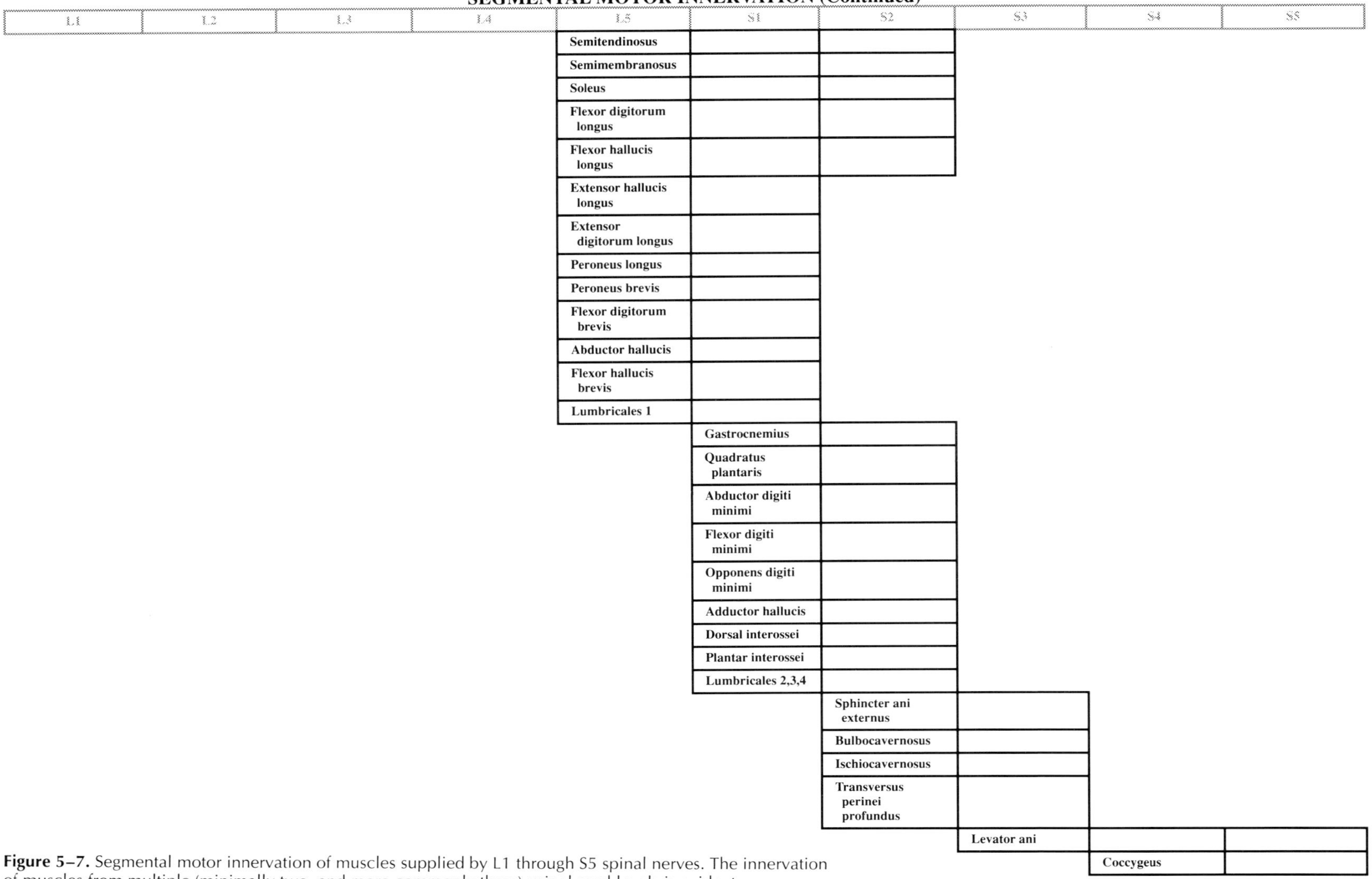

	L1	L2	L3	L4	L5	S1	S2	S3	S4	S5
Semitendinosus										
Semimembranosus										
Soleus										
Flexor digitorum longus										
Flexor hallucis longus										
Extensor hallucis longus										
Extensor digitorum longus										
Peroneus longus										
Peroneus brevis										
Flexor digitorum brevis										
Abductor hallucis										
Flexor hallucis brevis										
Lumbricales 1										
Gastrocnemius										
Quadratus plantaris										
Abductor digiti minimi										
Flexor digiti minimi										
Opponens digiti minimi										
Adductor hallucis										
Dorsal interossei										
Plantar interossei										
Lumbricales 2,3,4										
Sphincter ani externus										
Bulbocavernosus										
Ischiocavernosus										
Transversus perinei profundus										
Levator ani										
Coccygeus										

Figure 5–7. Segmental motor innervation of muscles supplied by L1 through S5 spinal nerves. The innervation of muscles from multiple (minimally two, and more commonly three) spinal cord levels is evident.

87

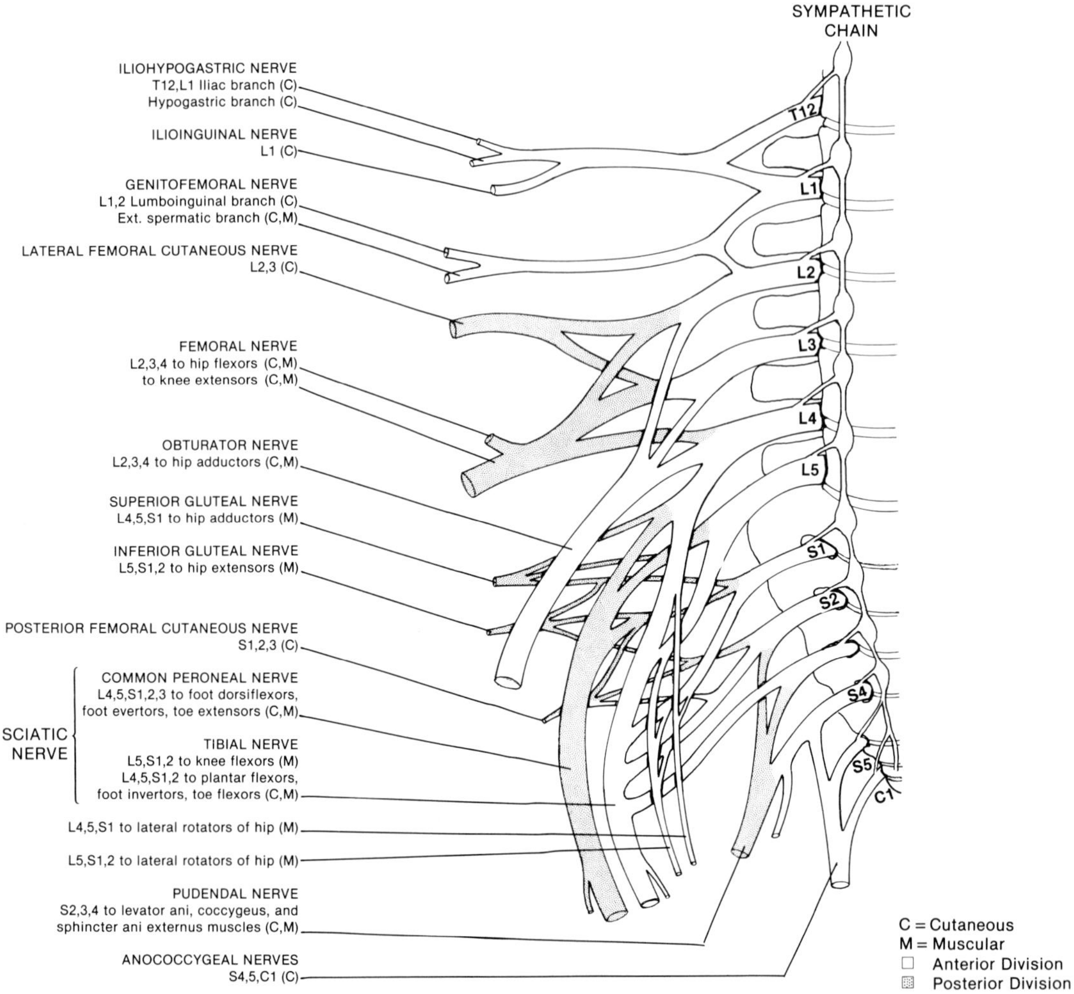

Figure 5–8. Nerves originating in the lumbosacral spine. The plexus, roots, branches, divisions (anterior and posterior), terminal branches, and autonomic nervous system components of the lumbosacral plexus are included. The cutaneous and motor components of the peripheral nerves are noted. The functions of muscles are listed under the associated nerves.

pain indicative of hip joint dysfunction. Patients with iliopsoas spasm are unable to lower the leg and may also experience groin pain with pressure. A negative test is indicated by the test leg's falling to the table or being parallel with the opposite leg.

The integrity of the sacroiliac joints is tested by applying pressure down and out on the anterior superior iliac spines. This pressure stresses the anterior sacroiliac ligaments, and the test is positive if the patient complains of buttock or posterior leg pain. Compression of the iliac wings toward the midline stresses the posterior iliac ligaments, and the test is positive when the patient complains of low back pain. Strain on the sacroiliac joint may also be elicited by asking the patient to flex the hip and knee maximally and adduct the leg, bring-

ing the knee toward the opposite shoulder. Pain in the stressed sacroiliac joint indicates a positive test. Gaenslen's test is another examination for abnormalities of the sacroiliac joint. The hip farthest from the edge of the examination table is flexed to the chest, while the test hip is extended by lowering it off the table. Pain that is localized to the low back is due to sacroiliac joint disease. Lesions of the hip joint and L4 nerve root must be differentiated from sacroiliac disease.

Neurologic function associated with abnormalities of the lumbosacral spine should be tested when the patient is in the supine position. The examination may be conducted according to systems (motor, sensory, reflexes) or to nerve root lesions (Table 5–1). When the first sacral root is compressed, the patient can

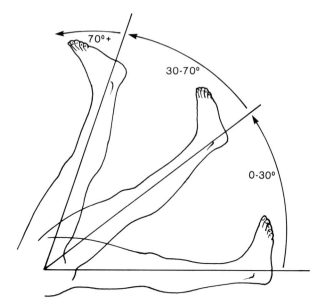

Figure 5–9. Dynamics of the single straight leg raising test. Tension is applied to the sciatic roots at 30° of elevation. Sciatic roots are maximally tightened over a herniated disc between 30° and 70°. No additional tension is generated with angles greater than 70°. Pain elicited at this height of elevation may be articular or muscular in origin.

have gastrocnemius weakness. The Achilles reflex (ankle jerk) often is diminished or absent, and atrophy of the calf may be apparent. Another muscle innervated by the first sacral root is the gluteus maximus. It can be tested with the patient lying supine with the knee on the involved side flexed at 90°. The strength of the gluteus maximus as well as the integrity of the S1 nerve can be evaluated unilaterally by having the patient raise his buttocks off the examining table 5 or 6 times. The affected side will be weaker as compared with the normal side. Sensory loss for the S1 root is confined to the posterior aspect of the calf and/or lateral side of the foot.

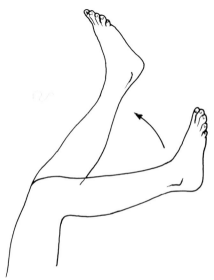

Figure 5–10. The Lasègue test.

Compression of the fifth lumbar nerve root may lead to weakness in extension of the great toe and, less often, to weakness of the everters and dorsiflexors of the foot. The sensory deficit may occur over the anterior tibia and the dorsomedial aspect of the foot down to the great toe. Primary reflex changes are uncommon, but sometimes a change in the posterior tibial reflex can be elicited. The absence of this reflex, however, must be asymmetric for it to have any clinical significance. A superficial reflex associated with L5 lesions is the gluteal reflex; stroking the skin over the buttock will result in contraction of the gluteal muscles.

Involvement of the fourth lumbar nerve root may lead to quadriceps muscle weakness. This can present as weakness of knee extension and/or the complaint of an unstable knee. Atrophy of the thigh musculature can be marked, and the sensory loss will be over the anteromedial aspect of the thigh. The patellar tendon reflex is affected.

When testing muscle power, it is important to test the muscles with the intervening joints in a neutral position. Pressure is applied by the examiner to a nonarticular structure for a minimum of 5 seconds. Where feasible, it is preferable to test both sides simultaneously. The innervation of muscles follows a sequential pattern starting with the hip and ending with the ankle (Fig. 5–15). Hip flexion is supplied by L2 and L3 and hip extension by L4 and L5. Knee extension (forward movement) is a function of L3 and L4 and knee flexion (backward movement) of L5 and S1. Ankle dorsiflexion is associated with L4 and L5 and ankle plantar

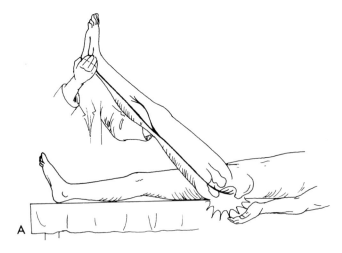

Figure 5–11. Confirmatory straight leg raising test. *A,* The leg is raised until radicular symptoms are elicited. *B,* The leg is lowered until pain is relieved. The foot is then dorsiflexed; if this recreates radicular pain, the test result is considered positive. (From Reilly BM: Practical Strategies in Outpatient Medicine. Philadelphia, WB Saunders Co, 1984.)

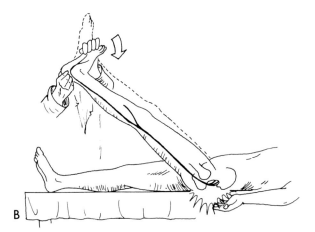

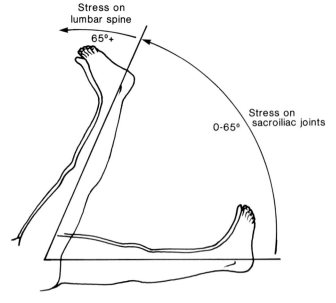

Figure 5–12. Bilateral straight leg raising test. The movement from 0° to 65° or 70° places stress on the sacroiliac joints. Above 70°, stress is placed on structures in the lumbar spine. Patients with psychogenic pain and a positive single straight leg raising test frequently develop pain at a smaller degree of elevation during the bilateral test.

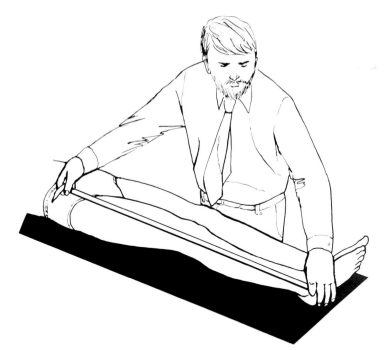

Figure 5–13. Measuring leg length.

flexion with S1 and S2. Ankle inversion is a function of L4. Ankle eversion is associated with L5 and S1.

The presence of tender motor points in the lower extremity in patients with sciatic pain has diagnostic and prognostic importance (Fig. 5–16). The points represent the main neuromuscular junctions for the involved muscle groups and remain reliably constant in location from patient to patient. Patients with radiculopathy and tender motor points have a segmental nerve root lesion at the corresponding level within the affected myotome. In addition, patients with tender motor points remain symptomatic longer than those without them.[13]

Other superficial and deep reflexes may be tested in the supine position in addition to the patellar and Achilles reflexes. The bulbocavernous reflex is an indication of S3 and S4 nerve root function and is tested by pinching the skin over the dorsum of the glans penis. A normal response is contraction of the bulbous urethra. The superficial abdominal reflex is elicited by rubbing a sharp object in a rhomboid shape on the abdomen. A positive reflex results in the retraction of the umbilicus in the direction of the quadrant stroked. Unilateral absence of the reflex suggests a lesion of an ipsilateral nerve root between T7 and L2, depending on the quadrant affected. Total absence of the reflex is seen in normal or obese patients as well as in those with upper motor neuron lesions. If a positive Babinski reflex is present, the absence of abdominal reflexes takes on greater significance. The adductor re-

Figure 5–14. Patrick's test ("faber" maneuver). The test is done by stabilizing the pelvis with downward pressure on the contralateral iliac wing (*small arrow*—arm not drawn) while lowering the ipsilateral flexed, abducted, and rotated leg. Rapid lowering tests the status of the sacroiliac joint, while slow lowering tests the hip.

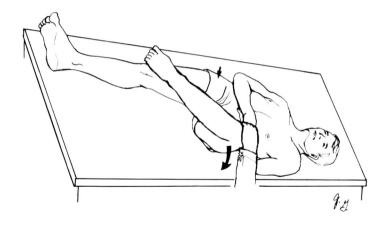

TABLE 5–1. LUMBOSACRAL ROOT SYNDROMES

ROOT	DERMATOME	MUSCLE INNERVATION	MUSCLE ACTION	ASSOCIATED REFLEX
L1	Back to trochanter Groin	Iliopsoas	Hip flexion	Cremasteric
L2	Back Anterior thigh to level of knee	Iliopsoas Sartorius Hip adductors (longus, brevis, pectineus, magnus, gracilis)	Hip flexion Hip adduction	Cremasteric Adductor
L3	Back Upper buttock to anterior thigh Medial lower leg	Iliopsoas Quadriceps femoris Sartorius Hip adductors	Hip flexion Hip adduction Knee extension	Patellar
L4	Inner calf to medial portion of foot (first 2 toes)	Tibialis anterior Gluteus medius Gluteus minimus Tensor fasciae latae Quadratus femoris	Knee extension	Patellar Gluteal
L5	Lateral lower leg Dorsum of foot First 2 toes	Extensor hallucis Tibialis posterior Hamstrings	Toe extension Ankle dorsiflexion	Tibilias posterior Gluteal
S1	Sole Heel Lateral edge of foot	Gastrocnemius Gluteus maximus Hamstrings Peroneus	Ankle plantar flexion Knee flexion	Ankle Hamstring
S2	Posterior and medial upper leg	Flexor digitorum longus Flexor hallucis longus	Ankle plantar flexion Toe flexion	None
S3	Medial portion of buttocks	—	—	Bulbocavernosus
S4	Perirectal	—	—	Bulbocavernosus
S5	Perirectal	—	—	Anal
C1	Tip of coccyx	—	—	Anal

flex indicates L2 function. The examiner's hand is placed over the medial femoral condyle and is struck with a reflex hammer. A normal response is adduction of the leg. The cremasteric reflex is elicited in males by stroking the inner aspect of the thigh with a sharp object. Upward retraction of the scrotal sac is the normal response. Lesions of L1 or L2 will result in unilateral absence of the reflex.

Gross sensory function may be surveyed by running the examiner's hands lightly over all the exposed areas on the anterior and lateral

NERVE ROOT ORGANIZATION OF MUSCLE FUNCTION

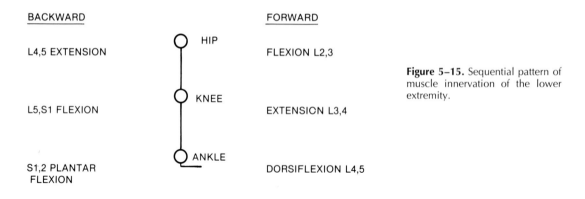

BACKWARD

L4,5 EXTENSION

L5,S1 FLEXION

S1,2 PLANTAR FLEXION

HIP

KNEE

ANKLE

FORWARD

FLEXION L2,3

EXTENSION L3,4

DORSIFLEXION L4,5

Figure 5–15. Sequential pattern of muscle innervation of the lower extremity.

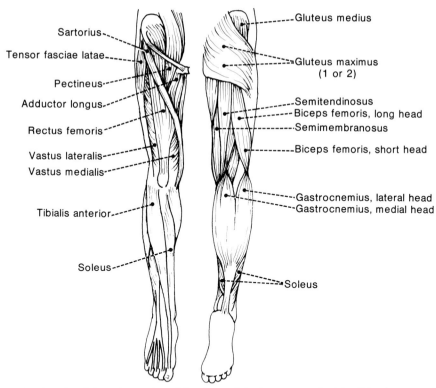

Figure 5–16. Anterior *(left)* and posterior *(right)* views of the lower extremity identifying location of motor points that become tender in association with corresponding nerve root lesions.

aspects of the thighs, lower legs, and feet. If the patient describes differences in sensation, a careful examination differentiating dermatomal abnormalities from peripheral nerve dysfunction must be completed testing pinprick, light touch, and vibratory function.

In the *lateral* position, the sacroiliac joints and hip abductors are tested. Pressure is applied to the iliac wing compressing the sacroiliac joint. This test causes forward pressure on the sacroiliac joint. Pain is felt in the sacroiliac joint suggestive of an intraarticular process or a strain of the posterior sacroiliac ligaments. Hip abduction, predominantly an L5 function, is tested as the patient elevates the upper leg against downward pressure applied below the knee by the examiner. The hip should be in a neutral position, not flexed or extended. The neutral position allows for sole testing of the hip abductors. These tests are repeated on the other side in a similar fashion.

In the *prone* position, the neurologic examination may be completed. For ''high'' discs (L2-3 and L3-4), dural irritability is checked by the femoral stretch test, which assesses irritation of the roots of the femoral nerve—L2, L3, and L4.[14] With the patient prone, the femoral nerve is stretched by bending the knee and

passively elevating the thigh up from the examining table. The maneuver tethers the femoral nerve over the anterior portion of the pelvis. The test is positive if pain is reproduced in the front of the thigh (L2 and L3) or the medial aspect of the leg (L4). Pain that is localized to the back occurs secondary to the extension of the lumbosacral spine associated with extending the hip. The significance of the location of pain in the leg should not be overlooked.[15] Pain produced by leg extension, limited to an area just lateral to the midline, is frequently localized to vertebral apophyseal joints. This sign may occur in patients with early degenerative joint disease before spinal stenosis occurs.

The muscle power of the gluteus maximus (S1 root) should be tested in the prone position. The patient is asked to squeeze the buttocks tightly together while the examiner palpates the muscles to assess muscle tone. Inability to tense one side is objective evidence of a neurologic deficit. This test is another check on the patient's cooperation, since it is difficult to tighten only one buttock voluntarily. The gluteus maximus may be affected to the degree that it atrophies. The examiner observing the buttocks at the level of the feet may

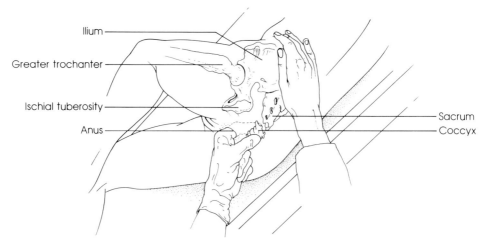

Figure 5–17. Palpation of the coccyx. (From Magee DJ: Orthopedic Physical Assessment. Philadelphia, WB Saunders Co, 1987, p 199.)

discover flattening that is secondary to atrophy. This is secondary to an L5, S1, or S2 inferior gluteal nerve lesion. This observation is a gluteal skyline test.[16]

The medial and lateral hamstring reflexes should be obtained. The knee is flexed and the lower leg is held by the examiner's arm. The hamstrings are supplied by L5 and S1. A loss of reflex may occur with lesions at either level. The findings from other tests (ankle reflex) may help localize the lesion.

Sensory examination of the skin over the lower legs, buttocks, and perianal area is important in determining the integrity of the upper (S1, S2) and lower (S3, S4) sacral nerve roots. The area tested is the perineum (saddle area). If saddle anesthesia is present, additional tests, including the well leg raising test and a test of anal sphincter tone, must be completed. If results of these tests are abnormal, the patient must be evaluated for a massive central disc protrusion. These patients require immediate evaluation because expeditious operative decompression of the disc is necessary to preserve bladder and bowel continence. (Parasympathetic nerves have cell bodies in the lower part of the spinal cord and send peripheral fibers to supply the bladder and rectum through the S2, S3, and S4 roots.)

The final part of the evaluation is the genital and rectal examination. The testicles should be palpated for any nodules or masses. The patient is then placed on his side. The gloved finger is well lubricated and inserted into the rectum with gentle but persistent pressure. Rectal tone is determined by the pressure exerted on the inserted finger. The circumference of the rectum should be palpated. In men, the prostate is felt on the anterior wall of the rectum. A hard prostate suggests the presence of a malignancy. In women, the vagina is contiguous to the anterior wall of the rectum. The presence of firm nonfixed nodules suggests the presence of endometriosis. The examining finger should then move around the rectum, palpating the pelvic musculature. Increased tension, manifested by firmness in the palpated muscles (piriformis, coccygeus), may be determined. Finally, the coccyx and sacrum are palpated (Fig. 5–17). External pressure from the thumb on the sacrum will test for any abnormal motion in this portion of the spine. Sacral masses are palpated anterior to the sacrum through the posterior wall of the rectum. These masses will not be palpated unless the rectal examination is done. If the clinical history suggests a gynecologic source for back pain in a female patient, a complete pelvic examination is indicated. The examiner should palpate the uterus, cervix, and ovaries for any masses or adhesions associated with neoplastic or inflammatory lesions.

Commonly Used Low Back Tests

There are a number of other tests that may be added to the physical examination just described. For the most part these are just variations of tests previously described, but they need to be presented since they are commonly used to confirm positive test findings.

Schober Test (Fig. 5–18). The Schober test measures the amount of flexion in the lumbar spine. Patients with spondyloarthropathies have decreased lumbar flexion and abnormal

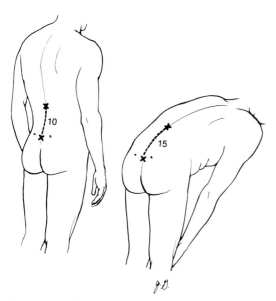

Figure 5–18. Schober test measuring forward flexion of the lumbar spine. Normal expansion is 5 cm. This test is used in patients with spondyloarthropathies to monitor response to therapy.

Schober tests. A point between the sacroiliac dimples is marked along with another mark 10 cm above the lower one. The patient is asked to bend forward and the increased distance measured. Patients with normal lumbar flexion increase the distance 4 to 5 cm. Patients with limited flexion will have distances less than 4 cm. The validity of this test has recently been questioned.[17] The test may not accurately measure lumbar flexion. The test is also non-specific being positive in chronic back pain, spondyloarthropathies, and spinal tumors.[18] However, in another study, the modified Schober test was the most repeatable test of four tests assessing lumbar spinal motion.[19]

Contralateral or Well Leg Straight Leg Raising Test (Fajersztajn Test) (Fig. 5–19). This test is positive when pain is reproduced in the involved leg below the knee as the straight leg raising test is performed on the opposite or uninvolved side.[20–22] This test is quite specific and sensitive to pressure on the nerve root; when positive, surgery is usually indicated to relieve the pain.

Voluntary Release. This test is used to differentiate the patient with true organic nerve damage from the one with an extensive emotional overlay. On attempting a sustained muscle contraction, such as dorsiflexion of the ankle, the patient with a functional problem holds up the ankle with intermittent quivering, breaking, contraction, and release in a jerky

manner as opposed to the smooth release seen in a patient with an organic disorder. When this occurs, it is strongly suggestive of nonorganic pathology.

Bow String Sign (Cram Test). The patient is seated with the knee flexed 70° and the body bent forward so as to lengthen the course of the sciatic nerve. The examiner's finger is then pressed into the popliteal space to increase tension on the nerve. A positive test occurs when pain is increased down the leg and suggests the presence of a radiculopathy.[23]

Naffziger Test. This test is done by compressing the jugular veins in the neck for approximately 10 seconds until the patient's face begins to flush. The patient is then asked to cough to increase the intrathecal pressure; sciatic pain will be aggravated if there is dural sensitivity.

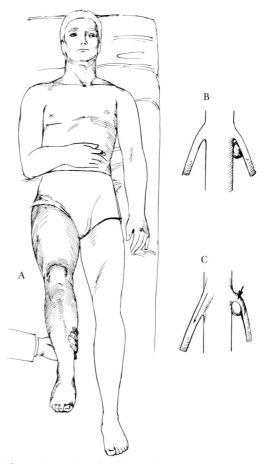

Figure 5–19. Contralateral or well leg test of Fajersztajn. Movement of nerve roots when the leg on the contralateral side is raised. When the leg is raised on the unaffected side *(A)*, the roots on the opposite side slide downward and toward the midline *(B)*. In the presence of a medial disc herniation, this movement increases nerve root tension *(C)*. (Modified from DePalma AF, Rothman RH: The Intervertebral Disc. Philadelphia, WB Saunders Co, 1970.)

Valsalva Test. This test increases intrathecal pressure when the patient is asked to bear down like he is trying to move his bowels. Sciatic pain will occur in the presence of dural irritation. Coughing and sneezing also raise intraabdominal pressure and can be used as a modification of this test since leg pain will be produced in the same way.

Brudzinski/Kernig Test. With the patient lying supine, the head is passively flexed down upon the chest. A positive test is reproduction of the patients' leg pain. The occurrence of neck pain is not significant. A positive Kernig test occurs when the supine patient extends his knee on a hip that is flexed at 90° and develops back pain. Pain is secondary to meningeal nerve root or dural irritation.[24, 25]

Milgram Test. This is a further modification of the tension test. While in the supine position, the patient is asked to raise both extended legs about 1 to 3 inches from the examining table. This is another way to increase intraabdominal pressure, and thus intrathecal pressure. The patient is asked to hold the position for 30 seconds. The test is considered positive if the maneuver creates leg pain. Just as in the straight leg raising test, however, a complaint of back pain does not make it significant.

Hoover Test. This test checks the validity of a patient's attempt to raise one leg off the examining table. Normally as a patient attempts to raise one outstretched leg, he must simultaneously press down with the opposite leg. Thus the downward pressure of the normal leg is a good indication of how hard he is trying. The examiner can check the sincerity of his effort by keeping a hand under the foot.[26]

Kneeling Bench Test. The patient, kneeling on a 12 inch high bench, is asked to bend forward and touch the floor. Flexion at the hips is the only requisite to accomplish this. If the hips are normal and the fingers do not reach the floor, nonorganic back pain must be suspected.

Stoop Test. This test evaluates the association of intermittent claudication of neurogenic origin with exercise and position.[27] The patient is asked to walk briskly for 1 to 2 minutes. When back, posterior thigh, and lower limb pain appear, the patient sits and flexes forward. A positive test occurs if the pain is relieved with flexion. Reflexes may be absent during a period of neurogenic claudication. The reflexes must be examined expeditiously, since recovery of reflex function corresponds with the relief of pain, which may occur within 3 to 4 minutes.[28]

Oppenheim Test. This test is used to detect upper motor neuron lesions. A dull object is run down the anterior portion of the tibia. A positive response is similar to that of the Babinski test, with extension of the big toe and splaying of the other toes. A positive test is secondary to an upper motor neuron lesion.

Functional Disorders

In some cases, the objective findings associated with the low back problem do not match the subjective complaints. This is especially true in cases associated with compensation and/or litigation. These cases are termed "functional," which is used medically in contradistinction to "organic." For these functional cases there is usually a psychologic component as well as secondary gain involved.

Watching the patient attempt a sit-up on the examination table provides useful information. Patients with pain secondary to symptomatic lumbar segmental instability will be unable to complete one sit-up. Patients with discogenic disease have increased pain with flexion and will not assume an upright position without rolling to one side and pushing themselves up with their arms. Patients with severe lumbar muscle spasm will also have difficulty doing a sit-up. They will also roll to their side in order to get off the examination table. Patients with posterior element and psychogenic disease will have no difficulty with arising from a supine position.

Accentuation of symptoms for greater effect may be a sign of a patient with psychogenic difficulties. Lurching from one piece of office furniture to another associated with sudden paroxysms of twitching and pain in the lumbar spine is unusual behavior for the patient with organic back disease.

To evaluate patients with these functional disorders a list of physical signs was developed by Waddell.[29] This provides a simple and rapid screen to help identify the few patients who require more detailed investigation. Any of the following individual signs count as one if positive; a finding of three or more of the five types is clinically significant. Isolated positive signs are ignored (Fig. 5–20).

1. Tenderness—when related to physical disease, tenderness is usually localized to a particular skeletal or neuromuscular structure. Nonorganic tenderness is nonspecific and diffuse.
   a. Superficial—the skin is tender to light pinch over a wide area of lumbar skin.

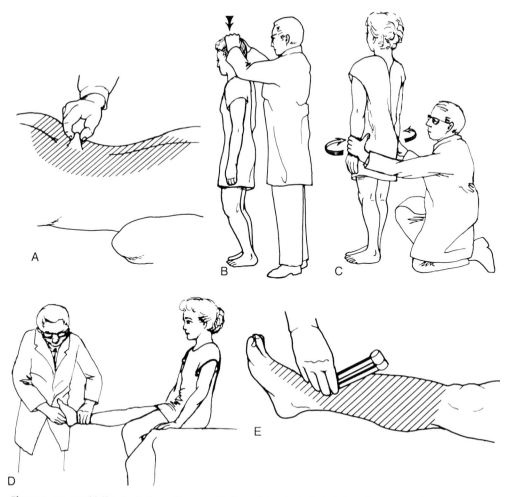

Figure 5–20. Waddell tests. *A,* Superficial sensitivity to light pinch. *B,* Axial loading causing low back pain. *C,* Passive rotation of the shoulders and pelvis in the same plane causing back pain. *D,* Straight leg raising test in the seated position. Stroking the skin on the bottom of the foot distracts the patient. *E,* Stocking distribution of sensory deficit.

b. Nonanatomic—deep tenderness is felt over a wide area and is not localized to one structure; it often extends to the thoracic spine, sacrum, or pelvis.
2. Simulation tests—these should not be uncomfortable; so, if pain is reported, a nonorganic influence is suggested.
   a. Axial loading—there is a complaint of low back pain with vertical pressure on the skull of a patient who is standing.
   b. Rotation—back pain is reported when the shoulders and pelvis are passively rotated in the same plane.
3. Distraction tests—first, a positive finding is demonstrated in the usual manner; next this finding is rechecked while the patient's attention is distracted. Findings that are present only on formal examination and disappear at other times are considered positive.

4. Regional disturbances—findings that involve a divergence from accepted neuroanatomy.
   a. Weakness—nonanatomic "voluntary release" or unexplained "giving way" of muscle groups.
   b. Sensory—sensory abnormalities fit a "stocking" rather than a dermatomal pattern.
5. Overreaction—this may take the form of disproportionate verbalization, jumping, cringing, excessive facial expression, etc. Judgement should, however, be made with caution, as it is very easy to introduce observer bias.

The above standardized group of nonorganic physical signs is easily learned and can be incorporated unobtrusively to add less than 1 minute to the routine physical examination.

These tests are extremely important, and when three are positive the finding should be followed up.

Reproducibility of Physical Signs

Compared with physical signs in other fields of medicine, the physical findings associated with the examination of the lumbosacral spine are poorly defined in regard to performance and measurement.[30] The lack of definition makes it difficult for physicians to reproduce an abnormal physical finding in patients over time. Another concern is the reliability of physical signs to identify normal function and the presence of pathology.[31]

McCombe and associates[32] evaluated the reproducibility between observers of 54 physical signs used in the evaluation of low back pain. Three health professionals examined 83 back pain patients for specifically defined abnormalities of pain pattern, posture, movement, tenderness, sacroiliac and piriformis dysfunction, root tension signs, root compression signs, and inappropriate signs. Reliable signs consisted of measurements of lordosis, flexion range, determination of pain location on flexion and lateral bend, measurements associated with straight leg raising test, determination of pain location in the thighs and legs, and sensory changes in the legs. Describing the location of pain increased the reliability of nerve root tension signs. Reproducibility of bone tenderness over the sacroiliac joint, spinous processes, and iliac crest was greater than that associated with soft tissue structures. Measurement of movement with a tape is a worthwhile way of reproducing results. Constant reexamination is needed to correlate the validity and reproducibility of physical findings with other components of patient evaluation for low back pain.

SUMMARY

With conclusion of the history and physical examination, the examining physician should have the answers to important questions concerning prior surgery, pre-existing back injury, the presence of a malignancy or systemic illness, the presence of nerve root irritation, and the possibility of the patient's being a malingerer. The physician should gather these facts together and construct a list of diseases for the differential diagnosis. The diagnosis of low back pain of undetermined etiology is inadequate. Patients may have muscle strain, facet joint disease, discogenic disease with or without nerve root irritation, or a systemic illness. In patients with mechanical abnormalities, no additional evaluation is necessary with the initial visit. Other patients with systemic symptoms and signs may require additional evaluation. Appropriate laboratory evaluation is useful in differentiating some of the myriad of systemic illnesses associated with low back pain (see Chapter 6).

References

1. Hall H: Examination of the patient with low back pain. Bull Rheum Dis 33:1, 1983.
2. McKenzie RA: Prophylaxis in recurrent low back pain. NZ Med J 89:22, 1979.
3. Mayer TG, Tencer AF, Kristoferson S, Mooney V: Use of noninvasive techniques for quantification of spinal range of motion in normal subjects and chronic low back pain dysfunction patients. Spine 9:588, 1984.
4. Moll JMH, Wright V: Normal range of spinal mobility. An objective clinical study. Ann Rheum Dis 30:381, 1971.
5. Blower PW, Griffin AJ: Clinical sacroiliac tests in ankylosing spondylitis and other causes of back pain. Ann Rheum Dis 43:192, 1984.
6. Spengler DM, Freeman CW: Patient selection for lumbar discectomy. Spine 4:129, 1979.
7. Blower PW: Neurological pattern in unilateral sciatica. Spine 6:175, 1981.
8. Nehemkis AM, Carver DW, Evanski PM: The predictive utility of the orthopedic examination in identifying the low back pain patient with hysterical personality features. Clin Orthop 145:158, 1979.
9. Finneson BE: Examination of the patient. In Finneson BE (ed): Low Back Pain. 2nd ed. Philadelphia: JB Lippincott, 1981, p 54.
10. Fahrni WH: Observations on straight-leg-raising with special reference to nerve root adhesions. Can J Surg 9:44, 1966.
11. Kosteljanetz M, Espersen JO, Halaburt H, Miletic T: Predictive value of clinical and surgical findings in patients with lumbago-sciatica. A prospective study (Part 1). Acta Neurochir (Wien) 73:67, 1984.
12. Shiqing X, Quanzhi Z, Dehao F: Significance of straight-leg-raising test in the diagnosis and clinical evaluation of lower lumbar intervertebral disc protrusion. J Bone Joint Surg 69:517, 1987.
13. Gunn CC, Chir B, Milbrand WE: Tenderness at motor points. A diagnostic and prognostic aid to low back injury. J Bone Joint Surg 58A:815, 1976.
14. Dyck P: The femoral nerve traction test with lumbar disc protrusion. Surg Neurol 6:163, 1976.
15. Herron LD, Pheasant HC: Prone knee-flex provocative testing for lumbar disc protrusion. Spine 5:65, 1980.
16. Katznelson A, Nerubay J, Level A: Gluteal skyline (G.S.L.): A search for an objective sign in the diagnosis of disc lesions of the lower lumbar spine. Spine 7:74, 1982.
17. Miller SA, Mayer TG, Cox R, Gatchel RJ: Reliability problems associated with the modified Schober technique for true lumbar flexion measurement. Spine 17:345, 1992.

18. Rae PS, Waddell G, Venner RM: A simple technique for measuring lumbar spinal flexion. J R Coll Surg Edin 29:281, 1984.
19. Gill K, Krag MH, Johnson GB, et al.: Repeatability of four clinical methods for assessment of lumbar spinal motion. Spine 13:50, 1988.
20. Hudgins RW: The crossed straight leg raising test: a diagnostic sign of herniated disc. J Occup Med 21:407, 1979.
21. Hudgins WR: The crossed-straight-leg-raising test. N Engl J Med 297:1127, 1977.
22. Woodhall R, Hayes GJ: The well-leg raising test of Fajersztajn in the diagnosis of ruptured lumbar intervertebral disc. J Bone J Surg 32A:786, 1950.
23. Cram RH: A sign of sciatic nerve root pressure. J Bone Joint Surg 35B:192, 1953.
24. Brudzinski J: A new sign of the lower extremities in meningitis of children (neck sign). Arch Neurol 21:217, 1969.
25. Kernig W: Concerning a little noted sign of meningitis. Arch Neurol 21:217, 1969.
26. Archibald KC, Wiechec F: A reappraisal of Hoover's test. Arch Phys Med Rehabil 51:234, 1970.
27. Dyck P: The stoop-test in lumbar entrapment radiculopathy. Spine 4:89, 1979.
28. Joffe R, Appleby A, Arjona V: Intermittent ischemia of the cauda equina due to stenosis of the lumbar canal. J Neurol Neurosurg Psychiatry 29:315, 1966.
29. Waddell G, McCullogh JA, Kummel E, Venner RM: Nonorganic physical signs in low back pain. Spine 5:117, 1980.
30. Deyo RA: Measuring the functional status of patients with low back pain. Arch Phys Med Rehabil 69:1044, 1988.
31. Waddell G, Main CJ, et al.: Normality and reliability in the clinical assessment of backache. Br Med J 284:1519, 1982.
32. McCombe PF, Fairbank JCT, Cockersole BC, Pysent PB: Reproducibility of physical signs in low back pain. Spine 14:908, 1988.

6

Laboratory Tests

The availability and expense of an ever-expanding variety of laboratory tests have complicated the professional life of the practicing physician. In the period of time when the laboratory evaluation was limited to blood counts, urinalysis, sedimentation rates, and serum chemistry, the physician obtained basic useful information about a patient for an inexpensive price. Our present state of affairs is quite different. The number of available tests has grown at a great rate without a corresponding increase in diagnostic accuracy but with an appreciable increment in cost. In fact, the results of tests done at an inappropriate time or interpreted incorrectly may only confuse the physician and hide the true diagnosis. For example, a patient with cryoglobulinemia secondary to multiple myeloma will have an inappropriately "normal" erythrocyte sedimentation rate. The cryoglobulins conceal the presence of increased plasma proteins caused by the malignant disease, which is usually associated with an abnormal sedimentation rate. Another example would be the interpretation of an elevated acid phosphatase after palpation of the prostate gland during a rectal examination for metastic prostatic carcinoma. Therefore, laboratory tests should be used in the situation in which a physician has developed a differential diagnosis through his history and physical examination for which laboratory data are needed to confirm or reject specific diagnoses.

In general, laboratory tests play a minor role in the diagnosis of low back pain. They are rarely needed on an emergent basis. They do have a role in separating mechanical from systemic diseases and are also useful in distinguishing metabolic-endocrinologic disorders from those with more inflammatory characteristics.

The vast majority of individuals with low back pain do not require laboratory studies with their initial evaluation. This is particularly true of a patient with a history of acute onset of pain related to physical activity. These patients may be given therapy for their back pain without additional tests. They are candidates for laboratory evaluation if they fail to respond to back pain therapy. The threshold for obtaining a laboratory evaluation at an initial visit is lower for new-onset low back pain in an elderly individual. Since medical etiologies for back pain occur commonly in older individuals, evaluation for systemic pathology should be pursued earlier in the diagnostic process in this group. Occasionally younger individuals will present with severe, systemic symptoms (fever, chills, eye inflammation) that strongly suggest a local (infection) or systemic (spondyloarthropathy) inflammatory process as the source of their back pain. Laboratory evaluation during the initial evaluation may help confirm the inflammatory nature of their disease. Laboratory tests that are important in the study of low back syndromes include blood counts, blood chemistry tests, urinalysis, immunologic studies (cellular and humoral), body fluid analysis, cultures, and tissue biopsy. (For laboratory abnormalities associated with specific illnesses, refer to the corresponding chapter in Section III or the appropriate listing in the Appendix).

HEMATOLOGIC TESTS

Erythrocyte Sedimentation Rate (ESR)

The most useful test in helping to differentiate medical from mechanical low back pain is measurement of the erythrocyte sedimentation rate (ESR). The ESR mirrors the state of activity of the acute phase response. The acute phase response is a reaction by the body to tissue injury. With tissue necrosis, a systemic response is initiated that results in an increase in concentration of glycoproteins of hepatic origin that affect complement and coagulation cascades. The acute phase response has a beneficial effect of limiting the spread of tissue damage and facilitating wound healing. The increased concentration of plasma proteins causes an increased aggregation of erythrocytes, which form a stack of discs (rouleaux). With rouleaux formation, erythrocyte mass is increased in relationship to cell surface area, resulting in an increased rate of fall of the cells.

The test is done by collecting anticoagulated blood from a patient and placing it in a specialized tube. The decrease in height of the column of erythrocytes is measured over an hour. The Wintrobe method uses a 100 mm long tube and cannot measure ESR values greater than the patient's hematocrit.[1] The Wintrobe method is most useful for mild elevations of ESR and may be more sensitive than the Westergren method for minimal elevations.[2] The Westergren method is the standard method for measuring ESR and involves diluting blood and using a 200 mm tube.[3] This method allows for the fall of erythrocytes to a distance greater than the packed height of the red cells. Larger ESRs are more accurately determined by the Westergren method.

In general, an elevated ESR suggests the presence of inflammation in the body. The ESR will be elevated with tissue injury, whatever the source (Table 6–1). It is used to screen for inflammatory diseases and to follow the response to therapy. For example, the spondyloarthropathies (ankylosing spondylitis,

Reiter's syndrome) frequently produce ESR elevation. The ESR is normal in mechanical low back pain (muscle strain and osteoarthritis).

It is important to remember that the ESR value must be interpreted according to the sex and age of the patient. The Westergren upper limits of normal are 15 mm/hr for men under 50 years of age and 20 mm/hr for men older than 50. For women, the upper limit is 25 mm/hr under 50 years of age and up to 30 mm/hr over age 50. The upper limit continues to rise as patients grow older. In patients over 70 years of age, an ESR of 50 mm/hr or higher may be normal.[4] The change in ESR may be more important than the absolute value when a patient is evaluated by a clinician. A 70-year-old patient who had a Westergren ESR of 10 mm/hr and now has an ESR of 48 mm/hr is worthy of additional evaluation even though the ESR value is in the normal range.

ESR may be "falsely" normal with any process that, by altering red blood cell (RBC) morphology, inhibits rouleaux formation and slows the decline of erythrocytes despite the presence of increased concentrations of acute phase reactants. Sickle cell anemia is associated with a normal ESR despite extensive tissue injury.

Markedly elevated ESRs (100 mm/hr or greater) are most commonly associated with malignancies, particularly with metastases.[5] Other diseases associated with markedly increased ESR include connective tissue disease (polymyalgia rheumatica-temporal arteritis) and acute bacterial infection (pneumonia).

The ESR is the most valuable screening test for the detection of medical spinal pathology. In one series, an ESR of over 25 mm/hour had a false positive rate of only 6%.[6]

The test has a number of flaws.[7] ESR is seldom the sole clue to systemic disease and is

TABLE 6–1.   CAUSES OF ELEVATED ERYTHROCYTE SEDIMENTATION RATE

RHEUMATIC DISEASES	ACUTE INFECTIONS
Spondyloarthropathies	Bacterial, including endocarditis, pyelonephritis
Rheumatoid arthritis	Tuberculosis
Rheumatic fever	
Polymyalgia rheumatica	**TISSUE NECROSIS**
Systemic lupus erythematosus	Surgery
	Myocardial infarction
MALIGNANT DISEASES	
Multiple myeloma	**MISCELLANEOUS**
Solid tumors (colon, breast)	Endocrinopathies
Metastases	Pregnancy
	Vaccinations
ABDOMINAL DISEASES	
Cholecystitis	
Pancreatitis	
Inflammatory bowel disease	

not a useful tool in asymptomatic individuals.[8] The ESR may be normal in patients with systemic diseases including cancer. Red cell morphology, a factor independent of the concentration of acute phase reactants, influences the rate of cell sedimentation. ESR is an indirect measure of the concentration of acute phase reactants. The activity of an illness is not always mirrored in the rise or fall of the ESR.[9]

Despite its shortcomings, ESR remains the primary test for screening for systemic illness in low back pain patients. The continued use is based on its availability in a wide variety of office and hospital laboratories, its simplicity, and the broad experience with test results in a multitude of medical conditions.

C-Reactive Protein

C-reactive protein (CRP), first described in 1930, is an acute phase protein synthesized by hepatocytes.[10] It was named for its property of precipitating the somatic C-polysaccharide of the pneumococcus. The protein is an aggregate of five identical subunits that are arranged in a planar, cyclic pentagon.[7] CRP may recognize inflammatory tissue damage by binding to phosphocholine, a cell membrane-based compound. Phosphocholine is part of endogenous damaged tissues and exogenous tissues, such as bacteria. The exact function of CRP in acute phase response is not known. It does activate the complement pathway and interacts with phagocytic cells. CRP modulates neutrophils thereby suppressing superoxide production and degranulation and reducing phosphorylation of intracellular proteins. CRP also interacts with monocytes, platelets, and lymphocytes.

Levels of CRP in normal adult humans are less than 0.2 mg/100 ml. Slight variations occur with minor injuries. Concentrations of less than 1 mg/100 ml are regarded as normal or insignificant elevations, between 1 and 10 mg/100 ml are moderate increases, and over 10 mg/100 ml are marked increases. CRP increases within hours of an inflammatory stimulus, usually reaches a peak in 2 to 3 days, and then recedes over 3 to 4 days. It may remain elevated in chronic inflammatory states such as rheumatoid arthritis and tuberculosis.

CRP may be measured to levels as low as 0.2 mg/100 ml by a number of methods including laser nephelometry, enzyme immunoassay, radial immunodiffusion, and radioimmunoassay. Latex agglutination, a test that has been the measurement standard in the past, is not adequately sensitive for the current clinical setting. CRP is more accurate than ESR in detection of infections after spinal surgery.[11, 12] Serial determinations of CRP may also be helpful in following the course of acute and chronic illnesses.[13] With greater availability and accuracy, CRP can be used more frequently in detecting inflammatory states in patients with low back pain.

Hematocrit

The hematocrit (Hct) is normal in patients with mechanical back pain, including those with herniated nucleus pulposus, spinal stenosis, and muscle strain. The presence of anemia suggests an inflammatory process of a systemic variety that involves diminished erythrocyte production or hastened RBC destruction. Rheumatologic disorders cause chronic inflammation and frequently cause "anemia of chronic disease," which is associated with inadequate production of red cells. Malignancies, particularly those of hematologic origin (multiple myeloma), characteristically cause anemia. Hematologic disorders, including hemoglobinopathies, and myelofibrosis are also associated with decreased Hct.

Most laboratories determine Hct indirectly. Coulter machines measure mean corpuscular volume (MCV) and hemoglobin concentration (Hgb) and derive the Hct from these measurements. Changes in the MCV may have a significant effect on the Hct value. On serial determinations Hct may vary widely, and the variation may be disconcerting to the physician. In these circumstances, following the measured Hgb concentration is helpful. A drop in Hgb signifies a true change in the number of erythrocytes and requires further investigation.

Not all decreases in Hct are related to primary disorders of the lumbosacral spine. Many patients will ingest nonsteroidal anti-inflammatory drugs (NSAIDs) for back pain. Many of these preparations are sold "over the counter" and contain aspirin. Patients may not mention these drugs to the physician, thinking that the medications are unimportant since they are nonprescription. However, these medications, as well as other NSAIDs, irritate the gastric mucosa, causing bleeding. In some patients, the amount of NSAID-associated bleeding is appreciable, causing a drop in the Hct. Therefore, a falling Hct may be more closely associated with therapy than the lesion causing the pain. Decreased Hct should be evaluated with red blood cell indices, reticulocyte count, serum iron, total iron binding capacity, haptoglobin, and examination of the stool for occult blood.

In addition to the determination of Hct, levels of iron and transferrin saturation may be helpful in determining the cause of anemia. Low serum ferritin and low transferrin saturation suggest iron deficiency anemia. Elevated levels of ferritin above 400 μg/L and transferrin saturation of more than 55% are suggestive of hemochromatosis.[14] This determination may be useful in the patient with low back pain and chondrocalcinosis.

White Blood Cell Count and Differential

The white blood cell count (WBC) is normal in mechanical low back pain as well as in many forms of medical low back pain. An elevated WBC (leukocytosis) suggests the presence of an infection, particularly if early forms of polymorphonuclear leukocytes (bands) are present. Increased numbers of white blood cells are also seen in malignancies, particularly those of bone marrow or lymphatic origin. Elevations of WBC occur less commonly in the spondyloarthropathies.

Drugs may alter the number and distribution of white blood cells in the differential. Corticosteroids loosen the white cells that line blood vessels (marginated pool). The pool is predominantly polymorphonuclear leukocytes. Corticosteroids are also lympholytic. Patients on corticosteroids have increased WBC in the 12,000 to 20,000 range (depending on the dose of medication). Polymorphonuclear leukocytes are present in greater number than lymphocytes in the WBC differential in the presence of corticosteroids. A rare toxic effect of some of the drugs used in the treatment of low back pain (e.g., phenylbutazone) is agranulocytosis or aplastic anemia. A WBC obtained before the institution of therapy helps determine the patient's "normal" WBC. A drop in WBC after the institution of therapy requires close monitoring and may necessitate discontinuing the patient's drug regimen.

Platelets

Platelets are normal in mechanical low back pain and most medical causes. In malignancies, platelets are commonly abnormal and may be elevated (thrombocytosis).[15] Platelets are frequently decreased (thrombocytopenia) in bone marrow and lymphatic tumors. Platelet counts may also be modified by drug therapy. A complete blood count (CBC) obtained at the initiation of drug therapy will establish the patient's usual platelet count.

Blood Chemistry Tests

Blood chemistry is usually evaluated with a battery of 12 or more tests (SMA 12). There is nothing especially mystical about the selection of tests included in the chemistry profile other than the fact that they are frequently ordered and the process for their measurement is automated. Although the groupings of tests seem haphazard, combinations of tests help identify abnormalities associated with dysfunction in specific organ systems.[16] Disorders may be associated with specific tests as follows: *renal*—blood urea nitrogen, uric acid, creatinine, glucose; *hepatic*—total bilirubin, alkaline phosphatase, lactic dehydrogenase, serum glutamic oxaloacetic transaminase (SGOT) or aspartate aminotransferase (AST); *parathyroid*—calcium, phosphorus; *bone*—calcium; *tumor*—total protein, albumin, lactic dehydrogenase; and *hematologic*—lactic dehydrogenase, total protein.

Serum Calcium and Phosphorus

An increase in serum calcium and decrease in serum phosphorus reflect activity of parathormone on bone and kidney. Patients with primary hyperparathyroidism have this altered relationship of calcium to phosphorus. Malignancies are associated with hypercalcemia. Malignancies with elevated serum calcium include those with parathormone activity (oat cell carcinoma of the lung), bone metastases, or multiple myeloma.

Metabolic bone disease may be associated with altered serum calcium and phosphorus concentrations. Osteomalacia (diminished vitamin D effect on bone) results in decreased serum calcium and a spectrum of changes in phosphorus levels. Phosphorus levels may be elevated in renal disease and acromegaly or diminished as occurs in hereditary disorders, including familial vitamin D–resistant rickets with hypophosphatemia. Osteoporosis is not associated with any alterations of serum calcium or phosphorus concentrations. Calcium and phosphorus are also unaltered in osteoarthritis and mechanical causes of low back pain.

Serum Alkaline Phosphatase

Alkaline phosphatase (ALP) is produced to the greatest degree by osteoblasts. Any condition that increases osteoblastic activity will increase ALP.[17] Disorders associated with ALP elevations include Paget's disease, metastatic carcinoma, hyperparathyroidism, osteomalacia, and fractures during healing phase. Of the illnesses that cause low back pain, metastatic tumors and Paget's disease cause the greatest increases (2 to 30 times normal). Up to 86% of patients with metastatic prostate carcinoma and 77% with metastatic breast cancer to bone have ALP elevations.[18] Not all bone tumors cause ALP elevations. Multiple myeloma, which causes little osteoblastic activity, is associated with increased ALP activity in fewer than 20% of patients. The ALP abnormalities in these myeloma patients may reflect healing bone fractures and may persist for several weeks.

The increase in ALP associated with Paget's disease is proportional to the activity of osteoblasts, which are activated by increased osteoclastic resorption of bone. The degree of enzyme elevation is proportional to the extent of skeletal involvement. ALP increases over time in patients who are untreated. A rapid and marked elevation of enzyme activity occurs in some patients who develop sarcomatous degeneration of a Paget's lesion.

Metabolic bone disease, particularly osteomalacia, is associated with abnormal ALP. Osteomalacia is associated with increased enzyme levels with accompanying low normal or decreased serum calcium concentration. Hyperparathyroidism is associated with increased ALP if the disease has caused bone disease. Radiographic changes of hyperparathyroidism may be present in the hands before serum elevations of ALP.[19]

Decreased levels of ALP are associated with an inherited deficiency of the enzyme (hypophosphatasia). The disease clinically resembles osteomalacia.

Not all elevations of ALP are associated with bone disease. Disease of the hepatobiliary system may be associated with marked increases of ALP activity. This is particularly evident in patients with obstructive lesions of the biliary system who may have concomitant abnormalities in other serum parameters of liver damage (gamma glutamyl transpeptidase [gamma GT], serum glutamic oxaloacetic transaminase [SGOT] or aspartate aminotransferase [AST], serum glutamic pyruvic transaminase [SGPT] or alanine aminotransferase [ALT], bilirubin, and cholesterol). Women who frequently have back pain during the course of a pregnancy may develop increased ALP levels of placental origin during the second and third trimesters. Diseases of the intestinal mucosa, such as peptic ulcer or ulcerative colitis, may also cause enzyme elevations.

Serum Uric Acid

Uric acid determination is normal in the vast majority of patients with low back pain. Serum uric acid may be elevated in patients with sacroiliac gout. These patients usually have extensive gouty disease in peripheral joints. The diagnosis of gout is documented by the demonstration of sodium urate crystals in synovial fluid or from a tophus. Hyperuricemia alone is insufficient evidence for a diagnosis of gout. Increased uric acid concentrations are also associated with any process that causes rapid cell turnover. Lactate dehydrogenase may also be increased in these circumstances. These disease states include myeloproliferative and lymphoproliferative disorders, psoriasis, hypothyroidism, hyperparathyroidism, and Paget's disease. Chronic renal failure as well as a variety of drugs, including thiazide diuretics, furosemide, low-dose salicylate, phenothiazines, phenylbutazone, and corticosteroids, can cause hyperuricemia.

Serum Glucose

The serum glucose determination obtained on a chemical profile has significance only if obtained with the patient in a fasting state. Elevations of glucose in the fasting state require formal testing of glucose metabolism, including a 2-hour glucose tolerance test. A number of drugs may either increase or decrease serum glucose concentrations. The drug history of the patient may help clarify abnormalities of glucose concentration observed with screening chemical evaluations.

Total Protein and Serum Albumin

Total protein and serum albumin concentrations are determined in most screening chemistry profile tests. In most patients with back pain, these tests are normal. However, in patients with chronic, systemic inflammatory diseases, the total protein concentrations may be altered. With chronic inflammation or infection (subacute bacterial endocarditis), the total globulins or the total protein may be increased. Marked increase in total protein associated with elevated globulin levels should raise the possibility of multiple myeloma.

Patients with increased total protein should be evaluated with a serum protein electrophoresis. An increase in gamma globulins requires a serum immunoelectrophoresis test. An increase in globulins requires serum immunoelectrophoresis to characterize the increased protein component. Increased monoclonal immunoglobulins may occur with benign (monoclonal gammopathies) or malignant (multiple myeloma) disorders. A diffuse elevation of gamma globulins (polyclonal increase) suggests the presence of a chronic inflammatory process.

Blood Urea Nitrogen and Serum Creatinine

Elevations in blood urea nitrogen and serum creatinine are associated with decreased renal function. Patients with visceral back pain of genitourinary origin may have elevations of these parameters. Additional evaluations, in the form of 24-hour urine collection for creatinine clearance and radiographic or sonographic examination, are helpful in defining the parenchymal or obstructive origin of the renal impairment. The drug history is important in a patient with abnormalities of blood urea nitrogen and creatinine. A number of drugs, including corticosteroids and nonsteroidal anti-inflammatory agents, may cause elevations of these tests.[20, 21]

Serum Acid Phosphatase

Acid phosphatase (ACP) has a role similar to that of ALP but is active at a lower pH. ACP is most closely associated with acinar cells of the prostate gland and prostatic metastases to bones. However, ACP is not produced solely in the prostate gland. The nonprostatic portion of ACP is present in bone, platelets, erythrocytes, and spleen. In a man over 50 years of age, an elevation of prostatic ACP is strong evidence of metastatic prostatic carcinoma. Nonprostatic ACP is elevated in a wide variety of diseases affecting bone, including Paget's disease, hyperparathyroidism, multiple myeloma, and primary bone tumors.[17] Gaucher's disease is also associated with elevations of nonprostatic ACP.

Serum Prostate-Specific Antigen

Prostate-specific antigen (PSA) is a serine protease produced only by prostatic epithelial cells.[22] Both normal and malignant prostate cells produce PSA. Benign prostatic hyperplasia (BPH) may increase serum PSA moderately while prostate cancer elevates levels markedly. There is considerable overlap between BPH and prostate cancer confined to the prostate gland.[23] However, the specificity of PSA for prostate cancer is 92% when PSA is more than 10.0 ng/ml.[24] Levels between 4.1 and 10.0 ng/ml are difficult to interpret. PSA is a more effective serum marker of prostate cancer than serum acid phosphatase.[25]

Another important concept concerning the use of PSA is the rate of change of serum concentration per year. When PSA increases 0.75 ng/ml/year, the specificity for prostate cancer is 90%.[26] The normalization of elevated PSA is being evaluated as a measure of successful outcome of therapy for prostate cancer.[27] However, PSA has remained elevated in a small percentage of patients who have no evidence of metastatic disease. Additional time will be necessary to determine if these individuals develop a recurrence of tumor, signifying the detection of PSA to be an accurate marker of occult tumor.

IMMUNOLOGIC TESTS

Histocompatibility Typing

The human leukocyte antigens (HLA) are present on all human nucleated cells.[28] HLA typing determines A, B, C, and D locus antigens. Specific haplotypes associated with the different loci are found in a wide variety of disorders. In regard to disorders of the lumbosacral spine, class I B antigens are most closely associated with the spondyloarthropathies. The histocompatibility antigen, HLA B27, is present in over 90% of patients with ankylosing spondylitis and 80% with Reiter's syndrome, compared with 8% of normal Caucasians and 4% of the normal black population. The HLA B27 test is performed in vitro using the patient's lymphocytes and antisera directed against specific HLA antigens. The presence of HLA B27 is not diagnostic for any specific spondyloarthropathy. In general, the overwhelming majority of patients with ankylosing spondylitis are more readily diagnosed on the basis of history, physical examination, and roentgenographic findings of sacroiliitis. HLA B27 is usually a superfluous test. The test is most helpful in the young patient who presents with back pain and equivocal sacroiliitis on radiographs. HLA B27 positivity in a patient with back pain and equivocal radiographs is additional evidence for the diagnosis of ankylosing spondylitis.

It is important to remember that between 4% and 8% of normal people in the United States are HLA-B27 positive. The presence of HLA B27 in a patient with noninflammatory back pain of bone or muscle origin is of no consequence.[29]

The HLA class II molecules are encoded in the HLA-D region. DR, DQ, and DP are the major subregions of the D region. HLA class II molecules are expressed on a limited number of cells in the immune system, such as B lymphocytes and macrophages. Class II molecules play a central role in antigen recognition and effective collaboration between immunocompetent cells for an efficient immune response.[30] Histocompatibility testing for class II molecules is primarily used for research purposes. Like class I antigens, class II antigens are not found exclusively in patients with specific illnesses. A proportion of normal individuals will have certain class II antigens.

Rheumatoid Factor

Rheumatoid factors (RF) are a group of autoantibodies to human IgG. RF may be of IgM, IgG, IgA, IgD, and IgE varieties. The classic RF is IgM antibody. RF occur in a wide spectrum of autoimmune and chronic infectious diseases. The disease most closely associated with RF is rheumatoid arthritis. Approximately 80% of patients with rheumatoid arthritis are seropositive for RF. The chance that the RF titer will be of importance in determining the cause of pain in a patient with lumbosacral spine dysfunction is very small. The rare patient with rheumatoid arthritis with back pain has such severe disease that the factor would have been obtained much earlier in the course of the disease.

The presence of RF activity may be important in the evaluation of a patient with back pain secondary to subacute bacterial endocarditis. Patients with chronic endocarditis develop RF after 6 weeks of infection in the setting of hypocomplementemia and immune complex deposition manifested by glomerulonephritis.[31] RF titers play a greater role in following the response to therapy than in diagnosing endocarditis. RF diminishes in titer as the patient's infection responds to antibiotic therapy.

RF, in low titer, may also be identified in an increasing proportion of normal individuals as they grow older. Over 40% of healthy individuals who are 75 years of age will have detectable RF.[32] Therefore, RF determinations add very little information to the evaluation of the patient with low back pain and should not be included in the laboratory examination of these individuals.

RF may appear as part of a "panel" of tests combined to facilitate more accurate diagnosis when screening patients with musculoskeletal complaints. The three tests most commonly offered are the RF, antinuclear antibody, and uric acid level. The predictive value of these tests is only 35% in individuals with joint disease and an estimated combined prevalence of the three illnesses of 10%.[33] Therefore, 66% of individuals with a positive test would not have one of these illnesses. The use of "panels" of tests in the evaluation of low back pain patients is not useful.

URINALYSIS

Abnormalities detected during a routine urinalysis are most helpful in identifying individuals with viscerogenic referred back pain of genitourinary origin. The presence of erythrocytes in urine suggests the presence of a significant lesion in either the upper or lower urinary tract. Erythrocytes may be related to a renal cell carcinoma, bladder carcinoma, nephrolithiasis, or chronic urinary tract infection. The presence of hematuria in a male necessitates a more thorough evaluation of the urinary tract. Hematuria in women may not be of as great significance owing to the presence of erythrocytes in urine during menstrual periods. However, the persistence of hematuria in a woman also requires further evaluation. Numerous white blood cells in the microscopic urine sediment may indicate infection of the kidney (pyelonephritis) or bladder (cystitis). Culture of a clean-catch urine specimen is helpful in documenting urinary tract infection. Proteinuria is also associated with infections, tumors, and inflammatory diseases of the glomerulus. The presence of proteinuria on a dipstick determination requires further evaluation. If the concentration of urinary protein is small, repeat urinalysis may detect no additional protein. If proteinuria persists, quantification of a 24-hour collection of urine is necessary. If multiple myeloma is suspected, a negative dipstick protein does not rule out the diagnosis since myeloma proteins are not detected by dipstick methods. The presence of myeloma proteins in urine is detected by adding sulfasalicylic acid to urine, a nonspecific test for protein that turns urine turbid, or immunoelectrophoresis of urine, which will identify the specific protein present in increased concentration.

In patients with metabolic bone disease, 24-hour urine collections may be helpful. Urine collection for calcium helps determine calcium excretion, degree of calcium absorption, and patient compliance with ingestion of calcium supplements. The value of the test result is only as good as the completeness of the collection. Partial collections are of no clinical value.

MISCELLANEOUS TESTS

Cerebrospinal fluid (CSF) is obtained from patients who undergo lumbar puncture. Abnormalities in CSF cells, protein, or pressure are noted in patients with infection, tumors, or other inflammatory lesions of the spinal cord or nerve roots. In most patients, diagnostic methods other than CSF, such as roentgenograms or CT scans, identify abnormalities of the low back with greater accuracy. Abnormalities identified with evaluation of CSF are rarely pathognomonic of a disease entity but rather confirm diagnoses suggested by other clinical and diagnostic test parameters.

Synovial fluid is rarely obtained from joints in the lumbosacral spine. On occasion, a patient with suspected septic arthritis of the sacroiliac joint may have an arthrocentesis. The amount of fluid obtained from the sacroiliac joint is usually small so that the usual tests completed for synovial fluid analysis, including cell counts and glucose determinations, cannot be done. The most important test is culture of fluid for organisms. Any remaining fluid may be sent for crystal analysis, cell count, and protein and glucose determinations.

BIOPSY SPECIMENS

In certain patients with low back pain, the diagnosis cannot be determined without histologic examination of tissue from the lumbosacral spine. Biopsy specimens are helpful in identifying benign and malignant tumors and for culture to confirm the presence of infection. Tissue biopsy is indicated after noninvasive tests have been completed if the cause of the patient's pain remains in doubt and examination of tissue is necessary to establish the diagnosis. Close cooperation is needed among the clinicians, radiologists, and surgeons in order to choose the appropriate site and method of biopsy. Some lesions are accessible to needle biopsy and do not require an operation. Other lesions, particularly those in the anterior portion of lumbar vertebrae, are inaccessible to the biopsy needle and require an open biopsy. Careful handling of the biopsy material is necessary so that the greatest amount of information is obtained from the invasive procedure.

SUMMARY

Laboratory test results should never replace a careful history and physical examination in the evaluation of the patient with low back pain. In the vast majority of circumstances the laboratory results help separate patients' disorders into categories (inflammatory vs. noninflammatory, bone vs. liver), but they rarely establish specific diagnoses. The clinician may place too much significance on laboratory findings, which results in inaccurate diagnoses. Laboratory tests are helpful when used appropriately. If their relative importance is kept in mind, the clinician will not be misled.

References

1. Wintrobe MM, Landsberg JW: A standardized technique for the blood sedimentation test. Am J Med Sci 189:102, 1935.
2. Pepys MB: Acute phase phenomena. In Cohen AS (ed): Rheumatology and Immunology. Orlando: Grune & Stratton, 1979, p 85.
3. International Committee for Standardization in Hematology: Recommendation for measurement of erythrocyte sedimentation rate of human blood. Am J Clin Pathol 68:505, 1977.
4. Hayes GS, Stinson IN: Erythrocyte sedimentation rate and age. Arch Ophthalmol 94:939, 1976.
5. Zacharski LR, Kyle RA: Significance of extreme elevation of erythrocyte sedimentation rate. JAMA 202:264, 1967.
6. Waddell G: An approach to backache. Br J Hosp Med 28:187, 1982.
7. Ballou SP, Kushner I: Laboratory evaluation of inflammation. In Kelley WN, Harris ED Jr, Ruddy S, Sledge

CB (eds): Textbook of Rheumatology, 4th ed. Philadelphia: WB Saunders Co, 1993, pp 671–679.

8. Sox HC Jr, Liang MH: The erythrocyte sedimentation rate. Guidelines for rational use. Ann Intern Med 104:515, 1986.

9. Malkiewitz A, Kushner I: Biochemical markers of inflammation in spondylitis. Spine State Art Rev 3:553, 1991.

10. Tillet WS, Francis T Jr: Serological reactions in pneumonia with a non-protein somatic fraction of pneumococcus. J Exp Med 52:561, 1930.

11. Thelander U, Larsson S: Quantitation of C-reactive protein levels and erythocyte sedimentation rate after spinal surgery. Spine 17:400, 1992.

12. Mustard RA Jr, Bohnen JMA, Haseeb S, Kasina R: C-reactive protein levels predict postoperative septic complications. Arch Surg 122:69, 1987.

13. Okamura JM, Miyagi JM, Terada K, Hokama Y: Potential clinical applications of C-reactive protein. J Clin Lab Anal 4:231, 1990.

14. Edwards CQ, Kushner JP: Screening for hemochromatosis. N Engl J Med 328:1616, 1993.

15. Levin H, Conley CL: Thrombocytosis associated with malignant disease. Arch Intern Med 114:497, 1964.

16. Ward PCJ: Chemical profiles of disease. Orthop Clin North Am 10:405, 1979.

17. Van Lente F: Alkaline and acid phosphatase determinations in bone disease. Orthop Clin North Am 10:437, 1979.

18. Schwartz MK: Enzymes in cancer. Clin Chem 19:10, 1973.

19. Goldsmith RS: Laboratory aids in the diagnosis of metabolic bone disease. Orthop Clin North Am 3:545, 1972.

20. Galen RS: The effects of drugs on laboratory tests. Orthop Clin North Am 10:465, 1979.

21. Clive DM, Stoff JS: Renal syndromes associated with nonsteroidal antiinflammatory drugs. N Engl J Med 310:563, 1984.

22. Cupp MR, Oesterling JE: Prostate-specific antigen, digital rectal examination, and transrectal ultrasonography: their roles in diagnosing early prostate cancer. Mayo Clin Proc 68:297, 1993.

23. Partin AW, Carter HB, Chan DW, et al.: Prostate specific antigen in the staging of localized prostate cancer: influence of tumor differentiation, tumor volume and benign hyperplasia. J Urol 143:747, 1990.

24. Catalona WJ, Smith DS, Ratliff TL, et al.: Measurement of prostate-specific antigen in serum as a screening test for prostate cancer. N Engl J Med 324:1156, 1991.

25. Cooke RR, Nacey JN, Beeston RE, Delahunt B: The efficacy of serum prostate specific antigen as a tumor marker in prostatic carcinoma: a comparison with serum acid phosphatase. N Z Med J 105:345, 1992.

26. Carter HB, Pearson JD, Metter EJ, et al.: Longitudinal evaluation of prostate-specific antigen levels in men with and without prostate disease. JAMA 267:2215, 1992.

27. Frazier HA, Robertson JE, Humphrey PA, Paulson DF: Is prostate specific antigen of clinical importance in evaluating outcome after radical prostatectomy? J Urol 149:516, 1993.

28. Brenner MB, Glass DN: HLA polymorphisms and rheumatic disease. In Cohen AS (ed): Laboratory Diagnostic Procedures in the Rheumatic Diseases. 3rd ed. Orlando: Grune & Stratton, 1985, pp 249–271.

29. Kahn MA, Khan MI: Diagnostic value of HLA-B27 testing in ankylosing spondylitis and Reiter's syndrome. Ann Intern Med 90:70, 1982.

30. Strominger JL: Biology of the human histocompatibility leukocyte antigen (HLA) system and a hypothesis regarding the generation of autoimmune disease. J Clin Invest 77:1411, 1986.

31. Williams RC Jr, Kunkel HG: Rheumatoid factor, complement, and conglutinin aberrations in patients with subacute bacterial endocarditis. J Clin Invest 41:666, 1962.

32. Heimer R, Levin FM, Rudd E: Globulins resembling rheumatoid factor in serum of the aged. Am J Med 35:175, 1963.

33. Lichtenstein MJ, Pincus T: How useful are combinations of blood tests in "rheumatic panels" in diagnosis of rheumatic diseases? J Gen Intern Med 3:435, 1988.

Radiographic Evaluation

7

The evaluation of patients with low back pain frequently includes the use of radiographic techniques to visualize the structures of the lumbosacral spine. When obtained at the appropriate time in the diagnostic evaluation, and when interpreted correctly in the setting of the patient's clinical history and physical examination, the radiographic images of the spine are extremely helpful in confirming the possible location and source of a patient's back pain (vertebral fracture, tumor). On the other hand, radiographic images that are obtained too soon in the diagnostic process or are interpreted incorrectly may delay the determination of the true diagnosis. For example, the presence of degenerative disc disease on a roentgenograph may dissuade the clinician from fully evaluating a patient with new-onset back pain. The physician may ascribe the patient's pain to radiographic changes found in the lumbar spine associated with degenerative disc disease. The patient may not respond to therapy and pain may persist. Does the physician continue therapy or take another roentgenogram? The patient may not like being exposed to additional radiation and may be resistant to re-evaluation. Only the persistence of pain persuades the patient to undergo radiographic evaluation again at a later date. At this time, the process (infection, tumor, joint inflammation) has destroyed enough bone for its presence to be detected with a plain roentgenogram. In this scenario, a roentgenogram taken in a time period between the initial and subsequent examination may have detected the lesion at an earlier stage of development.

The underlying fact that complicates the relationship of back pain, particularly of a mechanical nature, and radiographic findings is the progressive anatomic change that occurs naturally in the lumbosacral spine over time that is unassociated with pain. By age 50, up to 95% of adults who come to autopsy show evidence of aging changes in the lumbosacral spine with disc space narrowing, calcification, or marginal sclerosis (lumbar spondylosis).[1] Roentgenograms taken of living patients of a similar age demonstrate degenerative changes in 87%. The prevalence of roentgenographic changes increases with age. Only 5% or less of people under 20 years of age have spondylosis. In a comparison of 238 patients with back pain with 66 patients without pain, there was no difference between the two groups in regard to the prevalence of spondylosis and disc degeneration.[2] Another study has demonstrated increased prevalence of roentgenographic findings of disc degeneration in individuals who are involved in heavy labor.[3] Although an anatomic change is present and is identifiable, it is not necessarily the cause of the patient's pain.

On the other hand, radiographic evaluation of the lumbosacral spine may be very helpful at detecting specific abnormalities (lytic or blastic bone lesions, spinal cord tumors) that may be directly related to a patient's clinical symptoms and signs. Radiographic techniques are able to identify anatomic abnormalities associated with local destructive processes or systemic inflammatory illnesses that affect the skeletal system in general. The closest correlation between anatomic changes discovered with radiographic techniques and clinical symptoms occurs with medical diseases of the lumbar spine. The physician must not make the mistake of assuming the same very close correlation between anatomy and symptoms for mechanical lesions of the lumbar spine.

Most neurodiagnostic imaging studies have a high sensitivity (the ability to detect anatomic abnormalities) but a low specificity (the ability to remain negative in the absence of clinical disease). The poor correlation between anatomic changes and clinical symptoms has been associated with computerized tomography (CT) scan of the lumbosacral spine.[4] A study designed with neuroradiologists reading CT scans blinded to patients' symptoms reported a prevalence of 19% of patients under 40 years of age with a herniated nucleus pulposus. Diagnoses of canal stenosis and facet degeneration were reported in 50% of patients over 40 years of age. Despite the scan "abnormalities," both groups of patients were asymptomatic without neurologic signs except for 6 of the 52 studied patients with surgically proven spine disease. In essence, the CT scan of the lumbosacral spine detects anatomic changes that are unassociated with symptoms in a significant proportion of patients.

Magnetic resonance (MR) is another technique that visualizes soft tissues in and around the spinal column. MR scan has been reported to detect herniated discs, epidural scar tissue, and spinal cord tumors.[5] The sensitivity of MR is equal to or greater than that of myelography. As with the CT scan, MR may identify structural abnormalities of the lumbosacral spine that are unassociated with clinical symptoms.

This introduction is presented with the hope that physicians who evaluate patients with back pain will temper their enthusiasm for radiographic evaluation as an easy way to diagnose the cause of the pain. Radiographic studies of the lumbosacral spine play an important role in the evaluation of back pain but the limitations of the techniques must be remembered. Imaging studies should never be used as a screening test but rather to confirm the anatomic localization and extent of spinal disease as suspected from a careful history and physical examination. The presence of degenerative disease in the lumbar spine may or may not be the cause of the patient's symptoms. Radiographic changes associated with systemic illnesses have greater diagnostic importance.

PLAIN ROENTGENOGRAMS OF THE LUMBOSACRAL SPINE

Plain roentgenograms remain the initial step in radiographic diagnosis of the lumbosacral spine because of their availability, speed, relatively low exposure of tissue to radiation,

and reasonable cost. Conventional radiographs offer good spatial and contrast resolution of bony structures but are unable to image soft tissue structures clearly. In general, three roentgenographic views are all that are required to assess the lumbosacral spine. An anteroposterior (AP) view, a large port lateral view, and a small port lateral view to better visualize the lower two interspaces are needed. Two oblique views are also frequently taken because they occasionally help identify subtle spondylolysis. However, oblique views provide limited information and should not be routinely included.

The normal roentgenographic anatomy of the lumbar spine in the AP projection is shown in Figure 7–1. In this projection, the spinous and transverse processes, the pedicles, the facet joints, and the laminae are seen. The spinous processes are aligned in the middle of the vertebral bodies. The five lumbar processes should be counted. Rotation or lateral movement of the lumbar spine will appear as a deviation in the alignment of the spinous proc-

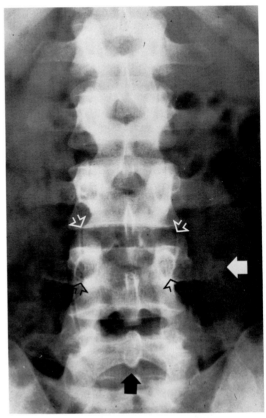

Figure 7–1. Anteroposterior view of a normal lumbar spine showing spinous process *(black arrow)*, transverse process *(white arrow)*, facet joints *(white open arrow)*, and pedicles *(black open arrow)*. (Courtesy of Anne Brower, M.D.)

esses.[6] The transverse processes project laterally from the middle of each vertebral body in a symmetric fashion. Lytic or sclerotic lesions of the transverse processes are identified preferentially in the AP projection. The pedicles are perpendicular to the vertebral body and are projected end-on in the AP view. They appear as a dense cortical rim of bone in the superior and lateral portions of the vertebral bodies. The loss of a pedicle ("winking-owl" sign) is frequently seen in patients with metastatic disease to the spine. A short interpediculate distance may be associated with constriction of neural elements, while widening of the distance at a single level may indicate an expanding intraspinal lesion. The facet joints run in a vertical orientation and are located close to the pedicles. Sclerosis may be seen surrounding facet joints but may be difficult to see in the AP projection. The primary soft tissue structure seen in the AP projection is the psoas muscle. The psoas forms a triangular shape with the top at the transverse process of L1 and the base on the iliac crests. Asymmetric visualization of the psoas muscle indicates clinical pathology in a minority of patients since positioning, muscle contraction, and spine rotation may affect the definition of the muscle border.

The lateral roentgenographic views visualize the lumbar and sacral spine and the L4-S1 area in a separate view. The normal roentgenographic anatomy of the lumbosacral spine is seen in Figure 7–2. In this projection, the bodies of the vertebrae, the pedicles, the spinous processes, and the intervertebral disc spaces are seen. The normal lumbar lordosis is observed with the posterior borders of the vertebral bodies lining up to form a smooth curve. Movement of a vertebral body in a horizontal plane in a forward or backward direction will be noted as a disruption of the curve and may be indicative of spinal instability. The slight concavity of the posterior surface of the vertebral bodies is noted. The disc spaces increase in size from L1 to L4. The L5-S1 disc space and intervertebral foramina are narrower than the spaces between the other lumbar vertebrae. The lumbar intervertebral foramina are best visualized in the lateral projection. Overlying shadows obscure posterior elements of the vertebral bodies. Soft tissues anterior to the spine may not be visualized well. However, examination of the area may discover calcification of structures, particularly of the aorta, which may have clinical significance.

The close-up view of the L5-S1 area provides information about the status of the interverte-

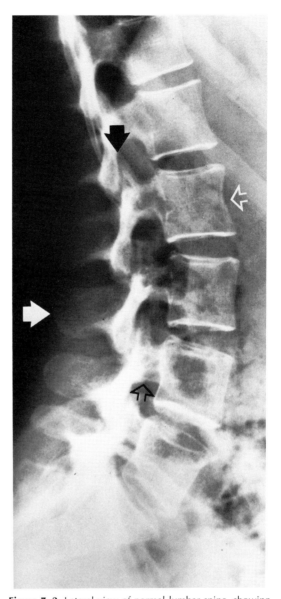

Figure 7–2. Lateral view of normal lumbar spine, showing spinous process *(white arrow)*, facet joint *(black arrow)*, laminae *(black open arrow)*, and vertebral body *(white open arrow)*. (Courtesy of Anne Brower, M.D.)

bral disc spaces and bone in the upper portion of the sacrum. An example is found in Figure 7–3.

The oblique projection is obtained to demonstrate the facet joints and pars interarticularis. In this view (Fig. 7–4), the posterior elements outline a shape that is reminiscent of a "Scotty dog." The nose is the transverse process, the eye the pedicle, the ear the superior articular process, the neck the pars interarticularis, the front legs the inferior articular process, and the body the laminae. A collar on the

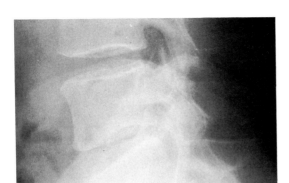

Figure 7–3. Coned-down view of a normal lumbosacral junction. The intervertebral disc between L5 and S1 may appear narrow compared with the other lumbar intervertebral discs.

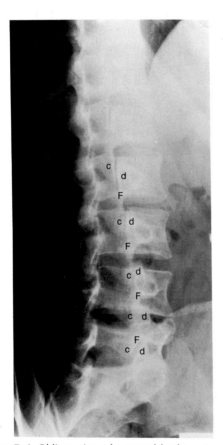

Figure 7–4. Oblique view of a normal lumbar spine. The inferior facet (c), the superior facets (d), and the pars interarticularis (F) are visualized on this view. (From Wiesel SW, Bernini P, Rothman RH: The Aging Lumbar Spine. Philadelphia, WB Saunders Co, 1982.)

"dog" suggests the presence of spondylolysis. Other specialized views of the lumbosacral spine may be obtained. These include flexion (Fig. 7–5), extension (Fig. 7–6), and Ferguson (Fig. 7–7) views of the pelvis. These views are not obtained on a routine basis but are reserved for patients with specific symptoms and signs. The chapters describing certain disease entities include information about those special roentgenographic evaluations that are helpful in making specific diagnoses.

Plain roentgenograms are easy to obtain, available to most physicians, and inexpensive compared with other radiographic techniques. The radiation exposure, cost, and applicability for the diagnosis of specific disease entities are listed in Table 7–1. The plain films are useful for surveying all levels of the lumbosacral spine and associated paraspinous soft tissues. These examinations, however, do not visualize the contents of the spinal canal, including the spinal cord, dural structures, or spinal ligaments. Plain films may not be sensitive enough to identify bony lesions unless 50% of the medullary portion of the bone has been destroyed.[6]

Usually plain roentgenograms of the lumbosacral spine will not add any information to the evaluation of many patients with mechanical low back pain but must be obtained if there is a suspicion of other pathology such as infec-

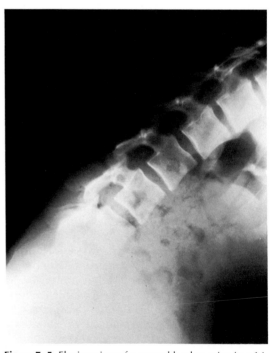

Figure 7–5. Flexion view of a normal lumbar spine in a 14-year-old female.

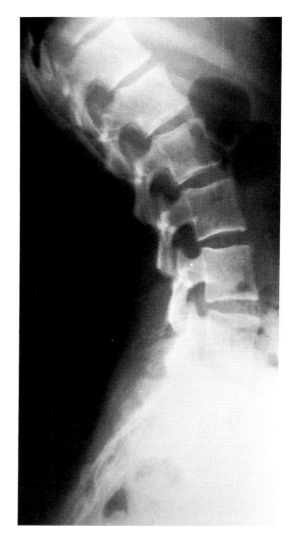

Figure 7–6. Extension view of a normal lumbar spine in a 14-year-old female.

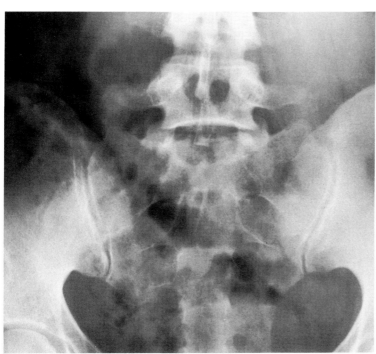

Figure 7–7. Ferguson view of normal sacroiliac joints in a 32-year-old female.

113

TABLE 7–1. RADIOGRAPHIC STUDIES AND DISEASE CATEGORIES
OF THE LUMBOSACRAL SPINE

RADIOGRAPHS	HERNIATED NUCLEUS PULPOSUS	SPINAL STENOSIS (OSTEO-ARTHRITIS)	SPONDYLO-LISTHESIS	SPONDYLOAR-THROPATHY	INFECTION
Plain Radiation 2.6 rads Cost: $180		1	1 (Motion)	1 (Sacroiliitis)	1
Tomogram Radiation: 5 rads Cost: $245					
Bone Scan Radiation: 0.15 rads Cost: $595				2	2*
Computed Tomography Radition: 3–5 rads Cost: $800	2	3	2	3	
Magnetic Resonance Radiation: None Cost: $1300	1†	2			3
Myelogram Radiation: 6–7 rads Cost: $1200	3†	4			
Discography Radiation: 2 rads (variable) Cost: $617	+/− (Disc degeneration)				
Epidural Venography Radiation: 2 rads Cost: $537	+/− (L5 lateral disc)				
Ultrasonography Radiation: None Cost: $383					
(Normal Background) Radiation: 0.6 rads/year					

*Best method.
†Costs include mean technical and professional fees.

tion, tumor, hip arthritis, or urologic disease. Therefore, not everyone with acute low back pain requires a set of plain roentgenograms. If one is comfortable with diagnosis of an acute low back strain in a young patient (up to 50 years of age), treatment may proceed without radiographic evaluation for the first 4 to 6 weeks after the onset of pain.[7] Roentgenograms are indicated if there is no response to the treatment. On the other hand, roentgenograms are indicated on the first visit if the patient is older (over 50 years of age) or there is additional medical information that requires investigation. Roentgenograms are too often misread, or more specifically, "overread." Normal asymptomatic people approaching 50 years of age will frequently have disc narrowing. As previously described, the intervertebral disc has an 88% water content. It contains a gelatinous nucleus pulposus confined under great pressure between two cartilaginous end-plates and by an elastic annulus fibrosus. The disc inevitably dehydrates with age. Numerous microscopic injuries occur with everyday wear and tear, which permits a certain amount of leakage of nuclear material from the central portion of the disc. As this occurs insidiously and gradually, the process evolves without symptomatology or impairment. Consequently, as the years pass, the disc spaces will narrow from repeated microtrauma and usually will remain symptom free. Thus the narrowing of a disc space on roentgenogram per se is not necessarily the etiology of the patient's complaint.

RADIONUCLIDE IMAGING (BONE SCAN)

Radionuclide imaging addresses function and tissue metabolism of organs by delivering

**TABLE 7–1. RADIOGRAPHIC STUDIES AND DISEASE CATEGORIES
OF THE LUMBOSACRAL SPINE (Continued)**

RADIOGRAPHS	TUMOR	ENDOCRINOLOGIC DISORDER	HEMATO- LOGIC DISORDER	TRAUMA	OTHER
Plain Radiation 2.6 rads Cost: $180	1	1 (Osteoporosis))	1	1	1
Tomogram Radiation: 5 rads Cost: $245					5 (Post-op fusion mass)
Bone Scan Radiation: 0.15 rads Cost: $595	2* (Metastatic)	2 (Osteomalacia)	2 (Hemoglobin- opathy)	3	4
Computed Tomography Radition: 3–5 rads Cost: $800	4 (Myeloma)	3 (Mineral quantification)		2* (Intraspinal)	3* (Retroperitoneum)
Magnetic Resonance Radiation: None Cost: $1300	3* (Intraspinal)				
Myelogram Radiation: 6–7 rads Cost: $1200	5* (Cord compression)				
Discography Radiation: 2 rads (variable) Cost: $617					
Epidural Venography Radiation: 2 rads Cost: $537					
Ultrasonography Radiation: None Cost: $383					2 (Aneurysm)
(Normal Background) Radiation: 0.6 rads/year					

Numbers include sequence of radiographic studies used for diagnosis.

to target structures a very small dose of radio-isotope material. This tracer emits radiation in proportion to its attachment to the target structure. These studies are noninvasive and associated with low risk but are relatively expensive.

Radionuclide imaging is a very good technique for the detection of bone abnormalities. Bone is living tissue containing osteoblasts and osteoclasts. In normal situations the activity of these cells is balanced. Any process that disturbs the normal balance of bone production and resorption can produce an abnormality on bone scan. Increased osteoblastic activity is associated with greater concentration of radionuclide tracer on the bone scan. Interruption of blood flow to the bone will result in an absence (cold spot) of tracer on the scan. Interruption of metabolic activity will also result in decreased activity on bone scan.

In addition to blood flow to bone, a number of other factors affect the distribution of radionuclide in the normal adult skeleton. Bone turnover is an important factor. In children the epiphyseal and metaphyseal growth plates are sites of active bone turnover and areas of increased radionuclide concentration. In adults, metaphyses of tubular bones may show more activity than diaphyses. Other factors, including the surface absorption to bone, diffusion of tracer within bone tissue, and ion exchange between ionic tracers and the ions within bone also play a role.

The most commonly used radiopharmaceutical for bone scanning is technetium-99m (^{99m}Tc). This radiopharmaceutical is ideal for bone scan since it has a half-life of 6 hours, emits gamma rays, but has low radiation exposure of approximately 150 millirads.[8] The ^{99m}Tc compounds used for bone imaging are phosphates (inorganic compounds) or phosphonates (organic compounds). The phosphates have a greater propensity for protein binding, while diphosphonates are chemically more stable.[9] Examples of these compounds are methylene diphosphate (MDP) or ethylene hydroxydiphosphonate (EHDP). Pertechnetate may also be attached to technetium and may be used for radionuclide angiographic studies of bone. ^{99m}Tc pertechnetate binds primarily to serum albumin and will be taken up rapidly by organs with increased blood flow.[10] Bone scan images must be taken within 5 to 15 minutes after injection of pertechnetate to allow this effect to be seen.

Gallium-67 (^{67}Ga) citrate is another radionuclide that is occasionally utilized in the evaluation of patients with low back pain. ^{67}Ga binds to human polymorphonuclear leukocytes. Those pathologic processes associated with localization of polymorphonuclear cells are associated with the accumulation of gallium. Therefore, ^{67}Ga scanning has been used to complement ^{99}Tc studies, particularly in the evaluation of vertebral osteomyelitis and sacroiliac septic arthritis.[11, 12]

Bone scan images are obtained with scintillation cameras that detect the production of

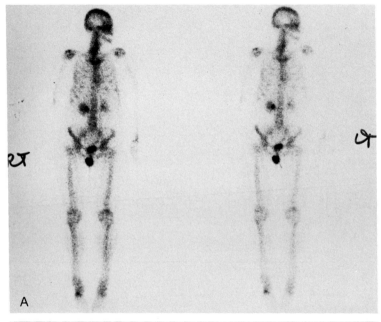

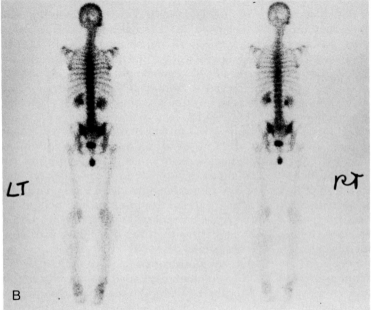

Figure 7–8. Normal bone scan using ^{99m}Tc MDP. *A,* Anterior view—early image *(right),* late image *(left). B,* Posterior view—early image *(right),* late image *(left).*

gamma rays from different locations in the body. A large field-of-view camera surveys the entire skeleton, while close-up spot views are reserved for regions of clinical concern or suspicious areas seen on the total body image. For example, lesions that involve the pelvis may be obscured by activity in the bladder, since 50% of radionuclide activity is lost in the urine. Lateral views of the pelvis may allow visualization of posterior structures unaffected by activity in the bladder.

Bone scan images can be taken at different times after the injection of radionuclide. An immediate blood pool image is obtained by sequential images, 3 to 5 seconds apart. Images are then obtained 2 to 4 hours after injection. Occasionally a delayed scan at 24 hours is obtained to detect residual increased bone activity.

The normal bone scan image mirrors the response of normal bone to mechanical pressure, the thickness of bone, and excretion of 50% of the radionuclide in the kidney and bladder (Fig. 7–8). On the anterior view, normal concentrations of radionuclide are present over the calvarium, facial bones, sternum, humeral heads and acromioclavicular joints, pelvis (particularly iliac wings), bladder, and, to a lesser degree, the knees and ankles. On the posterior view, the calvarium, axial spine, kidneys, and sacroiliac joints are prominent. Bone scans of reduced quality may occur secondary to dehydration, marked obesity, therapeutic agents (corticosteroids), increased age (patients over 30 years of age have progressively diminished uptake), or defective radionuclide preparations.[13]

In the clinical situation, radionuclide imaging is a useful technique to screen the entire skeletal system for abnormal activity. Bone scan is particularly useful in circumstances of roentgenographic changes lagging behind increased bone activity. Bone scan has been utilized most commonly for detection of metastatic disease (Fig. 7–9). Approximately 80% of metastatic lesions are found in the axial skeleton.[14] Between 10% and 40% of patients with metastatic disease with normal radiographs will have abnormalities on bone scan including areas that are painless.[15] One notable exception to early detection by bone scan is multiple myeloma. The neoplastic plasma cells do not induce an osteoblastic response by bone. Therefore the lytic lesions of myeloma will not cause increased activity on bone scan until a fracture occurs.[16]

A lack of correlation between radiographic findings and bone scan activity also occurs in

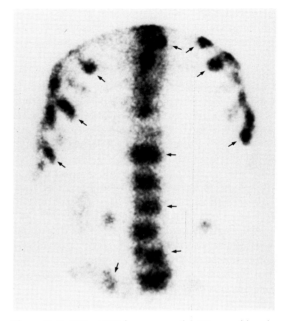

Figure 7–9. ^{99m}Tc MDP bone scan of a 70-year-old male with metastatic prostatic carcinoma. Increased uptake is noted in the ribs, vertebral column, and pelvis *(black arrows).*

osteomyelitis. Radiographs may not be positive for 10 to 14 days after the onset of the disease, whereas bone scan may be abnormal within 1 day.[17]

Radionuclide bone imaging is also useful to detect the early stages of septic arthritis. The bone scan images demonstrate increased activity on the blood flow and delayed static scans before radiographs show changes of infection other than capsular distention.

Trauma to bone, particularly stress fractures, may be difficult to detect by conventional radiography. Bone scintigraphy can detect lesions within 3 days of fracture. Activity of the fracture site may remain increased for an extended period of time but with a diminished level of intensity on scan. The older the fracture, the milder the increase in uptake. This fact may be useful in determining the age of compression fractures of the spine.[18]

The generalized bone disease associated with metabolic abnormalities is associated with diffuse increased uptake on bone scan. Bone scan is more sensitive than radiography in the detection of primary hyperparathyroidism, renal osteodystrophy, and osteomalacia. Osteoporosis is associated with normal scans unless compression fractures occur.[19]

Arthritis may be detected by bone scan. Noninflammatory joint disease (osteoarthritis) is associated with osteoblastic activity in the form of sclerosis and osteophyte formation. Inflammatory arthropathies are associated with increased blood flow and increased activity on bone scan. The bone scan can quantitate increased activity in portions of the sacroiliac joints in patients with spondyloarthropathies.[20]

Other diseases associated with abnormal bone scans include Paget's disease, hemoglobinopathies, and aseptic necrosis of bone. Paget's disease is a generalized disease of bone associated with increased blood flow to bone. The correlation between plain roentgenograms and bone scan abnormalities is close. The activity of disease is reflected in the degree of intensity of the bone lesions.

Patients with sickle cell anemia have positive bone scans. In patients with acute infarcts of bone, the bone scan may demonstrate a cold spot. Within a few days, blood flow is restored and increased uptake appears.

Aseptic necrosis of bone is associated with bone death, which may occur by a number of different mechanisms. Interruption of blood flow occurs secondary to disruption of vessels, increased pressure, or intraluminal occlusion. Early in the course of this lesion, blood flow is halted and an absence of radionuclide is noted on scan. With revascularization, reparative processes are initiated and increased blood flow is noted.

In general, radionuclide imaging is a useful technique for the evaluation of bone abnormalities in patients with low back pain. Although the bone scan is a highly sensitive test, the resolution of its image is relatively low. It also has less specificity than other radiographic techniques for diagnosing pathologic processes affecting the lumbosacral spine.

MYELOGRAPHY

The myelogram is the "bench mark" for evaluating pressure on the neural elements when an invasive spinal procedure is contemplated. At this time iohexol, a water-based, nonionic dye, is the contrast agent of choice. The newer agents are reported to have fewer side effects, such as seizures, nausea, and vomiting, while still giving excellent definition to the neural elements and their relationship to the surrounding structures. Oil-based contrast dye (Pantopaque) is rarely used. Although the myelogram is a very useful test, it requires a lumbar puncture, significant radiation exposure, and sometimes hospitalization. The test should not be done unless an invasive therapeutic procedure (surgery) is contemplated.

Lumbar myelography may be performed with the patient hospitalized or on an outpatient basis. In most circumstances, a water-soluble, nonionic contrast medium is injected via a small, 22-gauge lumbar puncture needle. Approximately 10 to 15 ml of dye is injected. The radiographs need to be completed 20 to 30 minutes after the injection because of dilution of the dye.

Certain precautions are necessary before and after myelography. Any drugs that lower seizure thresholds (e.g., phenothiazine derivatives) should be discontinued for 48 hours before the procedure. Patients with epilepsy should be maintained on their anticonvulsants. Patients should not eat for 4 hours before the procedure.

After the procedure, patients should be in a semisitting position in bed for 2 hours. After that period, the patient may lie down in bed with the head raised 10 degrees. This procedure helps prevent contrast reaching the upper subarachnoid space. The most common complication is headache in 68% of patients. Nausea and vomiting occurs in 38%, back pain in 26%, and seizures in 0.4%.[21] These complications may be treated with analgesics along with caffeine, antiemetics, intravenous fluids, and intravenous diazepam for acute seizures.

The normal myelogram of the lumbar spine consists of one frontal, one lateral, and two oblique projections. The frontal view demonstrates the cauda equina and the nerve roots exiting along the inferior surface of the pedicles. The oblique view highlights the nerve roots surrounded by the nerve root sheath (Fig. 7–10). The lateral radiograph in the prone position shows the relationship of the subarachnoid space and dura to the posterior portions of the vertebral bodies and intervertebral discs. It should be remembered that the caudal limit of the subarachnoid spaces varies in position. It may end at the L5-S1 disc interspace or at the S3 level. At the L5-S1 interspace the interposition of epidural fat between the subarachnoid and vertebral bodies may limit the utility of myelography in detecting an L5-S1 disc herniation.

The possible locations for lesions are extradural, intradural-extramedullary, or intramedullary. A prime example of an extradural lesion is a herniated nucleus pulposus. Other extradural lesions include osteophytes, abscesses, tumors, and hematomas. Neurofibromatosis causes intradural-extramedullary lesions, as do arachnoiditis and infection. Intramedullary lesions are spinal cord tumors, vascular malformations, and syringomyelia. Ex-

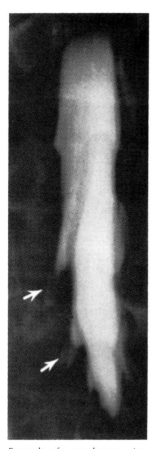

Figure 7–10. Example of a myelogram. An oblique view demonstrating nerve root sleeves (sheaths) *(arrows)* containing the exiting nerve roots (the linear filling defects) during a metrizamide myelogram. (From Resnick D, Niwayama G: Diagnosis of Bone and Joint Disorders. Philadelphia, WB Saunders Co, 1981.)

tradural lesions will push the cord and subarachnoid space away from their normal course and will interrupt the column of contrast. Intradural-extramedullary lesions push the cord away from the dura. Intramedullary tumors cause expansion of the cord with symmetric obliteration of the subarachnoid space.

The myelogram should be employed strictly as a confirmatory study. An abnormal myelogram without anatomic correlation with history and physical findings is not meaningful. It has been shown that 24% of asymptomatic people will have an abnormal myelogram (with Pantopaque contrast).[22] The experienced spine surgeon usually reserves the myelogram for preoperative assurance to confirm the location of the damaged disc or to check for a congenitally anomalous nerve root, tumor, or double disc. If the myelogram is used as a "screening test" in the absence of objective clinical findings, exploratory surgery and

disaster are the frequent results. Patients who undergo a myelogram without positive physical findings (tension sign or motor weakness) are reported to have a significantly higher chance of developing side effects from the procedure itself (nausea, vomiting, or increased back pain).

A particular advantage of the myelogram is that it can evaluate the lower thoracic spine. Intradural-extramedullary tumors in the lower thoracic area can present as acute radiculopathies. When appropriate pathology is not found in the lumbosacral area, the lower thoracic spine should be scrutinized for the existence of an occult spinal tumor by moving the dye rostrally to the thoracic spine.

Above all, it should not be forgotten that the myelogram is an invasive procedure and should not be taken lightly. The dye that is injected is a foreign material that can cause an adverse reaction. Fortunately, the water-soluble agent that is generally used currently is only a short-lived irritant, since it is rapidly excreted. Pantopaque, on the other hand, the dye used in the past and occasionally still used for pan-myelography (imaging of the entire spine), cannot always be removed entirely and has been known to cause arachnoiditis, which is an inflammation of the arachnoid in the spinal canal.

The metrizamide myelogram compares favorably with the CT scan in specificity and sensitivity as regards the diagnosis of herniated lumbar discs. A group of patients with surgically confirmed pathology of herniated lumbar discs underwent both preoperative metrizamide myelograms and CT scans. Each test was then evaluated by a neuroradiologist blinded to the patient's symptoms. Results indicated that myelography was more accurate than computerized tomography by 83% versus 72%.[23]

The reliability of other techniques, such as CT, in the evaluation of the postoperative lumbar spine patient is questioned. This is particularly true for the evaluation of patients with arachnoiditis. Myelography remains the diagnostic study of choice in patients with suspected arachnoiditis with metal artifact; otherwise MR may be used.

The myelogram is a very useful test in identifying lesions within the spinal canal, but it has its limitations. It is an invasive procedure associated with many more side effects than the other imaging techniques. The invasiveness and potential toxicity of the procedure explain, in part, the enthusiasm of radiologists for noninvasive techniques, such as MR, for imaging the same spinal cord structures. MR is more sensitive than myelography in detecting herniated intervertebral discs.[24]

COMPUTERIZED TOMOGRAPHY (CT)

Computerized tomography (CT) has become quite useful for evaluating abnormalities of the lumbosacral spine, where the spatial anatomy is complex.[25] CT creates cross-sectional (axial) images of the internal structure of the spine at various levels and, with reformatting, coronal and sagittal sections can be obtained. The CT scan assesses not only the bony configuration and structure-space relationship but also the soft tissue in graded shadings so that ligaments, nerve roots, free fat, and intervertebral disc protrusions can be evaluated as they relate to their bony environment in a single scan. CT also permits excellent visualization of paraspinal soft tissues.

The CT scan can be an extremely valuable diagnostic tool if used appropriately to confirm clinical findings derived from the history and physical examination. It is important to understand that the scan should be used for confirmation, not for primary diagnosis or general screening.

As with the myelogram, careful study has revealed the potential pitfalls of making clinical decisions based on CT scan findings isolated from the patient's complete clinical picture.[4] CT scans of the lumbar area of 53 normal subjects with no history of back trouble and six with back pain were submitted to three neuroradiologists who were unaware of the subjects' symptoms. Of the scans reviewed, 34.5% were read as abnormal and there was agreement among the interpreters in only 11% of the cases. The implication is that a patient with no history and physical findings indicative of spinal pathology has a 1 in 3 chance of having an abnormal CT scan. If a major therapeutic decision (to perform surgery) is made based only on the scan results, there is a 30% chance that the patient will be considered for unnecessary surgery. However, if the patient's history and physical findings correlate with the imaging findings of spine pathology, the CT scan frequently can be a helpful confirming diagnostic tool. The CT scan has the great advantage of being noninvasive and safely administered as an outpatient procedure. The radiation associated with a CT scan is 3 to 5 rads (Table 7–1). Radiation exposure is increased with high-resolution, slow-speed scanning.

As opposed to bone scintigraphy, which generates a survey of the entire skeleton on one view, the CT scan is able to assess only one slice of the skeleton per view. Lesions that are not contained in the plane will not be viewed by the CT scanner. The machine takes slices every 0.5 cm. It is important to tell the radiologist which area of the skeleton needs to be examined so that the duration of the test and exposure of the patient to radiation are limited.

A CT image of the lumbar spine will contain different anatomic structures depending on the level of the cross-section (Fig. 7–11). A scan through the superior portion of the L4 vertebral body will show the transverse and spinous processes, laminae, inferior facet of L3, superior facet of L4, pedicles, and vertebral body (Fig. 7–12). A view in the middle of the vertebra demonstrates cancellous bone in the vertebral body along with the normal bone defect in the center of the posterior surface of the vertebral body caused by the basivertebral veins, pedicles, and laminae—a complete bony ring of the spinal canal (Fig. 7–13). The intervertebral foramina are shown in a view of the lower third of L4 (Fig. 7–14). A section through the intervertebral disc demonstrates the inferior facet of L4, the superior facet of L5, the spinous process, and the intervertebral disc (Fig. 7–15).

The strength of CT scan as a radiographic technique in the evaluation of the lumbosacral spine is not its resolution of structures, but its definition of spatial relationships of anatomic

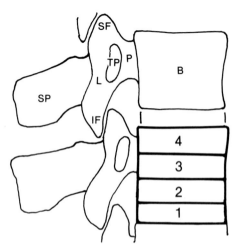

Figure 7–11. The four basic CT sections of the lumbar spine. The structures imaged by the scan include the spinous process (SP), inferior articular facet (IF), laminae (L), transverse process (TP), superior articular facet (SF), pedicle (P), and body (B).

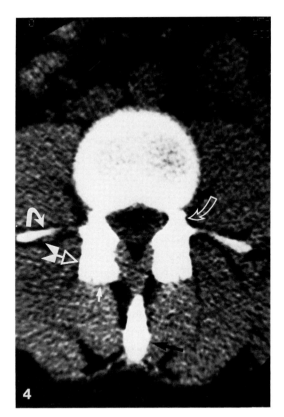

Figure 7-12. Section 4 contains the superior third of the vertebral body, the pedicles *(open curved arrow)*, the transverse processes *(curved arrow)*, the superior facets *(arrow with tail)*, the spinous process *(black arrow)*, and the inferior facet of the next higher vertebra *(short arrow)*.

relationship with surrounding vital structures.[31] Plain roentgenographs may be better for spatial resolution but are unable to detect soft tissue extension. CT scan also may be able to detect intramedullary bone loss from multiple myeloma, for example, which may not be detectable by plain roentgenograms or bone scintiscan.

CT is useful in the diagnosis and assessment of trauma since the patient is stationary during the procedure, limiting the hazards of moving the patient. Fragments of bone that may not be detectable by plain roentgenograms are localized to the spinal canal by CT techniques.[32]

The use of myelography as an adjunct to the CT scan can significantly improve the assessment of neural compression. CT scan immediately following myelography allows an axial view with intrathecal contrast highlighting the precise edge of the dural sac. Bone or soft tissue can be evaluated in light of the degree of neural impingement on the dye column.[33]

The question of the ability of CT to identify a clinically significant herniated nucleus pulposus without the aid of a myelogram has not been answered. CT scans detect intervertebral discs that have expanded into the spinal canal.

structures. CT is helpful in the evaluation of spinal stenosis, infections with paraspinal abscesses, postsurgical epidural scarring, facet and sacroiliac joint arthritis, primary metastatic tumors of the lumbar spine and pelvis, and trauma to the spinal column. Degenerative enlargement of facet joints may produce symptoms of spinal stenosis and is readily examined by CT.[26, 27] CT scan can visualize the medullary portion of the vertebral body and can detect bone destruction before changes are visible on plain radiographs.[28] CT with or without contrast can detect the presence of epidural fibrosis, which can be differentiated from a recurrent herniated nucleus pulposus.[29] CT scan is able to visualize the sacroiliac joint in patients with sacroiliitis. This technique can be used with patients whose conventional radiographs of the sacroiliac joints reveal equivocal findings of arthritis.[30]

CT is useful in the diagnosis of tumors of the lumbosacral spine for localizing the lesion, determining the intramedullary and extraosseous extent of the tumor, and defining its

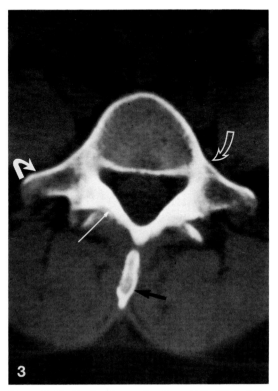

Figure 7-13. Section 3 contains the middle third of the vertebral body, the pedicles *(open curved arrow)*, the laminae *(long arrow)*, and the spinous process *(black arrow)*.

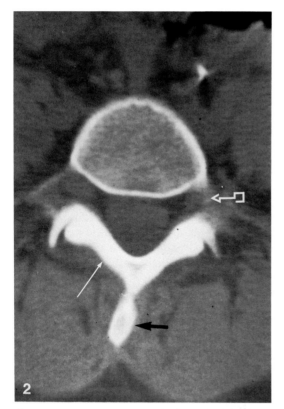

Figure 7–14. Section 2 contains the lower third of the vertebral body, the neural foramina and nerve roots *(arrow with square)*, the laminae *(long arrow)*, and the spinous process *(black arrow)*.

The CT can also identify compression of the dural sac, spinal nerves, root ganglia, and spinal veins. CT may be particularly helpful for lateral disc herniation beyond the dural sleeve, which may not cause an impression on the contrast column of the myelogram. Whether CT can totally replace the myelogram as the diagnostic test for herniated disc remains to be determined but their use together exceeds the value of either alone.[34]

MR has many advantages that may supersede both CT and myelography for the diagnosis of damaged discs.

MR is more sensitive than CT for the diagnosis of herniated discs.[35] In 25 patients who underwent surgery at 31 levels for a herniated nucleus pulposus and who were evaluated by MR and simultaneous contrast CT scan, surgical findings supported the MR diagnosis at 28 of 31 levels (90.3% accuracy); whereas the CT diagnosis correctly reflected only 24 of 31 levels (77.4% accuracy). At 10 levels where MR and CT scanning had a discrepancy, MR was incorrect at three levels and CT scan at seven levels. This study demonstrated the superiority

of MR over CT scan for evaluation of acute lumbar disc herniation.

MR and contrast CT were similar in accuracy in detecting spinal stenosis in central canal, lateral recess, and foraminal locations.[36] In a retrospective study of 41 patients visualized by MR and contrast CT, a 96.6% agreement was demonstrated for level of stenosis. However, MR detected disc degeneration in 74 of 123 segments; whereas only 27 of 123 segments were designated on CT scan.

MAGNETIC RESONANCE (MR) SCAN

Magnetic resonance (MR) imaging is the newest neurodiagnostic technique that displays small differences in tissue density with sharp contrast without exposing the patient to radiation or contrast material. MR has been

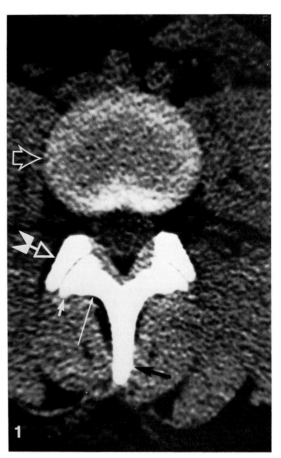

Figure 7–15. Section 1 contains the intervertebral disc *(open white arrow)* and the facet joints. The imaged osseous structures include the superior facet of the vertebra below the disc *(arrow with tail)* and the inferior facet *(short arrow)*, the laminae *(long arrow)*, and the spinous process *(black arrow)* of the vertebra above the disc.

clinically available since 1985. Over this period, MR has been increasingly used for the evaluation of musculoskeletal disorders, including low back pain and sciatica.[37] It has become the diagnostic procedure of choice for certain disorders, including intramedullary tumors of the spinal cord. MR technology for use in the lumbar spine is still being developed. At present, only a few systematic, prospective studies have been performed to compare the results of MR with more conventional techniques and confirmed pathology.[38, 39]

The principle behind MR involves the generation of a magnetic field by the nuclei of atoms with an odd number of protons. When placed between the poles of a strong magnet (up to 20,000 times the earth's magnetic field) the protons line up between the magnetic poles and vibrate at a frequency specific to each type of atom. Transmitting radio waves equal to the specific frequency of the target atoms and directed at a right angle to the static magnetic field causes the atoms to vibrate at an angle away from the vertical orientation. When the transmission of the radio waves is discontinued, the protons return to a state of relaxation (vertical position) by releasing radio waves. The radio waves generated by the atoms are detected by radio antennas and the information is analyzed by computer to generate cross-sectional images of the body. Variations in proton density, radio frequency, and the time to return to the state of relaxation (relaxation time) will modify the image produced by the MR scanner.

Proton density refers to the number of nuclei per unit volume of the structure to be examined. The most commonly measured atom is hydrogen. The hydrogen in water will generate a different amplitude of image if it is loosely bound to tissue molecules or tightly bound to specific molecules. Therefore, the amount and binding of water in the target structure will have a direct effect on the image generated by the MR scanner.

The proton relaxation times also play a major role in the generation of the MR. When the aligned protons are deflected by a radio wave, they achieve a level of increased excitation by their axes spinning in the shape of a cone. The time it takes for the proton to regain its magnetization in its vertical position is the T_1 relaxation time. The time it takes for the proton to lose its magnetization in the horizontal plane is the T_2 relaxation time. It is possible to change the pulse sequences of radio waves to accentuate differences in T_1 and T_2 relaxation times. The weighting of the images to T_1 or T_2 relaxation time will have a marked effect on the appearance of the MR images. With T_1 weighted images, nerve tissue is white and cerebrospinal fluid (CSF) gray; with more T_2 weighted images, CSF is white and nerve tissue is gray.

The MR includes a sagittal and axial view of the lumbar spine with both T_1 and T_2 weighted images. Patients who are on life support systems (metal machines) or have cardiac pacemakers or metal clips on intracranial aneurysms are not suitable candidates for MR. Pacemakers may revert from the demand mode to a fixed rate mode of operation. Metal clips may twist or loosen. Although nonferromagnetic implants, such as stainless steel appliances, are not attracted to the magnets, these objects cause artifacts that degrade the image. Claustrophobic individuals may have great difficulty in the closed space in the scanner and may need to be sedated with medications, such as oral diazepam, in order to complete the study.

The normal MR of the lumbosacral spine visualizes the vertebral column, intervertebral discs, and the spinal canal along with the spinal cord in the sagittal view (Fig. 7–16). The axial view shows the paravertebral soft tissue structures, the disc or vertebral body, the spinal canal, and the spinal cord (Fig. 7–17). The choice of relaxation times (T_1 or T_2) and pulse sequences, among other factors, may be modified to highlight specific structures or produce contrast that accentuates abnormalities associated with certain pathologic states.

MR is an excellent technique to view the spinal cord within the spinal canal.[40] MR is the preferred imaging modality for syringomyelia, atrophy, cord infarction, traumatic injury, intramedullary tumors, or multiple sclerosis affecting the spinal cord. MR may be more accurate than CT scan at characterizing extramedullary tumors. MR delineates the extent of extradural tumor invasion of the spinal canal and compression or displacement of the spinal cord. MR can identify the vertebral bodies in which bone marrow has been replaced with tumor.[41] MR also shows early changes in discs and vertebral endplates with infectious discitis.[42] The importance of MR as a diagnostic tool for mechanical and systemic disorders has been further advanced by the availability of gadolinium-diethylenetriamine pentaacetic acid (Gd-DTPA) as an intravenous paramagnetic contrast agent. Epidural scar and recurrent herniated discs have similar appearances on unenhanced MRs. Gd-DTPA does not cross an intact blood-brain barrier. Pathologic proc-

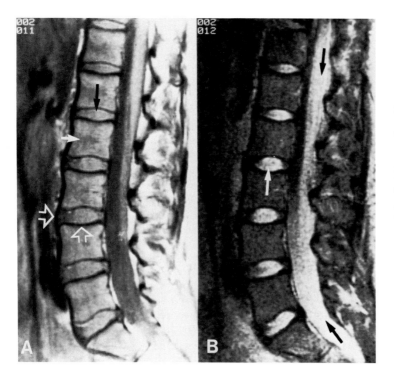

Figure 7–16. Normal MR scan of the lumbar spine, sagittal view. *A,* The T₁ weighted image demonstrates bone marrow and fat as whiter structures *(white arrow)* with vertebral endplates (cortical bone) and ligaments as blacker images *(open white arrows).* The intervertebral discs *(black arrow)* are intermediate in intensity. *B,* T₂ weighted image demonstrates CSF *(black arrows)* and nucleus pulposus *(white arrow)* as whiter structures. The nucleus pulposus can be separated from surrounding annular fibers and longitudinal ligaments.

esses (epidural scar, intramedullary tumors) that disrupt the blood-brain barrier result in leakage of Gd-DTPA and enhancement on MR.[42a–42c] CT scan continues to offer better definition of the bony architecture of the spinal canal than does MR. CT scan has been the radiographic method of choice for neural foraminal stenosis, posterior facet joint disease, and spinal stenosis.[43]

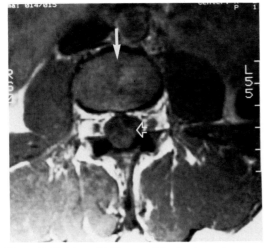

Figure 7–17. Normal MR scan of the lumbar spine, transaxial view. T₁ weighted image demonstrates surrounding soft tissue structures, intervertebral disc *(white arrow),* and the cauda equina *(open arrow)* surrounded by the spinal canal.

Numerous studies are under way to determine the sensitivity and specificity of MR in the diagnosis of lumbar spine disorders. Early studies that used MR scanners with poor resolution due to smaller magnets and body coils that did not allow thin imaging slices failed to demonstrate superiority of MR.[44] With the advent of surface coils, stronger magnets, and newer pulse sequences, MR scan resolution continues to improve and acquisition time continues to decrease. Most studies suggest that MR is more accurate in the detection of degenerative disc disease than discography or myelography.[45, 46] Compared to CT, MR is at least as accurate in making the diagnosis of spinal stenosis, sequestered lumbar intervertebral discs, and far lateral disc herniation.[36, 47, 48] MR, especially when used with gadolinium, has clear advantages for demonstrating intraspinal tumors, detecting disc space infection, and distinguishing recurrent disc herniation from postoperative scar.[49–52] In a prospective investigation of operative low back pain patients, the greatest correlation of imaging studies (myelography, CT, MR) with surgical findings was 93%, achieved by the combination of CT and MR.[47]

As with the other diagnostic imaging modalities, MR also has been shown to have a high frequency of abnormalities in asymptomatic individuals. In a prospective and blinded study, 22% of the asymptomatic subjects under age 60 and 57% of those over age 60 had significantly abnormal scans.[53] In addition, the prevalence of disc degeneration on the T_2 weighted images was found to approach 98% in subjects over age 60. It is essential to understand the frequency and spectrum of imaging abnormalities which may exist without causing clinical symptoms to better interpret these studies in symptomatic patients.

MR is still a relatively new technique with continuing development. The potential for this procedure as a diagnostic tool in the evaluation of patients with low back pain and sciatica is well established. Like CT scan, the sophistication of the radiologists using these machines will increase and the improvement in MR hardware and software will advance. However, our enthusiasm for the technique must be tempered by its high sensitivity for detecting asymptomatic as well as symptomatic spine pathology.[54] Despite the relatively high financial cost of an MR, the temptation to overutilize this noninvasive imaging modality as a screening test must also be tempered.

OTHER RADIOGRAPHIC TECHNIQUES

Tomography

In the period prior to CT and MR, conventional tomography was a preferred method to detect abnormalities in bones that were difficult to evaluate with routine roentgenograms because of their size, location, or orientation in the skeleton or surrounding tissues. Some of these areas included the sacroiliac joints and apophyseal joints of the spine.[55, 56] Tomography was particularly helpful in the patient with suspected infection of the spine. Tomographic slices through vertebral bodies helped define abnormalities of subchondral bone in vertebral bodies that raised the suspicion of osteomyelitis or discitis. Tomography also detected the presence of vertebral fractures, benign tumors (nidus of an osteoid osteoma), or soft tissue extension of malignant tumors.

Currently, the tomogram should not be dismissed as a useless technique because of the availability of CT and MR. Not all physicians have access to a CT or MR machine. Some patients are not good candidates for evaluation by these newer techniques, such as those with claustrophobia, metal implants, or inability to remain in a supine position. In these circumstances, tomography is a useful alternative to MR or CT techniques. Tomography is

useful to assess the amount and extent of new bone formation that is present following an attempt at spinal fusion. Also worthy of some consideration is the relatively modest cost of tomography in contrast to that of CT or MR scans.

Discography

Discography is a radiographic technique that is performed by placing a fine-gauge spinal needle into a disc space followed by the injection of radiopaque dye. The amount of dye accepted into the disc (normal 1 ml, abnormal 3 ml), the injection pressure, the radiographic appearance of the dye, and the reproduction of the patient's pain are important data generated during the test. The test has been used predominantly in patients in whom a diagnosis of the cause of radicular pain is unknown and other radiographic techniques have generated equivocal findings. Alternatively, this test has been used to provoke referred back pain from degenerative discs or annular tears. Although some reports have suggested a close correlation among abnormal discograms, degenerative disc disease, and chronic low back pain, other studies have reported little correlation between abnormal discograms and the local source of a patient's pain.[57, 58] Although a discographic study may reproduce a patient's spinal pain, results of spinal surgery for relief of back pain alone, without radicular symptoms of disc herniations caused by degenerative disease, have been unreliable.[59] A more recent study of discograms in normal, asymptomatic subjects demonstrated anatomic abnormalities in 17% of discs examined. If pain with injection was the criterion for a positive test, only symptomatic patients had positive results. Discography revealed abnormal findings in 13 of the 20 discs studied in symptomatic individuals.[60] Discograms are less sensitive in identifying abnormal discs than MR or CT. Therefore, reliance on data generated regarding the status of lumbar discs by noninvasive radiographic techniques (MR and CT) is usually adequate to define the integrity of the intervertebral space.[61] Discograms are less commonly indicated.

Epidural Venography

Opacification of the venous system surrounding the spinal column has been achieved through selected catheterization of the ascending lumbar veins in patients with disc herniations and intraspinous lesions.[62] The basic concept behind this invasive technique is based upon the consistent and reliable proximity of epidural veins to neural structures at risk of impingement. Abnormal venous filling is presumed to reflect an encroachment of the nerve by some anatomic structure. The utility of venography was greatest in patients in whom myelograms did not adequately define anatomy in the L4-L5 and L5-S1 disc spaces. Interruption, increased accumulation, or deviation of the column of dye was indicative of a disc herniation.[63] Patients with previous lumbar spine surgery, history of thrombophlebitis, and significant dye allergy could not undergo this examination. The utility of this invasive test in the setting of CT and MR technology has been greatly diminished. CT and MR can identify abnormalities (lateral disc herniations) that were missed by myelography. A shortened dural sac was one of the prime indications for epidural venography. Venography may be done if these other radiographic techniques are unavailable or if the patient is unable to undergo CT or MR because of contraindications.

Ultrasonography

Ultrasonography is used infrequently in the evaluation of the bony structures of the lumbar spine. The principle of diagnostic ultrasound is the same as used in radar, in which sound waves are generated by a transducer, bounced off an object, and returned to a receiver. Ultrasonography uses sound waves at 2 million to 10 million cycles per second to bounce off structures within the body. The transducer is able to generate the pulse of sound waves and then acts as the receiver of the reflected waves. The pattern of waves is altered whenever the sound beam encounters an interface between tissues of different densities. Cystic areas allow relatively unimpeded passage of waves as compared with solid structures, for example. Gray scale and real time ultrasonography are newer techniques that allow for detection of greater detail of structures and recording dynamic events inside the body, respectively. The major limitation for ultrasonography in the lumbar spine is that the sound beam does not transmit well through bone. Occasionally, ultrasonography has been utilized in the preoperative evaluation of spinal stenosis and intraoperatively for assessment of spinal cord compression in traumatic injuries.[64, 65] Ultrasonography is better able to establish the existence of a paraspinous abscess than conventional radiography. Ultrasonography is also useful in needle guidance for aspiration and drainage of accessible abscesses.[66, 67] Patients with abdominal aneurysms may be evaluated expeditiously by ultrasonography. The test is a noninvasive method to identify the presence and extent of an aneurysm.[68] Ultrasonography is also a useful technique for evaluating the status of structures in the pelvis and retroperitoneum.[69]

The role of diagnostic ultrasound is greatest in the evaluation of patients with low back pain with a medical etiology. This is particularly true for those individuals with viscerogenic referred pain. In these patients, ultrasonography offers significant information with less discomfort, radiation exposure, and cost than other radiologic procedures.

Spinal Angiography

Selective angiography of the blood supply to the vertebral column and spinal cord is now technically possible. Most spinal angiography is performed using mild sedation and local anesthesia. A femoral approach is used for most lumbar studies. Selective arterial catheterization is performed for vessels at least one level above and below the abnormality. Intra-arterial digital subtraction angiography reduces procedure time, contrast dosages, and patient discomfort.[70] Common uses for spinal angiography include mapping of the blood supply to the spinal cord and localization of feeder vessels for arteriovenous malformation.[71] Angiography is also used for preoperative planning of anterior approaches to the spine or preoperative embolization of vessels supplying a spinal tumor (Fig. 7–18).[72] Complications are rare but can include arterial spasm with subsequent spinal cord injury. The complications are sufficiently frequent, neurologic, 8.2% and nonneurologic, 3.7%, that the procedure is performed only when absolutely necessary.[73]

Closed Biopsy of the Lumbar Spine

With the advent of more sophisticated technology, closed needle biopsy of the lumbar spine has become a readily available procedure.[74] A successful closed biopsy obviates the need for open surgical biopsy, which is associated with the attendant risks, time, and ex-

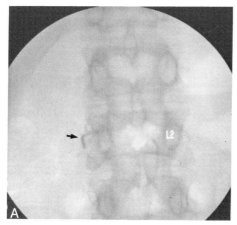

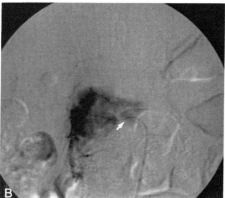

Figure 7-18. Spinal angiogram. A 31-year-old woman developed low back pain localized to second lumbar vertebra. *A,* Anteroposterior view of the second lumbar vertebra prior to injection. A gel foam has been placed in the right muscular radicular artery *(arrow). B,* Digital subtraction angiogram. A microcatheter has been placed in vessels feeding a vertebral tumor prior to preoperative embolization to decrease bleeding *(arrow).* The tumor was removed after embolization. The tissue diagnosis of the tumor was hemangioendothelioma.

pense. Closed needle biopsy may utilize a thin needle for aspiration for cytologic or culture material or a cutting needle to obtain an intact section of tissue for histologic review.[75, 76]

Advantages and disadvantages exist with closed biopsy in comparison to open biopsy. The closed procedure uses local anesthesia. The potential for infectious complications is limited. The time to complete the procedure is short and diminishes the period of hospitalization. The location of the lesion can be permanently recorded by radiographs taken at the time of biopsy. A major disadvantage of trocar biopsy is the size of the tissue specimen obtained for histologic evaluation. The amount of tissue recovered with a trocar is relatively small and may be insufficient for the pathologist to provide a specific diagnosis. Experience

with the procedure on the part of the radiologist and pathologist helps in the decision regarding adequacy of the specimen for making specific diagnoses. Closed biopsy may also be a potential problem for sampling of malignant tumors. Theoretically tumor cells may be implanted along the withdrawal path of the needle. In the clinical situation tumor implantation rarely occurs. Open biopsy requires general anesthesia and creates a larger wound. These are clear disadvantages. However, this approach is much more certain to provide sufficient biopsy material for diagnosis. Open biopsy also provides the surgeon the opportunity to visualize the extent of the lesion, which may not be apparent on radiographs.

Biopsy of a vertebra in the lumbar spine is indicated for lesions that are exclusively in the axial skeleton. Disease entities that may be diagnosed by closed needle biopsy include metastatic lesions, infectious diseases, and articular or osseous abnormalities, including aseptic necrosis of bone. Metabolic bone disease usually causes generalized bone abnormalities. Bone in the iliac crest is easily accessible to percutaneous biopsy, obviating the need for vertebral body biopsy in bone diseases of a generalized nature. Other diseases that may cause localized lesions that may be diagnosed by histologic examination of a closed biopsy specimen include sarcoidosis, fibrous dysplasia, eosinophilic granuloma, and Paget's disease.

Contraindications to closed biopsy are vertebral lesions with extensive destruction where biopsy may be associated with hemorrhage and spinal instability. Lesions that may be associated with increased vascularity may bleed excessively when a closed biopsy sample is taken. Very vascular tumors, both benign (e.g., hemangioma) and malignant (e.g., renal cell carcinoma and thyroid carcinoma), may bleed with biopsy. Closed biopsy of the lumbar spine is also contraindicated if a lesion more accessible to percutaneous biopsy is present. Radionuclide studies are helpful in identifying lesions more accessible to closed needle biopsy than those located in the spine.[77]

The procedure for closed biopsy of the lumbar spine requires hospitalization. Patients should not eat on the morning of the examination and require a sedative and pain medication. The radionuclide and radiographic studies of the biopsy site are reviewed to determine the location for the biopsy. Biplanar fluoroscopy is utilized to localize the lesion. Local anesthesia to the area all the way down to the periosteum of the bone to be sampled is needed to allow for adequate pain control.

The choice of biopsy needle is determined by the condition and type of lesion (soft vs. hard, vascular vs. nonvascular) to be biopsied. The Craig needle is used most frequently.[78] A right lateral approach is preferred at the appropriate level of the axial skeleton. The right lateral approach helps to lessen the possibility of contacting the aorta. The patient is placed in a prone position and a point 6.5 cm from the spinous process of the vertebra to be sampled is identified. At an angle of 145°, a spinal needle is inserted until bone is contacted (Fig. 7–19). A fluoroscopic image is taken to determine appropriate needle position. For biopsy of the posterior elements a greater angle is needed.[79] After the biopsy sample is taken the patient should be observed at bed rest for 24 hours.

Open surgical biopsy of the lumbar spine is a more complicated procedure. Posterior elements of the vertebral bodies may be visualized through a midline or paramedian incision. Biopsy samples from anterior portions of L1-L4 may be taken using a posterior approach through a longitudinal incision just lateral to the paraspinous musculature. Dissection through the muscles leads to the transverse process, which may be followed onto the vertebral body. The lower lumbar segments and anterior lesions of the sacrum require an anterior approach through the retroperitoneum. Posterior lesions of the lower lumbar segments and sacrum may be reached through a posterior approach.[80]

Needle biopsy is an effective method to diagnose lesions of the skeletal system. Debnam

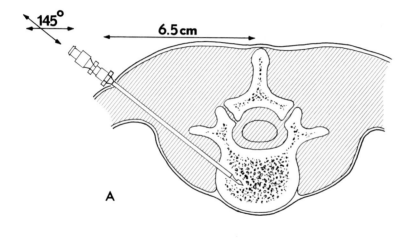

A

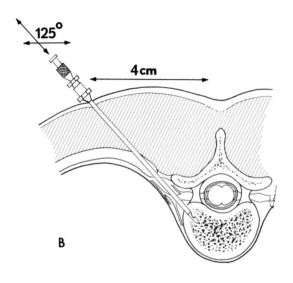

B

Figure 7–19. Technique of spinal biopsy. *A*, In the lumbar spine, the needle is inserted 6.5 cm from the spinous process at an angle of 145° from the horizontal. Biopsy of the posterior elements requires an angle greater than 145°. *B*, In the thoracic spine, needle placement is less lateral and directed more perpendicular to the skin. (From Resnick D, Niwayama G: Diagnosis of Bone and Joint Disorders, 2nd ed. Philadelphia, WB Saunders Co, 1988.)

and Staple reported an 81% rate of correct diagnoses in patients with bone lesions.[81] The high rate of success was related to a number of factors. These authors carefully selected patients for biopsy. Patients had careful roentgenographic and radionuclide investigation of their lesions, careful selection of the biopsy site, and careful histologic examination of the biopsy specimen. The need for biopsy of lesions of the lumbosacral spine is relatively uncommon. When necessary, closed needle biopsy is a helpful diagnostic technique for physicians who are familiar with its advantages and disadvantages. Open biopsy should be undertaken if closed biopsy is contraindicated or if equivocal results are obtained with percutaneous methods.

Bone Densitometry

Four general methods are available for measuring bone mineral density in various anatomic sites including the axial skeleton.[82] Single-photon absorptiometry is a technique limited to measurements of the peripheral skeleton and is not used for the spine. Dual-photon absorptiometry (DPA) uses two sources of photon energy to separate soft and bone tissue components of bone and surrounding tissues. DPA is used to measure the bone mineral density of the lumbar spine and long bones. The precision (reproducibility) of DPA spinal measurements is between 2% to 4% with accuracy variability of 5% to 10%.[83, 84] Quantitative computed tomography (QCT) measures bone calcium in trabecular bone in cross-sectional images of three to four vertebral bodies. The quantification of bone mineral is determined by comparison to a number of calibration phantoms containing mineral equivalents of known density. The precision error of QCT is 2% to 4% with accuracy variability of 10% to 15%.[85, 86] Dual energy radiography (DER) is based on the same principle as DPA but makes use of a dual energy source of x-ray, rather than a dual photon source. The precision of DER for bone mineral density of the vertebral spine is 1% with accuracy variability of 4% to 8%.[87, 88]

Each technique is limited by technical factors. DPA long-term precision is affected by the decay of the radioactive source. DPA is also affected by anatomic abnormalities of the spine and vascular calcifications. QCT has increased levels of radiation exposure compared to other methods and the accuracy is significantly affected by intravertebral marrow fat.

DER may be less sensitive than QCT in predicting vertebral fractures.[88]

The determination of bone mineral has progressed with more accurate assessment with less exposure to x-ray. The important determination that remains to be ascertained is the risk for fracture that is associated with specific amounts of vertebral body bone mineral. A combination of techniques (QCT for the diagnosis of osteoporosis and DER for sequential determinations and response to therapy) may be found to be the best way for quantifying bone mineral calcium and risk for fracture.[89]

NORMAL VARIANTS

Normal radiographic variation is a common finding when investigation of large groups of asymptomatic individuals is undertaken. Radiographic variations may be a consequence of skeletal changes that occur during growth and development or may be positional artifacts. This is particularly true in the sacroiliac joints (Fig. 7–20). The margins of the sacroiliac joints are normally indistinct during ado-

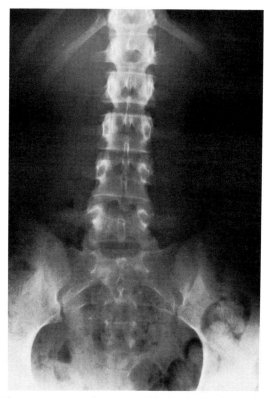

Figure 7–20. Normal AP view of the lumbosacral spine in a 14-year-old female. The joint margins are less well defined than joint margins found in adults (see Fig. 7–7).

lescence and may be confused with changes consistent with those of the spondyloarthropathies. Obliquity of the joints may obscure them on an anteroposterior view. An oblique view of the sacroiliac joints will demonstrate the normal state of the joint. In women exclusively, the bilateral indentation of the inferior portion of the iliac side of the sacroiliac joint (paraglenoid sulci) is a normal variant.

Normal variation may also be noted in the lumbar spine. Radiographic changes of the vertebral bodies may mimic findings associated with significant abnormalities including infection and tumor. However, careful clinical and repeated radiographic evaluation of the patient demonstrates the benign nature of these x-ray changes. A few examples of these findings might include limbus vertebra, nondiscogenic sclerosis, and bone islands.[90, 91]

PITFALLS OF RADIOGRAPHIC EVALUATION

The following case study is presented to temper the enthusiasm of clinicians for radiographic techniques as the method of choice in the diagnosis of low back pain.

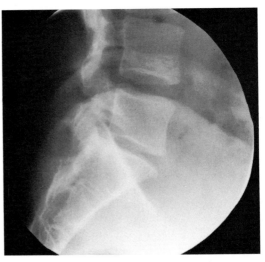

Figure 7–22. Coned-down view of the lumbosacral junction revealing an unremarkable L5-S1 intervertebral disc space.

Case Study: A 54-year-old white man was evaluated for a chief complaint of a recurrence of severe low back pain. The patient first noted symptoms of left-sided sacroiliac pain at age 20. At age 26, he developed right-sided sacroiliac pain. Back pain was most severe in the morning and improved with activity. He developed abdominal pain with cramps and a diagnosis of Crohn's disease was made. An intravenous pyelogram at that time demonstrated bilateral sacroiliitis with fusion (Fig. 7–21). A lateral view of the lumbosacral spine revealed no syndesmophytes and a normal L5-S1 disc space (Fig. 7–22). The patient was started on indomethacin 25 mg t.i.d. with good relief of his symptoms.

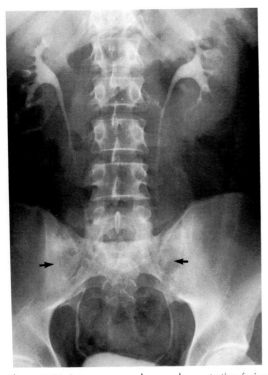

Figure 7–21. Intravenous pyelogram demonstrating fusion of both sacroiliac joints *(black arrows).*

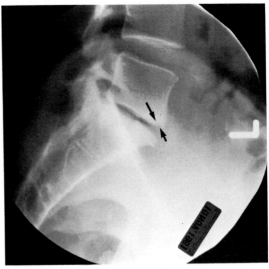

Figure 7–23. Coned-down view of the lumbosacral junction demonstrating disc space narrowing, bony sclerosis, and possible endplate erosion *(arrows).*

The patient did well until 2 years later, when he developed sudden onset of severe midline low back pain radiating from the right buttock to the knee. Coughing or sneezing increased pain in the same distribution. Physical examination revealed normal vital signs. Moderate paraspinous muscle spasm along with a loss of lumbar lordosis was noted on examination of the axial skeleton. The sacroiliac joints were not tender to percussion. The straight leg raising test was negative bilaterally. Motor strength and reflexes were normal. The patient had great difficulty arising from a supine position.

Plain roentgenograms demonstrated L5-S1 disc space narrowing and vertebral body sclerosis along with the possibility of vertebral endplate erosions (Fig. 7–23). A radionuclide scan was obtained when symptoms persisted and demonstrated markedly increased uptake over the L5-S1 region consistent with infection. Tomograms were obtained to better investigate the area for the presence of an infection. The tomograms demonstrated marked narrowing of the L5-S1 disc space with subchondral endplate sclerosis without destructive changes (Fig. 7–24). The radiologist suggested a gallium scan for detection of possible early osteomyelitis. The scan was normal. At this time the patient's radicular symptoms became more prominent. An electromyogram suggested the presence of very mild radiculopathy. A CT scan of the lumbosacral spine was obtained for detection of a herniated disc. The CT scan demon-

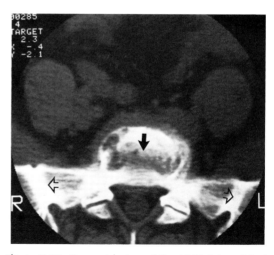

Figure 7–25. Transaxial view of the L5-S1 intervertebral disc space demonstrating a vacuum phenomenon in the disc proper *(arrow)*. Fused sacroiliac joints are also present *(open arrows)*.

strated a degenerative L5-S1 disc with a vacuum phenomenon (Fig. 7–25). The patient underwent lumbar myelography since surgical intervention for a correctable lesion was contemplated. The myelogram demonstrated a mild protrusion at the L4-L5 level (Fig. 7–26). The L5-S1 disc level showed no

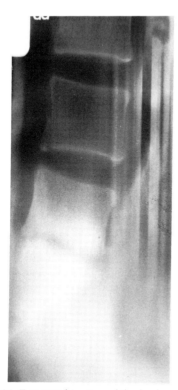

Figure 7–24. Tomographic view of the lumbosacral junction revealing marked disc space narrowing and surrounding bony sclerosis. No definite area of bony erosion was detected.

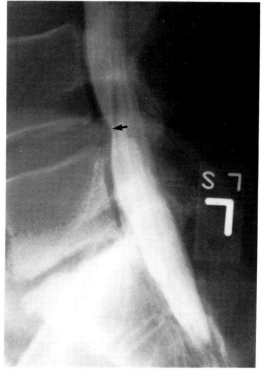

Figure 7–26. Lumbar myelogram, lateral view. The L4-L5 intervertebral disc is mildly protruded *(arrow)*. The L5-S1 disc is unassociated with any impingement of neural elements.

impingement of the neural elements. The patient refused any additional diagnostic tests. The possibilities of degenerative disc disease, spondylitis, and infection were reviewed with the patient. He decided on a therapeutic trial for radiculopathy including corticosteroids (prednisone, 25 mg/day) for 2 weeks, followed by indomethacin and a lumbosacral corset. Over the next month, the patient's symptoms resolved.

In 1992, 6 years after the episode of radicular pain, the patient was admitted to the hospital for severe diffuse back pain with radiating pain from the left buttock to the mid-thigh. In 1991, the patient developed biopsy-proven gastric cancer. An MR was obtained to determine the presence and extent of metastatic disease. The MR demonstrated findings that had been discovered on the plain roentgenograms, tomogram, CT scan, and myelogram. The L4-L5 disc was protruded as demonstrated on the myelogram, while the L5-S1 disc was severely degenerated. The new MR finding in all of the vertebral bodies was abnormal, a signal indicative of diffuse metastatic disease (Fig. 7–27).

We believe this case highlights the difficulties a physician may be faced with when obtaining too many diagnostic tests with conflicting results and the impact of MR on the radiographic evaluation of the lumbar spine. Radiologists may read films accurately describing the abnormalities they see. MR is a sensitive radiographic technique that is able to identify abnormalities that, in the past, required a number of different examinations to detect. This patient would not have undergone the number of evaluations he did if MR had been available in 1986. However, MR, like other radiographic techniques, may identify anatomic abnormalities that have little clinical importance. Radiographic findings only become significant when corroborating what is suspected by the history and physical examination of the patient.

The technology that is the basis of MR continues to improve.[92] In the future, improved imaging will be obtained through the use of perfusion imaging with new intravascular contrast agents, dynamic studies of CSF motion, and MR spectroscopy. These technologies will have to be evaluated as they become available to determine their appropriate place in the evaluation of low back pain patients.

The clinician is faced with choosing the best imaging procedure that is cost-efficient. Each medical center will have radiology departments with greater familiarity, or greater levels of competence, with certain procedures. It is important for the clinician to maintain a dialogue with the radiologist in regard to the method of choice for a specific clinical situation. A radiologist who knows the diagnostic

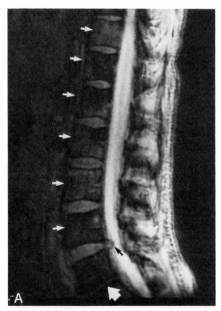

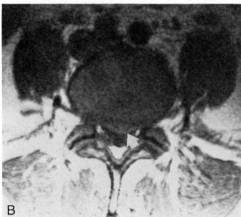

Figure 7–27. Lumbar MR. *A,* Sagittal view of T$_1$ weighted image demonstrating disc herniation *(black arrow)* and severe disc space loss at the L5-S1 interspace *(large white arrow).* Signal abnormalities are noted in most vertebral bodies indicative of metastatic disease *(small white arrows).* *B,* Axial view of L4-L5 interspace demonstrating diffuse central disc protrusion *(arrow).*

problem faced by the clinician has a much greater opportunity to make an interpretation that pertains specifically to the physician's dilemma. Only through communication between the clinician and the radiologist can the patient's needs truly be best served.

References

1. Hult L: The Munkfors investigation: a study of the frequency and causes of the stiff-neck-brachialgia and lumbago-sciatica syndromes, as well as observations on certain signs and symptoms from the dorsal spine and the joints of the extremities in industrial

and forest workers. Acta Orthop Scand (Suppl) 16:1, 1954.

2. Witt I, Vestergaard A, Rosenklint A: A comparative analysis of X-ray findings of the lumbar spine in patients with and without lumbar pain. Spine 9:298, 1984.

3. Lawrence JS: Disc degeneration: its frequency and relationship to symptoms. Ann Rheum Dis 28:121, 1969.

4. Wiesel SW, Tsourmas N, Feffer HL, et al.: A study of computer assisted tomography. 1. The incidence of positive CT scans in an asymptomatic group of patients. Spine 9:549, 1984.

5. Modic MT, Masaryk JT, Paushter D: Magnetic resonance imaging of the spine. Radiol Clin North Am 24:229, 1986.

6. Ardan GM: Bone destruction not demonstrable by radiography. Br J Radiol 24:107, 1951.

7. Liang M, Komaroff AL: Roentgenograms in primary care patients with acute low back pain: a cost-effective analysis. Arch Intern Med 142:1108, 1982.

8. Davis M, Jones A: Comparison of ^{99m}Tc-labeled phosphate agents for skeletal imaging. Semin Nucl Med 7:19, 1976.

9. Pendergrass H, Potsaid M, Costronovo F: The clinical use of ^{99m}Tc-diphosphonate (HEDSPA). Radiology 109:557, 1973.

10. Weiss TE, Shuler SE: I. New techniques for identification of synovitis and evaluation of joint disease. II. Joint imaging as a clinical aid in diagnosis and therapy. Bull Rheum Dis 25:786, 1974.

11. Staab EV, McCartney W: Role of gallium 67 in inflammatory disease. Semin Nucl Med 8:219, 1978.

12. Namey TC, Halla J: Radiographic and nucleographic techniques in the diagnosis of septic arthritis and osteomyelitis. Clin Rheum Dis 4:95, 1978.

13. Wilson MA: The effect of age on the quality of bone scans using ^{99m}Tc-pyrophosphate. Radiology 139:703, 1981.

14. McNeil BJ: Rationale for the use of bone scans in selected metastatic and primary bone tumors. Semin Nucl Med 8:336, 1978.

15. De Nardo GL, Jacobson SJ, Raventos A: [85]Sr bone scan in neoplastic disease. Semin Nucl Med 2:18, 1972.

16. Woolfenden JM, Pitt MJ, Durie BGM, Moon TE: Comparison of bone scintigraphy and radiography in multiple myeloma. Radiology 134:723, 1980.

17. Handmaker H, Leonards R: The bone scan in inflammatory osseous disease. Semin Nucl Med 6:95, 1976.

18. Marty R, Denney J, McKamey MR, Rowley MJ: Bone trauma and related benign disease: assessment by bone scanning. Semin Nucl Med 6:107, 1976.

19. Fogelman I, Bessent RG, Turner JG, et al.: The use of whole-body retention of Tc-99m diphosphonate in the diagnosis of metabolic bone disease. J Nucl Med 19:270, 1978.

20. Goldberg RP, Genant HK, Shimshak R, Shames D: Applications and limitations of quantitative sacroiliac joint scintigraphy. Radiology 128:683, 1978.

21. Baker RA, Hillman BJ, McLennan JE, Strand R, Kaufman S: Sequelae of metrizamide myelography in 200 examinations. AJR 130:499, 1978.

22. Hitselberger WE, Witten RM: Abnormal myelograms in asymptomatic patients. J Neurosurg 28:204, 1968.

23. Bell GR, Rothman RH, Booth RE, et al.: A study of computer assisted tomography. II. Comparison of metrizamide myelography and computed tomography in the diagnosis of herniated lumbar disc and spinal stenosis. Spine 9:552, 1984.

24. Szypryt EP, Twining P, Wilde GP, et al.: Diagnosis of lumbar disc protrusion: a comparison between magnetic resonance imaging and radiculography. J Bone Joint Surg Br 70:717, 1988.

25. Rosenthal DI, Mankin HJ, Bauman RA: Musculoskeletal applications for computed tomography. Bull Rheum Dis 33:1, 1983.

26. Ullrich CG, Binet EF, Sanecki MG, Kieffer SA: Quantitative assessment of the lumbar spinal canal by computed tomography. Radiology 134:137, 1980.

27. Carrera GF, Haughton VM, Syversten A, Williams AL: Computed tomography of the lumbar facet joints. Radiology 134:145, 1980.

28. Kattapuram SV, Phillips WC, Boyd R: CT in pyogenic osteomyelitis of the spine. AJR 140:1199, 1983.

29. Teplick JG, Haskin ME: CT of the postoperative lumbar spine. Radiol Clin North Am 21:395, 1983.

30. Carrera GF, Foley WD, Kozin F, et al.: CT of sacroiliitis. AJR 136:41, 1981.

31. Lukens JA, McLeod RA, Sim FH: Computed tomographic evaluation of primary osseous malignant neoplasms. AJR 139:45, 1982.

32. Colley DP, Dunsker SB: Traumatic narrowing of the dorsolumbar spinal canal demonstrated by computed tomography. Radiology 129:95, 1978.

33. Voelker JL, Mealey J Jr, Eskridge JM, Gilmor RL: Metrizamide-enhanced computed tomography as an adjunct to metrizamide myelography in the evaluation of lumbar disc herniation and spondylosis. Neurosurgery 20:379, 1987.

34. Williams AL, Haughton VM, Syvertsen A: Computed tomography in the diagnosis of herniated nucleus pulposus. Radiology 135:95, 1980.

35. Forrestall RM, Marsh HO, Pay NT: Magnetic resonance imaging and contrast CT of the lumbar spine: comparison of diagnostic methods and correlation with surgical findings. Spine 13:1049, 1988.

36. Schnebel B, Kingston S, Watkins R, Dillin W: Comparison of MRI to contrast CT in the diagnosis of spinal stenosis. Spine 14:332, 1989.

37. Han JS, Kaufman B, El Yousef SJ, et al.: NMR imaging of the spine. AJR 141:136, 1983.

38. Pech P, Haughton VM: Lumbar intervertebral disc: correlative MR and anatomic study. Radiology 156:699, 1985.

39. Schneiderman G, Flannigan B, Kingston S, et al.: Magnetic resonance imaging in the diagnosis of disc degeneration: correlation with discography. Spine 12:276, 1987.

40. Paushter DM, Modic MT, Masaryk TJ: Magnetic resonance imaging of the spine: applications and limitations. Radiol Clin North Am 23:551, 1985.

41. Porter BA, Shields AF, Olson DO: Magnetic resonance imaging of bone marrow disorders. Radiol Clin North Am 24:269, 1986.

42. Modic MT, Pflanze W, Feiglin DHI, Belhobek G: Magnetic resonance imaging of musculoskeletal infections. Radiol Clin North Am 24:247, 1986.

42a. Sze G, Stimac GK, Bartlett C, et al.: Multicenter study of gadopentetate dimeglumine as an MR contrast agent: evaluation in patients with spinal tumors. AJNR 11:967, 1990.

42b. Lim V, Sobel DF, Zyroff J: Spinal cord pial metastases: MR imaging with gadopentetate dimeglumine. AJNR 11:975, 1990.

42c. Gero B, Sze G, Sharif H: MR imaging of intradural inflammatory diseases of the spine. AJNR 12:1009, 1991.

43. Maravilla KR, Lesh P, Weinreb JC, et al.: Magnetic

resonance imaging of the lumbar spine with CT correlation. AJNR 6:237, 1985.

44. Modic MT, Masaryk T, Boumphrey F, et al.: Lumbar herniated disk disease and canal stenosis: prospective evaluation by surface coil MR, CT, and myelography. AJNR 7:709, 1986.

45. Gibson MJ, Buckley J, Mawhinney R, et al: Magnetic resonance imaging and discography in the diagnosis of disc degeneration. A comparative study of 50 discs. J Bone Joint Surg Br 68:369, 1986.

46. Weisz GM, Lamond TS, Kitchener PN: Spinal imaging: will MRI replace myelography? Spine 13:65, 1988.

47. Modic MT, Masaryk T, Boumphrey F, et al.: Lumbar herniated disk disease and canal stenosis: prospective evaluation by surface coil MR, CT, and myelography. Am J Neuroradiol 7:709, 1986.

48. Osborn AG, Hood RS, Sherry RG, et al.: CT/MR spectrum of far lateral and anterior lumbosacral disk herniations. Am J Neuroradiol 9:775, 1988.

49. Breger RK, Williams AL, Daniels DL, et al.: Contrast enhancement in spinal MR imaging. Am J Neuroradiol 10:633, 1989.

50. Nguyen CM, Ho KC, Yu S, et al.: An experimental model to study contrast enhancement in MR imaging of the intervertebral disc. Am J Neuroradiol 10:811, 1989.

51. Boden SD, Davis DO, Dina TS, et al.: Contrast-enhanced MR imaging after successful lumbar disc surgery: prospective study. Radiology 182:59, 1992.

52. Boden SD, Davis DO, Dina TS, et al.: Postoperative discitis: distinguishing early MR findings from normal postoperative disc space changes. Radiology 184:765, 1992.

53. Boden SD, Davis DO, Dina TS, et al.: Abnormal magnetic-resonance scans of the lumbar spine in asymptomatic subjects: a prospective investigation. J Bone Joint Surg Am 72:403, 1990.

54. Kent DL, Larson EB: Magnetic resonance imaging of the brain and spine: Is clinical efficacy established after the first decade? Ann Intern Med 108:402, 1988.

55. Wilkinson M, Meikle JAK: Tomography of the sacroiliac joint. Ann Rheum Dis 25:433, 1966.

56. Reichmann S: Tomography of the lumbar intervertebral joints. Acta Radiol 12:641, 1972.

57. Holt E: The question of lumbar discography. J Bone Joint Surg 50:720, 1968.

58. Simmons EH, Segil CM: An evaluation of discography in the localization of symptomatic levels in discogenic disease of the spine. Clin Orthop 108:57, 1975.

59. Spangfort EV: The lumbar disc herniation. A computer aided analysis of 2504 operations. Acta Orthop Scand (Suppl) 61:142, 1972.

60. Walsh TR, Weinstein JN, Spratt KF, et al.: Lumbar discography in normal subjects. A controlled, prospective study. J Bone Joint Surg Am 72:1081, 1990.

61. Schneiderman G, Flannigan B, Kingston S, et al.: Magnetic resonance imaging in the diagnosis of disc degeneration: correlation with discography. Spine 12:276, 1987.

62. Gargano FP, Mexer JD, Sheldon JJ: Transfemoral ascending lumbar catheterization of the epidural veins in lumbar disk disease. Radiology 111:329, 1974.

63. Gershater R, St. Louis EL: Lumbar epidural venography. Radiology 131:409, 1979.

64. Asztely M, Kadziolka R, Nachemson A: A comparison of sonography and myelography in clinically suspected spinal stenosis. Spine 8:885, 1983.

65. Eismont FJ, Green BA, Berkowitz BM, et al.: The role of intraoperative ultrasonography in the treatment of thoracic and lumbar spine fractures. Spine 9:782, 1984.

66. Allen EH, Cosgrove D, Millard JC: The radiological changes in infections of the spine and their diagnostic value. Clin Radiol 29:31, 1978.

67. Holm HH, Pedersen JF, Kristensen JK, et al.: Ultrasonically guided percutaneous puncture. Radiol Clin North Am 13:493, 1975.

68. Wheeler WE, Beachley MC, Ranniger K: Angiography and ultrasonography: a comparative study of abdominal aortic aneurysms. AJR 126:95, 1976.

69. Yamanaka T, Kimura K: Differential diagnosis of pancreatic mass lesion with percutaneous fine-needle aspiration biopsy under ultrasonic guidance. Dig Dis Sci 24:694, 1979.

70. Yeates A, Drayer B, Heinz ER, Osborne D: Intra-arterial digital subtraction angiography of the spinal cord. Radiology 155:387, 1985.

71. Merland JJ, Reizine D: Treatment of arteriovenous spinal cord malformations. Semin Intervent Radiol 4:281, 1987.

72. Eskridge JM: Interventional neuroradiology. Radiology 172:991, 1989.

73. Forbes G, Nichols DA, Jack CR, et al.: Complications of spinal cord arteriography: prospective assessment of risk for diagnostic procedures. Radiology 169:479, 1988.

74. Ottolenghi CE: Aspiration biopsy of the spine. J Bone Joint Surg Am 51:1531, 1969.

75. Adler O, Rosenberger A: Fine needle aspiration biopsy of osteolytic metastatic lesions. AJR 133:15, 1979.

76. Moore TM, Meyers MH, Patzakis MJ, et al.: Closed biopsy of musculoskeletal lesions. J Bone Joint Surg Am 61:375, 1979.

77. Collins JD, Bassett L, Main GD, Kagan C: Percutaneous biopsy following positive bone scans. Radiology 132:439, 1979.

78. Craig FS: Vertebral body biopsy. J Bone Joint Surg Am 38:93, 1956.

79. Resnick D: Needle biopsy of bone. In: Resnick D, Niwayama G (eds): Diagnosis of Bone and Joint Disorders. Philadelphia: W B Saunders Co, 1981, pp 692-701.

80. Friedlaender GE, Southwick WO: Tumors of the spine. In: Rothman RH, Simeone FA (eds): The Spine. Philadelphia: W B Saunders Co, 1982, pp 1024-1025.

81. Debnam JW, Staple TW: Trephine bone biopsy by radiologists. Results of 73 procedures. Radiology 116:607, 1975.

82. Genant HK, Faulker KG, Gluer C: Measurement of bone mineral density: current status. Am J Med 91:49S, 1991.

83. Nilas L, Borg J, Gotfredsen A, Christiansen C: Comparison of single- and dual-photon absorptiometry in postmenopausal bone mineral loss. J Nucl Med 26:1257, 1985.

84. Siemenda CW, Johnston CC: Bone mass measurement: which site to measure? Am J Med 84:643, 1988.

85. Steiger P, Block JE, Steiger S, et al.: Spinal bone mineral density by quantitative computed tomography: effect of region of interest, vertebral level, and technique. Radiology 175:537, 1990.

86. Gluer CC, Genant HK: Impact of marrow fat on accu-

racy of quantitative CT. J Comput Assist Tomogr 13:1023, 1989.

87. Wahner HW, Dunn WL, Brown ML, et al.: Comparison of dual-energy x-ray absorptiometry and dual photon absorptiometry for bone mineral measurements of the lumbar spine. Mayo Clin Proc 63:1075, 1988.

88. Sartoris DJ, Resnick D: Dual energy radiographic absorptiometry for bone densitometry: current status and perspective. AJR 152:241, 1989.

89. Pacifici R, Rupich R, Griffin M, et al.: Dual energy radiography versus quantitative computer tomography for the diagnosis of osteoporosis. J Clin Endocrinol Metab 70:705, 1990.

90. Feldman F: The symptomatic spine: relevant and irrelevant roentgen variant and variations. Orthop Clin North Am 14:119, 1983.

91. Keats TE: An Atlas of Normal Roentgen Variants That May Simulate Disease. Chicago: Year Book Medical Publishers, 1984, pp 236–264.

92. Bates D, Ruggieri P: Imaging modalities for evaluation of the spine. Radiol Clin North Am 29:675, 1991.

Miscellaneous Tests

ELECTRODIAGNOSTIC STUDIES

Electrodiagnostic studies are commonly used in the evaluation of diseases affecting the peripheral nervous system. These studies are extensions of the neurologic examination and provide a means to categorize muscle and nerve damage. They can confirm the clinical impression of nerve root compression, define the severity and distribution of involvement, and document or exclude other illnesses of nerves or muscles that could contribute to the patient's symptoms and signs. It is important to remember that electrodiagnostic tests measure the integrity of the nerve-muscle relationship and do not, by themselves, offer a specific etiologic diagnosis or quantify the degree of nerve damage. For patients with back and leg pain, electrodiagnostic studies are helpful in documenting radiculopathy (disease located at the level of the spinal roots) and excluding peripheral neuropathy caused by systemic diseases, such as diabetes, as the cause of the patient's complaints.

Electrodiagnostic studies include evaluation of electrical activity generated by muscle fibers at rest and during contraction (electromyogram) and speed of conduction of impulses electrically generated in peripheral nerves (nerve conduction studies). Studies of the integrity of the neuromuscular junction are not done in the evaluation of patients with spinal disease but are reserved for patients with neuromuscular abnormalities like myasthenia gravis.

Electromyography (EMG) is a test that measures the action potentials of muscle fibers. The EMG machine consists of an amplifier, oscilloscope, audio system, and recording electrode. The recording electrodes are needles ranging from 18 to 26 gauge that are inserted into muscles. The procedure consists of inserting needle electrodes through the skin to varying depths of each muscle to be studied. Each muscle is examined at two or more locations and in three or more directions. The multiple locations and directions are needed because abnormalities may be focal in distribution. The test is painful but usually does not require sedation or analgesics. The test takes over an hour to complete and may cost up to $600.

Nerve conduction studies of motor and sensory nerves may also be done as part of an electrodiagnostic study of a patient with neurologic symptoms. When motor nerves are evaluated, surface electrodes are attached to the skin over a foot muscle, and electric shocks of increasing voltage are generated until the largest electrical potential response of the muscle is recorded. A point distal in the nerve is stimulated, and the time required for the wave of depolarization to reach the recording site is termed the distal latency. Proximal latency is determined by stimulation of the same nerve at a proximal site. The distance between the points of stimulation is divided by the difference between the proximal and distal latencies to compute the conduction velocity of the tested peripheral nerve. Conduction is measured in the fastest conducting fibers only. Conduction in slower fibers is masked by the faster velocity in the fast fibers. Sensory conduction velocities are of low amplitude and are difficult to detect in the lower extremities. They are of limited value in the evaluation of nerve root disease affecting the legs.

EMG and nerve conduction studies do not detect spinal cord lesions or sensory radiculopathy. Evoked potentials (EP) are electrical responses of the nervous system to external sensory stimuli.[1] EP testing demonstrates abnormalities of the sensory system when clinical signs and symptoms are ambiguous. EPs may identify the location of unsuspected lesions in the central nervous system and may monitor the response of the lesion to therapy.

EPs generate low amplitude electrical activity between 0.1 to 20 microvolts (μV). These low amplitude potentials are obscured by the background noise produced by muscle artifact, electroencephalogram activity, and environmental interference. The EP occurs at the same time interval following a stimulus. Averaging of the signal response after repeated stimulation identifies the EP that can be separated from background noise. The evoked response is characterized by peaks and waves that are identified by their polarity, latency, amplitude, and configuration. Normal values are influenced by patient factors, including gender, age, body size, and temperature.[2]

Somatosensory evoked potentials (SEPs) are a means to determine the conduction of potentials generated by stimulation of peripheral structures to the spinal cord or cerebral cortex. A stimulus is generated peripherally, travels through the dorsal root ganglion, and ascends in the ipsilateral dorsal column. The stimulus then ascends to the contralateral ventroposterolateral nucleus of the thalamus and then to the primary sensory cortex. The stimulus can be measured over the spinal cord or scalp overlying the cortex. A computer is able to average the small potentials generated by peripheral stimulation and determine the latency associated with the peripheral site. SEPs may test large mixed nerves, small sensory nerves, a single dermatome, or sacral roots below S1 by stimulating organs supplied by the pudendal nerve.[3]

To understand the significance of abnormal electrodiagnostic findings, a review of basic EMG and nerve conduction concepts is worthwhile.

EMG Studies

1. *Motor unit.* The motor unit includes an anterior horn cell, axon terminal arborization, myoneural junction, and all the muscle fibers supplied by that single nerve cell.

2. *Motor unit potential.* The motor unit potential is a summation of electrical activity associated with the fibers in one motor unit. Motor unit fiber size varies from few to thousands of fibers. Therefore, motor unit potentials vary in amplitude and duration. Normal motor unit potentials have 2 to 4 spikes, an amplitude up to 4.0 millivolts (mV), and a duration up to 15 milliseconds (ms).

In a partially denervated muscle (commonly the circumstance with disc herniations), the remaining normal axons from unaffected nerve roots grow to innervate more of the muscle fibers than composed the original motor unit (Fig. 8–1). The increase in the number of muscle fibers per motor unit results in a longer duration and asynchronous depolarization of muscle fibers. The result is a motor unit potential of increased amplitude and longer duration. The slightly different time intervals of stimulation result in a polyphasic response with multiple spikes. The amplitude may vary up to 20 mV or greater.

Fibrillations are action potentials that arise spontaneously from small clusters of denervated, healthy muscle fibers awaiting reinnervation. Fibrillations have an amplitude of 20 to 300 μV and a short duration of less than 5.0 ms. They may fire up to 30 times per second. Once present, fibrillations may persist for months until the muscle fibers are reinnervated. The amplitude of fibrillations diminishes with time. Fibrillations are abnormal but are a nonspecific finding (myopathies also are associated with fibrillations).

Positive sharp waves are thought to come from healthy denervated muscle fibers injured by the entry of the electrode needle. The amplitude of these waves is similar or slightly greater than that of fibrillations and their du-

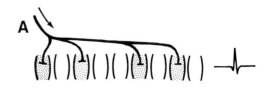

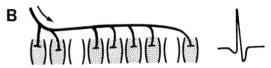

Figure 8–1. Schematic of a motor unit. The shaded muscle fibers are functional members of one motor unit with an axon that branches terminally to innervate the appropriate muscle fibers. The action potential produced by each motor unit is seen on the right. The unshaded muscle fibers belong to other motor units. *A,* A normal motor unit with four innervated muscle fibers, with corresponding action potential. *B,* Fibers that belonged to other motor units and had been denervated have been reinnervated by terminal sprouting from a normal, undamaged axon. The corresponding action potential has greater amplitude and duration.

ration is 10 ms. Like fibrillations, positive waves are abnormal but a nonspecific finding (Fig. 8–2).

"Giant" motor unit potentials are extremely high-voltage and long-duration motor unit potentials. In patients with denervated muscles, these potentials appear after reinnervation.

Fasciculation potentials are attributed to the spontaneous discharge of a group of muscle fibers belonging to a single motor unit. The amplitude of the waves is up to 5 mV and the duration is 15 ms. Fasciculation potentials may be seen in normal muscle, but is more frequently noted in muscles affected by chronic radiculopathies and anterior horn cell disorders.

3. *Interference.* As muscle contraction increases, greater numbers of individual motor units are brought into play, resulting in generation of greater numbers of unit potentials. The potentials obscure individual patterns on the oscilloscope screen, resulting in a blur of activity near the baseline level. This is normal and is referred to as interference.

4. *Insertional activity.* The insertion of the needle electrode damages nerve fibers, which results in electrical activity. The activity is present only with movement of the needle. In normal fibers, action potential generation ceases once the needle electrode comes to rest.

In radiculopathies, the insertional activity persists with decreased intensity for a number of seconds. This phenomenon is termed prolonged insertional activity and may be the only indication of an abnormality. However, increased insertional activity is a subjective evaluation dependent on observer criteria. This abnormality becomes significant only with other supporting EMG evidence.

Nerve Conduction Studies

1. *H-reflex.* An H-reflex is an electrically elicited analogue of the tendon reflex (Fig. 8–3). By electrical stimulation of large afferent fibers in a mixed nerve that synapses with alpha motor neurons, a monosynaptic reflex is evoked. The H-reflex is commonly used in the evaluation of S1 root lesions. The time latency (the period from time of stimulation until the impulse has traveled through the spinal cord to produce the reflex in the associated muscle) is standardized for age and the length of the limb or height of the patient. The difference between latencies of the lower extremities is 2 ms or less.

2. *F-response.* Antidromic activation of motor neurons following supramaximal stimulation of a peripheral nerve gives rise to an F-response (Fig. 8–4). The F-response travels along the motor nerve that supplies the innervation of the muscle. It is not a reflex, since it does not involve sensory fibers. It is dependent on integrity of only the motor unit. Unlike the H-reflex, the F-response is variable in latency and a number of repeated responses must be recorded. The most commonly reported result of the F-response is the minimum response time or latency. The difference in the minimal latency between two extremities is usually less than 2 ms.

A normal EMG with the muscle relaxed generates normal insertional activity only with electrode movement. Background fasciculations may be present. Motor unit potentials are normal in size, shape, and number. Maximum intensity of muscle contraction results in an interference pattern that obscures individual action potentials.

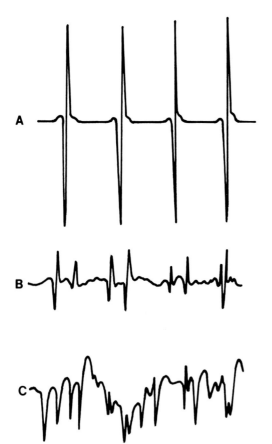

Figure 8–2. Electromyographic signals. *A,* Normal motor unit potential with 4 spikes, amplitude of 4.0 mV and duration of 15 ms. *B,* Fibrillations consisting of small clusters of spikes with diminished duration and amplitude (200 μV). *C,* Positive sharp waves (amplitude 250 μV).

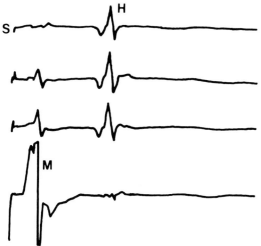

Figure 8–3. The H-reflex. The H-wave (H) appears and becomes maximum as the intensity of the stimulus (S) increases and disappears at supraphysiologic levels of stimulation when the M-wave is maximum.

Magnetic coil stimulation (MCS) is a method to activate nerve roots without the need for electrical stimulation. MCS is painless and is able to stimulate deep nerves that are not easily accessible to electrical activation. This technique may complement the H-reflex for S1 radiculopathy.[20]

Electrodiagnostic Abnormalities Associated with Nerve Root Compression

In the first 3 days after compression, a decreased number of motor unit action poten-

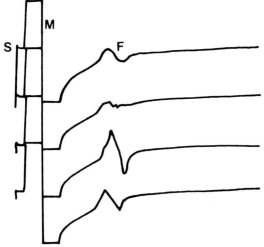

Figure 8–4. The F-response. The F-wave (F) is recorded after supraphysiologic stimulation (S). The amplitude, shape, and latency change with each stimulation.

tials are noted during muscle contraction (Table 8–1). Also within the first week, H-reflex latency differences may appear in S1 radiculopathy before EMG changes are noted.[4] At day 7 to 10, the paraspinous muscles show the presence of positive waves along with polyphasic waves. Changes in the paraspinous muscles will occur before changes in the extremities supplied by the same nerve root.[5] In about one third of patients with radiculopathy, EMG abnormalities were found solely in the paraspinous muscles. Soon after the appearance of positive waves and fibrillations, an increasing proportion of polyphasic waves is noted in limb muscles supplied by the corresponding nerve root.

Evaluation of the paraspinous muscles is helpful in localizing the area of nerve impingement. The paraspinous muscles are supplied by the posterior primary rami, which branch off a mixed peripheral nerve soon after its formation by the coalescence of the dorsal and ventral nerve root. There is marked anatomic segmental overlap in the superficial erector spinae muscles. The deepest layer, the multifidus layer, has the least degree of overlap. EMG studies done with electrodes placed 3 to 5 cm within the paraspinal muscle mass test the multifidus. Lesions of a single nerve root will have abnormalities found at one level only. Lesions that affect the anterior primary ramus, plexus, or peripheral nerve will have no effect on the paraspinous muscles.

Lesions that occur proximal to the branching off of the primary rami will result in abnormalities in both anterior and posterior divisions. Abnormalities may be limited to the paraspinous muscles in nerve root disease without anterior division abnormalities.

The most frequent abnormality found on an EMG for radiculopathy is the presence of positive waves. This is followed by an increased proportion of polyphasics and fibrillation potentials and a decreased number of motor units per contraction.[6]

TABLE 8–1. ELECTROPHYSIOLOGIC ABNORMALITIES IN NERVE ROOT LESIONS

Day 3	Reduced muscle action potentials
	H-reflex delayed (S1)
	F-response delayed (S1)
Day 7	Paraspinal fibrillations
Day 14	Paraspinal positive waves
	Associated proximal limb muscle positive waves
Day 21	Positive waves in entire myotome
Day 28	Fasciculations
Day 42	Prolonged polyphasic motor unit potentials

By the third week, paraspinous muscle fibrillation potentials are noted along with the emergence of positive waves in nerve root–associated limb muscles. The diagnosis of root involvement is supported by the documentation of abnormal EMG findings in at least three muscles supplied by three different peripheral nerves having a common root of origin. With continued injury of 2 months or longer, motor unit amplitude and duration increase. It is important to remember that in many patients, electrical signs of nerve damage will not appear for 21 days after the initial insult. EMG examination done too quickly in the course of events will miss the lesion. An experienced electromyographer should be aware of this occurrence and should counsel the attending clinician on the appropriate time for electrodiagnostic studies.

EMG may not be helpful in chronic radiculopathies. Muscles may become reinnervated and will not show spontaneous fibrillation potentials noted in acute radiculopathies. The severity of nerve dysfunction cannot be accurately determined by EMG. The cause of abnormal EMG findings cannot be specified by electrodiagnostic testing. Nerve root compression caused by a tumor, osteophyte, or herniated disc will have similar findings. The level of a radicular injury can be localized to within one or two segments by EMG. The exact disc level can only be estimated.[7]

Relative contraindications for EMG examination is a patient with a bleeding tendency (hemophilia, thrombocytopenia) and those on anticoagulant therapy. The placement of needles through the skin may increase the possibility of cellulitis in individuals susceptible to infection. An EMG should be limited to one side of the body if a muscle biopsy is considered since inflammation is associated with needle placement.

Electrodiagnostic Results

Electrodiagnostic examination has a degree of accuracy in identifying patients with nerve root compression similar to that of myelography and clinical examination. In studies comparing EMG and Pantopaque myelographic findings in patients undergoing surgery, EMG identified a root lesion and its level in 78% to 92% of patients, while the accuracy of myelography was 76% to 88%.[8–10] EMG was equally accurate in identifying root lesions at all lumbosacral levels, while myelography had greater accuracy at L4-L5 (85%) than at the L5-S1 level (60%).[11]

Motor nerve conduction and sensory nerve conduction velocities are normal in nerve root disease, since peripheral nerves contain fibers from several roots and root lesions from disc disease rarely produce complete loss of conduction through the involved roots. Damage to sensory nerves proximal to the dorsal root ganglia produces no change in the peripheral sensory fibers. Conduction studies are of value in patients with suspected root disease by excluding peripheral nerve disease as a potential cause of denervation changes.

H-reflexes are most sensitive to lesions of the sensory fibers in the S1 roots. Unilateral reduction of H-reflexes may be the sole electrophysiologic abnormality in some patients with S1 radiculopathy. The absence of an H-reflex correlates with an S1 radiculopathy with associated loss of ankle reflex.[4] H-reflex has an advantage over EMG in that H-reflex is abnormal almost immediately and is abnormal with sensory lesions. Milder S1 radiculopathies may be associated with subtle alterations in latency and amplitude that may be easily overlooked. These abnormalities may be missed by the experienced electromyographer. An abnormal H-reflex is sensitive but not specific in determining the site of the lesion. Any abnormality of sensory roots, motor roots, spinal cord, sacral plexus, or sciatic nerve will demonstrate similar abnormalities. H-reflex has also been determined for L4 radiculopathies.[12]

One benefit of F-responses is that they become abnormal almost immediately after injury. Asymmetric F-response in the gastrocnemius muscle also has been reported with S1 motor root disease.[12] However, F-responses are relatively insensitive in detecting radiculopathy. The reliance on motor fibers alone may play a role in the relative insensitivity of F-responses. Like H-reflex, abnormal F-responses are not synonymous with radiculopathy. Any lesion along the length of the affected nerve will result in an abnormal F-response. Acute and chronic radiculopathies cannot be distinguished by F-responses.

A normal electrophysiologic examination does not exclude the possibility of a radiculopathy causing neurologic symptoms, but a definite abnormality points toward an organic origin of a patient's symptoms. This may be of particular importance in patients claiming disability or applying for worker's compensation benefits.

Some non-neurologic disorders may be associated with EMG abnormalities. Metabolic disorders, particularly diabetes, may cause diffuse paraspinal abnormalities (profuse spontaneous activity) with no evidence of radiculopathy. Patients may improve with control of their diabetes. Paraspinal fibrillations and positive waves have been reported with metastatic disease.[14] EMG examination demonstrating marked segmental compromise of the posterior primary ramus distal to the spinal root with relative sparing of the anterior ramus may be the earliest evidence of paraspinal muscle metastases. Although CT scan may be unable to identify the presence of metastases, MR is able to detect paraspinal lesions. Although a pattern of posterior primary ramus segmental compromise is not diagnostic of metastases, the abnormal EMG pattern may suggest MR examination.[15] Spinal stenosis is associated with bilateral EMG abnormalities in a majority of patients.[16] Patients with arachnoiditis have also been associated with abnormal paraspinal electrophysiologic studies.[17] Mechanical abnormalities like muscle strains, ligamentous injury, and degenerative disc disease without nerve root compression should be associated with a normal EMG.

The role of serial EMG determinations in the management of patients with radicular pain is not well established compared with therapeutic decisions based upon the patient's symptoms and clinical findings. Once EMG changes of reinnervation occur, they may persist indefinitely. Denervation changes may also persist for many years following injury to the motor nerve, even when there is no evidence of continuing injury. It is difficult to determine the age or activity of a lesion once reinnervation changes appear. In addition, the degree of EMG abnormalities does not necessarily correlate with the extent of nerve damage.

Electrophysiologic studies obtained after laminectomy present particular difficulty in interpretation because of the injury to paraspinous muscles associated with ischemia from retractors during surgery. In addition, up to 24% of patients may develop a recurrent herniated disc after surgery.[18] In 25% of all patients with root lesions from disc disease, denervation changes persist after surgery even in the absence of persistent impingement.[19] EMG abnormalities, particularly in the paraspinous muscles, will be significant for a new lesion in a post-laminectomy patient if the patient has acute recurrence of symptomatology and EMG abnormalities at a level different from the level affected during the previous episode of radiculopathy.

Somatosensory Evoked Potentials

SEPs of large mixed nerves measure motor and sensory function of peripheral nerves. The most common nerves stimulated in the lower extremity are the posterior tibial and peroneal nerves. Mixed nerve SEPs are not helpful for detecting single level sensory radiculopathies since large mixed nerves carry nerves from multiple nerve roots. However, mixed nerve SEPs are sensitive in detecting spinal cord abnormalities that affect cord pathways. Spinal cord tumors and multiple sclerosis are two types of pathologic pathways that result in abnormal mixed nerve SEPs.

Small sensory nerve evoked potentials (SSEPs) are measured in the lower extremity. L4, L5, and S1 radiculopathies are detected by abnormalities in the distribution of the saphenous, superficial peroneal, and sural nerves. Lower extremity SEPs are more sensitive than EMGs in some patients with lumbosacral radiculopathy. In a study of 59 patients with radiculopathy, 38 had an abnormal CT/myelogram, 32 had abnormal SEPs, while 11 had abnormal EMGs.[21] All 21 patients with normal CT/myelograms had normal SEPs. SEP was less sensitive in patients in whom spinal stenosis was the only radiographic finding. The intermittent nature of nerve compression with spinal stenosis may explain the lessened sensitivity of SEPs in patients with spinal stenosis. SEP may be most helpful in patients with nondiagnostic EMG.

A dermatomal somatosensory evoked potential (DSEPs) is generated by direct stimulation of skin and recording cortical responses. The accuracy of the test is dependent on the placement of stimulating electrodes. In the lower extremity, S1 is tested by stimulating the lateral foot, L5 by testing the dorsum of the big and second toe, and L4 by testing the medial aspect of the calf above the ankle. The recording of DSEPs is technically demanding requiring an experienced technician. DSEPs are complementary to other electrodiagnostic tests. DSEPs do not evaluate motor nerve function and are not as sensitive as EMG for the diagnosis of nerve root lesions.[3]

Sacral roots below S1 are tested by pudendal evoked potentials (PEPs). PEPs are generated by stimulating the dorsal nerve of the penis or clitoris using surface electrodes or by stimulating the urethra and anal sphincter using catheter electrodes. The major limitation of PEPs is that only sensory nerve fibers of the pudendal nerve are tested.[22] Bulbocavernosus reflex is needed to measure muscle function.

In summary, electrodiagnostic studies are helpful in the evaluation of patients with neurologic dysfunction, although they do not pinpoint specific diagnoses. The procedures do not require hospitalization of the patient and are performed in the outpatient department. These studies may identify a specific nerve root lesion when clinical symptoms suggest abnormalities at two different levels. EMG tests may be abnormal when the corresponding myelogram is normal. MR tends to be more closely associated with electrodiagnostic abnormalities than myelograms. An abnormal EMG is corroborative evidence of organic disease and helps the surgeon select patients who are candidates for surgery. EMG changes may recede after resolution of nerve impingement. In patients with non-neurologic disorders, EMG findings are normal. Electrodiagnostic tests help differentiate peripheral nerve lesions from radiculopathy. When used in the appropriate setting and with the limitations of the tests in mind, the clinician may rely on these procedures to supply information that is useful in both diagnosis and management of patients with low back pain.

THERMOGRAPHY

Thermography is a noninvasive procedure that images the infrared radiation (heat) emitted from the body surfaces. Thermography is based on the principle that alterations in a variety of body functions will alter the cutaneous vascular supply that heats the skin. Postganglionic sympathetic cell bodies involved in the control of cutaneous vessels are located in the sympathetic chain ganglia that are connected to the spinal nerves distal to the dorsal root ganglia by the rami communicantes. The postganglionic nerve fibers from these cells travel to the cutaneous blood vessels by way of the peripheral nerves. Since the postganglionic nerves travel with peripheral nerves composed of fibers from multiple nerve roots, sympathetic abnormalities spread beyond a single dermatome. Stimulation of peripheral sensory nerves may affect sympathetic nerve fibers at the same or contiguous segment levels, resulting in alterations of blood flow to the skin. Factors that are associated with sensory nerve activation of nociceptive fibers (substance P) may also have an effect on cutaneous blood flow. However, pain is a complex phenomenon that cannot be simplified to a direct correlation with cutaneous heat production.

Thermography does not take a picture of pain itself, but does reveal pathophysiologic conditions associated with neurovascular, soft tissue, circulatory, and musculoskeletal disorders.

The two types of thermography equipment are liquid crystal (contact) and electronic (noncontact). Contact thermography utilizes cholesterol crystals that change color with variations of surface temperature. The crystals are placed inside inflatable transparent boxes, each of which has one flexible thermosensitive side that is applied to the body. Each box has a limited temperature range. An examination with liquid crystals requires the selection of the box with the appropriate temperature range. A picture is taken of the box to record the pattern of surface temperature. The box is chosen by trial and error. The advantages of liquid crystal thermography include the absence of radiation exposure, ease of use, and lower cost as compared with electronic thermography.

Electronic thermography utilizes an infrared radiation sensor that converts heat readings to electrical signals, which are displayed on a black-and-white or color monitor. A picture can be taken of the video screen or the image can be stored on computer discs. This system has the advantage of viewing large areas of the body during a single examination.

The examination must be performed in an air conditioned, draft-free room. The ambient temperature must be between 68° and 72° F. The patient should have refrained from smoking the day of the test. In addition, the patient should refrain from pain medications, physical therapy, and exposure to strong sunlight for at least 24 hours before the examination. The patient must disrobe and be in equilibrium with room temperature for 30 to 60 minutes before the examination is started. The patient's temperature must be normal. If the patient is febrile, the examination must be postponed.

Examination of the lumbosacral spine and lower legs with liquid crystals consists of separate images of buttocks; anterior, lateral, and posterior thighs; lower legs; dorsa of the feet; and toes.[23] The examination requires 1 to 2 hours to complete.

The assessment of a thermogram is based upon the distribution and temperature range of the skin. Both sides of the body have a temperature within 0.17° to 0.45° C in the healthy state.[24] The degree of thermal asymmetry between opposite sides of the body varies in different locations but remains less than 0.5° C. Values are reproducible for a period of 5 years.

A thermogram is abnormal if a side-to-side difference of 1° C involving 25% of its evaluated area is present. Alterations in the physiologic temperature distribution patterns also indicate abnormalities.[25]

Acute pain is associated with increased heat, while chronic pain is linked with decreased temperatures. Increased temperature is found over areas involved with an inflammatory process. Increased muscle metabolism associated with spasm or tonic contraction can be detected as increased heat conveyed to the surface by circulation.

Artifacts are common. Skin folds conserve heat and will appear "hot" on thermogram. Sunburn will alter the skin pattern. Alterations of the skin associated with injections, tattoos or vaccinations will change the normal thermographic patterns as well.[26]

Thermographic Abnormalities Associated with Low Back Pain

Thermographic diagnosis of low back pain syndromes include evaluation of the lumbar spine and lower extremities as well as images of the lower thorax, trunk, gluteal region, thighs, legs, and feet. Thermal asymmetry in patients with low back pain is associated with a decrease in the affected limb's temperature. In one study, when the asymmetry of temperature exceeded 1 standard deviation from the mean temperature of homologous regions measured in 90 normal subjects, the positive predictive value of detecting root impingement was 94.7% and specificity was 87.5%.[27]

The utility of thermography has been studied in patients with lumbar disc disease. Studies have reported a close correlation of abnormal thermograms and surgically proven herniated discs.[28, 29] Investigators have also found that in patients with herniated discs thermography and myelography have accuracy rates of 95% and 84%, respectively.[25] Infrared thermographic imaging has been compared to MR, CT, and myelography in patients with chronic back pain. Thermographic findings correlated with MR, CT, and myelographic abnormalities 94%, 87%, and 80% of the time, respectively. Of 22 MR scans of patients with disc prolapses associated with nerve root lesions, 95% had leg abnormalities on thermography.[30] CT and thermographic findings were correlated in 15 asymptomatic volunteers and 19 patients with nerve root displacement.[31] The thermogram had 60% specificity and 100% sensitivity in detecting nerve root le-

sions. Thermographic accuracy in detecting nerve root irritation also has been reported to be greater than that of electromyography. This difference in sensitivity is thought to be related to thermographic capability to detect sensory nerve abnormalities.[27]

Psychogenic or functional low back pain is difficult to differentiate from structural disease. Hendler and associates tried to differentiate psychogenic pain and malingering from true organic pain syndromes.[32] Of 224 patients referred with a diagnosis of psychogenic pain, 43 (19%) had abnormal thermograms corresponding to the symptomatic area. The thermogram was positive when other diagnostic tests, including EMG, were normal.

Although a number of studies have reported on the utility and accuracy of thermography in low back pain and other musculoskeletal conditions, the procedure has not won acceptance by many physicians. The reasons for this lack of acceptance may be the need for special rooms to do the test, the array of equipment needed, and the necessity of extensive experience with the technique to evaluate test results. These factors certainly play a role. However, the most important factor that still remains is the reliability of the thermogram in diagnosis of low back pain problems. Large prospective studies including control patients must be completed before the scientific merit of this diagnostic technique can be determined.

While some studies have reported a positive correlation between thermography and radiculopathy, a number of studies have appeared in the literature questioning the accuracy of thermography in the diagnosis of lumbosacral radiculopathy. For example, Mahoney and associates have reported findings of an investigation of thermography in patients with sciatica. The thermograms of normal controls and patients with herniated disc were compared. The sensitivity of thermograms to identify the side with the herniated disc was 35%. The "normal" controls showed "abnormal" or "asymmetric" patterns in 75% of the individuals studied. The thermogram was considered of no diagnostic value in evaluation of sciatica.[33] In a comparison study, thermography was unable to document a correlation between pain and alteration in body temperature.[34] A critique of this study by Uematsu and associates suggested that the poor results of the study were related to the lack of adherence to appropriate procedure in obtaining thermograms in the study patients. They stated that poor equipment, poor focusing, inadequate contrasts, improper patient positioning, and preparation all played a role in the poor results of the study.[35] Harper and So, in independent studies, were unable to demonstrate the reliability of thermography in the diagnosis of radiculopathy.[36, 37] In the Harper study of 55 patients with radiculopathy and 37 normal controls, 5 readers reviewed thermograms in a blinded fashion. The specificity of thermography ranged from 20% to 44%. Thermography predicted the level of the radiculopathy correctly in less than 50% of cases. In the So study, thermographic abnormalities did not follow a dermatomal distribution and did not identify the clinical or electrophysiologic level of radiculopathy.

In a meta-analysis for diagnostic accuracy and clinical utility of thermography for lumbar radiculopathy, significant methodologic flaws were identified in 27 of 28 studies reviewed.[38] The one study of high quality found no discriminant value for liquid-crystal thermography. The authors concluded that thermography could not be recommended for routine clinical investigation of low back pain.[38]

At present thermograms are not recommended for use in the routine decision making for diagnosis of low back patients. Thermograms detect autonomic dysfunction in different parts of the body. In the vast majority of individuals, determination of autonomic function is not necessary to adequately treat patients for their low back pain. Interpretation of thermograms needs to be standardized. Additional prospective studies must be conducted to correlate the findings of thermography with the most sensitive radiographic techniques. The specificity and sensitivity of the thermogram needs further definition. The value and role of thermography will be clarified as well-designed studies are completed demonstrating diagnostic significance and effects on therapy. The technique will become a more significant test as it becomes more widely available and well-trained physicians are accessible to interpret thermographic results.

DIFFERENTIAL NERVE BLOCKS

In patients who have intractable and chronic low back pain, identification of the source of pain, whether somatic, sympathetic, or psychogenic, is essential in planning an appropriate treatment regimen. Differential nerve blocks are an invasive means to examine the central and peripheral components of a patient's pain. They are particularly helpful in localizing the source of pain in patients who have undergone multiple operations on the lumbosacral spine and continue to experience back pain.

The different susceptibilities of sensory fibers to anesthesia is the physiology upon which differential blocks are based.[39] The different peripheral sensory fibers are classified as A (alpha and delta), B (preganglionic autonomic), and C (unmyelinated). Different concentrations of local anesthetics have selective sensitivity for these fibers.[40] Fiber sensitivity is greatest in B fibers, followed in decreasing order by C and then A fibers.[41] The sensitivity is related in part to the amount of myelination of fibers. Unmyelinated fibers have exposure of the entire surface of the axon membrane to local anesthetics. In myelinated nerves the membrane is exposed only at Ranvier's nodes, since the myelin layer insulates the rest of the axon. Higher concentrations of local anesthetics are needed to penetrate the nerve to block transmission. Alternative explanations have suggested that large, fast-conducting fibers are more susceptible to conduction blockade than smaller, slower-conducting fibers.[42] They concluded that conduction velocity is directly proportional to distance between nodes of Ranvier. The fastest fibers with the longest internodal distances should be affected before small diameter fibers. The discrepancy between these conflicting findings may be explained by the location of nerve fibers in neural bundles. Small-diameter fibers are more superficial and surround large-diameter fibers in dorsal spinal roots. Anesthetics injected as part of a spinal block would reach the small fibers first and would affect their function before the large fibers.

Anesthetics may also be given that block sensory fibers but leave motor nerve function intact. The local anesthetics with rapid onset, short duration of action, and ability to selectively block sympathetic, sensory, and then motor fibers with increasing concentrations are lidocaine and procaine. Fiber size, degree of myelination, nerve fiber location, length of nerve fiber exposed to anesthetic, neuropathologic state of the nerve, and the concentration and lipid solubility of the anesthetic all play a role in the effects of spinal blockade on nerve function.[43]

Differential Block Procedure

Antegrade spinal block requires three concentrations (0.25%, 0.5%, and 1.0%) of local anesthetic (procaine) that are prepared prior to starting the procedure. The patient must have pain at the time of the procedure. If pain is absent, the procedure is postponed. Other contraindications include anticoagulation and local skin infection at the injection site. The patient is told that he will receive a series of medications that may or may not relieve the pain. A lumbar needle is placed into the subarachnoid space. A placebo is injected as the patient is told that he is receiving one of the drugs. After 20 minutes of no pain relief, a 5-ml injection of 0.25% procaine is administered. At this concentration of anesthetic, the sympathetic fibers are blocked. If there is pain relief without loss of sensory function other than sympathetic nerve function, a sympathetic mechanism of pain production is confirmed. If there is no pain relief despite sympathetic blockade, 5 ml of 0.5% procaine is injected. If there is no pain relief despite loss of pinprick sensation, 1% solution is injected for motor blockade. If pain continues despite sensory and motor paralysis, the site of the lesion is proximal to the site of the blocks. The pain may be related to malingering, psychogenic pain or a central nervous system lesion.[44] Patients who continue to experience pain despite nerve blocks will not benefit from surgery or nerve blocks directed at peripheral structures.

The procedure for retrograde spinal block is slightly different. The patient receives the full dose of anesthetic after the placebo is injected. The benefit of doing the procedure in this fashion is that a catheter does not need to be left in the subarachnoid space for repeated injection. The patient will develop total motor and sensory loss. If pain persists, it is proximal to the site of the blockade. If pain is relieved, it is due to somatic or sympathetic mechanisms. If pain relief continues after sensation returns, the mechanism of pain is sympathetic in origin.

The results of the test are most dramatic when the patient is completely relieved of pain with only saline or when no relief is obtained with 1% anesthetic that produces motor paralysis or affects a sensory level several dermatomes above the pain site. In these circumstances, a central nervous system defect, structural or psychiatric, is present.[45]

In one study, nerve blocks were helpful in making an appropriate diagnosis of organic versus functional disease in 35 (87.5%) of 40 patients. The results of the block helped the physicians plan appropriate therapy (medical and/or surgical versus psychiatric) for the appropriate patients.[46]

Differential blocks may also be given in the epidural space as opposed to the subarachnoid space. Cherry described a technique utilizing an epidural catheter that was useful in differentiating psychogenic from organic pain.[47] Three injections were administered—normal saline placebo, 1 µg/kg fentanyl active injection, and 0.5 mg intravenous naloxone reversing injection 20 minutes later. Pain that was relieved by fentanyl and worsened by naloxone was of organic origin. Pain that was unaffected by naloxone was of psychogenic or central origin. This procedure did not differentiate sympathetic versus sensory pathways of pain but was limited to psychogenic or central versus somatic pain.

Patients who do not experience any pain relief from differential spinal blockade have pain of central or psychogenic origin. Techniques that affect central neurologic function are used to differentiate origins of pain central to the level of spinal blockade and those of psychiatric origin.[43] The tests are based on the assumption that patients in a light plane of sleep will respond to pain in a similar pattern as when fully awake. Conversely, if the low back pain resolves and the individual responds to other painful stimuli over other body locations, such as the anterior tibia, the implication is that the pain is of psychogenic origin. Sodium pentothal is slowly infused until the patient falls into a light plane of sleep. The infusion is stopped and the patient is allowed to wake up while being periodically tested for typical pain responses in areas other than the low back. When the patient responds to the pain stimulus, a stimulus that causes their typical back pain is given. If the stimulus does not cause typical back pain, the origin of the pain is psychogenic. Intravenous lidocaine, 1.2 to 2.0 mg/kg, is given until tingling is reported by the patient. Two minutes later, the patient's pain is assessed. A relief of pain that has been resistent to peripheral injections suggests a central origin. No relief suggests a psychogenic origin. Few studies have been completed proving the validity of these intravenous tests for determining the source of back pain.[48, 49]

Nerve blocks are invasive procedures with the potential for significant morbidity. They are undertaken by experienced anesthesiologists in the evaluation of pain in patients with complicated symptomatology. In those difficult patients, the risks of surgery outweigh the risks associated with differential nerve block.

The blocks should be undertaken if an unnecessary operation can be prevented based upon the results of the procedure.

References

1. Chiappa KH (ed): Evoked Potentials in Clinical Medicine, 2nd ed. New York: Raven Press, 1990.
2. Waldman HJ: Evoked potentials. In Raj PP (ed): Practical Management of Pain, 2nd ed. St Louis: Mosby-Yearbook, 1992, pp 155–167.
3. Glantz RH, Haldeman S: Other diagnostic studies: electrodiagnosis. In Frymoyer JW, Tucker TB, Hadler NM, et al. (eds): The Adult Spine: Principles and Practice. New York: Raven Press, 1991, pp 541–548.
4. Schuchmann JA: Evaluation of H-reflex latency in radiculopathy. Arch Phys Med Rehabil 58:560, 1976.
5. Johnsson B: Morphology, innervation and electromyographic study of the erector spinae. Arch Phys Med Rehabil 50:638, 1969.
6. Johnson EW, Melvin JL: Value of electromyography in lumbar radiculopathy. Arch Phys Med Rehabil 52:239, 1971.
7. Haldeman S: The electrodiagnostic evaluation of nerve root function. Spine 9:42, 1984.
8. Shea PA, Woods WW, Weden DH: Electromyography in diagnosis of nerve root compression syndrome. Arch Neurol Psychiat 64:93, 1950.
9. Knuttsoni B: Comparative studies of electromyographic, myelographic and clinical-neurological examinations in the diagnosis of lumbar root compression syndrome. Acta Orthop Scand (Suppl) 49:1, 1961.
10. Brady LP, Parker LB, Vaughn J: An evaluation of the electromyogram in the diagnosis of the lumbar disc lesion. J Bone Joint Surg Am 51:539, 1969.
11. Knuttson B: Electromyographic studies in the diagnosis of lumbar disc herniations. Acta Orthop Scand 28:290, 1959.
12. Sabbahi MA, Khalil M: Segmental H-reflex studies in upper and lower limbs of patients with radiculopathy. Arch Phys Med Rehabil 71:223, 1990.
13. Eisen A, Schomer D, Melmed C: An electrophysiological method for examining lumbosacral root compression. Can J Neurol Sci 4:117, 1977.
14. Watson R, Waylonis GW: Paraspinal electromyographic abnormalities as a predictor of occult metastatic carcinoma. Arch Phys Med Rehabil 56:216, 1975.
15. LaBan MM, Tamler MS, Wang AM, Meerschaert JR: Electromyographic detection of paraspinal muscle metastasis. Correlation with magnetic resonance imaging. Spine 17:1144, 1992.
16. Jacobson RE: Lumbar stenosis—an electromyographic evaluation. Clin Orthop 115:68, 1976.
17. Grue BL, Pudenz RH, Sheldon CH: Observations on the value of clinical electromyography. J Bone Joint Surg Am 39:492, 1957.
18. Epstein JA, Lavine LS, Epstein BS: Recurrent herniation of lumbar intervertebral disc. Clin Orthop 52:169, 1967.
19. Blom S, Lemperg R: Electromyographic analysis of the lumbar musculature in patients operated on for lumbar rhizopathy. J Neurosurg 26:25, 1967.
20. Chokroverty S, Flynn D, Picone MA, et al.: Magnetic coil stimulation of the human lumbosacral vertebral column: site of stimulation and clinical application. Electroencephalogr Clin Neurophysiol 89:54, 1993.
21. Walk D, Fisher MA, Doundoulakis SH, Hemmati M: Somatosensory evoked potentials in the evaluation of lumbosacral radiculopathy. Neurology 42:1197, 1992.
22. Haldeman S, Bradley WE, Bhatia N: Evoked responses from the pudendal evoked responses. Arch Neurol 39:280, 1982.
23. Pochaczevsky R: The value of liquid crystal thermography in the diagnosis of spinal root compression syndromes. Orthop Clin North Am 14:271, 1983.
24. Uematsu S, Edwin DH, Jankel WR, et al.: Quantification of thermal asymmetry. Part 1: Normal values and reproducibility. J Neurosurg 69:552, 1988.
25. Pochaczevsky R, Wexler CE, Myers PH, et al.: Liquid crystal thermography of the spine and extremities. J Neurosurg 56:386, 1982.
26. LeRoy PL, Bruner WM, Christian CR, et al.: Thermography as a diagnostic aid in the management of chronic pain. In Aronoff GM (ed): Evaluation and Treatment of Chronic Pain. Baltimore: Urban and Schwarzenberg, 1985, pp 232–250.
27. Uematsu S, Jankel WR, Edwin DH, et al.: Quantification of thermal asymmetry. Part 2: Application in low back pain and sciatica. J Neurosurg 69:556, 1988.
28. Albert SM, Glickman M, Kallish M: Thermography in orthopaedics. Ann NY Acad Sci 121:157, 1964.
29. Edeiken J, Wallace JD, Curley RF, Lee S: Thermography and herniated lumbar disks. AJR 102:790, 1968.
30. Thomas D, Cullum D, Siahamis G, Langlois S: Infrared thermographic imaging, magnetic resonance imaging, CT scan and myelography in low back pain. Br J Rheumatol 29:268, 1990.
31. Chafetz N, Wexler CE, Kaiser JA: Neuromuscular thermography of the lumbar spine with CT correlation. Spine 13:922, 1988.
32. Hendler W, Uematsu S, Long D: Thermographic validation of physical complaints in "psychogenic pain" patients. Psychosomatics 23:283, 1982.
33. Mahoney L, McCullock J, Csima A: Thermography in back pain: 1. Thermography as a diagnostic aid in sciatica. Thermology 1:43, 1985.
34. Mahoney L, Patt N, McCulloch J, Csima A: Thermography in back pain: 2. Relation of thermography to back pain. Thermography 1:51, 1985.
35. Uematsu S, Haberman J, Pochaczevsky R, et al.: A commentary on experimental methods, data interpretation and conclusion. Thermology 1:55, 1985.
36. Harper Cm Jr, Low PA, Fealev RD, et al.: Utility of thermography in the diagnosis of lumbosacral radiculopathy. Neurology 41:1010, 1991.
37. So YT, Aminoff MJ, Olney RK: The role of thermography in the evaluation of lumbosacral radiculopathy Neurology 39:1154, 1989.
38. Hoffman RM, Kent DL, Deyo RA: Diagnostic accuracy and clinical utility of thermography for lumbar radiculopathy: A meta-analysis. Spine 16:623, 1991.
39. Gasser HS, Erlanger J: Role of fiber size in establishment of nerve block by pressure or cocaine. Am J Physiol 88:581, 1929.
40. Nathan PW, Sears TA: Some factors concerned in differential nerve block by local anesthetics. J Physiol 157:565, 1961.
41. McCollum DE, Stephen CR: Use of graduated spinal anesthesia in the differential diagnosis of pain of the back and lower extremities. South Med J 57:410, 1964.
42. Gissen AJ, Covino B, Gregus J: Differential sensitivities of mammalian nerve fibers to local anesthetic agents. Anesthesiology 53:467, 1980.

43. Nehme AE, Warfield CA: Diagnostic measures. In Warfield CA (ed): Principles and Practice of Pain Management. New York: McGraw-Hill, 1993, pp 53–61.
44. Raj PP, Ramamurthy S: Differential nerve block studies. In Raj PP (ed): Practical Management of Pain. St Louis: Mosby-Yearbook, 1986, pp 173–177.
45. Winnie Ap, Collins VS: Differential neural blockade in pain syndrome of questionable etiology. Med Clin North Am 52:123, 1968.
46. Ahlgren EW, Stephen R, Lloyd AC, McCollen DE: Diagnosis of pain with a graduated spinal block technique. JAMA 195:83, 1966.
47. Cherry DA, Gourlay GK, McLachlan M, Cousins MJ: Diagnostic epidural opioid blockade and chronic pain: preliminary report. Pain 21:143, 1985.
48. Boas RA, Covino RB, Shahnarian A: Analgesic responses to I.V. lignocaine. Br J Anaesth 54:501, 1982.
49. Schoichet RP: Sodium amytal in the diagnosis of chronic pain. Can Psychiatr Assoc J 23:219, 1978.

9

A Standardized Approach to the Diagnosis and Treatment of Low Back Pain

A patient with back pain will present to a physician complaining of a set of symptoms. Patients do not come labeled with specific diagnoses, such as ankylosing spondylitis or subacute bacterial endocarditis. The problem confronting the examining physician is to integrate the patient's symptoms, physical signs, and x-ray findings into a logical diagnosis and subsequent treatment plan. With the myriad of symptoms, signs, laboratory tests, radiographic methods, and possible diagnoses to choose from, the clinician may be disorganized in his approach to the patient with low back pain, resulting in delay in establishing a diagnosis and in instituting appropriate therapy. The information that has been presented in the preceding chapters of Section II can be assembled into a thoughtful approach to the patient with low back pain. This chapter presents a standardized approach to the diagnosis and treatment of patients with low back pain. This approach helps organize the thought processes of the clinician, helping to expedite the appropriate and timely evaluation of patients. As with any protocol, there will be exceptions to the rule. Not all patients will fit easily into the categories to be discussed. Common sense helps the examining physician individualize the evaluation of the unusual patient. This protocol has been utilized in the evaluation of over 5000 patients and has proved to be useful in the vast majority of those individuals.[1]

A number of algorithmic approaches have been presented for the diagnosis and treat-

ment of low back pain patients. The development of some algorithms has been based on the experience of a single institution. For example, "The Pennsylvania Plan" is based on the experience of Rothman and associates at the Pennsylvania Hospital.[2] This algorithm concentrates on the mechanical disorders associated with alterations in the intervertebral disc and avoids discussion of medical causes of low back pain.

Another algorithm was published by the Quebec Task Force on spinal disorders. In 1983, this multidisciplinary group was established to formulate guidelines for the diagnosis and treatment of painful spinal disorders.[3] The algorithm was formulated in the context of occupation-related injury and disability. The data used for the algorithm was based on data from the Quebec Worker's Compensation Board and review of 469 publications in the medical literature. The report ranked scientific support for a variety of diagnostic measures and therapies for low back pain. In an effort to simplify diagnoses, the task force classified activity-related spinal disorders into 11 categories (Table 9–1). In addition, the categories were qualified by duration of symptoms and work status. The algorithm was formulated based on the scientific support and the classification system.

The first four categories of the classification system describe pain symptoms and radiation without associated specific pathology causing the symptoms. Categories 5 through 9 are associated with specific pathologic entities. Cat-

TABLE 9–1. QUEBEC TASK FORCE CLASSIFICATION OF LOW BACK PAIN

1. Pain without radiation
   a,b,c w or i
2. Pain + radiation to extremity, proximally
   a,b,c w or i
3. Pain + radiation to extremity, distally
   a,b,c w or i
4. Pain + radiation to lower limb neurologic
   a,b,c w or i
5. Presumptive compression of a spinal nerve root on a simple roentgenogram (spinal instability or fracture)
6. Compression of a spinal nerve root confirmed by specific imaging techniques (CT, MR, myelogram), EMG or venography
7. Spinal stenosis
8. Postsurgical status 1–6 months after intervention
9. Postsurgical status > 6 months after intervention
10. Chronic pain syndrome
11. Other diagnoses

a = <7 days, b = 7 days–7 weeks, c = > 7 weeks, w = working, i = idle.

Modified from Spitzer WO, et al.: Scientific approach to the assessment and management of activity-related spinal disorders: report of the Quebec Task Force on Spinal Disorders. Spine 12:S17, 1987.

egory 10 included patients with no specific identifiable disease and chronic pain. The final category includes all individuals with medical causes for low back pain. The algorithm allows for the evaluation of individuals who are less than 20 or over 50 years of age, have severe trauma, recurrent symptoms, neoplasm, fever, or neurologic deficit using a few simple diagnostic tests. These tests include plain lumbar spine films and an "inflammatory screen" (blood test) that is not well defined for specific disorders. Most patients receive conservative therapy without diagnostic tests. Referral to consultants and more expensive diagnostic tests are reserved for individuals who do not improve after 7 weeks of therapy. Surgery is limited to those with specific radicular symptoms and is not indicated for back pain alone. One of the strengths of this algorithm is the emphasis on a return to work as part of the treatment and measurement of outcome of low back pain patients. The only therapies considered useful in randomized, controlled trials include bed rest for 2 days, back school for individuals in categories 1 through 4, and surgical decompression for patients with confirmed neural compression with radiculopathy.

Although the Quebec Task Force algorithm is based on scientific literature and the outcomes of a large number of patients, it concentrates on the evaluation of mechanical disorders primarily. The medical causes of low back pain are briefly mentioned.

The revised algorithm in this chapter incorporates some of the work-related issues associated with the Quebec algorithm, while updating those factors important for the evaluation of patients with back pain associated with medical disorders. The specificity and sensitivity of historic, physical, and laboratory findings must be considered in deciding on those factors that are most helpful and cost effective in determining the diagnosis of a patient.[4] These statistical probabilities are important in guiding evaluations, but they do not negate the importance of sound clinical judgment based on experience with low back pain patients.

DIAGNOSTIC AND TREATMENT PROTOCOL

The protocol is organized into the format of an algorithm (see Algorithm, Part I, pages 166 and 167). Webster defines an algorithm as "a set of rules for solving a particular problem in a finite number of steps."[5] This algorithm is an organized pattern of decision-making and thought processes that have proved useful in caring for patients with low back pain.

Each patient will have an associated set of unique circumstances surrounding his case. There are, however, a number of common factors a physician should keep in mind when managing this population of patients. The primary objective for the physician is to return the patient with acute low back pain to regular activity as quickly as possible. In achieving this goal the physician must be concerned with making efficient and precise use of diagnostic studies, avoiding ineffectual surgical procedures, and making therapy available at a reasonable cost to the patient and society. Although scientifically proven data demonstrating efficacy for every aspect of low back care are not available, there is a large body of information to guide physicians in handling these patients. The algorithm follows well-delineated rules established as the consensus of a broad segment of physicians. It allows the patient to receive the most helpful diagnostic and therapeutic measures at optimal times. For example, not every patient who presents with clinical findings of a herniated disc requires an MR; only after initial treatment fails is this study appropriate.

Cauda Equina Compression (CEC)

The protocol begins with the universe of patients who present with signs and symptoms of a low back problem. They will have undergone an initial medical history and physical examination. The first major decision is to rule in or out the presence of cauda equina compression (CEC) syndrome. Significant compression of the cauda equina or truly progressive motor weakness is the only major surgical emergency to be found in patients with an acute mechanical low back problem.[6]

The compression usually is due to extrinsic pressure on the caudal sac by a massive, centrally herniated disc. Epidural abscesses and/or tumor masses are other examples of disorders causing CEC. Other causes for acute onset cauda equina syndrome include epidural hematoma and trauma. The symptom complex includes low back pain, bilateral motor weakness of the lower extremities, bilateral sciatica, saddle anesthesia, and even frank paraplegia with bowel and bladder incontinence.

Once this diagnosis is suspected, the patient should undergo an immediate myelogram, CT scan, or a MR and, if it is positive, subsequent emergency surgical decompression. The major reason for prompt surgical intervention is to arrest the progression of neurologic loss. The chance of actual return of neurologic function following surgery is unpredictable. Although the incidence of CEC syndrome in the total population of low back pain patients is very low, less than 1%, it is the only entity affecting structures in the spine that requires immediate operative intervention.

Medical Illness

The patients who do not have a CEC syndrome should then be evaluated for acute, severe symptoms suggestive of underlying medical illness as the cause of their back pain. These groups include individuals with constitutional symptoms of fever or weight loss suggestive of a tumor or infection. Patients with pain that is increased with recumbency may have a tumor of the spinal column. Patients with prolonged morning stiffness may have a spondyloarthropathy. Acute severe, localized back pain is frequently associated with a vertebral crush fracture secondary to a systemic, generalized process (metabolic bone disease) or a local tumor. Patients with viscerogenic pain (renal colic, dyspepsia, pulsatile

pain of an aneurysm, for example) have symptoms associated with the organ system affected. Patients with a prior history of a neoplasm are at greater risk of having a medical cause for low back pain.

Patients with marked neurologic deficits, signs of severe systemic disease, and vascular collapse are frequently evaluated in emergency rooms. Also, women with ectopic pregnancies may present to an emergency room with low back and pelvic pain. The emergency room physician plays a key role in the appropriate care of these patients. Thoughtful evaluation of these gravely ill patients with expedited admission to the hospital can be very important in the rare patient with life-threatening back disease.[7] Simple tests, such as an HCG level or ultrasound of the abdomen for ectopic pregnancy or expanding abdominal aneurysm, may be very helpful in determining those low back pain patients with specific, life-threatening causes for their symptoms.

Medical evaluation, including laboratory and radiographic tests, of patients with low back pain should be initiated only if they have significant symptoms and signs of an underlying medical illness with initial presentation. Simple tests that may be helpful in patients with new onset back pain who are 50 years of age or older include plain roentgenogram of the lumbar spine and an ESR.[8] These patients need to be evaluated by the medical algorithm. If no definitive medical etiology can be determined after screening evaluation with history and physical examinations, these individuals should start receiving initial conservative treatment for their symptoms.

Another concern that may enter into the evaluation of patients with low back pain early in the algorithm is psychologic overlay affecting the presence and severity of pain. At the time of presentation to a physician, individuals may have experienced chronic pain in relationship to depression or a work-related injury. Patients with chronic pain frequently have no pathoanatomic cause for their symptoms.[9] The presence of continued back pain may be reinforced or perpetuated by social and psychologic factors. The concerns about the effects of pain on family relationships, income, and employment status may add significant stress that tends to perpetuate pain.[10] Somatic amplification of symptoms may become an essential part of economic survival. Patients receiving worker's compensation respond less well to therapy than those not receiving compensation.[11] In patients with work-related back pain, job dissatisfaction plays a significant role in individuals who had persistent low back pain resistant to therapy.[12]

In patients where psychologic factors or somatic amplification is suspected, components of the history (lack of response to all therapies) and positive "nonorganic" signs should identify patients with nonmechanical or nonmedical low back pain.[13] In these patients, the use of screening tools for depression may be helpful. However, before a patient is branded as having a "nonorganic" problem, they should be evaluated by the process presented in this algorithm. If no specific abnormalities can be identified and psychologic factors are present, psychiatric evaluation is appropriate after the initial evaluation and response to therapy has been determined.

Conservative Therapy

The remaining patients who do not have a CEC syndrome or acute, severe medical illness should be started on a course of conservative (nonoperative) therapy regardless of the diagnosis at this stage. The specific diagnosis, whether a herniated disc or a simple back strain, is not important at this stage because the entire population with back pain is treated the same way. Some of these patients eventually will need an invasive procedure (surgery), but at this point there is no way to predict which individuals will respond to conservative therapy and which will not.

The early treatment of acute low back pain is a waiting game. The passage of time, the use of anti-inflammatory and muscle relaxant medications, and rest (controlled physical activity) are the modalities that have proved safest and most effective.[14] The vast majority of these patients will respond to this approach. In today's society, with its emphasis on quick solutions, many patients are pushed too rapidly toward more complex treatment, especially invasive treatment. This "quick fix" has no place in the treatment of acute low back pain. In most cases surgery does not return people to heavy work, and in the long run the best chance of getting a patient back to full activity is the nonoperative approach.

The physician should treat the patient conservatively and wait up to 6 weeks for a response. Most of these patients will improve within 2 to 10 days; a few will take longer.[15] Once the patient has achieved approximately 80% relief he should be mobilized. A few of these patients will benefit from the help of a lightweight, flexible corset. After the patient is

more comfortable and has increased his activity level, he should begin a program of back exercises and return to a normal lifestyle. The pathway along this section of the algorithm is a 2-way street: should regression occur with exacerbation of symptoms, the physician can resort to more stringent conservative measures. The patient may require further controlled physical activity. Most patients with acute low back pain will proceed along this pathway, returning to their normal life patterns within 2 months of the onset of symptoms. Some will also benefit by attendance in a back school program.[16] Patients may also benefit from a work evaluation if physical conditions of employment place the individual at risk for recurrent back pain. This evaluation might include ergonomic review of the job site, work place modification, functional capacity examination, work hardening for the patient, and vocational rehabilitation to find alternative employment if the individual is unable to complete the tasks associated with his initial job. All these factors should be considered in order to return patients to work without restrictions. The combination of controlled physical activity, medications, back school, exercises, and work evaluation should be considered part of a conservative therapy protocol.

The vast majority in this initial group have nonradiating low back pain, termed back strain. The etiology of back strain is not clear. There are several possibilities, including ligamentous or muscular strain, continuous mechanical stress from poor posture, or a small tear in the annulus fibrosus. Patients usually complain of pain in the low back, often localized to a single area. On physical examination they demonstrate a decreased range of lumbar spine motion, tenderness to palpation over the involved area, and muscle spasm. Their roentgenographic examinations usually are normal, but if therapy is not rapidly successful, films should be obtained to rule out other possible etiologic factors such as an infection or tumor. The mainstay of successful treatment for back strain is controlled physical activity. Anti-inflammatory and muscle relaxant medications give patients symptomatic relief of their pain but do not hasten healing.

After 6 weeks, patients in whom the initial treatment regimen fails are sorted into 4 groups. The first group is composed of people with pain localized to the low back. The second group includes those who complain mainly of leg pain, defined as pain radiating below the knee and commonly referred to as sciatica. Patients in the third group have anterior thigh pain, and those in the fourth group have posterior thigh pain. Each group follows a separate diagnostic path.

Localized Low Back Pain

The first group of patients will complain predominantly of low back pain despite 6 weeks of conservative care. This group should have their plain x-rays carefully examined for structural abnormalities. Flexion and extension views may be obtained but a debate exists whether these views actually demonstrate spinal instability. Spondylolysis with or without spondylolisthesis is the most common structural abnormality to cause significant low back pain.

Spondylolysis can be defined as a break in the continuity of the pars interarticularis in the lamina.[17] Approximately 5% of the population have this defect, which is thought to be caused by a combination of genetic structural abnormalities and environmental stress (Fig. 9–1). If the defect permits displacement of one vertebra on another, it is termed spondylolisthesis. Most people with this defect are able to perform their activities of daily living

with little discomfort. These patients usually will respond to nonoperative measures, including a thorough explanation of the problem, a back support, and exercises. In a small percentage of such cases, conservative treatment fails and a fusion of the involved spinal segments becomes necessary.[18] This is one of the few times primary fusion of the lumbar spine is indicated in a nontraumatic situation, and it must be stressed that it is a relatively infrequent occurrence. Most patients with spondylolisthesis do not need surgery.

Fusion surgery for spondylolisthesis is a successful operation in most circumstances. Patients with postoperative pain should be evaluated by the multioperated spine algorithm. Patients who fail to obtain pain relief with this algorithm should be treated with chronic pain therapy. In addition to changes of spondylolysis, plain roentgenograms may show intervertebral disc changes in patients with low back pain. It is important to remember that decreased disc height and associated changes of the surrounding vertebral bodies (traction osteophytes) may be present in patients who are asymptomatic (Figs. 9–2 and 9–3). However, articular degeneration with facet joint sclerosis may be associated with decreased back motion and back pain. Osteoarthritis of the facet joints

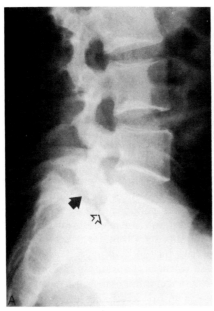

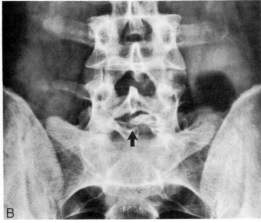

Figure 9–1. A 34-year-old man presented with low back pain that was exacerbated with extension. Conservative therapy was only mildly effective at decreasing low back pain. Plain roentgenograms, lateral view *(A)* reveals a grade 2 isthmic spondylolisthesis (open black arrow). Defect is present in the pars interarticularis (black arrow). Posteroanterior view *(B)* reveals a spina bifida occulta (black arrow) in addition to the spondylolisthesis. He responded to a change in his nonsteroidal therapy and an intensive flexion exercise program. *(A* from Borenstein DG: Low back pain. In Klippel JH, Dieppe P (eds): Rheumatology. St Louis, Mosby, 1994.)

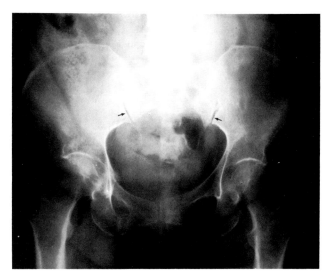

Figure 9–2. Posteroanterior view of the pelvis revealing vacuum phenomenon (black arrows) in both sacroiliac joints. The presence of vacuum signs is indicative of early degenerative changes in the joints. (Courtesy of Anne Brower, M.D.)

is the diagnosis most often associated with these roentgenographic changes. In the patient with disc degeneration, other sources of back pain may need to be investigated before the physician ascribes the patient's pain to osteoarthritis of the spine. Acromegaly also causes degenerative changes of intervertebral discs, but these changes occur over a short

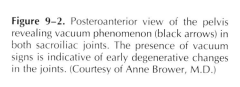

Figure 9–3. Posteroanterior view of the lumbar spine and pelvis revealing osteophyte formation in the lumbar spine (open black arrows) and the inferior border of the sacroiliac joints (black arrows). (Courtesy of Anne Brower, M.D.)

period of time in comparison with those of primary osteoarthritis.

On occasion, disc calcifications are noted on plain roentgenograms in patients with low back pain. Disc calcification is associated with ochronosis, calcium pyrophosphate dihydrate disease, hemochromatosis, hyperparathyroidism, and acromegaly. Evaluation with specific laboratory tests will help discriminate among the disease entities that cause disc calcifications. In these diseases, once roentgenographic abnormalities are present, lumbosacral spine disease is progressive even with effective therapy that rectifies hormonal imbalance or excessive iron stores.

Patients who fail to respond to an initial course of conservative therapy may respond to a local injection of a combination of an anesthetic and a long-acting corticosteroid preparation into the area of maximal tenderness (trigger point injection).[19] If this is unsuccessful, the patient should undergo a thorough medical evaluation. This may be done by the physician who initially evaluated the patient. However, it may be in the patient's interest to be evaluated by another physician who has a different approach to the problem. Evaluation and treatment by two different physicians has proved helpful in patients who have experienced acute or chronic low back pain.[20]

The back strain protocol includes a review of the patient's history and physical examination as well as specific diagnostic and therapeutic interventions. Without x-ray findings of spine instability or disc calcification, the medical evaluation of the patient with low back pain limited to the back must start with a review of the patient's history and physical examination. The time spent in the review of the patient's symptoms and signs is extremely important. The patient may have forgotten to list an important symptom during the initial evaluation. The symptoms may have changed in character or intensity. Constitutional symptoms of weight loss or occasional fever may have appeared. The areas of pain that were ill-defined have now localized to a vertebral body. The emergence of these symptoms and signs alerts the physician to a potential medical cause of the patient's back pain.

The histories of patients with medical low back pain may be divided according to symptoms into five groups (see Algorithm, pages 168 and 169):

1. *Fever and/or weight loss.* Patients with a history of fever, weight loss, or other constitutional symptoms frequently will have an infection or tumor as the cause of their pain. Occasionally, patients with a spondyloarthropathy will develop fever in association with their arthritis of the spine.

2. *Pain at night or with recumbency.* Patients who have a marked increase in back pain at night may have a benign or malignant neoplasm affecting tissues in or near the spinal column or cord. As opposed to patients with spondyloarthropathy, who develop increased pain at night after they have been recumbent in bed for hours, patients with malignancies have pain that is increased soon after they become recumbent.

3. *Morning stiffness.* Morning stiffness lasting for hours is a hallmark symptom of patients who have an inflammatory arthropathy of the spine. Patients with ankylosing spondylitis have great difficulty getting out of bed and are unable to "loosen up" until midday. Patients with osteoarthritis of the lumbosacral spine also have difficulty getting out of bed, but their stiffness rarely lasts more than 30 minutes.

4. *Acute, localized bone pain.* Patients who develop acute, localized bone pain with no or an insignificant history of trauma have sustained an acute fracture of a vertebra. In the absence of trauma, the development of vertebral fractures suggests decreased strength of bone structure secondary to diminished bone mineralization (osteopenia). Acute, localized bone pain may also be secondary to death of bone cells (avascular necrosis of bone). Tumors and granulomatous processes may replace bone calcium, resulting in abnormal bone architecture and pathologic fracture.

5. *Visceral pain.* Visceral pain occurs in patients with back pain who have symptoms of dysfunction in another organ system. Colicky back pain is suggestive of spasm in a hollow viscus, such as the ureter or cystic duct. Severe, tearing back pain associated with dizziness or syncope is very suggestive of an expanding abdominal aneurysm. Back pain that occurs at regular daily intervals and is associated with eating may be indicative of ulcer disease. Women who complain of back pain that is monthly and associated with their menstrual periods may have endometriosis.

The medical evaluation of each group of patients is different. It is helpful to identify the appropriate group of medical symptoms when first seeing the patient so that an appropriate evaluation is completed thoughtfully and expeditiously.

FEVER AND WEIGHT LOSS

The plain roentgenograms of the patients with fever and weight loss should be reviewed. What seemed normal initially may not appear so in the face of constitutional symptoms. If the roentgenograms are unrevealing, a bone scan is indicated. The bone scan will identify areas of increased bone cell activity of any source. Therefore, it is a sensitive but nonspecific test. Patients with early osteomyelitis or tumor may have increased uptake on bone scan without any corresponding roentgenographic changes. Over 30% of bone mineral must be lost before the radiologist detects it on a plain roentgenogram. A negative bone scan does not eliminate the possibility of a tumor causing back pain. Multiple myeloma does not cause an osteoblastic response by bone. There is no increased bone activity on bone scan. If the physician is suspicious of this possibility, a CT or MR scan of the lumbar spine should be ordered along with serum protein tests to evaluate for myeloma (Fig. 9–4). If any of these tests are positive, the patient should undergo appropriate evaluation with cultures for infection and/or biopsy of the detected lesion when infection or tumor is suspected. Antibiotics are the treatment of choice for infections. Surgical excision is preferred if tumors, particularly of the benign variety, are accessible to total removal. Radiotherapy and chemotherapy are utilized occasionally with benign tumors but more commonly with malignant lesions. In postsurgical patients who develop fever, C-reactive protein (CRP), if available, or an ESR are useful tests to identify patients with infection. CRP is more sensitive than ESR for determination of individuals with postoperative infections.[21]

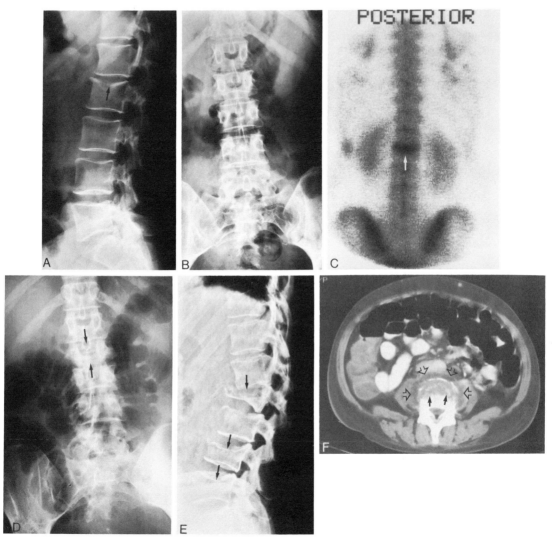

Figure 9–4. A 46-year-old woman with systemic lupus erythematosus manifested by severe skin and joint disease was treated with prednisone in doses ranging from 20 to 40 mg/day along with hydroxychloroquine 400 mg/day. She developed abdominal pain in association with intermittent, low grade fever. Plain roentgenograms of the lumbar spine on 1/27/88, posteroanterior view *(A)* and lateral *(B)* revealed no specific abnormality except for slight indentation of the superior endplate of the L2 vertebral body (black arrow). Localized back pain developed and she underwent bone scintiscan on 2/11/88. *C,* The scan revealed increased tracer in the L2 vertebral body (white arrow) compatible with compression fracture. Repeated blood cultures were negative for any growth. She received a 2-week course of antibiotics with some improvement in her abdominal pain. Over the next month, her back pain became more persistent and diffuse with increasing abdominal symptoms. She was readmitted to the hospital and repeat posterioanterior *(D)* and lateral *(E)* views of the lumbar spine on 4/28/88 revealed marked destruction of the L2 vertebral body. Also affected were the endplates of L4 and L5 vertebral bodies (black arrows). *F,* CT scan of the L2 vertebra revealed marked destruction of the body of the vertebra (black arrows) with an associated soft tissue abscess (open black arrows). The abscess extended from the L2 to L5 vertebral level. The patient expired from sepsis despite maximum antibiotic therapy. *(F* from Borenstein DG: Low back pain. In Klippel JH, Dieppe P (eds): Rheumatology. St Louis, Mosby, 1994.)

PAIN AT NIGHT OR WITH RECUMBENCY

Tumors of the spinal column or cord are of prime concern in the patient with nocturnal pain. After the re-evaluation of the patient's history and physical examination, the plain roentgenograms should be reviewed. If no abnormality is detected, the patient should undergo a bone scan. Bone scan is a sensitive test for detecting spinal column neoplasms but is not as useful for identifying spinal cord tumors. CT or MR scan is indicated if the bone scan is negative but multiple myeloma is suspected.

The alterations of bony architecture associated with spinal bone tumors are detectable by CT scan. However, subtle soft tissue changes may be missed by this technique. MR is a useful radiographic technique using no radiation or contrast dye to visualize the spinal cord. Extradural and intramedullary lesions are detectable by this technique (Fig. 9–5).

Patients with positive findings need a tissue diagnosis before therapy is instituted. If a primary source for the tumor other than the spinal column is detected, a tissue specimen for biopsy may be obtained from the most convenient location. Therapy is tailored to the specific neoplastic lesion. A combination of surgical, chemotherapeutic, and radiotherapeutic techniques may be effective at containing the growth of neoplasms.

MORNING STIFFNESS

Morning stiffness that lasts for hours in association with low back pain is a very common symptom of patients with a spondyloarthropathy. Occasionally, patients present with additional symptoms, such as iritis or keratodermia blennorrhagica, which help raise the suspicion of the possibility of a specific spondyloarthropathy. After completion of the examination for articular and extra-articular manifestations of

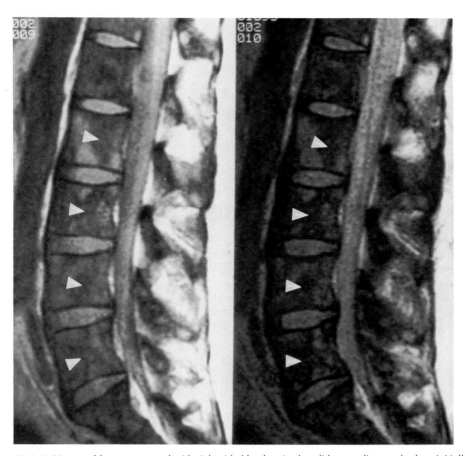

Figure 9–5. A 52-year-old man presented with right-sided back pain that did not radiate to the legs initially. He was treated with conservative therapy for 6 weeks. His pain increased to include the left side of his back and right hip and became persistent. He had to sleep in a chair at night. His hematocrit fell to 29. MRI of the lumbar spine reveals on proton density *(left)* and T₂-weighted sequence *(right)* decreased signal intensity in multiple vertebral bodies indicative of diffuse marrow replacement (white arrows). A diagnosis of prostate cancer was made with biopsy of the prostate gland.

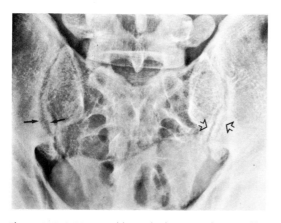

Figure 9–6. A 35-year-old man had a 5-year history of low back pain and morning stiffness. He previously had not sought medical care for back pain. A posteroanterior view of the sacroiliac joints revealed early joint margin erosions on both sides of the joints (black arrows) and sclerosis (open black arrows). Bilateral sacroiliac joint disease was compatible with a diagnosis of ankylosing spondylitis. The patient responded to nonsteroidal drug therapy.

disease, the physician should review the plain roentgenograms for early changes of spondyloarthropathy, including loss of lumbar lordosis, joint erosion in the lower one third of the sacroiliac joints, and squaring of the vertebral bodies (Fig. 9–6). If the plain views are normal, tilting the x-ray tube 30° will line up the face of the sacroiliac joint in one plane (Ferguson view). This view is helpful in detecting early changes of sacroiliitis. A normal sacroiliac examination does not eliminate the possibility of a spondyloarthropathy causing the patient's symptoms. A bone scan can detect the pattern of joint involvement in other parts of the axial and peripheral skeleton. Areas of active inflammation over the axial and peripheral skeleton may be detected by this technique. A specific diagnosis is not established by the presence of increased scintigraphic activity (metastatic tumor is also "hot" on bone scan). Osteoarthritis also may be associated with widespread areas of increased uptake. However, the patient's symptoms, signs, and laboratory tests (normal ESR, for example) should separate patients with osteoarthritis from those with inflammatory arthropathy.

Patients with spondyloarthropathy are usually treated with a combination of nonsteroidal anti-inflammatory drugs along with physical therapy. Occasionally, patients with specific forms of spondyloarthropathy (Whipple's disease, hidradenitis suppurativa) may require antibiotics as part of their treatment regimen.

ACUTE LOCALIZED BONE PAIN

Acute localized bone pain is usually associated with either fracture or expansion of bone. Any process that increases mineral loss from bone (osteoporosis, osteomalacia, hyperparathyroidism), causes bone death (hemoglobinopathy), or replaces bone with abnormal cells (tumor, sarcoidosis) will weaken the bone to the point where fracture may occur spontaneously or with minimal trauma. Patients with acute fractures experience acute onset of pain in the area of the back that corresponds to the fractured bone. Palpation over bone during the physical examination may localize the specific vertebra affected. After the physical examination elicits localized bone pain, review of the plain roentgenogram in the painful area may help to identify abnormalities in affected skeletal structures that were initially thought to be normal. Bone scan is useful to detect increased bone activity soon after a fracture at a time when the plain roentgenogram is unremarkable. CT scan may identify the location of a fracture, undetected by a plain roentgenogram, that is localized by increased tracer on bone scan. Finding an abnormality tells the clinician that a pathologic process is present but is not sufficient to define the specific cause of the bony change. MR may detect alterations in intravertebral bone marrow indicative of an inflammatory process, such as an infection, or a process that has replaced normal bone marrow (Fig. 9–7). Additional evaluation is necessary. Screening tests that are helpful in detecting systemic illnesses include an ESR along with a complete blood count. Abnormalities in any of these tests should heighten the physician's suspicion of a systemic illness causing the patient's symptoms. The differential diagnosis of the diseases associated with this symptom complex is quite broad. Further evaluation of these patients must be tailored to the specific situation. For example, evaluation for sickle cell anemia and sarcoidosis would be more appropriate in a black patient than in a Caucasian. An acid phosphatase determination is more appropriate in an older man than in a young woman. The diagnostic evaluation and therapeutic regimen for each disease process is reviewed in Section III.

If the laboratory evaluation of the patient is entirely normal and decreased bone mineral is noted on roentgenograms, the patient's diagnosis is osteopenia, most likely osteoporosis. The therapy for osteoporosis involves increased activity and calcium supplements,

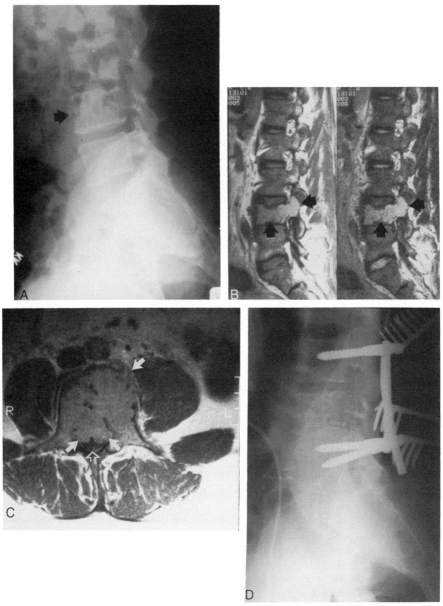

Figure 9–7. A 43-year-old man described the onset of left-sided low back pain after participating in a session of karate exercises. His examination revealed decreased range of motion of the lumbar spine without any neurologic deficits. He was treated with conservative therapy and was told to return in 2 weeks. During that period he had an increase in pain directly over the spine with radiation into the right anterior thigh. Lateral roentgenograph of the lumbar spine *(A)* reveals a loss of trabecular markings and integrity of the anterior vertebral body border (black arrow). *B,* MR of a sagittal proton density (left) and T$_2$-weighted image (right) reveals increased signal intensity involving the body and pedicle of the L4 vertebra (black arrows). *C,* MR of an axial T$_2$-weighted image reveals increased signal in the vertebral body with expansion beyond the vertebral body anteriorly and posteriorly (white arrows) with compression of the thecal sac. Marginal room remains in the canal for the cauda equina (open white arrow). *D,* Postoperative lateral roentgenogram of the lumbar spine. The plasmacytoma was removed with decompression of the spinal canal. Rods were placed to stabilize the spine to prevent neurologic damage. He was discharged from the hospital 10 days after his surgery with normal neurologic function and only mild postoperative back pain. (Views B, C, D from Borenstein DG: Progressive low back pain. In Klippel JH, Dieppe P (eds) Rheumatology. St. Louis, Mosby, 1994.)

along with estrogens, calcitonin, vitamin D, or etidronate in the appropriate patient.

VISCERAL PAIN

Patients with visceral pain have back pain in association with symptoms of gastrointestinal or genitourinary disease. These patients have symptoms of dyspepsia, abdominal pain, or change in bowel habits. They may have hematuria, polyuria, or flank pain. Patients with visceral pain may have colicky, severe tearing, or episodic low back pain.

Patients with colicky pain have spasm in a hollow viscus. Two structures in the abdomen that cause colicky back pain associated with obstruction are the ureters and the cystic duct. Patients with colicky back pain should have a urinalysis and an intravenous pyelogram. If these tests are normal and the patient continues to have colicky pain, a gallbladder scan may help document decreased function and the presence of gallstones.

Patients with severe tearing pain may be particularly problematic. Severe tearing pain may be a sign of an expanding abdominal aneurysm. If these patients complain of syncope or are hypotensive, they must be evaluated for an aneurysm on an emergency basis. Their hematocrit can be checked as blood is drawn for typing and cross-match for possible transfusion. Patients with an aneurysm may be evaluated with ultrasonography, depending on their hemodynamic status. Patients with an expanding aneurysm usually require vascular surgery to repair the aortic defect. Patients who are candidates for surgical correction of expanding aneurysms should undergo CT scan if hemodynamically stable. The timing of surgery depends on a number of factors, including the size and location of the aneurysm. The surgeon and the evaluating physician work together to determine the time for surgery to maximize the potential for a good outcome.

Patients with visceral pain may have a recurrence of pain on a regular basis. The frequency may be daily, associated with eating (gastrointestinal—pancreatitis, peptic ulcer disease), or monthly, associated with menstrual periods (endometriosis). These patients have a history of low back pain that is not particularly modified by changes of position. Examination of the abdomen demonstrates tenderness with palpation that may be localized to the right upper quadrant (ulcer disease), epigastrium (pancreas), or lower quadrants (uterus and ovaries). Careful gynecologic examination demonstrates masses, nodules, or adhesions, which suggest the presence of an inflammatory intrapelvic process. Serum tests for pancreatic injury (amylase, trypsin) may identify those individuals with gastrointestinal-associated back pain. Rectal examination may identify abnormalities in the colon associated with defecation that may cause low back or sacral pain (Fig. 9–8).

Therapy for these entities is directed at decreasing inflammation in the affected organ system. Hormonal therapy is effective in endometriosis, while antiulcer therapy is helpful in patients with peptic ulcer disease.

If patients do not fit into any of the five categories, they should be evaluated for muscle stiffness and pain. Patients who are over 50 years of age with proximal stiffness, particularly in the morning, may have polymyalgia rheumatica. Younger patients also may have muscle pain. In contrast to the diffuse areas of pain in polymyalgia rheumatica, local areas of tenderness are problematic in patients with fibromyalgia. "Tender points" are found in characteristic locations throughout the muscular system. There are no diagnostic tests for these diseases. The diagnosis is a clinical one. One laboratory test that is helpful in distinguishing between these two entities is measurement of the ESR. Polymyalgia rheumatica is associated with an elevated sedimentation rate, while fibromyalgia is not. If a patient has not had a sedimentation rate test in the evaluation, the test should be done. Therapy for the two illnesses is quite different. Polymyalgia rheumatica is treated with low-dose corticosteroids (prednisone, 15 mg per day). Fibromyalgia is treated with mild exercise, injections, and moderate doses of tricyclic antidepressants.

Some patients will go through the entire medical evaluation without any detectable abnormalities. A surreptitious illness may be present that has not progressed to the point of detectability by the physician's diagnostic tests. These patients need to be watched carefully while they continue therapy for localized low back pain as part of the back strain protocol. Re-evaluation is indicated if these patients complain of any new symptoms. A repeat sedimentation rate test is a cost-effective method to identify those individuals who require close scrutiny. The development of an elevation in the sedimentation rate suggests an inflammatory process that has gone undetected. The presence of an elevated sedimentation rate helps separate those individual with a systemic inflammatory disease from those with a mechanical process.

If the medical work-up is unrevealing, the patient should undergo a thorough psychoso-

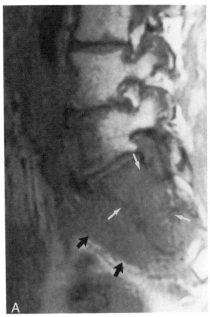

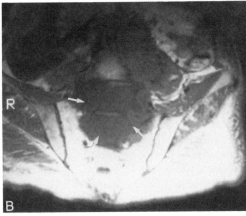

Figure 9–8. A 59-year-man had a history of bladder transitional cell carcinoma. He had a cystectomy and ileal loop placed. He had resolution of colicky low back pain. Approximately 2 years later, he experienced increasing back pain and difficulty defecating. MR of the lumbar spine revealed on proton density sagittal *(A)* and coronal T₁-weighted *(B)* views decreased signal intensity in the sacrum compatible with diffuse metastatic disease (white arrows). Anterior soft tissue mass is also present (black arrows). He died of metastatic disease within 1 year of the MR examination.

cial evaluation in an attempt to explain the failure of the previous treatment. This is predicated on the knowledge and belief that a patient's disability is related not only to his pathologic anatomy but also to his perception of pain and his mental stability in relation to his social environment. It is quite common to see a patient with a frank herniated disc continue working, regarding his disability as only a minor problem, while at the other end of the spectrum the hysterical patient takes to his bed at the slightest twinge of low back discomfort.

Drug habituation, depression, alcoholism, and other psychiatric problems are seen frequently in association with back pain. If the evaluation suggests any of these problems, proper measures should be instituted. There are a surprising number of ambulatory patients addicted to commonly prescribed medications who use back pain as an excuse to obtain these drugs. Narcotics and tranquilizers, alone or in combination, are common offenders. Narcotics are truly addictive, while tranquilizers have the potential for habituation and depression. Since the complaint of low back pain may be a manifestation of depression, it is counterproductive to treat such patients with agents that may exacerbate depression.

Those patients who do not show evidence of a systemic medical problem or psychiatric difficulties are referred to the "low back school."[22] This concept has as its basis the belief that patients with low back pain, given proper education and understanding of their disease, often can return to a productive and functional life. Ergonomics, the proper and efficient use of the body in work and recreation, is stressed, particularly as it relates to the spine. Back school need not be an expensive proposition. It can be as simple as a one time classroom session with a review of back problems and a demonstration of exercises with patient participation. This type of educational process has proved very effective. It is most important, however, that a patient be thoroughly screened before referral to this type of facility. One does not want to be in the position of treating a metastatic tumor in a classroom.

Individuals who continue to experience pain after 12 weeks of evaluation and therapy are considered as chronic pain patients. Recent investigations have suggested that defining pain as acute, subacute, and chronic may not be a helpful classification in the identification of those individuals with the potential for improvement.[23] The pain intensity, disability, and depression experienced by an individual is a better determinant of potential for improvement than the duration of pain. Decreasing pain intensity and the perception of disability and depression are key factors in patient improvement at any point in a treatment program.

Chronic pain therapy may include a number of treatment modalities: medications, physical therapy, TENS, biofeedback, relaxation therapy. The combination of two or more of these therapies simultaneously may be effective at modifying pain while the patient increases their physical function. Some patients remain resistant to therapy. These individuals may benefit from a referral to a multidisciplinary pain clinic.

Sciatica (Leg Pain Below the Knee)

The next group of patients consists of those with sciatica, which is defined in this instance as pain radiating below the knee. These people usually experience their symptoms secondary to mechanical pressure and inflammation of the nerve roots that originate between L4-5 (L5 nerve root) and L5-S1 (S1 nerve root). Pain, numbness, and tingling can then travel down the leg along the anatomic course of the particular nerve involved. The etiology of the mechanical pressure can be soft tissue (herniated disc), bone, or a combination of the two.

At this juncture, these patients have had up to 6 weeks of controlled physical activity and anti-inflammatory medication but still have persistent leg pain. The next therapeutic step is an epidural steroid injection.[24] This may be performed on an outpatient basis. The anti-inflammatory medication (steroids) is injected directly into the epidural space, close to the location of the actual compression of the nerve root. Epidural injections are usually prescribed after visualization of the lumbar spine by MR or CT scan. If symptoms and signs are classic for nerve impingement, the epidural injection may be given without radiographic tests. If the patient does not improve, radiographic evaluation of the lumbar spine is essential. Epidural injections have proved 40% effective in relieving leg pain. The maximum benefit from a single injection is achieved within 2 weeks. The injection may have to be repeated one or two times, and another 4 to 6 weeks should pass before its success or failure is determined. It should be pointed out that there are alternative conservative treatments available (such as traction, passive physical therapy, and manipulation). Each will be discussed in Section IV as to their efficacy. Unfortunately, these methods in general have not stood the test of scientific scrutiny, so they should not become a routine part of the treatment program.[25]

If epidural steroids are effective in alleviating the patient's leg pain or sciatica, the patient starts on a program of exercises and is encouraged to return promptly to a normal lifestyle. Heavy work (lifting more than 50 pounds regularly) is not recommended because these patients will be prone to recurrences of disc herniation. Those who have sustained a disc herniation should be placed on some type of restricted work. This treatment pathway usually will be completed in less than 3 months, and most patients with sciatica will not have to undergo any major invasive treatment. Thus, a radiculopathy in and of itself is not a contraindication to nonoperative therapy.

Should the epidural steroid injections prove ineffective and if 3 months have passed since the onset of pain, some type of invasive treatment should be considered. The patient group at this point is divided into those with probable herniated discs and those with symptoms secondary to spinal stenosis.

Patients with herniated discs have symptoms secondary to the nucleus pulposus herniating through the annulus fibrosus and causing pressure and inflammation of an individual nerve root. As already mentioned, the L5 and S1 nerve roots are those most commonly involved. The pain will radiate along the anatomic pathway of the nerves that travel below the knee and into the foot. The highest incidence of this entity occurs in the fourth decade of life but also can be seen in older patients.

The physician must now carefully re-evaluate the patient for a neurologic deficit and for a positive tension sign (straight leg raising test). For those with either a neurologic deficit or positive tension sign along with continued leg pain, a MR or CT scan should be obtained. MR is preferred as the inital study because of better vizualization of soft tissue structures (intervertebral discs) while offering adequate imaging of bony structures, (Fig. 9–9). If MR or CT is clearly positive and correlates with the clinical findings, myelography need not be performed since the test is invasive. If there is any question about the radiographic findings of the MR or CT, a metrizamide myelogram should be obtained.

There is repeated documentation that for surgery to be effective for the treatment of a herniated disc, the surgeon must find unequivocal preoperative evidence of nerve root compression.[26] Thus the more precise the preoperative diagnosis, the better the outcome. Mechanical nerve root compression must be firmly substantiated not only by neurologic examination but also by radiographic data before laminectomy. There is no place for "explora-

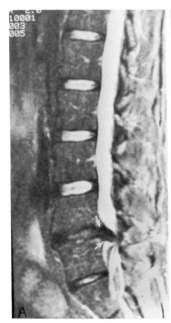
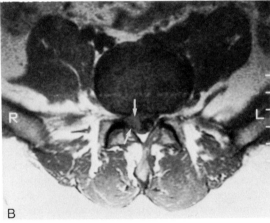

Figure 9–9. A 37-year-old man developed back pain after a piece of furniture fell on him while at work. He had back pain for about 2 years when he developed radicular right leg pain. MR of the lumbar spine revealed on a T_2-weighted sagittal (A) and T_1-weighted axial (B) images a large herniated nucleus pulposus at the L5-S1 level (white arrows). His leg pain resolved after three epidural corticosteroid injections.

tory" back surgery. If the patient has neither a neurologic deficit nor a positive straight leg raising test, then regardless of radiographic findings, there is not enough evidence of nerve root compression to undertake surgery. Twenty-five percent of asymptomatic patients have positive myelograms and 35% have positive CT scans.[27] A similar proportion of patients have MR findings for anatomic abnormalities that are unassociated with symptoms.[28] Normal patients also may have equivocal EMG findings. These patients without objective findings are the ones who have poor results and have given back surgery such a bad reputation.

If there are no objective findings of radiculopathy, the physician should avoid surgery and proceed to a psychosocial evaluation. Exceptions should be few and far between. When sympathy for the patient's complaints outweighs the objective evaluation, treatment is fraught with difficulties. Of those who meet these specific criteria for lumbar laminectomy, 95% can expect good to excellent results.[29]

The second group of patients whose symptoms are based on mechanical pressure on the neural elements are those with spinal stenosis.[30] Spinal stenosis is a narrowing of the spinal canal secondary to increased bone formation, a natural occurrence with age. Patients over 60 years of age are most affected by spinal stenosis. If the spinal canal is small to start with and then decreases further, pressure develops on the nerve which may cause radia-

tion of pain into the legs. These patients may or may not have a positive neurologic examination or straight leg raising test. Ambulation may result in mechanical irritation, poor excursion of the spinal nerves due to entrapment, edema, and neural ischemia. Accordingly, if these patients ambulate until their symptoms are reproduced, such as with a "stress test", the initially negative neurologic and tension signs may become positive. A stress test may include the patient walk some stairs or a distance in the office.

The diagnosis of spinal stenosis usually can be made from the plain roentgenograms, which will demonstrate facet degeneration, disc degeneration, and decreased interpedicular and sagittal canal diameter. Myelogram, CT, or MR will better define the involved areas than plain films (Fig. 9–10) and may be helpful to delineate the extent of surgery required for decompression. If symptoms are severe and there is radiographic evidence of spinal stenosis, surgery is appropriate. Age alone is not a deterrent to surgery. Many elderly people who are in good health except for a narrow spinal canal will benefit greatly from adequate decompression of the lumbar spine. Patients who have continued pain after surgery for a herniated intervertebral disc or spinal stenosis should be evaluated by the multioperated spine algorithm. Patients who fail to obtain pain relief with this algorithm should be treated with chronic pain therapy.

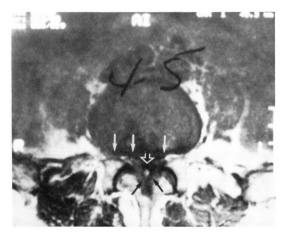

Figure 9–10. A 78-year-old woman developed increasing low back and leg pain associated with walking. She had a partial response to nonsteroidal therapy. MR was obtained in anticipation of lumbar epidural corticosteroid injection. MR of the lumbar spine axial view reveals marked spinal stenosis with osteophytes, bulging disc (white arrows), and ligamentum flavum hypertrophy (black arrows) compressing the cauda equina (open white arrow). She responded to epidural injections. She refused decompression surgery. (From Borenstein DG: Low back pain. In Klippel J, Dieppe P (eds): Rheumatology. St Louis, Mosby, 1994.)

Anterior Thigh Pain

A small percentage of patients will have pain that radiates from the back into the anterior thigh. This pain usually is relieved by rest and anti-inflammatory medications. If, after 6 weeks of treatment, the discomfort persists, a work-up should be initiated to search for underlying pathology. Several entities must be considered.

An inguinal hernia causes anterior thigh pain. Occasionally, hernia patients may experience pain in the lateral aspect of the low back. Careful physical examination is essential to identify those individuals with a direct or indirect inguinal hernia.

Hip arthritis causes pain that classically radiates to the groin. However, the peripheral nerves that supply the hip joint also innervate muscles in the low back and anterior thigh. Hip disease may present as lateral low back and anterior thigh pain. Once again, a careful physical examination will identify those individuals with decreased hip motion that may recreate their back pain. Roentgenograms of the hip demonstrate joint disease (Fig. 9–11).

An abdominal aneurysm may cause pain which radiates into the anterior thigh. Ultrasonography is a useful technique for visualization of the abdominal aorta and determining its integrity. CT scan is necessary if surgical intervention is contemplated.

Kidney disease should also be considered in a patient with anterior thigh pain. Stones in the kidney may cause pain that radiates from the back into the genitalia or anterior thigh. A urinalysis will reveal hematuria. An intravenous pyelogram (IVP) may be considered to evaluate the urinary tract.

Peripheral neuropathy, most commonly caused by diabetes, also can present initially as back pain with radiation to the anterior thigh. An elevation in fasting blood sugar should raise the possibility of glucose intolerance. Raised values on a formal oral glucose tolerance test confirm the diagnosis. Patients with femoral neuropathy associated with diabetes may have improvement in their symptoms with normalization of their glucose concentrations.

Retroperitoneal processes secondary to expanding structures cause back and anterior thigh pain. Retroperitoneal tumors cause symptoms including anterior thigh pain as well as back pain. Expanding structures in the retroperitoneum either compress or stretch the

Figure 9–11. A 64-year-old woman had a history of right-sided low back pain with radiation into the anterior thigh. An evaluation of her lumbar spine, including MR, was unrevealing. Physical examination of her hips revealed marked decrease in range of motion. A posteroanterior view of the pelvis revealed severe joint space narrowing along with sclerosis and subchondral cysts. She underwent right hip joint arthroplasty with resolution of her back and leg pain. She has refused left joint replacement. Two years after her operation she remains ambulatory without significant left hip pain on maximum nonsteroidal therapy.

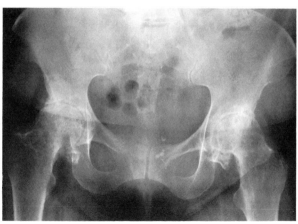

splanchnic nerves, which contain visceral afferents that share a common origin with those cutaneous nerves that innervate the anterior thigh. MR evaluation of the retroperitoneum is indicated if retroperitoneal tumors are suspected.

Patients with an L3-4 disc herniation may experience anterior thigh weakness, sensory loss, or, to a lesser degree, pain. Radiographic evaluation of the spinal canal, including CT or MR scan, can identify these individuals with a herniated disc.

If any of the entities listed above are discovered, the patient is treated accordingly. If no physical cause can be found for the anterior thigh pain, the patient is treated for recalcitrant back strain by following the algorithm.

Posterior Thigh Pain

The final group of patients will complain of back pain with radiation into the buttocks and posterior thigh. Most of them will be relieved of their symptoms with 6 weeks of conservative therapy. However, if their pain persists after the initial treatment period, they are considered to have back strain and are given a local injection of steroids and local anesthetic in the area of maximum tenderness. If the injection is unsuccessful, the next decision point is to distinguish between referred and radicular pain.

Referred pain is pain in mesodermal tissues of the same embryologic origin. The muscles, tendons, and ligaments of the buttocks, the sacroiliac joints, and posterior thigh have the same embryologic origin as those of the low back. When the low back is injured, pain may be referred to the posterior thigh, where it is perceived by the patient. Referred pain cannot be cured with a surgical procedure.

Radicular pain is caused by compression of an inflamed nerve root along the anatomic course of the nerve. A herniated disc or spinal stenosis in the high lumbar area (e.g., at the L2-3 or L3-4 interspace) could cause radiation of pain into the posterolateral thigh. An MR is used in this situation. If it is normal, the patient is considered to have referred pain and the diagnosis of back strain. If either test is abnormal, the patient is diagnosed as having mechanical root compression from either a herniated disc or spinal stenosis. Epidural steroids should be tried first; if these do not give adequate relief, a MR of the lumbar spine concentrating on the upper lumbar disc levels is

indicated (Fig. 9–12). If the patient has an identifiable lesion and a lack of response to therapy, surgical intervention is recommended. Patients who have continued pain after surgery for a herniated intervertebral disc should be evaluated by the multioperated

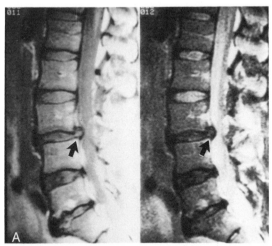

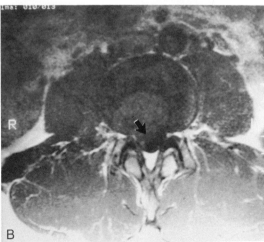

Figure 9–12. A 37-year-old man with a history of localized testicular carcinoma presented with right lateral thigh pain. Pain was localized to the trochanteric area initially but spread to the knee after an extended bicycle trip. Local trochanteric injection was helpful in decreasing the local pain but did not help the leg pain. MR of the lumbar spine reveals on proton density *(A, left side)* and T_2-weighted sagittal *(A)* and T_1-weighted axial *(B)* views a large posterolateral L3–L4 herniation (black arrows). The disc is impinging the right L3 and L4 nerve roots. A slight anterior spondylolisthesis of 3 mm of L3 on L4 is present. Also noted is degenerative disc signal at L4–L5 and L5–S1. Subsequently, the patient underwent hemilaminectomy and discectomy at L3–L4 and foraminotomies at L5–S1. Postoperatively, the posterolateral leg pain to the knee improved. Subsequently, he developed a second primary testicular tumor with metastatic disease. He is currently receiving radiation and chemotherapy.

spine algorithm. Patients who fail to obtain pain relief with this algorithm should be treated with chronic pain therapy.

This group of patients is very difficult to evaluate. The most common mistake is the performance of surgery on people thought to have radicular pain who actually have referred pain. Again, referred pain is not responsive to surgery.

In the majority of cases the diagnosis and management of low back pain is not necessarily a mystery. Approximately 20% of patients with low back pain have a specific pathoanatomic diagnosis.[31] The algorithm presents a series of easy-to-follow and clearly defined decision-making processes to identify those patients with specific diagnoses. Use of this algorithm provides patients with the most helpful, expeditious evaluation and does not subject them to procedures that are useless technical exercises.

In the next section, the low back pain and medical evaluation algorithms are presented. In the section following the algorithms, a clinical evaluation form including historic, physical, laboratory, and radiographic components of the diagnostic examination is presented. All or part of this form, as the physician thinks appropriate, may be used in the evaluation of the patient with back pain. A similar form has been published as part of the Quebec Spinal Task Force Report.[3]

Additional aids for differential diagnosis may be found in the appendix at the end of the book, which includes a truth table of differential diagnosis of low back pain and clinical data associated with specific disease entities that cause back pain.

LOW BACK PAIN (LBP) ALGORITHM

166

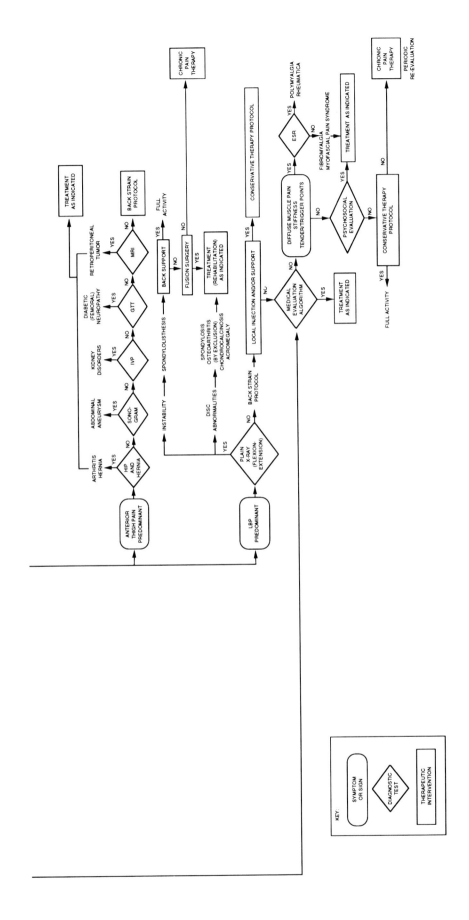

LOW BACK PAIN EVALUATION

MEDICAL HISTORY
Name: Sex: M_____ F_____   Date:

Address: Date of Birth:

Occupation: Workmen's Compensation: Y_____ N_____
                                         Self-employed: Y_____ N_____

FAMILY HISTORY
Family members with back pain: Y_____ N_____

Describe:

Other familial illness:

SOCIAL HISTORY
Working Y_____ N_____   Labor: Heavy_____ Moderate_____
                                                Sedentary_____ Light_____

Smoking: Alcohol: Recreational Drugs:

Leisure time activities: Hobbies: Sports:

Education:

PAST MEDICAL HISTORY
Current Medical Illnesses:

               Diabetes _____   Vascular/Hypertension _____

               Arthritis _____   Cancer _____   Other _____

Current Medications:

Severe injuries: Hospitalizations/Operations:

1

REVIEW OF SYSTEMS

Constitutional: Fever _____ Weight loss_____

Anorexia _____ Severe fatigue_____

Skin: Psoriasis_____ Nail changes_____ Nodules_____

Head/Neck: Conjunctivitis _____ Iritis_____

Oral ulcers_____ Thyroid _____

Cardiopulmonary: Dyspnea_____ Cough_____

Hemoptysis _____ Chest pain _____

Gastrointestinal: Abdominal pain_____ Blood in stool_____

Nausea/Vomiting____ Change in bowel _____ Ulcers _____
habits

Genitourinary: Frequency_____ Burning _____ Hematuria _____

Hesitancy _____ Sexual _____ Menses_____
dysfunction

Hematologic: Anemia_____ Bleeding disorder _____

Neurologic: Mental status_____ Muscle weakness_____ Sensation _____

Personality: Obsessive _____ Passive _____

Depressive _____ Anxious_____

Musculoskeletal: Arthritis _____

2

CHIEF COMPLAINT:

BACK PAIN:

Onset: Acute _____ Gradual _____ With activity _____

Twist _____ Fall _____ Bending _____

Lifting _____ Pulling/pushing _____

Increasing _____ Decreasing _____ Same _____

Direct blow/trauma _____

Duration: Days _____ Weeks _____ Months _____

Frequency: Daily _____ Episodic _____
Weekly _____ Continuous _____
Monthly _____
Other _____

Location and Radiation:
Paraspinous R _____ L _____
Sacroiliac R _____ L _____
Buttocks R _____ L _____
Thighs Anterior _____ Posterior _____
Lower leg R _____ L _____
Leg paresthesias _____ Leg weakness _____

Time of Day: AM _____ PM _____

3

AGGRAVATING FACTORS:

	Standing _____	Walking _____
	Sitting _____	Driving _____
Recumbency:	Supine _____	Prone _____
AM Stiffness:	Y_____ N_____	Duration_____
Movements:	Flexion _____	Extension_____
Other:	Coughing _____	Valsalva _____
	Sneezing _____	

ALLEVIATING FACTORS:

	Standing _____	Walking _____
	Sitting _____	
Recumbency:	Supine _____	Prone _____
Movements:	Flexion _____	Extension _____
Medications:	Antiinflammatories_____	Narcotics _____
	Muscle relaxants _____	
Supports:	Brace _____	

VISUAL PAIN SCALE

Severe ├──────────────────────────────────────┤ None

⊞ Numbness   ⬲ Pins & Needles

⊠ Burning   ⬚ Stabbing

■ Dull

4

PHYSICAL EXAMINATION

Vital Signs: T_____ P_____ R_____ BP_____ Weight_____ Height_____

General Description

Skin: Rash _____   Nodules _____

                    Vesicles _____   Petechiae _____

                    Ulcers _____

Head/   Conjunctivitis _____   Iritis _____
Neck

                    Fundi   _____   Oral ulcers _____

                    Thyromegaly _____

Lymph: Lymphadenopathy _____

Lungs: Chest expansion _____cm

                    Breath sounds _____

Heart: Cardiomegaly_____   Gallops _____

                    Murmurs   _____

Abdomen: Quadrant tenderness _____

                    Organomegaly_____

                    Masses—pulsatile _____

                    Bowel sounds _____

                    Hernia _____   CVA tenderness _____

Vessels: Pulses: Dorsalis pedis _____   Posterior tibial _____

                            Other _____

Bone/Muscle:

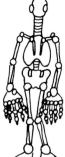

5

LUMBOSACRAL SPINE

STANDING:

Posterior view:

Pigmentation _____   Hair tufts _____

Scoliosis _____   Bone prominence___

Sacroiliac joint motion R_____ L_____

Trendelenburg sign R _____ L _____

Lateral view: Lordosis: Normal _____   Decreased _____   Increased_____

Kyphosis: Normal_____   Decreased _____   Increased_____

Lower extremity deformities_____

Anterior view: Pelvic tilt_____

Motion: Flexion _____ ^{0} Finger to floor_____cm

Extension _____ ^{0}

Lumbosacral rhythm   Normal_____   Reversed _____

Lateral bending   R _____ ^{0} L_____ ^{0}

Rotation   R _____ ^{0} L_____ ^{0}

Toe walking_____   Heel walking_____   Squat_____

Tenderness: Midline _____   Paraspinous _____   Iliac crest_____

Posterior iliac spine_____   Greater trochanter_____

Sciatic notch_____   Posterior thigh_____   Spasm_____

KNEELING: Ankle reflex   R_____   L_____

Forward flexion_____ ^{0}

SEATED IN CHAIR: Foot dorsiflexor strength   R_____   L _____

BENT FORWARD OVER EXAM TABLE: Gait: Normal _____   Abnormal _____

Antalgic_____   Shuffling_____   Wide based_____

Sacroiliac tenderness   R _____   L_____

6

SEATED-LEGS DANGLING:

Tripod sign   R_____   L _____
Knee reflex   R_____   L _____
Thigh pain _____   Knee pain_____

SUPINE: Leg lengths   R_____   L _____

Passive straight leg   R_____^{0} L_____^{0}
Lasègue test   R_____   L_____
Bilateral straight leg

Hip motion Flexion   R_____^{0} L_____^{0}
               Extension   R_____^{0} L_____^{0}
               Abduction   R_____^{0} L_____^{0}
               Adduction   R_____^{0} L_____^{0}
               Int. Rot.   R_____^{0} L_____^{0}
               Ext. Rot.   R_____^{0} L_____^{0}

Patrick test   R_____   L_____

Hoover test_____

Pelvic compression   Inward_____   Outward_____

Reflexes: Abdominal (T12-L2)
           Cremasteric (L1-L2)   R_____   L_____
           Adductor (L2)   R_____   L_____
           Patellar (L4)   R_____   L_____
           Ankle (S1)   R_____   L_____
           Bulbocavernosus (S2-S3)   R_____   L_____

Sensory: Medial thigh (L4)   R_____   L_____
           Anterior tibia (L5)   R_____   L_____
           First web space (L5)   R_____   L_____
           Posterior calf (S1)   R_____   L_____
           Lateral foot (S1)   R_____   L_____
           Perineum (S2-S5)   R_____   L_____

Motor strength: (0-5, 5 = Normal)
           Hip flexion (L2-L3)   R_____   L_____
           Hip extension (L4-L5)   R_____   L_____
           Knee flexion (L3-L4)   R_____   L_____
           Knee extension (L5-S1)   R_____   L_____
           Ankle dorsiflexion (L4-L5)   R_____   L_____
           Ankle plantar flexion (S1-S2)   R_____   L_____
           Ankle inversion (L4)   R_____   L_____
           Ankle eversion (L5-S1)   R_____   L_____

Long tract signs:

	Babinski sign	R _____	L _____
	Oppenheim's sign	R _____	L _____
	Clonus	R _____	L _____

PRONE:	Femoral stretch test (L2-L4)	R _____	L _____
	Gluteus maximus strength (L5-S1)	R _____	L _____
	Sensory: Posterior upper leg (S1-S2)	R _____	L _____
	Posterior lower leg (S3-S4)	R _____	L _____
	Perianal (S4-S5)	R _____	L _____

Rectal exam: Rectal tone_____   Rectal masses _____

Testicles_____   Pelvic organs _____

OTHER
TESTS: Schober's test _____ cm   Voluntary release _____

Well leg straight leg raising_____ Bow-string sign _____

Naffziger test_____   Valsalva test _____

Milgram test _____   Kneeling bench test __ Stoop test ____

Waddell test:

	Appropriate	Inappropriate
1. Tenderness	_____	_____
2. Simulation: axial loading	_____	_____
rotation	_____	_____
3. Distraction: seated	_____	
straight leg	_____	_____
4. Regional disturbances	_____	_____
5. Overreaction	_____	_____

DIAGNOSTIC TESTS

CBC: HCT_____   WBC_____   Platelets_____   Differential_____

ESR: _____mm/h (Wintrobe or Westergren)

SMA-12: Ca_____ P_____ Uric acid_____ Cholesterol_____T Protein_____ Albumin_____
Bilirubin_____ Alk Phos_____ LDH_____ SGOT_____ Acid Phosphatase_____

URINALYSIS: Sp Gr_____ Blood_____ Bilirubin_____ Acetone_____ Glucose_____
Protein_____   pH_____   Microscopic_____

8

RADIOGRAPHS:
    Plain Roentgenograms _____

                                         _____

    Bone scan   _____

                                           _____

    CT scan   _____

                                           _____

    MRI scan   _____

                                           _____

ELECTRODIAGNOSTIC STUDIES:
    Electromyogram   _____

                                           _____

    Nerve conduction   _____

                                           _____

           Pain quality: Superficial somatic_____ Deep somatic_____

                                      Radicular _____ Visceral-Referred___

                                      Psychogenic_____

DIAGNOSIS:

THERAPY:
    Rest   _____

    Drugs   _____

    Physical therapy   _____

    Injection   _____

    Surgical consultation _____

9

References

1. Lonstein MB, Wiesel SW: Standardized approaches to the evaluation and treatment of industrial low back pain. Spine State Art Rev 2:147, 1987.
2. Holmes HE, Rothman RH: The Pennsylvania plan: an algorithm for the management of lumbar degenerative disc disease. Spine 4:156, 1979.
3. Spitzer WO, LeBlanc FE, Dupuis M, et al.: Scientific approach to the assessment and management of activity-related spinal disorders: report of the Quebec Task Force on spinal disorders. Spine 12:S1, 1987.
4. Deyo RA, Rainville J, Kent DL: What can the history and physical examination tell us about low back pain? JAMA 268:760, 1992.
5. Webster's Dictionary, Springfield, Massachusetts, F & C Merriam Co, 1982.
6. Floman Y, Wiesel SW, Rothman RH: Cauda equina syndrome presenting as a herniated lumbar disk. Clin Orthop 147:234, 1980.
7. Neidre A: Low Back Pain: evaluation and treatment in the emergency department setting. Em Med Clin North Am 2:441, 1984.
8. Deyo RA, Diehl AK: Cancer as a cause of back pain: frequency, clinical presentation, and diagnostic strategies. J Gen Intern Med 3:230, 1988.
9. Gatchel RJ, Mayer TG, Capra P, et al.: Quantification of lumbar function: VI. The use of psychological measures in guiding physical functional restoration. Spine 11:36, 1986.
10. Korbon GA, DeGood DE, Schroeder ME, et al.: The development of a somatic amplification rating scale for low-back pain. Spine 12:787, 1987.
11. Walsh NE, Dumitru D: The influence of compensation on recovery from low back pain. Spine State Art Rev 2:109, 1987.
12. Bigos SJ, Battie MC, Spengler DM, et al.: A prospective study of work perceptions and psychological factors affecting the report of back injury. Spine 16:1, 1991.
13. Waddell G, McCulloch JA, Kummell E, et al.: Nonorganic physical signs in low back pain. Spine 5:117, 1980.
14. Deyo RA: Conservative therapy for low back pain: distinguishing useful from useless therapy. JAMA 250:1057, 1983.
15. Deyo RA, Diehl AK, Rosenthal M: How many days of bed rest for acute low back pain? A randomized clinical trial. N Engl J Med 315:1064, 1986.
16. Hurri H: The Swedish back school in chronic low back pain. I. Benefits. Scand J Rehab Med 21:33, 1989.
17. Rothman RH, Simeone FA: The Spine, 2nd ed. Philadelphia: W. B. Saunders Co., 1982.
18. Rothman RH: Indications for lumbar fusion. Clin Neurosurg 71:215, 1973.
19. Garvey TA, Marks MR, Wiesel SW: A prospective, randomized, double-blind evaluation of trigger-point injection therapy for low-back pain. Spine 14:962, 1989.
20. Borenstein DG, Feffer HL, Wiesel SW: Low back pain: an orthopedic and medical approach. Clin Res 33:757A, 1985.
21. Thelander U, Larsson S: Quantification of C-reactive protein levels and erythrocyte sedimentation rate after spinal surgery. Spine 17:400, 1992.
22. Fisk JR, Dimonte P, Courington SM: Back schools: past, present, and future. Clin Orthop 179:18, 1983.
23. Von Korff M, Deyo RA, Cherkin D, et al.: Back pain in primary care. Outcomes at 1 year. Spine 18:855, 1993.
24. White AH, Derby R, Wynne G: Epidural injections for the diagnosis and treatment of low back pain. Spine 5:78, 1980.
25. Frymoyer JW: Back pain and sciatica. N Engl J Med 318:291, 1988.
26. Tile M: The role of surgery in nerve root compression. Spine 9:57, 1984.
27. Wiesel SW, Tsourmas N, Feffer HL, et al.: A study of computer-assisted tomography: I. The incidence of positive CAT scans in an asymptomatic group of patients (1984 Volvo Award in Clinical Sciences). Spine 9:549, 1984.
28. Boden SD, Davis DO, Dina TS, et al.: Abnormal magnetic-resonance scans of the lumbar spine in asymptomatic subjects: a prospective investigation. J Bone Joint Surg 72S:403, 1990.
29. Hakelius A: Long term follow-up on sciatica. Acta Orthop Scand (suppl) 129:33, 1972.
30. Wiesel SW, Bernini PH, Roth RH: The Aging Lumbar Spine. Philadelphia: W. B. Saunders Co. 1983.
31. Nachemsom AL: Advances in low-back pain. Clin Orthop 200:266, 1985.

DISEASES ASSOCIATED WITH LOW BACK PAIN

Section III is a review of the illnesses associated with back pain. The discussion of each illness opens with a capsule summary that lists the frequency, location, and quality of back pain; the associated symptoms, signs, laboratory data, and radiographic findings; and the forms of therapy that are effective. The specifics of therapy are contained in the body of the associated chapter and in Section IV.

The frequency of back pain associated with each illness is quantified by the terms very common, common, uncommon, and rare. The percentage of patients with back pain associated with each term is as follows:

Very common—76% or greater
Common—51% to 75%
Uncommon—26% to 50%
Rare—25% or less

Each chapter contains data concerning prevalence, pathogenesis, clinical history, physical examination, laboratory data, radiographic evaluation, differential diagnosis, therapy, and prognosis for each disease.

The emphasis of each chapter is geared toward a review of back pain as it pertains to each illness. The chapter should not be considered a complete listing of all clinical characteristics associated with each disease. The factors that help the clinician recognize the underlying cause of the patient's low back pain and make the appropriate diagnosis are listed.

The section is divided into chapters according to primary disease processes, which include:

Mechanical
Rheumatologic
Infectious
Tumor and Infiltrative
Endocrinologic and Metabolic
Hematologic
Neurologic and Psychiatric
Referred Pain
Miscellaneous

Discussions of diseases that are only very rarely associated with back pain and are not included among the major subheadings of these chapters may be found in the differential diagnosis section under each subheading. For example, hemochromatosis is included in the differential diagnosis of Microcrystalline diseases.

Referred pain, although not in itself a primary disease process, is another major source of patients' complaints of low back pain. The chapter on referred pain includes disorders of vascular, genitourinary, and gastrointestinal origin that are associated with low back pain.

10

Mechanical Disorders of the Lumbosacral Spine

Mechanical disorders of the lumbosacral spine are the most common cause of low back pain. Mechanical low back pain may be defined as pain secondary to overuse of a normal anatomic structure (muscle strain) or pain secondary to injury or deformity of an anatomic structure (herniated nucleus pulposus). Mechanical disorders are local disorders of the spine. That is, the processes that cause pain are limited to the structures of the lumbosacral spine. Mechanical disorders are truly musculoskeletal diseases. Systemic complications with involvement of other organ systems (except the nervous system) are not associated with mechanical disorders. The presence of systemic illness (e.g., fever, weight loss, or anemia) should make the clinician look for a disease other than a mechanical disorder as the cause of the patient's symptoms and signs.

Mechanical disorders characteristically are exacerbated by certain activities and relieved by others. The pattern of alleviating and aggravating factors helps localize the disorder to particular portions of the lumbosacral spine; for example, flexion exacerbates disc disease but alleviates facet joint disease. The physical examination helps identify those individuals with neurologic dysfunction and significant muscle damage but is not sufficient to pinpoint the exact location of the injury. Laboratory data, in the form of electrophysiologic tests, can confirm the clinical suspicion of nerve impingement. Through radiologic evaluation of a patient with a mechanical disorder the physician may be able to identify anatomic alterations in the lumbosacral spine but can not necessarily correlate those changes with the patient's symptoms. The physician must take all of the clinical data together and formulate a working diagnosis that is reasonable, based upon the collected information.

It is essential to remember that the vast majority of patients with mechanical disorders improve given enough time. The physician does not want to intervene and cause the patient harm (inappropriate surgery) nor overlook the possibility of a serious complication associated with a mechanical disorder (cauda equina syndrome). Common sense is what is needed in the evaluation and therapy of these patients. The vast majority of patients will improve with controlled physical activity, nonaddictive nonsteroidal anti-inflammatory drugs, and, in appropriate patients, muscle relaxants. Surgical intervention is reserved for the patient who has not shown improvement on conservative therapy and has undeniable symptoms and signs associated with a mechanical disorder that is correctable by surgical intervention.

BACK STRAIN

Capsule Summary

Frequency of back pain—very common
Location of back pain—low back, buttock, posterior thigh
Quality of back pain—ache, spasm
Symptoms and signs—pain increased with activity, increased muscle tension
Laboratory and x-ray tests—none
Treatment—controlled physical activity, medications

PREVALENCE AND PATHOGENESIS

Back strain can be defined as nonradiating low back pain associated with a mechanical stress to the lumbosacral spine. The exact number of patients with back strain is difficult to determine. Most people with back pain (90%) have it on a mechanical basis.[1] Of patients with mechanical low back pain, back strain may account for 60% to 70% of abnormalities.

The etiology of back strain is not always clear but may be related to ligamentous or muscular strain secondary to either a specific traumatic episode or continuous mechanical stress. It is important to remember that the lumbosacral spine has two major biomechanical functions. The lumbosacral spine supports the upper body in a balanced, upright position while allowing locomotion. In a static, upright position, maintenance of erect posture is achieved through a balance among the expansile pressure of the intervertebral discs, the stretch placed on the anterior and posterior longitudinal and facet joint ligaments, and the sustained involuntary tone generated by the surrounding lumbosacral and abdominal muscles. The balance of the spine is also related to the reciprocal physiologic curves in the cervical, thoracic, and lumbosacral areas of the vertebral column. The balance in curvature results in an individual's posture. The proper alignment is also influenced by structures in the pelvis and lower extremities, including the hip joint capsule and the hamstring and gluteal maximus muscles. An individual's posture is good if it can be maintained for extended periods of time in an effortless, nonfatiguing fashion.

The movement of the lumbar spine is associated with a lumbar pelvic rhythm that results in the simultaneous reversal of the lumbar lordosis and rotation of the hips. During flexion and extension of the lumbar spine, tension is produced in the paraspinous, hamstring, and gluteal muscles, the fasciae that surround the muscles, and the ligaments that support the vertebral bodies and discs. In addition to the normal stresses placed on these structures with lowering and raising of the torso, the stresses on these anatomic structures are increased to an even greater degree when an individual is required to lift a heavy object. With lateral bending, paraspinous muscle activity increases on both sides of the spine but primarily on the side toward the lateral flexion. During axial rotation of the spine, the erector spinae muscles on the ipsilateral side and the rotator and multifidus muscles on the contralateral side are active. Lateral bending is accomplished by contraction of the abdominal wall oblique muscles in conjunction with the ipsilateral quadratus lumborum and psoas major.

Low back pain that is associated with back strain may be related to anatomic structures that are tonically contracted in the resting position. Low back pain may also occur during motion if the stress is greater than the supporting structures can sustain or if the components of the lumbosacral spine are structurally abnormal.[2]

Pain related to posture (static position) is thought to be related to an increase in the lumbosacral angle resulting in an accentuation of the lumbar lordosis (hyperlordosis). Some authorities have suggested that as much as 75% of all postural back pain is related to hyperlordosis.[2] The increased angle of the L5 and S1 vertebrae increases the shear forces of the disc, resulting in approximation of the articular surfaces of the facet joints and modifying their function to that of weight-bearing units. This irritates the synovial membrane and joint capsule. Hyperlordosis also increases stress on the supporting ligaments of the spine. Extension of the spine in younger individuals may increase to the degree that the spinous processes approximate, forming a pseudoarthrosis (syndrome of Baastrup). In hyperextension, not only may the facet joints and spinous processes be stressed, but the nerve root or recurrent nerve may be irritated (Fig. 10–1). Patients with recurrent nerve irritation may have low back pain only, while nerve root irritation is associated with radiation of pain to the leg, as seen with spinal stenosis.

It should be noted, however, that not all patients with increased lumbar lordosis have back pain. In a recent study, the degree of lumbar lordosis as determined by radiographs was no different for individuals with or without low back pain.[3] Until this controversy is resolved, hyperlordosis should be considered as a source of symptoms only after other causes of back pain have been eliminated from a physician's differential diagnostic list.

Low back pain may also occur during motion of the lumbosacral spine or with physical stresses (weight) that are greater than the forces that can be supported by muscular and ligamentous structures. The lumbar spine is required to support forces many times body weight. When lifting an object, an individual initially contracts the appropriate muscles. If the force is too great to be resisted by the

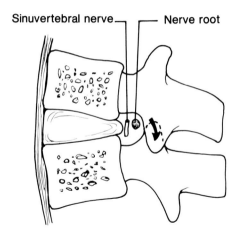

Figure 10–1. Nerve impingement with lumbosacral hyperextension. Extension approximates the articular surfaces of the facet joints *(arrow)* and narrows the neural foramen. Extension also causes the nucleus pulposus to move posteriorly, resulting in stretch of the annular fibers. Pain may result from the stretching of the annular fibers (back pain), or compression of the sinuvertebral nerve (back pain), nerve root (radicular pain), or facet joint (back and radicular pain).

muscle or if the muscle is fatigued, the stress is transferred to the ligaments. The intradiscal pressure increases and, if sufficiently strong, the force is passed on to the facet joints, which are not normally weight-bearing articulations. If the force is of a sufficient magnitude, damage can occur in muscle fibers, tendons, ligaments, annulus fibrosus, or facet joints.

If the lumbosacral spine or surrounding structures are anatomically abnormal, "normal" motion may result in strain pain. For example, patients with scoliosis have asymmetric orientation of their facet joints. The position of the facet joints does not allow free movement. The joint surfaces may be impacted to a greater degree in this orientation of the spine than joint surfaces found in a straight spine. Supporting structures may shorten in response to the curved configuration of the spine. Normal motions may be met with restriction because of limited excursion of ligaments and muscles. Tight hamstrings may limit full flexion of the lumbar spine, resulting in greater stretching forces being placed on the interspinous ligaments. In patients with normal hamstring motion but limited lumbar flexion, bending over will cause strain on the stretched posterior longitudinal ligaments and "tight" paraspinous muscles.

Damage may occur in lumbosacral spinal structures if the amount of force generated does not match the stress placed on the spine. Through experience, an individual will gauge

the amount of energy needed to complete a task, such as lifting a box. If the box is empty, a smaller amount of force is needed to lift the box. If the box is full and heavy, a greater amount of force is needed. If a great amount of force is generated in anticipation of a box being heavy when in fact it is empty, the extra force that has been generated may be dissipated through excessive movement of the spine, which may exceed the usual limits imposed by joint capsule and ligaments, resulting in tissue damage. On the other hand, if only a few muscle groups are recruited to lift an "empty" box when it is full, the force generated by the muscles will be inadequate to lift the object and the muscles will be damaged.[4] These scenarios may be further complicated if the lumbar spine is in a mechanically disadvantaged position (rotated, fully flexed). In these positions, the fibers of the annulus fibrosus are strained and may tear, causing fissures to occur. The disruption of these annular fibers causes degeneration of the disc and may be associated with production of pain.[5] The pain associated with annular tears may account for the history of frequent episodes of low back discomfort in patients who eventually rupture a nucleus pulposus.

A great deal of controversy surrounds the concept of skeletal muscle as the cause of low back pain. Evidence has been presented suggesting that low back spasm is a myth.[6] The lack of electromyographic evidence of increased muscle activity is used to support the argument that increased muscle contraction does not exist.[7] The presence of muscle edema is suggested as a reason for the physical changes in the muscle noticed on physical examination.[8]

Recent studies have demonstrated significant abnormalities in paraspinal muscle function. Dynamometry and postural endurance testing has demonstrated paraspinal weakness and excess fatigability in patients with low back pain.[9, 10] Muscle wasting and weakness can arise rapidly because of reduced motor unit recruitment owing to fear of pain or reflex inhibition. Muscle imbalance predisposes to mechanical disruption that perpetuates mechanical disadvantage. The endurance of back muscles related to a task is a more useful predictor of incidence of back pain than is the absolute strength of these muscles.[11]

Others have suggested that back strain is a manifestation of anxiety and is psychosomatic in origin.[12] Varying degrees of anxiety cause regional ischemia and altered states of muscle contractility and spasm mediated through the autonomic nervous system. However, review of a number of studies demonstrates no increased prevalence of neurotic symptoms in patients with back pain compared to those without back pain.[13]

In summary, muscle pain in low back pain patients may be caused by four different mechanisms.[14] 1. Pain is associated with muscle strain that is related to muscle disruption from indirect trauma such as excessive stretch or tension. First-degree strain is associated with microscopic disruption of muscle fibers. Second-degree strain causes macroscopic disruption of fibers but preserves structural integrity. Third-degree strain causes complete disruption of the muscle. An animal model of muscle strain reveals improved function by the seventh day after injury. A source of continued risk for recurrent injury is inelastic scar tissue. 2. Another possible source of muscle pain is muscle fatigue associated with overuse. Fatigue has a metabolic component manifested by increased concentrations of lactic acid, a byproduct of anaerobic metabolism. High loads requiring maximum effort of muscles causes ultrastructural damage to muscle with a delayed inflammatory response.[15] These alterations in muscle fibers cause release of inflammatory mediators associated with edema and pain receptor stimulation that results in pain. 3. Muscle spasm is associated with persistent contraction of muscle. The absence of blood flow with accumulation of metabolic byproducts may stimulate pain receptors within blood vessels. Studies with integrated electromyography demonstrates the increased central recruitment of paraspinal muscles.[9] 4. Paraspinous muscles become deconditioned after injury. Radiographic evaluation of cross-sectional views of patients with back pain demonstrate decreased muscle mass in paraspinous and psoas muscles.[16] Decreased muscle mass results in decreased muscle power that puts individuals at risk for persistent muscle injury. Determination of the cause of muscle pain in low back pain patients has implications for the choice of appropriate therapy.

CLINICAL HISTORY

Patients with muscle strain have back pain as their main complaint. The pain can be limited to a small local area or can cover a diffuse area of the lumbosacral spine but does not radiate to the lower extremities. At times, there may be a referral of pain to the buttocks or posterior thigh, since the mesenchymal structures in the lower back, buttocks, and posterior thigh all originate from the same embryonic tissue. Such referral of pain does not necessarily connote any mechanical compression of the neural elements and should not be called sciatica.

The patient may experience pain simultaneously with an injury. Subsequently, the pain increases in intensity and grows larger in its distribution after a few hours. The change in pain is associated with increasing edema in the injured structure along with the reflex contraction of surrounding muscles that limit motion. The patient may be able to continue to be active for a few hours. However, marked pain and stiffness occur the next day after sleeping. Flexion or extension of the spine may cause pain. Pain occurs with the motion that contracts the injured muscle. Certain motions may be painless, while others cause incapacitating pain. In general, muscle strain will be increased with activity and relieved with rest.

PHYSICAL EXAMINATION

Muscle strain results from overuse or overstretching of a muscle. On physical examination, any active motion of the involved muscle against resistance will cause pain. In one study of 429 patients with low back pain, 56 (13%) had contracted muscles on physical examination.[17] If a patient stands and is asked to bend laterally against resistance, resulting in muscle contraction without motion, he will complain of discomfort in the damaged muscle. The damaged muscle is tender on palpation. Passive stretching of the muscle will also cause pain. For example, backward bending against resistance will be instantaneously painful with muscle contraction, while forward flexion will become painful only after excursion is sufficient to stretch the muscle in a patient with erector spinae damage.

Patients with ligamentous sprains (disruption of the attachment of ligaments to bone) also develop localized back pain. Patients with supraspinous ligament sprains do not develop pain with active or passive extension but experience pain when the damaged ligament and its attachment to bone are stressed with flexion. Diagnosis of other ligamentous sprains is more difficult, since these structures are deep inside the back. Passive movements that put stress on the involved ligament will cause back pain, but identifying the specific location of injury is difficult.

Not infrequently, patients with muscle or ligamentous strain will develop pain in the low back in an area lateral to the fourth and fifth lumbar vertebrae and medial to the posterior iliac crest. This area of pain also spreads down to the sacrum. This area, referred to as the "multifidus triangle," contains a number of tissues, including facet joints, transversus ligament, quadratus lumborum and multifidus muscle, iliolumbar ligament, and dorsolumbar fascia, which may be sources of low back pain.[18] The greatest portion of stress placed upon the lumbosacral spine is concentrated in this area, making it a common location for tissue injury.

The usual physical findings are limited to local tenderness over the involved area with limited motion; however, the attacks will vary in intensity and can conveniently be divided into three categories: mild, moderate, and severe. The mild is associated with subjective pain without objective findings, and patients usually are able to return to customary activity in less than a week. The moderate is characterized by a limited range of spinal motion and paravertebral muscle spasm as well as pain, and patients frequently resume full activity in under 2 weeks. The severe may cause patients to tilt forward or list to one side. These patients have trouble ambulating and can take up to 3 weeks to recover full function.

Other than the abnormalities already described, the remainder of the physical exami-

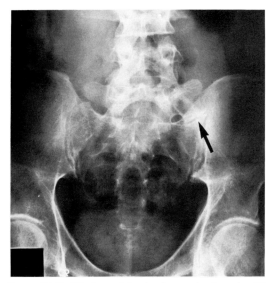

Figure 10–3. AP view of the lumbosacral spine of a 28-year-old man with systemic lupus erythematosus with abdominal pain of peritoneal origin. The roentgenogram revealed sacralization of the left part of the L5 vertebra with the formation of a pseudoarthrosis *(arrow)*.

nation is normal in patients with muscle strain. Specifically, the neurologic examination is normal in these individuals.

LABORATORY DATA

Laboratory tests are entirely normal in patients with back strain.

RADIOGRAPHIC EVALUATION

Low back strain does not cause or result from abnormalities that can be seen on radiographic evaluation of the lumbosacral spine. Thus, if the physician feels confident of the diagnosis of mechanical low back strain, a radiographic study during the initial evaluation is not necessary.[19]

Congenital abnormalities in the lumbar spine are a frequent finding noted in about 5% of the individuals in a normal population. The most common congenital abnormality is spina bifida occulta, which is found most frequently at the first sacral vertebra (Fig. 10–2). Another abnormality is sacralization or incorporation of the transverse process of the fifth lumbar vertebra into the sacrum (Fig. 10–3).[20] A sixth lumbar vertebra in addition to the normal number of five also is occasionally seen with lumbarization of the spine (Fig. 10–4). Most congenital abnormalities are asymptomatic. The recognition of a congenital abnor-

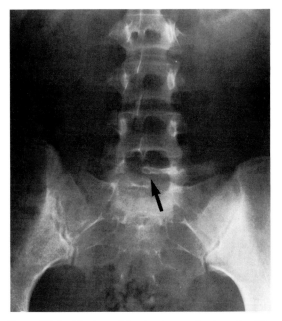

Figure 10–2. AP view of the lumbosacral spine of a 22-year-old asymptomatic woman with a congenital abnormality of the L5 vertebral body, including a spina bifida occulta *(arrow)*.

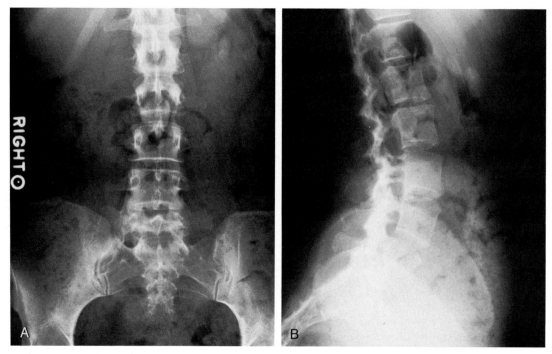

Figure 10–4. AP *(A)* and lateral *(B)* views of the lumbosacral spine of a 48-year-old woman. The patient has 6 lumbar vertebrae. A chest roentgenogram was obtained to verify the presence of 12 thoracic vertebrae.

mality occurs most frequently as a serendipitous event on a roentgenogram taken for another purpose (intravenous pyelogram, flat plate of the abdomen).

Theoretically, congenital abnormalities may be thought of as causing mechanical imbalances in the spine that may be associated with pain. The loss of a spinous process with spina bifida results in a loss of bony attachment for interspinous ligaments and paraspinous muscles and fascia. Sacralization of the fifth lumbar vertebra or lumbarization of the first sacral vertebra, particularly if unilateral, may cause an imbalance in motion, limiting rotation and increasing stress above the fused component. In the vast majority of patients, the fusions are extremely firm and are unassociated with symptoms. Low back pain should be ascribed to congenital abnormalities only after all other causes of back pain have been eliminated as possibilities.[21]

DIFFERENTIAL DIAGNOSIS

The diagnosis of back strain is based on the history of localized low back pain associated with a traumatic event, and a compatible physical examination demonstrating localized pain, muscle spasm, and a normal neurologic examination. The symptoms of back strain may be components of the list of complaints mentioned by patients with a wide variety of disease processes, including spondyloarthropathies and benign tumors of the lumbar spine. Muscle spasm is a reflex that occurs in response to bone or joint inflammation. The age of the patient, the presence of constitutional symptoms, or the persistence of pain should alert the physician to an alternative cause other than muscle strain (Table 10–1).

Trauma to the lumbosacral spine may also be associated with localized low back pain.[22] In a functional sense, there is little difference between apparent bone injuries and associated soft tissue disruptions. The functional effect of a sprain of the interspinous ligament is no different from that of a fracture or avulsion of a spinous process. Similarly, tearing of muscular attachments to the transverse process is functionally no different from an avulsion of that transverse process manifested as a fracture. The degree of trauma to the spine that is associated with muscle strain or sprain may limit motion but does not cause any instability. Trauma to the spine that results in facet dislocations, severe compression fractures, or Chance fracture (seatbelt injury) may cause instability of the spine and may damage neural elements. The treatment of patients with these injuries requires the expertise of a trained spine surgeon.

Patients with leg length discrepancies may

TABLE 10–1. MECHANICAL LOW BACK PAIN

	MUSCLE STRAIN	HERNIATED NUCLEUS PULPOSUS	OSTEO-ARTHRITIS	SPINAL STENOSIS	SPONDYLO-LISTHESIS	SCOLIOSIS
Age (years)	20–40	30–50	>50	>60	20	30
Pain pattern						
Location	Back (unilateral)	Back (unilateral)	Back (unilateral)	Leg (bilateral)	Back	Back
Onset	Acute	Acute (prior episodes)	Insidious	Insidious	Insidious	Insidious
Standing	↑	↓	↑	↑	↑	↑
Sitting	↓	↑	↓	↓	↓	↓
Bending	↑	↑	↓	↓	↑	↑
Straight leg	−	+	−	+ (stress)	−	−
Plain x-ray	−	−	+	+	+	+

complain of low back pain associated with muscular contraction. Patients may have low back pain, greater trochanteric bursitis, or degenerative hip disease. Pelvic obliquity resulting from a discrepancy of leg lengths may contribute to muscle pain and eventual degenerative changes in the lumbar spine. Measuring the lengths of leg with the patient in a supine position can determine the degree of leg length inequality. A simple heel lift can provide symptomatic relief of low back pain in the patient with significant leg length inequality.[23]

Controversy continues to surround the use of discography as a means to determine degenerative discs that are sources of low back pain. A controlled, prospective study reported on the accuracy of discography in detecting symptomatic intervertebral discs.[24] Discography revealed abnormal findings in 13 of the 20 discs in symptomatic individuals. In asymptomatic individuals, discogram was abnormal in 17%. A similar proportion (26%) was noted in a study by Holt.[25] Discography is not reliable and cannot be recommended as a specific test for the diagnosis of low back pain.

TREATMENT

The therapy of back strain includes controlled physical activity, nonsteroidal anti-inflammatory drugs, muscle relaxants, and physical therapy. Back strain is improved with controlled activity.[26] A period as short as 2 days has been shown to be effective at relieving back pain.[27] Continuing bed rest to 7 days did not appreciably decrease pain or hasten return to work. Convincing the patient to limit activities is a primary goal of therapy. Controlled physical activity allows the injured tissues to rest, permitting a greater opportunity for healing without reinjury. The time spent by the physician explaining the rationale for controlled physical activity to the patient is worth the effort. Bed rest is kept to a minimum. Increasing evidence supports the use of active exercise early in the course of back strain to maximize function. As soon as the very acute pain is diminished, patients should be encouraged to increase physical activity. A physical therapist may be used if the patients require encouragement to remain mobile.[28]

Non-narcotic analgesics in the form of nonsteroidal, anti-inflammatory drugs are helpful in making patients comfortable while their injury heals. Nonsteroidal drugs with a rapid onset of action are most helpful in patients with acute pain. These drugs may be continued until the patients' symptoms have resolved. Muscle relaxants may be helpful in the patient who has palpable spasms on physical examination or has difficulty sleeping at night because of muscle pain. Nonaddictive analgesics and muscle relaxants are preferred. The combination of nonsteroidal, anti-inflammatory drug with a muscle relaxant is better than a nonsteroidal alone in improving pain relief in low back pain patients with muscle spasm on physical examination.[29] Physical therapy modalities, in the form of cold (ice massage) initially or heat (warm bath) subsequently, may decrease pain and diminish spasm. Patients with very localized pain and severe spasm limiting mobility may benefit from an injection of local anesthetic with or without the addition of corticosteroid preparation. The injection relieves pain and blocks reflex spasm. These injections should be given to compliant patients who will limit their activity during the natural course of healing. Increased activity may cause additional damage to musculoligamentous structures, which may not be recognized by the patient in whom the protective mechanism of pain has been blocked by injection. Pressure over the maximum point of tenderness also may be effective in decreasing muscle spasm and pain.[30] Braces are reserved for patients who must remain active while healing continues. Braces may be recommended for subacute or chronic low back pain. A variety of therapies including traction, manipulation, and facet injection have been proposed for idiopathic low back pain. The scientific evidence to support the efficacy of many of these modalities is lacking.[31] (For additional information on therapy, see Section IV.)

PROGNOSIS

The course of patients with back strain is one of gradual improvement over a 2-week period. Almost 90% are cured in a 2-month period.[32] The recovery is total, without any lasting impairment.

Ten percent of patients may continue to experience low back pain associated with muscle strain. Pain may continue for months or years. This group of patients accounts for 70% to 80% of the costs associated with low back pain.[33] These patients are experiencing chronic low back pain, which must be evaluated and treated in a manner that takes into account the special difficulties of individuals with chronic pain. The goal of therapy in these individuals is to maximize function of the lumbosacral spine. These patients may receive drugs, physical therapy, psychiatric support, and vocational rehabilitation as part of their therapeutic program.

Another important consideration in the patient with low back strain is the likelihood of recurrence. The first episode of back pain is usually the briefest and least severe. However, the vast majority of individuals with an episode of back pain are at risk of developing another episode of back pain that will be more severe and of greater duration.[34] Of patients with occupationally related acute episodes of low back pain, 60% will have recurrent symptoms within 1 year.[35] The risk for an additional episode of back pain lessens after 2 years. The rate may be as high as 50% to 60% within 3 to 5 years.[34] These patients may have symptoms resistant to therapies that are beneficial in management of acute back pain, and therefore may require modifications in their work environment to limit the stress placed on the lumbosacral spine.

References

BACK STRAIN

1. Nachemson A: The lumbar spine—an orthopaedic challenge. Spine 1:59, 1976.
2. Cailliet R: Low Back Pain Syndrome, 3rd ed. Philadelphia: FA Davis Company, 1981, pp 53–68.
3. Hansson T, Bigos S, Beecher P, Wortley M: The lumbar lordosis in acute and chronic low-back pain. Spine 10:154, 1985.
4. Magora A: Investigation of the relation between low back pain and occupation: IV. Physical requirements: bending, rotation, reaching, and sudden maximal effort. Scand J Rehabil Med 5:186, 1973.
5. Farfan HF, Cossette JW, Robertson GW, et al.: Effects of torsion on lumbar intervertebral joints: the role of torsion in the production of disc degeneration. J Bone Joint Surg 52A:468, 1970.
6. Johnson EW: The myth of skeletal muscle spasm. Am J Phys Med Rehabil 68:1, 1989.
7. Harell A, Mead S, Mueller E: The problem of spasm in skeletal muscle: a clinical and laboratory study. JAMA 143:640, 1950.
8. Johnson EW: Editor's reply. Am J Phys Med Rehabil 68:256, 1989.
9. Cooper RG: Understanding paraspinal muscle dysfunction in low back pain: a way forward. Ann Rheum Dis 52:413, 1993.
10. Biering-Sorensoen F: Physical measurements as risk indicators for low back trouble over a one year period. Spine 9:106, 1984.
11. Parnianpour M, Nordin MA, Kahanovitz N, Frankel V: The triaxial coupling of torque generation of trunk muscles during isometric exertions and effect of fatiguing isoinertial movements on the motor output and movement. Spine 13:982, 1988.
12. Sarno JE: Etiology of neck and back pain: an autonomic myoneuralgia? J Nerv Mental Dis 169:55, 1981.
13. Cypress BK: Characteristics of physician visits for back symptoms: a national perspective. Am J Public Health 73:389, 1983.
14. Andersson GBJ: Evaluation of muscle function. In: Frymoyer JW, Ducker TB, Hadler NM, et al. (eds): The Adult Spine: Principles and Practice. New York: Raven Press, 1991, pp 241–274.
15. Newham DJ: The consequences of eccentric contractions and their relation to delayed onset muscle pain. Eur J Appl Physiol 57:353, 1988.
16. Cooper RG, Forbes W StC, Jayson MIV: Radiographic demonstration of paraspinal muscle wasting in patients with chronic low back pain. Br J Rheumatol 31:398, 1992.
17. Magora A: Investigation of the relation between low back pain and occupation. Scand J Rehabil Med 7:146, 1975.
18. Bauwens P, Cayer AB: The "multifidus triangle" syndrome as a cause of recurrent low back pain. Br Med J 2:1306, 1955.

19. Deyo RA, Diehl AK: Lumbar spine films in primary care: current use and selective ordering criteria. J Gen Intern Med 1:20, 1986.

20. Timmi PG, Wieser C, Zinn W. The transitional vertebra of the lumbosacral spine. Rheumatol Rehabil 16:180, 1977.

21. Keim HA, Durning RP: A new modified classification of transitional lumbosacral vertebrae and an analysis of Bertolotti's symptom-complex. Orthop Rev 11:(2)17, 1982.

22. Bucholz RW, Gill K: Classification of injuries to the thoracolumbar spine. Orthop Clin North Am 17:67, 1986.

23. Rothenberg RJ: Rheumatic disease aspects of leg length inequality. Semin Arthritis Rheum 17:196, 1988.

24. Walsh TR, Weinstein JN, Spratt KF, et al.: Lumbar discography in normal subjects: a controlled, prospective study. J Bone Joint Surg 72A:1081, 1990.

25. Holt EP Jr: The question of lumbar discography. J Bone Joint Surg 50A:720, 1968.

26. Wiesel SW, Cuckler JM, Deluca F, et al.: An objective analysis of conservative therapy. Spine 5:324, 1980.

27. Deyo RA, Diehl AK, Rosenthal M: How many days of bed rest for acute low back pain? N Engl J Med 315:1064, 1986.

28. Waddell G: Simple low back pain: Rest or active exercise? Ann Rheum Dis 52:317, 1993.

29. Borenstein DG, Lacks SL, Wiesel S: Cyclobenzaprine and naproxen versus naproxen alone in the treatment of acute low back pain and muscle spasm. Clin Ther 12:125, 1990.

30. Garvey TA, Marks MR, Wiesel SW: A prospective, randomized, double-blind evaluation of trigger-point injection therapy for low back pain. Spine 14:962, 1989.

31. Nachemson AL: Newest knowledge of low back pain: a critical look. Clin Orthop 279:8, 1992.

32. Dillane JB, Fry J, Kalton G: Acute back syndrome: a study from general practice. Br Med J 3:82, 1966.

33. Frymoyer JW: Back pain and sciatica. N Engl J Med 318:291, 1988.

34. Troup JDG, Martin JW, Lloyd DCEF: Backpain in industry: a prospective study. Spine 6:61, 1981.

35. Berquist-Ullman M, Larsson U: Acute low back pain in industry: a controlled prospective study with special reference to therapy and confounding factors. Acta Orthop Scand (Suppl) 170:1, 1977.

ACUTE HERNIATED NUCLEUS PULPOSUS

Capsule Summary

Frequency of back pain—very common

Location of back pain—low back to lower leg

Quality of back pain—sharp, shooting, burning, paresthesias in lower leg

Symptoms and signs—positive straight leg raising test, weakness, asymmetric reflexes

Laboratory and x-ray—CT, MR, myelogram—disc herniation. MR is the most sensitive test.

Treatment—controlled activity, medications, surgical excision of disc for conservative therapy failures

PREVALENCE AND PATHOGENESIS

A herniated disc can be defined as the herniation of the nucleus pulposus through the fibers of the annulus fibrosus.[1] Most disc ruptures occur during the third and fourth decade of life while the nucleus pulposus is still gelatinous. The time of the day a herniation occurs may relate to diurnal alterations in spinal anatomy. A cadaveric study of lumbar spine demonstrated changes of disc heights, water content, swelling pressure, compressive stiffness, bulging, loading of apophyseal joints, and forward and backward bending properties when loaded with compressive forces. The most likely time of the day associated with increased forces on the disc is in the morning.[2] The perforations usually arise through a defect just lateral to the posterior midline where the posterior longitudinal ligament is weakest. The two most common levels for disc herniation are L4–5 and L5–S1, accounting for 98% of lesions; pathology at the L2–3 and L3–4 can occur but is relatively uncommon.[3] Overall, 90% of disc herniations are at the L4–L5 and L5–S1 levels. Less than 10% of herniations occur at higher lumbar levels.

Approximately 80% of the population will experience significant back pain in the course of a herniated disc. The groups at greatest risk of developing herniations of intervertebral discs are younger individuals, with a mean age of 35 years.[4, 5] Only 35% of patients with disc herniation actually develop true sciatica. Not infrequently, sciatica develops 6 to 10 years after the onset of low back pain. The period of time of localized back pain may correspond to repeated damage to annular fibers that irritates the sinuvertebral nerve but does not result in disc herniation.

Disc herniations at L5-S1 will usually compromise the first sacral nerve root; a lesion at the L4–5 level will most often compress the fifth lumbar root, while a herniation at L3–4 more frequently involves the fourth lumbar root. It should be appreciated that variations in root configuration as well as in the position of the herniation itself can modify these relationships. Thus, an L4–5 disc rupture can at times affect the first sacral as well as the fifth lumbar root, and in extreme lateral herniations, the nerve existing at the same level as the disc will be involved.[6] These far lateral lumbar disk herniations may not be recognized for a number of months.[7]

Older patients may also develop disc herniation. Disc tissue that causes compression in elderly patients is composed of the annulus fibrosus and portions of the cartilaginous endplate. The cartilage is avulsed from the vertebral body.[8]

It is important to realize that not everyone with a disc herniation has significant discomfort. A large herniation in a capacious canal may not be clinically apparent, since there is no compression of the neural elements. On the other hand, a minor protrusion in a small canal may be crippling, since there is not enough room to accommodate both the disc and the nerve root.[9]

CLINICAL HISTORY

Clinically, the patients' major complaint is a sharp, lancinating pain. In many cases, there may be a prior history of intermittent episodes of localized low back pain. The pain not only is present in the back but also radiates down the leg in the anatomic distribution of the affected nerve root. It will usually be described as deep and sharp, progressing from above downward in the involved leg. Its onset may be insidious or sudden and associated with a tearing or snapping sensation in the spine. Occasionally when sciatica develops the back pain may resolve since once the annulus has ruptured, it may no longer be under tension. Disc herniation occurs with sudden physical effort when the trunk is flexed or rotated.

Finally, the sciatica may vary in intensity; it may be so severe that patients will be unable to ambulate and they will feel that their back is "locked." On the other hand, the pain may be limited to a dull ache which increases in intensity with ambulation. Pain is worsened in the flexed position and relieved in extension of the lumbar spine. Characteristically, patients with herniated discs have increased pain with sitting, driving, walking, coughing, sneezing, or straining.

PHYSICAL EXAMINATION

The physical examination will demonstrate a decrease in the range of motion of the lumbosacral spine, and patients may list to one side as they try to bend forward. On ambulation, patients walk with an antalgic gait, holding the involved leg flexed so as to put as little weight as possible on the extremity.

The neurologic examination is very important and may yield objective evidence of nerve root compression. It should be realized that there can be nerve root compression that causes pain but leaves the root enough room to function normally with no objective deficit. Also a nerve deficit may have little temporal

relevance, since it may be related to a prior attack at a different level.

When the first sacral root is compressed, the patient may have gastrocnemius-soleus weakness and be unable to repeatedly raise up on the toes of that foot. Atrophy of the calf may be apparent, and the ankle (Achilles) reflex is often diminished or absent. Sensory loss, if present, is usually confined to the posterior aspect of the calf and lateral side of the foot (see Fig. 3–14).

Involvement of the fifth lumbar nerve root can lead to weakness in extension of the great toe, and in a few cases to weakness of the everters and dorsiflexors of the foot. A sensory deficit can appear over the anterior leg and the dorsomedial aspect of the foot down to the great toe (see Fig. 3–13). There are usually no primary reflex changes, but on occasion, a diminution in the posterior tibial reflex can be elicited. There must be asymmetry in obtaining this reflex for it to have any clinical significance.

With compression of the fourth lumbar nerve root, the quadriceps muscle is affected; the patient may note weakness in knee extension, which is often associated with instability. Atrophy of the thigh musculature can be marked. A sensory loss may be apparent over the anteromedial aspect of the thigh, and the patellar tendon reflex can be diminished (see Fig. 3–12).

Nerve root sensitivity can be elicited by any method that creates tension. The straight leg raising test is the one most commonly employed. This test is performed with the patient supine. One of the examiner's hands is used to stabilize the pelvis while the other slowly raises the leg by the heel, keeping the knee fully extended. The test is considered positive only if pain develops in the leg below the knee or if the patient's radicular symptomatology is reproduced. Back pain alone does not indicate a positive test. As noted in Chapter 4, many variations of this test have been described and all can be useful as long as they are performed and interpreted correctly. One study correlated the location of the pain and the position of the protrusion of the disc. Central protrusions cause back pain, lateral protrusions cause leg pain, and intermediate protrusions cause pain in both locations.[10]

LABORATORY DATA

Medical screening laboratory tests (blood counts, chemistries, ESR) are normal in patients with a herniated disc. Electromyographic (EMG) findings may be positive in patients with nerve root impingement. Evidence of positive waves, giant potentials, and insertional irritability suggest radiculopathy associated with significant nerve root impingement. The EMG findings become much more significant in the presence of historical and physical findings consistent with herniation of a disc. Lower extremity somatosensory evoked potentials may be more sensitive than EMG in detecting abnormalities in patients who have sensory abnormalities alone.[11]

RADIOGRAPHIC EVALUATION

Plain roentgenograms may be entirely normal in a patient with symptoms and signs of nerve root impingement. Radiographic evaluation with CT scan may demonstrate disc bulging but may not correlate with the level of nerve damage (Fig. 10–5). Myelographic evaluation is better for identifying the exact level of nerve root impingement (Fig. 10–6).[12–14] MR also allows visualization of soft tissues, including discs in the lumbar spine[15] (Fig. 10–7). Herniated discs are easily detected with MR evaluation (Figs. 10–8 and 10–9). MR is a sensitive technique for the detection of far lateral and anterior disc herniations. Migratory fragments of discs that may be missed by other techniques are detectable by MR.[16] Contrast-enhanced MR may also be able to detect in-

flammation of nerve roots by the uptake of contrast in neural structures where the blood-brain barrier has been altered.[17] MR has become the radiographic technique of choice for detecting the presence of a herniated intervertebral disc. However, the radiographic finding of a herniation only becomes important in the clinical setting of a patient who has historic and physical findings of radiculopathy. MR abnormalities may be present in individuals who are asymptomatic.[18] MR with contrast is a sensitive technique for distinguishing between epidural scar and recurrent herniated disc in postoperative patients.[19, 20]

DIFFERENTIAL DIAGNOSIS

The initial diagnosis of a herniated disc is ordinarily made on the basis of the history and physical examination (see Table 10–1). Plain x-rays of the lumbosacral spine will rarely add to the diagnosis but should be obtained to help rule out other causes of pain, such as infection or tumor. Other tests such as the MR, CT, and myelogram are confirmatory by nature and can be misleading when used as screening tests.

Patients with spinal stenosis may also develop back pain that radiates into the lower extremities.[21] The patients with spinal stenosis tend to be older than those who develop herniated discs. Characteristically patients with

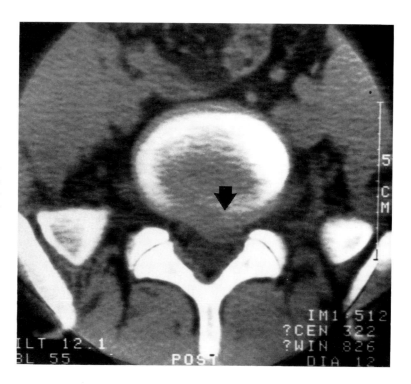

Figure 10–5. CT scan of lumbar spine demonstrating a nucleus pulposus herniating into the spinal canal (arrow) at the L5-S1 intervertebral disc space.

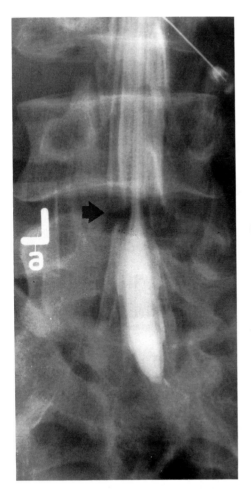

Figure 10–6. Lumbar myelogram with water-soluble dye demonstrating a large herniated nucleus disc (cutoff of nerve root sleeves) at the L4-5 intervertebral disc space *(arrow)*.

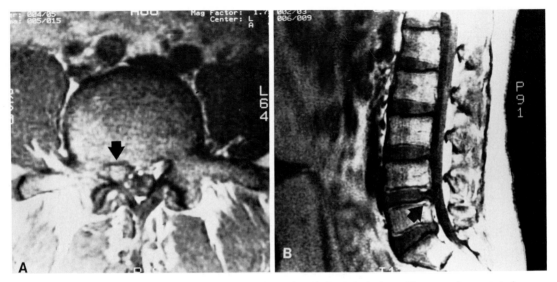

Figure 10–7. MR scan of the lumbar spine. *(A)* Coronal and *(B)* sagittal views. The scan demonstrated a herniated disc with protrusion into the spinal canal *(arrows)*.

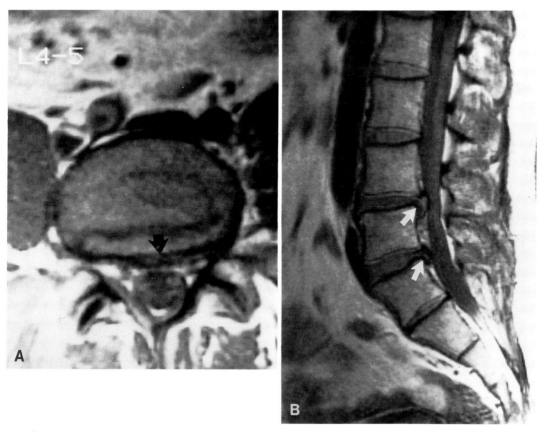

Figure 10–8. MR of the lumbar spine. *(A)* Coronal and *(B)* sagittal views of a 40-year-old man with chronic pain localized to the low back. The patient developed radicular symptoms. The MR demonstrates a large herniated disc at the L4–5 intervertebral disc space *(black arrow)*. The sagittal view reveals disc herniations at two disc levels *(white arrows)*.

Figure 10–9. MR of the lumbar spine. Axial view of lumbar spine demonstrating broad based disc herniation *(small white arrows)* with impingement of the corresponding nerve root posteriorly *(black arrow)*. The patient had left radicular pain with a positive straight leg raising test. His radiculopathy responded to conservative management.

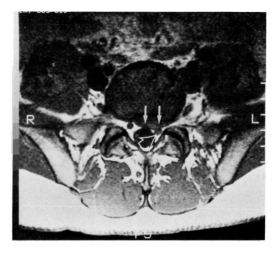

spinal stenosis develop lower extremity pain (pseudoclaudication) after walking for an unspecified distance. They also complain of pain that is exacerbated by standing or extending the spine. Radiographic evaluation is usually helpful in differentiating those individuals with disc herniation from those with bony hypertrophy associated with spinal stenosis. In a study of 1293 patients, lateral spinal stenosis and herniated intervertebral discs coexisted in 17.7% of individuals. Radicular pain may be caused by more than one pathologic process in an individual.[22]

Facet syndrome is another cause of low back pain that may be associated with radiation of pain to structures outside the confines of the lumbosacral spine.[23] Degeneration of articular structures in the facet joint causes pain to develop. In most circumstances, the pain is localized over the area of the affected joint and is aggravated with extension of the spine (standing). A deep, ill-defined, aching discomfort may also be noted in the sacroiliac joint, the buttocks, and the legs. The areas of sclerotome affected show the same embryonic origin as the degenerated facet joint. The direct association between facet joint disease and pain production is questioned by some investigators. Many individuals with arthritic changes in their facet joints visible on radiographic evaluation experience no symptoms. Patients with pain secondary to facet joint disease may have relief of symptoms with apophyseal injection of a long-acting local anesthetic.[24] The true role of facet joint disease in the production of back and leg pain remains to be determined.

Other mechanical causes of sciatica include congenital abnormalities of lumbar nerve roots, external compression of the sciatic nerve (wallet in a back pants pocket), or muscular compression of the nerve (piriformis syndrome). Medical causes of sciatica (neural tumors or infections, for example) are usually associated with systemic symptoms in addition to nerve pain in a sciatic distribution.

TREATMENT

The treatment for most patients with a herniated disc is nonoperative, since 80% of them will respond to conservative therapy when followed over a period of 5 years.[25] The efficacy of nonoperative treatment, however, depends on a healthy relationship between a capable physician and a well-informed patient. If patients have insight into the rationale for the prescribed treatment and follow instructions, the chances for success are greatly increased.

The primary element in the nonoperative treatment of acute disease is controlled physical activity.[26] For the first several days in the acute situation, bed rest may be necessary. This can usually be accomplished at home. The semi-Fowler's position, with hips and knees comfortably flexed, is ideal because it keeps intradiscal pressure down and reduces nerve root tension. After the first several days, the patient should be gradually mobilized. Walking should be encouraged, whereas sitting is prohibited since it causes excess pressure on the nerve root.

Drug therapy is another important part of the treatment, and three categories of pharmacologic agents are commonly used: anti-inflammatory drugs, analgesics, and muscle relaxants or tranquilizers. Inasmuch as the symptoms of low back pain and sciatica result from an inflammatory reaction as well as mechanical compression, anti-inflammatory medications are indicated. Adequate doses of aspirin have been found to work quite well, although other nonsteroidal anti-inflammatory medications are frequently used. The patient's pain will generally be relieved once the inflammation is brought under control. There may be residual numbness or tingling in the involved extremity, but this is usually tolerable. Some patients who fail to respond to anti-inflammatory medication may get dramatic relief from a short course of systemic steroids administered in decreasing dosages over a week.

Analgesic medication is administered to control pain if it is severe. Codeine is recommended for home use. If codeine does not work, hospitalization should be considered so that a stronger analgesic medication, such as morphine sulfate, can be strictly controlled. Long-term use of narcotics for these patients should be discouraged.

Muscle relaxants are utilized in patients with uncontrolled muscle contraction associated with nerve impingement. The mechanism of action of these agents is unknown. Most agents, other than diazepam, do not act directly on muscle fibers but act on the central nervous system by diminishing reflex contractions. The beneficial effects of this group of drugs may be related to their tranquilizing properties. In patients with severe muscle spasm, muscle relaxants do appear to be effective. It should be remembered, however, that use of diazepam for muscle spasm should be discouraged. When used on a chronic basis, diazepam may become a depressant. Diazepam will only add to the psychologic problems of patients with chronic pain. If other muscle relaxants without depressant properties are utilized from the outset, the problems related to depression, tolerance, and addiction can be prevented.

Surgical intervention is reserved for patients in whom conservative therapy fails. Patients with radicular pain, abnormal physical findings, and confirmatory radiographic tests are candidates for surgical intervention. The indications for surgery are listed in Chapter 20.

Scientific evidence confirms the efficacy of therapeutic interventions in the treatment of a herniated nucleus pulposus.[27] Some of the modalities that have been proven effective include bed rest for 1 week, medications, and surgical excision of the herniated disc fragment.[27]

PROGNOSIS

Eighty percent of those who follow the above regimen will be markedly improved. Although the noninvasive treatment of a herniated disc can be quite gratifying, it generally takes a significant period of controlled physical activity to improve. Patients must be aware of the time constraints from the onset of therapy in order to understand the rationale of the measures employed.

A prospective study of 11 patients with disc extrusions and radiculopathy followed the course of symptoms from 8 to 77 months. The extruded portion of the discs is resorbed without the need for surgical removal. All 11 patients had a decrease in neural impingement.[28] Surgical therapy is required for only a very small number of individuals with a herniated disc.

References

ACUTE HERNIATED NUCLEUS PULPOSUS

1. Mixter WJ, Barr JS: Rupture of the intervertebral disc with involvement of the spinal canal. N Engl J Med 211:210, 1934.
2. Adams MA, Dolan P, Hutton WC, Porter RW: Diurnal changes in spinal mechanics and their clinical significance. J Bone Joint Surg 72B:266, 1990.
3. Spangforth EV: The lumbar disk herniation: a computer-aided analysis of 2,504 operations. Acta Orthop Scand [Suppl] 142:1, 1972.
4. Nachemson AL: The lumbar spine: an orthopaedic challenge. Spine 1:59, 1976.
5. Kelsey JL: An epidemiological study of acute herniated lumbar intervertebral disc. Rheumatol Rehabil 14:144, 1975.
6. DePalma A, Rothman RH: The Intervertebral Disc. Philadelphia: WB Saunders Co, 1970.
7. Broom MJ: Foraminal and extraforaminal lumbar disk herniations. Clin Orthop 289:118, 1993.
8. Harada Y, Nakahara S: A pathologic study of lumbar disc herniation in the elderly. Spine 14:1020, 1989.
9. Kirkaldy-Willis WH: The relationship of structural pathology to the nerve root. Spine 9:49, 1984.
10. Shiqing X, Quanzhi Z, Dehao F: Significance of the straight-leg-raising test in the diagnosis and clinical evaluation of lower lumbar intervertebral disc protrusion. J Bone Joint Surg 69A:517, 1987.
11. Walk D, Fisher MA, Doundoulakis SH, Hemmati M: Somatosensory evoked potentials in the evaluation of lumbosacral radiculopathy. Neurology 42:1197, 1992.
12. Haughton VM, Eldevik OP, Magnaes B, Amundsen P: A prospective companion of computed tomography and myelography in diagnosis of herniated lumbar disks. Radiology 142:103, 1982.
13. Raskin SP, Keating JW: Recognition of lumbar disc disease: comparison of myelography and computed tomography. AJR 139:349, 1982.
14. Hitselberger WE, Witten RM: Abnormal myelograms in asymptomatic patients. J Neurosurg 28:204, 1968.
15. Modic MT, Masaryk T, Boumphrey F, Goormastic M, Bell G: Lumbar herniated disk disease and canal stenosis: prospective evaluation by surface coil MR, CT, and myelography. AJNR 7:709, 1986.
16. Osborn AG, Hood RS, Sherry RG, Smoker WRK, Harnsberger HR: CT/MR spectrum of far lateral and anterior lumbosacral disk herniations. AJNR 9:775, 1988.
17. Jinkins JR: MR of enhancing nerve roots in the unoperated lumbosacral spine. AJNR 14:193, 1993.
18. Boden SD, Davis DO, Dina TS, Patronas NJ, Wiesel SW: Abnormal magnetic-resonance scans of the lumbar spine in asymptomatic subjects: a prospective investigation. J Bone Joint Surg 72A:403, 1990.
19. Bundschuh CV, Stein L, Slusser JH, et al.: Distinguishing between scar and recurrent herniated disk in postoperative patients: value of contrast-enhanced CT and MR imaging. AJNR 11:949, 1990.
20. Hueftle MG, Modic MT, Ross JS, et al.: Lumbar spine: postoperative MR imaging with Gd-DTPA. Radiology 167:817, 1988.
21. Verbiest H: Pathomorphologic aspects of developmental lumbar stenosis. Orthop Clin North Am 1:177, 1975.
22. Bernard TN Jr, Kirkaldy-Willis WH: Recognizing specific characteristics of nonspecific low back pain. Clin Orthop 217:266, 1987.
23. Mooney V, Robertson J: The facet syndrome. Clin Orthop 115:149, 1976.
24. Fairbank JCT, Park WM, McCall IW, O'Brien JP: Apophyseal injection of local anesthetic as a diagnostic aid in primary low-back pain. Spine 6:598, 1981.
25. Weber H: Lumbar disc herniation: a prospective study of prognostic factors including a controlled trial. J Oslo City Hosp 28:36, 1978.
26. Wiesel SW: Lumbar spine: acute lumbar radicular syndromes. In Orthopaedic Knowledge Update, 2: Home Study Syllabus. Park Ridge, IL: American Academy of Orthopaedic Surgeons, 1987, pp 313, 323.
27. Nachemson AL: Newest knowledge of low back pain: a critical look. Clin Orthop 279:8, 1992.
28. Saal JA, Saal JS, Herzog RJ: The natural history of lumbar intervertebral disc extrusions treated nonoperatively. Spine 15:683, 1990.

OSTEOARTHRITIS/SPINAL STENOSIS

Capsule Summary

Frequency of back pain—very common

Location of back pain—low back to lower leg

Quality of back pain—ache, shooting, pins and needles

Symptoms and signs—pain with standing and walking, positive stress test

Laboratory and x-ray tests—osteophytes on plain roentgenograms, CT scan, myelogram

Treatment—medications, bracing, laminectomy for conservative therapy failures

PREVALENCE AND PATHOGENESIS

Osteoarthritis (degenerative joint disease) is a chronic, noninflammatory joint disease characterized by slowly developing joint pain, stiffness, deformity, and limitation of motion. The lumbosacral spine is only one of the many areas of the skeleton that are affected by this process. Osteoarthritis is the most common joint disease, with prevalence increasing with the age of population. Osteoarthritis is almost universally present in individuals over 75 years of age.[1] Men and women are affected by this illness. Among individuals under 45 years of age more men have the disease, while women develop the disease to a greater degree than men after 55 years of age.[2]

The etiology of osteoarthritis is multifactorial. Genetic, biochemical, and biomechanical factors play a role. Familial aggregation of generalized osteoarthritis, including involvement of the lumbar spine, has been reported. Thirty-six per cent of relatives of men with generalized osteoarthritis and 49% of relatives of women with the disorder showed the disease, as compared with expected values of 17% and 26%, respectively, for the same age group of the general population.[2]

Biochemical and metabolic alterations in cartilage play a role in the pathogenesis of osteoarthritis. Proteoglycans present in cartilage matrix develop altered composition over time. The glycosaminoglycans, which are part of the proteoglycans, act as sponges in the cartilage. They absorb water. The shock absorbency of cartilage is proportional to the proteoglycan content and its ability to bind water. In osteoarthritis, proteoglycan content is reduced along with a relative reduction of keratan sulfate and an increase in chondroitin sulfate (both glycosoaminoglycans).[3] Proteoglycans containing abnormal proportions of keratan and chondroitin sulfate form smaller subunits that retard glycosaminoglycan aggregation. The result of these alterations in the biochemical characteristics of osteoarthritic cartilage is retention of excess water in cartilage. In this state, the shock absorbency of cartilage is diminished and the collagen matrix of the cartilage is disrupted.[4, 5] Growth factors, including fibroblast, transforming, and insulin-like, have a role in the repair of damaged cartilage. Investigation of how growth factor synthesis is regulated in traumatized articular cartilage would be beneficial to the understanding of the underlying mechanisms central to the pathogenesis of osteoarthritis.[6]

Biomechanical factors may play a role in the development of osteoarthritis. Investigators have suggested that stiffening of subchondral bone associated with microfractures results in articular cartilage disruption.[7]

Whether a genetic, biochemical, or biomechanical abnormality, osteoarthritis causes articular cartilage degeneration. As the cartilage is worn away, chondrocytes attempt to replace the cartilage. Degradation is more rapid than repair, and erosion of the articular surface evolves. In response to abnormal mechanical stresses to joint surfaces, bony appendages (osteophytes) appear. In the lumbar spine, the location of osteoarthritis is primarily in the facet joints.

The degenerative changes that occur in the facet joints in association with alterations in intervertebral disc and soft tissue structures decrease the size of the spinal canal. The interaction of the two facet joints and the intervertebral articulation has been conceptualized into the "triple-joint complex" pathogenesis of spinal stenosis.[8] Narrowing of the spinal canal, whether on a congenital, developmental, or degenerative basis, is referred to as spinal stenosis. If the decrease in the spinal canal volume is severe, mechanical pressure on neural structures may occur.

In the first few decades of life, the gross appearance of the spine and its components will remain basically unchanged. The intervertebral discs will maintain their full height, with a thickened, laminated annulus fibrosus and a tense nucleus pulposus. The vertebrae are completely ossified except for their apophyseal rings and are essentially square in shape. The facets are well defined, with smooth capsules and normal articular cartilage. The ligamenta flava are only a few millimeters thick, and the space that is available for the neural elements within the canal and the foramina is capacious.

Symptoms are unusual even though some developmentally and congenitally narrow canals have much less space available even early in life.

Major changes occur in the lumbar spine between the third and fifth decades of life. The first manifestations of aging develop in the intervertebral discs. In the early years, the nucleus loses its vigor and the annulus fissures and degenerates. The first stage of lumbar stenosis is the degeneration of the intervertebral disc. In an evaluation of 330 discs and 390 facet joints with MR and CT, degenerative disc alterations on MR occur in the absence of facet joint changes on CT. Facet joint changes in the absence of disc alterations do not occur.[9] The resulting biomechanical insufficiency inevitably results in a transfer of stresses posteriorly to the facet joints and ligaments, which are ill suited to assume compressive, tensile, and shear loads. Capsular strains, hypermobility, and degenerative changes develop. These changes are often manifested radiologically by traction spurs, which form anteriorly, 1 to 2 millimeters from the disc. The ligamentum flavum is compelled to assume unnatural tensile loads in spite of having become redundant as the total spine length decreases with disc degeneration. The vertebrae themselves also tend to collapse and spread so as to further compromise the space available for the neural elements. Disc degeneration in and of itself may not be a painful process. Patients with disc degeneration may be asymptomatic until alterations in facet joint alignment result in the onset of articular pain. This stage of the illness may be characterized by pain localized to an area just lateral to the midline, over an apophyseal joint, and exacerbated by extension of the spine without radicular radiation of pain.

If a disc herniation occurs in a spinal canal that is relatively small, compression of the neural elements will result. The patient will experience symptoms not only of low back pain, as mediated through the sinuvertebral nerve supply to the outer margin of the annulus, but also of radiating pain in the distribution of the compressed neural elements. In pure terms, this can be thought of as a relative spinal stenosis, since the herniated nucleus pulposus is occupying space in an already small spinal canal. On the other hand, a similar-sized disc herniation in a large spinal canal may cause no symptoms at all because the neural elements have enough room to escape pressure. Thus, symptoms in this age group result from a combination of the disc hernia-

tion itself and the volume of the canal with which the person was born.

Patients in their 40s and older can show the hypermobile end-plate changes of the aging process. Degeneration both of the facet joints (osteoarthritis) and of the intervertebral discs leads to narrowing of the spinal canal. The canal is rimmed by large osteophytes that have developed as a result of the excessive load on the now incompetent intervertebral disc. The facets are hypertrophic and deformed by osteophytic spurs that are encased within the joint capsule. The ligamentum flavum becomes redundant and, in combination with the aforementioned changes, encroaches on the spinal canal and foramina. Although such distortion of the spinal canal occurs to some degree in all active people, not everyone suffers significant disability. The symptoms a person will have depend on the original size of the canal; if the spinal canal is small, the changes caused by aging of the disc and facet joints can lead to an absolute stenosis with compression of the neural elements. If, however, the spinal canal is large to begin with, the aging process will lead to only asymptomatic relative spinal stenosis without neural compression.[10]

In some individuals, the final pathologic end-stage of disc degeneration is a fibrous ankylosis between two adjacent vertebrae along with osteophyte formation and a marked narrowing of the disc space. If this is a stable phenomenon, the patient may be relatively free of symptoms or will be aware only of a sense of stiffness in the spine.

As the spine ages, one can also encounter postural alterations with reduction in lordosis. This is an attempt by the body to decompress the degenerated articular facets by maintaining a flexed rather than an extended posture; however, such postural alterations can lead to chronic muscle tension and become symptomatic. This flexed position also provides more room for the sensitive neural elements that are dynamically compressed in extension.

Although most of the described changes in the motor segment units progress from decade to decade, there is a wide range in the rate of deterioration. It is important to understand that these anatomic alterations do not necessarily dictate symptoms, define disability, or determine prognosis. As the spine ages, these phenomena appear to be tolerated to some degree by all.

The pathogenesis of the symptoms of spinal stenosis remains undetermined. Some authors suggest the symptoms associated with pseudoclaudication (leg pain) stem from compression of vascular structures, which results in diminished blood flow to the nerve roots. The compression may affect arteries, capillaries, or veins. Initially, the vascular abnormalities may result in no permanent change. However, over time, venous obstruction causes hypoxia that is associated with perineural fibrosis resulting in more persistent symptoms.[11] Others believe that the symptoms are related directly to mechanical compression of neural structures.[12] In the later stage of this disorder, patients develop increasing radicular pain with walking. The distance associated with the onset of radicular pain shortens with increasing severity of stenosis. The process may progress to the point that just standing upright without ambulation causes leg pain.

CLINICAL HISTORY

Patients with degenerative disease of the lumbosacral spine may complain of a broad variety of symptoms. Many patients with degenerative discs and osteoarthritis of the facet joints may be totally asymptomatic. Some may have mild discomfort in the low back, while others may have radiating leg pain with inability to walk. Patients with osteoarthritis of the facet joints develop pain primarily over the joints in the low back. Patients may have morning stiffness of short duration (30 minutes or less). Any body movements that compress the joints (extension) exacerbate symptoms of dull, aching pain. Patients may also be aware of decreased motion of the spine.

As the degenerative process continues, patients complain of symptoms associated with spinal stenosis. Patients with spinal stenosis most commonly have symptoms of pseudoclaudication.[13] Pseudoclaudication is associated with pain in the buttock, thigh, or leg that develops with standing or walking and is relieved by rest, in the presence of adequate blood flow to the lower extremities. Many patients develop leg pain with standing alone (94% in one study) in clear distinction from vascular claudication. Walking a distance as short as 200 yards also may bring on pain. Many patients may have bilateral leg pain. A majority of patients have back pain in combination with leg pain. However, it is important to remember that a small group of patients will have leg pain only, without any associated back pain. In addition to pain, patients may also complain of numbness, paresthesias, and weakness in the lower extremities.

Any positions that flex the lumbar spine are associated with resolution of symptoms. Characteristically, patients with spinal stenosis are able to ride a bicycle without difficulty. Walking up an incline or stairs does not cause symptoms, while walking down an incline or stairs (extension of the spine) does cause symptoms to appear.

There is an internationally accepted classification of the anatomic state and its clinical syndrome known as lumbar spinal stenosis, and the production of symptoms attributed to these changes can be either localized or generalized in origin. It is important to realize, however, that structural changes in the spinal and foraminal canals that are exaggerated with posture are anatomic changes and not absolute determinants of pain. The symptoms manifested may vary significantly among patients with similar pathomorphologic changes because of the temporal framework in which the neural compression has occurred, the susceptibility of the nerves involved, and the unique functional demands and pain tolerance of each patient.

PHYSICAL EXAMINATION

The physical findings associated with osteoarthritis of the lumbar spine may be unimpressive. Patients may have mild decreases in range of motion, particularly with extension. With more extensive degenerative disease associated with nerve impingement, objective signs of muscle weakness, atrophy, and asymmetric reflexes may be noted. With patients who develop symptoms with standing or walking, neurologic changes will occur only after the patient is stressed. The following stress tests can be used in an outpatient clinic: After a neurologic examination has been performed on the patient, he is asked to walk until his symptoms occur or he has walked 300 feet. A repeat examination is then done, and in some cases the second examination will reveal a neurologic deficit that was not present after the first examination.

LABORATORY DATA

Laboratory evaluation of patients with osteoarthritis and spinal stenosis is usually normal. Electromyography may be abnormal in some patients with persistent symptoms. The abnormal findings include changes associated with radiculopathies (positive waves, giant potentials).[13] Other neurophysiologic findings of spinal stenosis include bilateral and multisegmental neurogenic EMG abnormalities in the legs.[14] Somatosensory potentials may also be helpful preoperatively in identifying the level of cord compression and intraoperatively to assess the adequacy of neural decompression.[15]

RADIOGRAPHIC EVALUATION

Plain roentgenograms are very helpful in visualizing spinal stenosis and osteoarthritis. Disc spaces increase in size from the L1–2 interspace to L4–5. The L5-S1 interspace has a variable size. However, the parallel position of the endplates of L5 and S1 is evidence of degeneration in that interspace.

The roentgenograms will reveal intervertebral disc degeneration with loss of disc space height, traction osteophytes, decreased interpedicular distance, decreased sagittal canal diameter, and facet degeneration (Fig. 10–10).

The claw and traction osteophytes are two commonly observed abnormalities on the anterior aspects of the vertebral body observed on conventional radiographs of patients with osteoarthritis of the lumbar spine.[16] The traction osteophyte is horizontally oriented and arise from the margins of two adjacent vertebral bodies. The claw osteophyte is triangular and is curved at its tip. The traction osteophyte may be indicative of disc degeneration and an unstable discovertebral junction. These osetophytes form at the osseous site of attachment of the outer annular fibers to the anterior vertebral surface. With maturing of the lesion and less instability, periosteal deposition of bone convert the traction osteophyte to a claw osteophyte. These osteophytes may coexist in the same vertebral body and are indicative of the progression of the same pathologic process affecting the lumbar spine. The intervertebral disc anteriorly and the two facet joints posteriorly form a triangle with the neural elements in the center. These three structures are sometimes referred to as the "triple-joint complex," and their degeneration leads to loss of volume (area) in the triangle. As stated above, if the loss is severe enough, compression of the neural elements will take place (Fig. 10–11). The diagnosis of spinal stenosis depends less on the absolute measurement of the size of the canal but rather on the configuration of the canal and the relative amount of space at various levels of the spine.[17]

The technetium bone scan may supplement physical examination and plain roentgenograms in assessing the extent and severity of osteoarthritis.[18] The technetium bisphosphonate and phosphate agents preferentially chemabsorb to hydroxyapatite crystals, particularly

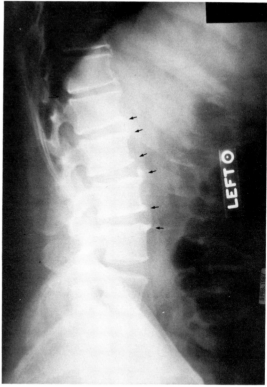

Figure 10–10. Lateral view illustrates traction osteophytes *(arrows)* at multiple levels associated with disc degeneration. Note that the osteophytes are horizontally oriented and emerge slightly above or below the disc space. A claw osteophyte is noted at the fourth arrow from the top while a traction osteophyte is located at the fifth arrow from the top.

newly formed crystals in new bone. Increased uptake occurs in areas of subchondral sclerosis. Specialized techniques are helpful in screening bone abnormalities in the lumbar spine including osteophytes (Fig. 10–12).[19]

CT scan is also a useful technique to identify the presence of facet joint disease along with disc degeneration. The CT scan can identify trefoil configuration of the spinal canal along with reduction in the dimensions of the bony canal (Fig. 10–13). High-resolution CT scans may be reformatted to reconstruct three-dimensional views of the lumbar spine.[18]

Myelography will demonstrate subtotal or total obstruction of the column of dye in the lumbar region in patients with spinal stenosis. The L4 and L5 vertebral body levels are the ones most commonly affected (Fig. 10–14).

Myelography is a dynamic study characterized by movement of the water-soluble dye up and down the spinal canal. The radiologist is able to actually visualize the locations in the spine that are the most severely compressed.

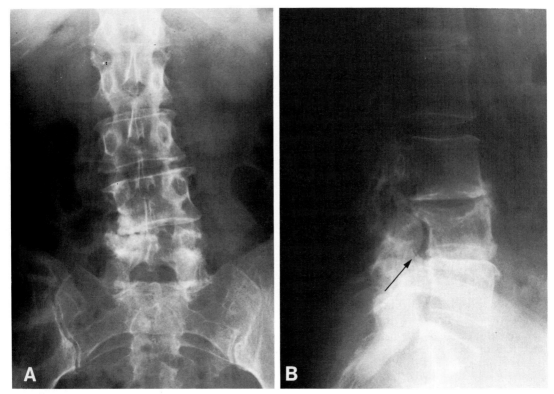

Figure 10–11. AP *(A)* and lateral *(B)* view of the lumbar spine in a patient with spinal stenosis at the L4–5 segment. A loss of area in the neural foramen is noted on the lateral view *(arrow).*

Myelography remains the diagnostic test of choice for spinal stenosis (CT and MR are static tests).

The role of MR continues to be modified with the development of this radiographic technique (Fig. 10–15). Three-dimensional imaging has been developed for MR. Different three-dimensional techniques are capable of providing either high or low signal intensity CSF that may act as its own contrast agent, thus allowing for myelographic images without the need for the injection of dye. Further development of this technique may result in images that are as good as a myelogram without the need for the injection of dye.[20]

The scientific data to support the accuracy of one radiographic technique versus another in the diagnosis of spinal stenosis is lacking.[21] A number of published studies that have had methodologic flaws that limited their usefulness as proof of the sensitivity and specificity for making the diagnosis of spinal stenosis.[21] At this time, the choice of technique depends on the issues of cost, reimbursement, access to equipment, and skill of radiologist. Determination of the most accurate technique will evolve as larger, more rigorous studies are

published and with improvements in imaging accuracy.

DIFFERENTIAL DIAGNOSIS

The diagnosis of osteoarthritis is suggested by the patient's age and a clinical history of back pain of long duration that increases with mechanical stresses, and is documented by characteristic changes on radiographic evaluation of the lumbosacral spine. The diagnosis of osteoarthritis is one made by exclusion of other possible diagnoses. The radiographic changes of osteoarthritis, including loss of disc height and traction osteophytes, occur as patients age. These changes are not necessarily associated with back pain.[22] Most patients with symptomatic osteoarthritis are in the same age group as most patients with tumors of the lumbosacral spine. The physician must feel confident about excluding the possibility of a more ominous cause of back pain before ascribing the patient's complaints to osteoarthritis of the spine.

Spinal stenosis may be caused by a number of processes that decrease space in the spinal canal for the neural elements.[23] The classifica-

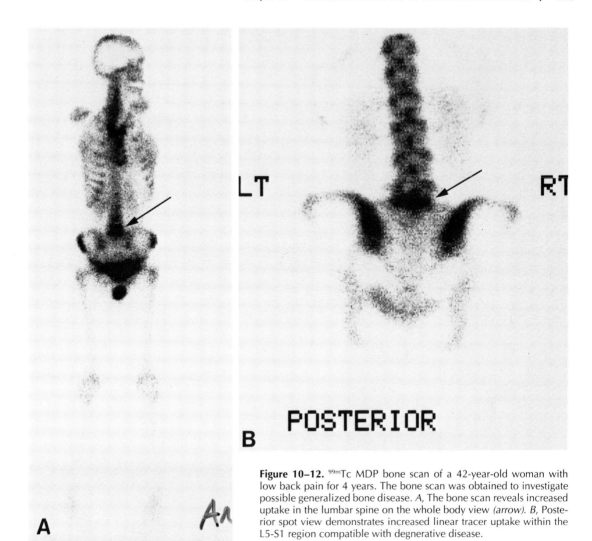

Figure 10–12. ^{99m}Tc MDP bone scan of a 42-year-old woman with low back pain for 4 years. The bone scan was obtained to investigate possible generalized bone disease. *A,* The bone scan reveals increased uptake in the lumbar spine on the whole body view *(arrow). B,* Posterior spot view demonstrates increased linear tracer uptake within the L5-S1 region compatible with degnerative disease.

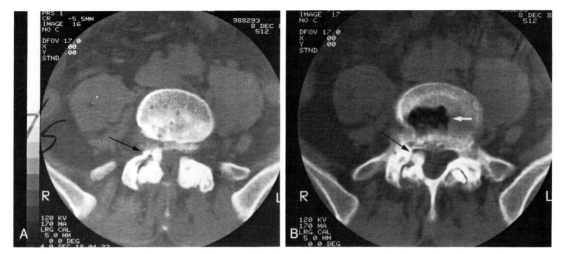

Figure 10–13. CT scan of a 68-year-old man with back pain that is exacerbated with standing. Cross-sectional views demonstrate vacuum phenomenon in intervertebral disc *(white arrow)* and facet hypertrophy (most prominent on the right), resulting in canal stenosis at multiple levels *(black arrows).* The patient's symptoms responded to epidural steroid injections.

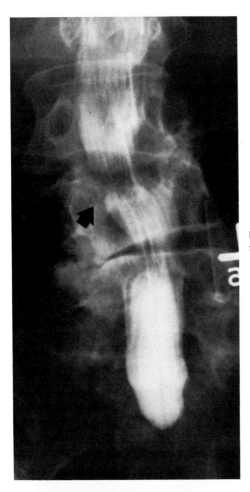

Figure 10–14. Myelogram of a 64-year-old patient with significant stenosis in the L3–4 region of the lumbar spine *(arrow)*.

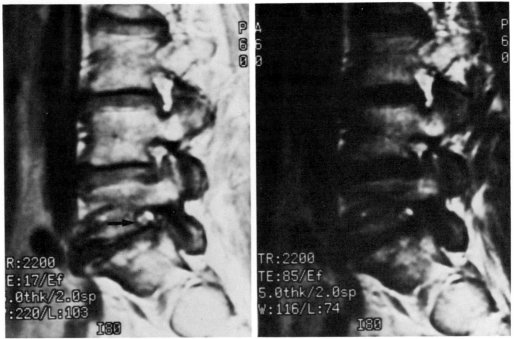

Figure 10–15. MR of the lumbar spine. Sagittal view of a T$_2$-weighted image demonstrating foramenal narrowing at L5-S1 interspace *(black arrow)* with associated intervertebral disc degeneration.

tion of spinal stenosis includes developmental and acquired forms (Table 10–2). Degenerative causes are responsible for the vast majority of individuals with lumbar spinal stenosis. A variety of medical disorders cause stenosis including calcium pyrophosphate crystal deposition, amyloid deposition, and intradural spinal tumors.[24–26] Patients may have both neurogenic and vascular claudication simultaneously. The alternate cause of claudication should be investigated if a partial improvement occurs with decompressive laminectomy or vascular surgery.[27]

Facet syndrome must also be considered in the differential diagnosis of patients with low back pain with lumbar spine extension. Pain may be localized over a single apophyseal joint early in the osteoarthritic process. As the proc-ess progresses, the apophyseal joint becomes increasingly irritated with referred pain into the buttock and posterior thigh. Patients with facet syndrome have referred pain into the leg with extension of the spine and ipsilateral side bending. Pain may also occur with rotation of the spine. Abnormal neurologic signs are seldom discovered on physical examination. Injection of local anesthetics has variable results with long-term relief in up to 60%.[28] Facet joint blocks are not always helpful in reducing pain. In one study, the diagnosis of facet syndrome could only be confirmed in 29% of referred patients.[29] No specific clinical finding could be identified that was specifically associated with a good response to injection. Another study of 109 patients with unilateral low back pain found improvement to be equal in the analgesic and placebo injection groups.[30] Similar outcome was also found in patients who received methylprednisolone injection versus placebo injection.[31] Another important point concerning facet joint injection is the lack of correlation between the response to injection and the outcome from posterior lumbar fusion. The clinical entity of facet joint syndrome and, thus, its appropriate treatment remains in question.[32]

TABLE 10–2. CLASSIFICATION OF LUMBAR SPINAL STENOSIS

A. Congenital/Developmental
  1. Idiopathic
  2. Genetic/Metabolic
      Achondroplasia
      Morquio's syndrome
      Hypophosphatemic vitamin D-resistant rickets
  3. Other
      Down's syndrome
      Scoliosis
B. Acquired
  1. Degenerative
      Spondylosis
      Isolated intervertebral disc resorption
      Lateral nerve entrapment
      Spondylolisthesis
      Adult scoliosis
      Calcification of the ligamentum flavum
      Intraspinal synovial cysts
      Spinal dysraphism
  2. Metabolic/Endocrine
      Osteoporosis with fracture
      Acromegaly
      Calcium pyrophosphate dihydrate crystal
        deposition disease
      Renal osteodystrophy
      Hypoparathyroidism
      Epidural lipomatosis
  3. Postoperative
      Postlaminectomy
      Postfusion
      Postdiscectomy
  4. Traumatic
      Fracture
  5. Miscellaneous
      Paget's disease
      Diffuse idiopathic skeletal hyperostosis
      Fluorosis
      Conjoined origin of lumbosacral nerve roots
      Amyloid

Modified from Moreland LW, Lopez-Mendez A, Larcon GS: Spinal stenosis: A comprehensive review of the literature. Semen Arthritis Rheum 19:127, 1989.

TREATMENT

The majority of patients with osteoarthritis and spinal stenosis of the lumbosacral spine can be treated nonsurgically. Nonsteroidal anti-inflammatory drugs are agents that are helpful in controlling symptoms. The toxicity of gastric irritation may be of greater concern in patients with osteoarthritis, since the group of people with this ailment are older. Gastric upset may occur more commonly in an older patient population. Medications may be given to protect the gastric mucosa in patients who are at risk for significant morbidity or mortality from a gastrointestinal bleed. Lumbosacral corsets are helpful in reminding the patient to avoid excessive spinal movement. Short courses of oral corticosteroids (Medrol [methylprednisolone acetate] Dosepak) are used on rare occasions in patients with severe symptoms of spinal stenosis who do not respond to nonsteroidal drugs. The use of oral corticosteroids must be given in only the most unusual circumstances. The potential risks of large doses of corticosteroids, including aseptic necrosis of bone, and hypertension must be weighed against the potential benefit that would only come with steroid use. Epidural corticosteroids should be considered before oral corticosteroids are given. Patients may require a course of three injections before they report relief of symptoms. The duration of benefit is variable. Some patients may have relief of symptoms that lasts months. With the return of symptoms, another course of injections may be given. Most patients who have responded to injections have been controlled with two courses of therapy per year. In a study of 249 patients with back pain of 3 months or longer, those who did not benefit 1 year after epidural injection had pain that interfered with activities, had unemployment due to pain, had a normal straight leg raising test, and had pain not decreased by medication.[34] Calcitonin also has been helpful in controlling symptoms of spinal stenosis.[35] Patients realizing the greatest degree of pain relief were those with moderate pain and walking capacity of more than 200 meters.[36] Operative therapy for spinal stenosis is reserved for patients who are totally incapacitated by their condition (see Chapter 20).

PROGNOSIS

Most patients with osteoarthritis and spinal stenosis have a relapsing course with recurrent episodes of back pain. Most patients respond to medical and physical therapy and do not require surgical intervention. A 4-year prospective study of spinal stenosis reported that conservative, nonsurgical therapy was effective in decreasing or controlling symptoms of spinal stenosis.[33] The natural course of lumbar stenosis is to improvement. A study of 32 patients who did not receive therapy revealed a decrease of symptoms in 15%, no change in 70%, and worsening in 15%. No severe deterioration requiring surgery occurred during the study period.

References

OSTEOARTHRITIS/SPINAL STENOSIS

1. Lawrence JS, Bremner JM, Bier F: Osteoarthrosis. Prevalence in the population and relationship between symptoms and x-ray changes. Ann Rheum Dis 25:1, 1966.
2. Kellgren JH, Lawrence JA, Bier F: Genetic factors in generalized osteoarthritis. Ann Rheum Dis 22:237, 1963.
3. Mankin HJ: The reaction of articular cartilage to injury and osteoarthritis. N Engl J Med 291:1285, 1335, 1974.
4. Mankin HJ, Thrasher ZA: Water content and binding in normal and osteoarthritic human cartilage. J Bone Joint Surg 57A:76, 1975.
5. Venn MF, Maroudas A: Chemical composition and swelling of normal and osteoarthritic femoral head cartilage. I. Chemical composition. Ann Rheum Dis 36:121, 1977.
6. Malemud CJ: The role of growth factors in cartilage metabolism. Rheum Dis Clin North Am 19:569, 1993.
7. Radin EL, Paul IL, Rose RM: Role of mechanical fractures in the pathogenesis of primary osteoarthritis. Lancet 1:519, 1976.
8. Farfan HS: Mechanical Disorders of the Low Back. Philadelphia: Lea and Febiger, 1973.
9. Butler D, Trafimow JH, Andersson GBJ, et al.: Discs degenerate before facets. Spine 15:111, 1990.
10. Arnoldi CC, Brodsky AE, Cauchoix J, et al.: Lumbar spinal stenosis and nerve root entrapment syndrome: definition and classification. Clin Orthop 115:4, 1976.
11. Jayson MIV: The role of vascular damage and fibrosis in the pathogenesis of nerve root damage. Clin Orthop 279:40, 1992.
12. Jellinger K, Neumayer E: Claudication of the spinal canal and cauda equina. In: Vinken PJ, Bruyn GW (eds): Handbook of Clinical Neurology. Vol 12. Vascular Diseases of the Nervous System. Amsterdam: North-Holland Publishing Company 1972, pp 507–547.
13. Hall S, Bartlesow JD, Onofrio BM, et al.: Lumbar spinal stenosis. Ann Intern Med 103:271, 1985.
14. Johnsson K, Rosen I, Uden A: Neurophysiologic investigation of patients with spinal stenosis. Spine 12:483, 1987.
15. Keim HA, Hajdu M, Gonzalez EG, et al.: Somatosensory evoked potentials as an aid in the diagnosis and intraoperative management of spinal stenosis. Spine 10:338, 1985.
16. Pate D, Goobar J, Resnick D, et al.: Traction osteophytes of the lumbar spine: radiographic-pathologic correlation. Radiology 166:843, 1988.
17. Schonstrom NS, Bolender NF, Spengler DM: The pathomorphology of spinal stenosis as seen on CT scans of the lumbar spine. Spine 10:806, 1985.
18. Durrault RG, Lander PH: Imaging of the facet joints. Radiol Clin North Am 28:1033, 1990.
19. Papanicolaou N, Wilkinson RH, Emans JB, et al.: Bone scintigraphy and radiography in young athletes with low back pain. AJR 145:1039, 1985.
20. Ross JS, Modic MT: Current assessment of spinal degenerative disease with magnetic resonance imaging. Clin Orthop 279:68, 1992.
21. Kent DL, Haynor DR, Larson EB, Deyo RA: Diagnosis of lumbar spinal stenosis in adults: a metaanalysis of the accuracy of CT, MR, and myelography. AJR 158:1135, 1992.
22. Frymoyer JW, Newberg A, Pope MH, et al.: Spine radiographs in patients with low-back pain: an epidemiological study in men. J Bone Joint Surg 66A:1048, 1984.
23. Moreland LW, López-Méndez A, Alarcón GS: Spinal stenosis: a comprehensive review of the literature. Semin Arthritis Rheum 19:127, 1989.
24. Delamarter RB, Sherman JE, Carr J: Lumbar spinal stenosis secondary to calcium pyrophosphate crystal deposition (pseudogout). Clin Orthop 289:127, 1993.
25. Honig S, Murali R: Spinal cord claudication from amyloid deposition. J Rheumatol 19:1988, 1992.
26. McGuire RA, Brown MD, Green BA: Intradural spinal tumors and spinal stenosis: report of two cases. Spine 12:1062, 1987.
27. Dodge LD, Bohlman HH, Rhodes RS: Concurrent lumbar spinal stenosis and peripheral vascular dis-

ease: a report of nine patients. Clin Orthop 230:141, 1988.

28. Moran R, O'Connell D, Walsh MG: The diagnostic value of facet joint injections. Spine 13:1407, 1988.
29. Jackson RP, Jacobs RR, Montesano PX: Facet joint injection in low back pain: A prospective statistical study. Spine 13:966, 1988.
30. Lilius G, Laasonen EM, Myllynen P, et al.: Lumbar facet joint syndrome: a randomised clinical trial. J Bone Joint Surg 71B:681, 1989.
31. Carette S, Marcoux S, Truchon R, et al.: A controlled trial of corticosteroid injections into facet joints for chronic low back pain. N Engl J Med 325:1002, 1991.
32. Jackson RP: The facet syndrome: myth or reality? Clin Orthop 279:110, 1992.
33. Onel D, Sari H, Donmerz C: Lumbar spinal stenosis: clinical/radiologic therapeutic evaluation in 145 patients. Spine 18:291, 1993.
34. Jamison RN, VadeBoncouer T, Ferrante FM: Low back pain patients unresponsive to an epidural steroid injection: identifying predictive factors. Clin J Pain 7:311, 1991.
35. Eskola A, Alaranta H, Pohjolainen T, et al.: Calcitonin treatment in lumbar stenosis: clinical observations. Calcif Tiss Int 45:372, 1989.
36. Eskola A, Pohjolainen T, Alaranta H, et al.: Calcitonin treatment in lumbar spinal stenosis: a randomized, placebo-controlled, double-blind, cross-order study with one-year follow-up. Calcif Tissue Int 50:400, 1992.

SPONDYLOLYSIS/SPONDYLOLISTHESIS

Capsule Summary

Frequency of back pain—common
Location of back pain—low back, posterior thigh, lower leg
Quality of back pain—ache
Symptoms and signs—pain increased with activity, lumbar "stepoff"
Laboratory and x-ray—lateral x-ray—pars abnormality on plain roentgenogram
Treatment—controlled activity, medications, bracing, surgical fusion

PREVALENCE AND PATHOGENESIS

Spondylolisthesis is a spinal condition in which all or part of a vertebra has slipped on another. The word is derived from the Greek "spondylos" meaning vertebra and "olisthesis" meaning to slip. There are five major types of this condition and the etiology of each is different (Table 10–3).[1]

Type I, dysplastic spondylolisthesis, is secondary to a congenital defect of either the superior sacral or inferior L5 facets or both with gradual slipping of the L5 vertebra. Type II, isthmic or spondylolytic, in which the lesion is in the isthmus or pars interarticularis, has the

TABLE 10–3. TYPES OF SPONDYLOLISTHESIS

I. Dysplastic—the upper sacrum or arch of L5 permits the listhesis to occur
II. Isthmic—the lesion is in the pars interarticularis. Three types can be recognized
  a. Lytic—fatigue fracture of the pars
  b. Elongated but intact pars
  c. Acute fracture
III. Degenerative—resulting from long-standing intersegmental instability
IV. Traumatic—resulting from fractures in other areas of the bony hook and the pars
V. Pathologic—generalized or localized bone disease

From Wiesel SW, Bernini, P, Rothman RH: The Aging Lumbar Spine. Philadelphia: W B Saunders Co, 1982.

greatest clinical importance in persons under the age of 50. If a defect in the pars interarticularis can be identified but no slipping has occurred, the condition is termed spondylolysis. If one vertebra has slipped forward on the other (horizontal translation), it is referred to as spondylolisthesis. Type II spondylolisthesis occurs secondary to a lytic process (fatigue fracture of the pars interarticularis), elongation (attenuated) of an intact pars, or acute fracture. Type III, or degenerative spondylolisthesis, occurs secondary to degeneration of the lumbar facet joints with alteration in the joint plane allowing forward or backward displacement. Degenerative spondylolisthesis is most common in an older age population. There is no pars defect and the vertebral body slippage is never greater than 30% (Table 10–4). Type IV, traumatic spondylolisthesis, is associated with acute fracture of a posterior element (pedicle, lamina, or facets) other than the pars interarticularis. Type V, pathologic spondylolisthesis, occurs because of a structural weakness of the bone secondary to a disease process such as a tumor.

TABLE 10–4. COMPARISON OF ISTHMIC AND DEGENERATIVE SPONDYLOLISTHESIS

	ISTHMIC	DEGENERATIVE
Spine level	L5	L4
Sex	Male	Female
Age at Onset	Under 20	Over 40
Race	White	Black
Sacralization	1%	22%

Modified from Rosenberg N: Degenerative Spondylolisthesis. Paper delivered at the meeting of the American Orthopedic Association, Hot Springs, VA, June 26, 1973. (Published in Wiltse LL: Spondylolisthesis and its treatment: conservative treatment, fusion with and without reduction. In: Ruge D, Wiltse LL: Spinal Disorders. Philadelphia: Lea and Febiger, 1977.)

The etiology of the defect in spondylolysis is not clear. Although there may be a hereditary component, the lesion is seldom seen in patients under the age of 5 and is found in 5% of people over the age of 7. The most attractive explanation is that although these children inherit a potential deficiency in the pars, they are not born with any identifiable defect. Between the ages of 5 and 7, however, they become more active and a stress fracture develops in the inherently weakened pars.[2] Some investigators have suggested that there is an increased incidence of sacral spina bifida in patients with spondylolysis. These abnormalities are found more commonly in dysplastic and isthmic spondylolisthesis than in the general population.[3] Young individuals involved in regular sports activities are at risk of developing structural abnormalities including spondylolysis. In a study of young athletes, back pain was reported most frequently in male gymnasts, while radiologic abnormalities occurred most frequently in wrestlers. Patients with the most severe back pain had radiographic evidence of spondylolysis, scoliosis, reduced disc height, Schmorl's nodes, or changes in vertebral body configuration.[4]

Spondylolisthesis is a very common cause of back pain in young individuals. Macnab, after studying 1000 patients with back pain, concluded that spondylolisthesis is the most likely cause of pain in patients under 26 years of age but rarely the sole cause of complaints after the age of 40.[5]

CLINICAL HISTORY

The most common clinical manifestation of spondylolisthesis is low back pain. Although the cause of this type of back pain in the adult has been studied extensively, its origin is not clear. There is no clear understanding of how so many patients develop this lesion between the ages of 5 and 7 but have no back complaints until perhaps age 35, when a sudden twisting or lifting motion will precipitate an acute episode of back and leg pain. The pain is improved with extension of the spine and exacerbated with flexion. The degree of slippage does not necessarily correlate with the degree of pain experienced by the patient.

A large number of patients with significant degrees of slippage will go through life with no discomfort, while other patients with a minimal degree of slip will have significant pain.

Fifty percent of patients will normally associate an injury with the onset of the symptoms. The physician should be aware that it is possible to sustain an acute fracture of the pars, but this is a very rare occurrence. When a case involving a fracture is suspected, a bone scan taken within 3 months of the injury can document the fracture. If the defect is longstanding, it will not be apparent on scintiscan.[2]

Besides back pain, these patients can also complain of leg pain. This occurs because there is frequently a buildup of a fibrocartilaginous mass at the site of the defect, which can cause pain by irritating the nerve root as it exits the neural foramen.

Once the symptoms begin, the patient usually has constant low-grade back discomfort that is aggravated by activity and relieved by rest. There are some periods during which the pain is more intense than others, but unless the picture is complicated by severe leg pain, total incapacitation is rare. The patients are seldom aware of any sensory or motor deficit. At this point it should be re-emphasized that in some people even severe displacement is asymptomatic and gives rise to no disability. It is not uncommon to pick up a previously unrecognized spondylolisthesis on a routine gastrointestinal radiologic study of a 50-year-old patient.

Patients with degenerative spondylolisthesis, spinal stenosis, and congestive heart failure may experience increased nocturnal back and leg pain. The proposed mechanism of pain production is increased venous volume and pressure in Batson's plexus. Improved cardiac function has the potential to lessen lumbar pain.[6]

PHYSICAL EXAMINATION

The physical findings of spondylolisthesis are fairly characteristic. In the absence of any radicular pain, the patient exhibits no postural scoliosis, but there is usually an exaggeration of the lumbar curve and a palpable "stepoff." The slip is usually apparent once it reaches three quarters of a vertebral body. There may also be a dimple at the site of the abnormality. Anteriorly, there maybe a transverse crease at the level of the umbilicus. Occasionally, mild muscle spasm is demonstrable and, in most instances, some local tenderness can be elicited. Although the range of motion is usually complete, some pain can be expected on hyperextension. Usually the neurologic examination is normal.

Hamstring tightness is commonly found in the symptomatic patient with spondylolysis or spondylolisthesis.[7] The mechanism of muscle tightness is not clear. Originally thought to be related to nerve root irritation, hamstring tightness is more closely associated with an attempt to stabilize the unstable L5-S1 junction.[7, 8] Patients with severe tightness have a typical position consisting of flexion of the hips and knees, backward-tilted pelvis, and flattening of the lumbar lordosis. The patients may have a stiff-legged gait with short strides referred to as a "pelvic waddle."[9]

LABORATORY DATA

Laboratory tests are normal in patients with spondylolysis and spondylolisthesis.

RADIOGRAPHIC EXAMINATION

Plain roentgenograms of the lumbar spine in any projection are usually adequate to localize the abnormality if the lesion is large enough. If the lesion is unilateral, as seen in 20% of patients, the lesion may be visible only on an oblique view of the lumbar spine.[10] Recognizing the "collar on the Scottie dog's neck" helps identify the local lesion. Patients with a dysplastic pars have an elongated interarticular region along with altered pedicles.

Forward subluxation of the body (spondylolisthesis) is best visualized on the lateral roentgenogram. The amount of slippage is graded by the system of Meyerding (Fig. 10–16).[11] The top of the sacrum is divided into four parallel quarters, posterior to anterior. A slip of 25% or less of the sacrum is Grade I, while movement of 75% or more of the sacrum is Grade IV (Figs. 10–17 and 10–18). The subluxation

occurs most commonly at the L5 level in isthmic spondylolisthesis but may occur at any of the lumbar vertebrae particularly with other types of spondylolisthesis (Fig. 10–19).

In some patients the static views of the lumbar spine may be unremarkable but the suspicion of spondylolisthesis is high. In these patients, flexion and extension views of the lumbosacral junction may be obtained to evaluate the presence of excessive motion. Measurement of dynamic vertebral translation, defined as the change in relative position from flexion to extension, rather than static displacement on a single view is preferred. Normal lumbar vertebral levels should have less than 3.0 mm of dynamic AP translation.[12]

Other radiographic techniques, including CT and myelography, are rarely indicated. Advances in bone scintigraphy in the form of single photon emission computed tomography (SPECT) allows for the identification of lesions not imaged by planar bone scan. SPECT is able to detect fractures in the pars interarticularis, transverse process, and vertebral body not detected by plain bone scan.[13] These lesions are usually detectable by CT. MR evaluation of individuals over 25 years of age with spondylolisthesis has demonstrated advanced degenerative disc disease at the level of the spondylolysis or spondylolisthesis compared to controls.[14] MR is able to detect entrapment and direct impingement of spinal nerve roots associated with spondylolisthesis.[15] It is able to detect the presence of a spondylolisthesis but may poorly delineate bone fragments around the defect or may detect alterations of the pars

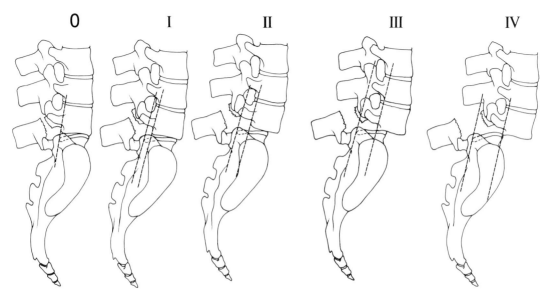

Figure 10–16. Grading system for spondylolisthesis.

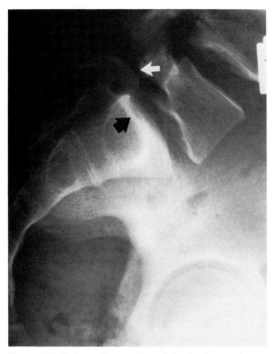

Figure 10–17. Lateral spot view of the lumbosacral junction. A Grade I spondylolisthesis is present with 25% slippage of the superior vertebral body *(black arrow)*. This view demonstrates a Type II spondylolisthesis with a pars defect *(white arrow)*.

rowing, vacuum phenomenon and vertebral body sclerosis.

Motion roentgenograms may not be helpful in identifying the unstable segment causing back pain. A recent study reported no statistical difference between the amount of motion at symptomatic segments and the motion at nonsymptomatic segments in patients with degenerative instability.[19]

In extreme degeneration of intervertebral discs, a retrolisthesis may occur. With decreased disc height, excess motion occurs in adjacent vertebral bodies, allowing posterior motion.[20] L1 and L2 vertebrae seem more commonly affected by this process. It is important to measure the anteroposterior diameter of adjacent vertebral bodies when diagnosing retrolisthesis. One of the vertebral bodies may be smaller in diameter, giving a false impression of abnormal motion.

DIFFERENTIAL DIAGNOSIS

The diagnosis of spondylolysis is confirmed by the discovery of a pars defect on a lateral roentgenogram and spondylolisthesis by the forward position of one vertebral body on another on flexion and extension views of the

interarticularis (osteoblastic metastases, sclerosis of the neck of the pars) that may be confused with spondylolisthesis.[16, 17]

Changes of degenerative spondylolisthesis are most common at the L4–5 interspace.[18] The stress on the lumbar spine may be maximum at L4. Comparing the anatomic structure of L4 and L5 may explain the increased stress on this vertebra. The L4 vertebra has relatively small transverse processes, less ligamentous support, and more mobility. This excess stress results in advanced degenerative changes in the facet joints at this level of the spine. The facets at the L4–5 level are directed more sagitally than those of the L5-S1 joints, allowing more anterior motion. In the presence of degenerative changes, the normal limitation of movement of one facet on the one in front becomes deficient, allowing forward displacement of L4. Slippage is never greater than 30% of the anteroposterior diameter of L5, since the spinous process of L4 hooks up on the body of the next lower vertebra. Radiographic findings associated with degenerative spondylolisthesis include signs of facet joint osteoarthritis—joint space narrowing, sclerosis, osteophytes, intervertebral disc space nar-

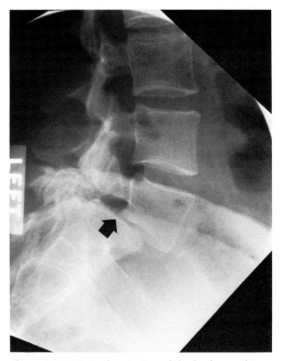

Figure 10–18. Lateral spot view of the lumbosacral junction. A Grade II spondylolisthesis is seen with a 50% slippage of the vertebral body.

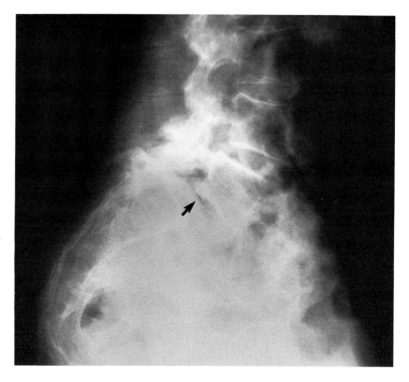

Figure 10–19. An 82-year-old woman was evaluated for low back pain of 2 months duration. The pain is constant, exacerbated by anterior flexion and relieved by lying supine. Lateral view of the lumbosacral spine reveals a Grade II degenerative spondylolisthesis at the L5-S1 interspace. A vacuum phenomenon is also present at the same interspace (arrow).

lumbosacral spine (see Table 10–1).[21] Fractures of the spine may cause abnormal motion of the lumbar spine. However, these fractures rarely occur spontaneously but more commonly in the setting of significant trauma to the lumbosacral spine.

It is important to remember that in adolescents or young adults, spondylolysis is usually asymptomatic. If back pain is present, a search should be made for other causes of back discomfort, including disc space infection, spinal cord tumor, osteoid osteoma, or early spondyloarthropathy. Disc herniation rarely occurs in this setting.

TREATMENT

The nonoperative treatment of the adult with spondylolisthesis is much the same as that used for backache from other causes. When the symptoms are acute, rest is indicated. If leg pain is a significant problem, anti-inflammatory medication can be quite beneficial. Exercises should be started once the patient is in a remission, and the patient is usually advised to wear a corset during occasional strenuous activity. Brace therapy may be helpful in decreasing symptoms in patients with spondylolisthesis. In a study of 28 patients who used antilordotic braces over 25 months, those with

spondylolisthesis had a significant reduction of lumbar lordosis and sacral inclination. At the conclusion of the period of brace treatment, all patients were pain-free and none had demonstrated a significant increase in slippage.[22] Flexion or extension exercises may be indicated for symptomatic spondylolisthesis. In a study of 48 patients with spondylolisthesis treated with flexion or extension exercises, after 3 years of therapy 62% of patients treated with flexion exercises had improvement while 0% of patients treated with extension exercises improved.[23] Flexion exercises are more effective than extension exercises for the treatment of spondylolisthesis.

Surgery in the form of fusion of the unstable segment is indicated only to relieve pain, not to prevent slippage. Not infrequently, patients whose spondylolisthesis progresses beyond Grade II need surgical intervention to decrease symptoms.[24] Surgical therapy may include spinal fusion for patients with low back symptoms and decompression with fusion for those with nerve root compression.[25]

PROGNOSIS

The identification of those adolescents who are at risk of developing symptomatically significant spondylolisthesis remains difficult. Adolescents with slips of greater than 50% are at risk for progression of the disease, according to some studies.[26] Patients diagnosed at a younger age, have a flattened lumbar lordosis, have minimal slip at initial evaluation, have spina bifida, and are male may develop progressive listhesis. Patients with these findings should have serial evaluations. In most studies of young patients with isthmic lumbar spondylolisthesis, radiologic progression of slippage is rare and occurs slowly.[27] In a study of 272 children and adolescents, 190 patients who had posterolateral surgical fusion had a similar amount of progression as those treated nonsurgically.[28] In a study of 40 patients with degenerative spondylolisthesis, progression of slippage was noted in 30%. No progression occurred in patients with restabilization of the spine characterized by narrowing of the intervertebral disc, spur formation, subcartilaginous sclerosis, or ossification of ligaments. No correlation existed between clinical symptoms and the progression of slippage.[29]

Once patients experience symptoms secondary to spondylolisthesis, it is unreasonable to expect them to perform heavy work or participate in high-performance athletics. These individuals should be restricted in regard to activities generally involving heavy lifting or repetitive bending. Surgical outcomes are good in patients who have fusions to relieve pain. The operation will not return people to strenuous activity and should not be undertaken with that expectation in mind.

References

SPONDYLOLYSIS/SPONDYLOLISTHESIS

1. Wiltse LL, Newman PH, Macnab I: Classification of spondylolisthesis. Clin Orthop 117:23, 1976.
2. Wiltse LL, Widell EH Jr, Jackson DW: Fatigue fractures: the basic lesion in isthmic spondylolisthesis. J Bone Joint Surg 57A:17, 1975.
3. Wynne-Davies R, Scott JHS: Inheritance and spondylolisthesis: a radiographic family survey. J Bone Joint Surg 61B:301, 1979.
4. Sward L, Hellstrom M, Jacobsson B, Peterson L: Back pain and radiologic changes in the thoracolumbar spine of athletes. Spine 15:124, 1990.
5. Macnab I: Spondylolisthesis with an intact neural arch—the so-called pseudospondylolisthesis. J Bone Joint Surg 32B:325, 1950.
6. LaBan MM, Wesolowski DP: Night pain associated with diminished cardiopulmonary compliance. A concomitant of lumbar spinal stenosis and degenerative spondylolisthesis. Am J Phys Med Rehabil 67:155, 1988.
7. Phalen GS, Dickson JA: Spondylolisthesis and tight hamstrings. J Bone Joint Surg 43A:5095, 1961.
8. Turner RH, Bianco AJ Jr: Spondylolysis and spondylolisthesis in children and teenagers. J Bone Joint Surg 53A:1298, 1971.
9. Newman PH: A clinical syndrome associated with severe lumbosacral subluxation. J Bone Joint Surg 47B:472, 1965.
10. Fredrickson BE, Baker D, McHolick WJ, et al.: The natural history of spondylolysis and spondylolisthesis. J Bone Joint Surg 66A:699, 1984.
11. Meyerding HW: Low backache and sciatic pain associated with spondylolisthesis and protruded intervertebral disc. J Bone Joint Surg 23:461, 1941.
12. Boden SD, Wiesel SW: Lumbosacral segmental motion in normal individuals: have we been measuring instability properly? Spine 15:571, 1990.
13. Ryan PJ, Evans PA, Gibson T, Fogelman I: Chronic low back pain: comparison of bone SPECT with radiography and CT. Radiology 182:849, 1992.
14. Szypryt EP, Twining P, Mulholland RC, Worthington BS: The prevalence of disc degeneration associated with neural arch defects of the lumbar spine assessed by magnetic resonance imaging. Spine 14:977, 1989.
15. Jinkins JR, Matthes JC, Sner RN, et al.: Spondylolysis, spondylolisthesis, and associated nerve root entrapment in the lumbosacral spine: MR evaluation. AJR 152:327, 1989.
16. Grenier N, Kressel HY, Schiebler ML, Grossman RI: Isthmic spondylolysis of the lumbar spine: MR imaging at 1.5T. Radiology 170:489, 1989.
17. Johnson DW, Farnum GN, Latchaw RE, Erba SM: MR imaging of the pars interarticularis. AJR 152:327, 1989.
18. Fitzgerald JAW, Newman PH: Degenerative spondylolesthesis. J Bone Joint Surg 58B:184, 1976.
19. Stokes IAF, Frymoyer JW: Segmental motion and instability. Spine 12:688, 1987.
20. Willis TA: Lumbosacral retrodisplacement. AJR 90:1263, 1963.
21. Laurent LE: Spondylolisthesis. Acta Orthop Scand (Suppl) 35:20, 1958.
22. Bell DF, Ehrlich MG, Zaleske DJ: Brace treatment for symptomatic spondylolisthesis. Clin Orthop 236:192, 1988.
23. Sinaki M, Lutness MP, Ilstrup DM, et al.: Lumbar spondylolisthesis: retrospective comparison and three-year follow-up of two conservative treatment programs. Arch Phys Med Rehabil 70:594, 1989.
24. Dandy DJ, Shannon MJ: Lumbosacral subluxation (Group I spondylolisthesis) J Bone Joint Surg 53B:578, 1971.
25. Johnson LP, Nasca RJ, Dunham WK: Surgical management of isthmic spondylolisthesis. Spine 13:93, 1988.
26. Bovall DW, Bradford DS, Moe JH, Winter RB: Management of severe spondylolisthesis (Grade III and IV) in children and adolescents. J Bone Joint Surg 61A:479, 1979.
27. Danielson BI, Frennered AK, Irstam LKH: Radiologic progression of isthmic lumbar spondylolisthesis in young patients. Spine 16:422, 1991.
28. Seitsalo S, Osterman K, Hyvarinen H, et al.: Progression of spondylolisthesis in children and adolescents: a long-term follow-up of 272 patients. Spine 16:417, 1991.
29. Matsunaga S, Sakou T, Morizono Y, et al.: Natural history of degenerative spondylolisthesis: pathogenesis and natural course of the slippage. Spine 15:1204, 1990.

ADULT SCOLIOSIS

Capsule Summary

Frequency of back pain—uncommon
Location of back pain—lumbar curve
Quality of back pain—ache
Symptoms and signs—lumbar curvature
Laboratory and x-ray tests—curvature on plain roentgenogram
Treatment—medications, physical therapy, braces, surgery

PREVALANCE AND PATHOGENESIS

Scoliosis is lateral curvature of the spine. The term is usually applied to curves in excess of 10°. The normal spine does curve in the lateral plane, but it should be straight (no lateral deviation) when viewed from the front or back. Many patients with lumbar or thoracolumbar curves are asymptomatic. It is felt by some that the incidence of low back pain found in scoliosis is no higher than that associated with the general population. However, others feel that pain is indirectly associated with scoliosis and that the larger the curve, the more severe the pain is likely to be. Scoliotic curves may be either structural (fixed), characterized by fixed rotation on forward bending, or compensatory, tending to maintain body alignment of the head over the pelvis and normal position on forward bending. When the apex of the curve is from L2 to L4, the curve is termed lumbar. When the apex is at L5 or the sacrum, the curve is termed lumbosacral. Kyphoscoliosis is lateral curvature of the spine associated with either increased posterior or decreased anterior angulation in the sagittal plane in excess of the accepted normal curve for that area. Kyphoscoliosis affects both the thoracic and lumbar spine. Studies of adults have recognized scoliosis between 3.9% to 6% of individuals.[1, 2]

In 1973, the Scoliosis Research Society developed a classification of spine deformity. The major categories include idiopathic, neuromuscular, congenital, neurofibromatosis, mesenchymal disorders, rheumatoid disease, trauma, extraspinal contractures, osteochondrodystrophies, infection of bone, metabolic disorders, disorders related to the lumbosacral joint, and tumors (Table 10–5). Nonstructural (compensatory) forms of scoliosis include those related to postural, hysterical, nerve root, inflammatory, leg length, and hip abnormalities. By far the largest group of cases of scoliosis are idiopathic, with over 90% falling in this category.[3]

CLINICAL HISTORY

The adult patient presenting with scoliosis typically is a woman between the ages of 20 and 40, though some patients may present as late as at 80 years of age. The patient initially is asymptomatic but gradually develops a feeling of tiredness at the end of the day in the lumbar area. The pain of scoliosis is mechanical in nature and is probably caused by disc and/or facet joint degeneration. In some instances, the pain is radicular in nature and is secondary to nerve root compression on the concave side of the lumbar curve. In severe cases, impingement of the ribs on the iliac crest may cause severe pain.

Patients will state that the pain becomes worse the longer they are ambulatory and the symptoms are rapidly relieved upon lying down. The site of the pain is at or just below the apex of the curve. As time passes, the pain occurs more frequently and is more severe.

Progression of the curve usually co-exists with increased pain. In the lumbar spine, a curve over 40° will generally lead to a constant rate of progression of 1° per year. The rate may increase to even a greater degree with pregnancy. Under 40°, in a skeletally mature individual, the curve will remain stable.

In taking the history of adolescents, the physician should inquire about family history and connective tissue, neuromuscular and traumatic disorders. Positive responses to these inquiries help identify those individuals who have specific reasons for developing scoliosis (neurofibromatosis, Marfan syndrome, muscular dystrophy) and do not belong in the idiopathic group. For example, spinal deformity is noted in 10% of individuals with neurofibromatosis.[4] Family history may give some insight into prognosis if a close relative has had progression with severe deformity.

Patients may complain of pain with certain motions of the spine. Patients with scoliosis do not have parallel facet joints. The planes of the facets are at an angle. The soft tissues on the concave side of the curve tend to shorten, resulting in a mechanical restriction of motion. With spinal flexion past a certain degree, ligamentous and capsular tissues are stretched, resulting in pain. In addition, extension of the spine may cause impingement of the asymmetric facet joints, resulting in low back pain.

PHYSICAL EXAMINATION

The patient should be undraped except for underwear. Specific examination should be done to identify scapular asymmetry and uni-

TABLE 10–5. CLASSIFICATION OF SCOLIOSIS

Structural Scoliosis
I. Idiopathic
   A. Infantile (0–3 years)
      1. Resolving
      2. Progressive
   B. Juvenile (3–10 years)
   C. Adolescent (> 10 years)
II. Neuromuscular
   A. Neuropathic
      1. Upper motor neuron
         a. Cerebral palsy
         b. Spinocerebellar degeneration
            i. Friedreich's disease
            ii. Charcot-Marie-Tooth disease
            iii. Roussy-Lévy disease
         c. Syringomyelia
         d. Spinal cord tumor
         e. Spinal cord trauma
         f. Other
      2. Lower motor neuron
         a. Poliomyelitis
         b. Other viral myelitides
         c. Traumatic
         d. Spinal muscular atrophy
            i. Werdnig-Hoffmann
            ii. Kugelberg-Welander
         e. Myelomeningocoele (paralytic)
      3. Dysautonomia (Riley-Day)
      4. Other
   B. Myopathic
      1. Arthrogryposis
      2. Muscular dystrophy
         a. Duchenne (pseudohypertrophic)
         b. Limb-girdle
         c. Facioscapulohumeral
      3. Fiber type disproportion
      4. Congenital hypotonia
      5. Myotonia dystrophica
      6. Other
III. Congenital
   A. Failure of formation
      1. Wedge vertebra
      2. Hemivertebra
   B. Failure of segmentation
      1. Unilateral (unsegmented bar)
      2. Bilateral
   C. Mixed
IV. Neurofibromatosis

V. Mesenchymal disorders
   A. Marfan's
   B. Ehlers-Danlos
   C. Others
VI. Rheumatoid disease
VII. Trauma
   A. Fracture
   B. Surgical
      1. Postlaminectomy
      2. Postthoracoplasty
   C. Irradiation
VIII. Extraspinal contractures
   A. Postempyema
   B. Post-burns
IX. Osteochondrodystrophies
   A. Diastrophic dwarfism
   B. Mucopolysaccharidoses (e.g., Morquio's syndrome)
   C. Spondyloepiphyseal dysplasia
   D. Multiple epiphyseal dysplasia
   E. Other
X. Infection of bone
   A. Acute
   B. Chronic
XI. Metabolic disorders
   A. Rickets
   B. Osteogenesis imperfecta
   C. Homocystinuria
   D. Others
XII. Related to lumbosacral joint
   A. Spondylolysis and spondylolisthesis
   B. Congenital anomalies of lumbosacral region
XIII. Tumors
   A. Vertebral column
      1. Osteoid osteoma
      2. Histiocytosis X
      3. Other
   B. Spinal cord (see neuromuscular)

Nonstructural Scoliosis
I. Postural scoliosis
II. Hysterical scoliosis
III. Nerve root irritation
   A. Herniation of nucleus puloposus
   B. Tumors
IV. Inflammatory (e.g., appendicitis)
V. Related to leg length discrepancy
VI. Related to contractures about the hip

From Bradford DS, Moe JH, Winter RB: Scoliosis and kyphosis. In: Rothman RH, Simeone FA (eds.): The Spine, 2nd ed. Philadelphia, WB Saunders Co, 1982.

lateral prominence, waist asymmetry, shoulder level, and asymmetry in the distance between the arms and the torso. As the patient bends over, prominence of one side of the rib cage is noted. From the rear, a measurement of the distance right or left from the gluteal cleft to a line drawn from C7 to the ground is a measurement of spinal imbalance. Inability to bend side to side may be secondary to intraspinal lesions such as a tumor, herniated disc, or osteoid osteoma, as well as scoliosis.

Lumbar scoliosis frequently involves the L1 vertebral body. Tilting of the lumbar spine at this level is associated with pelvic obliquity (unequal heights of the iliac wings), which is noted on physical examination.

A complete neurologic examination is useful to document those individuals who may be experiencing signs of nerve root compression. Muscle fatigue after exercise may be indicative of spinal stenosis associated with scoliosis.

LABORATORY DATA

Laboratory tests are normal in patients with idiopathic scoliosis.

RADIOGRAPHIC EVALUATION

Radiographic evaluation of scoliosis may be obtained with an erect AP and lateral view of the thoracolumbar spine. The AP view is used to measure the degree of curvature of the spine while the lateral detects the presence of spondylolisthesis. Additional views may be obtained to assess spinal flexibility. They should be obtained in a standardized manner so that progressive curvature can be measured.

Cobb's method is used to measure spine curvature (Fig. 10–20). The vertebrae forming the ends of the curve are those that are most severely tilted toward its concavity. Lines are drawn along the upper border of the superior end-vertebra and along the lower border of the inferior end-vertebra. Perpendiculars are erected from each of these lines and are extended to intersect. Cobb's angle is the angle formed by the intersection of these two perpendicular lines.[5] The severity of rotation of the vertebrae associated with scoliosis may be determined by the method of Nash and Moe,

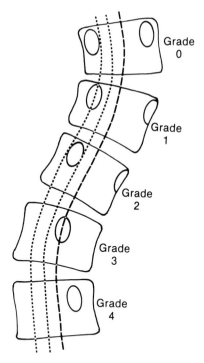

Figure 10–21. Grading of rotatory scoliosis.

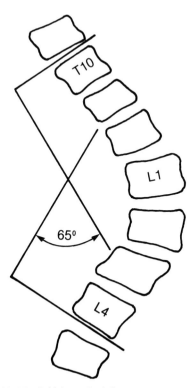

Figure 10–20. Cobb's method for measurement of spinal curvature. Lines are drawn along the superior end-vertebra at the uppermost extension of the vertebra and along the lower border of the inferior end-vertebra. The angle formed by the intersecting lines drawn perpendicular to the end-plates is Cobb's angle.

which is graded by the location of the pedicle on the concave side of the scoliosis. With Grades 1 and 2 the convex pedicle is visible on AP view. With Grades 3 and 4, the convex pedicle has twisted out of view (Fig. 10–21).[6] The use of other radiographic techniques, such as bone scintigraphy, CT, or MR, are limited to those individuals with neurologic dysfunction or those who are to undergo surgery. Radiographic studies of patients with neurologic dysfunction may identify a tumor or an area of nerve impingement.

To diagnose a progression of scoliosis, a definite increase of a curvature of greater than 5° must be seen on roentgenographic evaluation. The initial film taken in adulthood must be compared with the most current films to show progression.

DIFFERENTIAL DIAGNOSIS

The diagnosis of adult scoliosis is suspected during the physical examination and is confirmed by measurement of lumbar spine angulation observed on roentgenographic examination (see Table 10–1). The curve is significant in an adult if it is greater than 40°. Spinal angulation of less than 40° does not progress and rarely causes symptoms. Although the vast majority of individuals will have an idiopathic or degenerative form of adult scoliosis, some adults will develop spinal curvature secondary to specific medical or mechanical abnormalities. Patients with an osteoid osteoma may develop a reversible form of scoliosis secondary to muscle contraction.[7] Patients with osteomalacia of long duration develop weakening of bones, which may result in spinal curvature.[8]

Leg length disparity is a correctable but frequently overlooked cause of adult scoliosis.[9] Patients with this type of scoliosis frequently complain of pain with standing or walking that starts within 30 minutes of commencing the activity and resolves quickly on sitting down. Placing a lift in the shoe on the short leg, which partially corrects the length discrepancy, helps improve the scoliosis and relieves symptoms. Recognition of this abnormality and correction with equalization of leg length is worthwhile even if the individual has not recognized the leg length discrepancy for a number of years.[10]

TREATMENT

Treatment in the young adult is directed toward the prevention of future problems. If the curve is under 40° in the lumbar spine and the pain is not severe, nonoperative treatment can be employed. This includes analgesics and anti-inflammatory medication, local facet injections, physical therapy, and braces. The Milwaukee brace is a mainstay of nonoperative therapy in young individuals and is used to prevent progression of spinal curvature.[11] For the most part this form of bracing is rarely effective in the adult population. If discomfort cannot be controlled or the curve is progressive, surgery is indicated. The aim of surgery is to straighten the spine as much as is safely possible and to stabilize it in a corrected position.

In the older adult, treatment is directed toward the correction of existing problems. Besides pain and curve progression, the older adult is more likely to have compression of

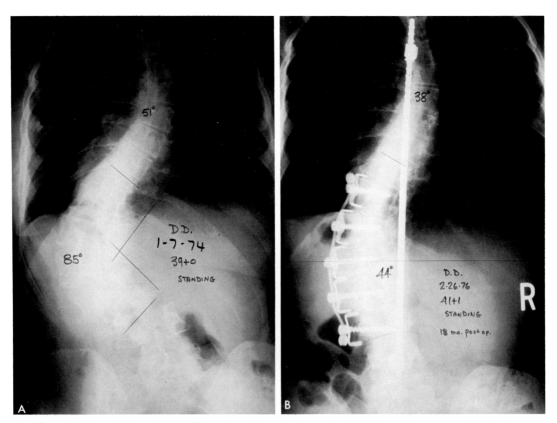

Figure 10–22. *A,* D.D., a 39-year-old female with progressive and painful idiopathic curvatures. The lumbar curve was the more progressive and more painful of the two curves. *B,* The same patient, 18 months after anterior Dwyer instrumentation, followed by fusion of the lumbar curve, posterior Harrington instrumentation, and fusion of both curves. Almost all her pain is gone. (From Rothman RH, Simeone FA [eds]: The Spine, 2nd Ed. Philadelphia, WB Saunders Co, 1982.)

neural elements. This occurs because of the degenerative changes associated with adult scoliosis of longer duration. The goal is to keep these patients functional. In most patients with a lumbar curve under 40°, this is possible without surgery. An operative procedure is indicated for unremitting pain, curve progression, or uncontrolled radiculopathy. With the newer internal fixation devices (e.g., Harrington rods and pedicule fixation) available, scoliosis surgery in the adult lumbar spine can be quite rewarding, resulting in spine stabilization and reduction in symptoms (Fig. 10–22).[12]

PROGNOSIS

Most patients with adult scoliosis do not require therapy, since their curvature is mild and nonprogressive. Patients with progressive curvature develop persistent pain at the apex of the curve, which may respond to medical therapy. Patients with even greater curvature may develop neurologic deficits and pulmonary insufficiency, particularly with thoracic scoliosis.[13]

Untreated scoliosis is associated with major disability and death. In the adult, pain may become progressive and severe as increasing degenerative changes occur in facet joints and intervertebral discs. Respiratory insufficiency may limit stamina and work potential in those with double curvature (thoracolumbar scoliosis).

Premature death may also be a complication of severe scoliosis. Nachemson reported a mortality twice that of the normal population at age 40 from cardiorespiratory causes in 130 nontreated scoliosis patients of all types.[14] Once again, this occurs in patients with double curvature.

Surgical intervention in the form of fusion and/or rods can halt further progression of spine curvature and relieve pain. Surgery is not without its complications, including pseudoarthrosis, infection, and curvature above the area of fusion. Location of the fusion and the configuration of the stabilizing device may result in complications after surgery. Patients over 30 with fusions at L3 or lower have more secondary surgeries for pseudoarthrosis, disc-

ectomy for disc herniation caudal to the fusion, and decompression for spinal stenosis. These individuals may also experience more back pain, interference with activities of daily living, and a greater requirement for regular pain medication.[15] Careful consideration must be given to the selection of surgical candidates. Scoliosis surgery is best done by physicians who have had extensive experience with the complexity of the surgical procedures and the special needs of the patients with this mechanical abnormality.

References

ADULT SCOLIOSIS

1. Kostuik JP, Bentivoglio J: The incidence of low back pain in adult scoliosis. Spine 6:268, 1981.
2. Vanderpool DW, James JIP, Wynne-Davies R: Scoliosis in the elderly. J Bone Joint Surg 51A:446, 1969.
3. Cobb JR: Outline for the study of scoliosis. Am Acad Orthop Surgeons Lect 5:261, 1948.
4. Akbarnia BA, Gabriel KR, Beckman E, Chalk D: Prevalence of scoliosis in neurofibromatosis. Spine 17:S244, 1992.
5. Bradford DS, Moe JH, Winter RB: Scoliosis and Kyphosis. In: Rothman RH, Simeone FA (eds): The Spine. 2nd Ed. Philadelphia: WB Saunders Co, 1982, pp 316–439.
6. Nash CL, Moe JH: A study of vertebral rotation. J Bone Joint Surg 51A:223, 1969.
7. Freiberger RH: Osteoid osteoma of the spine: a cause of backache and scoliosis in children and young adults. Radiology 75:232, 1960.
8. Steinbach HL, Noetzli M: Roentgen appearance of the skeleton in osteomalacia and rickets. AJR 91:955, 1964.
9. Gofton JP: Persistent low back pain and leg length disparity. J Rheumatol 12:747, 1985.
10. Rothenberg RJ: Rheumatic disease aspects of leg length inequality. Semin Arthritis Rheum 17:196, 1988.
11. Moe JH: Indication for Milwaukee brace nonoperative treatment in idiopathic scoliosis. Clin Orthop 93:38, 1973.
12. Harrington PR: An eleven year clinical investigation of Harrington instrumentation, a preliminary report on 578 cases. Orthop Clin North Am 3:113, 1972.
13. Nilsonne U, Lundgren KD: Long-term prognosis in idiopathic scoliosis. Acta Orthop Scand 39:456, 1968.
14. Nachemson A: A long-term follow-up study of nontreated scoliosis. Acta Orthop Scand 39:466, 1968.
15. Paonessa KJ, Engler GL: Back pain and disability after Harrington rod fusion to the lumbar spine for scoliosis. Spine 17:S249, 1992.

11

Rheumatologic Disorders of the Lumbosacral Spine

Rheumatologic disorders of the lumbosacral spine are common causes of back pain. These disorders affect the bones, joints, ligaments, tendons, and muscles, which are anatomic components of the lumbosacral spine. While mechanical disorders, such as muscle strain, disease of the intervertebral discs, and osteoarthritis of the lumbosacral spine, are frequent causes of low back pain, there are a number of other inflammatory and noninflammatory disorders associated with pain in the lumbosacral spine. The most important rheumatic disorders that cause inflammation of the joints of the axial skeleton are the seronegative spondyloarthropathies. This group of diseases is characterized by involvement of the sacroiliac joints, peripheral large joint disease, and the absence of rheumatoid factor. The seronegative spondyloarthropathies include ankylosing spondylitis (AS), Reiter's syndrome, psoriatic arthritis, enteropathic arthritis, familial Mediterranean fever, Behçet's syndrome, Whipple's disease, and arthritis associated with hidradenitis suppurativa. They are closely associated with genetic factors that predispose patients to these illnesses. Environmental factors play a role as the triggers of the inflammatory response in genetically predisposed individuals, but these factors have been only partially identified. Bacterial infection is associated with the onset of Reiter's syndrome and reactive arthritis. The role of trauma as an environmental trigger in AS, Reiter's syndrome, and psoriatic arthritis remains controversial.

In spondyloarthropathy, the history of pain, which is most severe in the morning and improves with activity, is characteristic. Physical examination demonstrates localized tenderness over the sacroiliac joints and vertebral column, with limitation of motion in all directions. Laboratory abnormalities are consistent with systemic inflammatory disease but are nonspecific. Radiographic evaluation is very useful in identifying characteristic joint space narrowing, sclerosis, and fusion in the sacroiliac joints, vertebral body squaring, and ligamentous calcification in the axial skeleton.

Rheumatoid arthritis, an inflammatory peripheral arthropathy, may involve the facet joints of the lumbar spine, but it more frequently affects the cervical spine and occurs in the setting of diffuse long-standing appendicular joint disease. Noninflammatory lesions affecting bone in the lumbosacral spine include diffuse idiopathic skeletal hyperostosis (DISH), osteochondritis, and osteitis condensans ilii. Muscle syndromes associated with low back pain include polymyalgia rheumatica and fibromyalgia.

In addition to drug therapy, treatment for these rheumatologic disorders involves a number of therapeutic modalities, which include patient education and physical and occupational therapy. Although there are no cures for these illnesses, medical therapy can be very effective in controlling symptoms.

ANKYLOSING SPONDYLITIS

Capsule Summary

Frequency of back pain—very common
Location of back pain—sacroiliac joints and lumbar spine

Quality of back pain—ache

Symptoms and signs—morning stiffness, decreased back motion, percussion tenderness over sacroiliac joints

Laboratory and x-ray tests—elevated sedimentation rate; bilateral symmetric sacroiliitis on plain roentgenograms

Treatment—range of motion exercises, nonsteroidal anti-inflammatory drugs, muscle relaxants

PREVALENCE AND PATHOGENESIS

Ankylosing spondylitis (AS) (Greek ankylos, bent; spondylos, vertebra) is a chronic inflammatory disease characterized by a variable symptomatic course and progressive involvement of the sacroiliac and axial skeletal joints. It is the prototype of the seronegative spondyloarthropathies. This disease complex is characterized by axial skeletal arthritis, the absence of rheumatoid factor in serum (seronegativity), the lack of rheumatoid nodules, and the presence of a tissue factor on host cells, HLA-B27. AS is a disease of antiquity, having been found in the remains of Egyptian mummies and having been known to Hippocrates.[1] A reappraisal of skeletal remains from a time period from Egyptian dynasties to the 19th century suggests that AS may not have been as common as once suspected. Forestier's disease (DISH), Reiter's syndrome, or psoriatic spondylitis may have occurred more commonly.[2] Over that period of time and to the present, AS has had many names, including rheumatoid spondylitis, Marie-Strümpell disease, von Bechterew's disease, and rheumatoid variant.

AS affects about 1% to 2% of the Caucasian population, a number equal to the prevalence for rheumatoid arthritis.[3, 4] Some studies have suggested that 6.7% of Caucasian adults in certain populations may have AS.[5] Initially, the male to female ratio was thought to be 10:1. More recent studies have demonstrated the ratio to be in the range of 3:1.[6] Women tend to be less symptomatic and develop less severe disease, and this may explain their small representation in earlier studies. In addition, the criteria necessary for diagnosis of AS also have an effect on the number of individuals found to have the illness.

The pathogenesis of AS is unknown. In the past, infections, trauma, and heredity were thought to be involved in the pathogenesis of this disease. A genetic predisposition to AS and to the seronegative spondyloarthropathies in general does exist. HLAs (human leukocyte antigens) are cell surface markers that are present on all nucleated mammalian cells. A portion of the short arm of the sixth chromosome of man that determines the expression of the HLA antigen contains the major histocompatibility complex (MHC), which is associated with control of the immune response of the host (Fig. 11–1). In the MHC region are loci that code for the A, B, C, and D HLA antigens. A, B, and C loci are class I antigens, which are serologically (antibody) defined. The antigen consists of 2 polypeptide chains, a large glycosylated chain that carries antigenic specificity and a small chain (beta-microglobulin) (Fig. 11–2). MHC class I genes are expressed on all nucleated cells. The heavy chain is divided into five distinct regions, three extracellular domains, a transmembrane region, and a cytoplasmic domain. There are many alleles for each locus (HLA-A—20 alleles, HLA-B—40 alleles, HLA-C—12 alleles).[7] The D locus or class II antigens are determined by interaction with

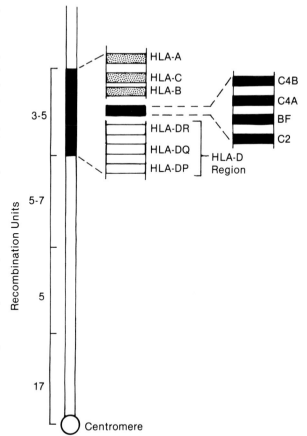

Figure 11–1. The short arm of the sixth chromosome of man containing the histocompatibility locus (HLA). Included in this area are the A, B, C, and D loci. The D locus includes 3 alleles (DR, DQ and DP). Interposed between the B and D loci is the genetic material which codes for some of the complement components (C4b, C4A, BF, C2).

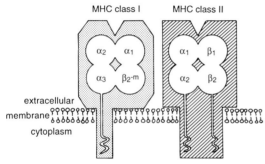

Figure 11–2. MHC class I molecules consist of a single alpha chain forming three domains along with beta-microglobulin that acts as a stabilizer for the alpha chain. MHC II molecules consist of two separate alpha and beta chains that form four extracellular domains.

specific lymphocytes (mixed lymphocyte reaction). The class II antigen consists of two membrane-inserted glycosylated polypeptides that are noncovalently bound (Fig. 11–2). Humans have at least three sets of genes for class II molecules: HLA-DR, HLA-DP, and HLA-DQ. Different alleles exist for each class II molecule. MHC class II antigens are expressed on cells that present antigens to CD4+ T lymphocytes. The class II molecules have an alpha and beta chain. Each chain has two domains, a transmembrane segment and an intracytoplasmic tail. Investigators have identified specific antigens associated with each locus.

A strikingly high association between HLA-B27 and AS has been demonstrated. HLA-B27 is present in over 90% of white patients with AS, compared with a frequency of 8% in a normal white population.[8] Approximately 2% of HLA-B27-positive whites have AS.[9] HLA-B27 is present in 50% of American blacks with AS, compared with a prevalence of 4% in the normal black population.[10] African blacks do not have the HLA-B27 antigen and rarely develop AS. Other ethnic groups such as the Haida and Pima Indian tribes have a large proportion of individuals affected by AS associated with an increased prevalence of HLA-B27. Approximately 20% of individuals who are HLA-B27 positive have evidence of spondylitis.[6] However, genetic factors alone will not result in the expression of the disease. Many individuals who are HLA-B27 positive have no evidence of a spondyloarthropathy. Identical twins who are HLA-B27 positive may be discordant for AS. One twin may have AS, while the other may be normal or develop symptoms and signs of a form of spondyloarthropathy other than AS.[11]

Part of this discordance may be related to the fact that there are at least three different epitopes (antigenic specificities) carried by

B27 (M_1, M_2^+, M_2^-). These HLA-B27 epitopes were defined by murine monoclonal antibodies. The antibody reacting with M_1 was an IgG, while the antibody reacting with M_2 was an IgM. Studies 12–15 of these B27 epitopes have shown the following:

1. B27 M_1 is shared by all B27 individuals.
2. M_2 is on most B27 molecules and cross-reacts with BW47.
3. B27 antigens are M_2-positive or M_2-negative.
4. M_2 variant is more commonly found in Orientals than in Caucasian populations.
5. B27 M_2-negative molecule is more strongly related to AS than other B27 variants.
6. B27 M_2-positive molecule may be associated with Reiter's syndrome.

Additional evidence for certain subclasses of B27 individuals being at increased risk of developing AS arises from the observation that spondylitis is more common among B27-positive relatives of spondylitics than in B27-positive relatives of healthy B27 control subjects. Susceptibility may be related to the B27 epitope or to the presence of additional or linked genes that increase susceptibility.[16–18] Since genetic information in the MHC region other than Class I antigen (complement components—Class III antigens) does not increase susceptibility to spondylitis, additional genetic information that predisposes to spondylitis is probably distant from the B27 locus.[19]

Since the report by Calin,[18] significant progress has been made in regard to understanding the heterogeneity of HLA-B27. HLA-B27 has been subdivided into at least six subtypes.[20] B*2705 is the major subtype of B27. This subtype is present in 90% of B27-positive Caucasians. B*2701 and B*2702 occur in 10% of B27 Caucasians. B*2703 is found only in American blacks.[21] The heterogeneity of HLA-B27 is apparent when its physical structure is examined.[22] The structure of the molecule forms an antigen-binding pocket. The floor of the antigen-binding site is formed by the beta strands and the margins are formed by alpha helices. Certain residues are highly variable and are associated with the subtypes of HLA-B27 (Fig. 11–3).[23] This binding site is the location for the attachment of antigen that is presented to the T-cell receptor for processing as an antigen.[24] The various B27 alleles differ from each other by one to six amino acids scattered throughout the peptide-binding groove of the class I molecule. Additional studies are being reported in regard to identification of HLA-B27 subtypes associated with the various spon-

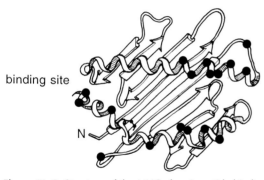

Figure 11–3. Structure of the MHC class I peptide-binding groove. The alpha 1 and 2 domains of the polypeptide chain form a beta-pleated sheet platform and two alpha helices that form the walls of groove into which the antigen peptides can bind. The filled circles correspond to residues critical in defining serologic epitopes on the alpha 1 and 2 domains.

dyloarthropathies.[25] Currently, the HLA-B27 subtypes are similar between groups.

The mechanism by which HLA-B27 antigen results in spondylitis is not known. The proposed hypotheses to explain this occurrence have included:

1. B27 as a receptor site for infectious agents.

2. B27 as a marker for an immune response gene that determines susceptibility to an environmental trigger.

3. B27 as a factor that induces tolerance to cross-reactive foreign antigens.[26, 27]

A genetically determined host response to an environmental factor(s) in genetically susceptible individuals seems to be the most likely basis for the pathogenesis of the spondyloarthropathies. B27 is not sufficient to develop AS and is supported by the fact that not all individuals with B27 develop disease, that B27 even in a homogeneous form does not cause disease, and that a small number of AS patients do not have B27. Recent studies in animals suggest that the HLA-B27 molecule itself plays a role in the pathogenesis of spondylitis. In transgenic rats made to express high levels of B27, an illness similar to AS develops.[28] The environmental component that may play a role in disease pathogenesis may be intestinal flora. Transgenic rats that are bacteria-free do not develop AS manifestations, while those exposed to bacteria subsequently develop disease. This illness provides direct evidence for the participation of the HLA-B27 molecule and environmental factors in disease pathogenesis.[29]

Although not frequently mentioned in the context of spondylitis, DR antigens may play a role in the appearance of certain disease manifestations. Miehle reported an increased prevalence of peripheral joint arthritis in HLA-DR4-positive patients with AS.[30]

The role of incidental trauma to the lumbosacral spine in the initiation of the inflammatory process of AS is unknown. Patients with AS may present with radicular back pain, which is thought to be secondary to a herniated lumbar disc. Some of these patients have laminectomies and have gone on to develop classic changes of AS in the axial skeleton. One of the potential complications of total hip joint replacement in a patient with AS is myositis ossificans, the calcification of soft tissues surrounding a joint. It may be possible that in the patients predisposed to this disease, significant tissue injury to the lumbosacral spine or peripheral joints can result in an inflammatory process that promotes tissue calcification and joint ankylosis.[31]

The difficulty of substantiating the role of lumbosacral spine trauma and the development of AS is illustrated by two histories. In the case of fraternal twin brothers, one was asymptomatic with no evidence of AS. The other brother, who was asymptomatic before a fall at work, developed low back pain. He had a decompression procedure (laminectomy) for a suspected herniated lumbar disc. Subsequently, he developed progressive fusion of the lumbar, thoracic, and cervical spine and peripheral arthritis of the hip. In another case, an Egyptian soldier who had symptoms of low back pain compatible with ankylosing spondylitis suffered a shrapnel wound in the lumbar spine and thighs. He was immobilized for an extended period and experienced marked limitation of axial skeletal motion. Radiographic evaluation demonstrated increased spondylitic changes in his axial skeleton. Did significant tissue damage to the axial skeleton or peripheral joints in those patients with active AS result in an exacerbation of symptoms and progression of disease in the injured area? Would AS have developed to the same degree in the absence of spinal surgery or tissue injury? Jacoby has reported on his experience with five patients who developed spondylitic symptoms after trauma. Radiographic evaluation of these patients revealed disease already present at the time of the injury. He suggests that trauma does not cause spondylitis but brings the patient to medical attention.[32]

Infective agents have also been proposed as initiators of the inflammatory process that causes AS. *Klebsiella pneumoniae* has been singled out as the most likely pathogen.[33] Immunologic abnormalities specific to B27-positive individuals have been described.[34] Certain bacteria (*Klebsiella, Shigella, Yersinia*) cause alterations in lymphocyte responses in patients who are B27 M_1 or M_2 positive.[35, 36] However, findings demonstrating the increased colonization of the gut and heightened lymphocyte sensitivity to *Klebsiella* organisms in AS patients have not been borne out in other investigations.[37, 38] Subsequent studies have not substantiated any increased sensitivity of lymphocytes from B27 patients with *K. pneumoniae nitrogenase* or *Yersinia* outer membrane protein.[39]

AS is a disease of the synovial and cartilaginous joints of the axial skeleton, sacroiliac joints, spinal apophyseal joints, and symphysis pubis. The large appendicular joints, hips, shoulders, knees, elbows, and ankles are also affected in 30% of patients. The inflammatory process is characterized by chondritis (inflammation of cartilage) or osteitis (inflammation of bone) at the junction of the cartilage and bone in the spine. An inflammatory granulation tissue forms and erodes the vertebral body margins. As opposed to rheumatoid arthritis, which is associated with osteoporosis as an early manifestation of disease, the inflammation of AS is characterized by ankylosis of joints and ossification of ligaments surrounding the vertebrae (syndesmophytes) and other musculotendinous structures such as the heels and pelvis.

CLINICAL HISTORY

The classic picture of AS is a man between the ages of 15 and 40 with intermittent, dull low back pain and stiffness slowly progressing over a period of months.[40] Back pain, which occurs over the course of the illness in 90% to 95% of patients, is greatest in the morning and is increased by periods of inactivity. Patients may have difficulty sleeping because of pain and stiffness. Patients may awaken at night and find it necessary to leave bed and move about for a few minutes before returning to sleep.[41] The back pain improves with exercise. The mode of onset is variable, with a majority of the patients developing pain in the lumbosacral region. In a small number of patients peripheral joints (hips, knees, and shoulders) are initially involved, and occasionally acute iridocyclitis (eye inflammation) or heel pain may be the first manifestation of disease. Rarely, patients may develop ankylosis of the spine without any back pain.[42] At the other end of the spectrum, back pain may be severe with radiation into the lower extremities, mimicking an acute lumbar disc herniation. These severe symptoms may be related to the piriformis syndrome.[43] The belly of the piriformis muscle crosses over the sciatic nerve. Inflammation in the sacroiliac joint, where the muscle attaches, results in muscle spasm and nerve compression. There are no abnormal, persistent neurologic signs associated with the sciatic pain. The symptoms are reversible with medical therapy that relieves joint inflammation. This symptom complex of radicular pain is referred to as pseudosciatica.

The usual patient has a moderate degree of intermittent aching pain that is localized to the lumbosacral area. Paraspinal musculoskeletal spasm may also contribute to the discomfort. With progression of the disease, pain develops in the dorsal and cervical spine and rib joints.

Spinal involvement is manifested by flattening of the lumbar spine and loss of normal lordosis. Thoracic spine disease causes decreased motion at the costovertebral joints, reduced chest expansion, and impaired pulmonary function. Involvement of the cervical spine causes the head to protrude forward, making it difficult to look straight ahead. Back pain, back stiffness, thigh, hip, or groin pain, and sciatica are the initial symptoms in 81% of patients. Pain in peripheral joints is the initial complaint in 13%, pain in the chest in 2%, and generalized aches in 1%.[44]

Peripheral joint arthritis (hips, knees, ankles, shoulders, elbows) occurs in 30% of patients within the first 10 years of disease.[45] Joint disease first appears as pain and stiffness. The inflammatory process may proceed to joint space narrowing and contractures. Fixed flexion contractures of the hips give rise to difficulty with walking and cause a rigid gait. Hip disease is the most frequent limiting factor in mobility rather than spinal stiffness. In fact, peripheral joint disease, particularly of the hips, which appears in the first 10 years of disease, is associated with greater disease activity and more extensive restriction of spinal motion.

Ankylosis also may occur in cartilaginous joints such as the symphysis pubic, sternomanubrial, and costosternal joints. Erosions of the plantar surface of the calcaneus at the attachment of the plantar fascia results in an enthesopathy (inflammation of an enthesis—attachment of tendon to bone).[46] This inflammation causes fasciitis and a periosteal reaction that causes heel pain and the formation of heel spurs. Achilles tendinitis is another enthesopathy associated with heel pain and AS.

AS also occurs in women but disease is underestimated.[47] There are a number of reasons to explain this fact. Women are not radiographed as often as men. They have a more benign course than men. Peripheral arthritis occurs more commonly in women suggesting an alternative diagnosis (rheumatoid arthritis). The disease has a slower progression in women. Women may have cervical spine disease characteristic of spondylitis with little lumbar spine involvement.[48]

AS is also associated with many nonarticular abnormalities. Constitutional manifestations of disease, such as fever, fatigue, and weight loss, are seen in a small number of patients with active disease, particularly in those with peripheral joint manifestations. Iritis, inflammation of the anterior uveal tract of the eye, may be the presenting complaint of 25% of the patients with AS and is present in up to 40% of patients over the course of the illness. It is usually unilateral and recurrent and is most often independent of the severity of the joint disease. Iritis is normally treated with topical corticosteroids along with the occasional use of systemic corticosteroids. Mild visual loss may be associated with iritis, but blindness is rare.

Neurologic complications of AS are secondary to nerve impingement or trauma to the spinal cord. In a study of 33 patients with AS and neurologic complications, cervical spine abnormalities were the most common cause of neurologic compromise.[49] In the lumbar spine, spinal stenosis was present in one patient. Patients with long-standing AS who develop new leg pain or urinary or bowel incontinence may be developing impingement of the nerves at the caudal end of the spinal cord, the cauda equina.[50, 51] As impingement progresses, sensory loss in the perineum develops along with thigh and leg weakness. The advent of more sensitive radiographic techniques has allowed a better understanding of the pathogenesis of this complication of AS.[52–54] The inflammation affecting ligaments causes dorsal meningeal inflammation with subsequent arachnoid adhesions (arachnoidits) resulting in erosions of the lamina. Hydrostatic pressure of cerebrospinal fluid adds to the modification of bony architecture. Nerve root injury is related to arachnoiditis in association with adhesion formation and tethering of the nerve roots. There is no effective therapy, although surgical intervention has been attempted in spondylitic patients who develop cauda equina secondary to degenerative processes (e.g., DISH).[55]

AS causes two significant changes to occur in the spine over time. Although the disease is associated with calcification of ligaments and joints, the loss of motion in the spine causes the vertebrae to become osteoporotic. Osteoporosis is a process in which there is a loss of bone calcium. Osteoporotic bones are weaker and are at greater risk of fracture.[56, 57] The other change is the loss of normal flexibility because of ankylosis of the spinal joints and ligaments. The spine in this ankylosed state is much more brittle and is prone to fracture even with minimal trauma. The most common location for fracture is the cervical spine, although dorsal and lumbar spine fractures also have been described. Patients who develop fractures may complain of nothing more than localized pain due to decreased and/or increased spinal motion, but severe sensory and motor functional loss corresponding to the location of the lesion may develop. Fracture in the lumbar spine may be associated with paralysis.[58] Therapy usually consists of external fixation with a brace when neurologic symptoms are minimal, but surgical decompression and fusion for severe neurologic abnormalities such as paraplegia may be required. Fractures that mend with external bracing or surgical fusion heal with normal bone formation.

Another complication of long-standing AS is spondylodiscitis, a destructive lesion of the disc and its surrounding vertebral bodies.[59–62] This lesion is associated with a new onset of localized pain in the spine, which, uncharacteristically for patients with AS, is improved with bed rest. The etiology of these lesions may be localized inflammation or minor trauma. In one study, patients with AS who did heavy manual labor were at greater risk of developing this abnormality than those who had sedentary occupations.[60] In most cases external immobilization was effective in controlling symptoms, while surgical fusion was reserved for the more severely affected patients.

Cardiac involvement occurs in 10% of patients when the duration of disease is 30 years or longer. Mild features include tachycardia, conduction defects, and pericarditis. The most serious cardiac abnormality is proximal aortitis, which can result in aortic valve insufficiency, heart failure, and death.[63] Aortic disease may be more common in patients with peripheral arthritis.[64] Prosthetic valve replacement may forestall cardiac deterioration. AS also may be a cause of cardiac conduction disturbances. In a study of patients with pacemakers, 8.5% of 223 men had evidence of sacroiliitis and spondylitis.[65] Patients may also have evidence of ventricular dyskinesia documented by two dimensional echocardiography.[66]

Pulmonary involvement is manifested by decreased chest expansion, which limits lung capacity. In addition, a fibrotic process affects the apical segments of the lung as a late and rare complication.[67, 68]

Amyloidosis, a deposition of a protein-like material in a number of visceral organs, is a very rare complication of AS.[69] Another form of proteinuria associated with AS patients is IgA nephropathy. Patients have raised IgA levels, proteinuria, and renal impairment.[70]

PHYSICAL EXAMINATION

A careful musculoskeletal examination, particularly of the lumbosacral spine, is necessary to discover the early findings of limitation of motion of the axial skeleton, which is especially noticeable with lateral bending or hyperextension. Percussion over the sacroiliac joints elicits pain in most circumstances. Other tests that may be helpful in identifying sacroiliac joint dysfunction place stress on the joint. The tests to be considered include a faber maneuver, Gaenslen test (pressure on a hyperextended thigh with a contralateral flexed hip), Yoeman test (hyperextension of the thigh with a prone patient), and distraction of the pelvic wings anteriorly and posteriorly.

Measurements of spinal motion, including Schober's test (lumbar spine motion) and measurements of lateral bending of the lumbosacral spine, occiput-to-wall distance (cervical spine motion), and chest expansion, are important in ascertaining limitations of motion and following the progression of the disease (Fig. 11–4). Paraspinous muscles may be tender on palpation and in spasm, resulting in limitation of back motion. Finger-to-floor measurements should be done but are intended mainly to determine flexibility, which is more closely associated with hip motion than with back mobility. Rotation may be checked with the patient seated. This fixes the pelvis, limiting pelvic rotation. Chest expansion is measured at the fourth intercostal space in men and below the breasts in women. The patient raises both hands over the head and is asked to take a deep inspiration. Normal expansion is 2.5 cm or greater. Peripheral joint examination is also indicated. Careful hip examination is necessary to determine the potential loss of function involved with simultaneous arthritis of the back and hip.[44] Examination of the eyes, heart, lungs, and nervous system may uncover unsuspected extra-articular disease.

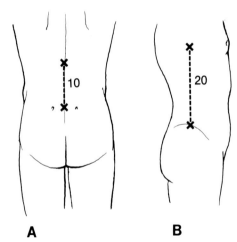

Figure 11–4. Measurement of anterior spinal flexion (A) and right and left lateral flexion (B). Figure depicts initial position before forward (A) or lateral (B) flexion.

LABORATORY DATA

Laboratory results are nonspecific and add little to the diagnosis of AS. A minority of patients (15%) have a mild anemia. ESR is raised in 80% of patients with active disease.[71] Patients with normal SRs with active arthritis may have elevated levels of C-reactive protein.[72] The rheumatoid factor and antinuclear antibody are characteristically absent.

Histocompatibility testing (for HLA) is positive in 90% of patients with AS but is also present in an increased percentage of patients with other spondyloarthropathies (Reiter's syndrome, psoriatic spondylitis, spondylitis with inflammatory bowel disease). It is not a diagnostic test for AS. HLA testing may be useful in the young patient with early disease, in whom the differential diagnosis may be narrowed by the presence of HLA-B27 positivity.[73] The presence of B27 homozygosity was evaluated in 100 patients with AS.[74] Homozygosity was associated with more severe disease but did not impart a greater risk for spondylitis in families of patients with AS.

RADIOLOGIC EVALUATION

Characteristic changes of AS in the sacroiliac joints and lumbosacral spine are very helpful in making a diagnosis but may be difficult to determine in the early stages of the disease.[75] The disease affects synovial and cartilaginous joints as well as sites of tendon and ligament attachment to bone (enthesis). The areas of the skeleton most frequently affected include the sacroiliac, apophyseal, discovertebral, and costovertebral joints.

The disease affects the sacroiliac joints initially and then appears in the upper lumbar and thoracolumbar areas.[76, 77] Subsequently, in an ascending order, the lower lumbar, thoracic, and cervical spine are involved. The radiographic progression of disease may be halted at any stage, although sacroiliitis alone is a rare finding except in some women with spondylitis or in men in the early stage of disease (Fig. 11–5).[41, 78] In the peripheral skeleton, the hips and shoulders (glenohumeral joints) are most commonly affected, followed by knees, hands, wrists, and feet including the heel.[79–81]

Evaluation of the sacroiliac joints is difficult on the conventional anteroposterior supine view of the pelvis because of bony overlap and the oblique orientation of the joint. A Ferguson view of the pelvis (x-ray tube tilted 15° to 30° in a cephalad direction) provides a useful view of the anterior portion of the joint, the initial area of inflammation in sacroiliitis. Radiographic evaluation of the sacroiliac joints is based on 5 observations: distribution, subchondral mineralization, cystic or erosive bony change, joint width, and osteophyte formation.[82] The corresponding areas of the sacroiliac joints, superior (fibrous), inferior (synovial), iliac (thinner cartilage), and sacral (thicker cartilage), must be compared to detect symmetry of involvement.

Sacroiliitis in AS is a bilateral, symmetric process. Early sacroiliitis appears in the inferior portion of the joint on the iliac side of the articulation. Patchy periarticular osteopenia appears along with areas of subchondral bony sclerosis. During the next stage, the articular space becomes "pseudowidened" secondary to joint surface erosions. With continued inflammation, the area of sclerosis widens and is joined by proliferative bony changes that cross the joint space. In the final stages of sacroiliitis, complete ankylosis with total obliteration of the joint space occurs (Fig. 11–6). Ligamentous structures surrounding the sacroiliac joint may also calcify. The radiographic changes as-

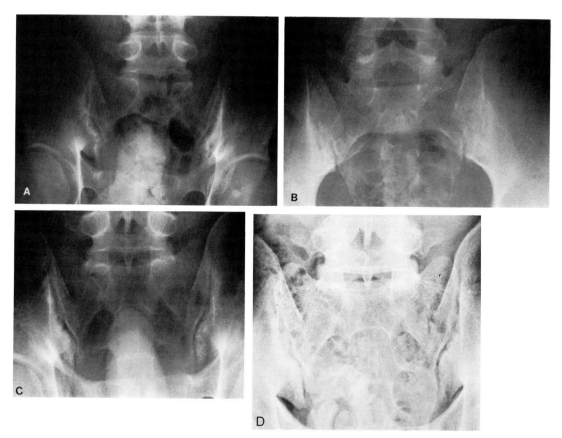

Figure 11–5. Serial views of the pelvis in a 30-year-old man with AS. *A,* 3/80, Sclerosis is noted primarily on the iliac sides of both sacroiliac joints with cystic erosions of the joint space. *B,* 10/83, Bilateral involvement with greater sclerosis in the right sacroiliac joint. *C,* 10/86, Degree of joint involvement has diminished with less sclerosis and greater definition of the joint margins. *D,* 10/88, Joint space remains intact with continuing resolution of erosions.

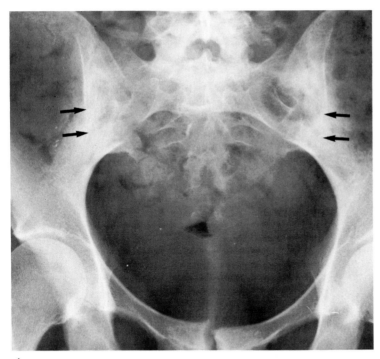

A

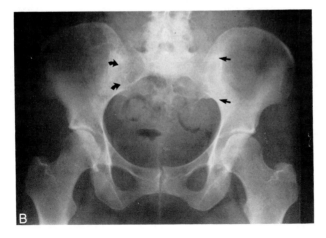

Figure 11–6. Ankylosing spondylitis. AP view of pelvis. *A,* A 44-year-old woman with persistent back pain since the age of 14, with recurrent iritis. Bilateral sacroiliitis is noted with fusion of those joints (*arrows*). *B,* 10/91, Seven years later, the left sacroiliac joint is obliterated (*black straight arrows*). The right sacroiliac is barely visible (*curved black arrows*).

TABLE 11–1. RADIOGRAPHIC GRADING OF SACROILIITIS

Grade 0 Normal—normal width, sharp joint margins

Grade 1 Suspicious changes—radiologist is uncertain whether grade 2 changes are present

Grade 2 Definite early changes—pseudowidening with erosion or sclerosis on both sides of the joint

Grade 3 Unequivocal abnormality—erosions, sclerosis, widening, narrowing, or partial ankylosis

Grade 4 Severe abnormalities—with narrowed joint space, ankylosis

Grade 5 Ankylosis of body joints with regression of surrounding sclerosis

Adapted from Dale K: Radiographic grading of sacroiliitis in Bechterew's syndrome and allied disorders. Scand J Rheumatol (Suppl) *32*:92, 1979.

sociated with sacroiliitis may be graded from 0 (normal) to 5 (complete ankylosis) (Table 11–1).[83]

It is important to realize that the inflammatory process associated with sacroiliitis does not always result in ankylosis. The inflammatory process may diminish and the joint may undergo healing associated with some resolution of the alterations associated with early disease (see Fig. 11–5).[84]

Abnormalities also occur in the lumbar, thoracic, and cervical spine. Classic AS causes vertebral column disease in association with sacroiliac disease. The occurrence of spondylitis without sacroiliitis in AS is an extremely rare finding.[85] This pattern of involvement is much more common in Reiter's syndrome or psoriatic spondylitis.

In the lumbar spine, osteitis affecting the anterior corners of vertebral bodies is an early finding. The inflammation associated with osteitis results in loss of the normal concavity of the anterior vertebral surface, resulting in a "squared" body (Fig. 11–7). As the inflammation heals, reactive sclerosis or "whitening" appears in the anterior portion of vertebral bodies. A simple method to assess vertebral squaring involves drawing a vertical line joining upper and lower margins of each lumbar vertebral body at the junction of the vertebral end plate and anterior surface of the vertebral body. The distance between this line and the anterior aspect of the vertebral body at its most concave point is then measured. This is the concavity measurement. The reference range for vertebral concavity is 1.1 to 4 mm based on measurements from 255 lumbar vertebrae. Squaring is associated with changes of 1 mm or less. This method may be helpful in following the course of the illness over time.[86]

While osteopenia of the bony structures ap-

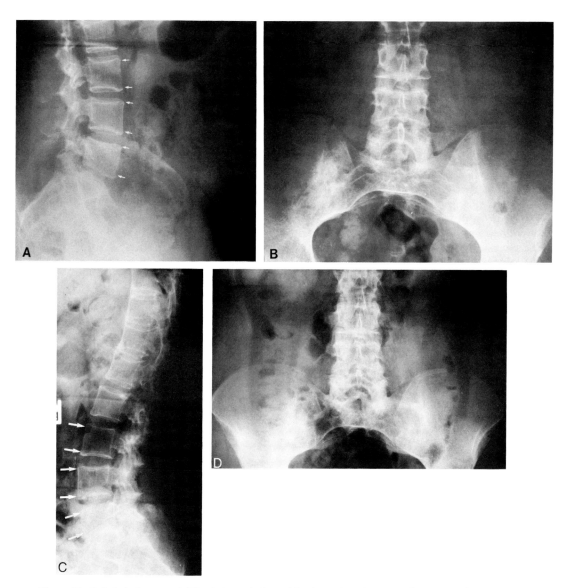

Figure 11–7. Ankylosing spondylitis. *A,* Lateral view of lumbar spine. Squaring of L3, L4, and L5 vertebral bodies with loss of concave contour is present (*arrows*). *B,* AP of pelvis reveals fusion of both sacroiliac joints. The extent of disease in the sacroiliac joints does not predict the degree of involvement in other areas of the axial skeleton. *C,* 10/90, Five years later, the squaring of vertebral bodies has stabilized (*arrows*). Syndesmophytes have not developed. *D,* AP of the pelvis reveals obliteration of the sacroiliac joints.

pears, calcification of disc and ligamentous structures emerges. Thin, vertically oriented calcifications of the annulus fibrosus and anterior and posterior longitudinal ligaments are termed syndesmophytes. "Bamboo spine" is the term used to describe the spine of a patient with AS with extensive syndesmophytes encasing the axial skeleton (Fig. 11–8).[87] Osteoporosis utilizing quantitative CT has been documented in AS patients.[88]

The discovertebral junction may be affected centrally, peripherally, or in combination.[61] Central erosions cause irregularity of the superior and inferior vertebral margins with surrounding sclerosis. Peripheral lesions cause erosions in the noncartilaginous portion of the junction. The radiographic findings include anterior or posterior bony erosion. Combined lesions affecting the central and peripheral portions of the discovertebral junction may cause ballooning of the disc space ("fish vertebrae") or narrowing of the disc space (spinal pseudoarthrosis).[89,90] This latter finding occurs most commonly in patients with AS of long duration who sustain trauma to the spine.

The apophyseal joints also are affected in the illness. As the disease progresses, fusion of the apophyseal joints occurs. Radiographs of the spine may demonstrate the loss of joint space and complete fusion of the joints.

The use of other radiographic techniques in the diagnosis of AS is of marginal additional benefit. Scintigraphic evaluation by bone scan may demonstrate increased activity over the sacroiliac joints in early disease prior to any detectable radiographic changes in the spinal joints.[91] However, quantitative scintigraphy is insufficiently discriminatory to be of consistent help clinically in differentiating spondylitis patients from normal individuals and from patients with other causes of back pain.[92] Scintigraphy also may not be adequately sensitive to follow the course of the illness over time.[93]

CT of the sacroiliac joint has been reported to be more sensitive and equally specific in the recognition of sacroiliitis when compared with conventional roentgenography.[94] However, CT should not be used for routine evaluation of the sacroiliac joints. The test should be reserved for patients with normal or equivocal roentgenographs in whom a diagnosis of spondyloarthropathy is suspected.[95] CT scan detects erosions on both sides of the joint that are frequently missed by plain roentgenograms.[96]

A number of MR studies have been reported demonstrating alterations of sacroiliac joints not noted by plain roentgenograms.[97] MR scan was better able to identify erosions, abnormalities of articular cartilage, and subchondral bone marrow. MR scan detects abnormalities of the spinal cord in patients with severe disease (Fig. 11–9), including those with pseudoarthroses (Fig. 11–10).[98] From a diagnostic and clinical perspective, plain roentgenograms normally provide adequate information at a reasonable cost. Plain roentgenograms remain the usual radiographic technique used for the diagnosis of AS.

DIFFERENTIAL DIAGNOSIS

Two sets of diagnostic criteria exist for AS. The Rome clinical criteria include bilateral sacroiliitis on radiologic examination plus low back pain for more than 3 months that is not relieved by rest, pain in the thoracic spine, limited motion in the lumbar spine, limited chest expansion, and iritis.[99] When these criteria proved to lack sensitivity in identifying patients with spondylitis, the Rome criteria were modified at a New York symposium in 1966 (Table 11–2). These criteria included a grading system for radiographs of the sacroiliac joints in addition to limited spine motion, limited chest expansion, and back pain.[100] Although these criteria are used mostly for studies of patient populations, they are helpful in the office setting. The criteria are not ideal for population surveys, since radiographic sacroiliitis may not be of the degree to satisfy criteria, thereby missing early disease.[101] Some of the measures of decreased mobility and chest expansion are imprecise. In the office setting, a physician typically makes the diagnosis of AS when the patient is a young male with bilateral sacroiliac pain, lumbar spine stiffness that is improved with activity, recurring radicular pain that alternates side to side, a history of iritis, and radiologic changes of spondylitis, and HLA-B27 status is determined in patients thought to have the disease. However, in the early stages of the disease, clinical symptoms may be mild or atypical and radiologic changes nonexistent, preventing early diagnosis. Suggestions have been made offering a weighting to individual characteristics of the illness to allow better codification of the diagnosis.[102] Others have also pointed out that the diagnostic criteria are too restrictive for certain patients with early disease or an undifferentiated spondyloarthropathy. The European Spondyloarthropathy Study Group has developed a preliminary classification system for spondyloarthropathy in general. (Table 11–3).[103]

Although spondyloarthropathies are a com-

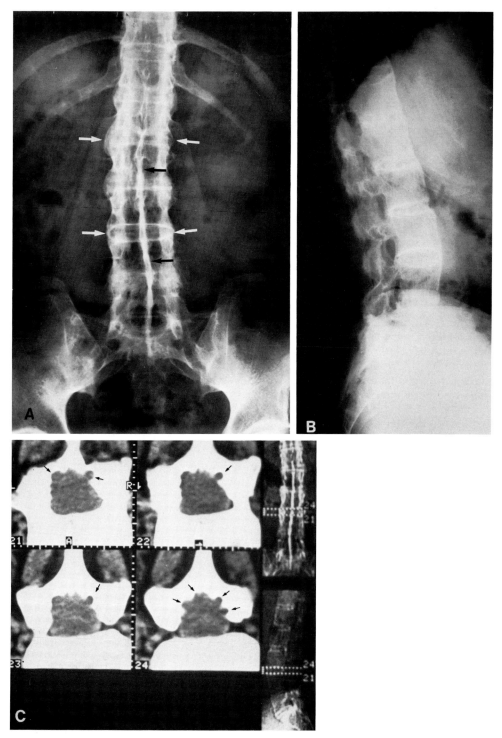

Figure 11–8. Ankylosing spondylitis. *A,* Bamboo spine with syndesmophytes involving the entire spine (*arrows*). interspinous ligaments have calcified (*black arrows*). The sacroiliac joints are fused. *B,* Lateral view reveals thin, vertically-oriented syndesmophytes and preservation of the intervertebral disc spaces. *C,* CT scan of the L3 vertebra of a 53-year-old man who developed cauda equina symptoms. The views reveal scalloping of the laminae of the vertebra. These erosions are secondary to dural ectasia or dural diverticula (*arrows*).

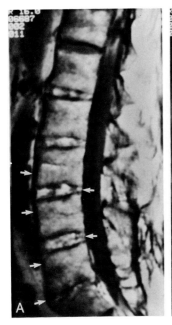
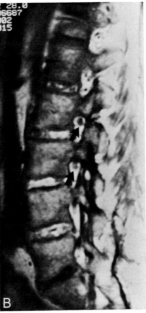

Figure 11–9. Ankylosing Spondylitis. A 67-year-old man with a 20-year history of AS. He has no range of motion in his axial skeleton and has a right hip replacement. *A,* MR scan of a T_1-weighted midline sagittal image with increased signal due to calcification in well maintained intervertebral discs. Syndesmophytes are present anteriorly and posteriorly (*white arrows*). *B,* MR scan of a T_1-weighted parasagittal image with intact neural foramina (nerve root = *black arrow*).

mon inflammatory musculoskeletal disorder, this group of illnesses is frequently overlooked by nonrheumatologists.[104] A delay in diagnosis from the onset of symptoms and referral to a rheumatologist ranged from 6 to 264 months.

The differential diagnosis of low back pain in the young patient includes other spondyloarthropathies, herniated lumbar disc, osteitis condensans ilii, osteoarthritis, rheumatoid arthritis, fibrositis, infection, and tumors. Characteristics of these specific diseases are listed in Table 11–4. The course of AS may be com-

plicated by other common arthritic diseases. AS and rheumatoid arthritis have developed in the same patient. The prevalence by sex (AS more common in men, RA in women) and the disease pattern are different, suggesting that the diseases are unassociated.[105] Another disease that may occur in the setting of spondylitis is diffuse idiopathic skeletal hyperostosis. The convergence of these two common diseases (Fig. 11–11) in the same patient, most commonly a middle-aged man, is likely. The occurrence of AS and DISH of the cervical

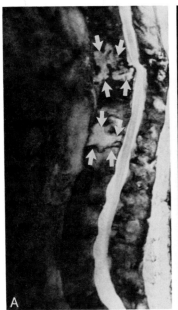
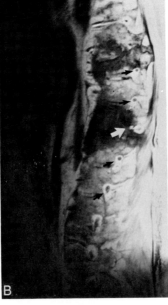

Figure 11–10. Ankylosing spondylitis. A 62-year-old man with a 30-year history of severe AS. He had a history of thoracic spine pain associated with a pseudoarthrosis at the T8 level. The patient had a falling accident with the onset of radicular pain in an L1 distribution. *A,* MR scan of a T_2-weighted sagittal image demonstrating two levels with pseudoarthrosis (*white arrows*). *B,* T_1-weighted image demonstrating intact neural foramena (*black arrows*). The L1 foramen is obliterated with inflammatory tissue associated with the pseudoarthrosis (*white arrow*).

TABLE 11–2. CLINICAL CRITERIA FOR ANKYLOSING SPONDYLITIS

ROME CRITERIA[98]

A. Clinical Criteria
1. Low back pain and stiffness more than 3 months not relieved by rest
2. Pain and stiffness in the thoracic region
3. Limited motion in the lumbar spine
4. Limited chest expansion
5. History of evidence of iritis or its sequelae

B. Radiologic Criterion
1. X-ray showing bilateral sacroiliac changes characteristic of ankylosing spondylitis
   Diagnosis: Criterion B + 1 clinical criterion
   or
   4 clinical criteria in absence of radiologic sacroiliitis

NEW YORK CRITERIA[99]

A. Clinical Criteria
1. Limitation of motion of the lumbar spine in anterior flexion, lateral flexion, and extension
2. History of or presence of pain at the dorsolumbar junction or in the lumbar spine
3. Limitation of chest expansion to 1 inch or less

B. Radiologic Criteria (Sacroiliitis)
Grade 3—unequivocal abnormality, moderate or advanced sacroiliitis with one or more erosions, sclerosis, widening, narrowing, or partial ankylosis.
Grade 4—severe abnormality, total ankylosis
Diagnosis:
Definite—Grade 3–4 bilateral sacroiliitis + 1 clinical criterion
   or
   Grade 3–4 unilateral or Grade 2 bilateral sacroiliitis with clinical criterion 1 or 2 and 3
Probable—Grade 3–4 bilateral sacroiliitis alone

---

spine has been reported.[106] Patients with AS and DISH should be easily differentiated by careful radiographic evaluation.[107] DISH may cause alterations of the sacroiliac joints.[108] CT scan of the SI joints differentiates the hyperostotic joint changes from those associated with joint erosion and fusion. Also of note is the occurrence of fracture in patients with DISH as well as those with AS.[109]

Patients may complain of low back pain located near the sacroiliac joints but the origin of the pain may be from contiguous structures. For example, the iliac crest near the sacroiliac joint may be painful with associated limitation of motion.[110] Local injection of anesthetic into the maximum point of tenderness may differentiate these patients with a soft tissue abnormality from those with sacroiliitis.[111]

TABLE 11–3. EUROPEAN SPONDYLOARTHROPATHY STUDY GROUP CLASSIFICATION CRITERIA FOR SPONDYLOARTHROPATHY

Inflammatory spinal pain or synovitis		
Asymmetrical		
Predominantly in the lower extremities		
And 1 of the following:		
Positive family history		
Psoriasis		
Inflammatory bowel disease	sensitivity	77%
Alternate buttock pain	specificity	89%
Enthesopathy		
Adding		
Sacroiliitis	sensitivity	86%
	specificity	87%

TREATMENT

The goals of therapy, as with other forms of inflammatory arthritis, are to control pain and stiffness, reduce inflammation, maintain function, and prevent deformity with avoidance of undue toxicity. Patients require a comprehensive program of education, physiotherapy, medications, and other measures. Patients are educated about their disease. They are told what they can reasonably expect from treatment and are encouraged to continue with as normal a lifestyle as possible. Patients are taught proper posture and mobilizing and breathing exercises to prevent the tendency to stoop forward and lose chest motion. Physical therapy in the form of range of motion exercises maintains and possibly improves motion.[112] The importance of a firm upright chair for sitting and a hard mattress with no pillows for sleeping is stressed. The physician gives encouragement and support to the patient to adapt his or her lifestyle to the disease. When the physician cannot give the patient adequate time to quell all concerns, the physician should arrange additional support for the patient in the form of a social worker, psychiatrist, or vocational counselor. The genetic im-

TABLE 11–4. DIFFERENTIAL DIAGNOSIS OF ANKYLOSING SPONDYLITIS

	ANKYLOSING SPONDYLITIS	REITER'S SYNDROME	PSORIATIC ARTHRITIS	ENTEROPATHIC ARTHRITIS	REACTIVE ARTHROPATHY	HERNIATED NUCLEUS PULPOSUS
Sex	Male	Male	=	=	=	=
Age at onset	15–40	20–30	30–40	15–45	Any age	20–40
Presentation	Back pain	Arthritis Urethritis Conjunctivitis	Extremity arthritis Psoriasis Back pain	Abdominal pain	GI, GU infection	Radicular pain
Sacroiliitis	Symmetric	Asymmetric	Asymmetric	Symmetric	Symmetric	–
Axial skeleton	+	+/–	+/–	+	+/–	–
Peripheral joints	Lower	Lower	Upper	Lower	Lower	–
Enthesopathy	+	+	+	–	+/–	–
Erythrocyte sedimentation rate	Elevated	Elevated	Elevated	Elevated	Elevated	Normal
Rheumatoid factor	–	–	–	–	–	–
HLA-B27	90%	80%	60% (Spondylitis)	50% (Spondylitis)	90%	8%
Course	Continuous	Relapsing	Continuous	Continuous	Self-limited or continuous	Episodic
Therapy	Nonsteroidals Exercise	Nonsteroidals Gold Methotrexate	Nonsteroidals Gold Methotrexate	Nonsteroidals Cortisteroids Antibiotics	Nonsteroidals Antibiotics	Nonsteroidals Epidural corticosteroids Surgery
Disability	Hip	Lower extremity	Lower extremity	Hip	–	Neurologic dysfunction

plications of the disease are placed in perspective. Offspring are at 10% risk of developing AS if a parent is positive for HLA-B27. Also, the importance of self-help groups, such as the Ankylosing Spondylitis Association located in Los Angeles, California, cannot be understated. These organizations offer medical literature, exercises, and other resources that are very useful to AS patients.

Medications to control pain and inflammation are useful in the patient with AS.[113] In the patient with mild spinal or peripheral joint disease, aspirin may be somewhat effective. However, in patients with more severe disease, aspirin is usually ineffective. If salicylates are used, anti-inflammatory salicylate serum concentrations (20 to 25 mg/dl) should be maintained. Other nonsteroidal anti-inflammatory drugs that have been demonstrated to decrease pain and inflammation in AS have been indomethacin and phenylbutazone. These drugs are effective in controlling spinal and peripheral joint disease but are associated with potentially serious side effects.[114] In a retrospective radiographic study, phenylbutazone decreased the rate of progression of axial skeletal disease in AS.[115] A follow-up study of 14

patients with AS who took indomethacin over an 18-year period reported a beneficial effect in a majority, including remission in 28% of patients.[116] Anti-inflammatory drugs, such as ibuprofen, tolmetin, fenoprofen, piroxicam, sulindac, and mefenamic acid also may be effective.[117] Sulindac has been compared with indomethacin and has comparable efficacy and a tolerance advantage of a twice-a-day dose regimen.[118] This drug has Federal Drug Administration (FDA) approval for use in AS. Naproxen also has FDA approval, and studies have shown efficacy of the drug in the treatment of AS.[119] As mentioned, other nonsteroidals may be useful for control of joint symptoms but are not approved by the FDA for use in patients with spondylitis. Some of the NSAIDS studied in AS include diclofenac, etodolac, flurbiprofen, and ketoprofen.[120]

Patients with acute ankylosing spondylitis may develop severe muscle spasm with associated limited motion, which may hinder patients' return to normal daily activities. In these patients, the addition of a muscle relaxant to a nonsteroidal drug helps decrease muscle pain and muscle spasm and improve back motion. Muscle relaxants at low dosage levels,

TABLE 11–4. DIFFERENTIAL DIAGNOSIS OF ANKYLOSING SPONDYLITIS (Continued)

	OSTEITIS CONDENSANS ILII	OSTEOARTHRITIS OF THE SPINE	RHEUMATOID ARTHRITIS	FIBROMYALGIA	INFECTION	TUMORS
Sex	Female	=	Female	Female	=	=
Age at onset	30–40	40–50	20–60	30–50	Any age	Young—benign Older—malignant
Presentation	Back pain	Back pain	Peripheral arthritis	Generalized fatigue Sleeplessness Tender points	Acute, severe unilateral back pain	Slowly progressive insidious pain
Sacroiliitis	Asymmetric	–	Symmetric (Cervical spine)	–	Asymmetric	Asymmetric
Axial skeleton	–	+		–	–	–
Peripheral joints	–	Lower	Upper and lower	–	–	–
Enthesopathy	–	–	–	–	–	–
Erythrocyte sedimentation rate	Normal	Normal	Elevated	Normal	Elevated	Elevated (malignant)
Rheumatoid factor	–	–	80%	–	–	–
HLA-B27	8%	8%	8%	8%	8%	8%
Course	Self-limited	Relapsing	Continuous	Continuous	Episodic	Continuous
Therapy	Bed rest Bracing Nonsteroidals	Nonsteroidals	Nonsteroidals Gold Methotrexate	Tricyclic antidepressants Nonsteroidals	Antibiotics Bracing	En bloc excision Chemotherapy Radiotherapy
Disability	–	Neurologic dysfunction	Generalized joint deformities (sacroiliitis late in disease)	Muscle pain	Neurologic dysfunction	Local invasion—benign Metastases—malignant

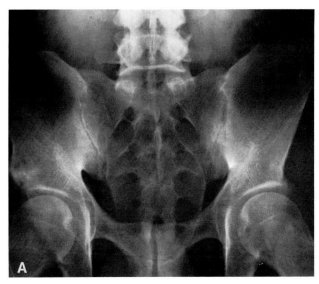

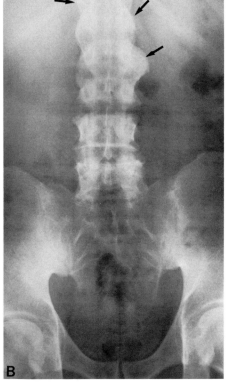

Figure 11–11. Ankylosing spondylitis and diffuse idiopathic skeletal hyperostosis in a 37-year-old man with a 17-year history of back pain. *A,* AP of pelvis reveals mild bilateral sacroiliitis with sclerosis and early joint erosions. *B,* AP view of the entire lumbosacral spine demonstrates large bony calcifications that flowed from the thoracic area to the first 3 lumbar vertebrae (*arrows*). L4 and L5 were spared. These flowing calcifications are characteristic of DISH.

such as cyclobenzaprine (10 mg once a day), are helpful while limiting possible drug toxicity. The sleepiness associated with muscle relaxants with long half-lives can be limited by giving the medication 2 hours before bedtime.

Systemic corticosteroids are rarely needed and are ineffective for the articular disease of AS. In the occasional patient who has continued joint symptoms while receiving maximum dose of nonsteroidal drugs, the addition of small doses of corticosteroids drugs (prednisone 5 mg/day) may prove to be useful. Larger doses of corticosteroids cause appreciably more toxicity without an increased benefit. Occasionally systemic corticosteroids are needed to control persistent iritis. Intra-articular injection of a long-acting steroid preparation is indicated if patients have peripheral joint disease with persistent effusions.

Pulse intravenous methylprednisolone has caused improvement in patients who failed to respond to nonsteroidal drugs. The use of IV pulses yielded dramatic responses lasting 14 months.[121] In another study, pulse methylprednisolone was helpful, but improvement in spinal motions lasted only 2 months.[122]

Intramuscular gold salt injections are not indicated for the axial skeletal disease of AS, but they may be helpful in the rare patient with peripheral joint disease who demonstrates persistent synovitis and joint destruction. Antimalarials and immunosuppressive medications are not indicated. A double-blind, placebo-controlled trial of penicillamine in AS detected no significant difference between the test drug and placebo in clinical and laboratory indices.[123] Methotrexate has been utilized in a few patients with AS with some success.[124, 125] However, additional studies are needed before any recommendation for use of this drug for AS can be given. Sulfasalazine also has been utilized in patients with AS, but, in general, the benefits have been mild. The benefit may be in those patients with gastrointestinal disorders with peripheral arthritis.[120, 126]

Orthopedic appliances, such as a heel cup for plantar fasciitis or a temporary spinal brace to prevent forward flexion, are useful in appropriate patients. Transcutaneous nerve stimulators, in addition to non-narcotic analgesics, are useful in reducing pain in patients with partial response to nonsteroidal drugs. In the patients with fixed flexion deformities of the hip, total joint replacement relieves pain and increases mobility.[127] Surgical procedures on the spine, such as lumbar spine osteotomy, are limited to patients who have such a degree of forward

flexion as to prevent them from looking up from the ground.[128] This operation has multiple potential complications and is viewed as a last resort procedure. Bradford has reported good outcome of spinal osteotomy in 20 of 21 patients, including two with progressive paraplegia.[129]

Radiotherapy was used frequently in patients with AS up to the 1960s and was effective at controlling pain and stiffness in the lumbosacral spine.[130] The effects of this therapy, however, were transient and did not prevent progression of the disease. In addition, long-term, follow-up studies on these patients demonstrated an increased mortality secondary to leukemia. A Canadian study has shown decreased survival of men who received radiotherapy to the spine after a 27-year follow-up period.[131] The therapy has been abandoned except for the rarest of patients who are intolerant of all other treatment.

PROGNOSIS

The general course of AS is benign and is characterized by exacerbations and remissions. Many patients with AS may have sacroiliitis with mild involvement of the lumbosacral spine. Limitation of lumbosacral motion may be mild. The disease can become quiescent at any time. Patients who go on to develop total fusion of the spine may feel better since ankylosis of the spinal joints is associated with decreased pain. In a study of 1492 patients followed over a 2-year period, the frequency of patients with a total remission of disease was small—less than 2% had a total remission.[132] These findings were independent of disease duration.

The role of HLA-B27 homozygosity on the course and severity of AS has been controversial. It has been suggested that homozygosity for HLA-B27 increases both the risk and the severity of AS and may be associated with severe peripheral arthritis along with axial disease.[133, 134] Other investigators have been unable to confirm this finding.[135, 136] Suarez-Almajor and Russell reported their experience of the effects of homozygosity on the severity of disease, and familial penetrance of spondylitis in association with HLA-B27. HLA-B27 was associated with statistically significantly increased severity of disease in homozygous patients but was not associated with earlier onset of disease or increased risk of family members to develop spondylitis.[137]

The prognosis of men and women with AS has been reported to be different.[138, 139] Women were reported to have a milder course, more peripheral disease, and less radiographic change in the axial skeleton. However, Gran compared 44 women and 82 men with AS and found no difference between the sexes in respect to age at onset, initial symptoms, work performance, restriction of spinal motion, or peripheral joint involvement.[140]

Most studies report that the majority of patients remain functional and employed over the course of the illness.[45] The prime predictor of more severe dysfunction is the presence of peripheral joint involvement, particularly in the hips, and this usually appears within the first 10 years of disease. A majority of these patients developed severe spinal restriction. Patients with fixed flexion contractures of the hips and ankylosis of the spine are severely limited in their functional capacity; however, total hip joint replacement may improve their mobility. Patients with spinal rigidity but normal hip function have minimal disability. However, they should avoid heavy labor, such as lifting objects heavier than 40 pounds.

References

ANKYLOSING SPONDYLITIS

1. Ruffer A: Arthritis deformans and spondylitis in ancient Egypt. J Pathol 22:159, 1918.
2. Rogers J, Watt I, Dieppe P: Paleopathology of spinal osteophytosis, vertebral ankylosis, ankylosing spondylitis and vertebral hyperostosis. Ann Rheum Dis 44:113, 1985.
3. Gran JT, Husby F, Hordvik M: Prevalence of ankylosing spondylitis in males and females in a young middle aged population of Tromso, Northern Norway. Ann Rheum Dis 44:359, 1985.
4. Hochberg MC: Epidemiology. In Calin A (ed): Spondyloarthropathies. Orlando: Grune & Stratton, 1984, pp 21–42.
5. Khan MA: An overview of clinical spectrum and heterogeneity of spondyloarthropathies. Rheum Dis Clin North Am 18:1, 1992.
6. Calin A, Fries JF: Striking prevalence of ankylosing spondylitis in "healthy" W27 positive males and females: a controlled study. N Engl J Med 293:835, 1975.
7. Engleman EG, Rosenbaum JT: HLA and disease: an overview. In Calin A (ed): Spondyloarthropathies. Orlando: Grune & Stratton, 1984, pp 279–296.
8. Schlosstein L, Terasaki PI, Bluestone R, Pearson CM: High association of an HL antigen, W27, with ankylosing spondylitis. N Engl J Med 288:704, 1973.
9. Khan MA, van der Linden SM: Ankylosing spondylitis and other spondyloarthropathies. Rheum Dis Clin North Am 16:551, 1990.
10. Good AE, Kawaniski H, Schultz JS: HLA-B27 in blacks with ankylosing spondylitis or Reiter's disease. N Engl J Med 294:166, 1976.
11. Hochberg MC, Bias WB, Arnett FC Jr: Family studies in HLA-B27 associated arthritis. Medicine 57:463, 1978.

12. Grumet FC, Calin A, Engleman EG, et al.: Studies of HLA-B27 using monoclonal antibodies: ethnic and disease associated variants. In Ziff M, Cohen SB (eds): The Spondyloarthropathies: Advances in Inflammation Research, Vol 9. New York: Raven Press, 1985, p 41.
13. Grumet FC, Fendly BM, Fish L, et al.: Monoclonal antibody (B27 M2) subdividing HLA-B27. Hum Immunol 5:61, 1982.
14. Karr RW, Hahn Y, Schwartz BD: Structural identity of human histocompatibility leukocyte antigen-B27 molecules from patients with ankylosing spondylitis and normal individuals. J Clin Invest 69:443, 1982.
15. Kaneoka H, Engleman EG, Grumet FC: Immunochemical variants of HLA-B27. J Immunol 130:1288, 1983.
16. Ebringer A, Shipley M (eds): Pathogenesis of HLA-B27–associated disease. Br J Rheumatol 2(Suppl): 1, 1983.
17. Engleman EG, Calin A, Grumet FC: Analysis of HLA-B27 antigen with monoclonal antibodies. J Rheumatol 10(Suppl 10):59, 1983.
18. Calin A, Marder A, Becks E, Burns T: Genetic differences between B27 positive patients with ankylosing spondylitis and B27 positive healthy controls. Arthritis Rheum 26:1460, 1983.
19. Gran JT, Teiberg P, Olaissen B, et al.: HLA-B27 and allotypes of complement components in ankylosing spondylitis. J Rheumatol 11:324, 1984.
20. Lopez de Castro JA, Bragado R, Lauzurica P, et al.: Structure and immune recognition of HLA-B27 antigens: implications for disease association. Scand J Rheumatol 87(suppl):21, 1990.
21. Hill AVS, Kwiatkowski D, Greenwood BM et al: HLA class I typing by PCR: HLA-B27 and an African B27 subtype. Lancet 337:640, 1991.
22. Matsumura M, Fremont DH, Peterson PA, Wilson IA: Emerging principles for the recognition of peptide antigens by MHC class I molecules. Science 257:927, 1992.
23. Bjorkman PJ, Saper MA, Samraoui B, et al.: Structure of the human class I histocompatibility antigen, HLA-A2. Nature 329:506, 1987.
24. Breur-Vriesendorp BS, Vingerhoed J, Kuijpers KC, et al.: Effect of a Tyr-to-His point-mutation at position 59 in the alpha-1 helix of the HLA-B27 class-I molecule on allospecific and virus-specific cytotoxic T-lymphocyte recognition. Scand J Rheumatol 87(suppl):36, 1990.
25. Maclean IL, Iqball S, Woo P, et al.: HLA-B27 subtypes in the spondyloarthropathies. Clin Exp Immunol 91:214, 1993.
26. Calin A: The relationship between genetics and environment in the pathogenesis of rheumatic diseases. West J Med 131:205, 1979.
27. Geczy AF, Prendergast JK, Sullivan JS, et al.: HLA-B27, molecular mimicry and ankylosing spondylitis: popular misconceptions. Ann Rheum Dis 46:171, 1987.
28. Hammer RE, Maika SD, Richardson JA, et al.: Spontaneous inflammatory disease in transgenic rats expressing HLA-B27 and human beta 2m: an animal model of HLA-B27-associated human disorders. Cell 63:1099, 1990.
29. Taurog JD: Molecular genetics of HLA-B27. Spine St Arts Rev 4:607, 1990.
30. Miehle W, Schattenkirchner M, Albert D, Bunge M: HLA-DR4 in ankylosing spondylitis with different patterns of joint involvement. Ann Rheum Dis 44:39, 1985.
31. Resnick D, Dwosh IL, Goergen TG, et al.: Clinical

and radiographic "reankylosis" following hip surgery in ankylosing spondylitis. AJR 126:1181, 1976.

32. Jacoby RK, Newell RLM, Hickling P: Ankylosing spondylitis and trauma: the medicolegal implications. A comparative study of patients with nonspecific back pain. Ann Rheum Dis 44:307, 1985.

33. Geczy AF, Alexander K, Bashir HV, et al.: HLA-B27, *Klebsiella,* and ankylosing spondylitis. Bacteriologic and chemical studies. Immunol Rev 70:23, 1983.

34. Sullivan JS, Geczy AF: The modification of HLA-B27 positive lymphocytes by the culture filtrate of *Klebsiella* 1243 BTS 1 is a metabolically active process. Clin Exp Immunol 62:672, 1985.

35. Van Bohemen GG, Grumet FC, Zanen HC: Identification of HLA B27 M1 and M2 cross-reactive antigens in *Klebsiella, Shigella,* and *Yersinia.* Immunology 52:607, 1984.

36. Sheldon PJ, Pell PA: Lymphocyte proliferative responses to bacterial antigens in B-27 associated arthropathies. J Rheumatol 24:11, 1985.

37. Warren RE, Brewerton DA: Faecal carriage of *Klebsiella* by patients with ankylosing spondylitis and rheumatoid arthritis. Ann Rheum Dis 39:37, 1980.

38. Edmonds J, Macauley D, Tyndall A, et al.: Lymphocytotoxicity of anti*Klebsiella* antisera in ankylosing spondylitis and related arthropathies: patient and family studies. Arthritis Rheum 24:1, 1981.

39. Lahesmaa R, Skurnik M, Gransfors K, et al.: Molecular mimicry in the pathogenesis of spondyloarthropathies. A critical appraisal of cross-reactivity between microbial antigens and HLA-B27. Br J Rheumatol 31:221, 1992.

40. Neustadt DH: Ankylosing spondylitis. Postgrad Med 61:124, 1977.

41. Wilkinson M, Bywaters EGL: Clinical features and course of ankylosing spondylitis as seen in a follow-up of 222 hospital referred cases. Ann Rheum Dis 17:209, 1958.

42. Hochberg MC, Borenstein DG, Arnett FC: The absence of back pain in classical ankylosing spondylitis. Johns Hopkins Med J 143:181, 1978.

43. Pace JB, Nagle D: Piriformis syndrome. West J Med 124:435, 1976.

44. Hart FD, MacLagen NF: Ankylosing spondylitis: a review of 184 cases. Ann Rheum Dis 34:87, 1975.

45. Carette S, Graham D, Little H, et al.: The natural disease course of ankylosing spondylitis. Arthritis Rheum 26:186, 1983.

46. Ball J: Enthesopathy of rheumatoid and ankylosing spondylitis. Ann Rheum Dis 30:213, 1971.

47. Gran JT, Husby G: Ankylosing spondylitis in women. Semin Arthritis Rheum 19:303, 1990.

48. Calin A, Elswood J: The relationship between pelvic, spinal and hip involvement in ankylosing spondylitis—one disease process or several? Br J Rheumatol 27:393, 1988.

49. Fox MW, Onofrio BM, Kilgore JE: Neurological complications of ankylosing spondylitis. J Neurosurg 78:871, 1993.

50. Russell ML, Gordon DA, Orgryzlo MA, McPhedran RS: The cauda equina syndrome of ankylosing spondylitis. Ann Intern Med 78:551, 1973.

51. Hassan I: Cauda equina syndrome in ankylosing spondylitis: a report of six cases. J Neurol Neurosurg Psychiatr 39:1172, 1976.

52. Mitchell MJ, Sartoris DJ, Moody D, et al.: Cauda equina syndrome complicating ankylosing spondylitis. Radiology 175:521, 1990.

53. Haddad FS, Sachdev JS, Bellapravalu M: Neuropathic bladder in ankylosing spondylitis with spinal diverticula. Urology 35:313, 1990.

54. Tullous MW, Skerhut HEI, Story JL, et al.: Cauda equina syndrome of long-standing ankylosing spondylitis: case report and review of the literature. J Neurosurg 873:441, 1990.

55. Rotes-Querol J, Tolosa E, Rosello R, Granados J: Progressive cauda equina syndrome and extensive calcification/ossification of the lumbosacral meninges. Ann Rheum Dis 44:227, 1985.

56. Hunter T, Dubo H: Spinal fractures complicating ankylosing spondylitis. Ann Intern Med 88:546, 1978.

57. Yau ACMC, Chan RNW: Stress fracture of the fused lumbo-dorsal spine in ankylosing spondylitis. J Bone Joint Surg 56B:681, 1974.

58. Fast A, Parikh S, Marin EL: Spine fractures in ankylosing spondylitis. Arch Phys Med Rehabil 67:595, 1986.

59. Wholey MH, Pugh DG, Bickel WH: Localized destructive lesions in rheumatoid spondylitis. Radiology 74:54, 1960.

60. Dihlmann W, Delling G: Discovertebral destructive lesions (so-called Andersson lesions) associated with ankylosing spondylitis. Skel Radiol 3:10, 1978.

61. Cawley MID, Chalmers TM, Kellgren JH, Ball J: Destructive lesions of vertebral bodies in ankylosing spondylitis. Ann Rheum Dis 31:345, 1972.

62. Dunn N, Preston B, Jones KL: Unexplained acute backache in longstanding ankylosing spondylitis. Br Med J 291:1632, 1985.

63. Bulkey BH, Roberts WC: Ankylosing spondylitis and aortic regurgitation: description of the characteristic cardiovascular lesion from study of eight necropsy patients. Circulation 48:1014, 1973.

64. Graham DC, Smythe HA: The carditis and aortitis of ankylosing spondylitis. Bull Rheum Dis 9:171, 1958.

65. Bergfeldt L, Edhag O, Vedin H, Vallin H: Ankylosing spondylitis: an important cause of severe disturbances of the cardiac conduction system. Prevalence among 223 pacemaker-treated men. Am J Med 73:187, 1982.

66. Gould BA, Turner J, Keeling DH et al.: Myocardial dysfunction in ankylosing spondylitis. Ann Rheum Dis 51:227, 1992.

67. Rosenow EC III, Strimlan CV, Muhm JR, Ferguson RH: Pleuropulmonary manifestations of ankylosing spondylitis. Mayo Clin Proc 52:641, 1977.

68. Applerouth D, Gottlieb NL: Pulmonary manifestations of ankylosing spondylitis. J Rheumatol 2:446, 1975.

69. Cruickshank B: Pathology of ankylosing spondylitis. Clin Orthop 74:43, 1971.

70. Lai KN, Li PKT, Hawkins B, et al.: IgA nephropathy associated with ankylosing spondylitis: occurrence in women as well as in men. Ann Rheum Dis 48:435, 1989.

71. Kendal MJ, Lawrence DS, Shuttleworth GR, Whitefield AGW: Hematology and biochemistry of ankylosing spondylitis. Br Med J 2:235, 1973.

72. Nashel DJ, Petrone DL, Ulmer CC, Sliwinski AJ: C-reactive protein: a marker for disease activity in ankylosing spondylitis and Reiter's syndrome. J Rheumatol 13:364, 1986.

73. Khan MA, Khan MK: Diagnostic value of HLA-B27, testing in ankylosing spondylitis and Reiter's syndrome. Ann Intern Med 906:70, 1982.

74. Suarez-Almazor ME, Russell AS: B27 homozygosity and ankylosing spondylitis. J Rheumatol 14:302, 1987.

75. McEwen C, DiTata D, Ling GC, et al.: Ankylosing spondylitis and spondylitis accompanying ulcerative colitis, regional enteritis, psoriasis and Reiter's disease: a comparative study. Arthritis Rheum 14:291, 1971.

76. Kinsella TD, MacDonald FR, Johnson LG: Ankylosing spondylitis: a late re-evaluation of 92 cases. Can Med Assoc J 95:1, 1966.

77. Rosen PS, Graham DC: Ankylosing (Strumpell-Marie) spondylitis (a clinical review of 128 cases) AIR 5:158, 1962.

78. Resnick D, Dwosh IL, Goergen TG, et al.: Clinical and radiographic abnormalities in ankylosing spondylitis: a comparison of men and women. Radiology 119:293, 1976.

79. Resnick D: Patterns of peripheral joint disease in ankylosing spondylitis. Radiology 110:523, 1974.

80. Ginsburg WW, Cohen MD: Peripheral arthritis in ankylosing spondylitis: a review of 209 patients followed up for more than 20 years. Mayo Clin Proc 58:593, 1983.

81. Dwosh IL, Resnick D, Becker MA: Hip involvement in ankylosing spondylitis. Arthritis Rheum 19:683, 1976.

82. Conc RD, Rcsnick D: Rocntgcnographic cvaluation of the sacroiliac joints. Orthopaedic Rev 12:95, 1983.

83. Dale K: Radiographic grading of sacroiliitis in Bechterew's syndrome and allied disorders. Scand J Rheumatol (Suppl)32:92, 1979.

84. Lindvall W: Early x-ray diagnosis of sacro-iliitis. Scand J Rheumatol (Suppl)32:98, 1979.

85. Cheatum DE: "Ankylosing spondylitis" without sacroiliitis in a woman without the HLA-B27 antigen. J Rheumatol 3:420, 1976.

86. Ralston SH, Urquhart GDK, Brzeski M, et al.: A new method for the radiological assessment of vertebral squaring in ankylosing spondylitis. Ann Rheum Dis 51:330, 1992.

87. Dale K: Radiographic changes of the spine in Bechterew's syndrome and allied disorders. Scand J Rheumatol (Suppl)32:103, 1979.

88. Devogelaer JP, Maldague B, Malghem J, et al.: Appendicular and vertebral bone mass in ankylosing spondylitis. Arthritis Rheum 35:1062, 1992.

89. Spencer DG, Park WM, Dick HM, et al.: Radiological manifestations in 200 patients with ankylosing spondylitis: correlation with clinical features and HLA-B27. J Rheumatol 6:305, 1979.

90. Martel W: Spinal pseudoarthrosis: a complication of ankylosing spondylitis. Arthritis Rheum 21:485, 1978.

91. Russell AS, Lentle BC, Percy JS: Investigation of sacroiliac disease: comparative evaluation of radiological and radionuclide techniques. J Rheumatol 2:45, 1975.

92. Esdaile JM, Rosenthall L, Terkeltaub R, Kloiber R: Prospective evaluation of sacroiliac scintigraphy in chronic inflammatory back pain. Arthritis Rheum 23:998, 1980.

93. Taylor HG, Gadd R, Beswick EJ, et al.: Quantitative radioisotope scanning in ankylosing spondylitis: a clinical, laboratory and computerized tomographic study. Scand J Rheumatol 20:274, 1991.

94. Carrera GF, Foley WD, Kozin F, et al.: CT of sacroiliitis. AJR 136:41, 1981.

95. Kozin F, Carrera GF, Ryan LM, et al.: Computed tomography in the diagnosis of sacroiliitis. Arthritis Rheum 24:1479, 1981.

96. Forrester DM: Imaging of the sacroiliac joint. Radiol Clin North Am 28:1054, 1990.

97. Ahlstrom H, Feltelius N, Nyman R, et al.: Magnetic resonance imaging of sacroiliac joint inflammation. Arthritis Rheum 33:1763, 1990.

98. Docherty P, Mitchell MJ, MacMillan L, et al.: Magnetic resonance imaging in the detection of sacroiliitis. J Rheumatol 19:393, 1992.

99. Kellgren JH: Diagnostic criteria for population studies. Bull Rheum Dis 13:291, 1962.

100. Bennett PH, Wood PHN: Population Studies of the Rheumatic Diseases. Proceedings of the 3rd International Symposium, New York, 1966. Amsterdam: Excerpta Medica, 1968, p 456.

101. Moll JMH, Wright V: New York clinical criteria for ankylosing spondylitis. Ann Rheum Dis 32:354, 1973.

102. Moll JM: Criteria for ankylosing spondylitis: facts and fallacies. Br J Rheumatol 27(suppl)34, 1988.

103. Khan MA, van der Linden SM: A wider spectrum of spondyloarthropathies. Semin Arthritis Rheum 20:107, 1990.

104. Kidd BL, Cawley MID: Delay in diagnosis of spondarthritis. Br J Rheumatol 27:230, 1988.

105. Clayman MD, Reinertsen JL: Ankylosing spondylitis with subsequent development of rheumatoid arthritis, Sjögren's syndrome, and rheumatoid vasculitis. Arthritis Rheum 21:383, 1978.

106. Williamson PK, Reginato AJ: Diffuse idiopathic skeletal hyperostosis of the cervical spine in a patient with ankylosing spondylitis. Arthritis Rheum 27:570, 1984.

107. Yagan R, Khan MA: Confusion of roentgenographic differential diagnosis of ankylosing hyperostosis (Forestier's disease) and ankylosing spondylitis. Spine St Art Rev 4:561, 1990.

108. Durback MA, Edelstein G, Schumacher HR Jr: Abnormalities of the sacroiliac joints in diffuse idiopathic skeletal hyperostosis: demonstration by computed tomography. J Rheumatol 15:1506, 1988.

109. Anas PP: Case records of the Massachusetts General Hospital. N Engl J Med 321:1178, 1989.

110. Collee G, Dijkmans BAC, Vandenbroucke JP, et al.: Iliac crest pain syndrome in low back pain: frequency and features. J Rheumatol 18:1064, 1991.

111. Collee G, Dijkmans BAC, Vandenbroucke JP, et al.: Iliac crest syndrome in low back pain: a double blind, randomized study of local injection therapy. J Rheumatol 18:1060, 1991.

112. Vitanen JV, Suni J, Kautiainen H, et al.: Effect of physiotherapy on spinal mobility in ankylosing spondylitis. Scand J Rheumatol 21:38, 1992.

113. Godfrey RG, Calabro JJ, Mills D, Matty BA: A double blind crossover trial of aspirin, indomethacin and phenylbutazone in ankylosing spondylitis. (Abstract.) Arthritis Rheum 15:110, 1972.

114. Fowler P: Phenylbutazone and indomethacin. Clin Rheum Dis 1:267, 1975.

115. Boersma JW: Retardation of ossification of the lumbar vertebral column in ankylosing spondylitis by means of phenylbutazone. Scand J Rheumatol 5:60, 1976.

116. Calabro JJ: Appraisal of efficacy and tolerability of Indocin (indomethacin, MSD) in acute gout and moderate to severe ankylosing spondylitis. Semin Arthritis Rheum 12(Suppl 1):112, 1982.

117. Simon LS, Mills JA: Nonsteroidal anti-inflammatory drugs. N Engl J Med 302:1179, 1237, 1980.

118. Calin A, Britton M: Sulindac in ankylosing spondylitis: Double-blind evaluation of sulindac and indomethacin. JAMA 242:1885, 1979.

119. Ansell BM, Major G, Liyanage G, et al.: A comparative study of Butacote and Naprosyn in ankylosing spondylitis. Ann Rheum Dis 37:436, 1978.

120. Gran JT, Husby G: Ankylosing spondylitis: current drug treatment. Drugs 44:585, 1992.

121. Mintz G, Enriquez RD, Mercado U, et al.: Intravenous methylprednisolone pulse therapy in severe ankylosing spondylitis. Arthritis Rheum 24:734, 1981.

122. Richter MB: Management of the seronegative spondyloarthropathies. Clin Rheum Dis 11:147, 1985.
123. Steven MM, Morrison M, Sturrock RD: Penicillamine in ankylosing spondylitis: a double blind placebo controlled trial. J Rheumatol 12:735, 1985.
124. Handler RP: Favorable results using methotrexate in the treatment of patients with ankylosing spondylitis. Arthritis Rheum 32:234, 1989.
125. Ferraz MB, da Silva HC, Altra E: Low dose methotrexate with leucovirin rescue in ankylosing spondylitis. J Rheumatol 18:146, 1991.
126. Dougados M, Maetzel A, Mijyawa M, et al.: Evaluation of sulphasalazine in the treatment of spondyloarthropathies. Ann Rheum Dis 51:955, 1992.
127. William F, Taylor AR, Arden GP, Edwards DH: Arthroplasty of the hip in ankylosing spondylitis. J Bone Joint Surg 59B:393, 1977.
128. Scudese VA, Calabro JJ: Vertebral wedge osteotomy: correction of rheumatoid (ankylosing) spondylitis. JAMA 186:627, 1963.
129. Bradford DS, Schumacher WL, Lonstein JE, Winter RB: Ankylosing spondylitis: experience in surgical management of 21 patients. Spine 12:238, 1987.
130. Brown WMC, Doll R: Mortality from cancer and other causes after radiotherapy for ankylosing spondylitis. Br Med J 2:1327, 1965.
131. Kaprove RE, Little AH, Graham DC, Rosen PS: Ankylosing spondylitis: survival in men with and without radiotherapy. Arthritis Rheum 23:57, 1980.
132. Kennedy LG, Edmunds L, Calin A: The natural history of ankylosing spondylitis. Does it burn out? J Rheumatol 20:688, 1993.
133. Kahn MA, Kushner I, Braun WE, et al.: HLA-B27 homozygosity in ankylosing spondylitis: relationship to risk and severity. Tissue Antigens 11:434, 1978.
134. Arnett FC, Schacter BZ, Hochberg M, et al.: Homozygosity for HLA-B27: impact on rheumatic disease expression in two families. Arthritis Rheum 20:797, 1977.
135. Spencer DG, Dick HM, Dick WC: Ankylosing spondylitis—the role of HLA-B27 homozygosity. Tissue Antigens 14:379, 1979.
136. Moller P, Berg K: Family studies in Bechterew's syndrome (ankylosing spondylitis) III: Genetics. Clin Genet 24:73, 1983.
137. Suarez-Almazor ME, Russell AS: B27 homozygosity and ankylosing spondylitis. J Rheumatol 14:302, 1987.
138. Hill HFH, Hill AGS, Bodmer JG: Clinical diagnosis of ankylosing spondylitis in women and relation to presence of HLA-B27. Ann Rheum Dis 35:267, 1976.
139. Jeannet M, Saudan Y, Bitter T: HL-A27 in female patients with ankylosing spondylitis. Tissue Antigens 6:262, 1975.
140. Gran JT, Ostensen M, Husby G: A clinical comparison between males and females with ankylosing spondylitis. J Rheumatol 12:126, 1985.

REITER'S SYNDROME

Capsule Summary

Frequency of back pain—very common
Location of back pain—sacroiliac joints and lumbar spine

Quality of back pain—ache
Symptoms and signs—morning stiffness, conjunctivitis, urethritis, decreased spinal motion, percussion tenderness of the sacroiliac joints
Laboratory and x-ray tests—increased sedimentation rate; sacroiliitis and/or spondylitis on plain roentgenograms
Treatment—exercises, nonsteroidal anti-inflammatory drugs

PREVALENCE AND PATHOGENESIS

Reiter's syndrome is a disease associated with the triad of urethritis (inflammation of the lower urinary tract), arthritis, and conjunctivitis. Reiter's syndrome is the most common cause of arthritis in young men and primarily affects the lower extremity joints and the low back. The disease results from the interaction of an environmental factor, usually a specific infection, and a genetically predisposed host. The course of the illness, while usually benign, may be chronic and remitting, resulting in significant disability.

Many physicians, including Hippocrates, have written about the apparent relation between venereal and gastrointestinal infections and the development of arthritis. In 1916, Reiter[1] and Fiessinger and Leroy[2] described young soldiers with an acute febrile illness that included conjunctivitis, urethritis, and polyarthritis appearing after dysenteric illness. However, the triad and the term Reiter's syndrome were not associated until Bauer and Engleman in 1942 referred to the findings of urethritis, conjunctivitis, and arthritis in World War II soldiers as Reiter's disease.[3]

Reiter's syndrome occurs in patients throughout the world with no racial or ethnic predisposition. Approximately 1% of patients with nongonococcal urethritis, a common infection, develop the syndrome.[4] A more recent study suggests that 3% of individuals with nonspecific urethritis develop Reiter's syndrome.[5] The syndrome develops in 0.2% to 3% of all patients with enteric infections secondary to *Shigella, Salmonella, Campylobacter,* and *Yersinia.*[6] The male to female ratio in venereal infection is in the range of 10:1, while the ratio is 1:1 in large outbreaks secondary to enteric infection. The ratio may also be 1:1 in patients with no antecedent infection or in whom urogenital symptoms may be a manifestation of the disease instead of a primary infection.[7, 8] In one study, the incidence was 3.5/100,000 men under the age of 50.[9]

The etiology of Reiter's syndrome is unknown. However, the interrelationship between the environment and genetics is crucial in the pathogenesis of illness.[10] The initiation of the disease is thought to be related to dysenteric (epidemic) or venereal (endemic) infections. The post-dysenteric form of Reiter's syndrome follows infections by *Shigella dysenteriae* and *flexneri*, *Salmonella enteritidis*, *Yersinia enterocolitica*, and *Campylobacter jejuni*.[11–16] For example, 19 of 260 (7.6%) individuals infected with *S. typhimurium* developed Reiter's syndrome.[17] The relationship of sexually acquired genital infections with *Chlamydia trachomatis* and *Ureaplasma urealyticum* and the precipitation of joint disease is not clearly established. Although the evidence for *Ureaplasma* is weak, there is increasing data in the medical literature connecting the pathogenesis of reactive arthritis with chlamydia infection.[18] The distinction of urethritis as an initiating event and as an integral manifestation of the syndrome is a difficult one to make. Patients with enteric infections develop urethritis without urethral infection.[11] *Chlamydia trachomatis* is cultured in 50% to 69% of patients with Reiter's syndrome at the onset of joint disease.[19, 20] Reiter's patients may also have higher prevalences and titers of antichlamydial antibodies than controls and demonstrate higher lymphocyte transformation stimulation indices than controls.[21] No correlation was found between Reiter's syndrome and *Mycoplasma hominis* or *Ureaplasma urealyticum* by the same authors.[21] The role of *Neisseria gonorrhoeae* in Reiter's syndrome is not clear, since 40% of patients with gonococcal infection also have chlamydial infection simultaneously.[22]

Reiter's syndrome may develop in patients who deny enteric or venereal infection. Some of these patients associate the onset of their disease with an episode of joint trauma.[23] The trauma is associated with swelling, stiffness, and pain in the traumatized joint, and this is followed by the emergence of additional joint symptoms, urethritis, conjunctivitis, or cutaneous lesions. Another possible manifestation of a response to trauma in these patients is the presence of bony bridging or nonmarginal syndesmophytes in the spine in the absence of sacroiliitis or back symptoms.[24, 25] However, there is no scientific evidence to substantiate the role of trauma as an initiator of Reiter's syndrome.

Characteristic of the spondyloarthropathies in general, Reiter's syndrome is associated with the HLA-B27 antigen. Between 60% and 80% of Caucasian patients are positive for HLA-B27. In blacks the prevalence of HLA-B27 has varied from 15% to 75%.[26–28] A majority of those who are negative for this antigen have HLA-B antigens that cross-react with B27, including B7, BW22, B40, and BW42.[26] HLA-B27 and related antigens may be linked to genes controlling the cellular immune response to certain infectious agents, and these genes cause an abnormal immune response. Alternately, HLA-B27 antigen may be immunologically cross-reactive with certain infectious agents (molecular mimicry).[29]

Despite its association with Reiter's syndrome, the HLA-B27 haplotype is not the only determinant for disease expression, since only a minority of HLA-B27 individuals develop Reiter's syndrome after exposure to infectious agents. In addition, HLA-B27 is associated with a wide range of diseases that cause spondyloarthropathy. There may be genetic material closely linked to HLA-B27 that actually determines the expression of Reiter's syndrome or other spondyloarthropathies.[30]

Evaluation of the HLA molecule reveals an antigen-binding groove that appears to serve the function of capturing appropriate corresponding antigen and presenting it to T-cell receptors of the CD8-positive cytotoxic cell. An explanation for the variability of HLA-B27 being associated with a variety of arthritides might be explained by the variability of key amino acid residues that affect the form of the binding site. HLA-B27 has been divided into six subtypes. These include B*2701 through B*2706. Different subtypes are associated with particular ethnic groups and susceptibility for spondyloarthropathy.[31]

CLINICAL FEATURES

The classic picture of Reiter's syndrome occurs in a young man about 25 years old who develops urethritis and a mild conjunctivitis, followed by the onset of a predominantly lower extremity oligoarthritis. The symptoms of urethritis are usually mild with a mucopurulent discharge and dysuria. Men may also develop acute or chronic prostatitis. Women may have vaginitis or cervicitis, although many with these manifestations of genitourinary tract involvement in Reiter's syndrome may be asymptomatic. This paucity of symptoms from the genitourinary tract may in part explain the infrequency of the diagnosis of Reiter's syndrome in women.[7] Urethritis occurs in both epidemic and endemic forms of the disease. Up to 93% of patients with Reiter's syndrome will have genitourinary symptoms during the course of their illness.[32]

The conjunctivitis is usually mild and is manifested by an erythema (redness) and crusting of the lids. Conjunctival inflammation is usually bilateral and gradually resolves over a few days, but it may recur spontaneously. Acute iritis occurs in 20% of Reiter's syndrome patients and is marked by severe pain, photophobia, and scleral injection.

Arthritis may occur 1 to 3 weeks after the initial infection. In many patients, arthritis is the only manifestation of disease.[33] The term reactive arthritis is used for patients who develop only the arthritis of Reiter's syndrome after an enteric or genitourinary infection. The weight-bearing joints—knees, ankles, and feet—are most frequently affected in an asymmetric manner. A minority of patients have a persistent monarthritis as their only articular abnormality. The involved joints are acutely inflamed, with some joints developing very large effusions.

Back pain is a frequent symptom of patients with Reiter's syndrome. During the acute course between 31% and 92% of the patients may develop pain in the lumbosacral region.[32, 34, 35] The pain is of an aching quality and is improved with activity. Occasionally the pain will radiate into the posterior thighs but rarely below the knees; it may be unilateral. This finding corresponds to the asymmetric involvement of the sacroiliac joints and contrasts with the symmetric involvement of AS.[36] Sacroiliitis is the cause of back pain in a majority of patients who, as determined by increased activity over the sacroiliac joints on scintiscan, are in the acute phase of the disease.[37] Radiographic evidence of sacroiliitis is usually restricted to those patients with severe disease. In retrospective studies, sacroiliitis can be detected radiographically in 9% of patients in the acute phase of illness and in up to 71% of patients who have had disease activity longer than 5 years.[4] Spondylitis affecting the lumbar, thoracic, and cervical spine occurs less commonly than sacroiliitis, with up to 23% of patients with severe disease showing such involvement.[38]

Another musculoskeletal manifestation of Reiter's syndrome is inflammation of the insertion of tendons and fascia (enthesopathy). Heel pain, "lover's heel," secondary to plantar fascia inflammation, is a common finding.[39] Other manifestations of enthesopathy in Reiter's syndrome patients are Achilles tendinitis, chest wall pain, dactylitis or "sausage digit," and low back pain with no evidence of active sacroiliitis.

Although not part of the classic triad of the disease, mucocutaneous lesions are very characteristic of Reiter's syndrome. Keratodermia blennorrhagica is a skin rash characterized by waxy, macular lesions that become vesicular and scale. They are found predominantly on the palms and soles. Histologically, they are indistinguishable from pustular psoriasis. Keratodermia that appears on the glans penis is referred to as circinate balanitis. It occurs in up to 31% of patients. Oral ulcers occur on the palate, tongue, buccal mucosa, and lips. These lesions are shallow and painless and occur in 33% of patients. Nail involvement is characterized by opacification and hyperkeratosis, but not pitting.

Constitutional symptoms occur in about a third of patients and are characterized by fever, anorexia, weight loss, and fatigue. Cardiac complications, including heart block and aortic regurgitation, occur as a late manifestation of disease in 2% of patients.[40] Neurologic disease occurs in 1% of patients and is associated with peripheral neuropathy, hemiplegia, and cranial nerve abnormalities.[41] Amyloidosis is also a rare and late complication of Reiter's syndrome.[42]

PHYSICAL EXAMINATION

Physical examination should include all organ systems that may be involved in the disease process. Many of the manifestations of Reiter's syndrome may be overlooked by patients. Important findings such as oral ulcers, circinate balanitis, and limitation of lumbosacral spine motion may be missed if not looked for by the physician. Conjunctivitis is manifested by erythema of the conjunctivae and crusting of the lids. Urethritis may be detected only by "milking" the urethra before urination for the presence of a mucopurulent discharge.

A complete musculoskeletal examination should include both upper and lower extremities as well as the axial skeleton. Men tend to have involvement in the knees, ankles, and feet, while women have more upper extremity disease.[7] The usual patient will have six or fewer joints affected. Percussion tenderness over the sacroiliac joints may be unilateral, correlating with asymmetric involvement in Reiter's syndrome. The mobility of the lumbosacral spine should be measured in all planes of motion. A search for evidence of enthesopathy, heel or Achilles tendon tenderness, is also required.

An examination of the oropharynx, genitals, palms, soles, and nails will cover the areas that are associated with the mucocutaneous lesions of Reiter's syndrome.

LABORATORY FINDINGS

Laboratory results are nonspecific and not helpful in making the diagnosis of Reiter's syndrome. A mild anemia of chronic disease, an elevated white blood cell count (leukocytosis), and an elevated platelet count (thrombocytosis) are demonstrated in about a third of the patients.[23] The ESR is elevated in 70% to 80% of patients, but the elevation does not follow the course of the disease. Synovial fluid analysis demonstrates an inflammatory fluid with no specific abnormalities. Rheumatoid factor and antinuclear antibodies are not present in this illness. HLA-B27 or one of the cross-reactive antigens is present in 80% of patients. HLA-B27 positivity is helpful in differentiating Reiter's syndrome from rheumatoid arthritis (this is more easily done by clinical examination). The test, however, is not helpful in differentiating Reiter's syndrome from the other spondyloarthropathies. Histocompatibility testing should not be regarded as a routine diagnostic test. Testing may be most helpful early in the course of an arthropathy when no typical extra-articular features are present.[43]

Since Reiter's syndrome is so closely associated with bacterial infection, laboratory investigation to discover a genitourinary or gastrointestinal infection is appropriate. Chlamydia testing should include urethral swabs or cervical brushings for direct fluorescent antibody and ELISA testing or, preferably, DNA-probe for chlamydial ribosomal RNA. Stool cultures may identify an unsuspected bacteria in the gastrointestinal tract. Synovial fluid may be tested by immunochemistry, polymerase chain reaction, or molecular hybridization for the presence of chlamydial antigens.[44]

RADIOGRAPHIC EVALUATION

In patients who do not manifest the complete triad of Reiter's syndrome, radiographic changes are helpful in confirming the diagnosis.[45] Joint destruction is most severe in the feet. The hips and shoulders are usually spared. The radiologic correlate of the enthesopathy of Reiter's syndrome is periosteal new bone formation at the attachments of the plantar fascia and Achilles tendon into the calcaneus. The incidence of sacroiliac disease increases with disease chronicity and may be more common in postvenereal, HLA-B27-positive patients.[36] Sacroiliac involvement may mimic AS (symmetric disease) or may be asymmetric in severity of joint changes (Figs. 11–12 and 11–13). Unilateral sacroiliac disease occurs early in the disease process.[34] Bone erosion is more common on the iliac than on the sacral side of the joint. Variable amounts of sclerosis are associated with erosions. Widening of the joint (erosions) followed by narrowing (fusion) will be the progression of radiographic changes. Fusion of the joints occurs less frequently than in AS. Sacroiliitis may be detected in 5% to 10% of individuals early in the illness, and up to 60% in prolonged illness.

Spondylitis is discontinuous in its involvement of the axial skeleton (skip lesions) and is characterized by nonmarginal bony bridging of vertebral bodies (Fig. 11–14). These verte-

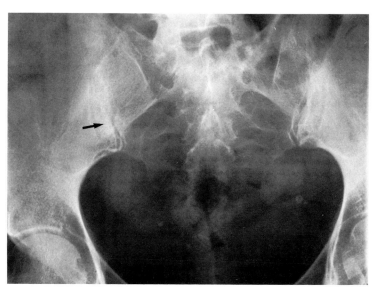

Figure 11–12. Reiter's syndrome. Spot view of the pelvis reveals greater involvement of the right sacroiliac joint characterized by joint sclerosis (*arrow*) predominate on the ilium.

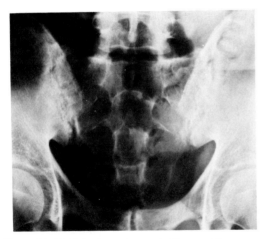

Figure 11–13. Reiter's syndrome. A 42-year-old man presented with left knee pain with persistent effusion over many years. He developed back pain after six years of knee pain. Ferguson view of the pelvis demonstrates bilateral sacroiliitis with more joint narrowing and sclerosis on the left.

DIFFERENTIAL DIAGNOSIS

Preliminary criteria for the diagnosis of acute Reiter's syndrome have been reported by the American Rheumatism Association.[50] Patients with Reiter's syndrome are distinguished from patients with other spondyloarthropathies and gonococcal arthritis by an episode of peripheral arthritis of more than 1 month's duration, occurring in association with urethritis and/or cervicitis.

Reactive arthritis may be considered a subset of Reiter's syndrome or a separate disease entity. Reactive arthritis refers to an inflammatory joint disease that follows an infection elsewhere in the body without microbial invasion of the synovial space.[51] Ahvonen introduced the term reactive arthritis to describe the nonpurulent joint inflammation associated with a *Yersinia enterocolitica* and *Y. pseudotuberculosis* enteric infection.[52] The reasons for the develop-

bral hyperostoses are markedly thickened compared with the thin syndesmophytes of AS.

Paravertebral ossification may appear about the lower 3 thoracic and upper 3 lumbar vertebrae.[46] This roentgenographic finding may antedate the appearance of sacroiliac or peripheral joint alterations.[47] Paravertebral ossification may be the source of nonmarginal syndesmophytes. Ossification may skip areas of the spine, in contradistinction to the continuous vertebral involvement of AS. Reiter's syndrome patients may also develop typical thin syndesmophytes similar to those of AS. The apophyseal joints may fuse, but the frequency of this finding is less than in classic AS.[48]

Whether spinal disease should be considered a complication of Reiter's syndrome or a manifestation of HLA-B27 disease is unclear. The differences in the appearance of spondylitis in Reiter's syndrome and AS suggest that the spondylitic process is dissimilar in the two conditions. The fact that spinal disease is often asymmetric, with skip areas and little squaring of vertebral bodies along with the finding of increased spinal involvement with severe, longstanding Reiter's disease, suggests that the process is related to Reiter's syndrome itself rather than HLA-B27. Spondylitis in Reiter's syndrome occurs in an older age group than in AS.

Increased uptake of tracer on bone scintigraphy can identify inflammatory involvement of the sacroiliac joint but is a nonspecific finding. CT scan also may be useful to identify inflammatory changes when changes on plain roentgenographs are minimal.[49]

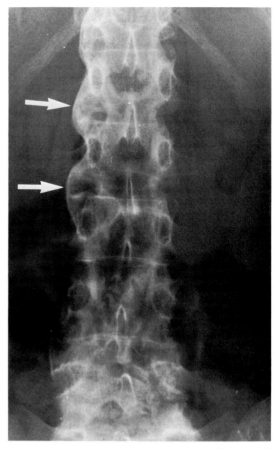

Figure 11–14. Reiter's Syndrome. A 35-year-old man with midline back pain has asymmetric nonmarginal syndesmophytes on the right side (more common on the nonaortic side) of the lumbar spine (*arrows*). A similar pattern may be seen with psoriatic spondylitis. (Courtesy of Anne Brower M.D.)

ment of arthropathy alone in reactive arthritis versus the full spectrum of Reiter's syndrome after exposure to infectious agents is unknown.[53] The infectious agents include *Salmonella*,[13] *Shigella*,[12] *Yersinia*,[14] *Campylobacter*,[16] and parasites, including *Giardia*,[54, 55] *Chlamydia*,[19] *Neisseria gonorrhea*,[56] *Streptococci*,[57] and nonspecific chronic urogenital infections.[58, 59] About 80% of patients with reactive arthritis are HLA-B27 positive.[60, 61] As with epidemic Reiter's syndrome, young men and women are equally affected. The onset and pattern of disease of reactive arthritis is similar to that of Reiter's syndrome. Approximately 30% of patients with reactive arthritis develop back pain.[61] Most of these patients are HLA-B27 positive. These patients also are at greater risk of developing radiographic evidence of sacroiliitis. Patients with reactive arthritis respond to the same therapy that is effective for Reiter's syndrome. At 5-year follow-up, a third of patients with reactive arthritis may continue to have back pain and show evidence of sacroiliitis.[61, 62]

The differential diagnosis of the patient who presents with low back pain and no other manifestation of Reiter's syndrome is the same as that presented for ankylosing spondylitis. This differential diagnosis includes the other spondyloarthropathies, herniated lumbar disc, DISH, and tumors (Table 11–4). In the patient who presents with acute monarticular disease after sexual intercourse, the diagnosis of infectious arthritis secondary to *Neisseria gonorrhoeae* must not be overlooked.[63] Bacterial cultures of the urethra, rectum, pharynx, and synovial fluid are necessary to detect the presence of the bacterium. Examination of synovial fluid for bacterial fatty acids, particularly succinic acid, helps differentiate those individuals with septic arthritis from those with effusions secondary to Reiter's syndrome.[64]

Human Immunodeficiency Virus

Human immunodeficiency virus (HIV) infection was first recognized during the early 1980s.[65] The disease is characterized by fever, weight loss, anorexia, lymphadenopathy, multiple infections, and Kaposi's sarcoma. The cause of the HIV infection is an RNA retrovirus that has a high affinity for the CD4 receptor that is expressed preferentially on T-helper/inducer lymphocytes. These cells are killed by the virus resulting in dysfunction in the surveillance function of the immune system. The absence of this function results in opportunistic infections and malignancies. Many organ systems are affected by the immune dysfunction and the persistent infections.[66] Compared with other organ systems, the musculoskeletal system is relatively spared. However, a range of musculoskeletal abnormalities are associated with HIV infection including arthralgias, myalgias, myopathy, and fibromyalgia. In a large study of 556 patients with HIV infection only 11% had musculoskeletal disorders and Reiter's syndrome was found in 0.5%.[67] Reiter's syndrome was the first distinct rheumatologic disorder described in association with HIV infection.[68] Reiter's syndrome may precede or follow the onset of AIDS. The usual articular symptoms are asymmetric oligoarthritis of large joints, enthesopathy, and skin lesions. Radiographic alterations of the spine occur and 66% of patients are HLA-B27. Therapy directed at controlling arthritis have the potential to exacerbate the underlying immunodeficiency.[69] Patients who develop Reiter's syndrome are severely ill. Debate remains regarding the association of AIDS with Reiter's syndrome. Reports have suggested a clear association,[70] while other studies have suggested that the increased risk is from risk behaviors associated with AIDS (bowel infections) and not to the virus itself.[71]

TREATMENT

The therapeutic regimen includes patient education, medications, and physical therapy. Patients are confused by the association of Reiter's syndrome and sexual relations. Many develop guilt or anxiety over sexual intercourse. The fact that urethritis may recur without any obvious cause must be made clear to the patient.

Acute joint symptoms are treated symptomatically with nonsteroidal anti-inflammatory drugs and the modalities of physical therapy. The drugs that are most effective for Reiter's syndrome are reviewed in Section IV. The joint and enthesopathic manifestations of Reiter's syndrome appear to respond better to indomethacin, phenylbutazone, or the other newer nonsteroidal anti-inflammatory drugs than to aspirin. The drugs are continued as long as the patient remains symptomatic. The effect of these agents on the long-term course of the disease is unknown. In patients with decreased range of motion of the spine associated with Reiter's syndrome, nonsteroidal anti-inflammatory drugs are useful to decrease pain. The addition of muscle relaxants in these patients can also be helpful in improving that component of immobility secondary to muscle tightness and spasm, which is associated with arthritis or enthesopathy.

The role of antibiotic therapy in the acute phase of Reiter's syndrome remains controversial. A recent study demonstrated that antibiotic therapy did not influence the appearance of Reiter's syndrome in patients with nonspecific urethritis.[19] A recent double-blind, placebo-controlled study of 3 months' duration evaluating the treatment with a lysine conjugate of tetracycline showed that those with chlamydia-associated reactive arthritis recovered more rapidly than those with post-Yersinia arthritis.[72] Antibiotic therapy should be considered for patients who present with Reiter's syndrome.

Gold salt therapy may be helpful in the patient with progressive, destructive peripheral joint disease. The immunosuppressive drug methotrexate is reserved for the patient with uncontrolled progression of joint disease and unresponsive, extensive skin involvement.[73] Azathioprine has been shown to be effective in controlling activity of intractable Reiter's syndrome in a placebo-controlled, cross-over study.[74] Corticosteroids are used as drops for iritis and as long-acting preparations for intra-articular injection. Systemic corticosteroids have less of an effect in Reiter's syndrome than they do in rheumatoid arthritis and are rarely used.

PROGNOSIS

Reiter's syndrome has no cure. The course of the illness is unpredictable. About 30% to 40% of patients have a self-limited illness, lasting 3 months to 1 year. Another 30% to 50% develop a relapsing pattern of illness with periods of complete remission. The final 10% to 25% develop chronic, unremitting disease associated with significant disability.[32, 75] C-reactive protein may be a better method to follow activity of disease than sedimentation rate in Reiter's syndrome in addition to clinical parameters (i.e., morning stiffness, joint swelling).[76] Patients who develop significant disability from Reiter's syndrome typically have painful or deformed feet or visual loss from iritis. A 5-year follow-up study of 131 consecutive patients with Reiter's syndrome revealed that 83% had some disease activity.[32] Fifty-one percent of patients had continued low back pain, while 45% had persistent foot or heel pain. Thirty-four percent had disease activity that interfered with their jobs, while 26% had to change jobs or were unemployed. Heel in-

volvement at the time of diagnosis was the finding most closely associated with a poor functional outcome. The presence of HLA-B27 did not correlate with functional outcome; however, a report from Finland suggested that the HLA-B27 status of the patient was associated with severity of disease.[61] Patients who were HLA-B27 positive had more frequent back pain and mucocutaneous and genitourinary symptoms. They also had a longer duration of disease and more frequent chronic low back pain and sacroiliitis. Chronic joint symptoms continued in 68% of 140 Reiter's syndrome patients studied, and 41% had chronic back pain. Most patients were able to lead normal lives, although 16% of the group had chronic destructive peripheral arthritis. Another report suggested that homozygosity for HLA-B27 may also be associated with more severe disease.[77]

In contrast, 55 Reiter's patients followed for 9.3 years had a 40% incidence of sacroiliitis. Sacroiliitis was rarely associated with spondylitis; 33 patients had mild limitation of back motion, but only 1 patient was functionally impaired by back disease.[78] The patients with sacroiliitis had more iritis, prolonged disease duration, and HLA-B27 positivity.

Reiter's syndrome is no longer considered a benign disease. Early therapy with nonsteroidal anti-inflammatory drugs, physical therapy, and appropriate shoes may have beneficial effects on patient function. Unfortunately, even aggressive therapy is unable to prevent disease activity and progressive disability in many Reiter's syndrome patients.

References

REITER'S SYNDROME

1. Reiter H: Uber eine bisher unerkannte Spirochaeten-infektion (Spirochaetosis arthritica). Dtsch Med Wochenschr 42:1535, 1916.
2. Fiessinger N, Leroy E: Contribution a l'etude d'une epidemic de dysenterie dans le somme. Bull Soc Med Hop Paris, 40:2030, 1916.
3. Bauer W, Engleman EP: A syndrome of unknown etiology characterized by urethritis, conjunctivitis, and arthritis (so-called Reiter's disease). Trans Assoc Am Phys 57:307, 1942.
4. Csonka GW: The course of Reiter's syndrome. Br Med J 1:1088, 1958.
5. Keat AC, Maini RN, Nkwazi GC, et al.: Role of *Chlamydia trachomatis* and HLA-B27 in sexually acquired reactive arthritis. Br Med J 1:605, 1978.
6. Noer HR: An "experimental" epidemic of Reiter's syndrome. JAMA 198:693, 1966.
7. Neuwelt CM, Borenstein DG, Jacobs RP: Reiter's syndrome: a male and female disease. J Rheumatol 9:268, 1982.

8. Yli-Kerttua UI: Clinical characteristics in male and female uro-arthritis or Reiter's syndrome. Clin Rheumatol 3:351, 1984.

9. Michet CJ, Machado EBV, Ballard DJ, et al.: Epidemiology of Reiter's syndrome in Rochester, Minnesota: 1950–1980. Arthritis Rheum 31:428, 1988.

10. Calin A: The relationship between genetics and environment in the pathogenesis of rheumatic diseases (medical progress). West J Med 131:205, 1979.

11. Paronen I: Reiter's disease: a study of 344 cases observed in Finland. Acta Med Scand (Suppl)212:1, 1948.

12. Good AE, Schultz JS: Reiter's syndrome following *Shigella flexneri* 2a. Arthritis Rheum 20:100, 1977.

13. Jones RAK: Reiter's disease after *Salmonella typhimurium* enteritis. Br Med J 1:1391, 1977.

14. Solem JH, Lassen J: Reiter's disease following *Yersinia enterocolitica* infection. Scand J Infect Dis 8:83, 1971.

15. Laitenen O, Leirisalo M, Skylv G: Relation between HLA-B27 and clinical features in patients with *Yersinia* arthritis. Arthritis Rheum 20:121, 1977.

16. Van de Putte LBA, Berden JHM, Boerbooms AM, et al.: Reactive arthritis after *Campylobacter jejuni* enteritis. J Rheumatol 7:531, 1980.

17. Inman RD, Johnston MEA, Hodge M, et al.: Post-dysenteric reactive arthritis: a clinical and immunogenetic study following an outbreak of salmonellosis. Arthritis Rheum 31:1377, 1988.

18. Rahman MU, Hudson AP, Schumacher HR Jr: Chlamydia and Reiter's syndrome (reactive arthritis). Rheum Dis Clin North Am 18:67, 1992.

19. Keat AC, Thomas BJ, Taylor-Robinson D, et al.: Evidence of *Chlamydia trachomatis* infection in sexually acquired reactive arthritis. Ann Rheum Dis 39:431, 1980.

20. Kousa M, Saikku P, Richmond S, Lassus A: Frequent association of chlamydial infection with Reiter's syndrome. Sex Transm Dis 5:57, 1978.

21. Martin DH, Pollock S, Kuo C, et al.: *Chlamydia trachomatis* infections in men with Reiter's Syndrome. Ann Intern Med 100:207, 1984.

22. Holmes KK, Handsfield HH, Wang SP, et al.: Etiology of nongonococcal arthritis. N Engl J Med 292:1199, 1975.

23. Arnett FC Jr: Reiter's syndrome. Johns Hopkins Med J 150:39, 1982.

24. Calin A, Fries JF: Striking prevalence of ankylosing spondylitis in "healthy" W27 positive males and females: a controlled study. N Engl J Med 293:835, 1975.

25. Cohen LM, Mittal KK, Schmid FR, et al.: Increased risk for spondylitis stigmata in apparently healthy HLA-W27 men. Ann Intern Med 84:1, 1976.

26. Arnett FC, Hochberg MD, Bias WB: Cross-reactive HLA antigens in B27-negative Reiter's syndrome and sacroiliitis. Johns Hopkins Med J 141:193, 1977.

27. Khan MA, Askari AD, Braun WE, Aponte CJ: Low association of HLA-B27 with Reiter's syndrome in blacks. Ann Intern Med 90:202, 1979.

28. Good AE, Kawaniski H, Schultz JS: HLA-B27 in blacks with ankylosing spondylitis or Reiter's disease. N Engl J Med 294:166, 1976.

29. McDevitt HO, Bodmer WF: HLA, immune response genes and disease. Lancet 1:1269, 1974.

30. Reveille JD, McDaniel DO, Barger BO, et al.: Restriction fragment length polymorphism (RFLP) analysis in familial ankylosing spondylitis. Independent segregation of a 9.2 Kb PVU II RFLP from B27 haplotypes. (Abstract.) Arthritis Rheum 30(Suppl 1):S36, 1987.

31. Khan MA: An overview of clinical spectrum and heterogeneity of spondyloarthropathies. Rheum Dis Clin North Am 18:1, 1992.

32. Fox R, Calin A, Gerber RC, Gibson D: The chronicity of symptoms and disability in Reiter's syndrome: an analysis of 131 consecutive patients. Ann Intern Med 91:190, 1979.

33. Arnett FC, McClusky E, Schacter BZ, Lordon RE: Incomplete Reiter's syndrome: discriminating features and HL-A W27 in diagnosis. Ann Intern Med 84:8, 1976.

34. Oates JK, Young AC: Sacroiliitis in Reiter's disease. Br Med J 1:1013, 1959.

35. Popert AJ, Gill AJ, Laird SM: A prospective study of Reiter's syndrome: an interim report on the first 82 cases. Br J Vener Dis 40:160, 1964.

36. Russell AS, Davis P, Percy JS, Lentle GC: The sacroiliitis of acute Reiter's syndrome. J Rheumatol 4:293, 1977.

37. Russell AS, Lentle BC, Percy JS: Investigation of sacroiliac disease: comparative evaluation of radiological and radionuclide techniques. J Rheumatol 2:45, 1975.

38. Good AE: Reiter's syndrome: long-term follow-up in relation to development of ankylosing spondylitis. Ann Rheum Dis 38:39, 1979.

39. Ball J: Enthesopathy of rheumatoid and ankylosing spondylitis. Ann Rheum Dis 30:213, 1971.

40. Ruppert GB, Lindsay J, Barth WF: Cardiac conduction abnormalities in Reiter's syndrome. Am J Med 73:335, 1982.

41. Good AE: Reiter's disease: a review with special attention to cardiovascular and neurologic sequelae. Semin Arthritis Rheum 3:253, 1974.

42. Miller LD, Brown EC, Arnett FC: Amyloidosis in Reiter's syndrome. J Rheumatol 6:225, 1979.

43. Calin A: HLA-B27: To type or not to type? Ann Intern Med 92:208, 1980.

44. Rahman MU, Cheema MA, Schumacher HR Jr: Molecular evidence for the presence of chlamydia in the synovium of patients with Reiter's syndrome. Arthritis Rheum 35:521, 1992.

45. Martel W, Braunstein EM, Borlaza G, et al.: Radiologic features of Reiter's disease. Radiology 132:1, 1979.

46. Cliff JM: Spinal bony bridging and carditis in Reiter's disease. Ann Rheum Dis 30:171, 1971.

47. Sundaram M, Patton JT: Paravertebral ossification in psoriasis and Reiter's disease. Br J Radiol 48:628, 1975.

48. Ford DK: Natural history of arthritis following venereal urethritis. Ann Rheum Dis 12:177, 1953.

49. Aliabadi P, Nikpoor N: Imaging evaluation of sacroiliitis. Rheum Dis Clin North Am 17:809, 1991.

50. Willkens RF, Arnett FC, Bitter T, et al.: Reiter's syndrome: evaluation of preliminary criteria for definite disease. Bull Rheum Dis 32:31, 1982.

51. Reactive arthritis. (Editorial.) Br Med J 281:311, 1980.

52. Ahvonen P, Sievers K, Aho K: Arthritis associated with *Yersinia enterocolitica* infection. Acta Rheum Scand 15:232, 1969.

53. Amor B: Reiter's syndrome and reactive arthritis. Clin Rheumatol 2:315, 1983.

54. Shaw RA, Stevens MB: The reactive arthritis of giardiasis. JAMA 258:2734, 1987.

55. Bocanegra TS, Espinoza LR, Bridgeford PH, et al.: Reactive arthritis induced by parasitic infestation. Ann Intern Med 94:207, 1981.

56. Rosenthal L, Olhagen B, Ek-S: Aseptic arthritis after gonorrhea. Ann Rheum Dis 39:141, 1980.

57. Hubbard WN, Hughes GRV: Streptococci and reactive arthritis. Ann Rheum Dis 41:435, 1982.

58. Olhagen B: Postinfective or reactive arthritis. Scand J Rheumatol 9:193, 1980.

59. Szanto E, Hagenfeldt K: Sacro-iliitis and salpingitis. Scand J Rheumatol 8:129, 1979.
60. Aho K, Ahvonen P, Lassus A, et al.: HLA 27 in reactive arthritis. A study of *Yersinia* arthritis and Reiter's disease. Arthritis Rheum 17:521, 1974.
61. Leirisalo M, Skylv G, Kousa M, et al.: Follow-up study on patients with Reiter's disease and reactive arthritis, with special reference to HLA-B27. Arthritis Rheum 25:249, 1982.
62. Marsal L, Winblad S, Wollheim FA: *Yersinia enterocolitica* arthritis in southern Sweden: a four-year follow-up study. Br Med J 283:101, 1981.
63. McCord WC, Nies KM, Louie JS: Acute venereal arthritis: comparative study of acute Reiter syndrome and acute gonococcal arthritis. Arch Intern Med 137:858, 1977.
64. Borenstein DG, Gibbs CA, Jacobs RP: Gas-liquid chromatographic analysis of synovial fluid. Arthritis Rheum 25:947, 1982.
65. Siegal FP, Lopez C, Hammer GS, et al.: Severe acquired immunodeficiency in male homosexuals, manifested by chronic perianal ulcerative herpes simplex lesions. N Engl J Med 305:1439, 1981.
66. Sande MA, Volberding PA: The Medical Management of AIDS, 3rd ed. Philadelphia: WB Saunders, 1992, p 525.
67. Fernanedez SM, Cardenal A, Balsa A, et al.: Rheumatic manifestations in 556 patients with human immunodeficiency virus infection. Semin Arthritis Rheum 21:30, 1991.
68. Winchester R, Bernstein DH, Fischer HD, et al.: The co-occurrence of Reiter's syndrome and acquired immunodeficiency. Ann Intern Med 106:19, 1987.
69. Keat A, Rowe I: Reiter's syndrome and associated arthritides. Rheum Dis Clin North Am 17:25, 1991.
70. Espinoza LR, Jara LJ, Espinoza CG, et al.: There is an association between human immunodeficiency virus infection and spondyloarthropathies. Rheum Dis Clin North Am 18:257, 1992.
71. Clark MR, Solinger AM, Hochberg MC: Human immunodeficiency virus is not associated with Reiter's syndrome: data from three large cohort studies. Rheum Dis Clin North Am 18:267, 1992.
72. Lauhio A, Leirisalo-Repo M, Lahdevirta J, et al.: Double-blind, placebo-controlled study of three-month treatment with lymecycline in reactive arthritis, with special reference to Chlamydia arthritis. Arthritis Rheum 34:6, 1991.
73. Farber GA, Forshner JG, O'Quinn SE: Reiter's syndrome: treatment with methotrexate. JAMA 200:171, 1967.
74. Calin A: A placebo controlled, crossover study of azathioprine in Reiter's syndrome. Ann Rheum Dis 45:653, 1986.
75. Good AE: Involvement of the back in Reiter's syndrome: follow-up study of thirty-four cases. Ann Intern Med 57:44, 1962.
76. Nashel DJ, Petrone DL, Ulmer CC, Sliwinski AJ: C-reactive protein: a marker for disease activity in ankylosing spondylitis and Reiter's syndrome. J Rheumatol 13:364, 1986.
77. Arnett FC, Schacter BZ, Hochberg MC, et al.: Homozygosity for HLA-B27. Impact on rheumatic disease expression in two families. Arthritis Rheum 20:797, 1977.
78. McGuigan LE, Hart HH, Gow PJ, et al.: The functional significance of sacroiliitis and ankylosing spondylitis in Reiter's syndrome. Clin Exp Rheumatol 3:311, 1985.

PSORIATIC ARTHRITIS

Capsule Summary

Frequency of back pain—rare

Location of back pain—sacroiliac joints and lumbar spine

Quality of back pain—ache

Symptoms and signs—morning stiffness, skin rash with plaques, back tenderness, decreased motion

Laboratory and x-ray tests—increased sedimentation rate; unilateral or bilateral sacroiliitis, nonmarginal syndesmophytes on plain roentgenograms

Treatment—topical drugs, nonsteroidal anti-inflammatory drugs, methotrexate

PREVALENCE AND PATHOGENESIS

Patients with psoriasis who develop a characteristic pattern of joint disease have psoriatic arthritis. French physicians, Bazin and Bourdillon, in the 1800s were the first to name the disease and describe it in detail.[1, 2] In the United States, there was hesitancy in ascribing joint disease to psoriasis. Many physicians thought that two common diseases were occurring in patients simultaneously, psoriasis and rheumatoid arthritis. More recent studies, however, have clearly demonstrated the association of psoriasis and arthritis.[3]

Precise data concerning the prevalence of psoriasis are not available. Many patients with mild disease may never be seen by physicians. Therefore, only estimates of prevalence have been made and have suggested that 1% to 3% of the population is affected by psoriasis. Psoriasis does, however, occur more commonly in people from temperate climate zones. Prevalence of psoriasis in the United States and Japan is similar. People from eastern and northern Africa are also similarly affected. Psoriasis is rare in southern and western Africa, and this is reflected in the low percentage of American blacks affected, most of whom originated from western Africa. Psoriatic arthritis occurs in 5% to 7% of individuals with psoriasis, and in 0.1% of the general population.[4, 5] More recent studies have reported a larger proportion with arthritis ranging from 20% to 34%.[6, 7] Psoriasis and psoriatic arthritis occur in equal frequency in both sexes. In a study of 220 patients with psoriatic arthritis, 47% were men and 53% women.[8]

The basic abnormality that results in the increased metabolic activity of the skin is unknown. Some investigators believe this abnormality resides in the most superficial layers of the skin (epidermis), while others believe that the inner layers of the skin (dermis) are the source of the increased metabolic activity. A psoriatic diathesis exists in patients who are at risk for disease. Abnormalities in protein synthesis, blood flow, and metabolism are present in normal-appearing skin, hair, and nails in these individuals. Recent experiments have shown a hyperproliferative effect on normal keratinocytes by psoriatic skin fibroblasts. These cells undergo unrestrained growth which reflects the condition of the skin in vivo.[9]

A genetic predisposition for the development of psoriasis and psoriatic arthritis does exist. Although a positive family history is obtained in about a third of patients with psoriasis, a definite pattern of inheritance has not been established. Psoriatic arthritis occurs more frequently in family members.[10] The skin disease of psoriasis has been associated with HLA-B13, HLA-BW17, HLA-CW6, and DRW6 antigens.[11] More recent population studies have identified B13, B17, B37, CW6, and DR7 as haplotypes associated with psoriasis.[12] Genetic factors also play a role in psoriatic arthritis. Patients with peripheral psoriatic arthritis have an increased frequency of HLA-BW38, HLA-DR4, and HLA-DR7 antigens.[13] Others have reported HLA-BW57, HLA-BW39, HLA-BW6, and HLA-BW7 associated with peripheral arthropathy.[14] Haplotypes associated with psoriatic arthritis most recently include B13, B17, B38, B39, DR4, and DR7.[15] Psoriatic spondylitis is associated with increased frequency of HLA-B27.[16]

Like AS and Reiter's syndrome, psoriatic arthritis may develop after exposure to a number of environmental factors. Trauma has been reported by a number of investigators as the initiator of arthritis or osteolysis (bone loss) in psoriasis.[17, 18] Chronic arthritis has developed after trauma to normal joints in patients with psoriasis uncomplicated by arthritis. Occasional anecdotal reports associating trauma and psoriatic arthritis continue to appear in the literature.[19, 20] Synovial joints in psoriasis patients may be more liable to damage owing to an enzyme deficiency of synovial fluid.[21] Other environmental factors, including infections with *Staphylococcus aureus* and *Clostridium perfringens,* and delayed hypersensitivity have been suggested as important elements in the development of psoriatic arthritis.[22, 23] Other abnormalities associated with psoriasis include increased levels of complement activation fragments, decreased T-cell subpopulations, and lipoxygenase products.[24–26]

CLINICAL FEATURES

Psoriatic arthritis has more than one clinical form, and this initially caused confusion in the description of the illness (Table 11–5).[27] Classic psoriatic arthritis is described as involving distal interphalangeal (DIP) joints and associated nail disease alone. This pattern occurs in 5% of patients. The most common form of disease, affecting 70% of patients with psoriatic arthritis, is an asymptomatic oligoarthritis; a few large or small joints are involved. Dactylitis, diffuse swelling of a digit, is most closely associated with this form of the disease. Skin activity and joint symptoms do not correlate, since patients with little skin activity may experience continued joint pain and stiffness. As opposed to rheumatoid arthritis, the clinical appearance of an involved joint does not necessarily correlate with symptoms. Patients with severely affected joints may be asymptomatic. Symmetric polyarthritis, which affects the small joints of the hands and feet and resembles rheumatoid arthritis, occurs in 15% of patients. Arthritis mutilans, characterized by extensive destruction of bone in hands, is found in 5% of patients. Spondylitis with or without peripheral joint disease occurs in 5% of patients.

In one report, clinical forms of psoriatic arthritis were divided into three major types—asymmetric, oligoarticular arthritis (54%); symmetric arthritis (25%); and spondyloarthritis (21%).[28] DIP involvement occurred most commonly in the group with asymmetric oligoarthritis and rarely in those with spondyloarthropathy. Arthritis mutilans occurred rarely in all groups.

Patients who develop axial skeletal disease, sacroiliitis or spondylitis, are men who have the onset of psoriasis later in life.[29] Patients who first develop psoriatic arthritis before the age of 20 may be more likely to develop arthri-

TABLE 11–5. CLASSIFICATION OF PSORIATRIC ARTHRITIS

FORM	INCIDENCE (%)
Asymmetric oligoarthritis	70
Symmetric "rheumatoid arthritis-like"	15
Distal interphalangeal predominant	5
Arthritis mutilans	5
Psoriatic spondylitis	5

tis mutilans. Low back pain, which is indistinguishable from the pain associated with the other spondyloarthropathies, is present in the vast majority of patients with axial skeletal disease. These patients may have back pain or peripheral joint symptoms as their initial complaint. Asymmetric or symmetric peripheral joint involvement may antedate the development of axial skeletal disease.

The typical patient with the symmetric or asymmetric form of psoriatic arthritis is a man or woman between the ages of 35 and 45. Patients with more severe disease have an onset of symptoms at an earlier age, manifested by inflammation in a few joints or by diffuse swelling of an entire digit. Psoriasis antedates the arthritis in a majority of patients (Table 11–6).[30] Between 10% and 20% of patients will have characteristic arthritis before the appearance of psoriatic lesions. Patients with severe skin involvement are more likely to develop arthritis.[31] However, even patients with minimal skin involvement still have some risk of developing joint disease. Nail involvement, characterized by pitting, horizontal ridging, onycholysis (opacification of the nail bed), and discoloration, occurs in 80% of patients with psoriatic arthritis, in contrast to a 30% incidence in patients with uncomplicated psoriasis. The activity of skin and nail disease does not necessarily correlate with joint symptoms, since any of the forms of psoriatic skin disease, whether guttate, pustular, seborrheic, or other, may be associated with joint involvement.[32, 33]

Although constitutional symptoms of fever, anorexia, and weight loss are rare in patients with psoriatic arthritis, fatigue and morning stiffness are common. Ocular involvement includes conjunctivitis in 20%, iritis in 10%, and scleritis in 2% of patients with psoriatic arthritis.[34] Iritis is more commonly seen in patients with axial skeletal disease. Cardiac complications, such as aortic insufficiency as seen in AS, are very rare and are usually associated with spondylitis.[35]

PHYSICAL EXAMINATION

An extensive examination of the skin is an essential part of the investigation of a patient with suspected psoriatic arthritis. The diagnosis of psoriasis is not difficult to make when the patient has the characteristic erythematous, raised, circumscribed, dry scaling lesions over the elbows, knees, and scalp and pitting of the nails. Skin lesions may be hidden in the scalp, gluteal folds, perineum, rectum, or umbilicus and may remain undetected unless a complete skin exam is done. Nails are examined for the presence of pitting, ridges, opacification, and hyperkeratosis.

A complete musculoskeletal examination is essential in determining the extent of joint involvement. Patients may be asymptomatic in a specific joint although physical examination demonstrates decreased function. They may have dactylitis of a toe and may be unaware of the change until it is pointed out by the physician. Examination of the axial skeleton should be completed even in the asymptomatic patient. A loss of spinal motion may be a manifestation of axial skeletal disease. Sacroiliac involvement may be unilateral or bilateral. Percussion over the sacroiliac joints can elicit symptoms over the affected side. Patients may develop spondylitis in the absence of sacroiliitis, and these patients have maximal tenderness with percussion over the spine above the sacrum.

LABORATORY DATA

The findings of anemia, mild leukocytosis, and elevated ESR occur in a minority of patients.[36] An elevated uric acid level (hyperuricemia) is detected in 20% of patients. This may be secondary to an increased metabolic rate and protein breakdown in patients with extensive skin involvement. These patients may develop secondary gout. Psoriatic synovial fluid is inflammatory but has no diagnostic features. Rheumatoid factor and antinuclear antibody (ANA) are usually absent. If they are present, the rheumatoid factor and ANA occur in the same frequency as found in age-matched controls. HLA-B27 is detected in approximately 35% to 60% of patients with axial skeletal disease.[37] In one study, patients with sacroiliitis and spondylitis had 90% positivity for HLA-B27, while in another study patients with spondylitis and normal sacroiliac joints had 43% positivity.[16, 29] In a study of 180 patients, 85% of patients with bilateral sacroiliitis were B27 positive, while 22% of those with asymmetric sacroiliitis were B27 positive.[38] Peripheral joint disease is associated with HLA-BW38, while psoriasis alone is associated with HLA-B13 and B17.[39]

TABLE 11–6. ONSET OF PSORIATRIC ARTHRITIS

	(%)
Psoriasis before arthritis	70
Psoriasis simultaneous with arthritis	20
Arthritis before psoriasis	10

RADIOGRAPHIC EVALUATION

While radiologic features of psoriatic arthritis and rheumatoid arthritis may be similar, certain features of DIP and PIP joints in psoriatic arthritis are distinctive.[40, 41] The joint involvement is oligoarticular with erosive changes in the DIP joint and terminal phalanx, especially the big toe. The "pencil-in-cup" deformity, osteolysis of the proximal phalanx and widening of the distal phalanx, is characteristic of psoriatic arthritis. Periosteal reaction occurs along the shafts of the long bones, as opposed to the periosteal changes in Reiter's syndrome, which are localized to the metatarsal bones and phalanges of the feet and hands.

Axial skeletal involvement was first emphasized by Dixon.[42] Up to 25% of patients have sacroiliac involvement manifested by sacroiliitis, which can be unilateral or bilateral.[43–45] Symmetric involvement, with balance in severity as well as location of disease, predominates over asymmetric disease. Sacroiliitis may occur without spondylitis (Fig. 11–15). Radiographic characteristics of sacroiliitis include erosions and sclerosis predominantly on the ilium, along with joint widening. Joint ankylosis occurs less commonly than in AS. Sacroiliitis with psoriasis has no radiographic changes that can be considered specific for the disease.[46] Spondylitis is characterized by asymmetric involvement of the vertebral bodies and nonmarginal syndesmophytes (Fig. 11–16). Spondylitis with normal sacroiliac joints may show up radiographically. Rare patients have been described with axial skeletal disease that mirrors the involvement characteristic of AS. Paravertebral ossification separated from the vertebral body may occur in the thoracolumbar region.[47] Squaring of vertebral bodies, osteitis of bone, and facet joint ankylosis occur less frequently in psoriatic spondylitis than in AS. Spinal disease progression occurs in a random rather than an orderly fashion ascending the spine as commonly noted in AS.

In psoriatic spondylitis, the cervical spine may also be affected, with joint space sclerosis and narrowing and anterior ligamentous calcification.[48] As with the other spondyloarthropathies, a scintiscan may demonstrate increased activity over the sacroiliac joints or axial skeleton before radiographic changes are detectable.[49]

DIFFERENTIAL DIAGNOSIS

The diagnosis of psoriatic arthritis is easily made when the patient has characteristic skin lesions and joint changes. The diagnosis is more difficult in the patient who presents with

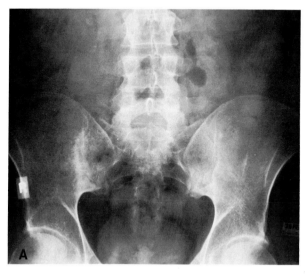

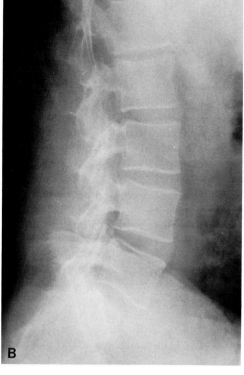

Figure 11–15. Psoriatic arthritis in a 36-year-old man with psoriasis, chronic back pain of 10 years' duration, and negative HLA-B27 antigen. *A,* AP of pelvis reveals sacroiliac joint space narrowing, erosions, and sclerosis more prominent on the right than on the left. *B,* Lateral view lumbar spine is unremarkable, with no changes of spondylitis.

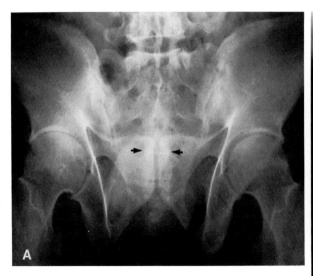
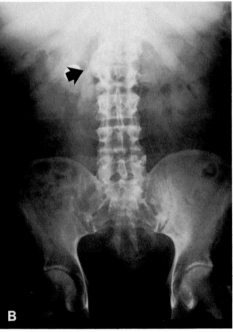

Figure 11–16. Psoriatic arthritis. A 55-year-old man with a 34-year history of psoriatic arthritis. *A,* Ferguson view of pelvis reveals bilateral sacroiliitis along with erosion and reactive sclerosis of the symphysis pubis (*arrows*). *B,* AP view of lumbosacral spine demonstrates a large nonmarginal syndesmophyte connecting L1 and L2 (*arrow*).

joint symptoms before the appearance of skin lesions. The differential diagnosis for such a patient should include Reiter's syndrome, gout, erosive osteoarthritis, and rheumatoid arthritis. Reiter's syndrome may be differentiated by urethritis, predominantly lower extremity involvement, and periosteal changes. Acute gout is confirmed by the detection of monosodium urate crystals in synovial fluid. Erosive osteoarthritis occurs in postmenopausal women and is characterized by inflammation in the DIP and PIP joints and radiographic findings of osteophytes, sclerosis, and cysts in these joints. The ESR remains normal. The clinical appearance of symmetric polyarthritis in psoriatic arthritis and rheumatoid arthritis is similar. The absence of rheumatoid nodules, rheumatoid factor, and the presence of DIP involvement and periostitis helps differentiate the patient with psoriatic arthritis from the one with rheumatoid arthritis (see Table 11–4).

TREATMENT

The goals of therapy are the maintenance and improvement in function through the reduction of inflammation. Therapy includes patient education, nonsteroidal anti-inflamma-

tory drugs, immunosuppressives, and physical therapy. The importance of appropriate skin care must be stressed. While in the past no correlation between improvement in skin and joint symptoms could be demonstrated, a recent study reported the improvement of nonspondylitic psoriatic arthritis in patients who responded to photochemotherapy for their skin disease.[50] Patients with refractory skin disease may be treated with methotrexate, PUVA, retinoic acid derivatives, and cyclosporine.[51] Nonsteroidal anti-inflammatory drugs, particularly indomethacin and phenylbutazone, are useful in controlling pain and stiffness in the peripheral and axial joints. Mefenamic acid also has been suggested as a useful drug for the control of joint symptoms. The nonsteroidals are given in maximum doses tolerated by the patient in order to better control the inflammation associated with their joint disease (indomethacin up to 150 mg/day, naproxen up to 1500 mg/day, sulindac up to 400 mg/day).

Drugs causing skin rash as a potential toxic effect have been contraindicated in the past; however, recent studies have demonstrated the efficacy and lack of skin toxicity of hydroxychloroquine and gold salts.[28, 52] These drugs are most helpful for the patient with refractory peripheral arthritis and may not have an effect on progressive axial skeletal arthritis. Oral gold also has been utilized for psoriatic arthritis.[53] However, intramuscular gold is more effective than the oral preparation.[54] Sulfasalazine has been shown to be effective in clinical trials.[55]

In patients with severe and extensive skin disease and destructive arthritis, immunosuppressive therapy with methotrexate, 6-mercaptopurine, and azathioprine is indicated.[56–58] Methotrexate is usually given orally (2.5 mg, q12h for a total dose of 7.5 mg). This is given once a week to limit toxicity. Liver fibrosis is the most common serious toxicity of methotrexate. Liver biopsy is recommended when the patient receives 2 gm of medicine.[59] The long-term benefits of methotrexate remain to be determined. In a multicenter study, methotrexate was helpful in patients with psoriasis as compared with controls only in skin lesion improvement and subjective physician assessment.[60] More recent studies have documented control of peripheral arthritis with methotrexate in a majority of patients.[61] These drugs have the potential for severe liver toxicity and leukopenia and should be reserved for the most severely affected patients. Methotrexate is safe with regard to liver toxicity in the majority of patients who receive low doses that are effective for control of psoriatic arthritis. Systemic corticosteroids are rarely used for skin or joint disease, since a rebound phenomenon appears when the drug is discontinued.[62] Intraarticular corticosteroids are useful in the patient with psoriatic monarthritis and persistent effusion. Once again, the immunosuppressives and corticosteroids are more effective for control of peripheral arthritis than for axial skeletal disease.

Retinoids (vitamin A) have been associated with improvement in psoriatic arthritis.[63] Maintenance therapy was required to prevent relapse. Of interest is the observation that less psoralen treatment was needed to achieve a clinical response when it was used in conjunction with retinoids. The need for less psoralen for control of psoriasis may decrease the incidence of squamous cell cancer of the skin, which has been noted in patients treated with psoralens for an average of 5.7 years.[64]

PROGNOSIS

The course of psoriatic arthritis is unpredictable.[30] A small percentage of patients develop destructive, disabling disease, while a majority have less pain and disability than is seen in rheumatoid arthritis. In one large study, 97% of psoriatic patients were able to work at their jobs, missing less than 12 months of work during a minimum 10-year follow-up period. Another survey found that women who developed symmetric large and small joint disease had more destructive arthritis.[28]

Patients who develop psoriatic spondylitis have varying degrees of restriction of spinal motion. There is no consistent correlation between the severity of peripheral joint disease and axial skeletal disease. A study of patients with AS, psoriatic spondylitis, and enteropathic spondylitis found the psoriatic patients to be the most severely affected.[65] Another study found AS patients to be more severely affected.[66] Other studies have demonstrated radiographic progression of spondylitis without an increase in symptoms or decreased spinal mobility.[67] The results of these studies leave the physician to follow each patient to identify their course. Progressive disease will require more aggressive therapy.

References

PSORIATIC ARTHRITIS

1. Bazin P: Lecons Theoriques et Cliniques sur les Affections Cutane et de Nature Arthritique et Darteux. Paris, Delahaye, 1860, pp 154–161.
2. Bourdillon C: Psoriasis et Arthropathies. These, Paris, 1888.
3. Wright V: Rheumatism and psoriasis: a re-evaluation. Am J Med 27:454, 1959.
4. Baker H: Epidemiological aspects of psoriasis and arthritis. Br J Dermatol 78:249, 1966.
5. Hellgren L: Association between rheumatoid arthritis and psoriasis in total populations. Acta Rheum Scand 15:316, 1969.
6. Scarpa R, Oriente P, Pulino A, et al.: Psoriatic arthritis in psoriatic patients. Br J Rheumatol 23:246, 1984.
7. Stern RS: The epidemiology of joint complaints in patients with psoriasis. J Rheumatol 12:315, 1985.
8. Gladman DD, Shuckett R, Russell ML, et al.: Psoriatic arthritis (PSA): an analysis of 220 patients. Q J Med 238:127, 1987.
9. Saiag P, Coulomb B, Lebreton C, et al.: Psoriatic fibroblasts induce hyperproliferation of normal keratinocytes in a skin equivalent model in vitro. Science 230:669, 1985.
10. Moll JMH, Wright V: Familial occurrence of psoriatic arthritis. Ann Rheum Dis 32:181, 1973.
11. McKendry RJR, Sengar DPS, DesGroseilliers JP, Dunne JV: Frequency of HLA antigens in patients with psoriasis or psoriatic arthritis. Can Med Assoc J 130:411, 1984.
12. Gladman DD: Psoriatic arthritis: recent advances in pathogenesis and treatment. Rheum Dis Clin North Am 18:247, 1992.
13. Espinoza LR, Vasey FB, Gaylord SW, et al.: Histocompatibility typing in the seronegative spondyloarthropathies: a survey. Semin Arthritis Rheum 11:375, 1982.

14. Beaulieu AD, Roy R, Mathon G, et al.: Psoriatic arthritis: risk factors for patients with psoriasis—a study based on histocompatibility antigen frequencies. J Rheumatol 10:633, 1983.

15. Sakkas LI, Loqueman N, Bird H, et al.: HLA class II and T-cell receptor gene polymorphisms in psoriatic arthritis and psoriasis. J Rheumatol 17:1487, 1990.

16. Metzger AL, Morris RI, Bluestone R, Terasaki PI: HLA-AW27 in psoriatic arthropathy. Arthritis Rheum 18:111, 1975.

17. Buckley WR, Raleigh RL: Psoriasis with acro-osteolysis. N Engl J Med 261:539, 1959.

18. Williams KA, Scott JT: Influence of trauma on the development of chronic inflammatory polyarthritis. Ann Rheum Dis 26:532, 1967.

19. Langevitz P, Buskila D, Gladman DD: Arthritis precipitated by physical trauma. J Rheumatol 17:695, 1990.

20. Pages M, Lassoued S, Fournile B, et al.: Psoriatic arthritis precipitated by physical trauma: destructive arthritis or associated with reflex sympathetic dystrophy? J Rheumatol 19:185, 1992.

21. Cotton DWK, Mier PD: An hypothesis on the aetiology of psoriasis. Br J Dermatol 76:519, 1969.

22. Landau JW, Gross BG, Newcomer VD, Wright ET: Immunologic response of patients with psoriasis. Arch Dermatol 91:607, 1965.

23. Mansson I, Olhagen B: Intestinal *Clostridium perfringens* in rheumatoid arthritis and other connective tissue disorders: studies of fecal flora, serum antitoxin levels, and skin hypersensitivity. Acta Rheum Scand 12:167, 1966.

24. Rosenberg EW, Noah PW, Wyatt RJ, et al.: Complement activation in psoriasis. Clin Exp Dermatol 15:16, 1990.

25. Rubins AY, Merson AG: Subpopulations of T lymphocytes on psoriasis patients and their changes during immunotherapy. J Am Acad Dermatol 17:972, 1987.

26. Voorhees JJ: Leukotrienes and other lipoxygenase products in the pathogenesis and therapy of psoriasis and other dermatoses. Arch Dermatol 119:541, 1983.

27. Moll JMH, Wright V: Psoriatic arthritis. Semin Arthritis Rheum 3:55, 1973.

28. Kammer GM, Soter WA, Gibson DJ, Schur PH: Psoriatic arthritis: a clinical, immunologic and HLA study of 100 patients. Semin Arthritis Rheum 9:75, 1979.

29. Lambert JR, Wright V: Psoriatic spondylitis: a clinical radiological description of the spine in psoriatic arthritis. J Med 46:411, 1977.

30. Roberts MET, Wright V, Hill AGS, Mehra AC: Psoriatic arthritis: follow-up study. Ann Rheum Dis 35:206, 1976.

31. Leczinsky CG: The incidence of arthropathy in a ten-year series of psoriasis cases. Acta Dermatol Venereol 28:483, 1948.

32. Wright V, Roberts MD, Hill AGS: Dermatologic manifestations in psoriatic arthritis: a follow-up study. Acta Dermatol Venereol 59:235, 1979.

33. Eastmoral CJ, Wright V: Nail dystrophy of psoriatic arthritis. Ann Rheum Dis 38:226, 1979.

34. Lambert JR, Wright V: Eye inflammation in psoriatic arthritis. Ann Rheum Dis 35:354, 1976.

35. Roller DH, Muna WF, Ross AM: Psoriasis, sacroiliitis and aortitis. Chest 75:641, 1979.

36. Baker H, Golding DH, Thompson M: Psoriasis and arthritis. Ann Intern Med 58:909, 1963.

37. Brewerton DA, Coffrey M, Nicholls A, et al.: HLA-B27 and arthropathies associated with ulcerative colitis and psoriasis. Lancet 1:956, 1974.

38. Torre Alonso JC, Rodriquez Perez A, Arribas Castrillo JM, et al.: Psoriatic arthritis (PA): a clinical, immunological and radiological study of 180 patients. Br J Rheumatol 30:245, 1991.

39. Espinoza LR, Vasey FB, Oh JH, et al.: Association between HLA-BW38 and peripheral psoriatic arthritis. Arthritis Rheum 21:72, 1978.

40. Avila R, Pugh DG, Slocumb CH, Winkelman RK: Psoriatic arthritis: a roentgenographic study. Radiology 75:691, 1960.

41. Wright V: Psoriatic arthritis: a comparative study of rheumatoid arthritis and arthritis associated with psoriasis. Ann Rheum Dis 20:123, 1961.

42. Dixon AS, Lience E: Sacroiliac joint in adult rheumatoid arthritis and psoriatic arthropathy. Ann Rheum Dis 20:247, 1961.

43. Harvie JN, Lester RS, Little AH: Sacroiliitis in severe psoriasis. AJR 127:579, 1976.

44. Maldonado-Cocco JA, Porrini A, Garcia-Morteo O: Prevalence of sacroiliitis and ankylosing spondylitis in psoriasis patients. J Rheumatol 5:311, 1978.

45. McEwen C, DiTata D, Lingg C, et al.: Ankylosing spondylitis and spondylitis accompanying ulcerative colitis, regional enteritis, psoriasis and Reiter's disease: a comparative study. Arthritis Rheum 14:291, 1971.

46. Molin L: Sacroiliitis in psoriasis. Scand J Rheumatol (Suppl) 32:133, 1979.

47. Bywaters EGL, Dixon ASJ: Paravertebral ossification in psoriatic arthritis. Ann Rheum Dis 24:313, 1965.

48. Kaplan D, Plotz CM, Nathanson L, Frank L: Cervical spine in psoriasis and in psoriatic arthritis. Ann Rheum Dis 23:50, 1964.

49. Barraclough D, Russell AS, Percy JS: Psoriatic spondylitis: a clinical radiological and scintiscan survey. J Rheumatol 4:282, 1977.

50. Perlman SG, Gerber LH, Roberts RM, et al.: Photochemotherapy and psoriatic arthritis: a prospective study. Ann Intern Med 91:717, 1979.

51. Ellis CN, Fradin MS, Messana JM, et al.: Cyclosporin for plaque-type psoriasis. Results of a multidose, double-blind trial. N Engl J Med 324:277, 1991.

52. Dorwart BB, Gall EP, Schumacher HR, Krauser RE: Chrysotherapy in psoriatic arthritis: efficacy and toxicity compared to rheumatoid arthritis. Arthritis Rheum 21:513, 1978.

53. Carrette S, Calin A: Evaluation of auranofin in psoriatic arthritis: a double-blind, placebo-controlled trial. Arthritis Rheum 32:158, 1989.

54. Palit J, Hill J, Capell HA, et al.: A multicentre double-blind comparison of auranofin, intramuscular gold thiomalate and placebo in patients with psoriatic arthritis. Br J Rheumatol 29:280, 1990.

55. Farr M, Kitas GD, Waterhouse L, et al.: Sulphasalazine in psoriatic arthritis: a double-blind, placebo-controlled study. Br J Rheumatol 29:46, 1990.

56. Black RL, O'Brien WM, Van Scott EJ, et al.: Methotrexate therapy in psoriatic arthritis: double-blind study in 21 patients. JAMA 189:743, 1964.

57. Baum J, Hurd E, Lewis D, et al.: Treatment of psoriatic arthritis with 6-mercaptopurine. Arthritis Rheum 16:139, 1973.

58. DuVivier A, Munro DD, Verbov J: Treatment of psoriasis with azathioprine. Br Med J 1:49, 1974.

59. Roenigk HH, Auerbach RM, Mailbach HI, Weinstein GD: Methotrexate guidelines—revised. J Am Acad Dermatol 6:145, 1982.

60. Wilkens RF, Williams JH, Ward JR, et al.: Randomized, double-blind, placebo controlled trial of low-dose pulse methotrexate in psoriatic arthritis. Arthritis Rheum 27:376, 1984.

61. Espinoza LR, Zakraoui L, Espinoza CG, et al.: Psoriatic arthritis: clinical response and side effects to methotrexate therapy. J Rheumatol 19:872, 1992.

62. Hollander JL, Brown EM, Jessar RA, et al.: The effect of triamcinolone on psoriatic arthritis: a two year study. Arthritis Rheum 2:513, 1959.
63. Farber EM, Abel EA, Charuworn A: Recent advances in the treatment of psoriasis. J Am Acad Dermatol 8:311, 1983.
64. Skern RS, Laud N, Melski J, et al.: Cutaneous squamous cell carcinoma in patients treated with PUVA. N Engl J Med 310:1156, 1984.
65. Edmunds L, Elswood J, Kennedy LG, et al.: Primary ankylosing spondylitis, psoriatic and enteropathic spondyloarthropathy: a controlled analysis. J Rheumatol 118:696, 1991.
66. Scarpa R, Oriente P, Pucino A, et al.: The clinical spectrum of psoriatic spondylitis. Br J Rheumatol 27:133, 1988.
67. Hanly JG, Russell ML, Gladman DD: Psoriatic spondyloarthropathy: a long term prospective study. Ann Rheum Dis 47:386, 1988.

ENTEROPATHIC ARTHRITIS

Capsule Summary

Frequency of back pain—rare
Location of back pain—sacroiliac joints
Quality of back pain—ache
Symptoms and signs—morning stiffness, abdominal pain or cramps
Laboratory and x-ray tests—increased sedimentation rate, blood in stool; bilateral sacroiliitis on plain roentgenograms
Treatment—exercises, nonsteroidal anti-inflammatory drugs

PREVALENCE AND PATHOGENESIS

Ulcerative colitis and Crohn's disease are inflammatory bowel diseases. Ulcerative colitis is limited to the colon, while Crohn's disease, or regional enteritis, may involve any part of the gastrointestinal tract. Inflammation of the gut results in numerous gastrointestinal symptoms, including abdominal pain, fever, and weight loss. These inflammatory diseases are also associated with extraintestinal manifestations, including arthritis. Articular involvement in these inflammatory bowel diseases includes both peripheral and axial skeletal joints. Peripheral arthritis is generally nondeforming and follows the activity of the underlying bowel disease. Axial skeletal disease is similar to AS and follows a course independent of activity of bowel inflammation.

The association of arthritis and ulcerative colitis was first elucidated by Bargen in the 1920s.[1] Crohn's disease was described by Crohn, Ginzburg, and Oppenheimer in 1932.[2] The association of arthritis and Crohn's disease was commented on by Van Patter and Steinberg in the 1950s.[3, 4]

Ulcerative colitis occurs four times more commonly in whites than nonwhites and more commonly among Jews than non-Jews. In a white population, the annual incidence of disease is up to 10 per 100,000 people.[5, 6] Symptomatic ulcerative colitis usually occurs between 25 and 45 years of age, and the disease is more common among women than men.

Crohn's disease occurs in all races and is distributed worldwide. In the United States, the annual incidence of the disease is 4 per 100,000 individuals.[5] The disease appears most often between the ages of 15 and 35. Men and women are equally affected. Patients from urban backgrounds and with high levels of education are at greater risk.

The frequency of peripheral arthritis is 11% in ulcerative colitis and 20% in Crohn's disease, and the occurrence of axial arthritis is equal in both sexes.[7, 8] Spondylitis occurs in 3% to 4% of both diseases and radiographic sacroiliitis in 10%.[9, 10] Women are equally affected in Crohn's disease and half as often as men in ulcerative colitis.

The etiology of both of these inflammatory bowel diseases is unknown.[6] Specific infections with bacteria, overproduction of enzymes, vascular disorders, and hypersensitivity to foods are but a few of the unproven theories suggested as possible causes. No specific genetic predisposition for these illnesses has been discovered, although there may be a familial predilection.[11, 12]

The pathogenesis of peripheral and axial arthritis may be different. Peripheral arthritis may evolve as a complication of active bowel disease. Hypothetically, endogenous or exogenous antigens may be absorbed through the bowel wall, initiating an immune response in which antigen-antibody complexes would collect in peripheral joints and cause synovitis. This scheme has clinical correlations in the close association of activity of bowel disease and peripheral arthritis and the association of peripheral arthritis and other extraintestinal manifestations of disease, including erythema nodosum and iritis.[13] A similar immune complex mechanism may also explain the arthritis associated with another bowel abnormality, intestinal bypass arthritis.[14, 15]

Axial arthritis of inflammatory bowel disease may be a hereditary accompaniment of the disease and not a manifestation of activity of bowel disease itself. Familial aggregation of spondylitis and sacroiliitis in relatives of patients with inflammatory bowel disease has been reported.[16, 17] Both non-HLA-related factors and HLA-B27 may play a role. Enlow reported an incidence of HLA-B27 in 30% of patients with axial arthritis and inflammatory bowel disease.[18] In the same study, when relatives of the HLA-B27-negative spondylitis patients were studied, four were found to have axial arthritis without inflammatory bowel disease. No specific HLA haplotype was associated with axial arthropathy. This study suggests that both HLA-B27 and non-HLA genetic determinants predispose to axial arthropathy in patients with inflammatory bowel disease. In patients with enteropathic spondylitis, HLA-B27 is positive in 50% to 75% of patients.[19] Although no association is reported between the activity of bowel disease and axial arthritis, Mielants and Veys have described silent inflammatory gut disease identified by colonoscopy.[20]

CLINICAL HISTORY

The early symptoms of ulcerative colitis are frequent bowel movements with blood or mucus. Mild disease is associated with some abdominal pain and a few bowel movements per day. Severe disease is characterized by fatigue, weight loss, fever, and extracolonic involvement. Crohn's disease is frequently an indolent illness characterized by generalized fatigue, mild nonbloody diarrhea, anorexia, weight loss, and cramping lower abdominal pain. Patients may have symptoms for years before the diagnosis is made.

Articular involvement in these inflammatory bowel diseases is divided into two forms, peripheral and spondylitic. In ulcerative colitis, peripheral arthritis starts as an acute monarticular or oligoarticular arthritis affecting the knee, ankle, elbow, PIP, wrist, or shoulder joints in patients with active bowel disease.[21] The attacks are painful, sometimes associated with effusions. They subside after 6 to 8 weeks and are nondeforming.[22] Joint symptoms follow the activity of the bowel disease. Patients with arthritis frequently demonstrate other extracolonic manifestations of ulcerative colitis, such as erythema nodosum, pyoderma gangrenosum, and uveitis, as well as extensive and chronic bowel disease with pseudopolyps and perianal disease.[23]

The peripheral joint involvement in Crohn's disease is similar in onset and distribution to that described above for ulcerative colitis.[24] However, the correlation of bowel inflammation and joint symptoms may continue while gastrointestinal complaints subside. The lack of association is probably secondary to the more scattered nature of Crohn's disease throughout the gut compared with the colonic involvement of ulcerative colitis and the difficulty in ascertaining complete remission of the illness.[17] Patients with colonic involvement with Crohn's disease may be at greater risk of developing peripheral arthritis.[25]

Axial skeletal involvement in ulcerative colitis and Crohn's disease is similar. Three groups of patients with inflammatory bowel disease and spondylitis have been described by Dekher-Saeys.[26] In about a third of patients, spondylitis antedates bowel disease. This interval may be as long as 10 to 20 years.[10] Seventy percent were HLA-B27 positive, 68% had radiographic changes of spondylitis, and 25% had iritis. An association between sacroiliitis and iritis in ulcerative colitis has also been reported by Wright.[27] One-fourth of the patients developed bowel symptoms before the onset of spondylitis. Thirteen percent were HLA-B27 positive, 36% had radiographic changes of spondylitis, and none had iritis. These patients had severe disease of the gut. The remaining fraction of patients had simultaneous onset of gut and spine disease. The spondylitis associated with inflammatory bowel disease has a course totally independent of that of the bowel disease. The clinical and radiographic findings are similar to those of AS, including involvement of shoulders and hips, although some have suggested that the spondylitis of inflammatory bowel disease is milder and that a higher proportion of patients are women.[28] Patients with spondylitis complain of aching low back pain with stiffness that is maximal in the early morning.[29] Occasional patients with Crohn's disease have been reported with severe back pain, limitation of lumbar motion, and decreased chest expansion even though they have no radiographic changes of spondylitis. In these patients, improvement in bowel disease was associated with improved musculoskeletal function.[26] Between 4% to 18% of patients have bilateral, symmetrical sacroiliitis that may not progress to clinical spondylitis.[30] Other musculoskeletal complications of inflammatory bowel disease include clubbing and periosteitis, avascular necrosis of bone, septic arthritis of the hips, and granulomatous inflammation of synovium, bone, and muscle.[31, 32]

PHYSICAL EXAMINATION

The general physical examination concentrates on the abdomen and gastrointestinal tract, including inspection of the oropharynx, perineum, and rectum. Examination for extraintestinal disease such as aphthous ulcers, iritis, erythema nodosum, and pyoderma gangrenosum is indicated. The musculoskeletal examination must include both peripheral joints and axial skeleton. Patients with spondyloarthropathy may have decreased motion of the spine in all planes and percussion tenderness over the sacroiliac joints. In rare circumstances, chest expansion is diminished. Also, in a small number of patients peripheral and axial skeletal disease may coexist.

LABORATORY DATA

Usual laboratory tests, such as decreased hematocrit, increased white blood cell count, increased platelet count, hypoalbuminemia, and hypokalemia, are abnormal, but are nonspecific. The inflammatory findings of increased WBC with poor mucin clot in the synovial fluid is also nondiagnostic. Rheumatoid factor and antinuclear antibodies are absent. No specific HLA antigen has been associated with ulcerative colitis, Crohn's disease, or peripheral joint disease. Approximately 50% of patients with symptomatic spondylitis and inflammatory bowel disease are HLA-B27 positive.[33]

RADIOGRAPHIC EVALUATION

Radiographs of peripheral joints demonstrate soft tissue swelling and occasionally joint effusions.[23, 34, 35] Findings of joint destruction, joint space narrowing, erosions, and periosteal proliferation are rare.[36] The radiographic changes of the spondylitis in inflammatory bowel disease are indistinguishable from those with classic AS (Fig. 11–17).[37] They include "squaring" of vertebral bodies, erosions, widening and fusion of the sacroiliac joints, symmetric involvement of sacroiliac joints, and marginal syndesmophytes (Fig. 11–18).[28] No correlation between colonic disease and spondylitis could be ascertained in a study of patients with Crohn's disease.[38] Asymptomatic radiographic sacroiliitis is demonstrated in up to 15% of patients with inflammatory bowel disease. In contrast to patients with classic AS, these patients have no association with HLA-B27, and women and men have equal involvement.[39] Scintigraphic evaluation of sacroiliac joints in inflammatory bowel disease patients has detected increased uptake of radiotracer in 52%.[40] The clinical significance of these findings remains to be determined.

CT scan is helpful in identifying sacroiliac joint abnormalities that may not be recognized by plain roentgenograms.[41] These abnormalities include joint erosions, loss of defined cortex, joint narrowing, joint widening, sclerosis, and bony ankylosis.

The clinical diagnosis of inflammatory bowel disease is suspected in an individual with diarrhea, rectal bleeding, abdominal cramps, abdominal pain, perianal fistula or abscess, and an abdominal pain, perianal fistula or abscess, and an abdominal mass along with erythema nodosum, iritis, or arthritis. Radiographic evaluation of ulcerative colitis reveals mucosal ulceration and edema affecting varying lengths of bowel. Crohn's disease causes deep ulcerations with strictures, fistulization, loop separation, and mass effect in a discontinuous pattern that may involve the small intestine as well as the colon.

DIFFERENTIAL DIAGNOSIS

A specific diagnosis of ulcerative colitis or Crohn's disease is made from the histologic examination of biopsy material from the gut. The inflammatory abnormalities of ulcerative colitis are limited to the superficial layers of the gut, mucosa, and submucosa. The most characteristic findings in ulcerative colitis are atrophy of mucosal glands and inflammatory cells in the crypts of the colon, causing crypt abscesses with no skip areas. Crohn's disease is characterized by a transluminal granulomatous inflammation. While biopsy material yields supportive evidence for one or the other illness, the final differentiation rests heavily on the history, clinical course, and barium contrast studies of the gut. The differential diagnosis for the bowel disease includes infectious colitis, diverticulitis, pseudomembranous colitis, and ischemic colitis. Infectious agents associated with colitis include *Shigella, Salmonella, Campylobacter fetus, Yersinia enterocolitica,* cytomegalovirus, amebas, and *Histoplasma.* Culture of an early morning stool specimen is an important part of the evaluation of a patient with chronic diarrhea. Special stains of biopsy material may discover an unsuspected organism. Diverticulitis will cause localized pain, fever, and diarrhea. Radiographic studies help identify the localized nature of the disorder caused by an infection of a colonic diverticulum. Patients who receive oral or parenteral antibiotics may develop, up to 4 weeks later, a nonbloody, watery diarrhea, which on endoscopic examination is associated with a yellowish-white pseudomembrane on the colonic surfaces. Stool cultures that grow *Clostridium difficile* or reveal *C. difficile* toxin virtually assure

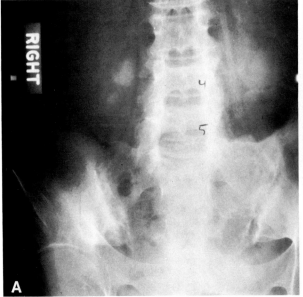

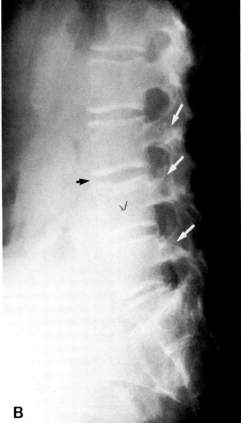

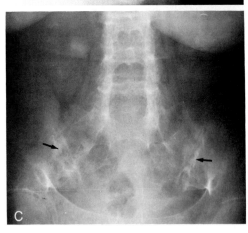

Figure 11–17. Crohn's disease. A 25-year-old woman with a 9-year history of Crohn's disease had a 4-year history of lower back pain and stiffness. The patient had a chest expansion of 2 cm and no movement of the lumbar spine with flexion. *A,* AP view of pelvis reveals bilateral symmetric sacroiliac joint abnormalities characterized by erosion and sclerosis. *B,* Lateral view of the lumbar spine demonstrates loss of lumbar lordosis, fusion of the facet joints (*white arrows*), and early syndesmophyte formation (*black arrow*). *C,* Five years later, AP view of pelvis on 7/3/90 reveals progressive joint erosion (*black arrows*) and generalized osteoporosis.

the diagnosis of pseudomembranous colitis. The abrupt onset of abdominal cramps with bleeding in a patient over 60 years of age with pre-existing atherosclerotic cardiovascular disease suggests an ischemic insult to the bowel. An abdominal flat plate film may demonstrate scalloping (''thumb printing'') of the wall. This finding is consistent with ischemic colitis. Of the various entities included in the preceding differential diagnosis of inflammatory bowel disease, bacterial infection of the gut is

the only entity associated with spondyloarthropathy (reactive arthritis)[42] (see the section on Reiter's syndrome earlier in this chapter).

The diagnosis of enteropathic arthritis is not difficult to make in the patient with ulcerative colitis or Crohn's disease with a nondeforming peripheral arthritis. Since most patients develop peripheral arthritis after the onset of gastrointestinal symptoms, the possibilities for the cause of their arthritis are limited. The real difficulty arises in diagnosis of the patient with

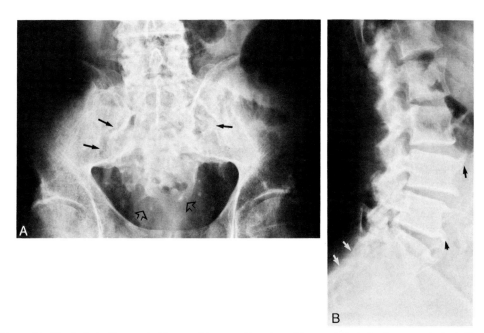

Figure 11–18. Crohn's disease. A 56-year-old man with a long history of Crohn's disease and alcoholism. Crohn's disease was manifested by rectal fistulae associated with sacral osteomyelitis. *A,* AP view of the pelvis reveals bilateral sacroiliitis (*black arrows*) and erosion of the inferior section of the sacrum (*open black arrows*). *B,* Lateral view reveals traction osteophytes (*black arrows*) (manifestation of intervertebral disc degeneration) and bony erosion of the dorsal portion of the sacrum (*white arrows*) (compatible with sacral osteomyelitis).

back symptoms before the onset of bowel disease; the differential diagnosis in such cases includes the other spondyloarthropathies, including AS and Reiter's syndrome. In a study of 1331 individuals with spondylitis, enteropathic spondylitis occurs in 6%, versus 85% for AS, and 9% for psoriatic spondylitis.[43] Enteropathic spondylitis occurs more commonly in women than the other forms of spondyloarthropathy. The severity of disease is greater than AS, but less than psoriatic spondylitis. The lower frequency of HLA-B27 may help differentiate enteropathic arthritis from AS. The absence of conjunctivitis, urethritis, and periosteitis, particularly in the heels, may help to distinguish it from Reiter's syndrome.

It is important to remember that the patient with enteropathic spondyloarthropathy commonly presents with back pain in the absence of gastrointestinal symptoms. The finding of morning stiffness should raise the suspicion of a spondyloarthropathy. The factors that help in making the diagnosis of enteropathic spondyloarthropathy are the pattern of peripheral arthritis, if present (upper extremity disease uncommon in AS and Reiter's syndrome, bilateral ankle arthritis uncommon in psoriatic disease), erythema nodosum, and iritis.

Patients with intestinal bypass surgery for morbid obesity may develop polyarthritis as a complication of this procedure. Most commonly patients are women who develop a polyarthritis after jejunocolostomy, probably secondary to a systemic reaction to bacterial products.[15, 44] The arthritis affects the knees, hands, feet, wrists, elbows, and hips. Involvement of the axial skeleton, particularly the sacroiliac joints, has only rarely been reported.[45] Radiographs of these patients reveal erosions, sclerosis, and articular space narrowing at the sacroiliac joint and syndesmophytes of the spine. HLA-B27 antigen may be detected in patients with axial joint involvement. Nonsteroidal anti-inflammatory drugs may be somewhat helpful in controlling joint pain. Patients with severe symptoms unresponsive to drugs may obtain improvement with revision of the bypass.[46]

TREATMENT

Treatment for peripheral arthritis must be directed toward control of the underlying bowel disease. Therapy might include sulfasalazine (Azulfidine, 4 to 6 gm/day), metronidazole, corticosteroid enemas, oral corticosteroids, and colectomy for the severe patient with ulcerative colitis.[47–49] A variety of therapies have been developed for the treatment of Crohn's disease. Newer forms of sulfasalazine, such as olsalazine and mesalamine, that have fewer side effects and may be given orally or as suppository are available.[50] In active, severe disease, the combination of sulfasalazine and corticosteroids is effective in 90% of patients.[51] Corticosteroids are effective when given orally or rectally.[52] Occasionally immunosuppressive drugs in the form of azathioprine or mercaptopurine are needed to control severe Crohn's disease. Mercaptopurine is given in doses of 50 mg/day. Clinical effect may take months to appear as a result of the slow-acting nature of the drug.[53, 54] Colectomized patients with ulcerative colitis do not have recurrences of peripheral joint disease.[21] Surgery is not nearly as effective in Crohn's disease, since it may have more extensive distribution through the gastrointestinal tract.

The therapeutic program for peripheral joint disease may also include nonsteroidal anti-inflammatory drugs, intra-articular injections of corticosteroids, and physical therapy. There is no evidence of increased gastrointestinal adverse effects with nonsteroidal anti-inflammatory drugs in these patients with inflammatory bowel disease. Initially lower therapeutic doses of the nonsteroidal anti-inflammatory drugs may be tried to test drug tolerability. Increased dosage of the medicine can be used if the patient tolerated the medicine but experiences inadequate relief of symptoms. If a patient has a good response to a nonsteroidal but develops gastrointestinal symptoms, the addition of medications to control those symptoms may be added to the patient's therapeutic program. In rare circumstances, nonsteroidals have been implicated as factors causing an exacerbation of inflammatory bowel disease.[55, 56]

Therapy for enteropathic spondylitis is similar to that for classic AS. This program includes patient education, nonsteroidal anti-inflammatory drugs, and physical therapy. Control of bowel disease does not necessarily correlate with improvement in back symptoms. In ulcerative colitis, colectomy should not be done with the expectation of resolution of spondylitic symptoms.

PROGNOSIS

The ultimate course and outcome of these patients is dependent on the severity of their bowel disease. Patients with severe ulcerative colitis have a mortality rate of 10% to 20% over 5 years. Patients with a severe initial attack, continuous clinical activity, involvement of the entire colon, and disease for 10 years or longer have a higher risk of developing cancer of the colon.[57] These patients may require colectomy. Although Crohn's disease is associated with frequent recurrences, the overall mortality rate of 5% for the first 5 years of disease is much less than in ulcerative colitis.[58]

Patients with peripheral enteropathic arthritis have nondeforming disease of short duration. These patients experience little disability from the arthritis and are able to work. The disability associated with enteropathic spondylitis is similar to that of AS in severely affected patients. The association of hip disease and spondylitis results in a marked decrease in mobility. Patients with spinal rigidity are at risk for fracture. These patients should not perform heavy labor associated with lifting.

References

ENTEROPATHIC ARTHRITIS

1. Bargen JA: Complications and sequelae of chronic ulcerative colitis. Ann Intern Med 3:335, 1929.
2. Crohn BB, Ginzburg L, Oppenheimer GD: Regional ileitis. A pathologic and clinical entity. JAMA 99:1323, 1932.
3. Van Patter WN, Bargen JA, Dockerty MB, et al.: Regional enteritis. Gastroenterology 26:347, 1954.
4. Steinberg VL, Storey G: Ankylosing spondylitis and chronic inflammatory lesions of the intestines. Br Med J 2:1157, 1957.
5. Monk M, Mendeloff AI, Siegel CI, Lilienfeld A: An epidemiological study of ulcerative colitis and regional enteritis among adults in Baltimore: hospital incidence and prevalence, 1960 to 1963. Gastroenterology 53:198, 1967.
6. Kirsner JB, Shorter RG: Recent developments in nonspecific inflammatory bowel disease. N Engl J Med 306:837, 1982.
7. Greenstein AJ, Janowitz HD, Sachar DB: The extraintestinal complications of Crohn's disease and ulcerative colitis: a study of 700 patients. Medicine 55:401, 1976.
8. Haslock F, Wright V: The musculoskeletal complications of Crohn's disease. Medicine 52:217, 1973.
9. Dekher-Saeys BJ, Meuwissen SGM, van den Berg-Loonen EM, et al.: Prevalence of peripheral arthritis, sacroiliitis and ankylosing spondylitis in patients suffering from inflammatory bowel disease. Ann Rheum Dis 37:33, 1978.
10. Acheson ED: An association between ulcerative colitis, regional enteritis and ankylosing spondylitis. Q J Med 29:489, 1960.
11. Almy TP, Sherlock P: Genetic aspects of ulcerative colitis and regional enteritis. Gastroenterology 51:757, 1966.
12. Paulley JW: Ulcerative colitis: a study of 173 cases. Gastroenterology 16:566, 1950.
13. Hochberg MC, Feinstein RS, Moser RL, Ryan MJ: Colitic arthritis. Johns Hopkins Med J 151:173, 1982.
14. Stein HB, Schlappner OLA, Boyko W, et al.: The intestinal bypass: arthritis-dermatitis syndrome. Arthritis Rheum 24:684, 1981.

15. Wands JR, Lamont JT, Mann E, Isselbacher KJ: Arthritis associated with intestinal-bypass procedure for morbid obesity. Complement activation and characterization of circulating cryoproteins. N Engl J Med 294:121, 1976.
16. Macrae I, Wright V: A family study of ulcerative colitis. Ann Rheum Dis 32:16, 1973.
17. Haslock I: Arthritis and Crohn's disease: a family study. Ann Rheum Dis 32:479, 1973.
18. Enlow RW, Bias WB, Arnett FC: The spondylitis of inflammatory bowel disease. Evidence for a non-HLA-linked axial arthropathy. Arthritis Rheum 23:1359, 1980.
19. Weiner SR, Clarke J, Taggart NA, et al.: Rheumatic manifestations of bowel disease. Semin Arthritis Rheum 20:353, 1991.
20. Mielants H, Veys EM: The gut in the spondyloarthropathies. J Rheumatol 17:7, 1990.
21. Wright V, Watkinson G: The arthritis of ulcerative colitis. Br Med J 2:670, 1965.
22. Palumbo PJ, Ward LE, Sauer WG, Scudamore HH: Musculoskeletal manifestations of inflammatory bowel disease: ulcerative and granulomatous colitis and ulcerative proctitis. Mayo Clin Proc 48:411, 1973.
23. McEwen C, Lingg C, Kirsner JB, Spencer JA: Arthritis accompanying ulcerative colitis. Am J Med 33:923, 1962.
24. Ansell BM, Wigley RAD: Arthritic manifestations in regional enteritis. Ann Rheum Dis 23:64, 1964.
25. Cornes JS, Stecher M: Primary Crohn's disease of the colon and rectum. Gut 2:189, 1961.
26. Dekher-Saeys BJ, Meuwissen SGM, van den Berg-Loonen EM, et al.: Clinical characteristics and results of histocompatability typing (HLA-B27) in 50 patients with both ankylosing spondylitis and inflammatory bowel disease. Ann Rheum Dis 37:36, 1978.
27. Wright R, Lumsden K, Luntz MH, et al.: Abnormalities of the sacro-iliac joints and uveitis in ulcerative colitis. Q J Med 134:229, 1965.
28. McEwen C, DiTata D, Lingg C, et al.: Ankylosing spondylitis and spondylitis accompanying ulcerative colitis, regional enteritis, psoriasis and Reiter's disease: a comparative study. Arthritis Rheum 14:291, 1968.
29. Bowen GE, Kirsner JB: The arthritis of ulcerative colitis and regional enteritis ("intestinal arthritis"). Med Clin North Am 49:17, 1965.
30. Gravallese EM, Kantrowitz FG: Arthritis manifestations of inflammatory bowel disease. Am J Gastroenterol 83:703, 1987.
31. Neale G, Kelsall AR, Doyle FH: Crohn's disease and diffuse symmetrical periostitis. Gut 9:383, 1968.
32. London D, Fitton JM: Acute septic arthritis complicating Crohn's disease. Br J Surg 57:536, 1970.
33. Morris RI, Metzger AL, Bluestone R, Terasaki PI: HLA-W27—a useful discriminator in the arthropathies of inflammatory bowel disease. N Engl J Med 290:1117, 1974.
34. Clark RL, Muhletaler CA, Margulies SI: Colitic arthritis: clinical and radiographic manifestations. Radiology 101:585, 1971.
35. Bywaters EGL, Ansell BM: Arthritis associated with ulcerative colitis: a clinical and pathological study. Ann Rheum Dis 17:169, 1958.
36. Frayha R, Stevens MB, Bayless TM: Destructive monoarthritis and granulomatous synovitis as the presenting manifestations of Crohn's disease. Johns Hopkins Med J 137:151, 1975.
37. Zvaifler NJ, Martel W: Spondylitis in chronic ulcerative colitis. Arthritis Rheum 3:76, 1960.
38. Mueller CE, Seeger JF, Martel W: Ankylosing spondylitis and regional enteritis. Radiology 112:579, 1974.
39. Hyla JF, Franck WA, Davis JS: Lack of association of HLA-B27 with radiographic sacroiliitis in inflammatory bowel disease. J Rheumatol 3:196, 1976.
40. Davis P, Thomson ABR, Lentle B: Quantitative sacroiliac scintigraphy in patients with Crohn's disease. Arthritis Rheum 21:234, 1978.
41. Scott WW Jr, Fishman EK, Kuhlman JE, et al.: Computed tomography evaluation of the sacroiliac joints in Crohn disease. Radiologic/clinical correlation. Skeletal Radiol 19:207, 1990.
42. Olhagen B: Postinfective or reactive arthritis. Scand J Rheumatol 9:193, 1980.
43. Edmunds L, Elswood J, Kennedy LG, et al.: Primary ankylosing spondylitis, psoriatic and enteropathic spondyloarthropathy: a controlled analysis. J Rheumatol 18:696, 1991.
44. Shagrin JW, Frame B, Duncan H: Polyarthritis in obese patients with intestinal bypass. Ann Intern Med 75:377, 1971.
45. Rose E, Espinoza LR, Osterland CK: Intestinal bypass arthritis. Association with circulating immune complexes. J Rheumatol 4:129, 1977.
46. Leff RD, Aldo-Benson MA, Madura JA: The effect of revision of the intestinal bypass on post-intestinal bypass arthritis. Arthritis Rheum 26:678, 1983.
47. Peppercorn MA: Sulfasalazine: pharmacology, clinical use, toxicity, and related new-drug development. Ann Intern Med 101:377, 1984.
48. Present DW, Korelitz BI, Wise HN, et al.: Treatment of Crohn's disease with 6-mercaptopurine. A long-term randomized double-blind study. N Engl J Med 302:981, 1980.
49. Summers RW, Switz DM, Session JT, et al.: National Cooperative Crohn's disease study: Results of drug treatment. Gastroenterology 77:847, 1979.
50. Jarnerot G: Newer 5-aminosalicylic acid-based drugs in chronic inflammatory bowel disease. Drugs 37:76, 1989.
51. Rijk MC, van Hogezand RA, van Lier HJ, et al.: Sulphasalazine and prednisone compared with sulphasalazine for treating active Crohn disease: a double-blind, randomized, multicenter trial. Ann Intern Med 114:445, 1991.
52. Linn FV, Peppercorn MA: Drug therapy for inflammatory bowel disease: Part I. Am J Surg 164:85, 1992.
53. Marsh JW, Vehe KL, White HM: Immunosuppressants. Gastroenterol Clin North Am 21:679, 1992.
54. Linn FV, Peppercorn MA: Drug therapy for inflammatory bowel disease: Part II. Am J Surg 164:178, 1992.
55. Kaufmann HJ, Taubin HL: Nonsteroidal anti-inflammatory drugs activate quiescent inflammatory bowel disease. Ann Intern Med 107:513, 1988.
56. Gran JT, Husby G: Ankylosing spondylitis: current drug treatment. Drugs 44:585, 1992.
57. Farmer RG, Hawk WA, Turnbull RB Jr: Carcinoma associated with mucosal ulcerative colitis, and with transmural colitis and enteritis (Crohn's disease). Cancer 28:289, 1971.
58. Lock MR, Farmer RG, Fazio VW, et al.: Recurrence and reoperation for Crohn's disease: the role of disease in prognosis. N Engl J Med 304:1586, 1981.

BEHÇET'S SYNDROME

Capsule Summary

Frequency of back pain—rare
Location of back pain—sacroiliac joints

Quality of back pain—ache

Symptoms and signs—morning stiffness, oral and genital ulcers, iritis, meningitis

Laboratory and x-ray tests—increased sedimentation rate; sacroiliitis on plain roentgenogram

Treatment—corticosteroids, thalidomide, colchicine

PREVALENCE AND PATHOGENESIS

Behçet's syndrome is a chronic relapsing systemic disease characterized by the triad of oral and genital ulcers and iritis. Additional features of the disease include vasculitis with aneurysms, erythema nodosum, meningoencephalitis, and arthritis with sacroiliitis. Disability from Behçet's syndrome occurs most commonly with loss of vision secondary to iritis and neurologic impairment secondary to meningoencephalitis and stroke. The disease was first described by Hulusi Behçet, a Turkish dermatologist, in 1937.[1] The triad of this syndrome has also been referred to as the mucocutaneous ocular syndrome.[2]

Behçet's syndrome occurs most commonly in people from eastern Mediterranean countries and Japan.[3, 4] The prevalence in Japan is approximately 1 in 7,500 population.[5] In Olmsted County, Minnesota, the prevalence is 1 in 25,000 population.[6] The disease affects men more commonly than women, except in North America where a study demonstrated an increased frequency in women.[7]

The etiology of Behçet's syndrome is unknown, although a number of immunologic abnormalities of a cellular and humoral variety have been described. These abnormalities include reduced T-lymphocyte reactivity and increased concentration of immunoglobulins.[7–9] However, no coherent pattern to these immunologic abnormalities has been ascertained. Recent studies have suggested that antibodies directed at heat shock proteins from streptococcal species are present in higher titers in Behçet's patients than normal controls.[10] Genetic factors may play a role in Japanese and Turkish patients, in whom an increased frequency of HLA-B5 has been associated with the disease.[11] HLA-B51 is a haplotype that is most frequently associated with Behçet's disease.[12, 13] HLA-B27 positivity is seen in patients with sacroiliitis.[14] HLA-B12 is found in a few patients with mucocutaneous involvement.[15]

CLINICAL HISTORY

The typical patient is 30 years old and presents with multiple, painful oral ulcers, which resolve over weeks. Genital ulcers, which are also painful, occur over the vulva, penis, or scrotum and are present in 80% of patients. Eye lesions, predominantly unilateral or bilateral iritis, occur in 66% of patients and may present with blurred vision and little ocular pain. Iritis may lead to blindness in these patients.[16] Skin manifestations, including ulceration, vasculitis, erythema nodosum, erythema multiforme, and the formation of pustules after the trauma of venipuncture (pathergy), occur in a majority of patients.[17] Central nervous system involvement occurs in 24% of patients. A multitude of neurologic manifestations have been described, including meningoencephalitis characterized by fever, headache, stiff neck, cerebrovascular accident or stroke, hemiparesis, seizures, loss of speech, and profound confusion.[18] Neurologic involvement is a bad prognostic sign, with a mortality rate of 31% to 41% in two studies.[19, 20] Vascular disease is associated with thrombophlebitis and arterial aneurysm. Gastrointestinal involvement includes colonic disease similar to ulcerative colitis.[17]

Articular involvement occurs in a majority of patients with Behçet's syndrome.[21, 22] Joint involvement has ranged from 18% to 64% in different studies.[23] Peripheral arthritis is usually polyarticular, involving the knees, ankles, wrists, or elbows. Monarticular disease occurs in the knees or ankles but is less common. Joint symptoms frequently occur after the onset of oral ulcerations.[24] The arthritis is asymmetric, recurrent, and nondeforming. Axial skeletal disease, with back pain and sacroiliitis, has been reported in a small proportion of patients with Behçet's syndrome.[25–27] In one study, 10 of 79 patients demonstrated radiographic changes of marked sacroiliitis. Spondylitis also has been described with the disease.[20]

PHYSICAL EXAMINATION

Examination of the oropharynx and genitourinary system is essential in Behçet's syndrome. Ophthalmologic examination is frequently necessary to demonstrate iritis, which may be mildly symptomatic. A complete neurologic examination is also indicated to document any abnormalities in mentation or neurologic function.

Examination of the back reveals percussion tenderness over the sacroiliac joints in patients with sacroiliitis. Range of motion of the lumbar spine may be diminished in these individuals.

LABORATORY DATA

Laboratory results are nonspecific in Behçet's syndrome. With active disease, ESR is elevated along with an increase in peripheral WBC. Synovial fluid is inflammatory in type, with an increase in WBC from 80,000 to 250,000, normal glucose, and poor mucin clotting.[22]

Pathologic evaluation of synovial tissue from Behçet's patients demonstrates a dense granulation tissue filled with inflammatory cells, including neutrophils, macrophages, lymphocytes, and macrophages. Inflammatory cells are also noted in the vasa vasorum of blood vessels associated with aneurysmal dilatation.

RADIOGRAPHIC EVALUATION

Bone and joint findings are usually mild and are characterized by osteoporosis and soft tissue swelling. Osseous erosions and joint space narrowing are rarely encountered.[28] Sacroiliitis, both unilateral and bilateral, has been noted in patients with Behçet's syndrome along with the rarer occurrence of spondylitis (Fig. 11–19).[27] Sacroiliitis is characterized by subchondral erosions and reactive sclerosis.[29] Patients who are HLA-B27 positive may be at greater risk for developing sacroiliitis and spondylitis. Patients with inflammatory disease of the bowel may develop sacroiliitis similar to that seen with ulcerative colitis or Crohn's disease.[17, 30]

Some radiographic studies of sacroiliitis in Behçet's patients have suggested that sacroiliitis is not found in increased frequency compared with controls.[31] However, CT evaluation of sacroiliac joints of Behçet's patients may increase the sensitivity of detecting the presence of sacroiliitis that may be missed by plain roentgenograms.[32]

DIFFERENTIAL DIAGNOSIS

The diagnosis of Behçet's syndrome is based on clinical features, since there are no pathognomonic laboratory findings. Diagnostic criteria that have been suggested include oral ulcers, genital ulcers, iritis, and skin lesions as a major group, and gastrointestinal, vascular, musculoskeletal, and central nervous system lesions and family history as a minor group.[33] The diagnosis is difficult to make, since the different manifestations of the illness may take years to appear. The diagnosis should be considered in a patient with recurrent oral ulcerations and one other manifestation of the disease. The differential diagnosis is very small when a patient has multisystem involvement with Behçet's syndrome. In patients with single organ system disease, the differential diagnosis is directed toward diseases that affect that organ system. For example, the differential diagnosis of oral ulcers would include herpes simplex infection; gastrointestinal disease, ulcerative colitis or Crohn's disease; and aseptic meningitis and Mollaret's meningitis. In patients with oral ulcers, back pain, and lower extremity arthritis, the diagnosis of Reiter's

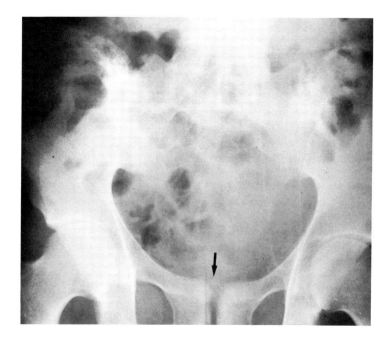

Figure 11–19. Behçet's syndrome. AP view of the pelvis of a 26-year-old man with Behçet's syndrome demonstrating bilateral sacroiliitis with obliteration of the joints along with "pseudowidening" of the symphysis pubis (*arrow*). (Courtesy of Theodor Schifter, M.D.)

syndrome must be excluded. Patients with Reiter's syndrome usually have painless oral ulcerations. Five sets of diagnostic criteria exist for the diagnosis for Behçet's disease.[34] A simplification of the criteria has been proposed. These new criteria are oral ulcerations in combination with any two manifestations including genital ulceration, typical defined eye lesions, typical defined skin lesions, or a positive pathergy test.[35]

TREATMENT

No specific therapy has been demonstrated to be effective in controlling the manifestations of Behçet's syndrome on a continued basis. Systemic corticosteroids suppress skin and joint inflammation. They are less effective on oral and genital ulcers and iritis. Recrudescence of disease activity is common during tapering of the amount of drug. Transfer factor, a component of blood that stimulates the immune system, has been effective in a small group of patients.[36] Cytotoxic drugs, particularly chlorambucil, are reserved for patients with severe iritis and central nervous system dysfunction.[37] Other experimental treatments used in uncontrolled trials that have produced some benefit have included administration of levamisole, thalidomide, and cyclosporine.[38–40] A number of medications are being studied for a variety of manifestations of Behçet's disease.[41] The eye disease in Behçet's syndrome is responsive to azathioprine at a dose of 2.5 mg/kg/day.[42] Cyclosporin A acts more rapidly than azathioprine in the treatment of eye disease. However, the toxicity of cyclosporin limits its utility for long-term use.[43] Colchicine is effective only in reducing the development of arthralgias.[41]

PROGNOSIS

Behçet's syndrome is characterized by frequent attacks early in the course of the illness. After 3 to 7 years, the frequency of attacks decreases. The disease is rarely disabling when the illness is limited to ulcerations, skin disease, and arthritis. Blindness is a major disability in patients with iritis. Severe ocular disease is more characteristic of Japanese patients with Behçet's syndrome than it is of patients from other geographic areas.[33] Central nervous system disease is associated with increased mortality. Death may be secondary to cranial nerve involvement, paraplegia, or encephalitis. Vascular disease is a late complication of Behçet's syndrome and is associated with severe disease.

Patients with arterial disease are at risk for the development of aneurysms and rupture, leading to death.[44]

References

BEHÇET'S SYNDROME

1. Behçet H: Über rezidivierende, aphthöse durch ein Virus verursachte Geschwüre am Mund, am Auge und an den Genitalien. Dermat Wchnschr 105:1152, 1937.
2. Robinson HM Jr, McCrumb FR Jr: Comparative analysis of the mucocutaneous-ocular syndromes: report of eleven cases and review of the literature. Arch Derm Syph 61:539, 1950.
3. Chajek T, Fainam M: Behçet's syndrome: report of 41 cases and a review of the literature. Medicine 54:179, 1975.
4. Oshima Y, Shimizu T, Yokakari R, et al.: Clinical studies on Behçet's syndrome. Ann Rheum Dis 22:36, 1963.
5. O'Duffy JD, Lehner T, Barnes CG: Summary of the Third International Conference on Behçet's disease, Tokyo, Japan, October 23–24, 1981. J Rheumatol 10:154, 1983.
6. O'Duffy JD: Behçet's disease. In Kelley WN, Harris ED Jr, Ruddy S, Sledge CB (eds): Textbook of Rheumatology, 2nd ed. Philadelphia: W B Saunders Co, 1985, pp 1174–1178.
7. O'Duffy JD, Carney JA, Deadhar S: Behçet's syndrome: report of 10 cases, 3 with new manifestations. Ann Intern Med 75:561, 1971.
8. Marquardt JL, Snyderman R, Oppenheim JJ: Depression of lymphocyte transformation and exacerbation of Behçet's syndrome by ingestion of English walnuts. Cell Immunol 9:263, 1973.
9. Lehner T: Behçet's syndrome and autoimmunity. Br Med J 1:465, 1967.
10. Lehner T, Lavery E, Smith R, et al.: Association between the 65-kilodalton heat shock protein, Streptococcus sanguis, and the corresponding antibodies in Behçet's syndrome. Infect Immun 59:1434, 1991.
11. Ohno S, Nakarayama E, Sugiura S, et al.: Specific histocompatibility antigens associated with Behçet's syndrome. Am J Ophthalmol 80:636, 1975.
12. Chajek-Shaul T, Pisanty S, Knobler H, et al.: HLA-B51 may serve as an immunogenetic marker for a subgroup of patients with Behçet's syndrome. Am J Med 83:666, 1987.
13. Arber N, Klein T, Meiner Z, et al.: Close association of HLA-B51 and B52 in Israeli patients with Behçet's syndrome. Ann Rheum Dis 50:351, 1991.
14. Chamberlain MA: Behçet's disease. Ann Rheum Dis 34(Suppl):53, 1975.
15. Lehner T, Batchelor JR, Challacombe SJ, Kennedy L: An immunogenetic basis for the tissue involvement in Behçet's syndrome. Immunology 37:895, 1979.
16. Colvard DM, Robertson DM, O'Duffy JD: The ocular manifestations of Behçet's disease. Arch Ophthalmol 95:1813, 1977.
17. Chamberlain MA: Behçet's syndrome in 32 patients in Yorkshire. Ann Rheum Dis 36:491, 1977.
18. Pallis CA, Fudge BJ: The neurological complications of Behçet's syndrome. Arch Neurol Psychiat 75:1, 1956.
19. Wolff SM, Schotland DL, Phillips LL: Involvement of nervous system in Behçet's syndrome. Arch Neurol 12:315, 1965.

20. Wright VA, Chamberlain MA, O'Duffy JD: Behçet's syndrome. Bull Rheum Dis 29:972, 1978–79.
21. Mason RM, Barnes CG: Behçet's syndrome with arthritis. Ann Rheum Dis 28:95, 1969.
22. Zizic TM, Stevens MB: The arthropathy of Behçet's disease. Johns Hopkins Med J 136:243, 1975.
23. Arbesfeld SJ, Kurban AK: Behçet's disease: new perspectives on an enigmatic syndrome. J Am Acad Dermatol 19:767, 1988.
24. Strachen RW, Wigzell FW: Polyarthritis in Behçet's multiple symptom complex. Ann Rheum Dis 22:26, 1963.
25. Perkins ES: Behçet's disease. Ophthalmological aspects. Proc R Soc Med 54:106, 1961.
26. Cooper DA, Penny R: Behçet's syndrome: clinical immunological and therapeutic evaluation of 17 patients. Aust NZ J Med 4:585, 1974.
27. Dilsen AN: Sacroiliitis and ankylosing spondylitis in Behçet's disease. (Abstract.) Scand J Rheum (Suppl)8:20, 1975.
28. Vernon-Roberts B, Barnes CG, Revell PA: Synovial pathology in Behçet's syndrome. Ann Rheum Dis 37:139, 1978.
29. Resnick D: Periodic, relapsing and recurrent disorders. In Resnick D, Niwayama G (eds): Diagnosis of Bone and Joint Disorders, 2nd ed. Philadelphia: WB Saunders, 1988, pp 1252–1264.
30. Empey DW, Hale JE: Rectal and colonic ulceration in Behçet's syndrome. Proc R Soc Med 65:163, 1972.
31. Chamberlain MA, Robertson RJ: A controlled study of sacroiliitis in Behçet's disease. Br J Rheumatol 32:693, 1993.
32. Olivieri I, Gemignani G, Camerini E, et al.: Computed tomography of the sacroiliac joints in four patients with Behçet's syndrome: confirmation of sacroiliitis. Br J Rheumatol 29:264, 1990.
33. Shimizu R, Ehrlich GE, Inaba G, Hayashi K: Behçet disease (Behçet syndrome). Semin Arthritis Rheum 8:223, 1979.
34. The International Study Group for Behçet's Disease. Evaluation of diagnostic (classification) criteria in Behçet's disease—towards internationally agreed criteria. Br J Rheumatol 31:299, 1992.
35. International Study Group for Behçet's Disease: Criteria for diagnosis of Behçet's disease. Lancet 335:1078, 1990.
36. Wolf RE, Fudenberg HH, Welch TM, et al.: Treatment of Behçet's syndrome with transfer factor. JAMA 238:869, 1977.
37. James DG: Behçet's syndrome. (Editorial.) N Engl J Med 301:431, 1979.
38. DeMerieux P, Spitler LE, Paulus HE: Treatment of Behçet's syndrome with levamisole. Arthritis Rheum 24:64, 1981.
39. Jenkins JS, Allen BR, Maurice PDL, et al.: Thalidomide in severe orogenital ulceration. Lancet 2:1424, 1984.
40. Nussenblatt RB, Palestine AG, Chan C, et al.: Effectiveness of cyclosporin therapy for Behçet's disease. Arthritis Rheum 28:671, 1985.
41. Yazici H, Barnes CG: Practical treatment recommendations for pharmacotherapy of Behçet's syndrome. Drugs 42:796, 1991.
42. Yazici H, Pazarli H, Barnes CG, et al.: A controlled trial of azathioprine in Behçet's syndrome. N Engl J Med 322:281, 1990.
43. Masuda K, Urayama A, Kogune M: Double-masked trial of cyclosporin versus colchicine and long-term open study of cyclosporin in Behçet's syndrome. Lancet I:1093, 1989.
44. Enoch BA, Castillo-Olivares JL, Khoo TCL, et al.: Major vascular complications in Behçet's syndrome. Postgrad Med J 44:453, 1968.

WHIPPLE'S DISEASE

Capsule Summary

Frequency of back pain—rare
Location of back pain—sacroiliac joint and lumbar spine
Quality of back pain—ache
Symptoms and signs—weight loss, diarrhea, arthralgias, lymphadenopathy, hypotension
Laboratory and x-ray tests—anemia, abnormal intestinal absorption tests; sacroiliitis on plain roentgenogram
Treatment—procaine penicillin G, streptomycin, trimethoprim-sulfamethoxazole

PREVALENCE AND PATHOGENESIS

Whipple's disease, or intestinal lipodystrophy, was first described by G. H. Whipple in 1907 and characterized by multiorgan system dysfunction.[1] Abnormalities of the musculoskeletal, gastrointestinal, cardiovascular, pulmonary, and nervous systems characterize the illness.

Whipple's disease is a rare illness, with approximately 741 cases reported in the world literature as of 1988.[2] The disease occurs most commonly in Caucasian men between the ages of 40 and 60. The male to female ratio is 10:1. Familial clustering of the disease has been reported.[3]

Whipple's disease has an infectious etiology. The organism that causes the disease has been identified by the use of molecular genetic techniques.[4] The organism is a gram-positive actinomycete, *Tropheryma whippelii*. The inflammation caused by these bacteria is granulomatous, manifested by macrophages filled with PAS-positive organisms in biopsy specimens. No information is currently available to identify this organism as a rare member of the normal human microbial flora or a rare organism in the environment.[5]

CLINICAL HISTORY

Musculoskeletal symptoms, arthralgias, joint pain without inflammation, or arthritis occur as the earliest manifestations of disease in a majority of patients.[6] Arthritis may antedate other manifestations of disease by as long as 20 to 35 years.[7] Peripheral joint involvement is marked by a migratory, oligoarticular or polyarticular arthritis affecting the knees, ankles, elbows, or fingers.[8] The joint disease is episodic and recurrent and rarely causes damage to articular structures, although cases of joint destruction have been reported.[9] Back pain and axial skeletal involvement, spondylitis or sacroiliitis, may occur in up to 19% of patients.[10] Many patients with axial skeletal arthritis have concomitant peripheral joint disease. Axial joint involvement may occur in the setting of a prolonged period of appendicular joint disease.[11]

The classic triad of malabsorption, diarrhea, and weight loss occurs at unspecified intervals after the onset of joint symptoms. In some patients, arthritic complaints remit after the onset of intestinal symptoms.[12] Some of the other protean manifestations of this illness include hypotension, lymphadenopathy, hyperpigmentation, fever, peripheral edema, and central nervous system dysfunction including headache, diplopia, depression, confusion, and personality change.[6, 13] Myopathy associated with periodic acid Schiff (PAS)-positive material infiltration, which responds to antibiotic therapy, also has been reported.[14]

PHYSICAL EXAMINATION

Patients may be febrile with hyperpigmented skin and lymphadenopathy. The abdominal examination may be normal. Patients with axial skeletal disease have tenderness over the spine with limitation in all planes of motion. Peripheral joints may be normal.

LABORATORY DATA

The hematologic findings are nonspecific, with 90% of patients developing anemia. Intestinal absorption studies of serum carotene, 5-hour D-xylose absorption, and 72-hour fecal fat demonstrate values consistent with malabsorption. Synovial fluid analysis shows an inflammatory exudate with a white blood cell count up to 36,000. The synovial tissue from biopsy specimens is hyperplastic, with PAS-positive bodies in synoviocytes.[15] Rheumatoid factor and antinuclear antibody are absent. The frequency of HLA-B27 in Whipple's disease patients has varied from 28% to 8% depending on the study population.[16, 17]

RADIOGRAPHIC EXAMINATION

Radiographic findings are infrequent in patients with peripheral joint disease. Rare instances of joint destruction and ankylosis have been reported.[9] Patients with spondylitis have changes in the sacroiliac joints and lumbar spine similar to those of AS.[18, 19]

DIFFERENTIAL DIAGNOSIS

The diagnosis of Whipple's disease is made by biopsy of the mucosa of the jejunum of the small intestine. The biopsy is accomplished by an oral route. The histologic material is stained with PAS to demonstrate the bacteria-like structures in granulomas. In the future, the identification of *T. whippelii* may be enhanced by the availability of polymerase chain reaction primers and oligonucleotide probes that will identify the organism without the need for culture of body tissues.[4] The differential diagnosis includes the other spondyloarthropathies, particularly Reiter's syndrome and enteropathic arthritis, Addison's disease, and lymphoma.

The presence of urethritis and/or conjunctivitis occurs in a large proportion of Reiter's disease patients. Biopsy of the small or large bowel in patients with inflammatory bowel disease will be positive for crypt abscesses in ulcerative colitis or for transmural inflammation in Crohn's disease. Addison's disease is associated with hyperpigmentation. Decreased response to ACTH will help identify those patients with Addison's disease. Lymphoma is diagnosed by lymph node biopsy.

TREATMENT

Prolonged antibiotic therapy with tetracycline has a favorable effect on the disease process.[20] Joint pain, diarrhea, and lymphadenopathy resolve within a few months. Relapses have occurred in the CNS approximately 2 years after the cessation of tetracycline therapy. These relapses probably occurred because of the persistence of organisms in the CNS, and the tetracycline did not penetrate adequately into the CNS to eradicate the organisms. An antibiotic regimen that will cross the blood-brain barrier includes parenterally administered procaine penicillin G, 1.2 million units/day and streptomycin, 1 gm/day, followed by a 1 year regimen of orally administered trimethoprim-sulfamethoxazole. Antibiotic therapy does have a beneficial effect on the gastric mucosa that has been documented by endoscopic observation.[21] The effect of antibiotic therapy on the progression of spondylitis is unknown.

PROGNOSIS

Early diagnosis is essential to the favorable outcome of this treatable illness. Patients may be ill for a number of years before it is correctly diagnosed. Antibiotic therapy has a beneficial effect on the manifestations of this illness. The joint disease is nondeforming and does not cause disability, but axial skeletal involvement is associated with some limitation of motion. Occasionally, severe manifestations, such as CNS disease, do occur in patients who are on continuous antibiotic therapy.[22]

References

WHIPPLE'S DISEASE

1. Whipple GH: A hitherto undescribed disease characterized anatomically by deposits of fat and fatty acids in the intestinal and mesenteric lymphatic tissues. Bull Johns Hopkins Hosp 18:382, 1907.
2. Dobbins WO: Whipple's disease. Mayo Clin Proc 63:623, 1988.
3. Puite RH, Tesluk H: Whipple's disease. Am J Med 19:383, 1955.
4. Relman DA, Schmidt TM, MacDermott RP, Falkow S: Identification of the uncultured bacillus of Whipple's disease. N Engl J Med 327:293, 1992.
5. Donaldson RM Jr: Whipple's disease: rare malady with uncommon potential. N Engl J Med 327:346, 1992.
6. LeVine ME, Dobbins WO: Joint changes in Whipple's disease. Semin Arthritis Rheum 3:79, 1973.
7. DeLuca RF, Silver TS, Rogers AI: Whipple disease: occurrence in a 76-year-old man with a 20-year prodrome of arthritis. JAMA 233:59, 1975.
8. Caughey DE, Bywaters EGL: The arthritis of Whipple's syndrome. Ann Rheum Dis 22:327, 1963.
9. Ayoub WT, Davis DE, Toreetti D, Viozzi FJ: Bone destruction and ankylosis in Whipple's disease. J Rheumatol, 9:930, 1982.
10. Kelley JJ, Weisiger BB: The arthritis of Whipple's disease. Arthritis Rheum 6:615, 1963.
11. Scheib JS, Quinet RJ: Whipple's disease with axial and peripheral joint destruction. South Med J 83, 684, 1990.
12. Hargrove MD Jr, Verner JV, Smith AG, et al.: Whipple's disease: report of two cases with intestinal biopsy before and after treatment. Gastroenterology 39:619, 1960.
13. Fleming JL, Wiesner RH, Shorter RG: Whipple's disease: clinical, biochemical, and histopathologic features and assessment of treatment in 29 patients. Mayo Clin Proc 63:539, 1988.
14. Swash M, Schwartz MS, Vandenburg MJ, Pollock DJ: Myopathy in Whipple's disease. Gut 18:800, 1977.
15. Hawkins CF, Farr M, Morris CJ, et al.: Detection by electron microscope of rod-shaped organisms in synovial membrane from a patient with the arthritis of Whipple's disease. Ann Rheum Dis 35:502, 1976.
16. Dobbins WO III: HLA antigens in Whipple's disease. Arthritis Rheum 30:102, 1987.
17. Bai JC, Mota AH, Maurino E, et al.: Class I and class II HLA antigens in a homogeneous Argentinian population with Whipple's disease: lack of association with HLA-B27. Am J Gastroenterol 86:992, 1991.
18. Canoso JJ, Saini M, Hermos JA: Whipple's disease and ankylosing spondylitis simultaneous occurrence in HLA-B27 positive male. J Rheumatol 5:79, 1978.
19. Khan MA: Axial arthropathy in Whipple's disease. J Rheumatol 9:928, 1982.
20. England MT, French JM, Brawson AB: Antibiotic control of diarrhea in Whipple's disease. A six year follow-up of a patient diagnosed by jejunal biopsy. Gastroenterology 39:219, 1960.
21. Geboes K, Ectors N, Heidbuchel H, et al.: Whipple's disease: endoscopic aspects before and after therapy. Gastroenterol Endo 36:247, 1990.
22. Knox DL, Bayless TM, Pittman FE: Neurological disease in patients with treated Whipple's disease. Medicine 55:467, 1976.

FAMILIAL MEDITERRANEAN FEVER

Capsule Summary

Frequency of back pain—rare
Location of back pain—sacroiliac joints
Quality of back pain—ache
Symptoms and signs—episodic abdominal pain
Laboratory and x-ray tests—leukocytosis, increased sedimentation rate with attacks; sacroiliitis on plain roentgenograms
Treatment—colchicine

PREVALENCE AND PATHOGENESIS

Familial Mediterranean fever (FMF) is a hereditary disorder characterized by recurrent, brief episodes of fever, serosal inflammation (peritonitis or pleuritis), and arthritis. Back symptoms and sacroiliitis have been described in a minority of patients with this disorder. Major disability occurs in the patient with FMF who develops persistent, destructive hip disease, and the disease can be fatal for those who develop amyloidosis and associated renal failure. FMF was first described in 1945 by Siegal,[1] and the name of FMF was associated with the illness in the 1950s.[2] The disease has also been called benign paroxysmal peritonitis and recurrent polyserositis.

The people most commonly affected are from eastern Mediterranean countries, including Sephardic Jews, Armenians, Turks, and some Arabs, but the disease may occur sporadically in other nationalities. A review stated that 1327 patients with FMF had been reported in the literature.[3] Large family studies suggest that the disease is transmitted by a single recessive gene, but no specific HLA antigen has been associated with the illness.[4] Investigation of both Armenians and non-Ashkenzi Jews have linked the gene for FMF to the alpha-globin complex on the short arm of the 16th human chromosome.[5, 6] Men are more frequently affected than women by a ratio of 3:2. The cause of the illness is unknown. A number of plasma components are increased during different phases of the disease, but no correlation with the pathogenesis of FMF has been made.[7, 8] Some of the factors that have been investigated include abnormalities of complement components, hydroxy-fatty acid metabolites, tumor necrosis factor, and lipocortin deficiency.[9, 10] Lipocortins inhibit phospholipase A2, the enzyme that releases arachidonic acid from phospholipids. Phospholipase A2 can activate cyclic adenosine monophosphate. The activation of adenyl cyclase in the absence of the inhibitory mechanisms of lipocortins can produce an attack of fever, pain, and inflammation. This phenomenon is in concert with the absence of response of FMF patients to corticosteroids.[10]

CLINICAL HISTORY

The disease is characterized by acute attacks of fever associated with peritonitis, pleuritis, or arthritis. The episodes of abdominal or chest pain are limited to a period of hours to days, while arthritis may persist much longer. Areas of painful erythema may also occur on the lower extremities below the knee. The onset of this illness is usually during childhood or adolescence.

The most frequent manifestation of FMF, occurring in 95% of patients, is peritonitis. Patients develop severe abdominal pain with absent bowel sounds suggestive of an acute abdominal crisis. Not uncommonly, they undergo a laparotomy that reveals no specific pathology. Within 24 to 48 hours, symptoms abate, leaving the patient in his usual state of health. Pleural pain, with difficulty in breathing and a minor effusion, occurs in 40% of FMF patients. Recurrences of abdominal or pleural pain occur irregularly, with remissions lasting months to years. Factors that have been suggested as possible initiators of attacks include menstruation, stress, heavy activity, and exposure to cold.[11]

Sacroiliitis, frequently asymptomatic, is another manifestation of FMF, with 10% to 17% of patients having either unilateral or bilateral disease.[12, 13] Sacroiliitis also has been described in children, in whom clinical symptoms of back pain are significant.[14] Lumbar spine changes consistent with spondylitis occur less commonly.

Articular manifestations of FMF occur in 75% of patients and are a presenting feature in 33%.[13] The joints most commonly affected are the knee, ankle, hip, shoulder, and, rarely, the sacroiliac. The usual joint attack has an abrupt onset, with rapidly intensifying pain affecting a single joint. An effusion may accompany the development of joint pain, and the attacks may last from a few days to a month. Most episodes of joint pain and swelling are not associated with residual joint damage. Occasionally, a patient with FMF may develop a protracted episode of arthritis affecting a single joint, such as a knee or hip, and this may last for a year or more.[13] These joints develop marked swelling and surrounding muscle atrophy. The sacroiliac joint is mostly affected when the arthritis becomes longstanding. Complete recovery of function may be expected in the patient with resolution of a protracted attack of arthritis in a knee. The outcome of hip arthritis, however, is more ominous, with residual limitation of motion and pain being the issue. Hip joint destruction also may occur.

Amyloidosis is the fatal complication of FMF because these patients have a deposition of amyloid in the kidneys. Nephrotic syndrome, characterized by proteinuria and peripheral edema, ensues, resulting in renal failure.[15] Most patients who develop amyloidosis die before they reach 40 years of age.[16]

PHYSICAL FINDINGS

Patients with FMF may have an entirely normal examination between attacks.[17] During attacks, examination of the abdomen, chest, skin and joints, including the back, is essential. Examination of the lower extremities for peripheral edema is helpful in detecting the presence of a nephrotic syndrome or the erysipelas-like erythema associated with acute attacks.

Patients with sacroiliitis on radiographs may have a normal lumbosacral spine examination. Others may have percussion tenderness over the involved joints.

LABORATORY DATA

Laboratory findings are nonspecific in FMF.[14] During attacks, WBC may be markedly elevated along with increases in ESR. Abnormal values quickly return to normal with resolution of the attack. Urinalysis may demonstrate protein and RBC indicative of renal amyloidosis. Rheumatoid factor and antinuclear antibody are absent. A number of studies have investigated the presence of autoantibodies in FMF patients compared with controls.[18, 19] The antibodies, including RNP, SSA/SSB, anti-DNA, and anticardiolipin, are not present in FMF patients. Synovial fluid may include increased WBC to one million, good mucin clot, increased proteins, and normal or low glucose.[16] HLA testing demonstrates no increased frequency of any specific antigen.

RADIOGRAPHIC EVALUATION

Sacroiliac joint changes include loss of cortical definition and sclerosis on both sides of the joint with or without erosions and fusions.[12] The involvement of the sacroiliac joints may be unilateral, or bilateral with asymmetric severity of involvement (Fig. 11–20). The changes in the lumbar spine include bony bridging between lumbar vertebrae.[13]

Soft tissue swelling and osteoporosis are seen in patients during brief attacks, but these changes are rapidly reversible with remission. Radiographic changes are more severe in patients with protracted attacks. When the knee is affected, osteoporosis may be widespread throughout the limb. On at least two occasions, resumption of weight-bearing has resulted in fractures of the tibia or femur secondary to the osteoporosis.[16] Other findings include sclerosis, joint space narrowing, and erosions. Marked joint space narrowing is a common finding after protracted attacks in a hip.

DIFFERENTIAL DIAGNOSIS

The diagnostic criteria for FMF include recurrent short attacks of fever with peritonitis, pleuritis, arthritis, erythema, and absence of data suggesting an alternative diagnosis. A Mediterranean ancestry is a helpful piece of data when a patient has his initial attack. A recent report has suggested that FMF attacks can be provoked in patients by metaraminol infusion. Noradrenaline has been associated with the precipitation of attacks of FMF. Metaraminol acts competitively to displace noradrenaline. Twenty-one patients developed attacks after receiving infusions. An equal number of controls did not have attacks. If confirmed, metaraminol infusion would become a useful diagnostic test.[20] This also suggests that FMF may be the result of an inborn error of catecholamine metabolism. Dopamine beta-hydroxylase is the enzyme responsible for the conversion of dopamine to noradrenaline. This enzyme has been found to be elevated in patients with FMF without treatment with colchicine.[21] Attempts at reproducing these findings in other populations of patients with FMF have not produced the same results.[22] Measurement of this enzyme cannot be recommended as a diagnostic test for FMF.

Sacroiliac joint involvement is similar to that associated with the seronegative spondyloarthropathies. Abdominal symptoms differentiate FMF from AS, Reiter's syndrome, and psoriatic arthritis. Patients with inflammatory bowel disease develop diarrhea, while FMF patients have normal bowel habits even during attacks. The absence of HLA-B27 antigen in FMF patients suggests that the pathogenesis of lumbosacral spine changes is different from those of the HLA-B27 positive spondyloarthropathies. The sacroiliitis of FMF patients is not related to a second disease, AS, but rather to some unspecified mechanism associated with FMF.

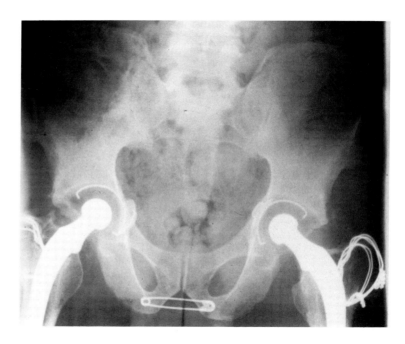

Figure 11–20. Familial Mediterranean fever. A 40-year-old man had active FMF since the age of 18. Bilateral hip arthritis required hip replacements at age 32. AP view of pelvis reveals bilateral sacroiliitis with asymmetric involvement, right greater than left. (Courtesy of Jacob Bar-Ziv, M.D., and Theodor Schifter, M.D.)

TREATMENT

An effective treatment for FMF is colchicine. A regimen of colchicine (0.6 mg orally twice a day) helps both in ameliorating the attacks and in reducing their frequency.[23] Colchicine also was shown to be beneficial in preventing amyloidosis in patients with FMF.[24] Articular involvement is less responsive to colchicine than the acute attacks of polyserositis. Colchicine has been utilized for extended periods of time to prevent attacks without significant toxicity.[25] Non-narcotic analgesics are useful in controlling pain. Bed rest, anti-inflammatory drugs, and corticosteroids may have no benefit for joint disease in FMF.[16] Prolonged immobilization may aggravate the osteoporosis and muscle atrophy. Joint replacement may be necessary for advanced disease of the hip. Therapy for renal failure is necessary for the patient who develops renal amyloidosis.

PROGNOSIS

The major morbidity from FMF, other than the frequency of acute attacks, is protracted disease of the hip. In one study, in 16 of 18 affected hips severe limitation of motion and pain developed.[16] Eight of these patients required joint arthroplasty and had a good outcome.

The major cause of mortality from FMF is amyloidosis and renal failure. This complication may be more common in patients in Israel than in the United States. Studies suggest that daily colchicine therapy may prevent the development or progression of amyloidosis in these patients, although not all patients, particularly those of European ethnicity, respond to colchicine therapy.[24, 26]

References

FAMILIAL MEDITERRANEAN FEVER

1. Siegal S: Benign paroxysmal peritonitis. Ann Intern Med 23:1, 1945.
2. Heller H, Sohar E, Kariv I, Sherf L: Familial Mediterranean fever. Harefuah 48:91, 1955.
3. Meyerhoff J: Familial Mediterranean fever: report of a large family, review of the literature and discussion of the frequency of amyloidosis. Medicine 59:66, 1980.
4. Sohar E, Pras M, Heller J, Heller H: Genetics of familial Mediterranean fever. A disorder with recessive inheritance in non-Ashkenazi Jews and Armenians. Arch Intern Med 107:529, 1961.
5. Shohat M, Bu X, Sholat T, et al.: The gene for familial Mediterranean fever in both Armenians and non-Ashkenazi Jews is linked to the alpha-globin complex on 16p: evidence for locus homogeneity. Am J Hum Genet 51:1349, 1992.
6. Pras E, Aksentijevich I, Gruberg L, et al.: Mapping of a gene causing familial Mediterranean fever to the short arm of chromosome 16. N Engl J Med 326:1508, 1992.
7. Shamir H, Pras M, Sohar E, Gafni J: Cryofibrinogen in familial Mediterranean fever. Arch Intern Med 134:125, 1974.
8. LeRoy EC, Sjoerdsma A: Clinical significance of hydroxyproline containing protein in human plasma. J Clin Invest 44:914, 1965.
9. Schattner A, Lachmi M, Livneh A, et al.: Tumor necrosis in familial Mediterranean fever. Am J Med 90:434, 1991.
10. Garcia-Gonzalez A, Weisman MH: The arthritis of familial Mediterranean fever. Semin Arthritis Rheum 22:139, 1992.
11. Schwartz J: Periodic peritonitis, onset simultaneously with menstruation. Ann Intern Med 53:407, 1960.
12. Brodey PA, Wolff SM: Radiographic changes in the sacroiliac joints in familial Mediterranean fever. Radiology 114:331, 1975.
13. Heller H, Gafni J, Michaeli D, et al.: The arthritis of familial Mediterranean fever. Arthritis Rheum 9:1, 1966.
14. Lehman TJA, Hanson V, Kornreich H, et al.: HLA-B27-negative sacroiliitis: a manifestation of familial Mediterranean fever in childhood. Pediatrics 61:423, 1978.
15. Sohar E, Gafni J, Pras M, Heller H: Familial Mediterranean fever: a survey of 470 cases and review of the literature. Am J Med 43:227, 1967.
16. Sohar E, Pras M, Gafni J: Familial Mediterranean fever and its articular manifestations. Clin Rheum Dis 1:195, 1975.
17. Siegal S: Familial paroxysmal peritonitis: analysis of fifty cases. Am J Med 36:893, 1964.
18. Ben-Chetrit E, Levy M: Autoantibodies in familial Mediterranean fever (recurrent polyserositis). Br J Rheumatol. 29:459, 1990.
19. Swissa M, Schul V, Korish S, et al.: Determination of autoantibodies in patients with familial Mediterranean fever and their degree relatives. J Rheumatol 18:606, 1991.
20. Barakat MH, El-Khawad AO, Gumaa KA, et al.: Metaraminol provocative test: a specific diagnostic test for familial Mediterranean fever. Lancet 1:656, 1984.
21. Barakat MH, Gumaa KA, Malhas LN, et al.: Plasma dopamine beta-hydroxylase: rapid diagnostic test for recurrent hereditary polyserositis. Lancet II:1280, 1988.
22. Courillon-Mallet A, Cauet N, Dervichian M, et al.: Plasma dopamine beta-hydroxylase activity in familial Mediterranean fever. Isr J Med Sci 28:427, 1992.
23. Dinarello CA, Wolff SM, Goldfinger SE, et al.: Colchicine therapy for familial Mediterranean fever: a double-blind trial. N Engl J Med 291:934, 1974.
24. Zemer D, Pras M, Sohar E, et al.: Colchicine in the prevention and treatment of the amyloidosis of familial Mediterranean fever. N Engl J Med 314:1001, 1986.
25. Ben-Chetrit E, Levy M: Colchicine prophylaxis in familial Mediterranean fever: reappraisal after 15 years. Semin Arthritis Rheum 20:241, 1991.
26. Gertz MA, Petitt RM, Perrault J, Kyle RA: Autosomal dominant familial Mediterranean fever-like syndrome with amyloidosis. Mayo Clin Proc 62:1095, 1987.

HIDRADENITIS SUPPURATIVA

Capsule Summary

Frequency of back pain—rare

Location of back pain—sacroiliac joints, lumbar spine

Quality of back pain—ache

Symptoms and signs—skin disease, lymphadenopathy, acne conglobata

Laboratory and x-ray tests—anemia, increased sedimentation rate; unilateral or bilateral sacroiliitis on plain roentgenograms

Treatment—antibiotics, incision and drainage

PREVALENCE AND PATHOGENESIS

Hidradenitis suppurativa and acne conglobata are chronic suppurative disorders of the skin. A recent report has described a group of patients with these skin diseases who have developed peripheral and axial skeletal arthritis similar to that of the seronegative spondyloarthropathies.[1]

These skin diseases are relatively uncommon conditions and their exact prevalence is unknown. Hidradenitis suppurativa is an infection of the apocrine sweat glands located in the axillae and inguinal regions. The disease is characterized by the development of recurrent inflammatory, suppurative nodules and sinus tracts. Acne conglobata is a form of acne characterized by the development of large abscesses and interconnecting sinuses in the skin; they form cysts that are similar to those of hidradenitis suppurativa. Acne conglobata is unassociated with signs of an acute illness and ulcerating lesions. The third component of the follicular occlusion triad is dissecting cellulitis of the scalp. The musculoskeletal abnormalities associated with the follicular occlusion triad are differentiable from those associated with acne fulminans, another severe form of acne. Acne fulminans is manifested by ulcerative, crusting lesions causing deep dermal involvement in the setting of an acute severe illness and usually associated with arthritis above the lumbosacral spine.[2]

The etiology of the arthritis associated with these skin conditions is unknown. Chronic cutaneous infections are components of the inflammatory process in hidradenitis suppurativa and acne conglobata. The joint disease that develops in these patients may be a reactive arthritis secondary to chronic infection, similar to the arthritis that develops in patients after a genitourinary or enteric infection; however, as opposed to other patients with reactive arthritis, patients with hidradenitis suppurativa or acne conglobata with arthritis do not have an increased frequency of HLA-B27 positivity.[2]

A number of factors suggest that this arthritis is a manifestation of chronic infection of the skin. The infections produce large quantities of bacterial products that are antigenic. These bacterial cellular fragments may cross-react with joint tissues, may be transported to joints where they lodge in synovial structures eliciting an inflammatory response, or a combination of both. The initiating factor may be the molecular mimicry of bacterial products, while the phlogistic characteristics of these products sustain the inflammation in the joint. The partial response of arthritic patients with this condition to antibiotics suggests that bacterial infection plays a significant role in the pathogenesis of this process.[3]

CLINICAL HISTORY

The typical patient is 32 years of age and black.[1, 2] Most have both hidradenitis suppurativa and acne conglobata. In the majority of patients, the skin disease precedes the onset of arthritis by 1 to 20 years. Peripheral arthritis affects the knees, elbows, wrists, and ankles most commonly, but small joints of the hands and feet may also be involved.[4] Attacks of arthritis last from weeks to months. Axial skeletal disease of the cervical and thoracic spine occurs less often. Joint symptoms frequently mirror the activity of skin disease.[5, 6]

PHYSICAL EXAMINATION

Skin examination is essential to document the extent and activity of the cutaneous disease. Musculoskeletal examination may show swelling, effusion, and warmth in peripheral joints, along with limitation of spinal movement and tenderness to percussion over the sacroiliac joints. The ankles and joints of the feet are most frequently affected. Peripheral joint involvement is symmetrical in 60% of the patients.[2]

LABORATORY DATA

A mild anemia occurs in a majority of patients along with occasional leukocytosis. The

ESR is usually elevated. Rheumatoid factor and antinuclear antibody are not present. Cultures of skin lesions are frequently sterile. There is no increased frequency of HLA-B27 or its cross-reactive antigens.

RADIOGRAPHIC EVALUATION

Radiographic findings in patients with peripheral arthritis include swelling, periarticular osteoporosis, periosteal new bone formation, and joint space erosions of finger joints. Axial skeletal abnormalities include sacroiliitis with narrowing, sclerosis, erosion, and fusion; the abnormalities are unilateral in most circumstances. Axial skeletal disease is associated with squaring of vertebral bodies, ligamentous calcification, and asymmetric syndesmophytes (Fig. 11–21). Sacroiliitis occurs in up to 80% of patients with the follicular occlusion triad.[2] The asymmetric syndesmophytes occur in any portion of the axial skeleton and have similar characteristics of those associated with Reiter's syndrome and psoriatic spondyloarthropathy.[7] Asymmetric sacroiliitis also has been described in a Caucasian patient with acne fulminans.[8]

DIFFERENTIAL DIAGNOSIS

The diagnosis of hidradenitis suppurativa or acne conglobata is based on the appearance and distribution of the skin lesions. These lesions must be differentiated from other suppurative infections of the skin, including Bartholin abscesses and actinomycosis. The associated arthritis must be differentiated from the other seronegative spondyloarthropathies (see the section on Reiter's syndrome earlier in this chapter).

The treatment of severe acne includes the use of synthetic vitamin A derivatives, including isotretinoin. Isotretinoin causes a number of side effects including skeletal hyperostosis.[9, 10] The location of the hyperostosis includes the axial skeleton. However, these skeletal changes are more frequently located in the cervical and thoracic spine. The patients develop small horizontal spurs extending from the anterior margin of the vertebral body. The sacroiliac joints are not affected.[9] The presence of these radiographic changes are not correlated with patient musculoskeletal signs or symptoms.[2] No consistent correlation has been made between the cessation of therapy and resolution of the hyperostoses, although

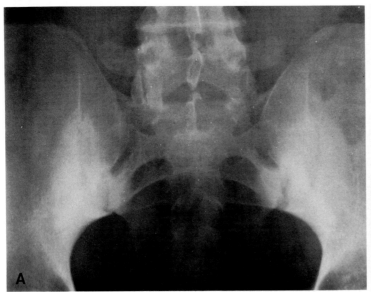
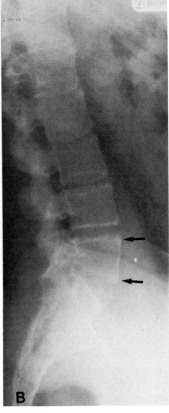

Figure 11–21. Hidradenitis suppurativa. A 24-year-old man had an 8-year history of hidradenitis suppurativa, acne conglobata, and dissecting cellulitis of the scalp, which responded to intermittent courses of antibiotics. The patient complained of bilateral back pain localized over the sacroiliac joints. *A,* Spot view of pelvis reveals bilateral sacroiliac joint involvement manifested by joint narrowing on the right and widening on the left along with extensive periarticular sclerosis. *B,* Lateral view of lumbar spine demonstrates early changes of spondylitis manifested by osseous erosion and sclerosis of the vertebral body, producing whitening of the corners of the L5 vertebra (*arrows*) along with early straightening of the anterior border.

improvement has been reported in some patients.[11]

TREATMENT

The therapy for hidradenitis suppurativa includes antibiotics and incision and drainage of skin tracts. Occasionally, corticosteroids or low-dose x-ray therapy is given to patients with persistent skin disease. Acne conglobata is effectively treated with corticosteroids but the drug is limited in utility because of side effects. Antibiotic therapy, tetracycline, is worthwhile on a long-term basis. Severe disease often requires the addition of retinoids including isotretinoin. Joint disease is responsive to nonsteroidal anti-inflammatory drugs. Rarely are corticosteroids needed for control of joint symptoms. Surgery for control of active skin disease may improve joint disease.

PROGNOSIS

Both skin diseases tend to be chronic and recurrent. They cause disfigurement in their severe forms but not physical disability. The joint disease associated with hidradenitis suppurativa and acne conglobata is associated with loss of range of motion in affected joints.[12] No significant disability has been reported; however, patients with severe axial skeletal and hip disease may be at the same risk for disability as reported in patients with other spondyloarthropathies.

References

HIDRADENITIS SUPPURATIVA

1. Rosner IA, Richter DE, Huettner TL, et al.: Spondyloarthropathy associated with hidradenitis suppurativa and acne conglobata. Ann Intern Med 97:520, 1982.
2. Knitzer RH, Needleman BW: Musculoskeletal syndromes associated with acne. Semin Arthritis Rheum 20:247: 1991.
3. Hellmann DB: Spondyloarthropathy with hidradenitis suppurativa. JAMA 267:2363, 1992.
4. Windom RE, Sanford JP, Ziff M: Acne conglobata and arthritis. Arthritis Rheum 4:632, 1961.
5. Golding DN: Acne and joint disease. J Roy Soc Med 78:(Suppl 10):19, 1985.
6. McKendry RJR, Hamdy H: Acne, arthritis, sacroiliitis. Can Med Assoc J 128:156, 1983.
7. Ellis BI, Shier CK, Leisen JJC, et al.: Acne-associated spondyloarthropathy: radiographic feature. Radiology 162:541, 1987.
8. Piazza I, Giunta G: Lytic bone lesions and polyarthritis associated with acne fulminans. Br J Rheumatol 30:387, 1991.
9. Gerber LH, Helfgott RK, Gross EG, et al.: Vertebral abnormalities associated with synthetic retinoid use. J Am Acad Dermatol 10:817, 1984.
10. Kilcoyne RF, Cope R, Cunningham W, et al.: Minimal spinal hyperostosis with low-dose isotretinoin therapy. Invest Radiol 21:41, 1986.
11. Carey BM, Parkin GJS, Cunliffe WJ, Pritlove J: Skeletal toxicity with isotretinoin therapy: a clinico-radiological evaluation. Brit J Dermatol 119:609, 1988.
12. Rosner IA, Burg CG, Wisnieski JJ, et al.: The clinical spectrum of the arthropathy associated with hidradenitis suppurativa and acne conglobata. J Rheumatol 20:684, 1993.

RHEUMATOID ARTHRITIS

Capsule Summary

Frequency of back pain—rare
Location of back pain—diffuse
Quality of back pain—ache
Symptoms and signs—joint disease of long duration, lumbosacral spine tenderness
Laboratory and x-ray tests—anemia, rheumatoid factor; unilateral or bilateral sacroiliitis without reactive sclerosis
Treatment—nonsteroidal anti-inflammatory drugs, anti-rheumatics, corticosteroids

PREVALENCE AND PATHOGENESIS

Rheumatoid arthritis (RA) is a chronic systemic inflammatory disease that causes pain, heat, swelling, and destruction in synovial joints. The joints characteristically affected by RA are small joints of the hands and feet, wrists, elbows, hips, knees, ankles, and cervical spine. The lumbar spine is rarely involved in the rheumatoid process. Patients who develop low back pain secondary to RA have long-standing, extensive disease in the usual joint locations associated with the illness. RA of the lumbosacral spine may be associated with apophyseal joint erosions and secondary intervertebral disc narrowing. Sacroiliac joint involvement is characterized by narrowing of the joint space without erosions or bony sclerosis. RA of the lumbosacral spine responds to the same therapy that is effective for joint disease in other locations.

The prevalence of RA is approximately 1% to 3% of the United States population.[1] Reevaluation of population data continues to suggest that a similar number of individuals are affected.[2] RA is found in all racial and ethnic groups. The condition occurs in all age groups. The male to female ratio is approximately 1:3. One study suggested that 5% of men and 3% of women with RA may have lumbar spine involvement.[3] Another study reported 4% of men and 5% of women had pronounced involvement of the sacroiliac joints.[4] In a study of RA patients with low back pain, 17% had sacroiliitis on radiographic evaluation.[5] These patients were almost evenly split between unilateral and bilateral disease.

The etiology of RA is probably multifactorial and is mediated through environmental and genetic factors. The combination of these factors results in an imbalance in immune function which results in the inflammation of synovial joints.[6] A possible environmental factor that may initiate RA is a virus.[7] After an initial flurry of scientific interest associating the presence of Epstein-Barr virus (EBV) with infection in RA, subsequent investigations have not found convincing evidence of a cause and effect relationship between the two processes.[8] Cross-reactivity may exist between EBV nuclear antigens and autoantigens, including collagen, actin, and cytokeratin, and synovial membrane antigens.[9] Cellular immunity is altered in RA. Increased numbers of T4 lymphocytes, which activate B lymphocytes to produce immunoglobulin, are frequently found in synovium from RA patients.[10] Many of the B and T lymphocytes and monocytes in rheumatoid synovium express histocompatibility antigens (DR and DQ), indicating increased cellular activity of these cells.[11] In addition, lymphocytes from RA patients demonstrate sensitivity to collagen present in the joints and eyes (Types II and III).[12]

A number of environmental antigens may be the initiating factors that are presented to antigen-presenting cells bearing major histocompatibility complex class II antigens.[13] The haplotypes associated with RA include HLA-DR4 and HLA-DR1.[14] Subtypes of DR4 associated with RA include DRB*0401, DRB1*0404/08, and DRB1*0405.[15] The appropriately presented antigen located in the peptide-binding grove formed by the HLA molecule activates lymphocytes that attract macrophages into synovium. The activation of macrophages results in the production of interleukin 1, tumor necrosis factor, platelet derived growth factor, and other cytokines. These factors attract additional lymphocytes and neutrophils. T lymphocytes accumulate in the synovial membrane. Helper-inducer T lymphocytes adhere better to the endothelial adhesive proteins than do suppressive-inducer subsets and gain access more easily to the extracellular matrix of the synovial membrane. There is an absence of suppressor-inducer T cells. Angiogenesis factors result in the growth of new capillaries. Activated metalloproteinases, including procollagenase and progelatinase, are released by

synovial cells and cause tissue destruction.[16] Arachidonic acid metabolites also are produced and affect components of the inflammatory response. This immune-mediated process becomes self-perpetuating even if the initiating factor is removed.[17]

The joints that are affected by the inflammation associated with RA are lined by a thin tissue layer, the synovial membrane, which produces synovial fluid that feeds the cartilage and lubricates the joint. Synovial membrane is not limited to joints alone but is found in many parts of the musculoskeletal system associated with motion, such as tendons, bursae, and ligaments. The inflammation associated with RA causes hypertrophy of this membrane along with the production of humoral factors that cause destruction of cartilage and bone cells. The end result of this inflammatory process, if left unchecked, is a destroyed joint with thinning cartilage, eroded bone, and disrupted supporting structures.

CLINICAL HISTORY

Patients with RA develop joint pain, heat, swelling, and tenderness. The joint involvement is additive and symmetric. The joints at greatest risk of being affected by the disease process include the proximal interphalangeal, metacarpal, carpal, elbow, hip, knee, ankle, and metatarsophalangeal. In the axial skeleton, the cervical spine is most frequently affected. Patients have joint pain and stiffness, which is most severe in the morning. Activity improves symptoms. This phenomenon, stiffness of a joint with rest, occurs frequently with active disease. As a component of systemic inflammation, afternoon fatigue is a common complaint.

Patients with RA of the lumbosacral spine usually have a history of extensive involvement of long duration. Low back pain appears along with increased synovitis in peripheral joints. The pain may be localized to the low back or may radiate into the thighs.[18] The sacroiliac joints are asymptomatic or mildly symptomatic.[4]

In a questionnaire study of 503 RA patients, 221 complained of back pain, with 167 complaining of pain of 3 months or longer. Most patients complained of more than one area of low back pain. The character of the pain was dull in 80% of patients. Radiating pain to the thigh occurred in 27% and to the lower leg in 10%. Pain was increased by certain positions including flexion (50%), sitting (52%), and with exercise (52%). In contrast to mechanical etiologies of back pain, pain was not exacerbated by inspiration (10%), cough (13%), and extension of the back (13%). Relief of pain was obtained by rest (75%), physiotherapy (28%), and analgesics (28%). A small minority had the combination of nocturnal pain, aggravation with rest, and relief with exercise.[5]

PHYSICAL EXAMINATION

Physical examination of a rheumatoid arthritis patient with lumbar spine involvement reveals diffuse peripheral joint involvement characterized by heat, swelling, tenderness, and loss of motion. Examination of the lumbar spine may show tenderness with palpation over the bony skeleton and limitation of all spinal movement. A number of patients may not demonstrate a significant decrease in back motion despite significant damage in peripheral joints. Neurologic examination, including a straight-leg raising test, is normal.

LABORATORY DATA

Abnormal laboratory findings include anemia, elevated ESR, and increases in serum globulins. Anemia (chronic disease type) is common and is related to disease activity.[19] Rheumatoid factors (antibodies directed against host antibodies) are present in 80% of patients with RA. The rheumatoid factors include IgM, IgG, and IgA subclasses. The presence of one class versus another does not usually predict the subsequent course of the illness.[20] Antinuclear antibodies are present in 30% of RA patients. Synovial fluid analysis demonstrates an inflammatory fluid characterized by poor viscosity, increased numbers of white blood cells, decreased glucose, and increased protein.

Histologic examination of the synovium from affected joints demonstrates an inflammatory, hyperplastic tissue characterized by mononuclear cell infiltration, synovial cell proliferation, fibrin deposition, and necrosis. Examination of lumbar spine apophyseal joints from RA patients at autopsy has shown similar hyperplastic changes consistent with those synovial alterations associated with the inflammatory disease.[3]

RADIOGRAPHIC FINDINGS

Characteristic radiographic changes of RA include soft tissue swelling, bony erosion without reactive sclerotic bone, joint space narrowing, and periarticular osteopenia. Radiographic examination of patients with lumbar spine RA demonstrates apophyseal joint erosion without sclerosis, secondary disc space narrowing with bony destruction secondary to rheumatoid nodules, and malalignment.[3, 18, 21–23] Some of the alteration in vertebral body configuration may be related to the presence of rheumatoid nodules.[24] The apophyseal joints are frequently affected in RA. However, unlike AS, joint fusion is rare.[5] Osteoporosis, secondary to the illness or corticosteroid therapy, also is a frequent finding in the spine of RA patients. Disc space narrowing, without osteophytosis, was commonly found in RA patients compared with age-matched controls.[5] Sacroiliac joint changes include asymmetric involvement with mild narrowing, iliac erosions, minimal sclerosis, and fibrous fusion.[25] The involvement of the sacroiliac joints with RA may be unilateral or bilateral. Ankylosis, if it develops, is not as sturdy as that associated with AS, and the site of the joint cleft usually persists as a linear density on the roentgenographic images of the joint. The sacroiliac margins above the synovial part of the joints are not affected.[26] On occasion, dislocation of the sacroiliac joint in RA patients may be noted.[27] As many as 35% of patients with long-standing disease may have sacroiliac changes.[28]

Patients with RA also may have a spondyloarthropathy such as AS or psoriatic arthritis. In these patients, the differentiation of radiographic findings may be difficult. Unless diagnostic criteria are followed carefully, an increased incidence of sacroiliac disease may be attributed to RA in surveys of patients with radiographic abnormalities in the lumbosacral spine, when in fact the accompanying disease process may be the source of the joint alterations.[4]

DIFFERENTIAL DIAGNOSIS

RA is a clinical diagnosis based on history of joint pain, distribution of joint involvement, and characteristic laboratory abnormalities (rheumatoid factor). In the patient who develops back pain in the setting of active disease of long duration, the diagnosis of RA of the lumbar spine is probable. However, since involvement of the lumbar spine in RA is unusual, other possibilities must be considered. These diseases include herniated intervertebral disc, spondyloarthropathies, and local infection.

Two illnesses that cause both peripheral and axial skeletal arthritis and may be confused with RA are multicentric reticulohistiocytosis and relapsing polychondritis. Multicentric reticulohistiocytosis, or lipoid dermatoarthritis, is a rare disorder of adults characterized by the presence of histiocytic nodules in the skin and severe, mutilating arthritis. A variety of lipids, including triglycerides, cholesterol esters, and phospholipids, are stored in histiocytes, which coalesce to form granulomas and which produce enzymes that destroy joint and other tissue structures.[29] In 70% of patients, the first sign of the disease is a symmetric polyarthritis that simulates the peripheral arthritis of rheumatoid disease.[30] The lumbosacral spine is affected less frequently. Patients develop skin nodules that are pigmented over the fingers, face, neck, and chest and are not associated with RA.[31] Patients with reticulohistiocytoses do not usually develop rheumatoid factor. Radiologic abnormalities occur in the hands, including circumscribed bone erosions, widened joint spaces, minimal periosteal reaction, and periarticular osteopenia.[32] Sacroiliac joint abnormalities include erosion and obliteration, with bony ankylosis of the articular space.[32, 33] The process may be bilateral but the lack of bony sclerosis helps differentiate this disease from AS. Therapy for this illness includes anti-inflammatory drugs. Corticosteroids and immunosuppressives, including cyclophosphamide, are used in patients with continued destructive disease.[34]

Relapsing Polychondritis

Relapsing polychondritis is a rare disease characterized by inflammation of cartilaginous structures, associated with peripheral arthritis that mimics RA. Patients with polychondritis produce antibodies against Type II collagen.[35] Patients develop acute swelling of cartilaginous structures (ears, nose) as well as swelling of the hand joints.[36] Between 12% and 30% of patients with relapsing polychondritis may have axial skeletal complaints.[37] Radiographic findings in the hands are usually those of a nondeforming, nonerosive arthropathy. On occasion, sacroiliac joint abnormalities are noted. These include unilateral or bilateral involvement, which may be asymmetric in regard to severity of disease. Relapsing polychondritis also may be complicated by spondyloarthropathy that resembles AS or Reiter's syndrome.[38] Abnormalities include absence of spondylitis, sacroiliac joint thinning, erosion, and surrounding sclerosis.[39] Therapy for relapsing polychondritis is high-dose prednisone (40 to 60 mg/day). Corticosteroids are usually effective for control of joint disease associated with polychondritis.

TREATMENT

The treatment for control of generalized RA includes a regimen of patient education, physical therapy, nonsteroidal anti-inflammatory drugs, remittive agents (gold, penicillamine, hydroxychloroquine), corticosteroids, and immunosuppressive agents.[8] The therapy has been organized into a therapeutic pyramid based on the use of less toxic therapies for all patients. Increasingly toxic therapies are added with increasing clinical severity of disease. A reassessment of the treatment regimen has been suggested.[40] This regimen initiates therapy with a multitude of drugs, with increased toxicity compared with nonsteroidals, in response to the morbidity and mortality associated with RA. Therapy is directed at the control of pain and stiffness, reduction of inflammation, maintenance of function, and prevention of deformity. Patients are educated about their disease so they may be active participants in their care. They are encouraged to continue with as normal a lifestyle as possible. Physical therapy provides temperature modalities (heat or cold) to relieve pain, exercises to maintain muscle strength, and assistive devices (canes, crutches, splints) to promote normal function and ambulation.

Medications to control pain and inflammation are useful in the patient with RA. Aspirin is a very effective agent if given in adequate doses to reach a serum concentration of 20 to 25 mg/dl. For patients who are unable to take the number of tablets necessary to reach that serum level, who are intolerant of the drug, or on whom it has no effect, other nonsteroidal anti-inflammatory medications are useful in controlling symptoms. These agents include ibuprofen, tolmetin, fenoprofen, naproxen, indomethacin, piroxicam, sulindac, mefenamic acid, and ketoprofen, etodolac, diclofenac, nabumetone, and oxaprozin. The choice of agent is dependent on a number of factors including drug half-life, formulation, dose range, and tolerability.[41]

Patients who continue with joint inflammation or who demonstrate joint damage (joint space narrowing, bony erosions, or cysts) despite adequate nonsteroidal therapy are candidates for remittive therapy. Remittive agents, such as hydroxychloroquine, gold salts, or penicillamine, have a delayed onset of action compared with that of nonsteroidal drugs. Hydroxychloroquine has a moderate, disease-suppressive action with few adverse reactions at doses of 400 mg/day or less.[42] Injectable gold salts (50 mg/week) alter the natural history of RA.[43] The combination of D-penicillamine

(125 to 750 mg/day) and sulfasalazine (2 gm/day) has been reported to have a beneficial effect on the inflammation in RA.[44] Methotrexate at doses between 7.5 mg to 15 mg/week is effective in decreasing the inflammation of RA and also may slow disease progression.[45] Methotrexate may be used for an extended period of time and may remain effective.[46] In a recent study using methotrexate, 587 RA patients were followed for 70 months; 76% of patients remained on methotrexate for that period of time. The drug remained effective in a majority of patients for the duration of the study.[47] However, the remittive agents are capable of slowing the progression of joint destruction and may allow for healing of damaged osseous structures.

Systemic corticosteroids are effective in controlling the inflammatory components of RA but are unable to slow the progression of disease. Corticosteroids are the most powerful and predictable remedy inducing immediate relief in RA.[48] They also are associated with a wide spectrum of toxicities, ranging from hypertension and diabetes to cataracts and osteonecrosis of bone. Glucocorticoid-induced osteoporosis is a significant complication of this therapy.[49] Intra-articular corticosteroid injections are used when a single joint remains active in the face of general control of the arthritic process.

Immunosuppressives are associated with severe toxic effects (aplastic anemia and cancer), which limit their benefit to the severely affected patient. Only a very small proportion of patients with RA require this therapy. Some of the immunosuppressives used in RA include azathioprine, chlorambucil, and cyclophosphamide.[50]

Experimental therapy of RA includes the use of total lymph node irradiation, cyclosporin A, and monoclonal antibodies. The studies of these agents are in the early stage of investigation, and additional time is needed to document their benefit in RA.[51–53]

PROGNOSIS

The course of RA cannot be predicted at time of onset. Some patients develop sustained disease, which is associated with joint destruction and resistance to therapy. Patients with rheumatoid factor, HLA-DR4, elevated ESR, and elevated C-reactive protein have a greater likelihood of poor outcome at two years as measured by radiographic progression.[54] Patients with HLA-DRB1, *0404, or *0408 haplotypes are at risk of developing nodules and

extra-articular manifestations of RA.[55] Patients with long-term disease are at risk of developing lumbar spine involvement. Although lumbar spine disease occurs in patients with a more active process, these particular symptoms are responsive to therapeutic measures. Patients with RA are not disabled specifically because of lumbar spine involvement. However, patients with lumbar spine disease have extensive generalized involvement, which usually affects their functional status and their ability to function in a job.

References

RHEUMATOID ARTHRITIS

1. O'Sullivan JB, Cathcart ES: The prevalence of rheumatoid arthritis: follow-up evaluation of the effect of criteria on rates in Sudbury, Massachusetts. Ann Intern Med 76:573, 1972.
2. Lawrence RC, Hochberg MM, Kelsey JL, et al.: Estimates of the prevalence of selected arthritic and musculoskeletal diseases in the United States. J Rheumatol 16:427, 1989.
3. Lawrence JS, Sharp J, Ball J, Bier F: Rheumatoid arthritis of the lumbar spine. Ann Rheum Dis 23:205, 1964.
4. Graudal H, de Carvalho A, Lassen L: The course of sacroiliac involvement in rheumatoid arthritis. Scand J Rheumatol (Suppl)32:34, 1979.
5. Helliwell PS, Zebouni LNP, Porter G, et al.: A clinical and radiological study of back pain in rheumatoid arthritis. Br J Rheumatol 32:16, 1993.
6. Stastny P: Immunogenetic factors in rheumatoid arthritis. Clin Rheum Dis 3:315, 1977.
7. Simpson RW, McGinty L, Simon L, et al.: Association of parvoviruses with rheumatoid arthritis of humans. Science 223:1425, 1984.
8. Decker JL: Rheumatoid arthritis: evolving concept of pathogenesis and treatment. Ann Intern Med 101:810, 1984.
9. Baboonian C, Venables PJW, Williams DG, et al.: Cross-reaction of antibodies to a glycine-alanine repeat sequence of Epstein-Barr virus nuclear antigen-1 with collagen, cytokeratin, and actin. Ann Rheum Dis 50:772, 1991.
10. Van Boxel JA, Paget SA: Predominantly T-cell infiltrate in rheumatoid synovial membranes. N Engl J Med 293:517, 1975.
11. Janossy G, Panayi G, Duke O, et al.: Rheumatoid arthritis: a disease of lymphocytes, macrophage immunoregulation. Lancet 2:839, 1981.
12. Trentham DE, Dynesius RA, Rocklin RE, David JR: Cellular sensitivity to collagen in rheumatoid arthritis. N Engl J Med 299:327, 1978.
13. Nepom GT, Byers P, Seyfried C, et al.: HLA genes associated with rheumatoid arthritis: identification of susceptibility alleles using specific oligonucleotide probes. Arthritis Rheum 32:15, 1989.
14. Harris ED Jr: Excitement in synovium: the rapid evolution of understanding of rheumatoid arthritis and expectations for therapy. J Rheumatol 19(Suppl 32):3, 1992.
15. Walport MJ, Ollier WER, Silman AJ: Immunogenetics of rheumatoid arthritis and the arthritis and rheu-

matism council's national repository. Br J Rheumatol 31:701, 1992.

16. Conca W, Kaplan PB, Krane SM: Increases in levels of procollagenase mRNA in human fibroblasts induced by interleukin-1, tumor necrosis factor, or serum follow c-jun expression and are dependent on new protein synthesis. Trans Assn Am Phys 102:195, 1989.

17. Harris ED Jr: Rheumatoid arthritis: pathophysiology and implications for therapy. N Engl J Med 322:1277, 1990.

18. Sims-Williams H, Jayson MIV, Baddeley H: Rheumatoid involvement of the lumbar spine. Ann Rheum Dis 36:524, 1977.

19. Baer AN, Dessypris EN, Krantz SB: The pathogenesis of anemia in rheumatoid arthritis: a clinical and laboratory analysis. Semin Arthritis Rheum 19:209, 1990.

20. Eberhardt KB, et al.: Disease activity and joint damage progression in early rheumatoid arthritis: relation to IgG, IgA, IgM rheumatoid factor. Ann Rheum Dis 49:906, 1990.

21. Dixon ASJ, Lience E: Sacro-iliac joint in adult rheumatoid arthritis and psoriatic arthropathy. Ann Rheum Dis 20:247, 1961.

22. Resnick D: Thoracolumbar spine abnormalities in rheumatoid arthritis. Ann Rheum Dis 37:389, 1978.

23. Pearson ME, Kosco M, Huffer W, et al.: Rheumatoid nodules of the spine: case report and review of the literature. Arthritis Rheum 30:709, 1987.

24. Heywood AWB, Meyers OL: Rheumatoid arthritis of the thoracic and lumbar spine. J Bone Joint Surg 68B:362, 1986.

25. Baggenstoss AH, Bidkel WH, Ward LE: Rheumatoid granulomatous nodules as destructive lesions of vertebrae. J Bone Joint Surg 34A:601, 1952.

26. Martel W: Radiologic differential diagnosis of ankylosing spondylitis (Bechterew's syndrome). Scand J Rheumatol (Suppl) 32:141, 1979.

27. Gersoff WK, Burkus JK: Dislocation of the sacroiliac joint associated with rheumatoid arthritis. A case report. Clin Orthop 209:219, 1986.

28. Sievers K, Laine V: The sacro-iliac joint in adult rheumatoid arthritis in adult females. Acta Rheumatol Scand 9:222, 1963.

29. Krey PR, Comerford FR, Cohen AS: Multicentric reticulohistiocytosis. Fine structural analysis of the synovium and synovial fluid cells. Arthritis Rheum 17:615, 1974.

30. Ehrlich GE, Young I, Rosherry SZ, Katz WA: Multicentric reticulo-histiocytosis (lipoid dermatoarthritis): a multi-system disorder. Am J Med 52:830, 1972.

31. Barrow MV, Holubar K: Multicentric reticulohistiocytosis: a review of 33 patients. Medicine 48:287, 1969.

32. Gold RH, Metzger AL, Miria JM, et al.: Multicentric reticulohistiocytosis (lipoid dermatoarthritis): an erosive polyarthritis with distinctive clinical, roentgenographic and pathologic features. AJR 124:610, 1975.

33. Johnson HM, Tilden IL: Reticulohistiocytic granulomas of skin associated with arthritis mutilans: report of a case followed fourteen years. Arch Dermatol 75:405, 1957.

34. Hanauer LB: Reticulohistiocytosis: Remission after cyclophosphamide therapy. Arthritis Rheum 15:636, 1972.

35. Foidart JM, Abe S, Martin GR, et al.: Antibodies to type II collagen in relapsing polychondritis. N Engl J Med 299:1203, 1978.

36. O'Hanlan M, McAdam LP, Bluestone R, Pearson CM: The arthropathy of relapsing polychondritis. Arthritis Rheum 19:191, 1976.

37. McAdam LP, O'Hanlan MA, Bluestone R, Pearson CM: Relapsing polychondritis: prospective study of 23 patients and review of the literature. Medicine 55:193, 1976.

38. Pazirandeh M, Ziran BH, Khandelwal BK, et al.: Relapsing polychondritis and spondyloarthropathies. J Rheumatol 15:630, 1988.

39. Braunstein EM, Martel W, Stillwell E, Kay D: Radiologic aspects of the arthropathy of relapsing polychondritis. Clin Radiol 30:441, 1979.

40. Wilske KR, Healey LA: Remodelling the pyramid, a concept whose time has come. J Rheumatol 16:565, 1989.

41. Brooks PM, Day RO: Nonsteroidal anti-inflammatory drugs—differences and similarities. N Engl J Med 324:1716, 1991.

42. Tett SE, Cutler D, Day RO: Antimalarials in rheumatic diseases. Clin Rheumatol 4:467, 1990.

43. Capell HA, Lewis D, Carey J: A three year follow-up of patients allocated to placebo, or oral or injectable gold therapy for rheumatoid arthritis. Ann Rheum Dis 45:705, 1986.

44. Taggart AJ, Hill J, Asbury C, et al.: Sulphasalazine alone or in combination with D-penicillamine in rheumatoid arthritis. Br J Rheumatol 26:32, 1987.

45. Scully CJ, Anderson CJ, Cannon GW: Long-term methotrexate therapy for rheumatoid arthritis. Semin Arthritis Rheum 20:317, 1991.

46. Sany J, Anaya JM, Lussiez V, et al.: Treatment of Rheumatoid arthritis with methotrexate: a prospective open long-term study of 191 cases. J Rheumatol 18:1323, 1991.

47. Buchbinder R, Hall S, Sambrook PN, et al.: Methotrexate therapy in rheumatoid arthritis: a life table review of 587 patients treated in community practice. J Rheumatol 20:639, 1993.

48. Harris ED Jr, Emkey RD, Nichols JE, et al.: Low dose prednisone therapy in rheumatoid arthritis: a double-blind study. J Rheumatol 10:713, 1983.

49. Lukert BP, Raisz LG: Glucocorticoid-induced osteoporosis: pathogenesis and management. Ann Intern Med 112:352, 1990.

50. Luqmani RA, Palmer RG, Bacon PA: Azathioprine, cyclophosphamide and chlorambucil. Clin Rheumatol 4:595, 1990.

51. Sodem M, et al.: Lymphoid irradiation in intractable rheumatoid arthritis. Arthritis Rheum 32:523, 1989.

52. Dougados M, Duchesne L, Awada H, et al.: Assessment of efficacy and acceptability of low dose cyclosporine in patients with rheumatoid arthritis. Ann Rheum Dis 48:550, 1989.

53. Horneff G, Burmester GR, Emrrich F, et al.: Treatment of rheumatoid arthritis with an anti-CD4 monoclonal antibody. Arthritis Rheum 34:129, 1991.

54. van der Heijde DMFM, van Riel PLCM, van Leeuween MA, et al.: Prognostic factors for radiographic damage and physical disability in early rheumatoid arthritis. A prospective follow-up study of 147 patients. Br J Rheumatol 31:519, 1992.

55. Weyand CM, Hicok KC, Conn DL, et al.: The influence of HLA-DRB1 genes on disease severity in rheumatoid arthritis. Ann Intern Med 117:801, 1992.

DIFFUSE IDIOPATHIC SKELETAL HYPEROSTOSIS (DISH)

Capsule Summary

Frequency of back pain—common
Location of back pain—thoracolumbar spine

Quality of back pain—ache

Symptoms and signs—dysphagia, decreased back motion

Laboratory and x-ray tests—flowing calcification of the anterolateral aspect of four contiguous vertebral bodies on plain roentgenogram

Treatment—nonsteroidal anti-inflammatory drugs, range of motion exercises

PREVALENCE AND PATHOGENESIS

Diffuse idiopathic skeletal hyperostosis (DISH) is a disease characterized clinically by spinal stiffness and pain and radiographically by exuberant calcification of spinal and extraspinal structures. Despite impressive radiographic abnormalities, patients rarely have significant loss of function or disability from the illness except for the rare individual who develops difficulty swallowing (dysphagia) secondary to cervical spine involvement. This disease has been known by many different names, including spondylitis ossificans ligamentosa, vertebral osteophytosis, ankylosing hyperostosis of Forestier and Rotés-Querol, and Forestier's disease. DISH was suggested in 1975 by Resnick as a more appropriate name in light of the diffuse bone growth that develops in both spinal and extraspinal locations.[1]

DISH is a common entity found in 6% to 28% of an autopsy population.[2-4] The usual patient is a man between the ages of 48 and 85 years.[5] The ratio of men to women is 2:1.[6] The disease occurs most commonly in Caucasians and rarely in blacks.

The etiology of DISH is unknown. In one series, occupational stress or spinal trauma was reported in 57% of patients with this condition.[1] The patients reporting such stress or trauma usually had occupations such as construction, ranching, or roofing that required at least a moderate degree of physical activity. Other individuals in the same study had no history of occupational or accidental trauma. Endocrinologic abnormalities associated with bony hyperostosis, acromegaly, and hypoparathyroidism, have been suggested as causes of DISH. No abnormalities in growth hormone (acromegaly) or parathormone (hypoparathyroidism) have been found.[5] Diabetes mellitus occurs in 30% of patients with the disease; however, this frequency of diabetes mellitus may be related to the age of the population rather than a true association of the two disorders.[1] Elevated levels of endogenous retinoic acids are present in DISH patients compared to controls.[7] The elevation in 13-cis and all-

trans-retinoic acid may be similar to the hyperostosis associated with retinoids used in the treatment of psoriasis and acne.

A specific genetic predisposition to the development of the problem has not been identified. HLA-B27 positivity was found in 34% of DISH patients in one study,[8] but a subsequent study found no significant association with HLA antigens.[9] Until further data are obtained to the contrary, DISH should not be classified with the HLA-B27-positive, seronegative spondyloarthropathies (AS, Reiter's syndrome).

CLINICAL FINDINGS

The principal musculoskeletal complaint in 80% of patients is spinal stiffness.[1] The duration of back stiffness before diagnosis may be 10 to 20 years, with onset when the patient's age is in the 40s. Morning stiffness dissipates within an hour, only to recur in the late evening.[6] Back pain in the thoracolumbar spine occurs in 57% of patients as their initial complaint.[1] Back pain is usually mild and intermittent and rarely radiating. In one study, 67% of DISH patients had lumbar spine pain.[10] In some study populations with DISH, back pain may occur with the same frequency as age matched controls.[11] DISH is clinically silent in some patients. Occasionally, patients will have cervical spine pain as their initial complaint. Dysphagia is seen in 17% to 28% of patients.[5] Dysphagia occurs secondary to constriction of the esophagus by anteriorly located cervical osteophytes.

Extraspinal manifestations of DISH occur in 37% of patients. In 20%, extraspinal pain was the initial or predominant complaint. The most common extraspinal skeletal areas involved include the shoulders, knees, elbows, and heels.

PHYSICAL EXAMINATION

Physical examination usually reveals mild limitation of motion in the lumbar spine.[12] Occasionally, a slight decrease in lumbar lordosis and a small increase in dorsal kyphosis may be present. Limitation of motion in the thoracic and cervical spine may also be found.[1] A minority of the patients will show tenderness to percussion over the sacroiliac joints.[5] A rare patient may develop neurologic signs from spinal cord compression secondary to DISH.[13] Patients with extraspinal disease may have diminished range of motion and pain on palpation over affected areas. Areas that may show

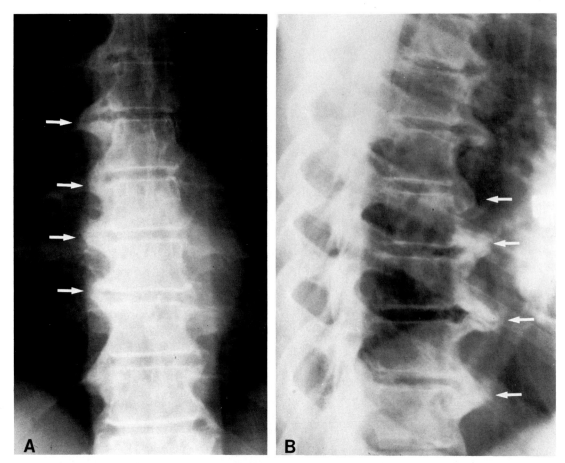

Figure 11–22. Diffuse idiopathic skeletal hyperostosis (DISH). AP (*A*) and lateral (*B*) views of thoracic spine demonstrating anterior, contiguous flowing ossification involving multiple vertebral bodies (*arrow*). The lucency of the disc space expands into the flowing ossification, creating a Y or T configuration. (Courtesy of Anne Brower, M.D.)

abnormalities include the hips, subtalar joints, shoulders, knees, elbows, and ankle joints.

LABORATORY DATA

Laboratory parameters are essentially normal in patients with DISH.[9] Occasionally, a mildly elevated ESR is noted. Since patients who develop the disease are elderly, laboratory abnormalities may be secondary to another illness affecting the patient. Therefore, elevations of fasting and 2-hour postprandial glucose levels are probably secondary to impending diabetes rather than to DISH.

Pathologic evaluation of the axial skeleton is not necessary for diagnosis of DISH. However, pathologic findings do correlate with the radiographic characteristics of DISH. These findings include (1) fibrous tissue separating anterior calcification and the annulus fibrosus of the intervertebral disc, (2) normal disc height, (3) close proximity of anterior calcifi-

cations, in most circumstances without fusion, and (4) widespread osteoporosis.[3]

RADIOGRAPHIC EVALUATION

DISH is diagnosed radiographically. It is made, not uncommonly, in asymptomatic people who happen to have characteristic bony changes in the thoracic spine on a chest radiograph (Fig. 11–22). The three criteria for spinal involvement include flowing calcification along the anterolateral aspect of four contiguous vertebral bodies; preservation of intervertebral disc height; and absence of apophyseal joint bony ankylosis and sacroiliac joint sclerosis, erosion, or fusion.[2] These criteria help differentiate it from spondylosis deformans, intervertebral disc degeneration, and AS. The fact that the posterior spinal elements are not affected permits almost normal range of motion on physical examination. Radiographic abnormalities are seen most frequently in the thoracic and lumbar spine (Fig. 11–23).[1] A majority of patients also develop cervical spine involvement.

In the lumbar spine, the upper vertebrae (first through third) are most commonly affected. Calcification occurs initially along the anterior aspect of the vertebral body. Bony excrescences are in an anterosuperior position near the disc margin and extend upward across the intervertebral disc space. The excrescences are thick in comparison to syndesmophytes. Careful observation will identify a thin radiolucent line that separates the vertebral body proper from the anterior calcification. The right-sided predilection of DISH in the thoracic spine is not continued in the lumbar spine, where bilateral or left-sided involvement is frequently seen.[14]

Extraspinal radiographic changes include bony proliferation or "whiskering," ligamentous calcification, and para-articular osteophytes.[6] Common locations for these changes are in the pelvis, heel, foot, patella, elbow, shoulder, and wrist. In the pelvis, the iliolumbar, sacrotuberous, and sacroiliac ligaments and iliopsoas tendon were locations for calcification. The calcification of ligaments was different from the pattern of pelvic involvement associated with spondylosis deformans, thus suggesting that DISH is a distinct entity independent of spondylosis deformans.[15]

Information concerning the presence of DISH may be a serendipitous piece of information obtained from abdominal CT scans performed for other diagnostic purposes. Degenerative alterations of the sacroiliac joints are most easily observed with CT evaluation. In a study of 100 abdominal CT scans in patients 55 years of age or older, patients with DISH had more severe degenerative alterations of the sacroiliac joints.[16] Some of the alterations noted in the sacroiliac joints include large bridging osteophytes at the anterior aspects of the joint.[17]

DIFFERENTIAL DIAGNOSIS

The diagnosis of DISH is based on the presence of characteristic radiographic changes and an absence of clinical abnormalities suggestive of another illness. Resnick[1] has proposed criteria for the diagnosis of DISH:

1. Flowing calcification and ossification along the anterolateral aspect of four contiguous vertebral bodies with or without associated localized pointed excrescences at the intervening vertebral body/intervertebral disc junctions.

2. Relative preservation of intervertebral disc height in the involved vertebral segment and the absence of radiographic evidence of degenerative disc disease.

3. Absence of apophyseal joint bony ankylosis and sacroiliac joint erosion, sclerosis, or intra-articular osseous fusion.

There are a number of causes of bony outgrowths of the spine, including spondyloarthropathies, acromegaly, hypoparathyroidism, fluorosis, ochronosis, neuropathic arthropathy, and trauma. Specific abnormalities associated with each of these entities, which are reviewed in other portions of this chapter, help differentiate these illnesses from DISH.

Spondyloarthropathies are frequently associated with sacroiliac joint disease. Acromegaly is associated with posterior scalloping of the vertebral body and increased intervertebral disc space height. Patients with hypoparathyroidism are hypocalcemic and develop tetany, which is not associated with DISH. Fluorosis causes generalized bone sclerosis to a greater

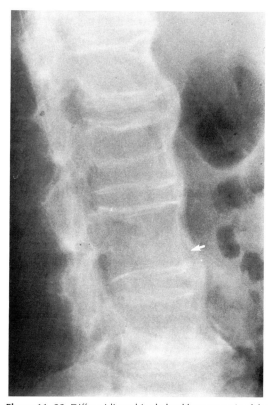

Figure 11–23. Diffuse idiopathic skeletal hyperostosis of the lumbar spine associated with "flowing" anterior ligament calcification involving five lumbar vertebrae. Notice clear area separating vertebral body and ligamentous calcification (*arrow*). Characteristic of the process, the disc spaces are spared. (Courtesy of Anne Brower, M.D.)

degree than that associated with DISH. Ochronotic involvement of the vertebral column is manifested by disc height loss and calcifications. Neuropathic arthropathy causes disorganization and destruction of bone in combination with bone formation. Trauma causes callus formation in localized areas of the spine. The simultaneous occurrence of DISH with other diseases does occur. For example, a patient with the diagnoses of DISH and AS has been reported.[18] The patient described in this paper had DISH in the cervical spine and spondylitis in the lumbosacral spine. Another patient has been described with dorsal spine DISH involvement and sacroiliitis associated with AS.[19] Currently, eight patients have been reported in the medical literature with coexistent DISH and AS. Of this group, only four are HLA-B27 positive.[20]

TREATMENT

Treatment is directed to relieving pain and maximizing function. In patients with back pain and stiffness, nonsteroidal anti-inflammatory agents may be helpful. Exercise programs are designed to encourage maximum ranges of motion throughout the axial skeleton. Local injections of lidocaine and corticosteroids are used in areas of bony overgrowth, such as the heel, for pain relief.

Patients with severe dysphagia may require removal of the offending hyperostosis.[21] A possible complication of surgical excision of exostoses is recurrence of bony overgrowth. Some patients with DISH who have had hip joint replacements have developed postoperative heterotopic ossification.[22]

PROGNOSIS

The course of DISH is usually benign. Confusion may occur in diagnosis of patients who present in their 40s with back pain with no physical findings or early radiographic changes. The differential diagnosis for such a patient requires investigation for a number of illnesses that affect the axial skeleton. The patients with DISH will have a very slow progressive course. They may have aching low back pain and stiffness for 20 years or longer but will rarely develop any limitations in their activities or morbidity from their illness.

Patients with DISH may develop symptoms of spinal stenosis. Ligamentous and capsular calcifications cause canal stenosis secondary to DISH. Hyperostotic stenosis differs from simple degenerative changes associated with osteoarthritic changes. The hyperostotic narrowing of the canal may be associated with neural compression.[23]

The course of patients with DISH may be complicated by other disease processes. For example, a patient with DISH developed an erosion of an area of hyperostosis in the lumbar spine. The erosion process was secondary to an expanding abdominal aneurysm.[24] Systemic symptoms or alterations in the radiographic appearance of DISH lesions should necessitate a medical evaluation for a complicating illness. Fractures of the spine may complicate patients with DISH.[25] Most locations for fractures are in the cervical and thoracic spine. Only a rare DISH patient has lumbar fracture.

References

DIFFUSE IDIOPATHIC SKELETAL HYPEROSTOSIS

1. Resnick D, Niwayama G: Radiographic and pathologic features of spinal involvement in diffuse idiopathic skeletal hyperostosis (DISH). Radiology 119:559, 1976.
2. Resnick D, Shaul SR, Robins JM: Diffuse idiopathic skeletal hyperostosis (DISH): Forestier's disease with extraspinal manifestations. Radiology 115:513, 1975.
3. Vernon-Roberts B, Pirie CJ, Trenwith V: Pathology of the dorsal spine in ankylosing hyperostosis. Ann Rheum Dis 33:281, 1974.
4. Boachie-Adjei O, Bullough PG: Incidence of ankylosing hyperostosis of the spine (Forestier's disease) at autopsy. Spine 12:739, 1987.
5. Utsinger PD, Resnick D, Shapiro R: Diffuse skeletal abnormalities in Forestier disease. Arch Intern Med 136:763, 1976.
6. Forestier J, Lagier R: Ankylosing hyperostosis of the spine. Clin Orthop 74:65, 1971.
7. Periquet B, Lambert W, Garcia J, et al.: Increased concentrations of endogenous 13-cis- and all-trans-retinoic acids in diffuse idiopathic skeletal hyperostosis, as demonstrated by HPLC. Clinica Chimica Acta 203:57, 1991.
8. Shapiro RF, Utsinger PD, Wiesner KB, et al.: The association of HLA-B27 with Forestier's disease (vertebral ankylosing hyperostosis). J Rheumatol 3:4, 1976.
9. Spagnola AM, Bennet PH, Terasaki PI: Vertebral ankylosing hyperostosis (Forestier's disease) and HLA antigens in Pima Indians. Arthritis Rheum 21:467, 1978.
10. Harris J, Carter AR, Glick EN, Storey GO: Ankylosing hyperostosis. I. Clinical and radiological features. Ann Rheum Dis 33:210, 1974.
11. Schlapbach P, Beyeler C, Gerber NJ, et al.: Diffuse idiopathic skeletal hyperostosis (DISH) of the spine: a cause of back pain: a controlled study. Br J Rheumatol 28:299, 1989.
12. Julkunen H, Heinonen OP, Pyorala K: Hyperostoses of the spine in an adult population, its relationship to hyperglycemia and obesity. Ann Rheum Dis 30:605, 1971.
13. Algenhat JP, Hallet M, Kido DK: Spinal cord compression in diffuse idiopathic skeletal hyperostosis. Radiology 142:119, 1982.

14. Resnick D, Niwayama G: Diffuse idiopathic skeletal hyperostosis (DISH): ankylosing hyperostosis of Forestier and Rotes-Querol. In Resnick D, Niwayama G (eds): Diagnosis of Bone and Joint Disorders, 2nd ed. Philadelphia: WB Saunders 1988, pp 1562–1602.

15. Haller J, Resnick D, Miller CW, et al.: Diffuse idiopathic skeletal hyperostosis: diagnostic significance of radiographic abnormalities of the pelvis. Radiology 172:835, 1989.

16. Yagan R, Ikhan MA, Marmolya G: Role of abdominal CT, when available in patients' records, in the evaluation of degenerative changes of the sacroiliac joints. Spine 12:1046, 1987.

17. Durback MA, Edelstein G, Schumacher HR: Abnormalities of the sacroiliac joints in diffuse idiopathic skeletal hyperostosis: demonstrated by computed tomography. J Rheumatol 15:1506, 1988.

18. Williamson PK, Reginato AJ: Diffuse idiopathic skeletal hyperostosis of the cervical spine in a patient with ankylosing spondylitis. Arthritis Rheum 27:570, 1984.

19. Olivieri I, Trippi D, Gherardi S, et al.: Coexistence of ankylosing spondylitis and diffuse idiopathic skeletal hyperostosis: another report. J Rheumatol 14:1058, 1987.

20. Maertens M, Mielants H, Verstraete K, et al.: Simultaneous occurrence of diffuse idiopathic skeletal hyperostosis and ankylosing spondylitis in the same patient. J Rheumatol 19:1978, 1992.

21. Meeks LW, Renshaw TS: Vertebral osteophytosis and dysphagia. J Bone Joint Surg 55A:197, 1973.

22. Resnick D, Linovitz RJ, Feingold ML: Postoperative heterotopic ossification in patients with ankylosing hyperostosis of the spine (Forestier's disease). J Rheumatol 3:313, 1976.

23. Kurihara A, Tanaka Y, Tsumura N, et al.: Hyperostotic lumbar spinal stenosis: a review of 12 surgically treated cases with roentgenographic survey of ossification of the yellow ligament at the lumbar spine. Spine 13:1308, 1988.

24. Chaiton A, Fam A, Charles B: Disappearing lumbar hyperostosis in a patient with Forestier's disease: an ominous sign. Arthritis Rheum 22:799, 1979.

25. Paley D, Schwartz M, Cooper P, et al.: Fractures of the spine in diffuse idiopathic skeletal hyperostosis. Clin Orthop 267, 1991.

VERTEBRAL OSTEOCHONDRITIS

Capsule Summary

Frequency of back pain—common

Location of back pain—midline, thoracolumbar junction

Quality of back pain—ache

Symptoms and signs—increased kyphosis, percussion tenderness

Laboratory and x-ray tests—vertebral body wedging, irregular endplates on plain roentgenograms

Treatment—exercises, bracing

PREVALENCE AND PATHOGENESIS

Vertebral osteochondritis (Scheuermann's disease) is a condition associated with an irregularity of ossification and endochondral growth, with pathologic changes developing at the junction of the vertebral body and intervertebral disc. This abnormality results in increasing wedging of vertebral bodies and progressive forward flexion of the spine (kyphosis). Vertebral osteochondritis primarily affects the thoracic spine in teenagers; however, a similar process has also been described as affecting the lumbar spine.[1] If left untreated, the illness may result in progressive kyphosis, persistent back pain, and signs of spinal cord compression. Scheuermann's disease, juvenile kyphosis, and osteochondritis deformans juvenilis dorsi are other names used interchangeably for this illness. Scheuermann first demonstrated the radiographic changes of wedged vertebrae in this disease in 1920.[2]

The prevalence of vertebral osteochondritis has been reported to vary from 0.4% to 8.3% of the general population, depending upon whether the diagnosis was based on radiographic or clinical criteria.[3] The male to female ratio is 1:2 for thoracic involvement, while the exact opposite ratio may be seen in disease of the lumbar spine.[4, 5]

The pathogenesis of vertebral osteochondritis is unknown. In the past, Scheuermann suggested that the wedge deformities associated with this illness are secondary to avascular necrosis of bone. Histologic examination of tissues from vertebral osteochondritic lesions has revealed no evidence of bone necrosis.[6] Schmorl suggested, instead, that disc material is extruded through the endplates into the cancellous bone of the body.[7] Alexander has postulated a similar mechanism.[8] Basically, during a period of rapid growth when the vertebral endplates are weakened, increased dynamic load through compression or shear forces causes disc material to move into vertebral bodies, resulting in an alteration of vertebral growth. The hereditary nature of the illness (increased familial occurrence) suggests a genetic predisposition to weakened vertebral endplates.[9] Other disease processes that result from compression forces (e.g., spondylolysis, intervertebral disc degeneration) are also associated with vertebral osteochondritis.[10] The radiographic abnormalities of intraosseous lucent areas and irregular contour of vertebral bodies fit into this pathogenetic schema. A cadaveric study of 103 spinal columns with Scheuermann's disease demonstrated anterior extension of vertebral bodies and the highest incidence of Schmorl's nodes at the vertebra with the greatest wedging, T8.[11] The location and histologic and radiographic characteristics of the lesions suggested a mechanical disorder. In the setting of late adolescence, with nearly complete posterior and posterolateral endplate growth, increased pressures from forward posture result in disruption of endochondral ossification in the anterior endplate resulting in anterior wedging and other manifestations of this illness.

Other possibilities seem unlikely. Scheuermann suggested that heavy labor at a young age may be associated with the development of vertebral osteochondritis.[12] However, vertebral osteochondritis usually occurs in young individuals with no history of heavy labor or trauma. Therefore, the effect of heavy labor on the development of vertebral osteochondritis is unknown. Endocrinologic dysfunction has not been discovered in enough patients to be of pathogenetic importance. Although Scheuermann's disease has been associated with osteoporosis, recent studies have demonstrated no significant difference in bone mineralization in patients with this illness compared with controls.[13, 14]

CLINICAL HISTORY

Patients with thoracic vertebral osteochondritis may present in three ways. They may complain of back pain, may demonstrate increasing kyphosis, or may be discovered to have vertebral osteochondritis by chance on a radiograph of the spine. Between 20% and 60% of the patients have back pain, and the pain is concentrated over the area of kyphosis. The pain may radiate down the back and is usually relieved with bed rest and exacerbated with activity.

Vertebral osteochondritis of the lumbar spine may occur independently or in conjunction with disease in the thoracic spine. The main symptoms of lumbar involvement include local pain and tenderness gradually increasing over weeks, radiation of pain to the hip, paravertebral muscle spasm, and limitation of back motion.

PHYSICAL EXAMINATION

Physical findings include a kyphotic deformity occasionally associated with scoliosis. The kyphosis occurs in the thoracic (75%), thoracolumbar (20%), and lumbar (5%) regions. Thoracic kyphosis is frequently associated with increased lumbar and cervical lordosis. Pain on palpation over the affected portion of the axial skeleton is not unusual, and paravertebral muscle spasm and tightness of the hamstrings does occur. Rarely, neurologic signs of cord compression may be elicited.[15, 16]

LABORATORY DATA

Laboratory parameters, such as hematocrit, white blood count, ESR, blood chemistries, rheumatoid factor, and antinuclear antibody are normal.

RADIOGRAPHIC EVALUATION

Radiographic abnormalities of vertebral osteochondritis include wedging of vertebral bodies, Schmorl's nodules (invasion of vertebral body by an intervertebral disc), irregular endplates, and increased kyphosis. Lumbar spine changes are similar (Fig. 11–24). In adult patients, the healed lesion results in characteristic radiographic changes, which include increased anteroposterior diameter of a vertebral body, disc space narrowing, loss of normal spine curvature, large Schmorl's nodules, and persistence of a separate fragment of bone anterosuperior to the front edge of a vertebral body (limbus vertebra). Over time, ossification of contiguous portions of the anterior aspects of intervertebral discs can lead to synostosis of neighboring vertebral bodies.[17] In younger patients with lumbar Scheuermann's disease, vertebral endplate irregularities, anterior Schmorl's nodes, and disc space narrowing may be identified without the 5° wedging of three consecutive vertebrae.[18] Some of these adolescents with lumbar involvement have a history of acute vertical compression injury associated with severe back pain and endplate fracture.

DIFFERENTIAL DIAGNOSIS

The diagnosis of thoracic vertebral osteochondritis is easily made when three contiguous vertebral bodies are wedged by 5° or more;[19] however, this criterion eliminates patients with fewer affected vertebrae or those with vertebral irregularity without wedging. No specific criteria have been suggested for lumbar involvement. Therefore, the diagnosis of vertebral osteochondritis should be suspected in a patient with characteristic radiographic changes of one or more thoracic or lumbar vertebrae. The lack of any constitutional symptoms, fever, weight loss, loss of appetite, and abnormal laboratory tests help differentiate vertebral osteochondritis in its early stages from infections (e.g., tuberculosis), neoplasm,

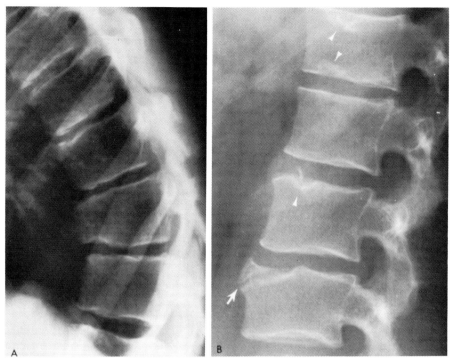

Figure 11–24. Vertebral osteochondritis (Scheuermann's disease). *A,* Thoracic spine. Findings include irregularity of vertebral contour, reactive sclerosis, intervertebral disc space narrowing, anterior vertebral wedging, and kyphosis. *B,* Lumbar spine. Observe the cartilaginous nodes (*arrowheads*) creating surface irregularity, lucent areas, and reactive sclerosis. An anterior discal herniation (*arrow*) has produced an irregular anterosuperior corner of a vertebral body, the limbus vertebra. (From Resnick D, Niwayama G: Diagnosis of Bone and Joint Disorders. Philadelphia: WB Saunders Co, 1988.)

hyperparathyroidism, Paget's disease, and rheumatoid arthritis.

TREATMENT

Treatment is directed at preventing deformity during the patient's rapid growth years and avoiding the development of poor body posture, associated back pain, and neurologic deficits as an adult. If the patient has a mild, reversible kyphosis, bed rest and daily exercises to strengthen the back extensor muscles are usually adequate to prevent further deformity. However, progression of kyphosis or radiographic changes of vertebral wedging require body casting or a Milwaukee brace. Milwaukee brace treatment, continued until growth is complete, has been effective at preventing the deformity in 40% of patients with vertebral osteochondritis.[4] A more recent followup study of patients treated with bracing reported a 69% improvement with reduced kyphosis and anterior vertebral wedging.[20] Surgical intervention is reserved for patients with severe kyphosis, intolerable back pain, visceral compromise (respiratory insufficiency), or

progressive neurologic deficit. A combination of anterior and posterior spine fusion was helpful in decreasing pain and deformity in 24 patients reported by Bradford.[21] Other surgical techniques utilizing a variety of rod instrumentation have been associated with improvement of vertebral deformity.[3]

PROGNOSIS

Patients with greater than 70° of kyphosis may develop increasing curvature after skeletal maturation is complete. Curvature of this degree can be associated with a marked increase in lumbar lordosis and persistent low back pain. Severe deformities also present a greater risk of neurologic compromise.

Lumbar spine osteochondritis may be associated with premature degeneration of intervertebral discs.[5] Butler has suggested that vertebral osteochondritis that results in loss of normal lumbar lordosis and mobility of the upper lumbar discs may make the lower lumbar discs more vulnerable to degeneration and protrusion. He believes that low back pain in middle-aged adults with this disorder is secondary to osteochondritis and disc degeneration that occurred in their youth. In a study of 67 patients who were followed for an average of 32 years, pulmonary dysfunction in the form of restrictive lung disease occurred in those with kyphotic angles greater than 100° curvature and with the apex of the curve between the first and eighth segments.[22] The limitations of the 67 patients were relatively minor with regard to physical functioning at work. From a social standpoint, those with curves greater than 85° were more likely to be single than married. In general, Scheuermann's kyphosis was considered a benign disorder. Surgical intervention is associated with significant complications and should be limited as a form of treatment for these patients.

References

VERTEBRAL OSTEOCHONDRITIS

1. Lamb DW: Localized osteochondritis of the lumbar spine. J Bone Joint Surg 36B:591, 1954.
2. Scheuermann HW: Kyfosis dorsalis juvenile. Ugesk Laeger, 82:385, 1920.
3. Lowe TG: Scheuermann's Disease. J Bone Joint Surg 72A:940, 1990.
4. Bradford DS, Moe JH, Montalvo FJ, Winter RB: Scheuermann's kyphosis and roundback deformity: results of Milwaukee brace treatment. J Bone Joint Surg 56A:740, 1974.
5. Butler RW: The nature and significance of vertebral osteochondritis. Proc Roy Soc Med 48:895, 1955.
6. Bradford DS, Moe JH: Scheuermann's juvenile kyphosis: a histologic study. Clin Orthop 110:45, 1975.
7. Schmorl G: Die Pathogenese der juvenilen Kyphose. Fortschr Geb Röntgenstr 41:359, 1930.
8. Alexander CT: Scheuermann's disease. A traumatic spondylodystrophy? Skel Radiol 1:209, 1977.
9. Halal F, Gledhill RB, Fraser FC: Dominant inheritance of Scheuermann's juvenile kyphosis. Am J Dis Child 132:1105, 1978.
10. Ogilvie JW, Sherman J: Spondylolysis in Scheuermann's disease. Spine 12:251, 1987.
11. Scoles PV, Latimer BM, DiGiovanni BF, et al.: Vertebral alterations in Scheuermann's kyphosis. Spine 16:509, 1991.
12. Scheuermann HW: Kyphosis Juvenilis (Scheuermann's Krankheit). Fortschr Geb Röntgenstr 53:1, 1936.
13. Lopez RA, Burke SW, Levine DB, Schneider R: Osteoporosis in Scheuermann's disease. Spine 13:1099, 1988.
14. Gilsanz V, Gibbens DT, Carlson M, King J: Vertebral bone density in Scheuermann's disease. J Bone Joint Surg 71A:894, 1989.
15. Bradford DS: Neurological complications in Scheuermann's disease: a case report and review of the literature. J Bone Surg 51A:567, 1969.
16. Ryan MD, Taylo TKF: Acute spinal cord compression in Scheuermann's disease. J Bone Joint Surg 64B:409, 1982.
17. Butler RW: Spontaneous anterior fusion of vertebral bodies. J Bone Joint Surg 53B:230, 1971.
18. Blumenthal SL, Roach J, Herring JA: Lumbar Scheuer-
mann's: a clinical series and classification. Spine 12:929, 1987.
19. Sorenson KH: Scheuermann's Juvenile Kyphosis. Munksgaard, Copenhagen, 1964.
20. Sachs B, Bradford D, Winter R, et al.: Scheuermann kyphosis: follow-up of Milwaukee-brace treatment. J Bone Joint Surg. 69A:50, 1987.
21. Bradford DS, Ahmed KB, Moe JH, et al.: The surgical management of patients with Scheuermann's disease. J Bone Joint Surg 62A:705, 1980.
22. Murray PM, Weinstein SL, Spratt KF: The natural history and long-term follow-up of Scheuermann kyphosis. J Bone Joint Surg 75A:236, 1993.

OSTEITIS CONDENSANS ILII

Capsule Summary

Frequency of back pain—uncommon
Location of back pain—sacroiliac joints
Quality of back pain—dull ache
Symptoms and signs—postpartum onset, percussion tenderness
Laboratory and x-ray tests—triangular area of sclerosis on iliac side of sacroiliac joint on plain roentgenogram
Treatment—exercises

PREVALENCE AND PATHOGENESIS

Osteitis condensans ilii is a disease characterized by mild back pain and unilateral or bilateral bony sclerosis of the lower ilium with sparing of the sacral portion of the sacroiliac joints. The illness is not progressive and is not associated with functional disability. The major difficulty with osteitis condensans ilii is that it is frequently confused with ankylosing spondylitis (AS).

The prevalence of osteitis condensans ilii has been estimated to be 1.6% in the Japanese and 3% in Scandinavians.[1, 2] The usual patient is a woman, 30 to 40 years of age. The ratio of women to men is 9:1 or greater.

The pathogenesis of osteitis condensans ilii is unknown. Urinary tract infections, inflammatory diseases of the sacroiliac joint, and abnormal mechanical stresses have been suggested as possible etiologies of this illness. Urinary tract infections may reach the ilium via nutrient arteries, resulting in reactive sclerosis.[3] The absence of a history of urinary tract infection in many individuals makes this mechanism unlikely. Others have suggested that osteitis condensans ilii is a subset of AS.[4] One study reported that a third of a population of women with osteitis subsequently developed AS. However, histocompatibility testing for HLA-B27 has not documented increased incidence of this antigen in osteitis patients.[5] In addition, part of the confusion of differentiating osteitis condensans ilii and AS is the milder form of the latter illness in women.[6] Careful review of the clinical symptoms and radiographic findings of the two groups of patients demonstrates the clear-cut differences that exist between the two illnesses (Table 11–7).

A more likely cause of osteitis condensans ilii is mechanical stress across the sacroiliac joint in association with pregnancy and diastasis of the symphysis pubis. Autopsy studies have suggested that a normal physiologic zone of hyperostosis on the anterior iliac margin of the sacroiliac joint may become exaggerated in response to abnormal stresses.[7] Abnormal stresses are placed across the sacroiliac joints during pregnancy.[5] However, this fact alone would not explain the occasional man with osteitis or woman who develops osteitis without having been pregnant. Therefore, the mechanical stresses that cause osteitis condensans ilii must be commonly but not exclusively associated with pregnancy. Diastasis of the symphysis pubis may explain this clinical occurrence. Diastasis of the pubis occurs frequently during pregnancy secondary to relaxin, a product of the corpus of pregnancy, which allows greater laxity of the supporting structures (ligaments) of the pelvis.[8] Patients may actually notice movement or a "popping" sensation in the sacroiliac joints and pubis. Diastasis may occur in as many as 1 in 600 deliveries.[9] Diastasis is not exclusively related to pregnancy but may occur secondary to trauma. Individuals with diastasis related to trauma, both men and women, may be at risk of developing osteitis condensans ilii.

CLINICAL HISTORY

The major symptom of osteitis condensans ilii is low back pain, which occurs in 30% of patients. The pain is dull, localized to one or the other side of the midline, with radiation into the buttock, on occasion. The pain is not exacerbated by coughing, sneezing, or straining at stool but may be increased with menstruation. Not uncommonly, women notice the onset of pain during pregnancy or the postpartum period. Morning stiffness is usually mild, lasting less than an hour. The episodes of pain may have a duration of weeks to months. The disease may then go into a complete or partial remission, which may last for years. A small proportion of patients may complain of fibrositic symptoms characterized by widespread musculoskeletal aching and local point tenderness.[10]

PHYSICAL EXAMINATION

Physical examination may demonstrate tenderness on sacroiliac joint percussion, pain with sacroiliac joint motion, and mild limitation of motion. The rest of the physical examination is normal.

LABORATORY DATA

Laboratory values are generally normal in patients with osteitis condensans ilii. Hematocrit, white blood count, platelets, urinalysis, and chemistry studies are normal. Rheumatoid factor and antinuclear antibody are negative.

RADIOGRAPHIC EVALUATION

The radiographic findings include an area of triangular sclerosis on the iliac aspect of the sacroiliac joint. The bony sclerosis is unassociated with joint erosions or extensive involvement of the sacrum (Figs. 11–25 and 11–26). The radiographic changes may resolve over time. There are no characteristic abnormali-

TABLE 11–7. SACROILIAC JOINT SCLEROSIS

	OSTEITIS CONDENSANS ILII	ANKYLOSING SPONDYLITIS	OSTEOARTHRITIS	METASTATIC TUMOR (PROSTATE)
Age	30–40	20–40	60	60
Sex	Women greater than men	Men greater than women	Equal	Men
Distribution	Bilateral or unilateral	Bilateral	Bilateral or unilateral	Unilateral
Erosions	Absent	Common	Absent	Uncommon
Osteophytes	Rare	Rare	Common	Absent
Ligamentous calcification	Absent	Common	Rare	Absent
Intra-articular bony ankylosis	Absent	Common	Rare	Absent

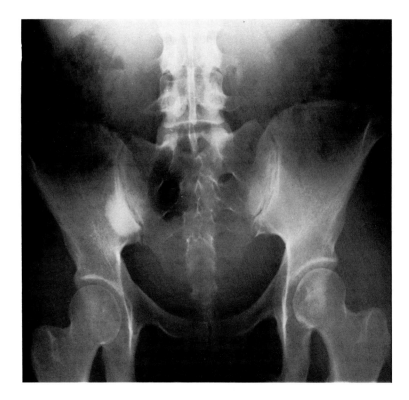

Figure 11–25. Osteitis condensans ilii. AP view of pelvis demonstrating a well-defined triangular shaped area of sclerosis limited to the iliac side of the sacroiliac joint. The joint space is well defined. Although these changes are usually bilateral, this woman had asymmetric involvement.

ties in other portions of the lumbar, thoracic, or cervical spine.[1]

DIFFERENTIAL DIAGNOSIS

The diagnosis of osteitis condensans ilii is based on the presence of radiographic changes on the iliac side of the sacroiliac joint and absence of findings consistent with spondylitis. Patients with spondyloarthropathy have more persistent low back pain associated with more stiffness and limitation of motion. Radiographic changes of spondyloarthropathy are characterized by erosion on both sides of the sacroiliac joints (Table 11–7).[11] CT scan may be helpful in differentiating the presence of sclerosis with joint space abnormalities from those with bony sclerosis alone.[12] Other processes that might cause confusion in diagnosis include septic arthritis with bacteria or tuberculosis, Paget's disease, or tumor. The clinical features of these illnesses and the associated radiographic changes help distinguish the specific diseases.

Septic arthritis secondary to tuberculosis or bacterial infection causes changes on both sides of the joint. Paget's disease is associated with lytic and blastic changes on roentgeno-

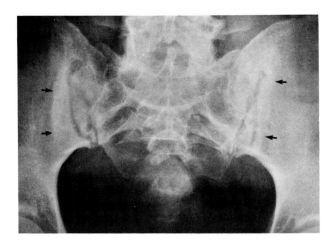

Figure 11–26. Osteitis condensans ilii. AP view of the pelvis of a 57-year-old woman demonstrating bilateral sclerosis of the iliac portions of the sacroiliac joints (*black arrows*). The woman was asymptomatic in regard to low back pain.

grams and increased serum alkaline phosphatase. Osteoblastic tumors, metastatic to the ilium, will increase in size on a rapid basis. The rapid rate of growth helps differentiate tumors from osteitis condensans ilii. Patients with metastatic lesions to the ilium with sclerosis that resembles osteitis condensans ilii frequently have persistent, progressive back pain that would be out of character for patients with primary osteitis.[13]

TREATMENT

The majority of patients benefit from a conservative regimen of a firm mattress for sleeping, local wet or dry heat, and exercises. Nonsteroidal anti-inflammatory drugs are rarely required. Surgical intervention for pelvic instability is reserved for patients with severe symptoms. Internal fixation of the sacroiliac joint and symphysis pubis may be necessary.[14]

PROGNOSIS

The course of osteitis condensans ilii is benign. In many circumstances the radiographic changes may reverse to normal.[2] Low back pain may persist for months but is responsive to therapy. Low back pain of osteitis condensans ilii does not cause decreased motion of the lumbosacral spine. This illness is not associated with disability, and patients are able to continue to work even though they experience symptoms of the illness.

References

OSTEITIS CONDENSANS ILII

1. Numaguchi Y: Osteitis condensans ilii, including its resolution. Radiology 98:1, 1971.
2. Wassman K: Osteitis condensans ilii. Acta Med Scand 151:151, 1955.
3. Wells J: Osteitis condensans ilii. AJR 76:1141, 1956.
4. Thompson M: Osteitis condensans ilii and its differentiation from ankylosing spondylitis. Ann Rheum Dis 13:147, 1954.
5. Singal DP, deBosset P, Gordon DA, et al.: HLA antigens in osteitis condensans ilii and ankylosing spondylitis. J Rheumatol 4(Suppl 3):105, 1977.
6. Resnick D, Dwosh I, Goergen TG, et al.: Clinical and radiographic abnormalities in ankylosing spondylitis. A comparison of men and women. Radiology 119:293, 1976.
7. Dihlmann W: Diagnostic Radiology of the Sacroiliac Joints. New York: Georg Thieme Verlag, 1980, p 104.
8. Szlachter BN, Quagliarello J, Jewelewicz R, et al.: Relaxin in normal and pathogenic pregnancies. Obstet Gynecol 59:167, 1982.
9. Taylor RW, Sonson RD: Separation of the pubic sym-

physis. An underrecognized peripartum complication. J Reprod Med 31:203, 1986.
10. DeBosset P, Gordon DA, Smythe HA, et al.: Comparison of osteitis condensans ilii and ankylosing spondylitis in female patients: clinical, radiological and HLA typing characteristics. J Chron Dis 31:171, 1978.
11. Withrington RH, Sturge RA, Mitchell N: Osteitis condensans ilii or sacro-iliitis? Scand J Rheumatol 14:163, 1985.
12. Olivieri I, Gemignani G, Camerini E, et al.: Differential diagnosis between osteitis condensans ilii and sacroiliitis. J Rheumatol 17:1504, 1990.
13. Parhami N, DiGiacomo R, Jouzevicius JL: Metastatic bone lesions of leiomyosarcoma mimicking osteitis condensans ilii. J Rheumatol 15:1035, 1988.
14. Jenkins DH, Young MH: The operative treatment of sacroiliac subluxation and disruption of the symphysis pubis. Injury 10:139, 1978.

POLYMYALGIA RHEUMATICA (PMR)

Capsule Summary

Frequency of back pain—uncommon

Location of back pain—buttocks, upper thighs

Quality of back pain—diffuse ache with stiffness

Symptoms and signs—morning stiffness, normal strength, diffuse muscle pain in proximal musculature

Laboratory and x-ray tests—elevated erythrocyte sedimentation rate, anemia

Treatment—corticosteroids, 15 to 25 mg daily initially, decreasing doses with improvement

PREVALENCE AND PATHOGENESIS

Polymyalgia rheumatica (PMR) is a clinical syndrome characterized by severe stiffness, tenderness, and aching of the proximal musculature of the upper and lower extremities. Individuals who are 50 years of age or older are most commonly affected by this syndrome. They have an elevated ESR as the primary abnormal laboratory finding. There is no pathognomonic pathologic abnormality that helps physicians diagnose this illness; therefore, other illnesses that may be associated with proximal muscle pain must be eliminated as possible causes of pain before a diagnosis of PMR is made.

The incidence of PMR depends to a great degree on the patient population studied. In one population study of Caucasians over 50 years of age, the incidence of PMR was 19.8 per 100,000 population of individuals 50 to 59 years of age and 112.2 per 100,000 in individuals 70 to 79 years of age. In the total population, the incidence rate was 11 per 100,000 population.[1] The prevalence of the disease increases in older age groups, with a majority of patients being over the age of 60.[2] The male to female ratio is 1:4. PMR is rare in blacks.[3] However, reports of temporal arteritis occurring in black patients have appeared in the literature.[4]

The pathogenesis of PMR is unknown.[5] No familial or genetic predisposition has been shown. Efforts to prove a viral etiology have not been successful.[6] A report of a married couple developing PMR simultaneously is supportive for an environmental pathogenesis of this illness.[7] Also, seasonal clustering associated with the onset of the illness during the summer months (May to August) suggests a temporal or environmental mechanism for the initiation of the illness.[8]

Some have suggested that PMR is an arthritic condition affecting the axial joints.[9, 10] The joints primarily affected include the sternoclavicular and humeroscapular. Synovitis has been demonstrated in these joints on bone scan. However, the relatively small proportion of patients with PMR and synovitis and the distribution of involved joints (relative absence in hip joints) make this mechanism unlikely. Additional studies have been reported supporting the presence or absence of joint disease in PMR patients. Investigations of PMR patients, including radiographic studies and necropsy, have been unable to demonstrate synovitis in patients with PMR.[12, 13] However, clinical reports have presented data describing patients with synovitis that may be confused with rheumatoid arthritis (RA) who develop classic PMR. Studies reporting increased presence of haplotype DR4 in PMR patients provide additional evidence for a relationship between PMR and RA.[14, 15] DR4 is increased in RA patients. This controversy may only be resolved once the etiology of PMR is discovered.

Immunologic mechanisms, including circulating immune complexes, cell-mediated immunity, and shifts in lymphocyte population, have been studied in patients with PMR. No consistent correlation in immune complex amount or composition or in the status of lymphocyte numbers or function has been clearly associated with disease pathogenesis.[16-18] Additional studies have demonstrated alteration in lymphocyte distribution and the elevation in a variety of cytokines, including interleukin-6, and interleukin-2 receptors.[19, 20] However, no consistent correlation has been reported demonstrating normalization of these abnormalities with patient clinical improvement.

A new area of study has been the investigation of muscle from PMR patients by the electron microscope. The mitochondria in affected muscle are abnormal. The mitochondria are enlarged, and, according to one study, 71% contain crystals that may impair their metabolic activity.[21]

From a historic perspective, Barber in 1957 was the first to propose the name of polymyalgia rheumatica for the clinical syndrome. PMR has had numerous names in the past, including senile rheumatic gout, polymyalgia arterica, and anarthritic rheumatoid disease.[22]

CLINICAL HISTORY

The classic picture of PMR is of a woman over 50 years of age who develops pain and stiffness symmetrically in the muscles of the shoulder girdle.[23] Discomfort in the low back, pelvic girdle, thighs, and neck is also commonly experienced. Pain appears initially in the shoulders more commonly than in the low back or pelvis. The pain is worse in the morning, such that getting out of bed is very difficult. Activity lessens the pain. Symptoms reappear when the patient becomes inactive. The onset of symptoms may be abrupt or gradual. There also may be constitutional symptoms, including fever, malaise, fatigue, anorexia, weight loss, and depression. In about a third of patients, a history of a prodromal viral illness may be elicited.

PHYSICAL EXAMINATION

Physical examination demonstrates muscle tenderness on palpation and muscle pain with motion, but atrophy and weakness are not present. Although active range of motion of joints may be limited by pain, passive motion is normal. Back motion is not limited. Occasionally joint swelling, particularly in the sternoclavicular area, may be seen.[24]

LABORATORY DATA

The characteristic laboratory finding is an elevated ESR, which is present in almost every case of PMR.[25] ESR is more sensitive than C-reactive protein for assessment of disease in PMR patients.[26] Patients with active disease also may develop a hypochromic anemia.[27] Increases in leukocytes and platelets may be more closely related to giant cell arteritis (GCA), which may accompany PMR, than to PMR itself.[28] Chemical studies are usually normal except in about a third of patients who have abnormal liver function tests, particularly alkaline phosphatase.[29] Rheumatoid factor and antinuclear antibody are usually negative or present in the same proportion as found in normal age-matched controls. Antimitochondrial antibodies have been reported in a minority of patients with PMR.[30] Their clinical significance remains in doubt. Muscle enzyme levels are normal. Anticardiolipin antibodies, IgG or IgM, are elevated in only 27% of PMR patients, while 80% of GCA patients have antibodies. GCA patients with both antibodies may be at risk for more severe vascular complications.[31]

Pathologic examination of muscle biopsy specimens from patients with PMR are unremarkable.[32] Synovial biopsy demonstrates nonspecific inflammation of the synovium.[33, 34]

RADIOLOGIC FINDINGS

Plain radiographs demonstrate typical changes in the skeleton that might be expected in patients of this age group. PMR is unassociated with any specific radiographic abnormality, but joint scans with technetium pertechnetate may demonstrate increased uptake in the shoulder joints.[35]

DIFFERENTIAL DIAGNOSIS

PMR is a diagnosis made after a number of other diseases with similar symptoms are excluded. Other diseases associated with proximal muscle pain include viral infections, subacute bacterial endocarditis, malignancy, osteoarthritis, RA, polymyositis, giant cell arteritis, fibromyalgia, thyroid dysfunction, and parathyroid dysfunction. A complete history, physical examination, and laboratory evaluation can usually differentiate these diseases. In some instances in which clinical symptoms or laboratory abnormalities are not absolutely characteristic, a tentative diagnosis of PMR is made and therapy is initiated. These patients are then continuously observed to be sure that another illness is not causing their muscle symptoms. When other diseases have been excluded and a patient demonstrates shoulder pain of a month's duration, is 50 years of age or older, has an elevated ESR, and responds to corticosteroid therapy, a diagnosis of PMR can be made.

The diagnosis of PMR should not be entertained until at least 6 weeks after onset of symptoms. Viral syndromes frequently resolve in this time period. Subacute bacterial endocarditis will cause cardiac abnormalities (murmur or change in heart size) that are not associated with PMR. Symptoms of malignancy do not usually respond to the dose of corticosteroids that is effective for PMR. For example, patients with renal cell carcinoma and lymphoma have presented with PMR symptoms resistant to therapy.[36, 37] Osteoarthritis causes symptoms that are maximum at the end of the day and is associated with a normal sedimentation rate. RA will affect more joints in the peripheral skeleton than is usually noted in PMR. In the initial states of RA in the elderly patient, symptoms of arthritis and muscle pain may be difficult to differentiate from those associated with PMR. The presence of rheumatoid nodules may be helpful in these circumstances. In one study, PMR patients were differentiated from RA patients by the presence of upper arm tenderness, the lack of rheumatoid factor, and normal ceruloplasmin levels.[38] Fibromyalgia causes muscle pain in specific locations and is associated with a normal ESR. Signs of thyroid disease (tachycardia, hyperreflexia) and parathyroid disease (polyuria, ulcer disease), for example, should help differentiate these endocrine abnormalities from PMR.

Patients with GCA, an inflammation of blood vessels, frequently have symptoms of PMR.[39] However, in addition to the symptoms of polymyalgia, these patients also have symptoms of headache, pain in the jaw with chewing (jaw claudication), and visual changes. The major complication of GCA is blindness caused by the occlusion of the artery that supplies the retina. The diagnosis of GCA is suspected in a patient with PMR who has headache, visual symptoms, or jaw claudication and has the diagnosis confirmed by biopsy of the temporal artery. GCA patients have ESR that are markedly elevated in almost all patients. In rare circumstances, the ESR may be normal or minimally elevated. This unusual presentation may occur when patients have received lowdose corticosteroids that may suppress the ESR without controlling their disease.[40]

Polymyositis is an inflammatory disease of muscle associated with muscle weakness. Muscle pain occurs in polymyositis in 50% of patients. Muscle weakness and pain occur in the shoulder and pelvic girdle, but low back pain can rarely be an associated symptom. A muscle biopsy showing inflammatory changes helps differentiate polymyositis from PMR.[41] The presence of increased serum creatine kinase concentrations also should raise the suspicion for a diagnosis of polymyositis.[42]

Bird has suggested seven criteria for the diagnosis of PMR. They include: (1) bilateral shoulder pain and stiffness, (2) onset of illness of less than 2 weeks' duration, (3) initial ESR greater than 40 mm/hour, (4) duration of morning stiffness exceeding 1 hour, (5) age 65 years or older, (6) depression and/or weight loss, and (7) bilateral tenderness of the upper arm. The diagnosis of PMR is probable if three or more criteria are met.[43]

TREATMENT

The generally accepted treatment for PMR is daily corticosteroids. Patients with PMR respond rapidly to corticosteroids with dramatic relief of symptoms. The prompt response is regarded as additional confirmation of the diagnosis. The use of steroids may also help relieve the vasculitis that may be associated with GCA. However, the doses needed to control GCA are higher, and patients have been reported to develop GCA while on corticosteroids for PMR.[44–46]

The dose of corticosteroids is usually 15 mg of prednisone every morning. Many patients will have a remarkable diminution of symptoms within 24 to 48 hours.[47] If the patient remains symptomatic, an increase to 25 mg is in order. Doses of 10 mg or less/day of prednisolone are inadequate to control symptoms.[48] If patients remain symptomatic at this dosage, splitting the dose in the morning and evening while limiting any further increase in prednisone dosage may be helpful. Alternate-day therapy is usually not effective.[45] Intramuscular injections of depot methylprednisolone also have been used to control PMR disease activity. An injection of 120 mg every 3 weeks followed by monthly injections resulted in disease control without suppression of the adrenal gland.[49]

The patient's response to therapy is monitored by a normalization of the sedimentation rate. The C-reactive protein (CRP) may fall more rapidly with therapy, and this may be a better indicator of acute response if it can be tested at a convenient clinical laboratory.[50] CRP is a most helpful monitoring response to therapy during the early stages of the illness. Subsequently, ESR is a more sensitive measure of disease activity. As the ESR or CRP normalizes, the prednisone dose may be slowly tapered. Initially the decrements may be made by 2.5 mg until 7.5 mg is reached. The usual time period between reductions is 1 month. Once 7.5 mg is reached, the reductions are 1 mg in magnitude. The goal is to have the patient off corticosteroids by the end of a year, if possible.

Approximately 30% of patients who discontinue steroids before a 2-year period of therapy has been concluded are at risk of a relapse.[51] Patients with an exacerbation of symptoms have an associated rise in ESR. The prednisone should be raised to the patient's initial dosage level. The level can be quickly tapered once symptoms are controlled. After an exacerbation of symptoms, the maintenance dose of prednisone should be kept at a higher level (10 mg) and the pace of tapering slowed to 1 mg every 2 to 3 months. In a study of 210 patients with PMR and GCA, the mean duration of treatment was 25.7 months for PMR and 30.9 months for GCA.[52] Return of hypothalamic-pituitary-adrenal axis function does not require alternate day corticosteroid therapy. Patients who are controlled with the equivalent of 5 mg of prednisone have return of function despite daily doses of medicine. The cumulative dose does not effect return of function.[53]

Corticosteroids have many toxic effects, including osteopenia, which may be particularly troublesome in elderly females. These same women are at greatest risk of developing PMR. Nonsteroidal anti-inflammatory drugs may be useful in diminishing symptoms in PMR patients. They may act as steroid-sparing agents. However, in general, they are useful only in patients with mild disease, whose diagnosis may be called into question. Deflazacort, another form of corticosteroid, is effective for controlling disease activity of PMR without the toxicities associated with prednisone. Cortisol secretion is not suppressed and calcium excretion is increased by deflazacort.[54] A very rare, but potentially serious, manifestation of corticosteroid toxicity is epidural lipomatosis.[55] A patient with epidural lipomatosis is at risk of developing neurologic deficits from neural compression. Immunosuppressive drugs, particularly azathioprine, have been used to decrease steroid dependence of patients with PMR.[56] This is particularly the case in patients with compression fractures secondary to chronic corticosteroid use. The immunosuppressives are not benign drugs and increase a patient's risk of developing an infection or a malignancy. Immunosuppressives should be used only after alternative therapies have been tried.

Patients with GCA require high-dose (60 mg or more) corticosteroids to control disease. These higher doses are necessary to diminish the risk of developing blindness.[44] The frequency of steroid toxicities may be as high as 66% of patients, if weight gain is included as a side effect, with doses of prednisolone of 30 mg/day or greater.[57]

PROGNOSIS

The course of PMR is usually benign. In most patients the disease is controlled. In one study of 76 patients, the mean prednisone dosage required was 22.8 mg/day.[58] Ayoub and coworkers suggest PMR may be divided into two patient populations. The first has limited disease that lasts about 2 years. The second group has disease that is active for 3 to 4 years. These patients require higher doses of corticosteroids for a longer period of time.[58] No specific characteristic could be ascertained that helped predict the classification of individual patients.

References

POLYMYALGIA RHEUMATICA

1. Chuang TY, Hunder GG, Ilbtrup DM, Kurland LT: Polymyalgia rheumatica: a 10-year epidemiologic and clinical study. Ann Intern Med 97:672, 1982.
2. Mowat AG, Hazelman BL: Polymyalgia rheumatica: a clinical study with particular reference to arterial disease. J Rheum 1:190, 1974.
3. Bell W, Klinefelter HF: Polymyalgia rheumatica. Johns Hopkins Med J 121:175, 1967.
4. Bielory L, Ogunkoya A, Frohman LP: Temporal arteritis in blacks. Am J Med 86:707, 1989.
5. Hunder GG, Hazelman BL: Giant cell arteritis and polymyalgia rheumatism. In Kelly W, Harris ED, Ruddy S, Sledge C (eds): Textbook of Rheumatology. Philadelphia: WB Saunders Co, 1981, pp 1189–1196.
6. Liang M, Greenberg H, Pincus T, Robinson WS: Hepatitis B antibodies in polymyalgia rheumatica. Lancet 1:43, 1976.
7. Faerk KK: Simultaneous occurrence of polymyalgia rheumatica in a married couple. J Intern Med 231:621, 1992.
8. Cimmino MA, Caporali R, Montecucco CM, et al.: A seasonal pattern in the onset of polymyalgia rheumatica. Ann Rheum Dis 49:521, 1990.
9. Coomes EN, Sharp J: Polymyalgia rheumatica—a misnomer? Lancet 2:1328, 1961.
10. Bruk MI: Articular and vascular manifestations of polymyalgia rheumatica. Ann Rheum Dis 26:103, 1967.
11. Kyle V, Tudor J, Wriaght EP, et al.: Rarity of synovitis in polymyalgia rheumatica. Ann Rheum Dis 49:155, 1990.
12. Fitzcharles MA, Esdaile JM: Atypical presentations of polymyalgia rheumatica. Arthritis Rheum 33:403, 1990.
13. Healy LA: Polymyalgia rheumatica and seronegative rheumatoid arthritis may be the same entity. J Rheumatol 19:270, 1992.
14. Cid MC, Ercilla G, Vilaseca J, et al.: Polymyalgia rheumatica: a syndrome associated with HLA-DR4 antigen. Arthritis Rheum 31:678, 1990.
15. Sakkas LI, Loqueman N, Panayi GS, et al.: Immunogenetics of polymyalgia rheumatica. Br J Rheumatol 29:331, 1990.
16. Park JR, Jones JG, Harkiss GD, Hazelman BL: Circulating immune complexes in polymyalgia and giant cell arteritis. Ann Rheum Dis 40:360, 1981.
17. Papaioannou CC, Hunder CG, McDuffie FC: Cellular immunity in polymyalgia rheumatica and giant cell arteritis: lack of response to muscles or artery homogenates. Arthritis Rheum 22:740, 1979.
18. Chelazzi G, Broggini M: Abnormalities of peripheral blood T lymphocyte subsets in polymyalgia rheumatica. Clin Exp Rheum 2:333, 1984.
19. Dasgupta D, Panayi GS: Interleukin-6 in serum of patients with polymyalgia rheumatica and giant cell arteritis. Br J Rheumatol 29:456, 1990.
20. Salvarini C, Macchioni P, Boiardi L, et al.: Soluble interleukin-2 receptors in polymyalgia rheumatica/giant cell arteritis. Clinical and laboratory correlations. J Rheumatol 19:1100, 1992.
21. Fassbender R, Simmling-Annefeld M: Ultrastructural examination of the skeletal muscles in polymyalgia rheumatica. J Pathol 137:181, 1982.
22. Barber HS: Myalgic syndrome with constitutional effects: polymyalgia rheumatica. Ann Rheum Dis 16:230, 1957.
23. Fernandez-Herlihy L: Polymyalgia rheumatica. Semin Arthritis Rheum 1:236, 1971.
24. Miller LD, Stevens MB: Skeletal manifestations of polymyalgia rheumatica. JAMA 240:27, 1978.
25. Healy LA, Parker F, Wilske KR: Polymyalgia rheumatica and giant cell arteritis. Arthritis Rheum 14:138, 1971.
26. Kyle V, Cawston TE, Hazelman BL: Erythrocyte sedimentation rate and C-reactive protein in the assessment of polymyalgia rheumatica/giant cell arteritis on presentation and during follow-up. Ann Rheum Dis 48:667, 1989.
27. Gordon I: Polymyalgia rheumatica: a clinical study of 21 cases. Q J Med 29:473, 1960.
28. Bengtsson BA, Malmvall BE: Giant cell arteritis. Acta Med Scand (Suppl)658:1, 1982.
29. Von Knorring, Wasastjerna C: Liver involvement in polymyalgia rheumatica. Scand J Rheum 8:197, 1976.
30. Sattar MA, Cawley MID, Hamblin TJ, Robertson JC: Polymyalgia rheumatica and antimitochondrial antibodies. Ann Rheum Dis 43:264, 1984.
31. Espinoza LR, Jara LJ, Silveira LH, et al.: Anticardiolipin antibodies in polymyalgia rheumatica-giant cell arteritis: association with severe vascular complications. Am J Med 90:474, 1991.
32. Brooke MH, Kaplan H: Muscle pathology in rheumatoid arthritis, polymyalgia rheumatica and polymyositis: a histochemical study. Arch Pathol 94:101, 1972.
33. Gordon I, Rennie AM, Branwood AW: Polymyalgia rheumatica: biopsy studies. Ann Rheum Dis 23:447, 1964.
34. Chou C, Schumacher HR Jr: Clinical and pathologic studies of synovitis in polymyalgia rheumatica. Arthritis Rheum 27:1107, 1984.
35. O'Duffy JD, Wahner HW, Hunder GG: Joint imaging in polymyalgia rheumatica. Mayo Clin Proc 51:519, 1976.
36. Sidhom DA, Basalaev M, Sigal LH: Renal cell carcinoma presenting as polymyalgia rheumatica. Resolution after nephrectomy. Arch Intern Med 153:2043, 1993.
37. Montanaro M, Bizzarri F: Non-Hodgin's lymphoma and subsequent acute lymphoblastic leukemia in a

patient with polymyalgia rheumatica. Br J Rheumatol 31:277, 1992.

38. Hantzschel H, Bird HA, Seidel W, et al.: Polymyalgia rheumatica and rheumatoid arthritis of the elderly: a clinical, laboratory, and scintigraphic comparison. Ann Rheum Dis 50:619, 1991.

39. Hamilton CR, Shelley WM, Tumulty PA: Giant cell arteritis including temporal arteritis and polymyalgia rheumatica. Medicine 50:1, 1971.

40. Wise CM, Agudelo CA, Chmelewski WL, et al.: Temporal arteritis with low erythrocyte sedimentation rate: a review of five cases. Arthritis Rheum 34:1571, 1991.

41. Bohan A, Peter JB, Bowman RL, Pearson CM: A computer-assisted analysis of 153 patients with polymyositis and dermatomyositis. Medicine 56:255, 1977.

42. Hopkinson ND, Shawe DJ, Gumpel JM: Polymyositis, not polymyalgia rheumatica. Ann Rheum Dis 50:321, 1991.

43. Bird HA, Esselinck W, Dixon AS, et al.: An evaluation of criteria for polymyalgia rheumatica. Ann Rheum Dis 38:434, 1979.

44. Hunder GG, Allen GL: Giant cell arteritis: a review. Bull Rheum Dis 29:980, 1978.

45. Hunder GG, Sheps SG, Allen GI, Joyce JW: Daily and alternate day corticosteroid regimens in treatment of giant cell arteritis: comparison in prospective study. Ann Intern Med 82:613, 1975.

46. Papadakis MA, Schwartz ND: Temporal arteritis after normalization of erythrocyte sedimentation rate in polymyalgia rheumatica. Arch Intern Med 146:2283, 1986.

47. Davison S, Spiera H: Concepts and treatment in polymyalgia rheumatica. J Mt Sinai Hosp NY 35:473, 1968.

48. Kyle V, Hazelman BL: Treatment of polymyalgia rheumatica and giant cell arteritis. I. Steroid regimens in the first two months. Ann Rheum Dis 48:658, 1989.

49. Dasgupta B, Gray J, Fernandes L, et al.: Treatment of polymyalgia rheumatica with intramuscular injection of depot methylprednisolone. Ann Rheum Dis 50:942, 1991.

50. Mallya RK, Hind CR, Berry H, Pepys MB: Serum C-reactive protein in polymyalgia rheumatica. A prospective serial study. Arthritis Rheum 28:383, 1985.

51. Fauchald P, Rygvold O, Ystsese B: Temporal arteritis and polymyalgia rheumatica: clinical and biopsy findings. Ann Intern Med 77:845, 1972.

52. Delecoeuillerie G, Joly P, Cohen de Lara A, et al.: Polymyalgia rheumatica and temporal arteritis: a retrospective analysis of prognostic features and different corticosteroid regimens (1 year survey of 210 patients). Ann Rheum Dis 47:733, 1989.

53. LaRochelle GE, LaRochelle AG, Ratner RE, et al.: Recovery of the hypothalamic-pituitary-adrenal (HPA) axis in patients with rheumatic disease receiving low dose prednisone. Am J Med 95:258, 1993.

54. Gray RE, Doherty GM, Galloway J, et al.: A double-blind study of deflazacort and prednisone in patients with chronic inflammatory disorders. Arthritis Rheum 34:287, 1991.

55. Taborn J: Epidural lipomatosis as a cause of spinal cord compression in polymyalgia rheumatica. J Rheumatol 18:286, 1991.

56. De Silva M, Hazelman BL: Azathioprine in giant cell arteritis polymyalgia rheumatica: a double-blind study. Ann Rheum Dis 45:136, 1986.

57. Kyle V, Hazelman BL: Treatment of polymyalgia rheumatica and giant cell arteritis. II. Relation between steroid dose and steroid associated side effects. Ann Rheum Dis 48:662, 1989.

58. Ayoub WT, Franklin CM, Torretti D: Polymyalgia rheumatica. Duration of therapy and long-term outcome. Am J Med 69:309, 1985.

FIBROMYALGIA

Capsule Summary

Frequency of back pain—common
Location of back pain—buttocks
Quality of back pain—general ache, sharp pain with pressure over tender points
Symptoms and signs—generalized fatigue "never rested," muscle soreness, multiple tender points
Laboratory and x-ray tests—normal
Treatment—rest, antidepressants, nonsteroidal anti-inflammatory drugs

PREVALENCE AND PATHOGENESIS

Fibromyalgia is a soft tissue, pain amplification syndrome. It is characterized by chronic pain in discrete tender point areas, and specific sleep disturbance that occurs in a perfectionist, compulsive individual. Fibromyalgia is unassociated with any structural abnormalities of muscle, bone, or cartilage. However, the persistent pain and chronic fatigue associated with the illness prevents patients from achieving their full potential.

The prevalence and incidence of fibromyalgia is unknown; however, many primary care physicians believe fibromyalgia to be a very common ailment with over 10 million Americans affected.[1] In the family practice setting 2.1% of patients have fibromyalgia.[2] The disease occurs most commonly in Caucasian women with a mean age of 29 years.[3]

The exact etiology of the disease is unknown. Moldofsky has suggested that specific disturbances in sleep may result in patients developing fibromyalgia. The abnormality in sleep is the superimposition of light stages of sleep, characterized by alpha waves on electroencephalogram, on deep stages of sleep, characterized by delta waves (non-REM sleep).[4] In a second study, Moldofsky produced fibrositic symptoms in healthy volunteers when their deep sleep was interrupted by loud noises over a 3-day period.[5] Sleep disturbances are frequent complaints of patients with fibromyalgia.[6, 7] Fibromyalgia may be a disorder of nonrestorative sleep in which a disorder of serotonin metabolism results in musculoskeletal pain. Chlorpromazine, a drug that increases delta sleep, decreased patients' pain and tender points in one study.[7] However, the role of sleep in the pathogenesis of fibromyalgia remains in question, since other studies have not been able to reproduce the findings of Moldofsky and other groups of patients (those with depression) have similar sleep disturbances without pain.[8–10]

Abnormalities with sleep are thought to disorder the processing of painful stimuli by the CNS.[11] These abnormalities can lower pain thresholds. Substance P levels in the CNS (not in serum) are higher in fibromyalgia patients than in normals.[12, 13] Other measures of CNS dysfunction include abnormal cortisol response, decreased somatomedin C levels, and decreased serotonin levels.[14–16] These abnormalities are not exclusive to fibromyalgia and may be of secondary importance and not the mechanism causing the disease.

Fowler has suggested that patients with fibromyalgia have increased muscle tone.[17] When performing a standardized task, they have 50% more electrical activity on electromyogram than do normal controls. In a study of fatigue characteristics as measured by surface integrated electromyographic activity, fibromyalgia patients had similar findings as normals.[18] Individuals with increased muscle tension and abnormal sleep patterns may be at risk of developing fibromyalgia. Muscle metabolism may be disordered in patients with fibromyalgia. A decrease in levels of adenosine triphosphate, adenosine diphosphate, and phosphoryl creatine and an increase in the levels of adenosine monophosphate and creatine were found in trapezius muscle of patients with fibromyalgia. These findings suggest that the source of pain in patients with fibromyalgia may be local tissue hypoxia.[19]

Smythe has suggested that trauma in a single incident or repeated episodes may be a cause of fibromyalgia.[20] In the anxious, perfectionist-type individual, trauma in areas of increased sensitivity may result in perpetuation of pain long after the injury and associated pain should have subsided. For example, cab drivers may develop cervical fibromyalgia, while bus drivers may develop fibromyalgia of the back. The association of trauma and fibromyalgia remains a conjecture at this time, since no prospective study has been completed that demonstrates this association. The relationship between trauma in the workplace and fibromyalgia remains to be determined.[21]

Fibromyalgia was also thought to be a psychogenic disorder and was classified with psychogenic rheumatism.[22] Most recent studies have shown no increased prevalence of psychologic disorders in patients with fibromyalgia compared with normal controls.[23] The majority of patients with fibromyalgia do not have any psychiatric disorder.[24] Some of the psychiatric difficulties associated with these patients may be related to chronic pain and dysfunction.[25]

The concept of fibromyalgia has evolved over many years. The central theme of the disease has been the tender point or fibrositic nodule, which was first described in 1824 by Balfour.[26] These areas were tender only with pressure. This was in contrast with trigger points, which were soft tissue regions that spontaneously caused radiating pain.[27] Myofascial pain syndromes were defined as muscle disorders with symptoms that were amplified by abnormalities in the CNS.[28] Subsequently, Gowers introduced the term fibrositis, although no inflammatory alterations could be identified in muscle.[29] More recently, a specific set of symptoms and signs have become associated with the disorder.[30] Although some authors do not believe that fibrositis or fibromyalgia, as it has been recently named, is a distinct entity, this disease has been reported by other rheumatologists to have a prevalence in the United States of 3 to 6 million.[31, 32]

CLINICAL HISTORY

Patients with fibromyalgia complain of generalized aching pain associated with profound stiffness and fatigue. Areas of pain are confined to articular and periarticular structures, including ligaments, tendons, muscles, and bony prominences. The pain may be unremitting with durations of 20 years or longer. Generalized stiffness is most notable in the morning, usually lasting up to an hour. A smaller percentage of patients have evening stiffness, while some patients have day-long stiffness. Fatigue is also a prominent feature. Characteristically, these patients arise in the morning after a restless sleep, feeling exhausted. Some patients complain of unrelenting fatigue. Other clinical features include polyarthralgias, occasionally associated with hand swelling, numbness, headaches, and anxiety.

Cold or humid weather, overactivity, total inactivity, and poor sleep exacerbate fibromyalgia. Patients with fibromyalgia have increased symptoms with changes in barometric pressure.[33] Factors that improve symptoms include moderate activity, warm, dry weather, and massage.

Fibromyalgia also occurs in older patients who have similar clinical findings as younger patients. In a study of 31 older patients with fibromyalgia, only 17% had the disease diagnosed before referral to a rheumatologist. A significant proportion of these patients were treated inappropriately with corticosteroids.[34]

PHYSICAL FINDINGS

Physical examination demonstrates specific areas that are tender to palpation. These areas are referred to as tender points and are localized to certain anatomic sites. The most commonly affected areas include the upper border of the trapezius, medial part of the knees, lateral border of the elbows, posterior iliac crest, and lumbar spine. Pressure over the area results in a pattern of local pain (Fig. 11–27). There is no tenderness outside the local area. In one study, patients had 4 to 33 tender points.[3] Usually patients with primary fibromyalgia have 12 or more discrete areas. The exact location that differentiates patients with fibromyalgia from controls continues to be evaluated. Some areas that may be useful include the anterior shoulder, anterior chest, posterior scapula, and medial knee.[35]

Patients with fibromyalgia may have "fibrositic" nodules located about the sacrum and posterior iliac crest. The nodules are mobile, firm, and tender to palpation. Biopsy of these nodules demonstrates fibrofatty tissue without inflammation. Besides the findings of tender points and nodules, the physical examination is normal, with full range of motion of the lumbosacral spine.

LABORATORY DATA

Laboratory parameters are normal. Blood chemistries, hematologic parameters, ESR, rheumatoid factor, and antinuclear antibody are all normal in primary fibromyalgia. Among the findings that are normal are serum tryptophan levels, absence of autoantibodies, and distribution of HLA antigens.[36–38]

Pathologic evaluation of muscle biopsies are unrevealing on histo-immuno-chemical and ultrastructural study. The biopsy may be only important to eliminate other disorders as the cause of muscle pain.[39]

RADIOGRAPHIC EVALUATION

Radiographic findings are normal in patients with fibromyalgia. The results of bone

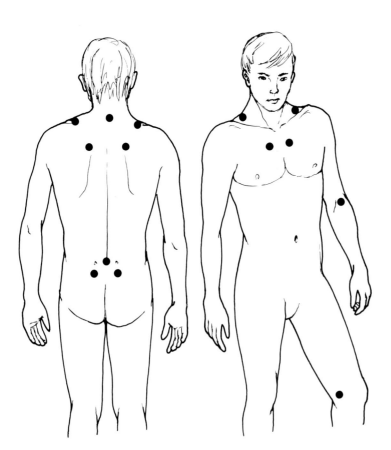

Figure 11–27. Diagram of common sites of tenderness on palpation in fibromyalgia patients.

scintiscans are no different in fibromyalgia patients than normals.[40]

DIFFERENTIAL DIAGNOSIS

The diagnosis of primary fibromyalgia is based on the presence of characteristic musculoskeletal abnormalities in the absence of stigmata of other diseases. Patients with diffuse aching and fatigue of at least 3 months' duration, at least 12 tender points, and disturbed sleep patterns probably have fibromyalgia. There are no specific physical or laboratory findings that are pathognomonic for this illness. Therefore, the diagnosis is one of exclusion, and these patients require constant re-evaluation. A variety of diagnostic criteria have been proposed.[3, 30] Goldenberg has divided the clinical characteristics of the disease into major and minor criteria (Table 11–8).[41] The presence of three major criteria and four of six minor criteria is necessary for the diagnosis of fibromyalgia by Goldenberg's approach. In 1990, a committee of the American College of Rheumatology presented classification criteria for fibromyalgia (Table 11–9).[42]

Repeat evaluation is necessary to detect early physical or laboratory findings that are indicative of an underlying disease process, such as rheumatoid arthritis or a malignancy. Patients with an underlying illness and muscle pain have secondary fibromyalgia. Other illnesses associated with secondary fibromyalgia include rheumatoid arthritis, osteoarthritis, spondyloarthropathies, connective tissue diseases, malignancies, hypothyroidism, hyperparathyroidism, chronic infections, and sarcoidosis.[43] Patients with HIV infection also may develop fibromyalgia.[44] Characteristic physical findings, inflammatory joint signs, laboratory abnormal-

TABLE 11–8. DIAGNOSTIC CRITERIA FOR FIBROMYALGIA

MAJOR CRITERIA
Chronic, generalized aches, pains, or stiffness (involving ≥ 3 anatomic sites for ≥ 3 mo)
Absence of other systemic condition to account for these symptoms
Multiple tender points at characteristic locations

MINOR CRITERIA
Disturbed sleep
Generalized fatigue or tiredness
Subjective swelling, numbness
Pain in neck, shoulders
Chronic headaches
Irritable bowel symptoms

Modified from Goldenberg DL: Fibromyalgia syndrome: an emerging but controversial condition. JAMA 257:2782, 1987.

TABLE 11–9. AMERICAN COLLEGE OF RHEUMATOLOGY CLASSIFICATION CRITERIA FOR FIBROMYALGIA

1. History of widespread pain. Pain is on both sides of the body and above and below the waist. Low back pain is considered lower segment pain.

2. Pain in 11 of 18 tender points on digital palpation—4 kg of force should be applied with digital pressure. The site must be painful not tender.

Widespread pain should be present for 3 months or more. A second clinical disorder does not exclude the diagnosis of fibromyalgia.

Modified from Wolfe F, et al: The American College of Rheumatology 1990 criteria for the classification of fibromyalgia: Report of the multicenter criteria committee. Arthritis Rheum 33:160, 1990.

ities, elevated ESR, and positive rheumatoid factor help differentiate these illnesses from primary fibromyalgia.

Fibromyalgia must also be differentiated from psychogenic rheumatism, which is characterized by significant anxiety, depression, or neurosis.[45] Patients with psychogenic rheumatism have severe pain of a burning or cutting quality. The pain is excruciating in intensity and without any recognizable anatomic boundaries. The patients usually deny stiffness. On examination, they have a marked response to minimal pressure on palpation. Their areas of tenderness do not correspond to the tender points of fibromyalgia. The laboratory evaluation of these patients is normal, and their complaints are resistant to all forms of therapy.

Chronic fatigue syndrome is another disorder that has a clinical spectrum that overlaps with fibromyalgia. This syndrome is associated with chronic fatigue that does not resolve with bed rest, no other complicating illness, mild fever, sore throat, painful lymph nodes, muscle weakness, headaches, arthralgias, and insomnia.[46] The severity of fatigue is greater in patients with chronic fatigue syndrome. In a review of patients with fibromyalgia only 20% fulfilled the criteria of fatigue.[47]

Myofascial Pain Syndrome

Myofascial pain syndrome (MPS) is a regional pain syndrome characterized by two major components: (1) a localized area of deep muscle tenderness (trigger point) that is accompanied by a palpable abnormality in muscle consistency (fibrositic nodule), and (2) a specific area of referral pain distant from the trigger point.[48] The muscles in MPS have the characteristics of being extremely tender to palpation, decreased flexibility, abnormal consistency, pain with contraction, and localized "twitch response" to rapid snapping of the trigger point or fibrositic nodule. Pressure over a trigger point results in a dull, aching pain in a referral pattern that does not follow any characteristic myotomal structure. Low back pain is a common symptom associated with MPS.[49] Pain location and muscles associated with MPS are listed in Table 11–10. MPS and fibromyalgia are not the same illness although superficially they seem quite similar. MPS is a localized pain syndrome, with sudden onset, and trigger points with distant referred pain. Fibromyalgia is a diffuse pain syndrome with gradual onset, multiple tender points, and disturbed sleep. Controversy remains in whether MPS exists as a separate clinical entity. The characteristic clinical findings of MPS, including trigger points, may not be differentiated in patients with MPS from patients with fibromyalgia or normal control subjects.[50] Therapy for MPS consists of local injection of trigger points along with the use of superficial cooling in association with muscle stretching.

TREATMENT

Treatment of fibromyalgia requires a multifactorial approach. In many circumstances, educating patients about their illness is reassuring and relieves some symptoms. Many patients are encouraged by having a specific diagnosis for their ailments. Their symptoms are no longer "in their head." They are told that their condition is not life-threatening, deforming, or degenerating but causes chronic pain.

The therapy of fibromyalgia is multifaceted.[51] Rest and relaxation are important for patients who are overworked. Patients are encouraged to remain at work, but they should not become excessively fatigued.[3] Some patients require a change in their job status to lighter-duty work. Range of motion and stretching exercises encourage improved mus-

cle function. Heat treatments are also useful. Drug therapy in the form of aspirin or other nonsteroidal anti-inflammatory agents is helpful in reducing the pain associated with fibrositis.[43] Injection of tender points with a combination of anesthetic agent and a long-acting corticosteroid is helpful in controlling localized pain.[52] Systemic corticosteroids are not used in patients with primary fibromyalgia. Narcotics are also not indicated for this disease.

With the thought that abnormal serotonin metabolism plays a role in the pathogenesis of fibromyalgia, antidepressants and muscle relaxants that increase serotonin levels have been studied in controlled short-term placebo-based drug trials. Cyclobenzaprine hydrochloride (Flexeril), a tricyclic muscle relaxant, at dosages of 10 to 40 mg/day caused significant improvement in pain, sleep, and tender points compared with placebo.[53] Improvement was also seen in a study with another tricyclic drug, amitriptyline hydrochloride (Elavil), at a dose of 50 mg at bedtime.[54] Amitriptyline, when effective, results in decreased symptoms within 2 weeks of starting therapy.[55] Imipramine hydrochloride at 50 to 75 mg/day had no beneficial effect on the symptoms of fibrositis.[56]

The basic program of therapy for a patient with fibromyalgia is a tricyclic agent along with patient education and controlled activity in a physical therapy program. The addition of a nonsteroidal agent is optional, dependent on the patient's muscle pain. Injection of tender points is useful if they are few in number.

All these modes of therapy do have a beneficial effect on the symptoms of fibromyalgia; however, fibromyalgia is a chronic illness that may be exacerbated by a number of factors, including increased tension, cold exposure, or sleep disturbances. Compliance with a program is essential for the long-term management of these individuals. Appropriate rest, exercise, and stress management may control disease symptoms without the need to use medications or injections.

TABLE 11–10. PAIN LOCATION AND MUSCLES ASSOCIATED WITH MYOFASCIAL PAIN SYNDROME

MUSCLE WITH TRIGGER POINT	REFERRED PAIN DISTRIBUTION
Quadratus lumborum	Buttock, sacrum, abdominal wall
Iliopsoas	Paravertebral lumbar spine, anterior thigh
Pelvic floor (obturator internus, levator ani)	Sacrum, posterior thigh
Gluteus maximus	Sacrum, buttock
Gluteus medius	Sacrum, buttock, lateral thigh
Gluteus minimus	Buttock, lateral thigh, lateral calf
Piriformis	Buttock, posterior thigh

Men with fibromyalgia may have sleep apnea as a cause of their chronic pain syndrome. These patients may benefit from therapy directed at improving their sleep apnea.[57]

PROGNOSIS

The course of fibromyalgia is one of exacerbations and remissions. The patients have low back, neck, knee, and chest pain that hinders their ability to perform up to their potential. Wood, in a study of English workers, reported that nonarticular rheumatism, which included patients with fibromyalgia, accounted for 10.9% of absences from work and corresponded to 10.5% of lost days from work.[58] Fibromyalgia may go unrecognized for an extended period. In such circumstances, the patients may be thought of as malingerers who are unwilling to do a full day's work. Fibromyalgia is a chronic condition. The illness is associated with functional disability and high levels of anxiety and depression despite therapy.[59]

Although fibromyalgia is not disabling in the same sense as the spondyloarthropathies, it is associated with reduced productivity and absenteeism. Recognition of the disease and institution of appropriate therapy can have a beneficial effect on the patient's outlook and work performance.

References

FIBROSITIS (FIBROMYALGIA)

1. The American Rheumatism Association Committee on Rheumatologic Practice: A description of rheumatology practice. Arthritis Rheum 20:1278, 1977.
2. Hartz A, Kirchdoerfer E: Undetected fibrositis in primary care practice. J Fam Pract 25:365, 1987.
3. Yunus M, Masi AT, Calabro JJ, et al.: Primary fibromyalgia (fibrositis): clinical study of 50 patients with matched normal controls. Semin Arthritis Rheum 11:151, 1981.
4. Moldofsky H, Scarisbrick P, England R, Smythe H: Musculoskeletal symptoms and non-REM sleep disturbance in patients with "fibrositis syndrome" and healthy subjects. Psychosom Med 37:341, 1975.
5. Moldofsky H, Scarisbrick P: Induction of neurasthenic musculoskeletal pain syndrome by selective sleep stage deprivation. Psychosom Med 38:35, 1976.
6. Campbell SM, Clark S, Tyndall EA, et al.: Clinical characteristics of fibrositis: I. A "blinded" controlled study of symptoms and tender points. Arthritis Rheum 26:817, 1983.
7. Moldofsky A, Lue FA: The relationship of alpha and delta EEG frequencies to pain and mood in fibrositis patients treated with chlorpromazine and L-tryptophan. Electroencephalogr Clin Neurophysiol 50:71, 1980.
8. Golden H, Weber SM, Bergen D: Sleep studies in patients with fibrositis syndrome. Arthritis Rheum 26:S32, 1983.
9. Moldofsky H: Workshop on sleep studies. Am J Med 81(Suppl 3A):107, 1986.
10. Wittig R, Zorick FJ, Blumer D, et al.: Disturbed sleep in patients complaining of chronic pain. J Nerv Ment Dis 170:429, 1982.
11. Yunus MB: Toward a model of pathophysiology of fibromyalgia—aberrant central pain mechanisms with peripheral modulation. J Rheumatol 19:846, 1992.
12. Vaeroy H, Helle R, Forre O, et al.: Elevated CSF levels of substance P and high incidence of Raynaud phenomenon in patients with fibromyalgia: new features for diagnosis. Pain 32:21, 1988.
13. Reynolds WJ, Chiu B, Inman RD: Plasma substance P levels in fibrositis. J Rheumatol 15:1802, 1988.
14. McCain GA, Tilbe KS: Diurnal hormone variation in fibromyalgia syndrome: a comparison with rheumatoid arthritis. J Rheumatol 19(Suppl):154, 1989.
15. Bennett RM, Clark SR, Campbell SM, et al.: Low levels of somatomedin C in patients with the fibromyalgia syndrome—a possible link between sleep and muscle pain. Arthritis Rheum 35:1113, 1992.
16. Russell IJ, Vaeroy H, Javors M, et al.: Cerebrospinal fluid biogenic amine metabolites in fibromyalgia/fibrositis syndrome and rheumatoid arthritis. Arthritis Rheum 35:550, 1992.
17. Fowler RS Jr, Kraft GH: Tension perception in patients having pain associated with chronic muscle tension. Arch Phys Med Rehabil 55:28, 1984.
18. Stokes MJ, Colter C, Klevstov A, et al.: Normal paraspinal muscle electromyographic fatigue characteristics in patients with primary fibromyalgia. Br J Rheumatol 32:71, 1993.
19. Bengtsson A, Henriksson KG, Larsson J: Reduced high-energy phosphate levels in the painful muscle of patients with primary fibromyalgia. Arthritis Rheum 24:817, 1986.
20. Smythe HA: Non-articular rheumatism and psychogenic musculoskeletal syndromes. In McCarty DJ Jr (ed): Arthritis and Allied Conditions, 10th ed. Philadelphia: Lea and Febiger, 1985, pp 1083–1094.
21. Littlejohn GO: Fibrositis/fibromyalgia syndrome in the workplace. Rheum Dis Clin North Am 15:45, 1989.
22. Savage O: Management of rheumatic diseases in the armed forces. Br Med J 2:336, 1942.
23. Clark S, Campbell SM, Forehand ME, et al.: Clinical characteristics of fibrosis. Arthritis Rheum 28:132, 1985.
24. Goldenberg DL: Psychiatric and psychologic aspects of fibromyalgia syndrome. Rheum Dis Clin North Am 15:105, 1989.
25. Merskey H: Physical and psychological considerations in the classification of fibromyalgia. J Rheumatol 16(Suppl) 72, 1989.
26. Balfour W: Observations with case illustrative of a new, simple, and expenditious mode of curing rheumatism and sprains. Lond Med Phys J 51:446, 1824.
27. Kellgren JH: Observations on referred pain arising from muscle. Clin Sci 3:175, 1938.
28. Travell J, Ringler SH: The myofascial genesis of pain. Postgrad Med 11:425, 1952.
29. Gowers WR: Lumbago: its lessons and analogues. Br Med J 1:117, 1904.
30. Wolfe F, Cathey MA: The epidemiology of tender points: a prospective study of 1520 patients. J Rheumatol 12:1164, 1985.
31. Hadler WM: Medical Management of the Regional Musculoskeletal Diseases. New York: Grune and Stratton, 1985.

32. Wallace DJ: Systemic lupus erythematosus, rheumatology, and medical literature: current trends. J Rheumatol 12:913, 1985.

33. Guedj D, Weinberger A: Effect of weather conditions on rheumatic patients. Ann Rheum Dis 49:158, 1990.

34. Yunus MB, Holt GS, Masi AT: Fibromyalgia syndrome among the elderly. Comparison with younger patients. J Am Geriatr Soc 36:987, 1988.

35. Simms RW, Goldenberg DL, Felson DT, et al.: Tenderness in 75 anatomic sites. Distinguishing fibromyalgia patients from controls. Arthritis Rheum 31:182, 1988.

36. Yunus MB, Dailey JW, Aldag JC, et al.: Plasma tryptophan and other amino acids in primary fibromyalgia: a controlled study. J Rheumatol 19:90, 1992.

37. Bengstsson A, Ernerudh J, Vrethem M, et al.: Absence of autoantibodies in primary fibromyalgia. J Rheumatol 17:1682, 1990.

38. Horven S, Stiles TC, Holst A, et al.: HLA antigens in primary fibromyalgia syndrome. J Rheumatol 19:1269, 1992.

39. Drewes Am, Andreasen A, Schnider HD, et al.: Pathology of skeletal muscle in fibromyalgia: a histo-immuno-chemical and ultrastructural study. Br J Rheumatol 32(Suppl):479, 1993.

40. Yunus MB, Berg BC, Masi AT: Multiphase skeletal scintigraphy in primary fibromyalgia syndrome: a blinded study. J Rheumatol 16:1466, 1989.

41. Goldenberg DL: Fibromyalgia syndrome: an emerging but controversial condition. JAMA 257:2782, 1987.

42. Wolfe F, Smythe HA, Yunus MB, et al.: The American College of Rheumatology 1990 criteria for the classification of fibromyalgia: report of the multicenter criteria committee. Arthritis Rheum 33:160, 1990.

43. Beetham WP Jr: Diagnosis and management of fibrositis syndrome and psychogenic rheumatism. Med Clin North Am 63:433, 1979.

44. Simms RW, Zerbini CA, Ferrante N, et al.: Fibromyalgia syndrome in patients infected with human immunodeficiency virus. The Boston City Hospital clinical AIDS team. Am J Med 92:368, 1992.

45. Rotes-Querol J: The syndromes of psychogenic rheumatism. Clin Rheum Dis 5:797, 1979.

46. Holmes GP, Kaplan JE, Gabtz NM, et al.: Chronic fatigue syndrome: A working case definition. Ann Intern Med 108:387, 1988.

47. Norregaard J, Bulow PM, Prescott E, et al.: A four-year follow-up study in fibromyalgia. Relationship to chronic fatigue syndrome. Scand J Rheumatol 22:35, 1993.

48. Travell JG, Simons DG: Myofascial Pain and Dysfunction. The Trigger Point Manual, The Lower Extremities Volume 2. Baltimore: Williams & Wilkins, 1992, pp 607.

49. Campbell SM: Regional myofascial pain syndromes. Rheum Dis Clin North Am 15:31, 1989.

50. Wolfe F, Simons D, Friction J, et al.: The fibromyalgia and myofascial pain syndromes: a study of tender points and trigger points in persons with fibromyalgia, myofascial pain syndrome and no disease (abstract). Arthritis Rheum 33(Suppl):S137, 1990.

51. Goldenberg DL: Treatment of fibromyalgia syndrome. Rheum Dis Clin North Am 15:61, 1989.

52. Kraus H: Triggerpoints. NY State J Med 73:1310, 1973.

53. Clark S, Tindall E, Bennett RM: A double blind cross-over trial of prednisone versus placebo in the treatment of fibrositis. J Rheumatol 12:980, 1985.

54. Carette S, McCain GA, Bell DA, Fam AG: Evaluation of amitriptyline in primary fibrositis. Arthritis Rheum 29:655, 1986.

55. Jaeschke R, Adachi J, Guyatt G, et al.: Clinical usefulness of amitriptyline in fibromyalgia: the results of 23 N-of-1 randomized controlled trials. J Rheumatol 18:447, 1991.

56. Wysenbeek AJ, Mor F, Lurie Y, Weinberger A: Imipramine for the treatment of fibrositis: a therapeutic trial. Ann Rheum Dis 44:752, 1985.

57. May KP, West SG, Baker MR, et al.: Sleep apnea in male patients with the fibromyalgia syndrome. Am J Med 94:505, 1993.

58. Wood PHN: Rheumatic complaints. Br Med Bull 27:82, 1971.

59. Ledingham J, Doherty S, Doherty M: Primary fibromyalgia syndrome—an outcome study. Br J Rheumatol 32:139, 1993.

60. Hudson JI, Goldenberg DL, Pope HG, et al.: Comorbidity of fibromyalgia with medical and psychiatric disorders. Am J Med 92:363, 1992.

12

Infections of the Lumbosacral Spine

Infections of the lumbar spine are uncommon causes of low back pain; however, these disorders must be included in the differential diagnosis of the patient with nonmechanical low back pain. This is particularly important because the prognosis of an infection is excellent if the disease process is recognized early and treated appropriately. When spinal infections are not promptly recognized, however, they can lead to catastrophic complications, including spinal deformity and spinal cord compression with associated paralysis and incontinence.

The clinical symptoms and course of spinal infections are dependent on the organism involved. Bacterial infections cause acute, toxic symptoms, while tuberculous and fungal diseases are more indolent in onset and course. The primary symptom of patients with spinal infection is back pain, which tends to be localized over the anatomic structure involved. Physical examination demonstrates decreased motion, muscle spasm, and percussion tenderness over the involved area. Results of common laboratory tests are nonspecific. Radiographic abnormalities, including vertebral body subchondral bone loss, disc space narrowing, and erosions of contiguous bony structures, are helpful in diagnosis when present but often lag behind clinical symptoms by weeks to months.

The definitive diagnosis of spinal infection requires identification of the offending organism by culturing aspirated and/or surgically excised biopsy material from the lesion. Treatment consists of antimicrobial drugs directed against the specific organism causing the infection, immobilization with bed rest to relieve pain, a cast if spinal instability is present, and surgical drainage of abscesses to relieve spinal cord compression. Patients who have a prompt diagnosis and appropriate antimicrobial therapy are able to combat the infection without residual disability. Significant disability from persistent pain, spinal instability, and spinal cord compression may occur when there has been a delay in diagnosing a persistent osteomyelitis or epidural abscess.

Herpes zoster is a viral infection of dorsal root ganglia that causes severe back pain in association with a skin rash. The diagnosis of this infection is easy in the presence of a dermatomal skin rash but quite difficult in the period before the rash appears. Postherpetic neuralgia, a complication of the infection, causes significant morbidity with persistent back pain particularly in the elderly population.

Lyme disease is a spirochettal infection caused by *Borrelia burgdorferi*. Early manifestations of the illness are back pain and the appearance of a skin rash, erythema chronicum migrans. In later stages, polyradiculitis affecting the lower extremities may develop. The diagnosis of Lyme disease is established by the presence of a history of tick exposure, characteristic symptoms and signs, and the presence of confirmatory laboratory tests. The illness is treated by the use of oral or intravenous antibiotics.

VERTEBRAL OSTEOMYELITIS

Capsule Summary

Frequency of back pain—very common
Location of back pain—lumbar spine or sacrum—involved bone

Quality of back pain—sharp ache

Symptoms and signs—general malaise, percussion tenderness, fever

Laboratory and x-ray tests—leukocytosis, elevated ESR, culture of bone and blood; subchondral bone loss on plain roentgenograms, soft tissue mass on CT scan, abnormal signal on MR

Treatment—antibiotics, immobilization

PREVALENCE AND PATHOGENESIS

Vertebral osteomyelitis is a disease process caused by the growth of a potentially wide variety of organisms in the bones that compose the axial skeleton. These organisms include bacteria—*Staphylococcus aureus, Escherichia coli,* and *Brucella abortus;* mycobacteria—*Mycobacterium tuberculosis;* fungi—*Coccidioides immitis;* spirochetes—*Treponema pallidum;* and parasites—*Echinococcus granulosus.* Vertebral osteomyelitis develops most commonly from hematogenous spread through the blood stream. The clinical symptoms and course are dependent on the infecting organism and the associated host inflammatory response. Bacterial infections are generally associated with an acute, toxic reaction, while granulomatous infections caused by tuberculous or fungal organisms are more indolent in onset and course. The diagnosis of vertebral osteomyelitis is frequently missed because patients' symptoms are ascribed to more common causes of low back pain, such as muscle strain, and radiographic changes lag behind the evolution of the infection. Over the past decade, 348 cases of vertebral osteomyelitis have been reported in the medical literature[1] and it has been found to account for 2% to 4% of all cases of osteomyelitis.[2] A more recent article was able to document 397 patients in the medical literature.[3] The mean range of adults reported with vertebral osteomyelitis was from 45 to 62. In one study, over 52% of patients with vertebral osteomyelitis were 50 years of age or older.[4] Those in their 60s represented the single largest group. The male to female ratio is up to 3:1.

Vertebral body bone is most frequently infected by hematogenous spread through the blood stream. It is supplied by the paravertebral venous system and nutrient arteries.[5, 6] The venous plexus of Batson is a network of valveless veins that lines the vertebral column. The flow in this venous system is modified by changes in intra-abdominal pressure. Increased pressure tends to force blood from infected areas in the pelvis (bladder, gastrointestinal tract) into the veins of the vertebral column. This fact might explain the predisposition of patients with urinary tract infections, rectosigmoid disease, or postpartum infection to vertebral osteomyelitis.[7–9] Although genitourinary infections are more frequent in women than in men, the incidence of vertebral osteomyelitis is higher in men. A possible explanation is the highly vascularized tissue around the longer urethra, which may develop metastatic infection after urologic manipulation.[4] Other potential hematogenous sources of infection include soft tissue infection, infective endocarditis, dental extraction, furunculosis, and intravenous drug abuse.[4, 10]

On the other hand, the localization of early foci of osteomyelitis in vertebral bodies in the subchondral region corresponds to an area richly supplied by nutrient arteries.[6] The spread of infection from extraspinal foci is associated with the constitutional symptoms of septicemia. It is probable that both routes may be involved in individual patients.

Infection from contiguous sources, direct implantation by lumbar puncture or disc operations, is relatively rare compared with infection caused by hematogenous spread. Occasionally, patients with vertebral osteomyelitis may have a history of prior trauma to the spine, but trauma usually does not play a role in the pathogenesis of hematogenous vertebral osteomyelitis.[11] Studies of patients with vertebral osteomyelitis and epidural abscess, however, report a significant percentage with a history of substantial trauma prior to the development of the infection.[12] A hematoma associated with trauma can become a culture medium for hematogenously spread organisms. The role of minor trauma, such as muscle strains, as a predisposing factor for vertebral osteomyelitis is uncertain. The importance of unrelated and coincident minor trauma may be overestimated in patients with vertebral osteomyelitis, thus confusing the diagnosis and delaying the initiation of appropriate antibiotic therapy to the disadvantage of the patient.

Approximately 40% or more of patients with vertebral osteomyelitis have an unequivocal extraspinal primary source for infection. The usual locations for these infections include the genitourinary tract, skin, and respiratory tract (Table 12–1).[13] Parenteral drug abusers also develop vertebral osteomyelitis, particularly with *Pseudomonas aeruginosa.*[14] Any patient with a chronic disease that decreases host immunity, such as diabetes mellitus, chronic alcoholism, malignancy, and sickle cell anemia, is also at risk of developing vertebral osteomyelitis.[3]

The organisms gain entrance into the vertebral bodies in the subchondral area, which is richly supplied by nutrient arterioles on the anterior surface and by the main nutrient artery entering through the posterior vertebral nutrient foramen.[6] The infection may spread across the periphery of the disc to involve the adjacent vertebra or may rupture through the endplates into the disc. The posterior elements are affected less often and later in the course of the infection. The infection spreads through the disc material to reach the opposite endplate and vertebra. The disc material is quickly destroyed by bacterial enzymes. This is in contrast to tuberculous infection, which causes bony destruction but little damage to the intervertebral disc.[15] Infection of three or more vertebral bodies is quite rare. Involvement of the posterior elements of the vertebrae is unusual.

An infection of a vertebral body may extend beyond the bone into the soft tissues. Infections in the lumbar spine can produce a psoas abscess, which can become very large. The infection may also drain into the spinal canal, causing an epidural abscess, or penetrate the dura, causing a picture of meningitis.[12] In addition, bone destruction may cause instability of the spine, which may result in compression of the spinal cord or nerve roots.

The lumbar spine is the most frequently affected area of the spine, followed by the thoracic spine, with the sacrum and cervical spine affected in equal frequencies.[11]

The most frequently encountered organism causing infection is *S. aureus*, which may be

TABLE 12–1. SOURCE OF INFECTION IN PYOGENIC VERTEBRAL OSTEOMYELITIS (n = 370 PATIENTS)

	NO. OF PATIENTS	PERCENT OF PATIENTS WITH SOURCE IDENTIFIED
Source identified	188	
Genitourinary tract	87	46
Skin	35	19
Respiratory tract	27	14
Spinal surgery	16	9
Bowel	7	4
Intravenous drug abuse	6	3
Intravenous catheter	5	3
Dental	4	2
Bacterial endocarditis	1	1
No. source identified	182	

From Schwartz ST, Spiegel M, Ho G, Jr: Bacterial vertebral osteomyelitis and epidural abscess. Semin Spine Surg 2:97, 1990.

TABLE 12–2. BACTERIOLOGY OF PYOGENIC VERTEBRAL OSTEOMYELITIS (n = 220 BACTERIA)

	NO. OF CASES	PERCENT OF BACTERIAL ISOLATES
Gram-positive aerobic cocci	159	72
Staphylococcus aureus	139	
Staphylococcus coagulase-negative	5	63
		2
Streptococcal sp	15	7
Gram-negative aerobic bacilli	55	24
Escherichia coli	35	16
Proteus sp	11	5
Pseudomonas sp	3	1
Klebsiella sp	3	1
Other*	3	1
Anaerobic bacteria†	6	3

Serratia species, *Enterobacter agglomerans, Eikenella corrodens*.
†*Corynebacterium diphtheroides, Bacteroides fragilis, Peptostreptococcus,* and *Propionibacterium.*
From Schwartz ST, Spiegel M, Ho G, Jr: Bacterial vertebral osteomyelitis and epidural abscess. Semin Spine Surg 2:98, 1990.

found in up to 60% of cases (Table 12–2). In rare circumstances, *S. epidermidis* may cause vertebral osteomyelitis in immunocompetent individuals.[16] Other gram-positive organisms include streptococci, including *S. pneumonia*. Group G streptococcal osteomyelitis of the spine has been reported in elderly individuals with malignancies.[17] Gram-negative organisms, including *E. coli, Pseudomoas, Klebsiella, Pasteurella,* and *Salmonella,* are relatively uncommon.[18] Other rare gram-negative organisms include *Proteus mirabilis,* and polymicrobial infections including *Bacteroides fragilis*.[19–21] Anaerobic organisms cause infection in 3% or less of patients.[3, 22] Even more infrequent as causes of infection are mycobacteria, fungi, spirochetes, and parasites.

CLINICAL HISTORY

The primary symptom of patients with vertebral osteomyelitis is low back pain. The pain may develop over 8 to 12 weeks before the diagnosis is established in patients.[13] A history of a recent primary infection, or an invasive diagnostic procedure, is common. The pain may be intermittent or constant, may be present at rest, and is exacerbated by motion. This group of symptoms is one of the four clinical syndromes of pyogenic vertebral osteomyelitis described by Guri.[23] The other three clinical syndromes include patients who may develop a hip joint syndrome characterized by acute pain in the hip with limited motion and flexion contracture. The patient with the abdominal syndrome presents with symptoms that are easily confused with those of appendicitis. Signs of acute meningitis, including positive Kernig and Brudzinski tests and positive straight leg raising tests, are components of the meningeal syndrome. Paraplegia without back pain is a very rare occurrence.[24]

Patients with certain underlying illnesses may develop vertebral osteomyelitis secondary to specific organisms. *S. aureus* is associated with soft tissue infection, endocarditis, or infected intravenous lines. Pneumococci are associated with respiratory infection. Those with diabetes mellitus or chronic urinary tract infections develop vertebral osteomyelitis secondary to gram-negative bacteria.[11] Parenteral drug abusers develop *Pseudomonas* and *Candida* osteomyelitis.[25] Patients with sickle-cell anemia may get *Salmonella* osteomyelitis.[26] Fungal osteomyelitis secondary to candida has been reported to complicate vertebral osteomyelitis previously infected with *Serratia marcescens.*[27]

Brucellosis, a disease caused by *Brucella* species, affects patients who ingest unpasteurized milk products or more commonly, since the advent of pasteurization, workers involved with meat processing.[26] The infection, passed from lower animals, cattle or hogs, to humans occurs in government meat inspectors, veterinarians, farmers, stockmen, rendering-plant workers, and laboratory personnel. The *Brucella* organism, *B. melitensis* (the most virulent), *B. suis, B. canis,* or *B. abortus,* penetrates the mucous membranes of the oropharynx or enters through breaks in the skin, traverses the lymph nodes, and enters the blood stream through which it spreads to the reticuloendothelial system. The clinical manifestations of brucellosis vary and may be classified into asymptomatic or serologic, acute systemic or localized, and chronic or relapsing forms.[28] The most common category of complications is osseous, occurring in up to 70% of cases. Patients with *Brucella* spondylitis usually are men over 50 years of age with pre-existing spinal disease.[29] The lumbosacral spine is affected most often.[30] The range of involvement in endemic areas is between 58% to 70%.[31, 32] The disease has an insidious onset with intermittent fever, chills, weakness, weight loss, and headache. Patients commonly complain of tenderness of pain over the vertebral bodies, which is worse with activity and relieved by rest.[33, 34] Radiation of pain is associated with nerve root irritation of a mechanical or inflammatory nature.[34]

Elderly patients, alcoholics, and drug abusers are at greatest risk of developing vertebral osteomyelitis secondary to *Mycobacterium tuber-* *culosis.*[35] Prior to antibiotic therapy children were most frequently affected, but more recent data from patients with skeletal tuberculosis in the United States show average ages of 40 to 51.[36, 37] Skeletal tuberculosis occurs as a result of hematogenous spread from another source, usually pulmonary, during an acute infection or as a reactivation of a quiescent focus present in bone for many years after initial seeding.[38, 39] Of patients with skeletal tuberculosis, 50% to 60% have axial skeletal disease.[38] This may be explained in part by the affinity of this organism to the relatively high oxygen concentrations that exist in the cancellous bone of the vertebral bodies. Tuberculous spondylitis begins in the subchondral area of the vertebral body adjacent to the intervertebral disc, and the organism creates an inflammatory process characterized by the formation of granulomas and caseation necrosis of bone. Initially, only the vertebral body is affected. However, the infection can spread to involve contiguous structures, which include the intervertebral disc, other vertebral bodies, and soft tissues such as muscle and ligaments, to form a paravertebral abscess or can spread to the spinal cord and meninges. The more extensive the destruction the greater the potential for deformity of the axial skeleton with kyphoscoliosis and associated spinal cord compression.[40]

The clinical presentation of a patient with tuberculous spondylitis consists of pain over the involved vertebrae radiating into a buttock or lower extremity, low-grade fever, and weight loss of varying duration. Patients with more advanced disease may present with neurologic symptoms and angular deformities of the spine with loss of height. The onset of symptoms is gradual, and the time before presentation to a physician may be as long as 3 years.[41] Paraplegia may be the first manifestation of tuberculous spondylitis even before any deformity of the spine is apparent.[42] In contrast, heroin addicts may present with a more toxic picture associated with back pain, fever, night sweats, weight loss, and neurologic dysfunction of rapid evolution.[35]

Infections secondary to *Actinomyces israelii* and fungal organisms—*Coccidioides immitis, Blastomyces dermatitidis,* and *Histoplasma duboisii*—are very rare causes of vertebral osteomyelitis. Patients with *Actinomyces* infection of the spine may develop lesions from extension of adjacent abscesses or from hematogenous spread.[43, 44] Actinomycosis may be the cause of anaerobic infection in patients with wound infections or pressure sores. The clinical course of these infections is very similar to that of tuberculosis. These patients present with a history of constitutional symptoms over an extended period of time and complain of localized pain over the affected vertebral body.[45–47] Coccidioidomycosis may affect the spine in half of the 0.5% of patients who have disseminated disease.[48]

Before the advent of penicillin, syphilis was a common cause of axial skeletal infection, but currently this is an extremely rare complication of syphilis.[49] Syphilis may affect the axial skeleton by direct infection of bone or by the loss of normal sensation.[51] Both forms are a result of tertiary syphilis, which is the form of the disease that occurs after the initial infection (primary) and hematogenous spread (secondary) of the organism. Back pain also has been reported in secondary syphilis.[51] The pain is associated with arthritis in larger joints. The growth of the organism in bone results in the formation of a gumma and bony destruction.[52] The cervical spine is most frequently affected, but the disease also has been detected in the lumbar area.[53] The most common symptom is pain in the involved area which is greatest at night and accompanied by stiffness and loss of normal spinal curvatures. Patients may develop neurologic symptoms, including radicular pain secondary to nerve root impingement.[54] Patients with neurosyphilis, on the other hand, lose normal sensation and without this protective awareness fractures and destruction of the bony skeleton result. This is called neuropathic arthropathy or Charcot's disease. These patients feel little pain and are frequently symptom-free. However, patients may have back pain with bone deformity. This is particularly true if patients develop nerve impingement secondary to spinal instability and collapse.[55] Patients with syphilis may also develop back pain on a muscular basis or on an osseous basis in the early stages of neurosyphilis.[56, 57]

Echinococcus granulosus is a cestode worm of the dog.[58] Intermediate hosts for the ova of this worm are sheep, cattle, hogs, and man. The ova attach to the intestinal mucosa and gain entrance to the blood stream where they disseminate, particularly to the liver and occasionally to bone and form cysts (hydatid disease). The skeleton is affected in about 3% of patients with hydatid disease, and 50% of those cases are found in the spine.[59] The disease produces a slowly destructive lesion of bone, which in the spine erodes through the vertebral bodies and can rupture into the neural canal. The cysts then migrate up and down the canal. Patients with hydatid disease of the spine have symptoms that can last from a few weeks to 5 years. Pain is a common symptom associated with swelling. Occasionally painless paraplegia of sudden onset may be the presenting sign of disease. Patients who develop paraplegia either die from the disease or are chronically disabled.[60]

PHYSICAL EXAMINATION

Physical findings in patients with vertebral osteomyelitis include a decreased range of motion, muscle spasm, and percussion tenderness over the involved bone. Patients with psoas muscle irritation may demonstrate decreased hip motion along with a flexion contracture. Those with thoracolumbar vertebral osteomyelitis may have abdominal tenderness on palpation. Some of the patients with bacterial vertebral osteomyelitis have a fever.[61, 62] Neurologic abnormalities, including paraplegia, are reported in a number of series of patients with vertebral osteomyelitis.[11, 63, 64] In one study, patients who develop paralysis have a time period between symptoms and diagnosis of 3 months and are diabetic or have a urinary tract infection.[65] Patients with the more indolent infections of tuberculosis and coccidioidomycosis usually have less fever but greater spinal deformity than those with pyogenic vertebral osteomyelitis.

LABORATORY DATA

The commonly ordered blood tests (CBC, ESR, and serum chemistries) yield results that are normal or nonspecific. The ESR is abnormal in the vast majority of patients with vertebral osteomyelitis, particularly during the acute phase.[11, 61] In a study by Joughin and associates, ESR was better than fever or leukocytosis as a marker of vertebral osteomyelitis.[66] Hematocrits may be normal, and there is a normal or slightly elevated white blood cell count. A small, but significant, number of patients have normal ESR and white blood cell counts.[67]

The most useful laboratory test for the diagnosis of vertebral osteomyelitis is the direct culture of blood and bone lesions. Blood cultures may be positive in 50% of patients with acute osteomyelitis and obviate the need for bone biopsy. In patients with negative blood cultures, bone aspiration or surgical biopsy produces material that on culture is often positive for the offending organism (Fig. 12–1).[39] *S. aureus* is the bacterium associated with vertebral osteomyelitis in up to 60% of pa-

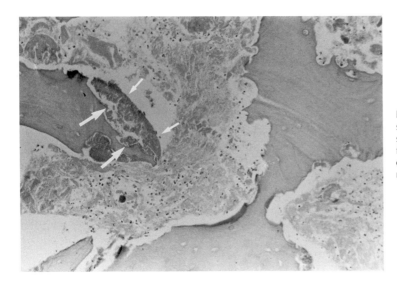

Figure 12–1. Osteomyelitis. Histologic section of acute osteomyelitis demonstrating necrotic bone, fibrin, acute inflammatory cells, and a collection of organisms (*arrows*). (Courtesy of Arnold Schwartz, M.D.)

tients.[61, 62] Gram-negative organisms (*E. coli, Proteus,* and *Pseudomonas*) are often grown from elderly patients and parenteral drug abusers with vertebral osteomyelitis. Cultures from peripheral sources of infection (urinary tract, skin, and respiratory tract) may be positive and should be obtained from the patient with suspected vertebral osteomyelitis. The diagnosis of brucellosis is associated with a positive bone culture or elevations in brucellar agglutinin titers of 1:32 or greater. Radioimmunoassay and enzyme-linked immunosorbent assay (ELISA) for *Brucella* antigens are also available.[68, 69] In general, IgM antibodies are associated with acute brucellosis and IgG are associated with chronic infection.[70]

The purified protein derivative (PPD) test is usually positive for patients with tuberculous spondylitis unless they are anergic secondary to miliary disease. The number of organisms in an infected spine is less than one million bacteria. Therefore, it is appropriate to culture both purulent material and biopsy specimens in order to improve the potential for a positive culture.[71] Histologic evidence of granulomas suggests tuberculous or fungal infection. The ESR is rarely elevated in tuberculous spondylitis. As far as fungal infections are concerned, antibody titers may be raised or skin tests reactive, but none of these tests are as specific as the growth of organisms from either aspirated material or biopsy specimens. The laboratory abnormalities of tertiary syphilis include the presence of antibodies to nontreponemal (Venereal Disease Research Laboratory [VDRL] test) and treponemal (fluorescent treponemal antibody absorption [FTA-ABS] test) antigens. Spirochetal organisms are not usually found in

tertiary lesions on histologic examination. The histologic changes include a granulomatous necrotizing process with a prominent obliterative endarteritis.

RADIOGRAPHIC EVALUATION

Radiographic changes follow the symptomatic onset of disease by 1 to 2 months (Table 12–3). The early abnormalities in pyogenic vertebral osteomyelitis include subchondral bone loss, narrowing of the disc space, and loss of definition of the vertebral body. Continued dissemination of infection may produce soft tissue swelling associated with paravertebral abscesses (loss of psoas shadow). Once the lesion starts to heal, bony regeneration appears and is characterized by osteosclerosis, which may finally result in bony fusion across the disc space (Fig. 12–2). The lumbar vertebrae, particularly the first and second, are the vertebral bodies in the axial skeleton most commonly affected.[11-13] Conventional tomograms may be done to obtain better bony and soft tissue details than plain films.

Brucellar spondylitis causes narrowing of the intervertebral disc space and destruction of the contiguous vertebrae, which may be associated with a large paravertebral abscess. Bone sclerosis with parrot-beak exostosis is a late roentgenographic sign and usually indicates the stage of healing.[34]

In tuberculous spondylitis the vertebral body is more commonly affected than posterior elements, which are affected in only 2% of spinal tuberculous cases. Pott's disease is much more common in the lower half of the spine between T6 and L4. The infection causes

TABLE 12–3. TIMETABLE FOR RADIOGRAPHIC FINDINGS IN BACTERIAL VERTEBRAL OSTEOMYELITIS

PERIOD	TIME OF APPEARANCE	OBSERVATIONS
1	3 to 6 weeks	Rarefaction of adjacent body endplates Widening of paraspinal lines Intervertebral space narrowing
2	6 to 10 weeks	Lytic scalloping and destruction of vertebral body endplates Compression of vertebral body as a result of central osteolysis Paravertebral soft tissue mass (abscess)
3	8 to 12 weeks	Reactive sclerosis
4	12 to 24 weeks	New bone formation with bony bridging of disc spaces
5	24 weeks or longer	Bony fusion of vertebral bodies

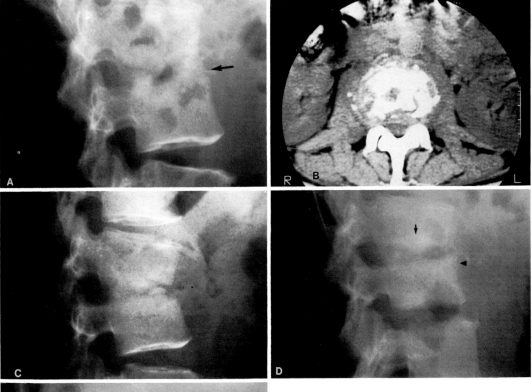

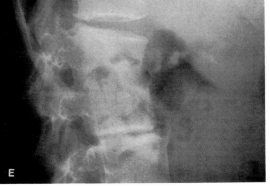

Figure 12–2. Serial roentgenograms of a 41-year-old man with staphylococcal osteomyelitis of the lumbar spine. *A,* 11/8/85. Erosion of the L2 and L3 endplates associated with destruction of the intervertebral disc (*arrow*). *B,* 11/20/85. CT scan reveals marked bony destruction associated with soft tissue extension of the infection. *C,* 11/27/85. Further collapse of the L2 vertebral body with reactive sclerosis. *D,* 11/4/86. Reactive sclerosis is noted in the vertebral body (*arrow*) and osteophytes are forming (*arrowhead*) at the body margin. *E,* 1/13/87. Total fusion of the L2 and L3 vertebral bodies. The duration of infection from onset to total fusion was approximately 12 to 14 months.

erosion of the subchondral bone and invades the disc space. These changes occur much less rapidly with tuberculous spondylitis than with pyogenic spondylitis. Patients who have back pain secondary to tuberculous spondylitis will usually present with readily identifiable destruction of vertebral bodies. This is in marked contrast with patients with pyogenic spondylitis, who develop back pain before roentgenographic alterations are noted in vertebral elements. The infection may also spread to soft tissue, forming paraspinal abscesses (Fig. 12–3). In this form, the anterior cortex of the vertebral body is destroyed. Severe angular deformities occur from marked destruction of vertebral bodies. Vertebral bodies may appear wedge-shaped, while the disc spaces are preserved. The lesion may look like a vertebra plana and may be confused with eosinophilic granuloma. The reactive sclerosis characteristic of healing pyogenic vertebral osteomyelitis

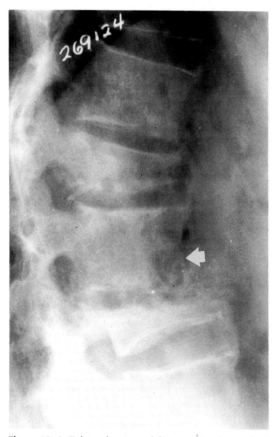

Figure 12–3. Tuberculous spondylitis resulting in vertebral and some discal destruction with collapsed vertebral bodies, loss of intervertebral disc height, reactive sclerosis, and anterior destruction. The *arrow* indicates subligamentous spread of infection. The multiple vertebral body involvement and the anterior destruction separate this process from pyogenic spondylitis. (Courtesy of Anne Brower, M.D.)

does not occur with tuberculous spondylitis. In many patients the disease is limited to two contiguous vertebrae, although four, five, or more segments may be involved (Fig. 12–4).

Fungal infections of the spine spare the intervertebral discs, involve the anterior and posterior elements of the vertebral body, and rarely cause vertebral collapse particularly with infections secondary to actinomycosis and coccidioidomycosis.[72] Actinomycoses causes lytic lesions of bone surrounded by a rim of sclerotic new bone. The disc is spared, although soft tissue abscesses may be present.[73] Coccidioidal spondylitis affects one or more vertebral bodies with paraspinal masses. This infection spares the discs and rarely causes vertebral collapse. The lesions are radiolucent and well demarcated. Periosteal new bone is seen, but sclerosis is infrequent.[74, 75]

Cryptococcal involvement of the spine is unusual. The infection is related to direct implantation at skeletal sites including the spine. Lesions are osteolytic with mild surrounding sclerosis and no periosteal reaction. The limited periostitis is characteristic of cryptococcosis.[76, 77] Disseminated blastomycosis affects bones in 50% of patients and has a radiographic appearance resembling that of tuberculosis of the spine. When the thoracolumbar area is affected, the anterior vertebral body is eroded with soft tissue masses and paravertebral extension.[78] Aspergillosis is a very rare cause of vertebral infection. However, recent reports have described vertebral involvement similar to that seen with tuberculosis secondary to *Aspergillus fumigatus* infection of an aortic bypass graft.[79]

Radiographic changes in the spine may include marked destruction and dissolution of bone in Charcot's arthropathy of the spine (neuropathic) and may show lysis and sclerosis in bone from gummatous osseous lesions (spirochetal infection).[50, 80] Periosteal changes may also be present.

In hydatid disease, the vertebral column is a common osseous location for this infection.[81] Hydatid disease is associated with single or multiple expansile osteolytic lesions containing altered trabeculae. Soft tissue calcification may also be seen, but periosteal new bone formation is unusual.[82]

Plain roentgenograms may be normal in patients with vertebral osteomyelitis. In an attempt to improve the cost effectiveness of plain roentgenograms, it has been suggested that only individuals who are 50 years or older with a long duration of symptoms, or vertebral lumbar point tenderness, have a lumbar roent-

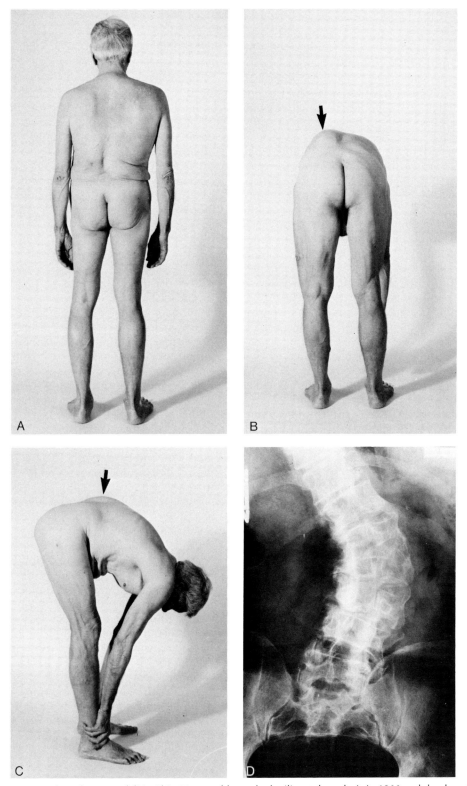

Figure 12–4. Tuberculous spondylitis. This 61-year-old man had miliary tuberculosis in 1966 and developed Pott's disease affecting his lumbar spine. *A,* In the upright position, the patient has a scoliosis centered in the lumbar area with convexity on the left. The right shoulder is higher than the left. In forward flexion, posterior (*B*) and lateral (*C*) views reveal a prominence in the left lumbar area compatible with a gibbus of the spine (*arrow*). *D,* Anteroposterior view of the lumbar spine taken 4/4/90 demonstrates a rotatory scoliosis with vertebral body loss of the L1, L2, and L3 bodies with reactive osteophytes at the L4 and L5 levels. MR examination revealed fusion of L1-L2, posterolateral disc herniations at the L2-L3 and L3-L4 levels with only mild spinal canal stenosis (not shown). (*D* from Borenstein DG: Low back pain. In Klippel J, Dieppe P (eds): Rheumatology. St Louis: CV Mosby, 1994.)

genogram.[83] Others have suggested that younger individuals with risk factors, such as intravenous drug abuse, are appropriate candidates for plain roentgenographic evaluation.[84] Once again, good clinical judgement should guide the physician to the use of appropriate tests.

Bone scintigraphy demonstrates abnormalities in the area of infection at an earlier stage of disease than does plain radiography. A bone scan may also demonstrate areas of involvement other than the one that is symptomatic. It must be kept in mind that false positives and negatives do occur and that increased uptake on bone scan may be caused by tumor, trauma, or arthritis as well. Negative bone scans also may occur if the test is completed too early in the course of the illness.[85] The combination of technetium and indium scans can add specificity to the 90% sensitivity in the diagnosis of osteomyelitis.[86]

CT may show bony changes prior to their appearance on routine radiographs (Fig. 12–5). The extent of soft tissue abscesses is also more easily visualized by this method.[87] CT may also be used to follow the course of illness after therapy is initiated. Difficulties in the CT diagnosis of vertebral osteomyelitis can occur when the radiographic features believed to be pathognomonic of specific disease entities, such as vertebral malignancy or severe degenerative disc disease, are present, which may be confused with characteristics of osteomyelitis.[86]

The role of MR in the diagnosis of vertebral infections is evolving.[88] MR changes correspond to the extent of the inflammatory process and increased water content in production of exudates containing white cells and fibrin. Variations in marrow signal also are noted with decreased T_1 weighted image and increased signal on T_2 weighted image. MR has a high sensitivity for inflammatory processes in soft tissue or bone. It has a sensitivity exceeding that of plain films and CT scan and approaches that of scintiscans.[89] MR is positive when other radiographic techniques, such as scintigraphic and CT scans, are normal.[90]

In patients with bacterial vertebral osteomyelitis, with the MR the involvement of the vertebral bodies, the intervening disc, and the extent of the extraosseous infection into the surrounding soft tissues can be determined.[90] The MR findings associated with tuberculous spondylitis that are different from bacterial vertebral osteomyelitis include the lack of abnormal signal of the intervertebral disc space, involvement of the posterior elements rather than the endplates, and the presence of large paraspinal soft-tissue masses.[91]These findings are not specific for tuberculosis. Patients with fungal infection of the spine may also demonstrate similar MR findings including preservation of disc height, destruction of posterior elements, and paravertebral masses.[92] Gadolinium-enhanced MR has advantages over nonenhanced MR in the evaluation of spinal infections.[93] Enhanced MR detects the presence of epidural abscesses. This technique also localizes the portion of a lesion that is most active, and documents a response to antibiotic therapy.

DIFFERENTIAL DIAGNOSIS

The definitive diagnosis of vertebral osteomyelitis is based upon the recovery and identification of the causative organism from aspirated material or biopsy.[94] Clinical history, physical examination, and laboratory investigation are too nonspecific to assure an accurate diagnosis.[95] Conditions confused with vertebral osteomyelitis include discitis, metastatic tumors, multiple myeloma, eosinophilic granuloma, aneurysmal bone cyst, giant cell tumor of bone, and sarcoidosis. Osteomyelitis may occur in bones in the pelvis and may be associated with severe low back pain or abdominal pain.[96] MR evaluation may help differentiate infection from other pathologic processes but culture evidence of the causative organism is required.[97] The appropriate diagnosis is reached by careful review of biopsy material. If there is doubt, biopsy must be performed on lesions of the vertebral body. Only after biopsy is it possible to differentiate tuberculosis from sarcoidosis, myeloma, other tumors, and osteomyelitis.

It is important to remember that on occasion more than one vertebral body is affected by osteomyelitis. While in most instances simultaneous involvement occurs in contiguous vertebral bodies, involvement of distant vertebrae and the entire lumbar spine may occur. A bone scan showing two or more areas of increased uptake in the spine may be inappropriately attributed to metastases, compression fractures, or osteoarthritis.[62, 98]

TREATMENT

Therapy of vertebral osteomyelitis includes antibiotics, bed rest, and immobilization. The choice of antibiotic therapy is based upon the organism causing the infection and its sensitivity to specific agents. Gram-positive bacteria such as *Staphylococcus* require penicillin or

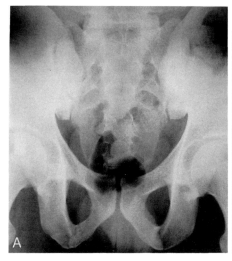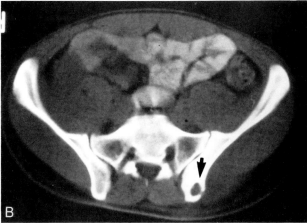

Figure 12–5. Osteomyelitis of the ilium. A 22-year-old man developed acute, severe pain over the left sacroiliac joint. *A*, Ferguson view of the pelvis revealed sclerosis of the iliac bone. The mineralization of the sacrum was difficult to determine. *B*, CT scan revealed a lytic area surrounded by reactive sclerosis limited to the left ilium (*arrow*). Biopsy and culture of the area was positive for *Staphylococcus aureus*.

semisynthetic penicillin (Nafcillin), while gram-negative bacteria are sensitive to aminoglycosides or a third generation cepholosprin. Patients are treated with 4 to 6 weeks of parenteral antibiotics followed by a course of oral antibiotics, which may have a duration of as long as 6 months. Bed rest is helpful in decreasing pain by limiting motion. Some patients require plaster casts or braces when there is major bone destruction or instability.

Brucellosis may be treated with oral tetracycline at a dose of 2 gm/day. Therapy should continue for 3 to 4 weeks. In severe cases, 0.5 gm of streptomycin is injected twice a day for a similar period.

The current recommendation for treatment of tuberculosis in the United States is a first-line, three-drug regimen including isoniazid (300 mg qd), rifampin (600 mg qd), and pyrazinamide (up to 2 gm qd) for 2 months. Two drugs (rifampin and isoniazid) are continued for an extended period, usually 18 months. Drug-resistant tuberculosis is becoming an increasingly frequent problem. Additional drugs for longer periods of time are required to control these infections. The actual duration of therapy depends on the clinical response of the patient with osseous tuberculosis.[99]

Fungal osteomyelitis requires parenteral amphotericin B therapy at a dose that the patient can tolerate without developing renal dysfunction. A total dose of 2.5 gm is usually employed as the initial course of therapy. Bone lesions, however, may be resistant to chemotherapy and may require surgical débridement. Immobilization is required for these patients as well.

Patients with tertiary syphilis without neurologic involvement are effectively treated with penicillin. Long-acting penicillin, benzathine penicillin G at 2.4 million units intramuscularly weekly for 3 weeks, is usually used. Patients who are allergic to penicillin may take tetracycline or erythromycin.

Hydatid disease has been resistant to most antihelminthic therapy. Mebendazole has shown some efficacy in preliminary studies. Definitive therapy requires surgical excision of cysts with care being taken to remove them in toto.[100] In patients with neurologic dysfunction and hydatid disease, anterior spinal decompression and fusion, along with mebendazole therapy, is associated with good neural recovery.[101]

Surgical procedures on the spine are needed in patients with vertebral osteomyelitis for: (1) abscess, (2) spinal cord compression and neurologic deficit, (3) severe deformity or instability, (4) persistent symptoms and elevated sedimentation rate, and (5) open biopsy to obtain culture material. Another indication for surgical intervention is the presence of spinal instability in association with osteomyelitis.[102] Many surgeons use an anterior approach to reach the spine. Laminectomy is not indicated in patients with vertebral osteomyelitis, since the removal of bone results in increased spinal column instability, dislocation, and spinal cord compression.[103] A number of surgeons include interbody fusion along with anterior debridement as a means to obtain neural decompression in combination with spinal stability.[65, 104, 105]

PROGNOSIS

The improvement in vertebral osteomyelitis may be monitored by following the decrease in patients' symptoms (pain, fever) and the return of the ESR to normal. With early diagnosis and the institution of appropriate therapy, vertebral osteomyelitis will resolve with minimal disability to the patient. However, when the diagnosis is delayed and the infection spreads to involve the spinal cord by compression (epidural abscess, granulation tissue) or direct extension (meningitis), potentially life-threatening complications may occur.[12, 41]

EPIDURAL ABSCESS

A number of studies have been published reviewing the clinical manifestations, diagnostic evaluation, treatment modalities, prognostic indicators, and final outcomes of a total of 112 patients with epidural abscesses.[106–108] In one series, epidural abscess occurred in 1.2 per 10,000 hospital admissions.[12] A lower rate of 0.8 cases per 10,000 admissions was noted in another study.[104] In most studies, epidural infection occurred more commonly in men. Predisposing disorders include diabetes mellitus, alcoholism, intravenous drug abuse, and cirrhosis. Although osteoarthritis of the spine is present in a number of patients with epidural abscess, the degenerative abnormalities are not a risk factor for infection.[3] While the source of an epidural infection may be distant (dental abscess) or local (decubitus ulcer), most often the source is unknown.[109] The posterior epidural space in the lumbar area is a common location for the infection. The anatomic correlation for these observations is that the extradural space is expanded posteriorly and laterally below L1 as well at T4-T9.[3]

The clinical manifestations of this infection occur secondary to direct compression by the abscess or granulation tissue or thrombosis of subarachnoid vessels. Back pain is very common but not universally seen in all patients who are unable to report their pain.[3] The progression of symptoms goes from local spinal pain to root pain, then weakness, and finally paralysis. Neurologic findings appear with the onset of radicular symptoms. Spinal tenderness is present in the vast majority of patients. Fever, sweats, or rigors occurs in a majority of

patients. The course of symptoms may be days to several months.[110]

Laboratory data in the form of peripheral white blood cell counts and ESR are not helpful since they are normal or nonspecifically elevated. Blood cultures are positive for the infecting organism about 50% to 95% of the time depending on the study group.[3, 117] The diagnosis is established by culture of CSF (at the time of myelogram). CSF is abnormal in 97% of patients including elevated protein concentrations, low glucose levels, or pleocytosis. CSF cultures may be positive for bacterial growth in the setting of a normal CSF white blood cell count.

Radiographic evaluation of the spine is helpful in identifying the location and extent of the abscess. Roentgenograms of the spine reveal vertebral changes of osteomyelitis in 44%.[111] Technetium bone scan may be positive in most patients, while gallium scan may miss the location of the abscess in about 33% of individuals. Scintiscans are positive if underlying osteomyelitis is present in the setting of the epidural abscess. CT with intrathecal contrast establishes the presence of spinal cord encroachment in a majority of cases. MR is superior to CT myelogram in defining the extent of the lesion.[107] The use of gadolinium contrast for MR helps to delineate lesions that may be equivocal with plain MR.[93]

Therapy includes the use of antibiotics and drainage of the abscess without causing instability of the spine. Speed in making the diagnosis is essential for obtaining a good outcome. Patients diagnosed within 36 hours of the onset of symptoms had minimal residual weakness. No recovery was observed in patients with paralysis for longer than 48 hour.[110] Mortality from epidural abscess ranges from 5% to 23%.[106, 108] These patients were significantly older than the rest of the patients who survived.

References

VERTEBRAL OSTEOMYELITIS

1. Waldvogel FA, Vasey H: Osteomyelitis: the past decade. N Engl J Med 303:360, 1980.
2. Kulowski J: Pyogenic osteomyelitis of the spine: an analysis and discussion of 102 cases. J Bone Joint Surg 18A:343, 1936.
3. Schwartz ST, Spiegel M, Ho G, Jr: Bacterial vertebral osteomyelitis and epidural abscess. Semin Spine Surg 2:95, 1990.
4. Sapico FL, Montgomerie JZ: Pyogenic vertebral osteomyelitis: report of nine cases and review of the literature. Rev Infect Dis 1:754, 1979.
5. Batson OV: The function of the vertebral veins and

their role in the spread of metastases. Ann Surg 112:138, 1940.

6. Wiley AM, Trueta J: The vascular anatomy of the spine and its relationship to pyogenic vertebral osteomyelitis. J Bone Joint Surg 41B:796, 1959.

7. Lame EL: Vertebral osteomyelitis following operation on the urinary tract or sigmoid: the third lesion of an uncommon syndrome. AJR 75:938, 1956.

8. Leigh TF, Kelley RP, Weens HS: Spinal osteomyelitis associated with urinary tract infections. Radiology 65:334, 1955.

9. Sherman M, Schneider GT: Vertebral osteomyelitis complicating postabortal and postpartum infection. South Med J 48:333, 1955.

10. Holzman RS, Bishko F: Osteomyelitis in heroin addicts. Ann Intern Med 75:693, 1971.

11. Garcia A Jr, Grantham SA: Hematogenous pyogenic vertebral osteomyelitis. J Bone Joint Surg 42A:429, 1960.

12. Baker AS, Ojemann RG, Swartz MN, Richardson EP Jr: Spinal epidural abscess. N Engl J Med 293:463, 1975.

13. Ross PM, Fleming JL: Vertebral body osteomyelitis: spectrum and natural history: a retrospective analysis of 37 cases. Clin Orthop 118:190, 1976.

14. Kido D, Bryan D, Halpern M: Hematogenous osteomyelitis in drug addicts. AJR 118:356, 1973.

15. Compere EL, Garrison M: Correlation of pathologic and roentgenologic findings in tuberculosis and pyogenic infections of the vertebrae. Ann Surg 104:1038, 1936.

16. De Wit D, Mulla R, Cowie MR, et al: Vertebral osteomyelitis due to *Staphylococcus epidermidis.* Brit J Rheumatol 32:339, 1993.

17. Hall M, Williams A: Group G streptococcal osteomyelitis of the spine. Brit J Rheumatol 32:342, 1993.

18. Byrne FD, Thrall TM, Wheat LJ: Hematogenous vertebral osteomyelitis: *Pasteurella multocida* as the causative agent. Arch Intern Med 139:1182, 1979.

19. Redfern RM, Cottam SN, Phillipson AP: Proteus infection of the spine. Spine 13:439, 1988.

20. Charles RW, Mody GM, Govender S: Pyogenic infection of the lumbar vertebral spine due to gas-forming organisms. Spine 14:541, 1989.

21. Feng J, Austin TW: Anaerobic vertebral osteomyelitis. Can Med Assoc J 145:132, 1991.

22. Incavo SJ, Muller DL, Krag MH, Gump D: Vertebral osteomyelitis caused by *Clostridium difficile.* Spine 13:111, 1988.

23. Guri JP: Pyogenic osteomyelitis of the spine: differential diagnosis through clinical roentgenographic observations. J Bone Joint Surg 28A:29, 1946.

24. Ling CM: Pyogenic osteomyelitis of the spine. Orthop Rev 4:23, 1975.

25. Sapico FL, Montgomerie JZ: Vertebral osteomyelitis in intravenous drug abusers: report of three cases and review of the literature. Rev Infect Dis 2:196, 1980.

26. Young EJ: Human brucellosis. Rev Infect Dis 5:821, 1983.

27. Ackerman G, Bayley JC: *Candida albicans* osteomyelitis in a vertebral body previously infected with *Serratia marcescens.* Spine 15:1362, 1990.

28. Maguire JH: Case 37–1986. N Engl J Med 315:748, 1986.

29. Ariza J, Gudiol F, Valverde J, et al.: *Brucella* spondylitis: a detailed analysis based on current findings. Rev Infect Dis 7:656, 1985.

30. Torres-Rojas J, Taddonio RF, Sanders CV: Spondylitis caused by *Brucella abortus.* South Med J 72:1166, 1979.

31. Colmenero JD, Reguera JM, Fernandez-Nebro A, Cabrera-Franquelo F: Osteoarticular complications of brucellosis. Ann Rheum Dis 50:23, 1991.

32. El-Desouki M: Skeletal brucellosis: assessment with bone scintigraphy. Radiology 181:415, 1991.

33. Keenan JD, Metz CW Jr: *Brucella* spondylitis: a brief review and case report. Clin Orthop 82:87, 1972.

34. Kelley PJ, Martin WJ, Schirger A, Weed LA: Brucellosis of the bones and joints: experience with 36 patients. JAMA 174:347, 1960.

35. Forlenza SW, Axelrod JL, Grieco MH: Pott's disease in heroin addicts. JAMA 241:379, 1979.

36. Brashear HR Jr, Rendleman DA: Pott's paraplegia. South Med J 71:1379, 1978.

37. Friedman B: Chemotherapy of tuberculosis of the spine. J Bone Joint Surg 48A:451, 1966.

38. Goldblatt M, Cremin BJ: Osteoarticular tuberculosis. Its presentation in the coloured races. Clin Radiol 29:669, 1978.

39. Chapman M, Murray RO, Stoker DJ: Tuberculosis of the bones and joints. Semin Roentgenol 14:266, 1979.

40. Seddon HJ: Pott's paraplegia: prognosis and treatment. Br J Surg 22:769, 1935.

41. Gorse GJ, Pais MJ, Kusske JA, Cesario TC: Tuberculous spondylitis: a report of six cases and a review of the literature. Medicine 62:178, 1983.

42. Reeder MM, Palmer PCS: The Radiology of Tropical Diseases with Epidemiological, Pathological, and Clinical Correlation. Baltimore: Williams & Wilkins, 1981.

43. Simpson WM, McIntosh CA: Actinomycosis of the vertebrae (actinomycotic Pott's disease). Arch Surg 14:1166, 1927.

44. Cope VZ: Actinomycosis of bone with special reference to infection of the vertebral column. J Bone Joint Surg 330:205, 1951.

45. Lane T, Goings S, Fraser D, et al: Disseminated actinomycosis with spinal cord compression: Report of two cases. Neurology 29:890, 1979.

46. Sarosi GA, Davies SF: Blastomycosis. Am Rev Respir Dis 120:911, 1979.

47. Wesselius LJ, Brooks RJ, Gall EP: Vertebral coccidioidomycosis presenting as Pott's disease. JAMA 238:1397, 1977.

48. McGahan JP, Graves DS, Palmer PES: Coccidioidal spondylitis: usual and unusual radiographic manifestations. Radiology 136:5, 1980.

49. Hunt JR: Syphilis of the vertebral column: its symptomatology and neural complications. Am J Med Sci 148:164, 1914.

50. Johns D: Syphilitic disorders of the spine: report of two cases. J Bone Joint Surg 52B:724, 1970.

51. Reginato AJ: Syphilitic arthritis and osteitis. Rheum Dis Clin North Am 19:379, 1993.

52. Freedman E, Meschan I: Syphilitic spondylitis. AJR 49:756, 1943.

53. Bingold AC: Luetic lumbar spondylosis. Proc R Soc Med 55:354, 1962.

54. Karaharju EO, Hannuksela M: Possible syphilitic spondylitis. Acta Orthop Scand 44:289, 1973.

55. Ramani PS, Sengupta RP: Cauda equina compression due to tabetic arthropathy of the spine. J Neurol Neurosurg Psychiatry 36:260, 1973.

56. Waught M: Syphilis as a cause of backache. Br Med J 1:803, 1972.

57. Roberts PW: Syphilis as a cause of backache. NY State J Med 19:20, 1919.

58. Alldred AJ, Nisbet NW: Hydatid disease of bone in Australia. J Bone Joint Surg 46B:260, 1964.

59. Morshed AA: Hydatid disease of the spine. Neurochirurgia 20:211, 1977.

60. Unger HS, Schneider LH, Sher J: Paraplegia secondary to hydatid disease: report of a case. J Bone Joint Surg 45A:1479, 1963.
61. Collert S: Osteomyelitis of the spine. Acta Orthop Scand 48:283, 1977.
62. Digby JM, Kersley JB: Pyogenic non-tuberculous spinal infection: an analysis of thirty cases. J Bone Joint Surg 61B:47, 1979.
63. Freehafer AA, Furey JG, Pierce DS: Pyogenic osteomyelitis of the spine: resulting in spinal paralysis. J Bone Joint Surg 44A:710, 1962.
64. Griffiths HED, Jones DM: Pyogenic infection of the spine: a review of twenty-eight cases. J Bone Joint Surg 53B:383, 1971.
65. Liebergall M, Chaimsky G, Lowe J, et al: Pyogenic vertebral osteomyelitis with paralysis: prognosis and treatment. Clin Orthop 289:142, 1991.
66. Joughin E, McDougall C, Parfitt C, et al: Causes and clinical management of vertebral osteomyelitis in Saskatchewan. Spine 16:1049, 1991.
67. Schofferman L, Schofferman J, Zucherman J, et al: Occult infections causing persistent low back pain. Spine 14:417, 1989.
68. Parrett D, Neilsen KH, White RG: Radioimmunoassay of IgM, IgG, and IgA *Brucella* antibodies. Lancet 1:1075, 1977.
69. Sippel JD, Masry NA, Farid Z: Diagnosis of human brucellosis with ELISA. Lancet 2:19, 1982.
70. Neinstein LS, Goldenring J: *Brucella* sacroiliitis. Clin Pediatr 22:645, 1983.
71. David PT, Horowitz T: Skeletal tuberculosis: a review with patient presentations and discussion. Am J Med 48:77, 1970.
72. Pritchard DJ: Granulomatous infections of bones and joints. Orthop Clin North Am 6:1029, 1975.
73. Young WB: Actinomycosis with involvement of the vertebral column: case report and review of the literature. Clin Radiol 11:175, 1960.
74. Dalinka MK, Greendyke WH: The spinal manifestations of coccidioidomycosis. J Can Assoc Radiol, 22:93, 1971.
75. Halpern AA, Rinsky LA, Fountains S, Nagel DA: Coccidioidomycosis of the spine: unusual roentgenographic presentation. Clin Orthop 140:78, 1979.
76. Litvinoff J, Nelson M: Extradural lumbar cryptococcosis. Case report. J Neurosurg 49:921, 1978.
77. Morris E, Wolinsky E: Localized osseous cryptococcosis: a case report. J Bone Joint Surg 47A:1027, 1965.
78. Baylin GJ, Wear JM: Blastomycosis and actinomycosis of spine. AJR 69:395, 1953.
79. Brandt SJ, Thompson RL, Wenzel RP: Mycotic pseudoaneurysm of an aortic bypass graft and contiguous vertebral osteomyelitis due to *Aspergillus fumigatus*. Am J Med 79:259, 1985.
80. Cleveland M, Wilson HJ: Charcot disease of the spine: a report of two cases treated by spine fusion. J Bone Joint Surg 41A:336, 1959.
81. Stewart GR, Loewenthal J: Vertebral hydatidosis. Aust NZ J Surg 36:175, 1967.
82. Hutchinson WF, Thompson WB, Derian PS: Osseous hydatid (*Echinococcus*) disease. JAMA 182:81, 1962.
83. Deyo RA: Plain roentgenography for low back pain: finding needles in a haystack. Arch Intern Med 149:27, 1989.
84. Chandrasekar P: Low back pain and intravenous abusers. Arch Intern Med 150:1125, 1990.
85. Schlaeffer F, Mikolich DJ, Mates SM: Technetium Tc 99m diphosphonate bone scan: false-normal findings in elderly patients with hematogenous vertebral osteomyelitis. Arch Intern Med 147:2024, 1987.
86. Smith AS, Blaser SI: Infectious and inflammatory processes of the spine. Radiol Clin North Am 29:809, 1991.
87. Kattapuram SV, Phillips WC, Boyd R: CT in pyogenic osteomyelitis of the spine. AJR 140:1199, 1983.
88. Modic MT, Pflanze W, Feiglin DHI, Belhobek G: Magnetic resonance imaging of musculoskeletal infections. Radiol Clin North Am 24:247, 1986.
89. Modic MT, Feiglin DH, Piraino DW, et al: Vertebral osteomyelitis: assessment using MR. Radiology 157:157, 1985.
90. Meyers SP, Weiner SN: Diagnosis of hematogenous pyogenic vertebral osteomyelitis by magnetic resonance imaging. Arch Intern Med 151:683, 1991.
91. Smith AS, Weinstein MA, Mizushima A, et al: MR imaging characteristics of tuberculous spondylitis vs vertebral osteomyelitis. AJR 153:399, 1989.
92. Cure JK, Mirich DR: MR imaging in cryptococcal spondylitis. AJNR 12:1111, 1991.
93. Post MJ, Sze G, Quencer RM, et al: Gadolinium-enhanced MR in spinal infection. J Comput Assist Tomogr 14:721, 1990.
94. Musher DM, Thorsteinsson SB, Minuth JN, Luchi RJ: Vertebra osteomyelitis: still a diagnostic pitfall. Arch Intern Med 136:105, 1976.
95. Kornberg M, Rechtine GR, Dupuy TE: Unusual presentation of spinal osteomyelitis in a patient taking propylthiouracil: a case report. Spine 10:104, 1985.
96. Weld PW: Osteomyelitis of the ilium masquerading as acute appendicitis. JAMA 173:634, 1960.
97. Borges LF: Case records of the Massachusetts General Hospital. N Engl J Med 320:1610, 1989.
98. Abdel Dayem HM, Tuason J: *Pseudomonas* osteomyelitis involving the entire lumbar spine. Clin Nucl Med 3:205, 1978.
99. Barnes PF, Barrows SA: Tuberculosis in the 1990s. Ann Intern Med 119:400, 1993.
100. Levack B, Kernohan J, Edgar MA, Ransford AO: Observations on the current and future surgical management of hydatid disease affecting the vertebre. Spine 11:583, 1986.
101. Charles RW, Govender CS, Naidoo KS: Echinococcal infection of the spine with neural involvement. Spine 13:47, 1988.
102. Patzakis MJ, Rao S, Wilkins J, et al: Analysis of 61 cases of vertebral osteomyelitis. Clin Orthop 264:178, 1991.
103. Kemp HBS, Shaw NC: Laminectomy in paraplegia due to infective spondylosis. Br J Surg 61:66, 1974.
104. Emery SE, Chan DPK, Woodward HR: Treatment of hematogenous pyogenic vertebral osteomyelitis with anterior debridement and primary bone grafting. Spine 14:284, 1989.
105. Lifeso RM: Pyogenic spinal sepsis in adults. Spine 15:1265, 1990.
106. Darouiche RO, Hamill RJ, Greenberg SB, et al: Bacterial spinal epidural abscess: review of 43 cases and literature survey. Medicine 71:369, 1992.
107. Curling OD, Gower DJ, McWhorter JM: Changing concepts in spinal epidural abscess: a report of 29 cases. Neurosurgery 27:185, 1990.
108. Hlavin ML, Kaminski HJ, Ross JS, Ganz E: Spinal epidural abscess: a ten-year perspective. Neurosurgery 27:177, 1990.
109. Guerrero IC, Slap GB, MacGregor RB, et al: Anaerobic spinal epidural abscess. J Neurosurg 48:465, 1978.
110. Eismont FJ, Montero C. Infections of the spine. In Davidoff RA (ed): Handbook of the Spinal Cord. New York: Marcel Dekker, Inc., 1987 pp, 411–449.
111. Heusner AP: Nontuberculous spinal epidural infections. N Engl J Med 239:845, 1948.

INTERVERTEBRAL DISC SPACE INFECTION

Capsule Summary

Frequency of back pain—very common
Location of back pain—lumbar spine—disc space
Quality of back pain—severe, sharp
Symptoms and signs—percussion tenderness, decreased motion
Laboratory and x-ray tests—elevated ESR, culture of disc and blood; disc space narrowing on plain radiographs; MR for early infection.
Treatment—antibiotics, immobilization

PREVALENCE AND PATHOGENESIS

Infection of the intervertebral disc (IVD) is an uncommon but potentially disabling cause of low back pain. While once thought to be exclusively a complication of vertebral osteomyelitis, IVD infection also can develop secondary to hematogenous invasion through the blood stream and by direct penetration during disc surgery. A significant clinical feature of this illness is the long delay between the onset of symptoms of low back pain, muscle spasm, and limitation of motion and the establishment of the diagnosis.

IVD infection is uncommon in adults, occurring with an incidence of 2 patients per year at an orthopedic hospital.[1] Approximately 2.8% of patients who have lumbar disc surgery develop disc space infection.[2] Men are more frequently affected, and the disease has been diagnosed in patients up to 63 years of age.

The pathogenesis of disc space infections in adults in the absence of a surgical or diagnostic procedure remains in doubt. In children, blood vessels supply the IVDs. Infection occurs secondary to hematogenous spread of organisms. Others have considered discitis in children a noninfectious disease, an inflammatory or traumatic disorder. The course in children is relatively benign.[3]

Although it is generally believed that the IVDs are avascular in adult life, a number of investigators have demonstrated some blood flow in adults.[4, 5] While there is a decrease in the number of vessels that enter the nucleus pulposus with aging, an adequate circumferential supply is maintained from the periphery.[6] The blood supply to IVDs is greater in children, which may explain the increased frequency of disc space infection in the pediatric age group as compared with adults.[3]

There is evidence supporting the impor-

tance of both the venous and arterial systems in the development of disc infections. Patients with pelvic and urinary tract infections may develop involvement of disc spaces with the identical organism, and it is postulated that these organisms may spread by means of the vertebral venous plexus of Batson.[7–9] Batson's plexus is a network of veins that surrounds the vertebral column and is connected to the major veins that return blood to the heart and the inferior and superior vena cava. However, other investigators believe that the reversal of flow in the venous system, which would allow infected blood to enter Batson's plexus, does not occur under usual circumstances. Instead, they suggest hematogenous spread through the arterial system as the source of infection.[5, 10] It is probable that either route may be involved in appropriate circumstances.

The intervertebral discs are infected by hematogenous spread, most commonly through the blood stream. However, other mechanisms may play a role in some circumstances. A few patients have been reported to have developed IVD infection following trauma or heavy physical labor.[11, 12] Trauma in the area of the IVD may result in the formation of a hematoma that is then infected by blood-borne organisms, but the likelihood of this occurrence is not great. In fact, most patients with IVD infections deny previous trauma.[1] Therefore, the association of this infection and trauma is unlikely. Patients who undergo operative procedures, needle biopsy, discography, or puncture of a disc during a lumbar puncture can develop infection by direct inoculation of the organism at the time of the procedure.[2] Spinal infection associated with lumbar disc surgery occurs less than 1% of the time whether an anterior, posterior, or percutaneous route is used.[13] Others may develop disc space infection from organisms which arise from contiguous abscesses.[14]

CLINICAL HISTORY

Patients with IVD infections of the lumbar spine have symptoms of localized low back pain. In some, the onset of the pain is acute and very severe. In other patients, the pain may be more insidious and milder. The duration of pain before diagnosis ranges from 1 month to 2 years.[12] It becomes chronic and may be associated with radiation into the flanks, abdomen, testes, or lower extremities. The pain is exacerbated by movement and relieved by absolute rest. Motion may initiate paroxysms of paravertebral muscle spasm, and the patients usually have great difficulty walking. Loss of motor strength or sensory symptoms may suggest spinal cord compression.

In one series, 77% of cases affected the lumbar disc, 15% the cervical spine, and 8% the thoracic spine.[12] In one group of patients, 3 of 13 had neurologic deficits at time of diagnosis. The two patients with lumbar infection had severe L5 root weakness and paraparesis.[12]

Discitis also may be a complication of invasive procedures including discography and disectomy. Patients who have postoperative infection develop a significant increase in back pain after a period of initial relief with no significant increase in radicular pain.

PHYSICAL EXAMINATION

Physical findings in patients with disc infection include localized tenderness on palpation, limitation of motion of the lumbar spine, and paravertebral muscle spasm. Fever is rarely present.[12] Patients prefer to remain motionless in bed. Examination of the skin, respiratory system, gastrointestinal system, and genitourinary system may demonstrate the primary source of infection.

LABORATORY DATA

The laboratory findings are nonspecific in disc space infections. The most commonly abnormal test is the ESR. It is elevated in up to 75% of patients.[1] The ESR is elevated in lumbar spine surgery patients for 2 to 4 weeks postoperatively. Rates remain elevated in patients with disc space infection for longer periods of time.[15] C-reactive protein (CRP) returns to normal more rapidly than ESR after uncomplicated lumbar spine surgery. A persistently elevated CRP may be associated with a postoperative infection.[15a] A mild leukocytosis with a normal differential is also seen.[12] Occasionally blood cultures are positive during the acute phases of the illness,[12] but culture of fluid obtained by needle aspiration or at surgery is usually positive.[12, 16] The most frequently cultured organism causing disc infection is *S. aureus*. Other gram positive organisms include *S. epidermidis*[17] and streptococcal species, including *S. milleri*.[18] Gram-negative organisms also have been implicated, particularly *P. aeruginosa*, in intravenous drug abusers.[16, 19] *Enterobacter cloacae* and *E. coli* have been the source of infection in other immunocompromised patients including the elderly and those with urosepsis.[20, 21] Gram-negative organisms,

including *Campylobacter fetus*, Group Ve-1, and *Kingella kingae*, have caused discitis in otherwise immunocompetent patients.[22–24] Anaerobic organisms have been implicated in rare circumstances,[25] as have fungal organisms.[26] The list of anaerobes and fungal organisms associated with discitis has been expanded to include *Eikenella corrodens* and *Aspergillus fumigatus*, respectively.[27–29]

RADIOGRAPHIC FINDINGS

The radiographic features of disc infection are distinctive and help to differentiate it from that of vertebral osteomyelitis; however, they may lag behind clinical symptoms by 6 weeks or more.[1] The earliest change is a decrease in the height of the affected intervertebral disc space (Fig. 12–6). Two months after the appearance of disc space narrowing, reactive sclerosis of subchondral bone appears in the adjoining vertebral bodies. Subsequently, progressive irregularity of the vertebral endplates develops and indicates a local extension of the inflammatory process and an osteomyelitis. At this juncture, the loss of vertebral bone may be associated with a "ballooning" of the IVD space.[1] This increase in apparent disc space is usually associated with involvement of the vertebral body posteriorly. Repair may occur at any stage of infection and is manifested by bony proliferation about the outside margin of the disc. The process may heal with bony ankylosis of the adjacent vertebral bodies across the affected disc space.

Bone scintiscans are very useful in rapidly identifying increased bone activity in areas contiguous to infected discs. The bone scan may be positive in an area of infection that appears normal on plain radiographs.[30] Both ^{99m}Tc and ^{67}Ga citrate scans are more sensitive than plain roentgenograms in detecting early disc infections.[31, 32]

MR is a sensitive method for the early detection of inflammation in infected tissues. It is able to detect early disc infection before changes occur on plain roentgenograms (Fig. 12–7).[33] MR with gadolinium enhancement is a useful test for the differentiation of normal postoperative healing changes from those related to septic discitis. Gadolinium-enhanced MR findings associated with infection include decreased signal intensity on T_1-weighted images in the bone marrow adjacent to the disc, increased signal intensity with loss of the intranuclear cleft in the disc space, and posterior anulus on T_2-weighted sequences.[34]

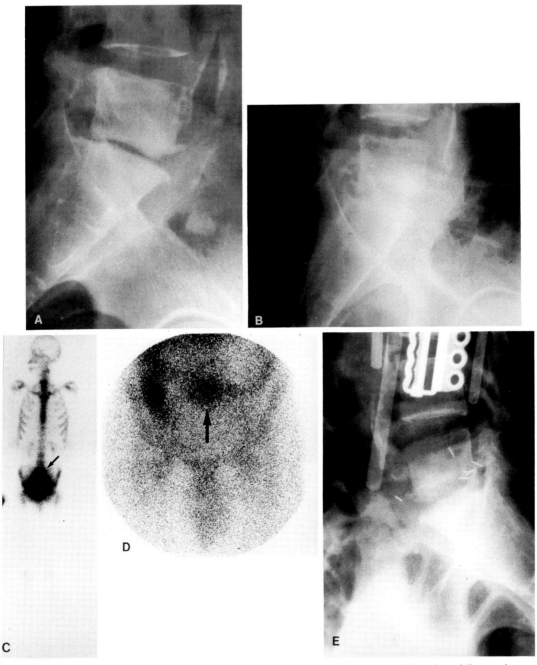

Figure 12–6. A 50-year-old man with a prior history of *S. aureus* endocarditis and drug abuse fell at work, striking his back. Roentgenograms were normal and the patient was given conservative therapy with a good response. Four months later, the patient complained of severe, localized lower lumbar pain. Percussion tenderness over the L5 vertebra was painful. *A*, 2/17/86. Lateral roentgenogram reveals marked disc space narrowing with early sclerosis of surrounding endplates. *B*, 3/4/86. Continued disc space dissolution has occurred with reactive bony sclerosis. *C*, 3/7/86. Bone scan revealed markedly increased uptake in the L5 region (*arrow*). *D*, 3/14/86. Gallium scan demonstrated increased uptake in the L5 vertebral area (*arrow*). *E*, 3/22/86. The patient admitted to intravenous drug use. Blood cultures grew *S. epidermidis*. Biopsy of the disc while the patient was on antibiotics obtained disc material that did not grow organisms on culture. The patient received antibiotics for staphylococcal infection and a lumbosacral brace. He was asymptomatic at time of discharge.

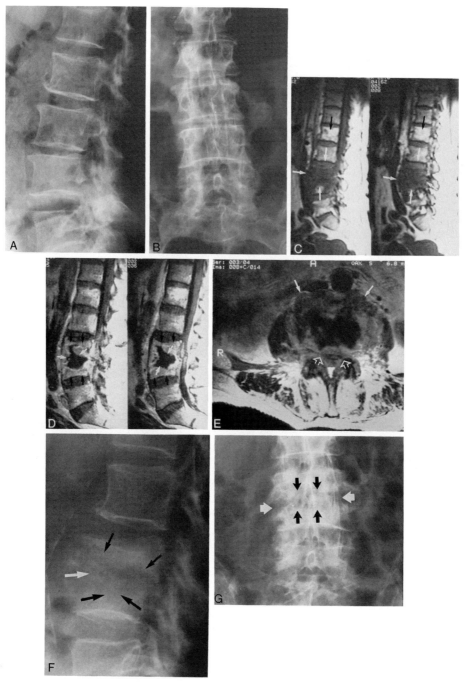

Figure 12–7. Discitis. A 86-year-old woman had an episode of *E. coli* urosepsis treated with antibiotics in 9/91. Lateral (*A*), and anterioposterior (*B*) plain roentgenograms were taken on 9/28/91 demonstrating intact IVD spaces in the lumbar area with the presence of small osteophytes. She developed low back pain and, then, leg pain over a 6-week-period. On 11/2/91, she was readmitted to the hospital. Blood cultures were positive for *E. coli*. MR examination was done on 11/5/91. Sagittal T_1 weighted images (*C*) reveal decreased signal in the area of the IVD and the bodies of L3 and L4 (*white arrows*) compatible with inflammatory tissue. Hemangioma was the cause of increased signal in L1 (*black arrow*). Sagittal (*D*) and axial (*E*) T_1 weighted gadolinium images demonstrate enhancement of the superior portion of L3 and the inferior portion of L4 (*black arrows*) and an irregular, nonenhancing area (*white arrows*) involving the disc and surrounding vertebral bodies compatible with an infectious process. Paraspinous (*white arrows*) and epidural (*white open arrows*) extension is best seen on axial view (*E*). Lateral (*F*) and anterioposterior (*G*) plain roentgenograms were taken on 11/28/91, which demonstrated vertebral body erosion (*black arrows*) and total desolution of the IVD space (*white arrow*). (Courtesy of Bernardo Kotelanski, M.D.)

TABLE 12–4. DIFFERENTIAL DIAGNOSIS OF DISORDERS PRODUCING NARROWING OF THE DISC IN THE LUMBAR SPINE

DISEASE	DISCOVERTEBRAL MARGIN	SCLEROSIS	"VACUUM PHENOMENA"	OSTEOPHYTES	OTHER FINDINGS
Infection	Poorly defined	Variable	Absent (except with gas-forming organisms)	Absent	Bone lysis, soft tissue mass
Intervertebral degenerative disease	Well defined	Prominent	Present	Variable	Cartilaginous nodes
Calcium pyrophosphate crystal deposition disease	Poorly or well defined	Prominent	Variable	Variable	Fragmentation, subluxation
Neuroarthropathy	Well defined	Prominent	Variable	Prominent	Disorganization
Trauma	Well defined	Prominent	Variable	Prominent	Fracture, soft tissue mass
Sarcoidosis	Poorly or well defined	Variable	Absent	Absent	Soft tissue mass

Modified from Resnick D, Niwayama G (eds): Diagnosis of Bone and Joint Disorders. 2nd ed. Philadelphia, WB Saunders Co, 1988.

DIFFERENTIAL DIAGNOSIS

The diagnosis of IVD infection is often overlooked because of nonspecific symptoms and its relative infrequency as a cause of back pain compared with mechanical disorders and the spondyloarthropathies. Nonetheless, physicians should be aware of this treatable entity so that the appropriate diagnosis will be made in an expeditious manner. The definitive diagnosis of a disc infection depends on the aspiration or biopsy of the infected site with subsequent confirmation by culture of the causative organism. A bone scan may help identify this entity in the patient who has normal radiographs.

The differential diagnosis of septic discitis and mechanical discitis is a problem in patients who have undergone invasive procedures (discography, discectomy) involving the intervertebral disc.[35, 36] The frequency of discitis occurring after discography ranges from 1% to 4% of procedures.[37] Patients with septic discitis (culture positive or negative) have elevated ESR and CRP levels and evidence of large infiltrates of lymphoplasmocytic cells.[35]

Other diseases that may be associated with IVD narrowing accompanied by lysis or sclerosis of adjacent vertebrae include osteomyelitis of a vertebral body, degenerative disease, calcium pyrophosphate dihydrate crystal deposition, neuroarthropathy, and trauma.[38] Sarcoidosis may cause similar changes on occasion. MR is able to detect the presence of sarcoid spondylodiscitis but can not differentiate pyogenic from granulomatous inflammation. Biopsy of the disc space is required.[39] Diagnosis of discitis including postoperative infections may be confirmed by the use of an automated percutaneous biopsy.[40] Patients with chronic renal failure may develop spinal erosive changes that simulate disc space infections. Disc changes range from superficial erosions at the anteriosuperior and anterioinferior margins of the vertebral bodies to large resorptive defects mimicking disc infection.[41] These changes occur after 3 years on dialysis. Table 12–4 describes the characteristic alterations that help differentiate these possible diagnoses. Primary or metastatic tumor in the spine does not lead to significant loss of IVD space. An intact disc space with adjacent vertebral body lysis is more characteristic of a tumor than of infection. On occasion, myeloma and chordoma can extend across or around the IVD to involve contiguous vertebrae.[42] It is also possible for intraosseous disc herniation to occur secondary to vertebral body bone weakening secondary to invasion.[43]

TREATMENT

Therapy of IVD infections includes antibiotics and immobilization by bed rest, casts, or bracing. There is little agreement in the literature as to just what component of therapy is most effective. Some authors suggest bed rest and immobilization are adequate and antibiotics are not necessary[44]; however, most patients receive a 4- to 6-week course of antibiotic therapy.[12] The response to treatment is monitored by a relief of pain, return of the sedimentation rate to normal, and radiographic evidence of disc space restoration or bony ankylosis of adjacent vertebral bodies. Five French immunosuppressed patients with Aspergillus discitis were treated with itraconazole alone or in combination with flucytosine and amphotericin B. Surgical débridement was not necessary in these patients.[45] Patients with severe pain may benefit from epidural morphine injection if the use of oral or parenteral narcotics needs to be limited.[46] Surgical exploration is not indicated unless there are signs of spinal cord compression, spinal instability, or severe deformity. Surgical fusion is usually unnecessary. Patients who develop a disc space infection after lumbar disc surgery may be treated with immobilization and antibiotics; surgical exploration is usually unnecessary.[2] Patients with fungal discitis may require surgical decompression, although resolution of the fungal infection has been reported with amphotericin B therapy alone.[47]

PROGNOSIS

Most patients with disc infections have a benign course and fully recover without disability. Back bracing may be required for a year or longer until ankylosis of adjacent vertebral bodies occurs. Patients usually have full range of motion with healing and are asymptomatic.[12]

When discitis is suspected early and antibiotics are given in high doses until normalization of ESR, discitis resolves in a few weeks and no or mild vertebral erosion occurs. When antibiotic therapy is delayed or is inadequate in regard to the sensitivity of the organism, dosage, or duration, infection may last months and be associated with marked destruction of the vertebral bodies.[48]

The most serious complication of disc space infection was reported by Kemp.[1] In his group of 13 patients, three were hemiplegic, three were paraplegic and all required surgical decompression. At operation, direct extension of inflammatory granulation tissue was identified growing posteriorly and involving the meninges and spinal cord. Cord damage was secondary to compression of the cord by edema, by inflammatory tissue, or from thrombosis of spinal cord vessels. Of the six patients with neurologic symptoms, two had complete recovery, two had partial recovery, and two had no recovery after surgical decompression. The appearance of neurologic symptoms was rapid in these patients, although most of them had back pain for longer than 4 months. Accurate diagnosis and the prompt institution of appropriate therapy should prevent the emergence of this complication of disc infection.

References

INTERVERTEBRAL DISC SPACE INFECTION

1. Kemp HBS, Jackson JW, Jeremiah JD, Hall AJ: Pyogenic infections occurring primarily in intervertebral discs. J Bone Joint Surg 55B:698, 1973.
2. Pilgaard S: Discitis (closed space infection) following removal of lumbar intervertebral disc. J Bone Joint Surg 51A:713, 1969.
3. Boston HC Jr, Bianco AJ Jr, Rhodes KH: Disc space infections in children. Orthop Clin North Am 6:953, 1975.
4. Smith NR: The intervertebral discs. Br J Surg 18:358, 1931.
5. Wiley AM, Trueta J: The vascular anatomy of the spine and its relationship to pyogenic vertebral osteomyelitis. J Bone Joint Surg 41B:796, 1959.
6. Hassler O: The human intervertebral disc. Acta Orthop Scand 40:765, 1970.
7. Batson OV: The function of the vertebral veins and their role in the spread of metastasis. Ann Surg 112:138, 1940.
8. Doyle JR: Narrowing of the intervertebral-disc space in children. J Bone Joint Surg 42A:1191, 1960.
9. Griffiths HED, Jones DM: Pyogenic infection of the spine. J Bone Joint Surg 53B:383, 1971.
10. Ghormley RK, Bickel WH, Dickson DD: A study of acute infectious lesions of the intervertebral discs. South Med J 33:347, 1940.
11. Ettinger WH Jr, Arnett FC Jr., Stevens MB: Intervertebral disc space infections: another low back syndrome of the young. Johns Hopkins Hosp Med J 141:23, 1977.
12. Onofrio BM: Intervertebral discitis: incidence, diagnosis and management. Clin Neurosurg 27:481, 1980.
13. Abramovitz JN: Complications of surgery for discogenic disease of the spine. Neurosurg Clin North Am 4:167, 1993.
14. Gordon EJ: Infection of disc space secondary to fistula from pelvic abscess. South Med J 70:114, 1977.
15. Jonsson B, Soderholm R, Stromqvist B: Erythrocyte sedimentation rate after lumbar spine surgery. Spine 16:1049, 1991.
15a. Thelander U, Larsson S: Quantitation of C-reactive levels and erythrocyte sedimentation rate after spinal surgery. Spine 17:400, 1992.
16. Scherbel AL, Gardner JW: Infections involving the intervertebral discs: diagnosis and management. JAMA 174:370, 1960.
17. Rawlings CE III, Wilkins RH, Gallis HA, et al.: Postoperative intervertebral disc space infection. Neurosurgery 13:371, 1983.
18. Meyes E, Flipo R, Van Bosterhaut B, et al.: Septic Streptococcus milleri spondylodiscitis. J Rheumatol 17:1421, 1990.
19. Selby RC, Pillary KV: Osteomyelitis and disc infection secondary to Pseudomonas aeruginosa in heroin addiction: case report. J Neurosurg 37:463, 1972.
20. Ponte CD, McDonald M: Septic discitis resulting from Escherichia coli urosepsis. J Fam Prac 34:767, 1992.
21. Solans R, Simeon P, Cuenca R, et al: Infectious discitis caused by Enterobacter cloacae. Ann Rheum Dis 51:906, 1992.
22. Mathieu E, Koeger A, Rozenberg S, Bourgeois P: Cam-

pylobacter spondylodiscitis and deficiency of cellular immunity. J Rheumatol 18:1929, 1991.

23. Levy DI, Bucci MN, Hoff JT: Discitis caused by the centers for Disease Control Microorganism Group Ve-1. Neurosurgery 25:655, 1989.

24. Meis JF, Sauerwein RW, Gyssens IC, et al.: Kingella kingae intervertebral diskitis in an adult. Clin Infect Dis 15:530, 1992.

25. Pate D, Katz A: Clostridia discitis: A case report. Arthritis Rheum 22:1039, 1979.

26. Pennisi AK, Davis DO, Wiesel S, Moskovitz P: CT appearance of Candida diskitis. J Comput Assist Tom 9:1050, 1985.

27. Noordeen MHH, Godfrey LW: Case report of an unusual cause of low back pain: intervertebral diskitis caused by Eikenella corrodens. Clin Orthop 280:175, 1992.

28. Sugar AM: Case records of the Massachusetts General Hospital. N Engl J Med 324:754, 1991.

29. Castelli C, Benazzo F, Minoli L, et al.: Aspergillus infection of the L3-L4 disc space in an immunosuppressed heart transplant patient. Spine 15:1369, 1988.

30. Norris S, Ehrlich MG, Keim DE, et al.: Early diagnosis of disc-space infection using Gallium-67. J Nucl Med 19:384, 1978.

31. Choong K, Monaghan P, McGuigan L, McLean R: Role of bone scintigraphy in the early diagnosis of discitis. Ann Rheum Dis 49:932, 1990.

32. Nolla-Sole JM, Mateo-Soria L, Rozadilla-Sacanell A, et al.: Role of technetium-99m diphosphonate and gallium-67 citrate bone scanning in the early diagnosis of infectious spondylodiscitis. A comparative study. Ann Rheum Dis 51:665, 1992.

33. Morgenlander JC, Rozear MP: Disc space infection: A case report with MRI diagnosis. Am Fam Phys 42:984, 1990.

34. Boden SD, David DO, Dina T, et al.: Postoperative diskitis: distinguishing early MR imaging findings from normal postoperative disk space changes. Radiology 184:765, 1992.

35. Guyer RD, Collier R, Stith WJ, et al.: Discitis after discography. Spine 13:1352, 1988.

36. Fouquet B, Goupille P, Jattiot F, et al.: Discitis after lumbar disc surgery: features of "aseptic" and "septic" forms. Spine 17:356, 1992.

37. Osti OL, Fraser RD, Vernon-Roberts B: Discitis after discography. J Bone Joint Surg 72B:271, 1990.

38. Patton JT: Differential diagnosis of inflammatory spondylitis. Skel Radiol 1:77, 1976.

39. Kenney CM III, Goldstein SJ: MRI of sarcoid spondylodiskitis. J Comput Assist Tomogr 16:660, 1992.

40. Onik G, Shang Y, Maroon JC: Automated percutaneous biopsy in postoperative diskitis: A new method. AJNR 11:391, 1990.

41. Sundaram M, Seelig R, Pohl D: Vertebral erosions in patients undergoing maintenance hemodialysis for chronic renal failure. AJR 149:323, 1987.

42. Resnick D, Niwayama G: Osteomyelitis, Septic Arthritis, and Soft-Tissue Infection: the Axial Skeleton. In Resnick D, Niwayama G (eds): Diagnosis of Bone and Joint Disorders. Philadelphia: WB Saunders, 1981, pp 2130–2153.

43. Resnick D, Niwayama G: Intervertebral disc abnormalities associated with vertebral metastais: observations in patients and cadavers with prostate cancer. Invest Radiol 13:182, 1978.

44. Sullivan CR: Diagnosis and treatment of pyogenic infections of the intervertebral disc. Surg Clin North Am 41:1077, 1961.

45. Cortet B, Deprez X, Trili R, et al.: Aspergillus discitis: a report of five cases. Rev Rheum[Engl] 60:38, 1993.

46. Zampella EJ, Zeiger HE: Epidural morphine as an adjunct in the treatment of intervertebral disc infection. Spine 12:825, 1987.

47. Holmes PF, Osterman DW, Tullos HS: Aspergillus discitis: report of two cases and review of the literature. Clin Orthop 226:240, 1988.

48. Postacchini F, Cinotti G: Iatrogenic lumbar discitis. J Bone Joint Surg 74B:(Suppl 1) 70, 1992.

PYOGENIC SACROILIITIS

Capsule Summary

Frequency of back pain—very common
Location of back pain—sacroiliac joint
Quality of back pain—severe, sharp
Symptoms and signs—buttock, thigh or calf tenderness, unwillingness to walk on affected leg, Patrick's test positive
Laboratory and x-ray tests—leukocytosis, blood cultures (positive in 50%); blurred joint margins on plain roentgenographs, MR for early infection
Treatment—antibiotics, abscess drainage

PREVALENCE AND PATHOGENESIS

Septic arthritis is a disease process caused by the direct invasion of a joint space by infectious agents, usually bacteria. Joints become infected by direct penetration, spread from contiguous structures, or more often by hematogenous invasion through the blood stream. Septic arthritis occurs more commonly in large peripheral joints (knees, shoulders) than in the lumbosacral spine; but when a joint of the axial skeleton is involved, the sacroiliac is the one most commonly affected.

Pyogenic sacroiliitis is an uncommon illness, accounting for 0.07% of hospital admissions in one study.[1] Approximately 80 patients with pyogenic sacroiliitis have been reported in the medical literature, although new cases continue to be reported, particularly with unusual organisms.[2–6] A recent article reviewed 166 patients with pyogenic sacroiliitis reported in the medical literature. This review excluded patients with sacroiliitis secondary to tuberculosis or brucellosis.[7] The disease occurs most commonly in young adult men. The range of ages is 20 to 66[1] and the male to female ratio is 3:2.[4] The average age of patients with pyogenic sacroiliitis is 22 years.[7]

The initial factor that may result in joint infection is entry of organisms into the sacroiliac joint. Most commonly, infectious agents reach the sacroiliac joint by traveling through the blood stream. They lodge in the vascular synovial membrane that lines the lower portion of the sacroiliac joint. The infectious agents grow in the synovium and invade the joint space. The organisms also might lodge in the ilium, the most frequently infected flat bone in the body, and grow into the sacroiliac joint. The relatively symmetric involvement of ilium and sacrum in pyogenic sacroiliitis suggests that the joint is the initial area affected.[1] Once an infection is established in a joint, rapid destruction may occur because of both the direct toxic effects of products of organisms on joint structures and the host's inflammatory response to them.

Any factor, such as intravenous drug abuse, skin infections, bone and urinary tract infections, endocarditis, pregnancy, and bowel disease,[1, 2, 8] that promotes blood-borne infection or inhibits the normal defense mechanisms of the synovial joint predisposes the host to infection. Although the role of trauma in the pathogenesis of pyogenic sacroiliitis is unclear, buttock or hip injuries have been reported in patients prior to development of pyogenic sacroiliitis.[2, 9] In one study in a rural population, 5 of 10 patients with pyogenic sacroiliitis had a history of pelvic trauma.[10] Most patients, however, deny a history of trauma, and its importance as a direct cause of infection is in question. In a significant number of patients, 41% in one review, no primary source of infection can be identified.[7] The histocompatibility typing associated with seronegative spondyloarthropathies, HLA-B27, is not associated with pyogenic sacroiliitis.[11]

Another mechanism of joint infection is contamination by local spread from a contiguous suppurative focus. Extension of a pelvic infectious process may cause disruption of the joint capsule or of the periosteum of the ilium or sacrum.[12] Infections spreading beneath the spinal ligaments may gain entry into the sacroiliac joints.[13] Another even more uncommon mechanism of joint infection is direct seeding of organisms into the joint during diagnostic or surgical procedures.

CLINICAL HISTORY

The typical patient with pyogenic sacroiliitis is a young man with fever who develops acute pain over the buttock.[4] Those who have subacute or chronic symptoms are frequently afebrile. The period of time between onset of symptoms and diagnosis may range from 12 to 20 days.[14] The pain is severe and may radiate to the low back, hip, thigh, abdomen, or calf.[1] Radiation of pain is related to irritation of the first two sacral, superior gluteal, and obturator nerves that cross anterior to the joint capsule. Abdominal pain associated with nausea and vomiting can confuse the diagnosis.[15, 16] A normal appendix was surgically removed because of the clinical impression of appendicitis in one patient.[14] Patients also complain of severe leg pain that prevents them from bearing weight on the affected limb. Irritation of the iliopsoas muscle as it passes anterior to the sacroiliac joint may cause persistent hip flexion and result in pain on motion of the hip. Pyogenic sacroiliitis is usually unilateral, although bilateral disease can occur.

PHYSICAL EXAMINATION

Physical examination demonstrates tenderness over the sacroiliac joint and pain on compression of the joint. Hyperextension of the hip, the Gaenslen's sign, stresses the sacroiliac joint capsule and causes pain in the buttock. Patrick's test, or the fabere sign—flexion, abduction, external rotation, and extension—of the hip, may be associated with sacroiliac joint pain. The test is done by placing the ankle of the affected side on the opposite knee and exerting downward pressure on the bent knee. If the maneuver is performed slowly, the hip may be taken through a full range of motion without producing sacroiliac pain. Therefore, the test should be done rapidly so that the sacroiliac joint will be stressed and become painful. Straight leg raising may be limited owing to stretching of inflamed sacral nerve roots over the anterior of the sacroiliac joint. A subgluteal abscess with swelling of the buttock and obliteration of the gluteal fold may also be seen. Infection may track along different fascial planes, presenting as masses in the inner thigh, posterior thigh, hip, lumbar spine, or abdomen.[15, 17] Rectal examination is important to detect the presence of these lesions. Muscle spasm of the gluteal and lumbar paravertebral muscles may be severe. The severity of the spasm may cause severe pain and scoliosis of the lumbar spine.[2] Fever and chills may be seen in the patient with an acute onset of disease.[3]

LABORATORY FINDINGS

Laboratory results demonstrate mild anemia, leukocytosis, and elevation in the ESR. Blood cultures may be positive in up to 50% of patients, eliminating the need for joint aspiration. Arthrocentesis of the sacroiliac joint under general anesthesia with fluoroscopic guidance is the most effective method of diagnosing pyogenic sacroiliitis.[18] Closed needle biopsy is of particular utility in patients with negative blood cultures.[19] Aspirations without fluoroscopy do not obtain adequate specimens.[4] Computed tomography has also been used for aspiration of the sacroiliac joint.

S. aureus and *S. epidermidis* account for a majority of infections of the sacroiliac joint.[1] *P. aeruginosa* is frequently cultured from sacroiliac joints in parenteral drug abusers.[20] Aerobic and anaerobic streptococci may also be cultured.[3] A wide variety of organisms have been associated with pyogenic sacroiliitis including *S. milleri, E. coli, N. gonorrhoea, P. mirabilis, Salmonella heidelberg,* and *Veillonella parvula.*[7, 21–25] Unilateral sacroiliitis also has been associated with syphilis during its secondary phase.[26]

Brucellosis is an infectious disease most commonly diagnosed in individuals in the Middle East, (an endemic area), those that consume raw milk, or those that attend infected animals. The most commonly affected joint is the sacroiliac joint. In a series of 214 patients, the sacroiliac joints were affected in 72.4%.[27] These individuals have low back pain with or without tenderness. Brucellar sacroiliitis has been reported in individuals who have emigrated to the United States.[28]

Tuberculosis also is associated with pyogenic sacroiliitis. Sacroiliac tuberculosis was a more common disease before the development of effective antituberculous antibiotic therapy. Strange reported 329 cases of sacroiliac tuberculosis.[29] The patients developed this complication as a manifestation of a generalized tubercular infection (Fig. 12–8). Sacroiliac joint involvement occurs in up to 9.7% of patients with skeletal tuberculosis. Patients have buttock pain and tenderness on direct palpation of the affected joint.[30] The onset of disease is insidious, the pain aching, and the course indolent. The diagnosis of tuberculous sacroiliitis may be confirmed by aspiration of fluid. The yield is improved by the simultaneous culture of synovial tissue. Therefore, open surgical biopsy may be required to confirm this diagnosis.[31] Closed biopsy may be adequate to yield tissue for culture and microscopic evaluation if open biopsy is too invasive.[30] Open biopsy also may be required from patients with fungal sacroiliitis as well, although aspiration may be adequate to obtain specimens that are subsequently positive on culture.[6]

RADIOGRAPHIC EVALUATION

The duration of symptoms before the appearance of radiographic changes in the sacro-iliac joints in bacterial sacroiliitis is 2 weeks (Fig. 12–9).[1] The radiographic findings include blurring of joint margins, pseudowidening of the joint space, erosions, and reactive sclerosis. The lower ilium is affected first, since the fibrocartilage is thinner on the iliac side compared with the sacral side of the joint. Healing is associated with bony ankylosis.

Bone scintiscans are very useful in rapidly identifying increased joint activity associated with infection, and localization is possible within 2 days of symptoms.[32] Shielding of radioactivity in the urinary bladder may allow detection of minimal asymmetry in tracer uptake early in the course of the illness. The 3-phase bone scan may be useful in differentiating osteomyelitis, septic arthritis, and cellulitis. The 3-phase bone scan consists of perfusion, blood pool, and delayed images. Blood pool is increased in all, while only osteomyelitis is associated with increased uptake on delayed bone images.[33] ^{99m}Tc[34] methylene diphosphonate or gallium scintiscans are more sensitive than plain roentgenograms in intravenous drug abusers.[34] CT may be more useful than plain radiographs in detection of early joint changes.[35] CT may identify subtle joint space widening, osseous erosion, or increased density of periarticular fat.[36]

MR is a sensitive radiographic technique for the detection of inflammatory conditions. A comparison of scintiscan, CT, and MR demonstrates a 100% sensitivity of MR compared to lesser sensitivities for the other techniques. MR demonstrated fluid in the sacroiliac joint, inflammation in bone marrow of the sacrum or ilium, swelling in the iliopsoas muscle, along with tracking of fluid posterior to the psoas muscle.[37] MR also is able to identify joint erosions in patients with disease of longer duration.[38]

DIFFERENTIAL DIAGNOSIS

The diagnosis of pyogenic sacroiliitis is frequently missed owing to a lack of physician awareness of this infection and the nonspecific low back symptoms of these patients, but it must be suspected in the appropriate host who presents with severe radiating low back pain. A bone scan will help localize the lesion to the sacroiliac joints. CT or MR may identify early changes of joint inflammation before plain roentgenograms are positive. Positive synovial fluid cultures from the sacroiliac joint confirm the diagnosis if blood cultures are negative. Biopsy is necessary if the diagnosis remains in

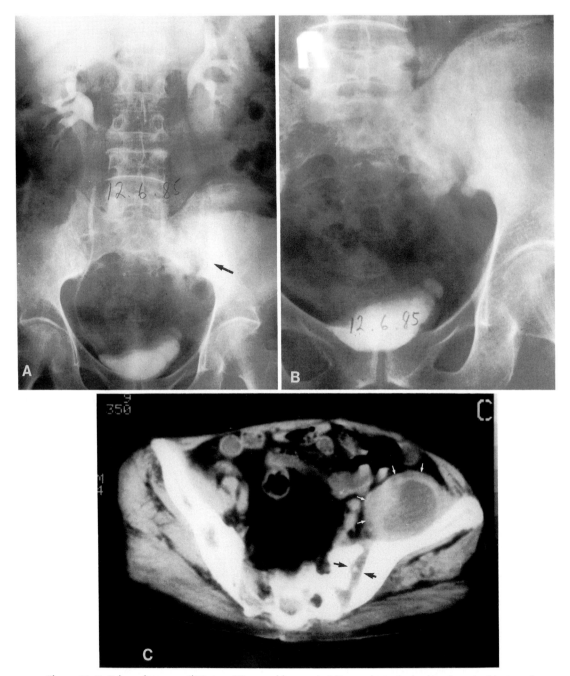

Figure 12–8. Tuberculous sacroiliitis in a 77-year-old man. *A,* IVP reveals marked sclerosis and widening of the left sacroiliac joint (*arrow*). *B,* Close-up view of the left sacroiliac joint. *C,* CT scan of pelvis demonstrating erosion of the left sacroiliac joint (*black arrows*) and associated soft tissue abscess (*white arrows*). (Courtesy of Theodor Schifter, M.D.)

doubt, cultures are negative, and granulomatous infection is being considered.

Unilateral sacroiliac joint infection must be differentiated from appendicitis, septic arthritis of the hip, gluteal abscess, psoas abscess, pyelonephritis, intervertebral disc herniation, intraspinal tumors, and metastatic disease.[39]

Osteomyelitis of the ilium may cause infection of a contiguous sacroiliac joint. The converse rarely occurs because of the tendency of primary infections of the sacroiliac joint to perforate the joint capsule anteriorly as opposed to invading surrounding bone.

Careful examination of the patient by physi-

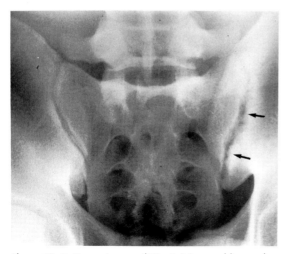

Figure 12–9. Pyogenic sacroiliitis. A 24-year-old man developed systemic lupus erythematosus requiring prednisone, 80 mg/day. The patient developed acute, severe, left-sided low back pain. The patient remained immobilized in bed because of pain. Aspiration of the sacroiliac joint yielded purulent fluid that grew *S. aureus* on culture. The patient improved with 6 weeks of vancomycin therapy. A roentgenogram of the pelvis at 17 months after hospitalization reveals unilateral involvement (*arrows*) with joint widening, erosion, and reactive sclerosis of the left sacroiliac joint.

cal and radiographic means should differentiate the patient with a local infection in the sacroiliac joint from those with infection in other areas in the axial skeleton and surrounding soft tissues. Cancer affecting bone usually has a more indolent course and multiple areas of involvement. Neoplasms of the sacrum include benign primary tumors, such as an aneurysmal bone cyst, osteoblastoma and giant cell tumor, and malignant primary tumors which include sarcomas, chordomas, myeloproliferative tumors, and metastatic tumors.[40]

The rare occurrence of bilateral disease must be differentiated from the seronegative spondyloarthropathies including ankylosing spondylitis, enteropathic arthritis, psoriatic arthritis, and Reiter's syndrome. These diseases have a much less explosive course. They are frequently associated with other systemic manifestations of disease (for example, skin rash, urethritis, and iritis), which help differentiate them from bilateral septic joint infection.

The vertebral apophyseal joints become infected in rare circumstances. Patients have localized back pain radiating into the buttock and lower extremity. Plain roentgenographs may not demonstrate an abnormality. Apophyseal joint infection should be considered if posterior elements of the vertebral bodies are affected. The abnormality may be suspected in

individuals with unilateral abnormalities on bone single photon emission CT, bone scintigraphy, or CT.[41, 42] Extension of the infection may cause extradural infection or epidural abscesses.[43]

TREATMENT

The therapy for septic arthritis of the sacroiliac joint consists of a high dose of parenteral antibiotics, which are chosen on the basis of susceptibility testing. The duration of the therapy is variable, but some studies have reported control of the infection in just days of antibiotic therapy.[1] Most studies have suggested that a minimum of 4 to 6 weeks of parenteral therapy is preferable,[2, 4] but oral antibiotics may be used if adequate bactericidal levels of antibiotics against the patient's organism are achieved at 1:8 dilution. Surgical drainage is required for periarticular abscesses and the débridement of necrotic bone and cartilage. Immobilization in a spica cast is unnecessary.

Tuberculous infection of the sacroiliac joint requires triple-drug therapy. This regimen includes isoniazid, ethambutol, and rifampin or streptomycin for 3 months. Two drugs are usually continued for 18 months.[44] Others have used two drugs for shorter periods of time.[45] Fungal infection may require amphotericin B and/or oral 5-fluorocytosine for at least a 6-week course.[6]

PROGNOSIS

With early diagnosis and adequate antibiotic therapy, septic arthritis of the sacroiliac joint has a good outcome. With therapy, patients can expect resolution of symptoms of pain, limitation of motion, and fever. The ESR returns to normal. Many patients have no radiographic changes and return to normal function. Even patients who have fusion of the sacroiliac joint as a result of an infection should expect no functional disability.

References

PYOGENIC SACROILIITIS

1. Delbarre F, Rondier J, Delrieu F, Evrard J, Cuyla J, Menkes CJ, Amor B: Pyogenic infection of the sacroiliac joint. J Bone Joint Surg 57A:819, 1975.
2. Lewkonia RM, Kinsella TD: Pyogenic sacroiliitis: diagnosis and significance. J Rheumatol 8:153, 1981.
3. Longoria RK, Carpenter JL: Anaerobic pyogenic sacroiliitis. South Med J 76:649, 1983.
4. Gordon G, Kabins SA: Pyogenic sacroiliitis. Am J Med 69:50, 1980.

5. Iczkovitz JM, Leek JC, Robbins DL: Pyogenic sacroiliitis. J Rheumatol 8:157, 1981.
6. Brand C, Warren R, Luxton M, Barraclough D: Cryptococcal sacroiliitis: case report. Ann Rheum Dis 44:126, 1985.
7. Vyskocil JJ, McIlroy MA, Brennan TA, Wilson FM: Pyogenic infection of the sacroiliac joint: case reports and review of the literature. Medicine 70:188, 1991.
8. Chandler FA: Pneumococcic infection of the sacroiliac joint complicating pregnancy. JAMA 101:114, 1933.
9. Dunn EJ, Bryan DM, Nugent JT, Robinson RA: Pyogenic infections of the sacroiliac joint. Clin Orthop 118:113, 1976.
10. Moyer RA, Bross JE, Harrington TM: Pyogenic sacroiliitis in a rural population. J Rheumatol 17:1364, 1990.
11. Veys EM, Govaerts A, Coigne E, et al.: HLA and infective sacroiliitis. Lancet 2:349, 1974.
12. Goldstein MJ, Nasr K, Singer HC, Anderson JG: Osteomyelitis complicating regional enteritis. Gut 10:264, 1969.
13. Oppenheimer A: Paravertebral abscesses associated with Strümpell-Marie diseases. J Bone Joint Surg 25:90, 1943.
14. Coy JT, Wolf CR, Brower TD, Winter WG Jr: Pyogenic arthritis of the sacroiliac joint: long-term follow-up. J Bone Joint Surg 58A:845, 1976.
15. L'Episcopo JB: Suppurative arthritis of the sacroiliac joint. Ann Surg 104:289, 1936.
16. Norman GF: Sacroiliac disease and its relationship to lower abdominal pain. Am J Surg 116:54, 1968.
17. Avila L: Primary pyogenic infections of the sacroiliac articulation. J Bone Joint Surg 23:922, 1941.
18. Hendrix RW, Lin PJP, Kane WJ: Simplified aspiration or injection technique for the sacroiliac joint. J Bone Joint Surg 64A: 1249, 1982.
19. Pouchot J, Vinceneux P: Usefulness of closed needle biopsy of sacroiliac joint in pyogenic sacroiliitis. J Rheumatol 18:1944, 1991.
20. Gifford DB, Patzakis M, Ivler D, Swezey RL: Septic arthritis due to *Pseudomonas* in heroin addicts. J Bone Joint Surg 57A:631, 1975.
21. Humphreys H, Keane CT, Marron P, Casey E: Infective sacroiliac arthritis and psoas abscess caused by *Streptococcus milleri*. J Infect 19:77, 1989.
22. Sacks-Berg A, Strampfer MJ, Cunha BA: *Escherichia coli* sacroiliitis: report of a case and review of the literature. Heart Lung 17:371, 1988.
23. Kerns SR, Dougherty K, Pope TL, Scheld WM: Septic sacroiliitis due to *Proteus mirabilis*. South Med J 83:589, 1990.
24. Mayall BC, Rodgers-Wilson S, Veit F: Sacroiliac joint infection by *Salmonella heidelberg*. Med J Aust 151:600, 1989.
25. Pouchot J, Vinceneux P, Michon C, et al.: Pyogenic sacroiliitis due to *Veillonella parvula*. Clin Infect Dis 15:175, 1992.
26. Reginato AJ, Ferreiro-Seoane JL, Falasca G: Unilateral sacroiliitis in secondary syphilis. J Rheumatol 15:717, 1988.
27. El-Desouki M: Skeletal brucellosis: assessment with bone scintigraphy. Radiology 181:415, 1991.
28. Abeles M, Mond CB: Sacroiliitis and brucellosis. J Rheumatol 16:136, 1989.
29. Strange FGS: The prognosis in sacroiliac tuberculosis. Brit J Surg 50:561, 1963.
30. Pouchot J, Vinceneux P, Barge J, et al.: Tuberculosis of the sacroiliac joint: clinical features, outcome, and evaluation of closed needle biopsy in 11 consecutive cases. Am J Med 84:622, 1988.
31. Wallace R, Cohen AS: Tuberculous arthritis: A report of two cases with review of biopsy and synovial fluid findings. Am J Med 61:277, 1976.
32. Berghs H, Remans J, Drieskens L, et al: Diagnostic value of sacroiliac joint scintigraphy with ^{99m}technetium pyrophosphate in sacroiliitis. Ann Rheum Dis 37:190, 1978.
33. Lisbona R, Rosenthall L: Observation on the sequential use of ^{99m}Tc-phosphate complex and ^{67}Ga imaging in osteomyelitis and septic arthritis. Radiology 123:123, 1977.
34. Guyot DR, Manoli A II, Kling GA: Pyogenic sacroiliitis in IV drug abusers. AJR 149:1209, 1987.
35. Carrera GF, Foley WD, Kozin F, et al.: CT of sacroiliitis. AJR 136:41, 1981.
36. Mitchell M, Howard B, Haller J, et al.: Septic arthritis. Radiol Clin North Am 26:1295, 1988.
37. Klein MA, Winalski CS, Wax MR, Piwnica-Worms DR: MR imaging of septic sacroiliitis. J Comput Assist Tomogr 15:126, 1991.
38. Murphey MD, Wetzel LH, Bramble JM, et al.: Sacroiliitis: MR imaging findings. Radiology 180:239, 1991.
39. Murphy ME: Primary pyogenic infection of sacroiliac joint. NY State J Med 77:1309, 1977.
40. Mansfield FL: Case records of the Massachusetts General Hospital. N Engl J Med 318:306, 1988.
41. Halpin DS, Gibson RD: Septic arthritis of a lumbar facet joint. J Bone Joint Surg 69B:457, 1987.
42. Swayne LC, Dorsky S, Caruana V, Kaplan IL: Septic arthritis of a lumbar facet joint: detection with bone SPECT imaging. J Nucl Med 30:1408, 1989.
43. Roberts WA: Pyogenic vertebral osteomyelitis of a lumbar facet joint with associated epidural abscess: a case report with review of the literature. Spine 13:948, 1988.
44. Gorse GJ, Pais MJ, Kusske JA, Cesario TC: Tuberculous spondylitis: a report of six cases and a review of the literature. Medicine 62:178, 1978.
45. Goldberg J, Kovarsky J: Tuberculous sacroiliitis. South Med J 76:1175, 1983.

HERPES ZOSTER

Capsule Summary

Frequency of back pain—very common

Location of back pain—lumbosacral dermatomes

Quality of back pain—burning, tingling, sharp, deep boring

Symptoms and signs—vesicular dermatomal rash, fever

Laboratory and x-ray tests—lymphocytosis, increased antibody response, lesional culture

Treatment—analgesics, corticosteroids, antiviral agents

PREVALENCE AND PATHOGENESIS

Herpes zoster (shingles) is a late complication of a varicella infection (chicken pox) during childhood. The disease is characterized by an erythematous, papular rash accompanied by pain in the distribution of a peripheral sensory nerve. The pain may antedate the skin lesions by 4 to 7 days and confuse the diagnosis. The process may resolve without any residual symptoms, but in older patients the infection may result in scarring and persistent pain that is resistant to treatment. In some patients, the pain is severe enough to cause considerable disability.

The varicella-zoster virus (VZV) belongs to the herpes virus group, which includes herpes simplex virus, cytomegalovirus, and Epstein-Barr virus. These viruses contain DNA in a viral capsid surrounded by an envelope that allows the virus to gain entrance into the host cells. The virus can replicate itself only within host cells. VZV incorporates variable amounts of host membrane into its envelope, allowing it to lie dormant in a "normal" cell. Clinical expression of the illness occurs when immune surveillance diminishes, allowing the virus to emerge from its hiding place.

The initial infection with VZV is varicella (chicken pox) at which time patients develop a viremia with dissemination of the virus throughout the body. The termination of this illness corresponds with the activation of both humoral and cellular immune mechanisms. The VZV is sequestered in the posterior spinal sensory ganglia in the spinal cord, where it remains dormant for an unspecified time. During a period of low host resistance, the viruses grow in a ganglion or nerve, resulting in skin lesions and pain. Patients with herpes zoster are infectious and can transmit a varicella infection to previously unexposed people. Evidence suggests that zoster is a reactivation of a previous infection and not due to a new exposure, since a varicella infection in a patient does not give zoster to someone who has previously had chicken pox.[1]

The factors that initiate the resurgence of infection are not known, but advancing age and diminished immune competence play a role. The incidence of herpes zoster is increased in patients over 50 years of age. Hope-Simpson reported in a study of 182 zoster patients a rate of 2 to 3 cases per 1000 for patients aged 20 to 50, 5 cases per 1000 for patients 50 years of age, and over 10 cases per 1000 for those 80 years old.[2] In another study, herpes zoster also occurred more frequently in an elderly population.[3] Herpes zoster occurs in 10% to 20% of the population.[4] It also is more common in patients with impaired immune function. This may be particularly true in patients with diminished cell-mediated immunity to VZV; lesional interferon concentrations are decreased in those with more widespread disease.[5] Herpes zoster was associated with lymphoreticular malignancies with VZV infection occurring in 25% of patients with Hodgkin's disease and 10% of non-Hodgkin's lymphoma patients over a 2-year study.[6] Patients who are receiving chemotherapy and/or radiotherapy also may have an increased risk of developing zoster. However, people who are otherwise normal who develop zoster are not more likely to develop a malignancy than any other healthy person.[7] Often, there is no identifiable precipitating cause for the reactivation of the virus, although trauma to an area of skin may precede the appearance of lesions. Zoster exhibits no sexual or racial predilection and has no seasonal variation or relation to varicella epidemics.

Herpes zoster starts in an individual with a history of chicken pox with replication of virus in the cell body of a cutaneous sensory neuron lying in the dorsal root ganglion. The virus spreads within the sensory nerve both centrally and peripherally. Histologic examination of the central nervous system will show inflammation, hemorrhage, and necrosis in the dorsal root ganglion, the posterior horn, and occasionally the corresponding motor neuron in the adjacent anterior horn. (This finding correlates with the occasional patient with motor loss associated with zoster lesions.) The large myelinated sensory fibers are preferentially affected; this results in a decreased ratio of large position to small pain fibers, diminishing pain modulation at the spinal cord level. The virus reaches the skin and replicates in the lower epidermal layers with ballooning degeneration of cells and development of multinucleated giant cells and intranuclear inclusion bodies. Inflammation in the skin causes erythema, edema, vesicular eruptions, hemorrhage, and necrosis. Healing in the skin results in depigmentation, atrophy, and permanent scarring. The virus can be grown from early vesicles but is unlikely once the lesion becomes pustular and develops a crust.

CLINICAL HISTORY

Herpes zoster presents with a 4- to 28-day prodrome of constitutional symptoms including fever, malaise, chills, lethargy, and gastrointestinal symptoms, particularly in the elderly. The first local symptom is usually pain in the nerve segment, which is burning or shooting in character and is often associated with dysesthesias in the area of skin supplied by the affected nerve root. Within a week after the onset of pain, an eruption appears as a series of localized erythematous papules that develop into vesicles grouped together upon an erythematous base and follow a segmental distribution (Fig. 12–10). Rarely, the pain may be followed by minimal erythema or no skin changes at all ("zoster sine herpete").[8] In this situation, the central nervous system is damaged without producing skin ulcers. This form of the disease may cause extensive neurologic disease and may be fatal in immunocompromised patients.[9] Within days, the eruption fades and the vesicles dry with crusts, leaving small scars in the skin. The skin may become partially or completely analgesic. Pain usually resolves with the skin lesion; however, it may persist for years. This postherpetic neuralgia is more likely to occur in elderly patients.

The course of the pain of zoster follows a characteristic pattern. Once the rash appears, the pain of the prodrome period recedes. As the rash evolves, the sensory and pain disturbances disappear, especially in those people under 40 years of age. In those over 50, the pain is more pronounced and is usually associated with unpleasant dysesthesias, the most distressing of which is pressure sensitivity of the skin to any touch. When the rash is at its greatest extent, the pain is minimal. As the rash crusts, the pain recurs, usually with an intense, lancinating quality. The pain becomes constant, deep, and boring. The skin feels increasingly tightened. The course of the rash and the pain are clearly not synchronous. Patients with resolution of the rash but continued pain are considered to have postherpetic neuralgia.

The frequency and severity of postherpetic neuralgia increases with age, with 35% of patients 60 years of age and 50% of patients over 70 years of age experiencing such pain.[10] The symptoms may last weeks to years. The pain has an unrelenting, deep, boring quality which is intensified by paroxyms of lancinating pain. To diminish the dysesthesias, patients often try to keep clothes off the affected area. Others may complain of a feeling of worms under the skin or ants crawling on the skin (formication). Patients may become clinically depressed because of the pain.

The dermatomes over the whole back are frequently affected. The thoracic spinal nerves are affected in 50% to 55% of cases, the cervical nerves in 15% to 20%, the lumbar and sacral nerves in 10% to 15%, and cranial nerves in 10% to 15%. The upper lumbar segments are more commonly affected than the lower segments.[11] The same segment may be involved with zoster on two or three occasions.[2] Herpes zoster infection is not associated with lumboradicular syndromes with or without a herniated disc.[12]

PHYSICAL EXAMINATION

The skin lesions may be found in any segmental sensory nerve distribution. They have a characteristic appearance that helps distinguish this lesion from other skin diseases. The lesions begin as an erythematous patch or indurated plaque. Scattered, grouped vesicles (1 to 3 mm) on an erythematous base are usual. The distal end of a skin dermatome is initially affected and new lesions appear in a more central location over a 1-week period. The lesions tend to coalesce, form a linear array, but remain unilateral and do not cross the midline. Occasionally, patients do develop bilateral disease and a few scattered extradermatomal vesicles. This is not necessarily a sign of disseminated disease associated with a worse prognosis.[13]

The vesicles are initially clear, then grow cloudy, crust, and desquamate over a 3-week period. Once crusts appear, the lesions are no longer contagious. The lesions heal with post-inflammatory hypopigmented macules or patches. If secondarily infected, lesions may

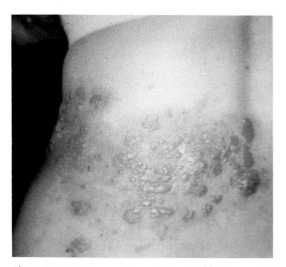

Figure 12–10. Herpes zoster. A 44-year-old woman with connective tissue disease on no medication developed severe, burning pain over the left side of her back. Four days after the onset of pain, the patient developed vesicular lesions in an T11 dermatomal pattern. The patient was treated with prednisone 40 mg/day for 3 weeks. She had no postherpetic neuralgia and her skin healed with residual hyperpigmentation. Over the following 5 years, her skin hyperpigmentation has lessened and she has experienced no postherpetic pain.

have depressed scars. Multiple areas of cutaneous lesions suggest disseminated disease.

In addition to cutaneous manifestations, patients with zoster may demonstrate other manifestations of neurologic dysfunction. Patients may have mild paresis in the motor nerve that corresponds to the spinal root level of the involved cutaneous nerve. The paresis is usually temporary.[14] Visceral involvement as well as autonomic nerve involvement occurs. Sacral zoster is sometimes associated with urinary retention and bladder paralysis. Cystoscopy reveals vesicles of the bladder neck, representing involvement of the autonomic supply of the bladder.[15] Other rare signs of central nervous system involvement included transverse myelitis, encephalitis, and cerebral vasculitis.[16, 17]

Physical examination may reveal fever and localized lymphadenopathy during the initial phase of disease. A non-immunosuppressed patient with no known underlying disease who develops disseminated lesions warrants a careful physical examination for lymphadenopathy and splenomegaly, and laboratory tests (CBC, renal function, anergy panel) to screen for a hidden lymphoproliferative malignancy.

LABORATORY DATA

Cerebrospinal fluid examination may demonstrate an increase in white blood cells in up to a third of patients with zoster. Viral cultures may be positive for virus if fluid from acute vesicular lesions is cultured. Gel-precipitin techniques can also be used to demonstrate specific antigens in fluid and crusts of lesions. Zoster antibodies may show a 4-fold rise during an infection.[18]

Dermal epithelial cells obtained from scraping the early lesions may show giant cells and intranuclear inclusion bodies. The Tzanck test findings are compatible but not diagnostic of zoster infection, since herpes simplex may show similar abnormalities.

RADIOGRAPHIC EVALUATION

Radiographs of the lumbar spine may demonstrate abnormalities such as fracture-dislocation, metastatic disease, or spinal tumor, which correspond to the location of the affected sensory root ganglion.

DIFFERENTIAL DIAGNOSIS

The diagnosis of herpes zoster is not difficult when the characteristic pain and vesicular eruption is present. The diagnosis is more difficult in the pre-eruptive stage. Zoster should be considered in the patient with sudden onset of burning pain in a segmental distribution. Following these patients for a short period until the appearance of vesicles helps establish the correct diagnosis. Herpes zoster should be considered in the differential diagnosis of radiculopathy even in the absence of skin rash.[19]

Other skin lesions may be confused with herpes zoster infection. Herpes simplex does not usually affect an entire dermatome as zoster does. Culture of lesions should help make the distinction. Contact dermatitis may appear in a linear band but lacks the painful prodrome. It is pruritic as opposed to painful, may cross the midline, and does not cause paresthesias. Superficial pyoderma, like impetigo, has fewer lesions, is not linear, and has no associated paresthesias. The radiation of pain may be confused with muscle strain or a herniated intervertebral disc.[20] The appearance of the skin rash helps differentiate zoster from these mechanical causes of back pain.

TREATMENT

The treatment of zoster is mainly supportive and is directed at controlling pain. Antibiotic therapy is indicated only for patients who develop bacterial superinfection. Patients with vesicles are infectious and should limit contact with individuals who have not had varicella. They are no longer infectious once the lesions crust over.

The therapeutic goals are to (1) limit segmental infection, (2) prevent general dissemination, (3) prevent tissue injury, and (4) prevent postherpetic neuralgia (Table 12–5). The first two goals deal with limiting viral replication, while the third deals with limiting inflammation, which causes tissue injury.[21] It is important to remember that herpes zoster is a self-limited illness, so treatment must be tailored specifically to the patient's age and status of immune function. In otherwise healthy patients under age 50, therapy may be limited to analgesics, mild sedatives, antipruritics, and antibacterial ointments. In the healthy individual over age 50, the goal is to prevent postherpetic neuralgia. Corticosteroids in short-course therapy have been shown to prevent the development of postherpetic pain in a significant percentage of patients.[22, 23] A study of oral high-dose acyclovir (an inhibitor of herpes virus DNA polymerase) in 205 immunocompetent patients over 60 years demonstrated faster healing when the drug was given early in the course of the eruption.[24] Patients receiving

**TABLE 12–5. THERAPY FOR
HERPES ZOSTER**

Immunocompetent	
Younger than 50	Analgesics
	Sedatives
	Topical antibacterial ointment for ulcerations
Older than 50	Corticosteroids (60 mg/day for 3-week period)
	Acyclovir?
	Adenosine monophosphate?
Immunocompromised	Intravenous acyclovir 500 mg/m² over 1 hour t.i.d. for 1 week
	or
	Oral acyclovir 800 mg 5 times daily for 1 week
Postherpetic neuralgia	Amitriptyline up to 100 mg daily
	Cutaneous nerve stimulation
	Local nerve blocks
	Capsaicin?

adenosine phosphate, 100 mg intramuscularly 3 times a week for 4 weeks, had improved healing and decreased pain as compared with a group receiving a placebo.[25] Additional studies are needed to clarify the role of these drugs in zoster infection in normal hosts. Epidural or sympathetic blockade in patients with zoster for 28 days or less does not prevent the onset of postherpetic neuralgia.[26, 27] Review of the studies of drugs used for the prevention of postherpetic neuralgia demonstrates deficiencies in study design.[28]

Appropriate therapy for immunocompromised patients, young and old, is associated with greater potential toxicities. The therapy is instituted to prevent the dissemination of virus beyond the primary dermatome. Administration of vidarabine, a purine analogue that blocks viral replication through its effects on viral DNA polymerase, given within 3 days of the onset of skin rash, has accelerated healing and decreased dissemination and postherpetic neuralgia as compared with the course of disease in controls.[29] The disadvantages of the drug include the need for 12-hour continuous intravenous infusion and renal toxicity. Zoster immune globulin (ZIG) has not been shown to be better than serum gamma globulin for prevention of dissemination and postherpetic neuralgia in immunocompromised patients and has not been recommended for this purpose.[30]

Intravenous acyclovir has become the recommended therapy for immunocompromised patients. The recommended intravenous dosage of 500 mg/m² of body surface adminis-

tered over 1 hour 3 times a week for 1 week at the earliest sign of the rash has reduced pain and dissemination and increased the rate of healing.[31] Acyclovir is a more selective antiviral agent and has less host toxicity. Oral acyclovir is used in ambulatory patients. Oral acyclovir, 800 mg 5 times/day for 7 days, is recommended for zoster in normal hosts.[32]

The role of corticosteroids in the immunocompromised group is limited. Corticosteroids may promote dissemination and not prevent postherpetic pain. Therefore, they have not been recommended for this group of patients.

Postherpetic neuralgia, once established, is a difficult problem to treat. Oral acyclovir is no better than placebo in relieving pain secondary to postherpetic neuralgia.[33] Therapy is directed at controlling pain, not at killing virus. Some of the therapies that have been tried include amitriptyline (25 mg nightly with maintenance dose of 100 mg), oral corticosteroids, intralesional triamcinolone, cutaneous nerve stimulation, anesthetic nerve blocks, and topical medications including capsaicin.[34] Niv and associates suggested that different components of postherpetic pain be treated with specific agents. Burning pain may best respond to tricyclic antidepressants, lancinating pain to anticonvulsant drugs (valproic acid), and dysesthetic pain to neuroleptic medication (fluphenazine). Patients with intact skin sensitivity respond to transcutaneous electrical nerve stimulation (TENS), and those with intact sensation may respond to dry needling to the level of the underlying muscle. The majority of the 97 consecutive patients treated with components of this conservative therapy had significant pain relief.[35]

A study of oral corticosteroids demonstrated no definite improvement compared to placebo for postherpetic neuraligia.[36] Antidepressants, amitriptyline, and desipramine, but not lorazepam, have been associated with relief of postherpetic pain.[37, 38] Topical capsaicin is more effective when applied daily for 6 weeks.[39] On a single dose basis, clonidine 0.2 mg has greater pain relief than codeine 120 mg, ibuprofen 800 mg, and placebo for postherpetic neuralgia.[40] Mexiletine, an oral lidocaine-like antiarrhythmic agent, has been helpful in the treatment of diabetic neuropathy.[41] Mexiletine, 450 to 900 mg in divided doses, has been effective in decreasing pain associated with peripheral nerve injuries.[26] This drug may have the potential to be effective for the treatment of neuralgia secondary to herpes virus reactivation. Studies involving zoster patients will need to be completed before the efficacy is documented. In general, many patients with neuralgia remain resistant to these therapies and continue to have pain.

PROGNOSIS

Herpes zoster is usually a disease of short duration causing little permanent disability. However, the patient who is older and has an underlying illness may be left with permanent residual effects. These may include postherpetic neuralgia, paralysis, and widespread dissemination. Postherpetic neuralgia is rare in patients under 40 years of age but occurs in up to 75% of patients over age 60.[23] Disseminated herpes zoster with at least 20 or more vesicles outside the primary dermatome occurs up to 10 days after the onset of skin rash and affects up to 10% of patients with zoster infections. Approximately 30% of these patients are immunocompromised, particularly those with lymphoproliferative malignancy,[42] immunosuppressive therapy, and poor cell-mediated immunity.[43] Most patients have resolution of disseminated zoster without sequelae. However, the immunocompromised patient has a worse prognosis.

Those patients left with persistent and intractable postherpetic pain may suffer significant disability. Available therapy to prevent this component of zoster infection or to manage its after-effects is inadequate.

References

HERPES ZOSTER

1. Miller LH, Brunell PA: Zoster, reinfection or activation of latent virus? Observations on the antibody response. Am J Med 49:480, 1970.
2. Hope-Simpson RE: The nature of herpes zoster: a long-term study and a new hypothesis. Proc R Soc Med 58:9, 1965.
3. Weller TH: Varicella and Herpes Zoster: changing concepts of the natural history, control, and importance of a not-so-benign virus. N Engl J Med 309:1362, 1434, 1983.
4. Strauss SE, Ostrove JM, Inchauspe G, et al.: Varicella-zoster virus infections: biology, natural history, treatment, and prevention. Ann Intern Med 108:221, 1988.
5. Stevens DA, Merigan TC: Interferon, antibody, and other host factors in herpes zoster. J Clin Invest 51:1170, 1972.
6. Schimpff S, Serpick A, Stoler B, et al.: Varicella-zoster infection in patients with cancer. Ann Intern Med 76:241, 1972.
7. Ragozzino MW, Melton LJ, Kurland LT, et al.: Risk of cancer after herpes zoster: a population-based study. N Engl J Med 307:393, 1982.
8. Burgoon CF, Burgoon JS, Baldridge GD: The natural history of herpes zoster. JAMA 164:265, 1957.
9. Dueland AN, Devlin M, Martin JR, et al.: Fatal varicella-zoster virus meningoradiculitis without skin involvement. Ann Neurol 29:569, 1991.
10. de Moragas JM, Kierland RR: The outcome of patients with herpes zoster. Ach Dermatol 75:193, 1957.
11. Watson CPN: Postherpetic neuralgia. Neurol Clin 7:231, 1989.
12. Jensen PK, Andersen EB, Boesen F, et al.: The incidence of herniated disc and varicella zoster virus infection in lumboradicular syndrome. Acta Neurol Scand 80:142, 1989.
13. Juel-Jensen BE: Herpes simplex and zoster. Br Med J 1:406, 1973.
14. Thomas JE, Howard FM Jr: Segmental zoster paresis—a disease profile. Neurology 22:459, 1972.
15. Frengley JD: Herpes zoster. A challenge in management. Primary Care 8:715, 1981.
16. Hogan EL, Krigman MR: Herpes zoster myelitis: evidence for viral invasion of the spinal cord. Arch Neurol 29:309, 1973.
17. Horte B, Price RW, Jiminez D: Multifocal varicella-zoster virus leukoencephaltis temporally remote from herpes zoster. Ann Neurol 9:251, 1981.
18. Williams V, Gershon A, Brunnel PA: Serologic response varicella-zoster membrane antigens measured by indirect immunofluorescence. J Infect Dis 130:669, 1974.
19. Burkman KA, Gaines RW Jr, Kashani SR, Smith RD: Herpes zoster: a consideration in the differential diagnosis of radiculopathy. Arch Phys Med Rehabil 69:132, 1988.
20. Rash MR: Herpes zoster complicating a herniated-thoracic disc. Orthop Review 11:91, 1982.
21. Price RW: Herpes zoster: an approach to systemic therapy. Med Clin North Am 66:1105, 1982.
22. Eaglestein WH, Katz R, Brown JA: The effects of early corticosteroid therapy on skin eruption and pain of herpes zoster. JAMA 211:1681, 1970.
23. Keczkes K, Basheer AM: Do corticosteroids prevent postherpetic neuralgia? Br J Dermatol 102:551, 1981.
24. Mc Kendrick MW, McGill JI, White JE, Wood MJ: Oral acyclovir in acute herpes zoster. Br J Med 293:1529, 1986.
25. Sklar SH, Blue WT, Alexander EJ, Bodian CA: Herpes zoster: the treatment and prevention of neuralgia with adenosine monophosphate. JAMA 253:1427, 1985.
26. Yanagida H, Suwa K, Corssen G: No prophylactic effect of early sympathetic blockade on postherpetic neuralgia. Anesthesiology 66:73, 1987.
27. Nurmikko TJ, Rasanen A, Hakkinen V: Clinical and neurophysiological observations on acute herpes zoster. Clin J Pain 6:284, 1990.
28. Schmader KE, Studenski S: Are current therapies useful for the prevention of postherpetic neuralgia? A critical analysis of the literature. J Gen Intern Med 4:83, 1989.
29. Whitley RJ, Soong SJ, Dolin R, et al: NIAID collaborative antiviral study group: early vidarabine therapy to control the complications of herpes zoster in immunocompromised patients. N Engl J Med 307:971, 1982.
30. Stevens D, Merigan T: Zoster immune globulin prophylaxis of disseminated zoster in compromised hosts. Arch Intern Med 140:52, 1980.
31. Bean B, Braun C, Balfour H: Acyclovir therapy for acute herpes zoster. Lancet 2:118, 1982.
32. Whitley RJ, Gnann JW Jr: Acyclovir: a decade later. N Engl J Med 327:782, 1992.
33. Surman OQ, Flynn T, Schooley, RT, et al.: A double-

blind, placebo-controlled study of oral acyclovir in postherpetic neuralgia. Psychosomatics 31:287, 1990.

34. Waston CP, Evans RJ, Reed K, et al.: Amtriptyline vs placebo in postherpetic neuralgia. Neurology 32:671, 1982.

35. Niv D, Ben-Ari S, Rappaport A, et al.: Postherpetic neuralgia: clinical experience with a conservative treatment. Clin J Pain 5:295, 1989.

36. Post BT, Philbrick JT: Do corticosteroids prevent postherpetic neuralgia? J Am Acad Dermatol 18:605, 1988.

37. Max MB, Schafer SC, Culnane M, et al.: Amitriptyline, but not lorazepam, relieves postherpetic neuralgia. Neurology 38:1427, 1988.

38. Kishore-Kumar R, Max MB, Schafer SC, et al.: Desipramine relieves postherpetic neuralgia. Clin Pharmacol Ther 47:305, 1990.

39. Bernstein JE, Korman NJ, Bickers DR, et al.: Topical capsaicin treatment of chronic postherpetic neuralgia. J Am Acad Dermatol 21:265, 1989.

40. Max MB, Schafer SC, Culnane M, et al.: Association of pain relief with drug side effects in postherpetic neuralgia: a single-dose study of clonidine, codeine, ibuprofen, and placebo. Clin Pharmacol Ther 43:363, 1988.

41. Dejgard A, Petersen P, Kastrup J: Mexiletine for the treatment of chronic painful diabetic neuropathy. Lancet I:9, 1988.

42. Merselis J, Kaye D, Hook E: Disseminated herpes zoster. A report of 17 cases. Arch Intern Med 113:679, 1964.

43. Mazur W, Whitley R, Dolin R: Serum antibody levels as risk factors in the dissemination of herpes zoster. Arch Intern Med 139:1341, 1979.

LYME DISEASE

Capsule Summary

Frequency of back pain—uncommon

Location of back pain—lumbar spine

Quality of back pain—ache

Symptoms and signs—erythema chronica migrans, general malaise, radiculoneuritis

Laboratory and x-ray tests—elevated ESR, borrelia antibodies, CSF pleocytosis

Treatment—antibiotics: oral for early disease, intravenous for late disease

PREVALENCE AND PATHOGENESIS

Lyme disease is an infectious illness caused by the spirochete, *Borrelia burgdorferi*, which was identified by Willie Burgdorfer in 1982.[1] The organism is transmitted to humans by a tick vector. The clinical manifestations of the illness appear as the *Borrelia* disseminate through the organs of the body and the immune system mounts a cellular and humoral response to the organism. A generalized malaise mimicking a flu-like state, including low back pain, occurs simultaneously with the appearance of a characteristic skin rash, erythema chronicum migrans. In later stages of the illness, cardiac and neurologic manifestations become prominent. Polyradiculitis, including the lower extremities, is associated with this stage. Chronic arthritis, chronic fatigue, and encephalomyelitis are potential manifestations of late disease. Lyme disease is suspected in an individual exposed to ticks and who develops an appropriate array of symptoms and signs. Diagnosis is confirmed by the presence of IgM or IgG antibodies to the *Borrelia*. All stages of the illness are treated with antibiotics, but they are most successful in early stages.

Lyme disease is the most common vector-transmitted disease in the United States.[2] Over 40,000 cases had been reported to the Centers for Disease Control from 1982 to 1991.[3] The illness is endemic in three areas of the United States: the Northeast from Maryland to Northern Massachusetts; the upper Midwest in Minnesota and Wisconsin; and the West, primarily the coast of California and Oregon. These locations correspond to areas with large deer populations. The deer are the primary hosts for the tick, *Ixodes dammini*, which is the vector for transmission of Lyme disease. However, the illness is not exclusive to these areas of the United States since cases have been reported in 43 states. The geographic spread of the illness in individual states has increased.[4] It also has been reported in Europe, Russia, Japan, and Australia. Lyme disease affects people in all age groups. A significant number of children are affected under the age of 9 years. Females and males are almost equally affected, 53% and 47%, respectively.[3] Lyme disease occurs primarily in caucasians, reflecting the exposure of this group to a nonurban setting.

The illness is spread to geographic areas by the tick vector. The tick, *Ixodes dammini*, is associated with the disease in the East and Midwest and in the West, *Ixodes pacificus*. The tick has a 3-stage, 2-year life cycle. The life cycle includes a larval, nymph, and adult stage of development. The usual host for the larval and nymph stage is the white-footed mouse, *Peromyscus leucopus*. The mouse is the primary reservoir for *B. burgdorferi*. The *Borrelia* parasitize the mice without causing illness, and the host is disease-free for the remainder of its life.

The life cycle of the tick is a complex process. Eggs are deposited in the early summer. Larvae do not hatch until July. Larvae that feed before September molt to become nymphs and those that do not feed will feed the following spring. Nymphs must feed again before they molt to become adults. Adult females attach to large vertebrates to feed and mate. After mating, the females are able to lay eggs to start a new cycle. White-tailed deer are the favorite host for the adult ticks. The frequency of Lyme disease infections relates, to a significant degree, to the size of the local deer population.

Larval or nymphal ticks feed on the mice and become infected with *B. burgdorferi*. The ticks become vectors of the illness for humans when they feed again in a later developmental stage. The *B. burgdorferi* reside in the midgut of the tick. With attachment of the tick to a host, the *Borrelia* are mobilized to the salivary glands where they infect the vertebrate.[5] This process requires approximately 24 hours to complete. Adult ticks do not transfer *B. burgdorferi* to their offspring. Larvae typically become infected with *Borrelia* by feeding on a reservoir host rather than from congenital transmission. The passage of *B. burgdorferi* between ticks and mice maintains the high rate of infection of the tick vectors in an endemic area.

The pathogenesis of Lyme disease is not entirely clear.[6] The currently accepted theory is that the organisms persist throughout the course of the illness. Organisms, although few in number, have been detected in affected organ systems long after the onset of the illness.[7, 8] Further evidence for the persistence of organisms is the variety of new IgG antibodies that emerge over time with prolonged illness. Amplification of the B-cell response would be unlikely without a changing antigenic stimulus.[9] In addition, antibiotics have a beneficial effect on the course of the illness at all stages of the disease.[10] In regard to genetic predisposition to particular manifestations of the illness, individuals with histocompatibility typing DR4 are susceptible to chronic Lyme arthritis.[11]

CLINICAL HISTORY

The clinical manifestations of Lyme disease may be dermatologic, cardiac, neurologic, or musculoskeletal during the course of the illness (Table 12–6). The disease is best described by a classification system that divides the illness into early and late infection. The affected organ systems manifest a variety of abnormalities depending on the duration of the infection.

Early infection is characterized by the emergence of pathognomonic skin lesions, localized lymphadenopathy, and a flu-like syndrome. This stage of the illness corresponds to the local invasion of the skin and associated lymph nodes by the organisms, along with systemic response manifested by a flu-like syndrome. Erythema chronicum migrans (ECM) is the most common and distinctive cutaneous manifestation of Lyme disease. ECM appears at the site of the tick bite. The lesions are identified in 60% to 80% of Lyme disease patients.[10, 12] The skin lesion appears between 2 to 28 days after the bite of an infected tick. The lesion starts as a single, expanding red macule, expands in an annular fashion, and may become 15 cm or larger. The central area may clear, forming a target lesion. The skin lesion is usually asymptomatic but may be tender, warm, or pruritic. *B. burgdorferi* may be isolated occasionally from skin biopsies obtained from the advancing front of the lesion but are rarely needed to identify the origin of the skin lesion.[13] The skin lesion appears most commonly on the trunk (38%), lower extremities (38%), upper extremities (11%), pelvic region (7%), and head and neck (6%).[14] Skin folds are preferred areas for tick attachment.

The flu-like syndrome is characterized by fatigue, fever, chills, malaise, headache, stiff neck, and arthralgias. Backache occurs in 26% of patients.[15] These symptoms may be the only clues to the diagnosis of Lyme disease when the skin lesion is absent. Less common manifestations include malar rash, sore throat, and nausea and vomiting.

As the *B. burgdorferi* organisms escape to the systemic circulation, the disseminated phase of early infection occurs. Additional organ systems are affected. Within a few weeks of disease onset, up to 48% of untreated patients develop multiple annular skin lesions.[16] Hematogenous spread of the *Borrelia* causes these lesions, that resemble ECM, to appear. The lesions may vary in number up to 20, are smaller than ECM lesions, and are less expansive.

Cardiac manifestations of early disseminated disease appear between 4 days to 7 months after the onset of disease.[17] Cardiac disease has been reported in 4% to 20% of Lyme disease patients. Heart block is the primary manifestation of cardiac involvement.[18] First-degree to complete heart blocks have been reported. Cardiac conduction abnormalities are temporary, lasting a few weeks. Temporary pacing is occasionally required for high-grade atrioventricular block. Atrial arrhythmias occur in association with Lyme pericarditis, while ventricular arrhythmias are associated with myocarditis.

TABLE 12–6. CLINICAL STAGES OF LYME DISEASE

EARLY INFECTION		LATE INFECTION
Localized	*Disseminated*	*Persistent*
Erythema chronicum migrans	Multiple annular lesions	Chronic arthritis
Local lymphadenopathy	Bell's palsy	Encephalomyelitis
	Meningitis	Chronic fatigue
	Radiculoneuritis	Acrodermatitis chronica atrophicans
	AV nodal block	
	Migratory arthralgias	
	Severe fatigue	
	Generalized lymphadenopathy	

Neurologic system involvement complicates early disseminated disease in 20% of patients.[19] Neurologic symptoms and signs develop weeks to 12 months after the resolution of ECM. The manifestations of nervous system disease include lymphocytic meningitis, cranial nerve palsies, peripheral neuritis, and radiculoneuritis.[20] Lyme meningitis, the most common CNS manifestation of Lyme disease, is associated with severe headache, stiff neck, photophobia, nausea and vomiting, and irritability.[21] Approximately 50% of patients with Lyme meningitis have associated encephalitis. Concentration deficits, emotional lability, and persistent fatigue are manifestations of encephalitis. The peripheral nervous system is involved. Peripheral neuritis; sensory radiculitis; brachial, lumbar, or sacral plexitis; and sensorimotor radiculoneuritis may occur within the first months of the illness.[1] These neurologic disorders may present with a variety of symptoms and signs including burning pain, paresthesia, loss of reflexes, and focal motor weakness. A majority of patients may develop facial (Bell's) palsy.[21] Other cranial nerves, including III, V, and VIII, also have been affected. A minority of patients (31% to 44%) develop radiculoneuritis, usually in the setting of cranial neuropathy.[20, 21] Upper extremity abnormalities are more common than lower. Involvement of the sensory and motor nerves of the lower extremities may occur in the setting of similar disease in the upper extremities. The patients with lower extremity disease have severe radicular pain, dysesthesias, sensory loss, leg weakness, and mononeuritis multiplex. Pain is the first symptom followed within 4 weeks by motor weakness. Weakness begins gradually and may progress to atrophy of the muscle. Sensory loss follows pain in a similar time frame in 50% of patients.[19] The sensory loss is dermatomal in distribution in the upper extremities. In the lower extremities, a symmetrical distal sensory loss may occur. The simultaneous occurrence

of radiculoneuritis and CSF pleocytosis is common in Europe and is know as Bannwarth's syndrome or tick-borne meningopolyneuritis.[22]

Musculoskeletal manifestations of early disease are primarily arthralgias and myalgias that occur within 8 weeks of infection.[22] Pain occurs in one or two sites at a time and migrate to other musculoskeletal structures. These locations may be affected for hours to days with spontaneous resolution of symptoms lasting for months. Fatigue is the most common symptom. Subsequently, a majority of untreated patients develop intermittent episodes of frank arthritis 4 days to 2 years after disease onset.[23] The large joints, particularly the knee, become swollen and warm but not significantly painful. The pattern of involvement is asymmetrical. Small joint involvement, independent of large joint disease, is unusual. The most frequently affected extra-articular locations are the back (14%) and neck (10%).[22] Periarticular involvement may occur interspersed with episodes of arthritis in other locations of the musculoskeletal system. In most circumstances, only one periarticular structure is affected at a time, with pain lasting weeks to months in a given location.

Late infection manifestations occur as the *Borrelia* persist in organ systems infected during earlier stages of the illness. Acrodermatitis chronica atrophicans is the skin manifestation of persistent infection in Lyme borreliosis.[24] The lesion occurs predominantly in women between 40 and 70 years of age. It begins insidiously with bluish-red discoloration and swollen skin on an extremity, usually the lower leg or foot. The inflammatory stage of the lesion may persist for years. Subsequently, the skin in the involved area becomes atrophic and develops a wrinkled appearance. ECM may have been present at the same site years earlier. *B. burgdorferi* may be cultured from these lesions for as long as 10 years after their onset.[25]

A spectrum of central and peripheral nervous system abnormalities has been described in late disease, which occurs more than 1 year after the onset of disease. These disease manifestations are uncommon. The most clearly defined is progressive encephalomyelitis characterized by spastic paresis, bladder dysfunction, ataxia, cranial nerve deficits, and dementia.[26] Late polyneuropathy may be manifested by sensory or motor abnormalities. Tingling paresthesias may occur in 50% of patients with late Lyme borreliosis.[27] The paresthesias are located distally in the arms, legs, or both, and are asymmetric and patchy in distribution. Radicular pain in the legs occurs in 25% of patients with onset corresponding with the onset of paresthesias.[28]

Monarticular or oligoarticular arthritis involving the knee is the most common musculoskeletal manifestation of late Lyme borreliosis.[23] Approximately 11% of untreated individuals with ECM will develop arthritis that will be persistent for 1 year or longer. Synovitis will appear between 4 months to 4 years after the appearance of ECM. In addition to the knee, the shoulder or hip are affected. Joint involvement is a more frequent manifestation of illness in Europe than in the United States. The arthritis may persist for 4 years or longer or spontaneously resolve.[29]

PHYSICAL EXAMINATION

Physical findings in the initial stages of the illness include the presence of ECM and regional lymphadenopathy. Musculoskeletal pain may occur at rest or with motion. The lumbar spine may be painful with palpation. Pain occurs only in one or two regions at a time. Episodes may resolve in hours to several days. This syndrome has been referred to as "localized, intermittent musculoskeletal pain" (LIMP).[30] Irregular pulse may be noticed in patients with cardiac involvement. Neurologic abnormalities may include cranial nerve dysfunction, sensory or motor nerve impairment (including sciatic nerve), and mental confusion or impaired memory. Patients with late disease may have patches of atrophic skin, persistent monarticular arthritis, spastic paresis, or organic brain syndrome.

LABORATORY DATA

The commonly ordered screening blood tests, including CBC, ESR, and serum chemistries, yield normal or nonspecific results during early disseminated disease.[31] The ESR is elevated in a majority of patients. A smaller proportion of patients have microscopic hematuria and abnormal levels of immunoglobulins, cryoglobulins, and liver enzymes.[32] In patients with neurologic involvement, the CSF has a lymphocytic pleocytosis and elevated protein concentration.[19] Antibodies against *Borrelia* also may be locally produced and detected in CSF. Synovial fluid analysis reveals findings consistent with an inflammatory arthropathy, including leukocyte counts of 5000 to $100,000/mm^3$ and predominantly polymorphonuclear leukocytes, with elevated protein and normal glucose concentrations.[10] Culture of skin, blood or synovial fluid rarely renders a positive result for *B. burgdorferi* and is rarely obtained in the clinical setting.

Histopathologic evaluation of tissue biopsies have the potential to identify the presence of organisms in affected organs.[33] The organisms are most easily identified in the skin at a time before dissemination when they are are most abundant. Inflammatory infiltrates may be identified in a variety of tissue samples but are not specific enough in the absence of organisms to make a definitive diagnosis. For example, synovial biopsy specimens reveal histopathologic changes that are similar to rheumatoid arthritis and Reiter's syndrome.[34]

Serologic tests are very helpful in detecting the antibody response, including IgM and IgG antibodies, to epitopes on the surface structures of *B. burgdorferi*.[35] Within the first 2 to 4 weeks of infection, IgM immunoglobulins directed against the flagellar antigen of *B. burgdorferi* appear. IgM antibodies peak after 6 to 8 weeks of illness. IgG immunoglobulins appear over the next few weeks corresponding with the gradual decrease in IgM antibody titer over 4 to 6 months. Patients with persistent disease have IgG antibodies exclusively, which remain indefinitely. Successful antibiotic therapy may result in a fall in IgG titer but only over a number of months. Some patients have persistently elevated antibodies despite eradication of the organism. These antibodies are most effectively detected by enzyme-linked immunosorbent assays (ELISA). The ELISA test is more sensitive and reproducible than immunofluorescence assays. Most ELISA tests use extracts of sonicated whole *B. burgdorferi* as antigen. The ELISA is associated with both false-negative and false-positive results. False-negative results occur during the first few weeks of infection before antibodies develop or in individuals who receive an inadequate course of antibiotic therapy early in the course of the illness but remain infected with live organisms. False-positive results occur in patients with a variety of spirochetal illnesses including gingivitis, syphilis, Rocky Mountain spotted fever, mononucleosis, and autoimmune disorders, such as rheumatoid arthritis and systemic lupus erythematosus (SLE). Although poor reproducibility of results is a major concern in interpreting Lyme antibody titers, the standardization of ELISA tests along with a relative high titer level has helped to differentiate true positive tests from sources of background cross-reactivity.

Western blot analysis is an immunoblotting technique used to confirm ELISA results or to detect antibody early in the clinical course of the illness that may not be detected by the ELISA method.[36] Western blot analysis detects antibodies to a number of specific *Borrelia* antigens. Although the ELISA and Western blot analyses are helpful, great diversity exists in the results of laboratories when testing the same samples.[37] These inconsistencies emphasize the utility of serologic tests as adjuncts in the clinical diagnosis of Lyme disease.

In rare circumstances, when the diagnosis of Lyme disease is suspected but serologic tests are inconclusive, T lymphocyte assays for reactivity to *Borrelia*-specific antigens may be helpful.[38] The subset of patients with late Lyme disease who have negative or indeterminate antibody responses are best candidates for the T-cell proliferative assay.[39] T-cells from infected patients proliferate when exposed to whole organisms. This assay is time consuming and should be completed in patients with a strong suspicion for the diagnosis without positive serologic tests.

A test that should be available soon for the diagnosis of Lyme disease utilizes polymerase chain reaction (PCR) technology.[40] PCR detects the presence of a very small amount of genomic DNA of *B. burgdorferi*. The PCR is superior to ELISA or the Western blot analysis since it relies on the presence of the organism itself for a positive result. PCR will become the diagnostic method of choice.

RADIOGRAPHIC EVALUATION

Radiographic findings of the lumbosacral spine are normal in patients with Lyme disease. Radiographic abnormalities, when they occur, are located in the peripheral joints, primarily the knee. Abnormalities include soft tissue swelling, loss of articular cartilage, chon-

drocalcinosis, and periarticular osseous erosions.[41]

DIFFERENTIAL DIAGNOSIS

The diagnosis of Lyme disease is based on the presentation of appropriate clinical symptoms in a patient who lives or has visited an endemic area. The history of a tick bite is helpful, but not essential, for the diagnosis. Culture of the organism from skin or its visualization on histologic sections of biopsies from affected organs is usually unrevealing. Serologic tests are useful adjuncts in diagnosis, but positive findings may be present in individuals previously exposed to the organisms but have cleared the infection. Basing a diagnosis solely on the presence of antibodies reactive to *B. burgdorferi* is to be discouraged.

The differential diagnosis as it affects back pain is related to the muscle pain syndromes and neurologic disorders that cause radiculopathy and plexopathy. Fibromyalgia has been associated with Lyme disease. Patients may develop tender points in the setting of Lyme disease.[42, 43] More often, patients develop the LIMP syndrome confined to one or two joint areas in clear distinction of the multiple areas affected with fibromyalgia.

The differential diagnosis of radiculopathy includes mechanical, neoplastic, and autoimmune disorders. Patients with mechanical disorders will describe radiating pain that is affected by body position. Assuming a comfortable position frequently relieves pain in patients with a mechanical cause of radiculopathy. Individuals with neoplastic disorders frequently have associated systemic symptoms that are rapidly progressive and disabling. Autoimmune disorders, such as SLE or systemic vasculitis, are associated with characteristic abnormalities in a variety of organ systems (malar rash, nodose lesions). These abnormalities help separate those patients with autoimmune disorders who may have false-positive serologic tests for Lyme disease from patients infected with *B. burgdorferi*.

THERAPY

The risk of tick bites can be reduced in endemic areas. Proper dress, by covering the skin, should be encouraged, including tucking trousers into socks to block attachment of ticks on the lower extremities. Clothes may be impregnated with N,N-diethylmetatoluamide or permethrin to deter ticks. However, exposure

TABLE 12–7. ANTIBIOTIC THERAPY FOR LYME DISEASE

Early Local Infection		
Erythema chronica migrans	tetracycline 500 mg q.i.d.	10–30 days
	doxycycline 100 mg b.i.d.	10–30 days
Children	amoxicillin 500 mg q.i.d.	10–30 days
Penicillin allergic	erythromycin 500 mg t.i.d.	10–30 days
Early Disseminated Infection		
Flu syndrome, Bell's palsy first-degree heart block	oral regimens	
Meningitis, radiculopathy, complete heart block, arthritis	ceftriaxone 2 gm IV q.d.	14–28 days
	cefotaxime 3 gm IV b.i.d.	14–28 days
or		
Late Persistent Infection	benzylpenicillin 5 million U IV q.i.d.	14–28 days

of the skin to these chemicals must be limited to decrease toxicities from these agents. During periods of feeding of the tick from spring to late summer, individuals should be examined daily for the presence of ticks. The transmission of disease is diminished by the daily removal of ticks since the inoculation of *B. burgdorferi* requires 24 hours or longer.

Randomized studies have demonstrated that the probability of developing symptoms of Lyme disease after an Ixodes tick bite is low and equals the rate of toxicity of the antibiotics used to treat the illness.[44] Prophylactic antibiotics should not be given routinely for tick bites.

Therapy for Lyme disease is based on antibiotics effective in eradicating *B. burgdorferi* from infected patients when clinical symptoms appear. *B. burgdorferi* is highly sensitive to tetracyclines, semisynthetic penicillins, and second- and third-generation cephalosporins. Erythromycin is an alternative agent but is less desirable than amoxicillin or doxycycline.[45] The actual choice of agent and its formulation, oral or intravenous, is dependent on the stage and organ involvement (Table 12–7).[46] The treatment of choice for early, local disease including ECM is doxycycline or tetracycline. Amoxicillin is used for children and pregnant women. Erythromycin is less effective but is an alternate choice in patients with penicillin allergy. The duration of therapy is 10 days. If patients have early disseminated disease, therapy may be continued for 30 days. Patients with facial palsy or first-degree heart block can be treated with oral antibiotics.

Patients with evidence of meningitis, radiculitis, or complete heart block have been treated with intravenous antibiotics. Intravenous antibiotics used to treat Lyme borreliosis include ceftriaxone and penicillin. Cefataxime is also effective for disseminated disease. Therapy is continued for 14 to 28 days. Patients with Lyme arthritis also are treated with intravenous antibiotics. Although no controlled studies have been completed for persistent late infection including central or peripheral nervous system disease, intravenous antibiotics are given for 28 days. The symptoms may not rapidly respond to the course of antibiotics. Clinical response may be delayed for as long as 6 to 8 months.[47] There is no scientific evidence to date supporting repeated courses of antibiotics for extended periods in the treatment of Lyme disease.

Major concern remains involving the use of parenteral antibiotic therapy for patients with nonspecific musculoskeletal pains and fatigue and a positive serologic test for Lyme disease. Lightfoot and coworkers suggest that costs and risks of intravenous antibiotic therapy outweigh the likelihood of improvement of nonspecific constitutional symptoms. Only when the value of patient anxiety about leaving a positive Lyme test untreated exceeds $3,500 for empiric antibiotic therapy is treatment cost-effective.[48]

PROGNOSIS

The prognosis of patients with Lyme disease with low back pain is excellent if they receive an appropriate course of antibiotics. They usually have no residual of back pain. Patients who have radiculopathy have neuroborreliosis. These patients may also respond to antibiotics but may require intravenous medications to improve. Clinical awareness of the symptoms and signs of Lyme disease in patients exposed to ticks should result in the rapid identification of the patient at risk for this illness. This is the most important way to prevent the dissemination of the organisms resulting in more serious forms of this illness. Radiculoneuropathy and peripheral neuropathy may resolve slowly over a 24-month period. The slow recovery may correspond to the slow healing of axonal damge. Prolonged courses of antibiotics do not influence the rate of recovery.

References

LYME DISEASE

1. Burgdorfer W, Barbour AG, Hayes SF, et al.: Lyme disease—a tick-borne spirochetosis? Science 216:1317, 1982.
2. Rahn DW: Lyme disease: Clinical manifestations, diagnosis, and treatment. Semin Arthritis Rheum 20:201, 1991.
3. Dennis DT: Epidemiology. In: Coyle PK (ed): Lyme Disease. St Louis: Mosby Yearbook, Inc., 1993, pp 27–37.
4. White DJ, Chang H, Benach JL, et al.: The geographic spread and temporal increase of the Lyme disease epidemic. JAMA 266:1230, 1991.
5. Burgdorfer W: Vector/host relationships of Lyme disease spirochete, *Borrelia burgdorferi*. Rheum Dis Clin North Am 15:775, 1989.
6. Garcia-Monco JC, Benach JL: The pathogenesis of Lyme disease. Rheum Dis Clin North Am 15:711, 1989.
7. Asbrink E, Hovmark A, Hederstedt B: The spirochetal etiology of acrodermatitis chronica atrophicans herxheimer. Acta Derm Venerol 64:506, 1984.
8. Johnston YE, Duray PH, Steere AC, et al.: Lyme arthritis: spirochetes found in synovial microangiopathic lesions. Am J Pathol 118:26, 1985.
9. Craft JE, Fischer DF, Shimamoto GT, Steere AC: Antigens of *Borrelia burgdorferi* recognized during Lyme disease: appearance of a new immunoglobulin M response and expansion of the immunoglobulin G response late in the illness. J Clin Invest 78:934, 1986.
10. Steere AC: Lyme disease. N Engl J Med 321:586, 1989.
11. Steere AC, Dwyer E, Winchester R: Association of chronic arthritis with increased DR4 and DR3. N Engl J Med 323:219, 1990.
12. Berger BW: Cutaneous manifestations of Lyme borreliosis. Rheum Dis Clin North Am 15:627, 1989.
13. Steere AC, Grodzicki RL, Kornblatt AN, et al.: The spirochetal etiology of Lyme disease. N Engl J Med 308:733, 1983.
14. Berger BW: Dermatologic aspects. In: Coyle PK (ed): Lyme Disease. St Louis: Mosby Yearbook, 1993, pp 69–72.
15. Steere AC, Bartenhagen NH, Craft JE, et al.: The early clinical manifestations of Lyme disease. Ann Intern Med 99:76, 1983.
16. Berger BW: Erythema chronicum migrans of Lyme disease. Arch Dermatol 120:1017, 1984.
17. Steere AC, Batsford WP, Weinberg M, et al.: Lyme carditis: cardiac abnormalities of Lyme disease. Ann Intern Med 93:8, 1980.
18. McAlister HF, Klementowicz PT, Andrews C, et al.: Lyme carditis: an important cause of reversible heart block. Ann Intern Med 110:339, 1989.
19. Reik L Jr: Neurologic aspects of North American Lyme

disease. In: Coyle PK (ed): Lyme Disease. St. Louis: Mosby Yearbook, 1993, pp 101–112.
20. Pachner AR, Steere AC: The triad of neurologic manifestations of Lyme disease: meningitis, cranial neuritis, and radiculoneuritis. Neurology 35:47, 1985.
21. Reik L, Steere AC, Bartenhagen, et al.: Neurologic abnormalities of Lyme disease. Medicine 58:281, 1993.
22. Ackerman R, Horstrup P, Schmidt R: Tick-borne meningopolyneuritis (Garin-Boujadoux, Bannwarth). Yale J Biol Med 57:485, 1984.
23. Steere AC, Schoen RT, Taylor E: The clinical evolution of Lyme arthritis. Ann Intern Med 197:725, 1987.
24. Asbrink E, Hovmark A: Early and late cutaneous manifestations of Ixodes-borne borreliosis (erythema migrans borreliosis. Lyme borreliosis). Ann NY Acad Sci 539:4, 1988.
25. Asbrink E, Hovmark A: Successful cultivation of spirochetes from skin lesions of patients with erythema chronica migrans and acrodermatitis chronica atrophicans. Acta Pathol Microbiol Immunol 66:161, 1985.
26. Ackermann R, Rehse-Kupper B, Gollmer E, Schmidt R. Chronic neurologic manifestations of erythema migrans borreliosis. Ann NY Acad Sci 539:16, 1988.
27. Logigian EL, Steere AC: Clinical and electrophysiologic findings in chronic neuropathy of Lyme disease. Neurology 42:303, 1992.
28. Logigian EL, Kaplan RF, Steere AC: Chronic neurologic manifestations of Lyme disease. N Engl J Med 323:1438, 1990.
29. Kaell AT, Bennett RS, Hamburger MI: Rheumatic manifestations. In: Coyle PK (ed) Lyme Disease. St. Louis: Mosby Yearbook, 1993, pp 73–85.
30. Kolstoe J, Messner RP: Lyme disease: musculoskeletal manifestations. Rheum Dis Clin North Am 15:649, 1989.
31. Rahn DW, Malawista SE: Lyme disease: recommendations for diagnosis and treatment. Ann Intern Med 114:472, 1991.
32. Kujala GA, Steere AC, Davis JS IV: IgM rheumatoid factor in Lyme disease: correlation with disease activity, total serum IgM and IgM antibody to *Borrelia burgdorferi*. J Rheumatol 14:772, 1987.
33. Duray PH: Histopathology of human borreliosis. In: Coyle PK (ed): Lyme Disease. St. Louis: Mosby Yearbook, 1993, pp 49–58.
34. Duray PH: The surgical pathology of human Lyme disease. An enlarging picture. Am J Surg Pathol 11(Suppl):47, 1987.
35. Magnarelli LA: Laboratory diagnosis of Lyme disease. Rheum Dis Clin North Am 15:735, 1989.
36. Ma B, Christen B, Leung D, Vigo-Pelfrey C: Serodiagnosis of Lyme borreliosis by western immunoblot: reactivity of various significant antibodies against *Borrelia burgdorferi*. J Clin Microbiol 30:370, 1992.
37. Corpuz M, Hilton E, Lardis P, et al.: Problems in the use of serologic tests for the diagnosis of Lyme disease. Arch Intern Med 151:1837, 1991.
38. Dattwyler RJ, Volkman DJ, Luft BJ, et al.: Seronegative Lyme disease: dissociation of specific T- and B-lymphocyte responses to *Borrelia burgdorferi*. N Engl J Med 319:1441, 1988.
39. Dressler F, Yoshinari NH, Steere AC: The T-cell proliferative assay in the diagnosis of Lyme disease. Ann Intern Med 115:533, 1991.
40. Rosa PA, Schwan TG: A specific and sensitive assay for the Lyme disease spirochete *Borrelia burgdorferi* using

defined area of dense sclerotic bone is virtually pathognomonic of osteoid osteoma. The amount of sclerosis is out of proportion to the small size of the nidus. Osteoid osteomas arise in the posterior elements of a vertebra (Fig. 13–3). The neural arch is affected in about 75% of vertebrae, articular facets in about 18%, and vertebral bodies in only about 7%.[20] The size and location of these lesions make them difficult to detect with plain roentgenograms (Fig. 13–4).

Bone scans are useful in localizing the lesion if plain roentgenograms are negative.[21] The nidus is demonstrated on radionuclide bone scan as an area of marked concentration of radioactivity.[22] Scintigraphy also may be used to monitor the occurrence of local tumor recurrence.[23] Computed tomography (CT) is also helpful in localizing the nidus and in detecting encroachment of the neoplasm on the spinal canal or the neural foramen (Fig. 13–5).[24] CT is the most useful for precise localization of the lesion and differentiating it from other bone lesions.[25] CT is the best technique for demonstrating subtle osseous detail, cortical penetration by a tumor, and matrix calcification and mineralization within a tumor.[26] In

rare circumstances, the intervertebral disc and surrounding bone may be altered if the tumor is located anteriorly in a vertebral body.[27] CT-guided percutaneous biopsy may be used to remove accessible lesions in the skeleton, including the lumbar spine.[28, 29] MR examination adds little in regard to clarifying bone architecture and is not used routinely in the evaluation of this primary bone tumor.[30]

DIFFERENTIAL DIAGNOSIS

The diagnosis of an osteoid osteoma is suggested by characteristic clinical and radiographic features and is confirmed by the histologic examination of biopsy material. Despite its characteristic appearance, osteoid osteoma of the spine remains an elusive diagnosis. Lumbosacral strain, psychogenic back pain, Scheuermann's disease, herniated nucleus pulposus, and nonspecific mechanical back pain are frequent prior diagnoses.[13, 31] In a large series, seven patients were clinically suspected of having herniated nucleus pulposus; three had undergone laminectomy.[2] Tomography and scintigraphy are extremely helpful in detecting lesions that are missed with

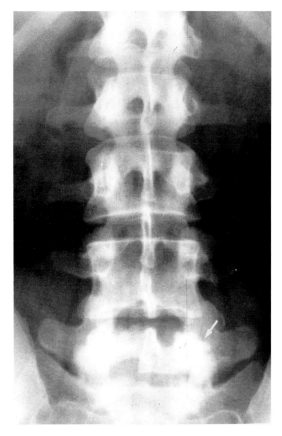

Figure 13–3. Osteoid osteoma. AP view of lumbar spine revealing a sclerotic pedicle of the L5 vertebra *(arrow)*. (Courtesy of Anne Brower, M.D.)

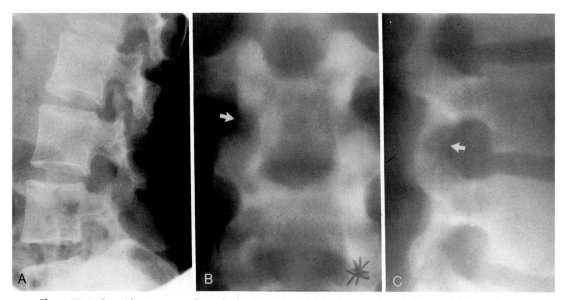

Figure 13–4. Osteoid osteoma involving the lamina of the third lumbar vertebra. *A,* Lateral plain film of spine is normal. Tomograms in AP *(B)* and lateral *(C)* directions reveal lucent nidus *(arrows)* with central calcific fleck. Minimal reactive bone surrounds the lucent nidus. (Courtesy of Anne Brower, M.D.)

screening roentgenograms. The physician's degree of suspicion should be raised when young adults with nontraumatic back pain have associated paravertebral muscle spasm and recent onset of scoliosis. Repeat evaluation and close follow-up are necessary in individuals with negative initial evaluations. These individuals may develop abnormal tests over a period of months.

Other diagnoses that need to be considered include osteoblastoma, osteosarcoma, osteomyelitis. Brodie's abscess, Ewing's sarcoma, eosinophilic granuloma, metastases, fracture, aseptic necrosis, osteochondritis, and aneurysmal bone cyst. Abnormalities in laboratory tests (elevated white blood cell count, erythrocyte sedimentation rate, bone chemistries) and characteristic histologic findings help differentiate these inflammatory, infectious, or malignant lesions from osteoid osteoma.

Osteosclerosis also is associated with the presence of bone islands or endostomas. A bone island is a homogeneous dense area of bone with distinct margins and no central lucent area. The absence of a nidus on pathologic section helps differentiate a bone island from an osteoid osteoma.[32] Bone islands are usually incidental roentgenographic findings and are clinically silent. Bone islands in the spine occur more commonly in the vertebral bodies. Rarely, they affect the posterior elements of the vertebrae and may expand over time.

In addition, histologic findings help differentiate the various lesions. For example, osteoblastoma is a larger lesion with less sclerosis. Ewing's sarcoma has no true nidus. Osteosarcoma may have "benign" areas that simulate osteoid osteoma, but careful examination will show areas of woven bone and osteoid of the malignant tumor infiltrating host lamellar bone. Osteoid osteoma may contain some atypical cells but does not infiltrate surrounding bone. Infiltration of any significant distance eliminates osteoid osteoma as a diagnostic consideration. The radiographic appearance of these lesions also helps differentiate them.

TREATMENT

Treatment of this benign lesion is simple excision of the nidus and surrounding sclerotic bone. If the nidus is not entirely removed, recurrence of the lesion is possible.[33] The pathologist should carefully examine the excisional biopsy to assure that the nidus has been fully removed.[14] Intraoperative bone scintiscans have been used to document the total removal of the nidus at the time of surgery.[34] The preoperative placement of a needle into the nidus under CT guidance is another method to identify the area of bone that must be surgically ablated.[35] Ablation of osteoid osteomas has been successful in accessible lesions with the use of a percutaneously placed electrode that heats the tip to 90° C for 4 minutes.[36] Total removal of the osteoma with surgical or percutaneous techniques may be a particular problem in poorly accessible areas of the spine. If the entire lesion is not removed, unroofing a cortical lesion with removal of some surrounding sclerotic bone may relieve symptoms.[37] Symptoms may persist when the nidus is not entirely removed. Even total removal of an osteoma does not guarantee prevention of a recurrence of the tumor. Osteoid osteomas have recurred in the same location after an asymptomatic interval of 10 years.[38] Medical therapy may alleviate symptoms but never to the same degree as is achieved with surgical removal of the neoplasm. Some patients may use nonsteroidal anti-inflammatory drugs to control tumor pain. However, unless the lesion spontaneously recedes, these patients do not obtain complete relief of symptoms without surgical ablation. It should also be noted that occasionally osteoid osteomas undergo spontaneous healing.[39]

PROGNOSIS

The course of osteoid osteoma is benign once the diagnosis is made and the lesion is excised. It may be a difficult diagnostic problem, however, because clinical symptoms may appear before it is radiographically evident. Low back pain and associated limitation of activities at work may be inappropriately ascribed to malingering or psychoneurosis. In the young adult with low back pain that is exacerbated at night and is relieved with aspirin, a thorough evaluation for the presence of this lesion is mandatory. Osteoid osteoma is a benign lesion without reported malignant transformation. Despite its benignity, osteoid osteoma should not be considered an innocuous lesion. Osteoid osteomas have been known to recur even after removal.[40] Persistent evaluation and appropriate surgery are necessary to prevent potential physical deformities and psychic stress in patients with this elusive neoplasm.

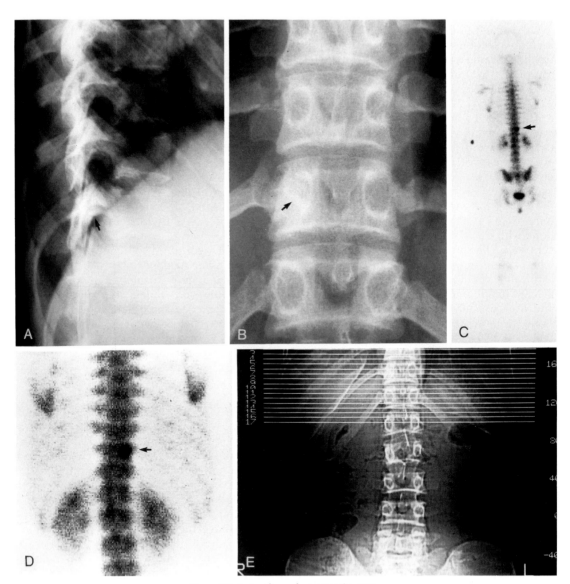

Figure 13–5. *See legend on opposite page*

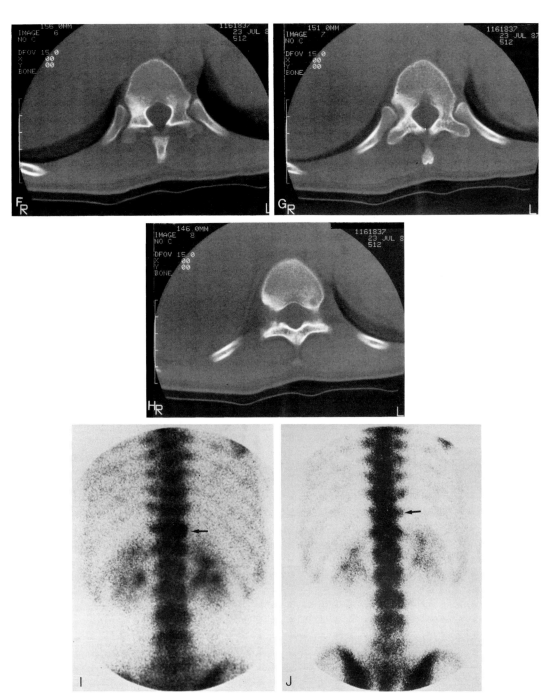

Figure 13–5. A 21-year-old woman gave a history of localized back pain over the thoracolumbar junction of 1 year's duration. The pain was increased at night and was responsive to salicylate therapy. *A,* Lateral view of the thoracolumbar junction reveals increased sclerosis in the pedicle of the T11 vertebra *(arrow). B,* Spot view of the lower thoracic vertebrae revealing an irregular border of the right pedicle *(arrow). C* and *D,* ^{99m}Tc MDP bone scan. *C,* Posterior view shows increased traces of accumulation in T11 *(arrow). D,* Spot view detects increased uptake in the lateral compartment of T11 *(arrows). E* to *H,* CT scan of the thoracolumbar junction. AP view *(E)* and views of levels 6 *(F),* 7 *(G),* and 8 *(H)* through T11, demonstrating reactive sclerosis around an area of central clearing without soft tissue extension. The diagnosis of osteoid osteoma was made and the patient's pain responded to diflunisal. The patient is being followed and is asymptomatic on the nonsteroidal drug 12 months later. She will have a biopsy of the lesion if it increases in size. The patient remained symptomatic despite 4 years of nonsteroidal therapy. *I,* ^{99m}Tc MDP bone scan completed one year before surgery reveals persistent accumulation of tracer in T11 *(arrow). J,* Repeat bone scan one day postoperatively reveals absence of increased uptake *(arrow)* one day after surgical removal of the osteoid osteoma confirmed on pathologic examination.

References

OSTEOID OSTEOMA

1. Mirra JM: Bone Tumors: Clinical, Radiologic, and Pathologic Correlations. Philadelphia: Lea & Febiger, 1989, pp 226–248.
2. Dahlin DC, Unni KK: Bone Tumors. General Aspects and Data on 8542 Cases, 4th ed. Springfield, IL. Charles C Thomas, 1986, pp 88–101.
3. Cohen MD, Harrington TM, Ginsburg WW: Osteoid Osteoma: 95 cases and a review of the literature. Semin Arthritis Rheum 12:265, 1983.
4. Freiberger RH: Osteoid osteoma of the spine: a cause of backache and scoliosis in children and young adults. Radiology 75:232, 1960.
5. Bettelli G, Capanna R, Van Horn Jr, et al.: Osteoid osteoma and osteoblastoma of the pelvis. Clin Orthop 247:261, 1989.
6. Huvos AG: Bone Tumors: Diagnosis, Treatment and Prognosis, 2nd ed. Philadelphia: WB Saunders, 1991, pp 49–66.
7. Jaffe, JL: Osteoid osteoma: a benign osteoblastic tumor composed of osteoid and atypical bone. Arch Surg 31:709, 1935.
8. Saville DP: A medical option for the treatment of osteoid osteoma. Arthritis Rheum 23:1409, 1981.
9. Sherman MS, McFarland G: Mechanism of pain in osteoid osteomas. South Med J 58:163, 1965.
10. Esquerdo J, Fernandez CF, Gomar F: Pain in osteoid osteoma. Histological facts. Acta Orthop Scand 47:520, 1976.
11. Byers PD: Solitary benign osteoblastic lesions of bone: osteoid osteoma and benign osteoblastoma. Cancer 22:43, 1968.
12. Lawrie TR, Aterman K, Sinclair AM: Painless osteoid osteoma. J Bone Joint Surg 52:1357, 1970.
13. Keim HA, Reina EG: Osteoid osteoma as a cause of scoliosis. J Bone Joint Surg 57:159, 1975.
14. Gitelis S, Schajowicz F: Osteoid osteoma and osteoblastoma. Orthop Clin North Am 20:313, 1989.
15. Haibach H, Farrell C, Gaines RW: Osteoid osteoma of the spine: surgically correctable cause of painful scoliosis. Can Med Assoc J 135:895, 1986.
16. Mehdian H, Summers B, Eisenstein S: Painful scoliosis secondary to an osteoid osteoma of the rib. Clin Orthop 230:273, 1988.
17. Silberman WW: Osteoid osteoma. J Inter Coll Surgeons 38:53, 1962.
18. Norman A, Dorfman HD: Osteoid osteoma inducing pronounced overgrowth and deformity of bone. Clin Orthop 110:233, 1975.
19. Schajowicz F, McGuire MH: Diagnostic difficulties in skeletal pathology. Clin Orthop 240:281, 1989.
20. Banna M: Clinical Radiology of the Spine and The Spinal Cord. Rockville, MD: Aspen Systems Corporation, 1985 pp 337–338.
21. Winter PF, Johnson PM, Hilal SK, Feldman F: Scintigraphic detection of osteoid osteoma. Radiology, 122:177, 1977.
22. Ghelman B: Radiology of bone tumors. Orthop Clin North Am 20:287, 1989.
23. Adams BK: Scintigraphy in benign bone tumours: a report of 4 cases. S Afr Med J 76:112, 1989.
24. Wedge HJ, Tchang S, MacFadyen DJ: Computed tomography in localization of spinal osteoid osteoma. Spine 6:423, 1981.
25. Bilchik T, Heyman S, Siegel A, Alavi A: Osteoid osteoma: the role of radionuclide bone imaging, conventional radiography and computed tomography in its management. J Nucl Med 33:269, 1992.
26. Heare TC, Enneking WF, Heare MM: Staging techniques and biopsy of bone tumors. Orthop Clin North Am 20:273, 1989.
27. Heiman ML, Cooley CJ, Bradford DS: Osteoid osteoma of a vertebral body: report of a case with extension across the intervertebral disc. Clin Orthop 118:159, 1976.
28. Mazoyer J, Kohler R, Bossard D: Osteoid osteoma: CT-guided percutaneous treatment. Radiology 181:269, 1991.
29. Poey C, Clement JL, Baunin C, et al.: Percutaneous extraction of osteoid osteoma of the lumbar spine under CT guidance. J Compt Assist Tomogr 15:1056, 1991.
30. Assoun J, Haldat FD, Richard G, et al.: Magnetic resonance imaging in osteoid osteoma. Rev Rhum [Engl Ed] 60:29, 1993.
31. MacLellan DF, Wilson FC Jr: Osteoid osteoma of the spine. J. Bone Joint Surg 49:111, 1967.
32. Gower DJ, Tytle T, Brumback R: Enlarging endostoma (bone island) of the spinous process. Neurosurgery 30:608, 1992.
33. Golding JSR: The natural history of osteoid osteoma with a report of 20 cases. J Bone Joint Surg 36B:218, 1954.
34. Lee DH, Malawer MM: Staging and treatment of primary and persistent (recurrent) osteoid osteoma. Clin Orthop 281:231, 1992.
35. Marcove RC, Heelan RT, Huvos AG, et al.: Osteoid osteoma: diagnosis, localization, and treatment. Clin Orthop 267:197, 1991.
36. Rosenthal DI, Alexander A, Rosenberg AE, Springfield D: Ablation of osteoid osteomas with a percutaneously placed electrode: a new procedure. Radiology 183:29, 1992.
37. Morrison GM, Hawes LE, Sacco JJ: Incomplete removal of osteoid osteoma. J Bone Joint Surg 33:166, 1951.
38. Regan MW, Galey JP, Oakeshott RD: Recurrent osteoid osteoma: case report with a ten-year asymptomatic interval. Clin Orthop 253:221, 1990.
39. Sim FH, Dahlin DC, Beabout JW: Osteoid osteoma. Diagnostic problems. J Bone Joint Surg 57A:154, 1975.
40. Dunlop JAY, Morton KS, Elliot GB: Recurrent osteoid osteoma. Report of a case with review of the literature. J Bone Joint Surg. 52B:128, 1980.

Osteoblastoma

Capsule Summary

Frequency of back pain—very common
Location of back pain—lumbar spine
Quality of back pain—dull, ache
Symptoms and signs—localized tenderness and pain
Laboratory and x-ray tests—posterior element expansile lesion on plain roentgenogram
Treatment—en-bloc or partial excision

PREVALENCE AND PATHOGENESIS

Osteoblastoma is a rare benign neoplasm of bone that accounts for about 3% of all benign bone tumors and about 0.5% of all bone tumors examined by biopsy.[1, 2] A majority of the lesions appear during the second or third decade of life. Nearly 90% of patients diagnosed with an osteoblastoma are 30 years of age or younger.[3] The tumor has a predilection for the spine. Approximately 40% of lesions are located in the axial skeleton.[4] The male to female ratio is 2.5 to 1.[5]

In the past, osteoblastoma has been referred to as an osteogenic fibroma, giant osteoid osteoma, spindle-cell variant of giant cell tumor, and osteoblastic osteoid tissue-forming tumor. Jaffe and Mayer in 1932 described a "benign" osteoblastic tumor of bone,[6] but it was Lichtenstein in 1956 who designated the lesion a benign osteoblastoma, which is now the accepted terminology.[7] The pathogenesis of osteoblastoma is unknown.

CLINICAL HISTORY

The major clinical symptom of osteoblastoma is dull, aching, localized pain over the involved bone. The pain is insidious in onset and may have a duration of months to years before diagnosis. As opposed to osteoid osteoma, the pain of an osteoblastoma is less severe, not nocturnal, and not relieved by salicylates. Pain may be aggravated by activity. Scoliosis may be a presenting feature. Osteoblastomas located in the lumbar spine may be associated with pain radiating into the legs, which may be accompanied by muscle spasm and limitation of motion. Pain was the presenting symptom in 81% of patients. Radicular pain was present in 29% of patients with spinal involvement.[5] Radicular pain and spinal cord

compression are more likely to occur in osteoblastoma than in osteoid osteoma because of its larger size. Osteoblastoma also may invade the spinal canal and completely encircle nerve roots.[8] It may cause abdominal symptoms when located in the sacrum.[9] The duration of pain before diagnosis averages about 14 months.

PHYSICAL EXAMINATION

Physical examination may demonstrate local tenderness on palpation with mild swelling over the spine. Pain may be exacerbated by spine extension.[10] A positive straight leg raising test is present in about 25% of patients.[7] Osteoblastomas associated with spinal cord compression will result in abnormalities on sensory and motor examination of the lower extremities. Reflexes may also be abnormal. Atrophy of surrounding muscles adjacent to the tumor may be seen.

LABORATORY DATA

This benign neoplasm does not have any associated abnormal screening blood tests. Characteristic abnormalities are present on pathologic examination. On gross examination, tumors are well circumscribed and composed of hemorrhagic granular tissue with variable calcification. The tumors range in size from 2 to 10 cm in length.

Histologically, an osteoblastoma may demonstrate cellular osteoblastic tissue with a large amount of osteoid material and the absence of chondrocytes and cartilage (Fig. 13–6). Multinucleated giant cells may be present. Mitotic

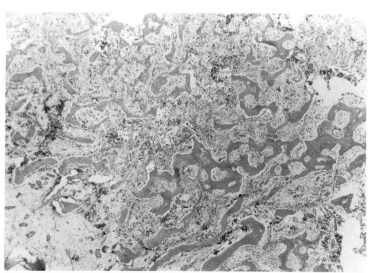

Figure 13–6. Osteoblastoma. Histologic section exhibiting a benign stroma, osteoblasts, and osteoclasts. The new osteoid matrix has a woven bone appearance. (Courtesy of Arnold Schwartz, M.D.)

figures may be seen, but atypical ones are not.[10] The tumor appears loosely arranged because of the large number of capillaries between the trabeculae of bone. The vascular character of the tumor shows features similar to those seen with aneurysmal bone cyst. The borders of the tumor are well demarcated and do not permeate the surrounding normal bone.

Difficulties exist in the differentiation of benign and aggressive, premalignant forms of osteoblastoma.[11] Flow cytometry may become more useful as a means of quantifying neoplastic cells harvested from the tumor. Additional studies will be needed to correlate the aneuploidy of cells and the biologic behavior of the tumor.[12]

RADIOGRAPHIC EVALUATION

Radiographic findings of osteoblastoma are variable and nonspecific. In the spine, lesions are most commonly located in the posterior elements of the vertebrae, including pedicles, laminae, and transverse and spinous processes

(Fig. 13–7).[13] The vertebral body is rarely primarily involved.[14] Osteoblastoma is located in the sacrum or lumbar spine in 40% of the lesions, in the cervical spine in 36%, and in the thoracic spine in 24%. In a study of 98 patients, 32 had spinal involvement. The distribution of lesions was 10 (31%) in the lumbar spine, 11 (34%) in the thoracic spine, 10 (31%) in the cervical spine, and 1 (3%) in the sacrum.[15] The lumbar spine was the site of an osteoblastoma in 53% of 65 patients with this bone tumor.[18] Osteoblastomas are expansile and may grow rapidly as measured by serial radiographic studies. Characteristically, the lesion is well delineated and is covered by a thin layer of periosteal new bone. The extent of reactive new bone formation is much less than that associated with osteoid osteoma (Fig. 13–8).[15] The center of the lesion may be radiolucent or radiopaque. A bone scan is helpful in localizing the lesion, but the finding of localized high uptake is nonspecific. Scoliosis may be noted in association with the tumor. The size of the tumor and the degree of scoliosis is not correlated. Bone scintigraphy may identify

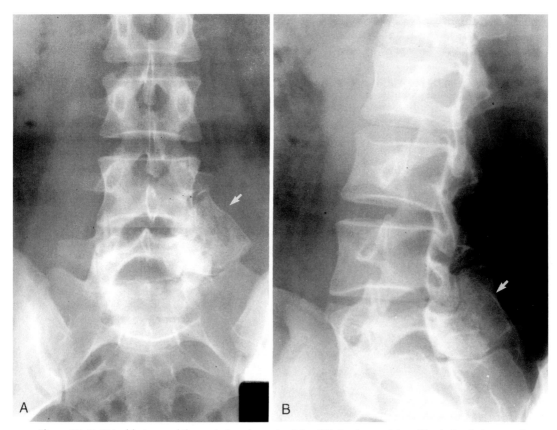

Figure 13–7. Osteoblastoma of the posterior elements of the fifth lumbar vertebra. The lesion is large and expansile, with well-circumscribed margins and homogeneous ossification *(arrows)* on AP *(A)* and oblique *(B)* views. (Courtesy of Anne Brower, M.D.)

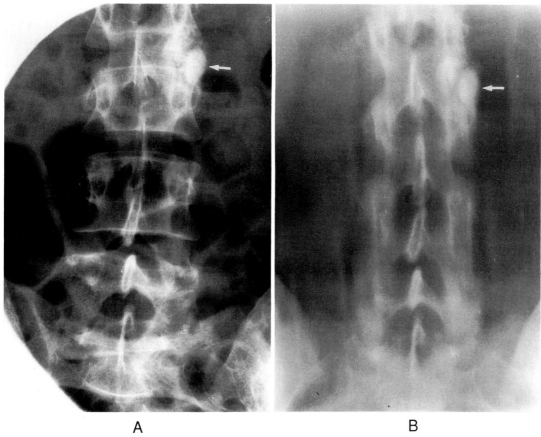

Figure 13–8. AP *(A)* and tomographic *(B)* views of the lumbar spine reveal an oval blastic lesion of the posterior elements of L2 *(arrows)*. The size, location, and configuration are consistent with an osteoblastoma. (Courtesy of Anne Brower, M.D.)

the location of an osteoblastoma even in the absence of abnormalities on plain roentgenograms.[16]

CT may provide better localization of the tumor, particularly when the lesion is obscured on plain roentgenograms.[17] CT helps determine the extent of the lesion and the degree of tumor matrix mineralization.[5] The relationship of the tumor to the spinal cord is better visualized in all circumstances with CT.[18] Angiography of the lesion does not help in making a specific diagnosis but highlights the vascular nature of the tumor.[19]

MR is better than CT in demonstrating the extension of bone sclerosis and in differentiating the tumor from adjacent structures and marrow.[20] Increased signal intensity in soft tissues surrounding the tumor is secondary to edema.[18] On occasion, low signal intensity is noted in a wide area beyond the osteoblastoma. This pattern may be confused with a malignant process. A marked inflammatory response to the tumor results in this MR appearance. The extent of the process was overestimated by the MR and a biopsy was taken from outside the tumor. This case is evidence for the use of CT as the modality of choice to determine the appropriate site for biopsy of a bone tumor.[21]

DIFFERENTIAL DIAGNOSIS

The diagnosis of an osteoblastoma is made by the thorough examination of biopsy samples. Osteogenic sarcoma, at presentation, may be easily confused clinically, radiographically, and histologically with osteoblastoma. The presence of an outer rim of bone on radiographic examination and the absence of cartilage and anaplastic cells on biopsy help differentiate osteoblastoma from a malignant process.

Osteosarcoma

Osteosarcoma is the most common primary bone tumor accounting for 20% of cases.[22] Approximately 1500 new cases are diagnosed each year in the United States. The second decade of life is associated with the peak incidence of this tumor. The other group of individuals at risk for osteosarcoma are over 50 years of age.[23] Osteosarcoma may occur as a complication of other pathologic conditions. The most common predisposing factor for secondary osteosarcoma is Paget's disease.[24] Osteosarcoma is classified as intramedullary, juxtacortical, and extraosseous.

The spine is an unusual location for the development of osteosarcoma. The incidence of tumors arising in the spine ranges between 0.85% and 3%.[22] Approximately 50% of these tumors are secondary to other conditions. However, in other studies of adults with osteosarcoma, the spine is spared.[25] Most patients develop localized pain with neurologic symptoms. The proximity of the tumor to the spinal cord and nerve roots results in the early onset of symptoms even with small tumors. The interval between the onset of symptoms and the confirmation of diagnosis is, on average, 6 months.[26, 27]

In the spine, plain roentgenograms reveal a mixed osteolytic and sclerotic bone lesion. The vertebral body is most frequently involved with 10% or less of lesions affecting the posterior elements. CT demonstrates the extent of expansion of the tumor into soft tissues. MR has an advantage of detecting the extension of tumor into the spinal canal (Fig. 13–9). Nonmineralized tumor has low signal intensity on T_1-weighted images and increased signal intensity on T_2-weighted images. Mineralized tumors appear dark on all sequences.

The diagnosis of osteosarcoma is confirmed by histologic evaluation of a biopsy specimen. Mirra has suggested five histologic aids that help differentiate osteoblastoma from osteosarcoma.[2]

1. Osteoblastomas do not produce cartilage.
2. Osteoblastomas produce thick trabeculae of osteoid with prominent capillaries and osteoclasts. Osteosarcoma produces extensive areas of poorly calcified bone with a paucity of prominent vessels.
3. The osteoid and woven bone of osteoblastoma are sharply delineated from surrounding lamellar bone. Osteosarcoma infiltrates surrounding bone. This has implications for biopsy, since it is best for the surgeon to obtain an intact wedge of bone that includes a margin of normal bone to allow for examination of the lesion–host bone relationship.
4. Osteoblastomas are rimmed by osteoblasts.

5. Osteoblastomas do not include areas that contain cells with bizarre nuclei, abnormal chromatin distribution, abnormal nucleoli, or atypical mitoses.

Therapy of osteosarcoma is directed at resection of the involved vertebral body. Subsequent therapy included chemotherapy and radiotherapy directed at the lesion.[28] The prognosis of these patients is poor with a 5-year survival of less than 50%. Ewing's sarcoma is a rare cause of disease in the lumbar spine. The importance in differentiating these lesions relates to the responsivity of Ewing's sarcoma to chemotherapy.[29] In Ewing's patients without neurologic involvement, chemotherapy can be attempted without surgical resection.

Osteoblastoma must also be differentiated from osteoid osteoma. Table 13–1 summarizes the features that differentiate these tumors. In brief, osteoid osteoma is associated with more intense, nocturnal pain, a lesion that is less than 2 cm in size, no associated soft tissue mass, and a histologic appearance demonstrating osteoid trabeculae with continuous and regular bone formation.

Giant cell tumor of bone may contain areas of woven bone. However, this lesion contains areas of solidly packed giant and stromal cells without intervening osteoid. Osteoblastoma contains areas of intervening bone and osteoid between collections of giant cells. Rarely, brown tumor of hyperparathyroidism may appear histologically like an osteoblastoma be-

TABLE 13–1. DIFFERENTIATION OF OSTEOBLASTOMA AND OSTEOID OSTEOMA

	OSTEOBLASTOMA	OSTEOID OSTEOMA
Clinical presentation	Moderate nocturnal pain	Intense nocturnal pain
	Lesion greater than 2 cm	Limited growth, less than 1.5 cm
	Rapid increase in size	Limited growth potential
Radiography	Minimal perifocal sclerosis	Marked perifocal sclerosis
	Associated soft tissue mass	No soft tissue mass
Histology	Osteoid trabeculae— discontinuous and irregular	Osteoid trabeculae— continuous and regular
	Stromal reaction— abundant	Stromal reaction— scant
	Osteoblastic giant cells—abundant	Osteoblastic giant cells—scant

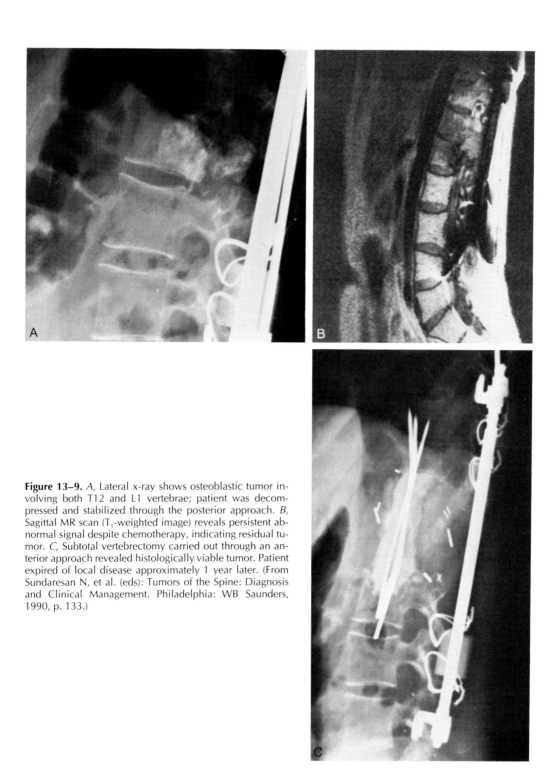

Figure 13–9. *A*, Lateral x-ray shows osteoblastic tumor involving both T12 and L1 vertebrae; patient was decompressed and stabilized through the posterior approach. *B*, Sagittal MR scan (T_1-weighted image) reveals persistent abnormal signal despite chemotherapy, indicating residual tumor. *C*, Subtotal vertebrectomy carried out through an anterior approach revealed histologically viable tumor. Patient expired of local disease approximately 1 year later. (From Sundaresan N, et al. (eds): Tumors of the Spine: Diagnosis and Clinical Management. Philadelphia: WB Saunders, 1990, p. 133.)

cause of the presence of giant cells. Serum determinations of calcium and phosphorus should differentiate elevated concentrations of these serum factors associated with hyperparathyroidism from the normal levels associated with osteoblastoma.

TREATMENT

Local excision of the entire lesion is the treatment of choice if bone can be sacrificed without loss of function or excessive risk of neurogenic dysfunction. Osteoblastoma in the posterior elements of the spine is usually inaccessible for complete excision in up to 40% of lesions in the spine. Partial curettage of these lesions may be associated with cessation of growth and relief of symptoms for an extended period of time.[4] Rapidly expanding or recurrent osteoblastomas may be controlled with radiation therapy. However, radiation therapy may be ineffective and is not completely free of risk in the form of malignant transformation, spinal cord necrosis, and aggravation of spinal cord compression.

PROGNOSIS

The course of osteoblastoma is usually benign. The lesion is responsive to partial curettage and low-dose radiation therapy. Marsh reported a series in which 1 of 13 patients with spinal osteoblastomas had a recurrence, which resulted in paraplegia 7 months after surgery.[4] Laminectomy and postoperative radiation was the treatment for this complication. Less than 5% of osteoblastomas recur; however, repeated recurrences have been described.[30] Malignant changes occur in a very few lesions considered to have been correctly diagnosed as benign osteoblastomas.[31]

References

OSTEOBLASTOMA

1. Dahlin DC, Unni KK: Bone Tumors: General Aspects and Data on 8542 cases, 4th ed. Springfield, IL: Charles C Thomas, 1986, pp 102–118.
2. Mirra JM: Bone Tumors: Clinical, Radiologic, and Pathologic Correlations. Philadelphia: Lea & Febiger, 1989, pp 389–430.
3. McLeod RA, Dahlin DC, Beabout JW: The spectrum of osteoblastoma. AJR 126:321, 1976.
4. Marsh BW, Bonfiglio M, Brady LP, Enneking WF: Benign osteoblastoma: range of manifestations. J Bone Joint Surg 57A:1, 1975.
5. Nemoto O, Moser RP, Van Dam BE, et al.: Osteoblastoma of the spine: a review of 75 cases. Spine 15:1272, 1990.
6. Jaffe HL, Mayer L: An osteoblastic osteoid tissue-forming tumor of a metacarpal bone. Arch Surg 24:550, 1932.
7. Lichtenstein L: Benign osteoblastoma—a category of osteoid and bone forming tumors other than classical osteoma, which may be mistaken for giant cell tumor or osteogenic sarcoma. Cancer 9:1044, 1956.
8. Boriani S, Capanna R, Donati D, et al.: Osteoblastoma of the spine. Clin Orthop 278:37, 1992.
9. Tate TC, Kim SS, Ogden L: Osteoblastoma of the sacrum with intraabdominal manifestation. Am J Surg 123:735, 1972.
10. Huvos AG: Bone Tumors: Diagnosis, Treatment, and Prognosis, 2nd ed. Philadelphia: WB Saunders, 1991, pp 67–83.
11. Gitelis S, Schajowicz F: Osteoid osteoma and osteoblastoma. Orthop Clin North Am 20:313, 1989.
12. Schajowicz F, McGuire MH: Diagnostic difficulties in skeletal pathology. Clin Orthop 240:281, 1989.
13. DeSouza-Dias L, Frost HM: Osteoblastoma of the spine: a review and report of eight new cases. Clin Orthop 91:141, 1973.
14. Alp H, Ceviker N, Baykaner K, et al.: Osteoblastoma of the third lumbar vertebra. Surg Neurol 19:276, 1983.
15. Pochaczevsky R, Yen YM, Sherman RS: The roentgen appearance of benign osteoblastoma. Radiology, 75:429, 1960.
16. Makhija MC, Stein IH: Bone imaging in osteoblastoma. Clin Nucl Med 8:141, 1983.
17. Tonai M, Campbell CT, Ahn GH, et al.: Osteoblastoma: classification and report of 16 patients. Clin Orthop 167:222, 1982.
18. Kroon HM, Schurmans J: Osteoblastoma: clinical and radiologic findings in 98 new cases. Radiology 175:783, 1990.
19. Banna M: Angiography of spinal osteoblastoma. J Can Assoc Radiol 30:118, 1974.
20. Syklawer R, Osborn RE, Kerber CW, Glass RF: Magnetic resonance imaging of vertebral osteoblastoma: a report of two cases. Surg Neurol 34:421, 1990.
21. Crim JR, Mirra JM, Eckardt JJ, Seeger LL: Widespread inflammatory response to osteoblastoma: the flare phenomenon. Radiology 177:835, 1990.
22. Sundaresan N, Schiller AL, Rosenthal DI: Osteosarcoma of the spine. In: Sundaresan N, Schmidek HH, Schiller AL, Rosenthal DI (eds): Tumors of the Spine: Diagnosis and Clinical Management. Philadelphia: WB Saunders 1990, pp 128–145.
23. Ghelman B: Radiology of bone tumors. Orthop Clin North Am 20:287, 1989.
24. Breton CL, Meziou M, Laredo JD, et al.: Sarcoma complicating Paget's disease of the spine. Rev Rhum [Engl ed] 60:17, 1993.
25. Siegel RD, Ryan LM, Antman KH: Osteosarcoma in adults: One institution's experience. Clin Orthop 240:263, 1989.
26. Shives TC, Dahlin DC, Sim FH, et al.: Osteosarcoma of the spine. J Bone Joint Surg 66A:660, 1986.
27. Sundaresan N, Rosen G, Huvos AG, Krol G: Combined modality treatment of osteosarcoma of the spine. Neurosurgery 23:714, 1988.
28. Jaffe N: Chemotherapy for malignant bone tumors. Orthop Clin North Am 20:487, 1989.
29. Sharafuddin MJA, Haddad FS, Hitchon PW, et al.: Treatment options in primary Ewing's sarcoma of the spine: report of seven cases and review of the literature. Neurosurgery 30:610, 1992.
30. Jackson RP: Recurrent osteoblastoma: a review. Clin Orthop 131:229, 1978.
31. Schajowicz F, Lemos C: Malignant osteoblastoma. J Bone Joint Surg 58B:202, 1976.

Osteochondroma

Capsule Summary

Frequency of back pain—uncommon
Location of back pain—lumbar spine
Quality of back pain—mild ache
Symptoms and signs—restricted motion
Laboratory and x-ray tests—exostosis—single or multiple on plain roentgenograms
Treatment—en-bloc excision for lesions that cause nerve impingement

PREVALENCE AND PATHOGENESIS

Osteochondroma is a common benign tumor of bone that occurs in single or multiple locations in the skeleton. Osteochondromas represent up to 36% of all benign bone tumors and 8% to 11% of all primary tumors of bone examined by biopsy.[1, 2] Approximately 60% of patients develop the lesion between the second and third decades of life. Patients with multiple osteochondromas develop lesions before they reach 20 years of age.[2] The male to female ratio is 2:1.[3]

The lesion was first described by Cooper in 1818.[4] Osteochondromas have been detected in skeletons dated between 3500 and 2000 B.C.[5] Exostosis and osteocartilaginous exostosis are two other names associated with this benign tumor. Mirra has proposed that the term exostosis be reserved for marginal osteophytes associated with osteoarthritis and that osteochondroma be reserved for the benign bone tumor since the two lesions occur in different areas of bone, occur at different ages of the skeleton, and have different pathogenetic mechanisms.[2]

The pathogenesis of osteochondroma is postulated to be related to an abnormality of cartilage growth. Keith thought that osteochondroma results from a defect in the periosteal cuff of bone that surrounds the lower end of the epiphyseal plate cartilage during embryogenesis.[6] The larger the defect is, the larger the tumor will be. A single defect results in a solitary tumor, while multiple defects cause hereditary multiple osteochondromatoses. Nests of cartilage in a periosteal location grow out from the epiphyseal growth plate and result in a bony prominence capped by a layer of cartilage that is continuous with the cortex of the underlying bone. Osteochondromas may be thought of as slow-growing developmental anomalies that cease to enlarge once growth has stopped. This progression correlates with the clinical history of recognition of the tumor

during childhood and its cessation of growth once the epiphyses close.[2]

Osteochondromas occur most commonly at the ends of tubular bones. Approximately 1% to 2% of osteochondromas are located in the spine. Approximately 50% are found in the lumbosacral spine, 30% in the thoracic spine, and 20% in the cervical spine.[1] Another review of 96 patients with solitary spinal osteochondromas reported the cervical spine to be the most commonly affected area with the lumbar spine involved in 23% of individuals.[7]

CLINICAL HISTORY

Osteochondroma is frequently asymptomatic and is discovered only as a painless prominence of bone or as a chance finding on a radiograph. If pain is present, it is mild, deep, and usually secondary to mechanical irritation of overlying soft tissue structures. Pain may increase with activity. An osteochondroma that continues to grow may cause loss of function and decreased motion. Osteochondromas attached to the spinal column have been associated with kyphosis and spondylolisthesis.[8] They may even grow large enough to cause nerve or spinal cord compression and may be associated with radicular pain, sensory abnormalities, motor weakness, and urinary and fecal incontinence.[9–12] The lesion grows slowly over months to years. The neurologic abnormality corresponds to the location of the tumor. Radiculopathy may be caused by this tumor.[13] Spinal stenosis also has been reported.[14]

PHYSICAL EXAMINATION

Physical examination may be normal without any neurologic deficit; however, osteochondromas near facet joints of the spine may cause some restriction in motion. Osteochondromas that grow close to the body surface may cause a palpable mass, which may be tender on palpation. Neurologic findings, when present, will correspond to the location of the lesion and related nerve root compression.

LABORATORY DATA

Screening laboratory tests are normal with this benign tumor of bone. Pathologically, a gross specimen of an osteochondroma may take the form of a pedunculated stalk or a flat prominence. The tumor's cortex and its periosteal covering are continuous with those of the underlying bone. The cartilage cap may cover the entire lesion or the rounded end of a stalked exostosis. The cap's cartilage is smooth and 2 to 3 mm thick. Actively growing lesions may have cartilage 1 cm thick. As the lesion grows older, the cartilaginous cap disappears. The lesion may vary in size up to 100 cm and is well circumscribed. Histologic examination of the tumor shows benign chondrocytes with small nuclei. The islands of cartilage and cartilage cells are embedded in the underlying cancellous bone. As the bone matures, the amount of cartilage decreases. However, residual microscopic foci of cartilage may be identified well into adult life.

RADIOGRAPHIC EVALUATION

The radiographic features of an osteochondroma are diagnostic. The lesion protrudes from the underlying bone on a sessile or pedunculated bony stalk that is continuous with the cortex and spongiosa of the underlying bone. The outer surface of the lesion may be smooth or irregular, but it is almost always well demarcated. If the cartilage cap is calcified, it may obscure the underlying stalk (Fig. 13–10).

In the spine, osteochondromas are located close to centers of secondary ossification, including the spinous process, pedicle, and neural arch.[15] CT and myelography are helpful in localizing the site of the lesion in the spinal column, its size, and its relationship to the nerve roots and spinal cord and in differentiating it from malignant lesions.[16, 17] Radionuclide bone scan reveals increased uptake at the site of the tumor. Malignant lesions may exhibit greater intensity of uptake, but this finding is not always a reliable distinguishing feature of

malignant transformation.[18, 19] The increased activity of a osteochondroma is related to endochondral ossification within the cartilaginous cap.

DIFFERENTIAL DIAGNOSIS

The diagnosis of an osteochondroma is based on its appearance on radiographs and the lack of clinical and laboratory findings. Chondrosarcomatous degeneration of osteochondroma occurs in less than 1% of patients. Adult patients with multiple lesions are at greater risk in this respect. Malignant transformation is usually heralded by increasing pain, enlarging soft tissue mass, and loss of definition of the outer border of the lesion on radiographs. However, the onset of pain in a previously asymptomatic osteochondroma is not always associated with malignant degeneration, since infarction of the cartilage cap or fracture through the base of an osteochondroma may also cause pain and new bone growth.[2]

Other non-neoplastic lesions to be considered in the differential diagnosis are callus associated with fractures, chondroid metaplasia, and osteophytes associated with osteoarthritis. The size and location of the benign tumor should help differentiate these non-neoplastic entities with similar histologic features.

TREATMENT

Osteochondromas require no therapy when they are asymptomatic.[20] Removal is indicated if the tumor is causing persistent pain or disability, has roentgenographic features sugges-

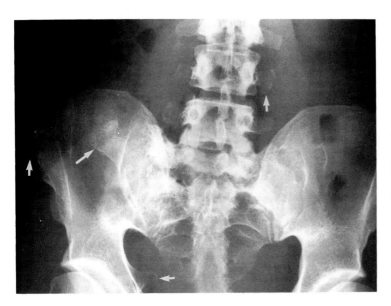

Figure 13–10. Osteochondromas. AP view of the lower lumbar spine and pelvis showing multiple osteochondromas *(arrows)*. The tumors have a bony cortex that is continuous with neighboring bone. (Courtesy of Anne Brower, M.D.)

tive of malignancy, or shows an abnormal increase in size. Patients with neurologic symptoms can be helped by removal of the lesion and decompression of the affected nerve root or spinal cord.[21]

Although chondrosarcoma is more common in patients with multiple osteochondromas, prophylactic removal of tumors in patients with multiple lesions is not practical. Patients must be followed closely for a change in symptoms or size of lesions. These lesions should be removed.

PROGNOSIS

The course of the solitary osteochondroma usually is benign and asymptomatic and is not associated with any dysfunction or inability to work. In the rare patient who has a vertebral osteochondroma and neurologic dysfunction, surgical decompression of the site should result in a return of function and complete cure.[22] There may be a recurrence of an osteochondroma if the tumor, particularly its cartilaginous cap and periosteum, is not completely removed. Continuous observation of the patients with osteochondromas is important, particularly for those with multiple lesions, because they can occasionally become malignant.

References

OSTEOCHONDROMA

1. Dahlin DC, Unni KK: Bone Tumors: General Aspects and Data on 8,542 cases. 4th ed. Springfield, Illinois: Charles C Thomas, 1986, pp 18–32.
2. Mirra JM: Bone Tumors: Clinical, Radiologic, and Pathologic Correlations. Philadelphia: Lea & Febiger, 1989, pp 1626–1659.
3. Huvos AG: Bone Tumors: Diagnosis, Treatment and Prognosis, 2nd ed. Philadelphia: WB Saunders, 1991, pp 253–291.
4. Cooper A: Exostosis. In: Cooper A, Travers B (eds): Surgical Essays. 3rd ed. London: Cox and Sone, 1818, pp 169–226.
5. Chamberlain AT, Rogers S, Romanowski CAJ: Osteochondroma in a British neolitic skeleton. Br J Hop Med 47:51, 1992.
6. Keith A: Studies on the anatomical changes which accompany certain growth disorders of the human body. J Anat 54:101, 1920.
7. Albrecht S, Crutchfield S, Segall GK: On spinal osteochondromas. J Neurosurg 77:247, 1992.
8. Blaauw G: Osteocartilaginous exostosis of the spine. In: Vinken PJ, Bruyn GW (eds): Handbook of Clinical Neurology. Tumors of the Spine and Spinal Cord, Part I. New York: American Elsevier, 1975, pp 313–319.
9. Borne G, Payrot C: Right lumbo-crural sciatica due to a vertebral osteochondroma. Neurochirurgie 22:301, 1976.
10. Palmer FJ, Blum PW: Osteochondroma with spinal cord compression. J Neurosurg 52:842, 1980.
11. Twersky J, Kassner EG, Tenner MS, Camera A: Vertebral and costal osteochondromas causing spinal cord compression. AJR 124:124, 1975.
12. O'Connon GA, Roberts TS: Spinal cord compression by an osteochondroma in a patient with multiple osteochondromatosis: case report. J Neurosurg 60:420, 1984.
13. van der Sluis R, Gurr K, Joseph MG: Osteochondroma of the lumbar spine: an unusual cause of sciatica. Spine 17:1519, 1992.
14. Royster RM, Kujawa P, Dryer RF: Multilevel osteochondroma of the lumbar spine presenting as spinal stenosis. Spine 16:992, 1991.
15. Inglis AE, Rubin RM, Lewis RJ, Villacin A: Osteochondroma of the cervical spine: Case report. Clin Orthop 126:127, 1977.
16. Kenney PJ, Gilula LA, Murphy WA: The use of computed tomography to distinguish osteochondroma and chondrosarcoma. Radiology 139:129, 1981.
17. Tigges S, Erb RE, Nance EP: Skeletal case of the day. AJR 158:1368, 1992.
18. Greenspan A: Tumors of cartilage origin. Orthop Clin North Am 20:347, 1989.
19. Edeling CJ: Bone scintigraphy in hereditary multiple exostoses. Eur J Nuc Med 14:207, 1988.
20. Chrisman OD, Goldenberg RR: Untreated solitary osteochondroma. Report of two cases. J Bone Joint Surg 50A:508, 1968.
21. Gokay H, Bucy PC: Osteochondroma of the lumbar spine: report of a case. J Neurosurg 12:72, 1955.
22. Esposito PW, Crawford AH, Vogler C: Solitary osteochondroma occurring on the transverse process of the lumbar spine. Spine 10:398, 1985.

Giant Cell Tumor

Capsule Summary

Frequency of back pain—common
Location of back pain—lumbar spine, sacrum
Quality of back pain—intermittent ache
Symptoms and signs—localized mass
Laboratory and x-ray tests—anterior vertebral body involvement on plain roentgenograms, MR–soft tissue extension
Treatment—en-bloc excision

PREVALENCE AND PATHOGENESIS

Giant cell tumor of bone is a common, locally aggressive lesion that may turn malignant. Giant cell tumors represent up to 21% of all benign tumors of bone and up to 5% of primary bone tumors examined by biopsy.[1, 2] Approximately 70% of patients are diagnosed between the ages of 20 and 40. The average age of patients with malignant giant cell tumors is more than that of patients with benign tumors. Patients with benign tumors are predominantly women, by a ratio of 3:2, while those with malignant tumors are predominantly men, by a ratio of 3:1.[3]

The first description of the benign characteristics of this tumor was by Cooper in 1818.[4] Bloodgood in 1919 was the first to refer to this neoplasm as a benign giant cell tumor.[5] Other names that have been associated with this perplexing neoplasm include myeloid sarcoma, medullary sarcoma, and osteoclastoma.

The pathogenesis of giant cell tumor is not known. The tumor starts after the skeleton has ceased to grow and has matured. The tumor arises from nonbone-forming supporting connective tissue of the bone marrow space. The factors that make this tumor inherently invasive or potentially malignant are unknown.

Most giant cell tumors occur at the ends of long bones, particularly around the knee. About 8% to 12% of giant cell tumors occur in the spine.[1, 6] The sacrum is the most frequently affected area in the spine. Approximately 68% of spinal giant cell tumors occur in the sacrum, 11% in the lumbar spine, 11% in the cervical spine, and 10% in the thoracic area. Other series have found frequencies of sacral involvement in the range of 3% to 8%.[7, 8] The ilium and ischium may also be involved in a small number of patients (0.05%).[9]

CLINICAL HISTORY

Giant cell tumor of bone causes intermittent, aching pain over the affected bone, which is almost always the predominant symptom. The duration of symptoms typically may vary from a few weeks to 6 months, but some patients have had pain over 2 years prior to diagnosis.[10] Patients with sacral or vertebral involvement may describe neurologic dysfunction, including paresthesias with radiation of pain into the lower extremities, muscle weakness, and urinary or rectal incontinence.[10, 11] In one study of 26 patients with sacral giant cell tumors, 88% had neurologic symptoms including neurogenic bladder dysfunction, sphincter weakness, and perineal hypesthesias.[12] Some patients are misdiagnosed as having a disc herniation with radiculopathy and undergo discectomy.

PHYSICAL EXAMINATION

Physical examination may demonstrate tenderness on palpation over the spine and sacrum. Localized swelling may be noted if the location of the giant cell tumor is superficial, that is, in the spinous process. Kyphosis, muscle spasm, and associated limitation of motion may also be noted. In a sacral lesion, an extracolonic mass may be found on rectal examination.[11] Neurologic findings may show sensory, motor, or reflex abnormalities depending on the level of nerve root compression.[13]

LABORATORY DATA

Laboratory results are normal in patients with benign giant cell tumors, but serum calcium, phosphorus, and alkaline phosphatase tests should be obtained to differentiate them from hyperparathyroidism, Paget's disease, and malignant giant cell tumor. Patients with malignant giant cell tumors may show abnormalities such as anemia and elevated sedimentation rate.

The tumor is a soft, friable, gray to red tumor mass on gross pathologic examination. Areas of the tumor may be cystic or necrotic, or may be filled with blood. This characteristic finding causes confusion with findings associated with aneurysmal bone cysts. The tumors cause expansion of host bone with cortical destruction. In most lesions the periosteum is relatively spared, with the tumor contained by a shell of new bone.

The histologic appearance of giant cell tumor of bone is not distinctively characteristic, since a number of other benign lesions may contain giant cells (Table 13–2). In general, giant cell tumors contain large numbers of osteoblast-like giant cells separated by inconspicuous mononuclear stromal cells (Fig. 13–11). The proliferating giant cells have round, oval, or spindle-shaped nuclei. Mitotic figures may be numerous. The nuclei lack the variations in size and shape that are characteristic of sarcoma. In a minority of lesions, small foci of osteoid and woven bone are seen. Thin-walled vessels with hemorrhages are also characteristic.

A great debate exists over the histologic grading of giant cell tumors. Some pathologists believe that the histologic grade is predictive of subsequent tumor behavior.[6] Others do not believe that grading, particularly at the benign end of the scale (Grades I and II), is predictive of any subsequent propensity to aggressive growth.[1, 2]

Cytogenic analysis of giant cell tumors reveals chromosomal abnormalities in tumor cells not detected in normal cells. Telomere-to-telomere chromosome translocations affecting the long arm of chromosomes 19 and 20 were noted in the tumors but were not predictive of the aggressiveness of the giant cell neoplasm.[14] The alteration in chromosome 19 may

TABLE 13–2. DIFFERENTIAL DIAGNOSIS OF GIANT CELL LESIONS OF BONE

	MOST COMMON AGE GROUP	LOCATION IN BONE	RADIOLOGIC APPEARANCE	GROSS FEATURES	MICROSCOPIC FEATURES	
					Giant Cells	*Stromal Cells*
Giant cell tumor	Third and fourth decades	Epiphysis or metaphysis	Eccentric expanded radiolucent area	Fleshy soft tissue	Abundant number uniformly distributed	Plump and polyhedral cells with abundant cytoplasm
Nonossifying fibroma	First decade	Metaphysis	Eccentric oval defects	Fleshy soft tissue	Focal distribution, small and few nuclei	Slender and spindly cells with little cytoplasm; whorled pattern
Aneurysmal bone cyst	First and second decades	Vertebral column or metaphysis of long bone	Eccentric blow out "soap bubble" appearance	Cavity filled with blood	Focal around vascular channels or hemorrhage	Large vascular channels; slender to plump cells with hemosiderin granules; metaplastic bone
Brown tumor of hyper- parathyroidism	Any age	Anywhere in bone	Subperiosteal, subchondral, and subligamentous resorption of bone	Fleshy tissue or cystic spaces	Focal around hemosiderin pigment or hemorrhage	Fibrous stroma with slender spindle cells
Simple bone cyst	First and second decades	Metaphysis	Trabeculations in radiolucent area	Cyst filled with clear fluid	Focal around cholesterol clefts	Cyst wall of fibrous tissue; metaplastic bone
Chondroblastoma	Second decade	Epiphysis	Radiolucency in spotty opacities	Firm to fleshy tissue	Few and focal	Plump and round or ovoid cells with pericellular calcifications
Fibrous dysplasia	First and second decades	Metaphysis	Ground-glass appearance	Firm and gritty	Few and focal	Woven bone and whorled fibrous tissue; no osteoblasts
Giant cell reparative granuloma	Second and third decades	Maxilla and mandible	Radiolucent focus	Soft fleshy tissue	Focal around hemosiderin pigment or hemorrhage	Slender or plump spindle cells
Ossifying fibroma	Second and third decades	Maxilla and mandible	Radiopaque	Firm and gritty	Few and focal	Lamellar bony trabeculae in fibrous tissue; osteoblastic rimming
Osteosarcoma	Second and third decades	Metaphysis	Radiolucent	Soft, firm, or hard	Focal distribution	Malignant cells with direct osteoid formation
Chondromyxoid fibroma	Second and third decades	Metaphysis	Eccentric with expanded cortex	Soft to firm	Focal distribution	Chondroid, myxoid, and fibrous lobules
Osteoblastoma	Second and third decades	Vertebral column, diaphysis of long bone	Radiolucent or dense	Hemorrhagic, gritty	Focal distribution	Abundant osteoid trabeculae with osteoblasts

From Resnick D, Niwayama G: Diagnosis of Bone and Joint Disorders. 2nd ed. Philadelphia, WB Saunders Co, 1988. Modified from Ghandur-Mnaymneh L, Mnaymneh WA: Bone lesions with giant cells: problems in differential diagnosis. J Med Liban 24:91, 1972.

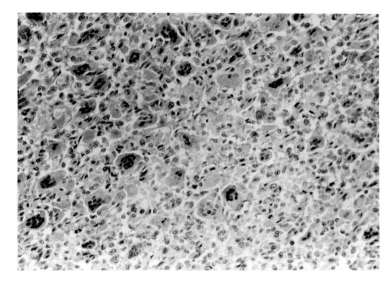

Figure 13–11. Giant cell tumor. Histologic section demonstrating an even distribution of a large number of giant cells with multiple nuclei. The tumor is very cellular but lacks fibrous or osteoid tissue. The histologic appearance of this tumor can not be differentiated from that of brown tumor of hyperparathyroidism. (Courtesy of Arnold Schwartz, M.D.)

affect the function of transforming growth factor-beta (TGF-β) on osteoclasts. Giant cell tumors may consist of osteoclasts that have been affected by TGF-β activity. Researchers in another study utilized flow cytometric DNA analysis of giant cell tumors in an attempt to predict the biologic behavior of these neoplasms. DNA analysis was unable to predict the likelihood of the tumor metastasizing.[15]

RADIOGRAPHIC EVALUATION

The radiographic findings of giant cell tumors are characteristic but not pathognomonic. The lesion is expansile, with irregular thinning of the cortical margin. It is lytic but may contain a delicate trabecular meshwork. Little bony reaction occurs in response to this lesion. Extensive sclerotic borders and periosteal reaction are not seen. In the spine, the vertebral body is frequently affected but the spinous and transverse processes also may be involved (Fig. 13–12).[16] The destruction of vertebral bone that is most commonly in the vertebral body, as opposed to the posterior elements in other benign tumors of the spine, results in lytic lesions without surrounding reactive sclerosis or matrix mineralization.[17] Radiographic changes of giant cell tumor in the sacrum may be subtle, and large tumors may be missed on plain radiographs. The lesion may be eccentrically located in the sacrum and may spread across the sacroiliac joint to involve the ilium. When located in the superior portion of the sacrum, they may erode through the L5-S1 disc space.[11]

If plain radiographs are insufficient to demonstrate abnormalities of the sacrum or spine,

a bone scan may be helpful in demonstrating abnormalities. However, radionuclide scintigraphy may exhibit increased tracer in bone across the adjacent joint and in other joints in the same extremity not involved with the tumor.[18] CT is useful in localizing the extent of a lesion in the sacrum. CT is superior to plain roentgenograms in detecting the extent of tu-

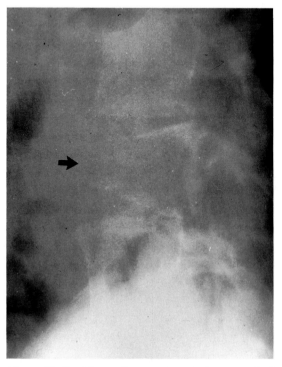

Figure 13–12. Giant cell tumor *(arrow)* shows vertebral body destruction characterized by collapse associated with loss of the anterior body margin. (Courtesy of Anne Brower, M.D.)

mor in the extraosseous space.[19] However, clear distinctions between tumor and muscle may be difficult to make with CT scan.

MR is the best imaging modality to study giant cell tumors and soft tissue extension because of superior contrast resolution. The tumor exhibits long T_1 and T_2 relaxation times that correspond to low intensity on T_1 images and high intensity on T_2 images. MR is better at determining the extraosseous extent of the tumor, while CT is better able to visualize mineralized structures including subtle cortical breaks.

DIFFERENTIAL DIAGNOSIS

A thorough review of the clinical, laboratory, pathologic, and radiologic data is necessary to make the diagnosis of a giant cell tumor of bone. This evaluation is required because a number of benign and malignant lesions are similar in pathology. Table 13–2 contains a list of benign and malignant lesions that contain giant cells that may mimic the findings of giant cell tumor of bone.[20] Not all of these neoplasms affect the lumbosacral spine. Aneurysmal bone cyst, brown tumor of hyperparathyroidism, chondroblastoma, fibrous dysplasia, osteogenic sarcoma, chondromyxoid fibroma, and osteoblastoma need to be included in the differential diagnosis of a giant cell-containing tumor located in the lumbosacral spine.

Aneurysmal bone cyst is a fibrous-walled structure filled with blood that occurs in association with other neoplasms, including giant cell tumor. A giant cell tumor with an aneurysmal bone cyst component should be treated as a giant cell tumor. Brown tumor of hyperparathyroidism contains cells that histologically are similar to those of a giant cell tumor. The elevation of serum calcium and decrease of serum phosphorus along with multiple locations of lesions help differentiate this entity. In addition, the giant cells of hyperparathyroidism are arranged in a more nodular pattern and are surrounded by areas of active bone.

Chondroblastoma is a benign lesion that affects men under 30 years of age and is located near epiphyseal cartilage. The tumor is most commonly found in long bones and is only rarely located in the pelvis or lumbar spine.[21] Radiographically, the lesion is a solitary lytic lesion with a surrounding sclerotic border and punctate calcification. Histologically, the tumor contains a variable number of giant cells with multiple nuclei, polygonal to round stromal cells with distinct borders, "chicken-

wire" calcification, and variable amounts of chondroid.[2]

Fibrous dysplasia is a benign process affecting either one bone or multiple bones in the skeleton. The disease is more common in women than in men and becomes prominent before the second decade of life. Fibrous dysplasia occasionally affects the pelvis, particularly the iliac wing, and to a lesser degree the lumbar spine. Radiologically, the medullary cavity of bone is replaced with fibrous tissue, which appears as a predominantly radiolucent, albeit hazy, matrix (often described as "ground glass") that may contain focal calcific deposits. Lesions appear matted, loculated, or trabeculated with well-defined, sclerotic margins. The affected bone may be expanded, bowed, and deformed.[22] Histologically, the lesion contains a benign fibrous tissue matrix with variable quantities of woven bone, little to no cartilage, and only small foci of giant cells, which are associated with areas of cystification or hemorrhage. The small number of these cells helps differentiate fibrous dysplasia from giant cell tumor.

Osteogenic sarcoma is a very rare tumor of the axial skeleton and pelvis. Approximately 1% to 2% of osteogenic sarcomas are located in the lumbar spine or pelvis.[23] It most commonly affects men between 10 and 30 years of age. The tumor may be osteoblastic or osteolytic. An osteoblastic lesion in a vertebral body affects one area of the body with dense sclerosis, which may extend into the neural arch. Irregular areas of calcification or ossification in the paravertebral soft tissues are usual. Osteolytic lesions are also associated with soft tissue masses and collapse of the anterior portion of a vertebra. Giant cell tumors when untreated are pure lytic lesions without any new bone formation. Histologic examination of osteosarcoma may demonstrate areas of osteoclast-like giant cells that superficially resemble giant cell tumor. However, close inspection of the specimen reveals frank anaplastic cells in areas away from bone-producing tissue.

Chondromyxoid fibroma is a very rare benign tumor, representing less than 1% of all primary bone neoplasms. The lesion occurs in men during the second and third decades of life. About 16% of these lesions occur in the ilium, ischium, or sacrum.[1] In the vertebral column, the lesion may affect the neural arch, vertebral body, or posterior elements. Radiographically, the tumor causes an area of osteolysis with bone expansion and variable calcification, which may be difficult to differentiate from other causes of bone damage.[24] On gross pathologic examination, this lesion is sharply delineated from surrounding bone. A thin sclerotic zone may be found in neighboring host bone. Histologically, the tumor contains different zones containing myxomatous, fibrous, and chondroid tissue. Nuclei of cells may be round, oval, or spindle-shaped. Giant cells, when present, are found in focal collections and are fewer in number than are those associated with giant cell tumor.

Osteoblastoma may be considered in the differential diagnosis, since a giant cell tumor rich in osteoid and woven bone may be mistaken for an osteoblastoma. However, concentrating on areas in giant cell tumors with no bone production will show masses of stromal and giant cells, which are not seen in osteoblastoma.

Giant cell tumors may also be associated with Paget's disease.[25] The lesions of Paget's disease are more common in the skull and facial bones than in the axial skeleton. The realization that giant cell tumors may complicate extensive Paget's disease is important. Not every expansion of a Pagetoid bone is sarcomatous degeneration. Lytic lesions with soft tissue extension in patients with Paget's disease does not necessarily imply a grave prognosis.[26, 27]

In very rare circumstances, pigmented villonodular synovitis may be confused with giant cell tumor of bone. Villonodular synovitis may proliferate and enter the spinal canal. The occasional multinucleated giant cells of this lesion should not be confused with giant cell tumor of bone or malignant processes.[28]

TREATMENT

The lesion must be staged before therapy is instituted.[29] Staging of a giant cell tumor includes CT scan to determine the exact extent of the tumor along with MR for the soft tissue distribution of the neoplasm in multiple planes. Angiography may be used to embolize the tumor prior to surgery.[8]

The therapy of choice for a giant cell tumor is en-bloc excision if the lesion is in an accessible location. Recurrence rates of 10% to 15% are reported following excision.[30] Curettage may control growth of the tumor, but the local recurrence rate is 50% within 5 years.[31] Radiation therapy is rarely curative, is associated with frequent recurrences, and may promote malignant transformation.[3] It is reserved for lesions that are inaccessible for surgical removal or curettage.[32] Lesions treated with radiation do not necessarily undergo malignant

degeneration. Patients who were followed up to 35 years after receiving radiation therapy had remission of their tumor.[33–36]

The ideal treatment for giant cell tumor of the spine is complete removal of accessible lesions.[37, 38] Decompression of the spine is necessary once neurologic symptoms appear. A delay of more than 3 months after the onset of nerve root symptoms may result in irreversible nerve deficits.[13] However, complete resection is frequently impossible because of the location and size of the lesions and the potential for critical blood loss with resection. In large sacral tumors, partial excision with irradiation or irradiation alone may be the only reasonable option.[39] More sensitive radiographic techniques and advanced surgical methods have increased the success of total resection and reconstruction of sacral and vertebral lesions.[40–41] Chemotherapy is not effective in controlling growth of this benign tumor.[19] Embolization of tumors in the spine may be used for inaccessible tumors. A potential risk associated with embolization of spinal lesions is ischemic injury to peripheral nerves and the spinal cord.[19]

PROGNOSIS

Giant cell tumors of bone are invasive, benign tumors and have a high local recurrence rate. Patients with benign giant cell tumors of the sacrum have died because of local invasion, malignant transformation, or secondary complications such as renal failure related to neurogenic bladder and obstruction.[11] Pulmonary metastases from benign giant cell tumors have been reported in patients with sacral tumors. The metastases occurred after a recurrence of the tumor and up to 10 years after diagnosis.[42] Regardless of treatment, the patients must continue to be examined for signs of recurrence. In some circumstances up to 5 courses of therapy were needed to successfully eradicate the disease.[3]

References

GIANT CELL TUMOR

1. Dahlin DC, Unni KK: Bone Tumors: General Aspects and Data on 8,542 cases. (4th ed) Springfield, Illinois: Charles C Thomas, 1986, pp 119–140.
2. Mirra JM: Bone Tumors: Clinical, Radiologic, and Pathologic Correlations. Philadelphia: Lea & Febiger 1989, pp 942–1020.
3. Hutter RVP, Worcester JW Jr, Francis KC, et al.: Benign and malignant giant cell tumors of bone: a clinicopathological analysis of the natural history of the disease. Cancer 15:653, 1962.

4. Cooper A, Travers B: Surgical Essays, 3rd ed. London: Cox and Son, 1818.

5. Bloodgood JG: Bone tumors. Central (medullary) giant cell tumor (sarcoma) of lower end of ulna, with evidence that complete destruction of the bony shell or perforation of the bony shell is not a sign of increased malignancy. Ann Surg 69:345, 1919.

6. Huvos AG: Bone Tumors: Diagnosis, Treatment and Prognosis, 2nd ed. Philadelphia: WB Saunders, 1991 pp 429–467.

7. Schajowicz F, Granato DB, McDonald DJ, Sundaram M: Clinical and radiological features of atypical giant cell tumours of bone. Br J Rad 64:877, 1991.

8. Campanacci M, Boriana S, Giunti A: Giant cell tumors of the spine. In: Sundaresan N, Schmidek HH, Schiller AL, Rosenthal DI (eds): Tumors of the Spine: Diagnosis and Clinical Management. Philadelphia: WB Saunders, 1990, pp 163–172.

9. Kuritzky AS, Joyce ST: Giant cell tumor in the ischium: a therapeutic dilemma. JAMA 238:2392, 1977.

10. Dahlin DC: Giant cell tumor of vertebrae above the sacrum: a review of 31 cases. Cancer 39:1350, 1977.

11. Smith J, Wixon D, Watson RC: Giant cell tumor of the sacrum: clinical and radiologic features in 13 patients. J Can Assoc Radiol 30:34, 1979.

12. Turcotte RE, Sim FH, Unni KK: Giant cell tumor of the sacrum. Clin Orthop 291:215, 1993.

13. Larrson SE, Lorentzon R, Boquist L: Giant cell tumors of the spine and sacrum causing neurological symptoms. Clin Orthop 111:201, 1975.

14. Schwartz HS, Jenkins RB, Dahl RJ, Dewald GW: Cytogenic analysis on giant cell tumors of bone. Clin Orthop 240:250, 1989.

15. Fukunaga M, Nikaido T, Shimoda T, et al: A flow cytometric DNA analysis of giant cell tumors of bone including two cases with malignant transformation. Cancer 70:1886, 1992.

16. DiLorenzo N, Spallone A, Nolletti A, Nardi P: Giant cell tumor of the spine: a clinical study of six cases, with emphasis on the radiological features, treatment, and follow-up. Neurosurgery 6:29, 1980.

17. Sim FJ, McDonald DJ, McLeod RA, Unni KK: Giant cell tumors: Mayo Clinic experience. In: Sundaresan N, Schmidek HH, Schiller AL, Rosenthal DI (eds): Tumors of the Spine: Diagnosis and Clinical Management. Philadelphia: WB Saunders, 1990, pp 173–180.

18. Van Nostrand D, Madewell JE, McNeish LM, et al.: Radionuclide bone scanning in giant cell tumor. J Nucl Med 27:329, 1986.

19. Carrasco CH, Murray JA: Giant cell tumors. Orthop Clin North Am 20:395, 1989.

20. Ghandur-Mnaymneh L, Mnaymneh WA: Bone lesions with giant cells: problems in differential diagnosis. J Med Liban 24:91, 1972.

21. Reyes CV, Kathuria S: Recurrent and aggressive chondroblastoma of the pelvis with late malignant neoplastic changes. Am J Surg Pathol 3:449, 1979.

22. Resnick CS, Lininger JR: Monostatic fibrous dysplasia of the cervical spine. Case report. Radiology 151:49, 1984.

23. Barwick KW, Huvos AG, Smith J: Primary osteogenic sarcoma of the column: a clinicopathologic correlation of ten patients. Cancer 46:595, 1980.

24. Mayer BS: Chondromyxoid fibroma of the lumbar spine. J Cand Assoc Radiol 29:271, 1978.

25. Hutter RVP, Foote FW, Frazell EL, Francis KC: Giant-cell tumors complicating Paget's disease of bone. Cancer 16:1044, 1963.

26. Potter HG, Schneider R, Ghelman B, et al.: Multiple giant cell tumors and Paget disease of bone: radiographic and clinical correlations. Radiology 180:261, 1991.

27. Bhambhani M, Lamberty BGH, Clements MR, et al.: Giant cell tumours in mandible and spine: a rare complication of Paget's disease of bone. Ann Rheum Dis 51:1335, 1992.

28. Kleinman GM, Dagi TF, Poletti CE: Villonodular synovitis in the spinal canal: case report. J Neuro Surg 52:846, 1980.

29. Heare TC, Enneking WF, Heare MM: Staging techniques and biopsy of bone tumors. Orthop Clin North Am 20:273, 1989.

30. Parrish F: Treatment of bone tumors by total excision and replacement with massive autologous and homologous grafts. J Bone Joint Surg 48A:968, 1966.

31. Johnson EW Jr, Gee VR, Dahlin DC: Giant cell tumors of bone. J Bone Joint Surg 41A:895, 1959.

32. Dahlin DC, Cupps RE, Johnson EW: Giant-cell tumor: a study of 195 cases. Cancer 25:106 1970.

33. Seider MJ, Rich TA, Ayala AG, Murray JA: Giant cell tumors of bone: treatment with radiation therapy. Radiology 161:537, 1986.

34. Bennett CJ, Marcus RB Jr, Million RR, Enneking WF: Radiation therapy for giant cell tumor of bone. Int J Radiation Oncology Biol Phys 26:299, 1993.

35. Schwartz LH, Okunieff PG, Rosenberg A, Suit HD: Radiation therapy in the treatment of difficult giant cell tumors. Int J Radiation Oncology Biol Phys 17:1085, 1989.

36. DeGroof E, Verdonk R, Vercauteren M, et al.: Giant-cell tumor involving a lumbar vertebra. Spine 15:835, 1990.

37. Johnson EW Jr, Gee VR, Dahlin DC: Giant cell tumors of the sacrum. Am J Orthop 4:302, 1962.

38. Stevens WW, Weaver EW: Giant cell tumors and aneurysmal bone cysts of the spine: report of 4 cases. South Med J 63:218, 1970.

39. Harwood AR, Fornasier VL, Rider WD: Supervoltage irradiation in the management of giant cell tumor of bone. Radiology 125:223, 1977.

40. Shikata J, Yamamuro T, Shimiyu K, et al.: Surgical treatment of giant-cell tumors of the spine. Clin Orthop 278:29, 1992.

41. Tomita K, Tsuchiya H: Total sacrectomy and reconstruction for huge sacral tumors. Spine 15:12, 1990.

42. Tubbs WS, Brown LR, Beabout JW, et al.: Bening giant-cell tumor of bone with pulmonary metastases: clinical findings and radiologic appearance of metastases in 13 cases. AJR 158:331, 1992.

Aneurysmal Bone Cyst

Capsule Summary

Frequency of back pain—common
Location of back pain—lumbar spine
Quality of back pain—acute onset, increasing severity
Symptoms and signs—localized bone tenderness, overlying skin erythema
Laborary and x-ray tests—expansile lesion of the posterior elements on plain roentgenograms
Therapy—en-bloc excision

PREVALENCE AND PATHOGENESIS

Aneurysmal bone cyst is a benign, non-neoplastic, cystic vascular lesion of bone that occurs de novo or in the setting of another bone condition such as giant cell tumor, chondroblastoma, chondromyxoid fibroma or fibrous dysplasia. Aneurysmal bone cyst represents about 1% to 2% of primary bone lesions.[1, 2] A more recent review reports aneurysmal bone cysts to be 6% of primary bone lesions.[3] The vast majority of young adults who develop them are under the age of 30. In contrast to the distribution of other primary bone tumors, most series report a slight female predominance.[4, 5] A review of 238 patients with aneurysmal bone cyst found a slight predominence of women at 54%.[6]

The first descriptions of the distinctive characteristics of this lesion are attributed to Jaffe and Lichtenstein in 1950.[7, 8] Other names that have been associated with aneurysmal bone cysts include ossifying hematoma, plain bone cysts, and atypical giant cell tumor.

The etiology of aneurysmal bone cyst remains uncertain. Trauma may play a role in its initiation, since injuries may induce the formation of arteriovenous malformations (AVM). These malformations consist of abnormal vascular channels. Several reports have suggested that trauma that initiated an AVM may have led to the development of an aneurysmal bone cyst.[9, 10]

In a third of the cases, aneurysmal bone cyst is superimposed on another pathologic process, which may be either a benign or a malignant bone tumor. Primary lesions that may be complicated by an aneurysmal bone cyst include giant cell tumor, chondroblastoma, chondromyxoid fibroma, nonossifying fibroma, osteoblastoma, fibrosarcoma, fibrous histiocytoma, osteosarcoma, and fibrous dysplasia.[11] The basic abnormality in both circumstances is a local change in intraosseous blood flow. The blood pools in bone, resulting in increasing intraosseous pressure followed by resorption, expansion, and cyst formation.[12] The recognition of an underlying causative process is important, since the clinical course of the patient may more closely follow that of the primary lesion.

While a majority of aneurysmal bone cysts occur in the long bones of the extremities, 15% to 25% of cases occur in the spine.[13, 14] The lumbosacral spine is affected in 36% of cases, the thoracic spine in 32%, and the cervical spine in 32%.

CLINICAL HISTORY

Patients with aneurysmal bone cysts usually present with symptoms of pain or swelling in the affected area. The pain is usually of acute onset and increases in severity over a short period of time. The duration of symptoms can range from months to several years. The patient may also experience limitation of motion.

The clinical manifestations of spinal aneurysmal bone cyst vary with the location and size of the lesion. A lesion of the spinous or transverse process may be entirely asymptomatic. Neurologic symptoms and signs include a spectrum of abnormalities from sensory changes to paraplegia and these may occur if the expansion of the lesion results in nerve root or cauda equina compression.[15, 16]

PHYSICAL EXAMINATION

Physical examination may demonstrate tenderness to palpation over the site of involvement. The overlying skin may be erythematous and warm if the aneurysmal bone cyst is close to the surface. Patients will demonstrate decreased range of motion with muscle spasm. Slightly over 10% of the patients may have associated scoliosis or kyphosis.[17] Neurologic findings correlate with the location of nerve root or cauda equina compression.

LABORATORY DATA

Screening blood tests are normal in this benign, vascular lesion of bone. Patients with secondary cysts will have abnormal tests that correspond to their underlying lesion (malignant tumor).

On gross inspection, the cyst contains anastomosing cavernous spaces that compose the bulk of lesion. The blood is unclotted. The presence of unclotted blood indicates that the lesion is a hemodynamically active lesion with pools of blood filling and draining. The pressure in the tumors is arterial.[3] Subperiosteal new bone that is eggshell thin separates the lesion from surrounding tissue.

Histologically, the cystic cavities are composed of vascular channels filled with fibrous connective tissue, osteoid, granulation tissue, and multinucleated giant cells (Fig. 13–13).[5] The solid portions of an aneurysmal bone cyst may be fibrous but may contain a lacework of osteoid trabeculae.

"Solid" variant of aneurysmal bone cyst occurs most commonly in long tubular bones but

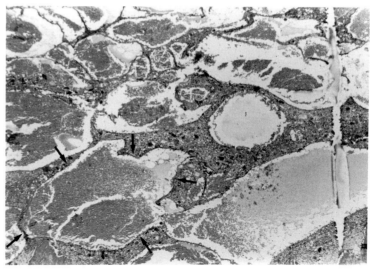

Figure 13–13. Aneurysmal bone cyst. Histologic section exhibiting large vascular channels *(arrows).* The intravascular stroma contains giant cells that are benign. As opposed to normal vessels, the vascular spaces are not lined by endothelial cells. This lesion must be differentiated from telangiectatic osteosarcoma, which will contain vascular channels but will also show atypical cells with bizarre mitotic figures within a sarcomatous stroma. (Courtesy of Arnold Schwartz, M.D.)

occasionally affects the axial skeleton. Histologically, the lesion is characterized by florid fibroblastic proliferation with osteoclast-like giant cell rich areas, stromal hemorrhage, and newly formed osteoid. The histology is similar to that of an aneurysmal bone cyst except for the presence of blood-filled spaces.[18]

RADIOGRAPHIC FINDINGS

The radiographic features of an aneurysmal bone cyst consist of a solitary, eccentrically located, osteolytic, expansile lesion that is sharply demarcated by a thin subperiosteal shell of bone. The cyst cavity is traversed by fine strands of bony cortex. A soft tissue mass may also be associated with the bony lesion. When in the spine, aneurysmal bone cysts occur most commonly in the lumbar and thoracic area and affect the posterior elements of the vertebrae, including pedicles, laminae, and spinous and transverse processes in 60% of lesions (Fig. 13–14). About 30% to 40% occur in vertebral bodies.[10] Lesion within the vertebral body may involve more than one vertebra by extension across the apophyseal joint or disc space.[19] The lesions may attain a considerable size. In the lumbar or sacral area, cysts may displace the kidney or ureter and may compress other pelvic organs.[20] The lesion may also expand to encroach on the neural canal.[21]

CT is useful in the diagnosis of aneurysmal bone cyst, especially for lesions in the axial skeleton. Multiple fluid levels (layering of solid blood components) on CT are suggestive but not diagnostic of an aneurysmal bone cyst.[22] MR may be useful in identifying the extent of lesions in bone and soft tissues.[23] MRs have an

expansile appearance of the lesion. The soft tissue extension of all cysts are well defined with a sharp interface. The fibrous tissue in the periphery of the tumor is highlighted by a low intensity signal in the rim of the lesion on both T_1- and T_2-weighted sequences. Increasing the T_2-weighting of sequences, fluid levels also are detected by MR evaluation.[24] Fluid lev-

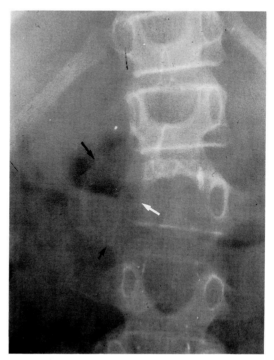

Figure 13–14. Aneurysmal bone cyst arising from the posterior elements of the second lumbar vertebra. Notice the loss of the pedicle *(white arrow)* and faint line of calcification lateral to the vertebral body *(black arrows).* (Courtesy of Anne Brower, M.D.)

els also may accompany telangiectatic osteogenic sarcomas, giant cell tumors, and chondroblastomas.

DIFFERENTIAL DIAGNOSIS

The characteristic radiographic appearance of the aneurysmal bone cyst helps differentiate it from other benign and malignant lesions. The posterior arch and the transverse or spinous process are the common locations of involvement in the spine. A solitary lytic lesion of the anterior body of a vertebra is more likely to be a metastasis, infection, or giant cell tumor. It is also important to remember that some primary bone tumors, including chondroblastoma and giant cell tumor, may have areas that histologically appear like aneurymal bone cysts. Careful evaluation of the entire specimen should alert the pathologist to the underlying lesion.

TREATMENT

Aneurysmal bone cysts can be treated by surgery, radiotherapy, or cryotherapy. Although they are benign lesions, they are highly prone to local recurrence after curettage. If the location of an aneurysmal bone cyst allows removal of a section of bone without loss of function, en-bloc resection is the treatment of choice, and lesions in the posterior elements of the spine may be treated with resection and bone grafting. Lesions that are too large or involve a vertebral body are treated with radiotherapy.[25] Radiation therapy controls the growth of lesions in inaccessible locations.[26] The benefit of radiotherapy must be weighed against the potential of radiation-induced sarcoma many years later. Cryosurgery, freezing the lesion, also has been reported to halt expansion of the cyst and prevent recurrence.[5, 27]

Embolization of the tumor with polyvinyl alcohol particles may slow the growth of tumors. Lesions may then calcify over months.[21] On occasion, spontaneous healing of a cyst may occur. Lesions may stabilize for extended periods of time. Older patients are more likely candidates for spontaneous tumor healing.[28]

PROGNOSIS

Aneurysmal bone cyst is a benign lesion but may cause severe dysfunction because of its expansile characteristics. If the lesion is diagnosed early and treated appropriately, dysfunction may be kept to a minimum. However, if it is located in the spine and is allowed to ex-

pand unchecked, serious neurologic deficits may result. In addition, an aneurysmal bone cyst weakens the bone and increases the risk of pathologic fracture. In rare circumstances, the cyst may transform into a malignant tumor.[29]

References

ANEURYSMAL BONE CYST

1. Mirra J: Bone Tumors: Clinical, Radiologic, and Pathologic Correlations. Philadelphia: Lea & Febiger, 1989, pp 1267–1312.
2. Dahlin DC, Unni KK: Bone Tumors. General Aspects and Data on 8,542 cases 4th ed. Springfield, Illinois: Charles C Thomas, 1986, pp 420–430.
3. Huvos AG: Bone Tumors: Diagnosis, Treatment, and Prognosis, 2nd ed. Philadelphia: WB Saunders, 1991, pp 727–743.
4. Dahlin DC, Besse BE, Pugh DG, Ghormley RK: Aneurysmal bone cysts. Radiology 64:56, 1955.
5. Biesecker JL, Marcove RC, Huvos AG, and Mike V: Aneurysmal bone cyst: a clinicopathologic study of 66 cases. Cancer 26:615, 1970.
6. Vergel AM, Bond JR, Shives TC, et al.: Aneurysmal bone cyst: a clinicopathologic study of 238 cases. Cancer 69:2921, 1991.
7. Jaffe HL: Aneurysmal bone cyst. Bull Hosp Joint Dis 11:3, 1950.
8. Lichtenstein L: Aneurysmal bone cyst: a pathological entity commonly mistaken for a giant cell tumor and occasionally for hemangioma and osteogenic sarcoma. Cancer 3:279, 1950.
9. Barnes R: Aneurysmal bone cyst. J Bone Joint Surg 38 B:301, 1956.
10. Donaldson, WF: Aneurysmal bone cyst. J Bone Joint Surg 44A:25, 1962.
11. Martinez V, Sissons HA: Aneurysmal bone cyst: a review of 123 cases including primary lesions and those secondary to other bone pathology. Cancer 81:2291, 1988.
12. Clough JR, Price CHG: Aneurysmal bone cyst: pathogenesis and long term results of treatment. Clin Orthop 97:52, 1973.
13. Lichtenstein L: Aneurysmal bone cyst: observations on fifty cases. J Bone Joint Surg 39A:873, 1957.
14. Dabska M, Buraczewski J: Aneurysmal bone cyst: pathology, clinical course and radiologic appearance. Cancer 23:371, 1969.
15. Hay MC, Patterson D, Taylor TKF: Aneurysmal bone cysts of the spine. J Bone Joint Surg 60B:406, 1978.
16. Dahlin DC, McLeod RA: Aneurysmal bone cyst and other non-neoplastic conditions. Skeletal Radiol 8:243, 1982.
17. Capanna R, Albisinni U, Picci P, et al.: Aneurysmal bone cyst of the spine. J Bone Joint Surg 67A:527, 1985.
18. Oda Y, Tsuneyoshi M, Shinohara N: Solid variant of aneurysmal bone cyst (extragnathic giant cell reparative granuloma) in the axial skeleton and long bones. Cancer 70:2642, 1992.
19. Banna M: Clinical Radiology of the Spine and the Spinal Cord. Rockville, Maryland: Aspen Systems Corp, 1985, pp 347–348.
20. Faure C, Boccon-Gibod L, Herve J, Pernin P: Case report 154. Skeletal Radiol 6:229, 1981.
21. Cory DA, Fritsch SA, Cohen MD, et al.: Aneurysmal

bone cysts: imaging findings and embolotherapy. AJR 153:369, 1989.

22. Hudson TM: Fluid levels in aneurysmal bone cysts: a CT feature. AJR 141:1001, 1984.

23. Zimmer WD, Berquist TH, Sim FH, et al.: Magnetic resonance imaging of aneurysmal bone cysts. Mayo Clin Proc 59:633, 1984.

24. Munk PL, Helms CA, Holt RG, et al.: MR imaging of aneurysmal bone cysts. AJR 153:99, 1989.

25. Slowick FA, Campbell CJ, Kettelkamp DB: Aneurysmal bone cyst. J Bone Joint Surg 50A:1142, 1968.

26. Maeda M, Tateishi H, Takaiwa H, et al.: High-energy, low-dose radiation therapy for aneurysmal bone cyst: report of a case. Clin Orthop 243:200, 1989.

27. Marcove RC, Miller TR: The treatment of primary and metastatic bone localized tumors by cryosurgery. Surg Clin North Am 49:421, 1969.

28. Malghem J, Maldague B, Esselinckx W, et al.: Spontaneous healing of aneurysmal bone cysts: a report of three cases. J Bone Joint Surg 71B:645, 1989.

29. Kyriakos M, Hardy D: Malignant transformation of aneurysmal bone cyst, with an analysis of the literature. Cancer 68:1770, 1991.

Hemangioma

Capsule Summary

Frequency of back pain—uncommon

Location of back pain—lumbar spine

Quality of back pain—throbbing, ache

Symptoms and signs—localized tenderness, decreased motion

Laboratory and x-ray tests—prominent vertical vertebral body striations on plain roentgenograms

Treatment—radiation for symptomatic lesions

PREVALENCE AND PATHOGENESIS

Hemangioma is a benign vascular lesion composed of cavernous, capillary, or venous blood vessels which may affect soft tissues or bone. Hemangiomas account for fewer than 1% of clinically symptomatic primary bone tumors.[1, 2] However, necropsy studies by a number of investigators have demonstrated that asymptomatic vertebral lesions are found in 12% of autopsies.[3, 4] The prevalence of hemangioma increases with age, with 25% of the lesions present in adults by the fifth decade of life. They are usually identified in patients between the fourth and fifth decades of life. Taking into account hemangiomas from all sites, women and men are equally affected.

The first reference to a hemangioma was reported by Toynbee in 1845.[5] A multitude of types of this vascular lesion have been described, including capillary, cavernous, venous, hypertrophic, juvenile, arteriovenous, intra-muscular, synovial, and histiocytic hemangioma.

The pathogenesis of hemangioma remains unknown. The lesions are considered as congenital vascular malformations by some or as benign neoplasms by others.

Approximately 50% of patients with a hemangioma will have the lesion in the spine or skull. The thoracic spine is the location for 65% of spinal lesions, cervical spine 25%, and lumbar spine 10%.[2]

CLINICAL HISTORY

The initial complaints of patients with symptomatic vertebral hemangiomas are localized pain and tenderness over the involved vertebra along with associated muscle spasm.[6] The pain usually starts as a vague, nondescript ache, which gradually increases in intensity and duration until it becomes constant and throbbing. Neurologic manifestations of cord compression by vertebral hemangioma may include sensory changes, motor weakness, radiculitis, and transverse myelitis.[7, 8]

Multiple hemangiomas may cause spinal cord compression resembling metastatic disease to the spine.[9] Neurologic symptoms tend to occur at time of expansion of the lesion in the vertebral body into the epidural space, pathologic fracture, or extradural hematoma.[10] These symptoms may include radicular pain, weakness or paralysis in a leg, or sensory deficits. When a lumbar vertebra is involved, patients may experience bilateral sciatica, sphincter, and sexual abnormalities.[11] Neurologic symptoms may occur acutely and recurrently.[12] Many of the hemangiomas that cause neurologic symptoms are located in the thoracic spine where the spinal canal is narrow. Women who are pregnant develop increased venous pressure that may result in hemangiomas becoming symptomatic and cause nerve compression secondary to bleeding.[13]

PHYSICAL EXAMINATION

Physical examination may demonstrate tenderness with palpation over the affected vertebral body. Limitation of motion may be present if related muscle spasm is severe.

Hemangiomas that expand bone may cause palpable swelling. Increased weakening of the vertebral body may result in fractures, which will markedly increase tenderness, and muscle spasm.[14] Increased pain and spasm also may result in kyphoscoliosis.[15] Hemangiomas may occur in the setting of systemic hemangiomatosis. In those circumstances, hemangiomas may be noted on the skin, mucous membranes, and other organs (multiple hemangiomatosis of bone or Osler-Weber-Rendu disease).[16, 17]

LABORATORY DATA

Screening blood tests are normal in this benign lesion of bone. Occasionally, the ESR is elevated.[18] Rarely, a consumptive coagulopathy with thrombocytopenia has been reported in patients with multiple vertebral hemangiomas.[19] This syndrome, Kasabach-Merritt syndrome, occurs with multiple hemangiomas and hemangioendotheliomas.[20]

On gross examination, the well-demarcated lesion is reddish-brown and either is confined to the vertebral body or extends into the surrounding soft tissue. The vertebral body is the preferential location of primary involvement with secondary extension into the arch or transverse process. Microscopically, a hemangioma is composed of numerous capillary and larger vascular channels contained in a fibrous stroma. The trabeculae that are not affected by the tumor are thickened in comparison to the lesional thinned osseous trabeculae.[6]

RADIOGRAPHIC EVALUATION

Vertebral hemangiomas primarily involve the vertebral bodies.[21] In an affected vertebral body, the vertical striations are prominent but horizontal striations are absent because of absorption. This gives rise to a "corduroy" appearance of the vertebral body (Fig. 13–15).

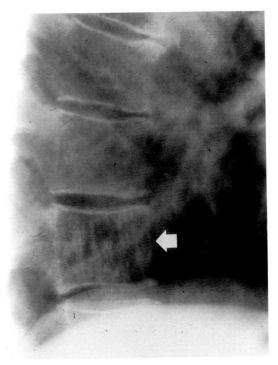

Figure 13–15. Hemangioma of a thoracic vertebra revealing radiolucency of the vertebral body and the accentuation of vertical trabeculation giving it a corduroy appearance *(arrow)*. (Courtesy of Anne Brower, M.D.)

This is most prominent on the lateral projection. The alteration of vertebral striations is diffuse and vertebral body configuration is usually unchanged (Fig. 13–16). Occasionally, vertebral body hemangiomas may extend from the body to the laminae, pedicles, or trans-

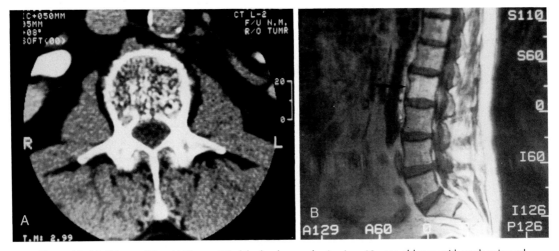

Figure 13–16. CT scan *(A)* and MR scan *(B)* of the lumbosacral spine in a 68-year-old man with neck pain and headaches secondary to osteoarthritis of the cervical spine. CT scan demonstrates loss of trabeculae in the vertebral body secondary to increased vascular channels. MR scan reveals increased signal in a T_1-weighted image of the same vertebral body *(arrow)*. This lesion was asymptomatic.

verse or spinous processes. Rarely, expansion or enlargement of a vertebra may occur.[8]

Symptomatic vertebral hemangiomas may have thinner and wider vertical striations. They may be associated with vertebral body collapse, hemorrhage, and soft tissue masses.[22] Hemangiomas rarely cause compression fractures because of the buttressing of the weaker components by the coarse, remaining trabeculations.[23] Radiologic study of 57 solitary vertebral hemangiomas identified six factors associated with a greater likelihood of compressing the spinal cord. These factors included location in the thoracic spine, involvement of the entire vertebral body, extension into the neural arch, an expanded cortex with indistinct margins, an irregular honeycomb pattern, and soft tissue mass. Only one hemangioma at the L3 level was associated with compressive signs.[24]

Bone scintigraphy demonstrates increased tracer uptake at the site of the vertebral hemangioma. The bone scan may demonstrate decreased uptake if the hemangioma has become thrombosed.[25]

Examination by CT demonstrates the bony changes of hemangioma including the expansion of the body and the involvement of the arch. Soft tissue extension is also noted by CT examination with or without contrast.[26]

MR examination of hemangiomas demonstrates increased signal intensity on both T_1- and T_2-weighted images. Increased signal intensity corresponds with fatty stroma (T_1) and vascularization (T_2) (Fig. 13–17). The aggressiveness of hemangiomas associated with expansion has been related to the absence of fat and increased degree of vascularity as measured by MR.[27]

Angiography may help identify the blood vessels that are feeding the tumor. Occasionally, hemorrhage may impede the filling of the tumor during angiography.[26] Angiography does not distinguish hemangioma from other vascular tumors.

DIFFERENTIAL DIAGNOSIS

The diagnosis of a vertebral hemangioma is uncomplicated when one vertebral body is affected with characteristic radiographic changes. It is more difficult when portions of a vertebra other than the body are affected. Bony resorption of a pedicle may mimic the destructive changes of metastatic cancer. A vertebral body fracture may occur with a hemangioma, but is more frequently seen in metastatic tumor.

Skeletal lymphangiomatosis may affect ver-

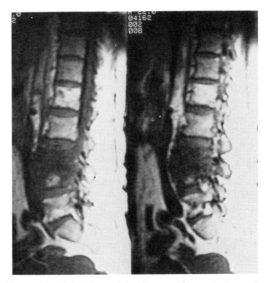

Figure 13–17. MR T_1-weighted image demonstrates an incidental finding of a hemangioma at L1 *(black arrow)* with discitis at L3-L4 level.

tebral bodies, causing increased striation, bony lysis with bone compression, and progressive scoliosis. Lymphangiography may be required to confirm this diagnosis. Histologically, lymphoid tissue is present to an increased degree in the vascular channels of the bone.[28]

A closely related but very rare cause of vertebral bone loss that may resemble hemangiomatosis is Gorham's disease (massive osteolysis).[2, 6] Multiple hemangiomas develop with total lysis of the affected bone and periosteum. The bone is replaced by fibrous tissue. The disease may either be self-limited or progress to a fatal outcome.[29] Hemangiopericytoma is also a very rare vascular tumor that may mimic hemangioma.[3] Angiolipoma is another tumor affecting vertebrae that may cause spinal cord compression that must be differentiated from a hemangioma.[30] Angiosarcoma is a very rare malignant tumor that may affect similar areas of the vertebral column as hemangiomas.[31]

Coarse trabeculation of a vertebral body also may be seen in Paget's disease. Abnormal laboratory tests (elevated ESR, serum alkaline phosphatase) should differentiate tumor and Paget's disease from a hemangioma.

TREATMENT

The treatment of choice for symptomatic vertebral hemangiomas is irradiation, since the lesions are radiosensitive. Radiation therapy effectively relieves symptoms even though the appearance of the lesion remains unchanged.[32] Surgical intervention in the form of laminectomy has an excessive morbidity and mortality due to profuse hemorrhage. Therefore, laminectomy should be reserved for those patients with neurologic deficits who require decompression of the spinal cord. Embolization of feeder vessels before surgery may render surgical decompression a safer procedure.[33] Embolization alone may be successful in controlling the growth of the tumor or may be used in combination with radiation therapy or surgery to reverse neurologic symptoms.[11, 34, 35]

PROGNOSIS

Vertebral hemangiomas are usually asymptomatic and have a benign course; however, when they become symptomatic, they require therapy to prevent expansion of the lesion. The major complication of a vertebral hemangioma is neural compression. Compression fractures may occur in vertebrae affected by a hemangioma. Hemangiomas may cause neural compression by compression fracture, expansion of an involved vertebra, direct extension of the hemangioma into the extradural space, or extradural hemorrhage. Appropriate diagnosis and treatment may help prevent this potentially disabling complication of this vascular neoplasm.

References

HEMANGIOMA

1. Mirra J: Bone Tumors: Clinical, Radiologic, and Pathologic Correlations. Philadelphia: WB Saunders, 1989, pp 1338–1377.
2. Dahlin DC, Unni KK: Bone Tumors: General Aspects and Data on 8,542 Cases, 4th ed. Springfield, Illinois: Charles C Thomas, 1986, pp 167–180.
3. Marcial-Rojas RA: Primary hemangiopericytoma of bone: review of the literature and report of the first case with metastasis. Cancer 13:308, 1960.
4. Schmorl G, Junghanns H: The Human Spine in Health and Disease, 2nd ed. New York: Grune and Stratton, 1971, p 325.
5. Toynbee J: An account of two vascular tumors developed in the substance of bone. Lancet 2:676, 1845.
6. Huvos AG: Bone Tumors: Diagnosis, Treatment and Prognosis, 2nd ed. Philadelphia: WB Saunders, 1991, pp 553–578.
7. Barnard L, Von Nuys RG: Primary hemangioma of the spine. Ann Surg 97:19, 1933.
8. McAllister VL, Kendall BE, Bull JWD: Symptomatic vertebral hemangiomas. Brain 98:71, 1975.
9. Zito G, Kadis GW: Multiple vertebral hemangiomas resembling metastases with spinal cord compression. Arch Neurol 37:247, 1980.
10. Mohan V, Gupta SK, Tuli SM, Sanyal B: Symptomatic vertebral hemangiomas. Clin Radiol 31:575, 1980.
11. Raco A, Ciappetta P, Artico M, et al.: Vertebral hemangiomas with cord compression: the role of embolization in five cases. Surg Neurol 34:164, 1990.

12. Newmark J, Jones HR Jr, Thomas CB, et al.: Vertebral hemangioma causing acute recurrent spinal cord compression. J Neurol Neurosurg Psychiatry 54:471, 1991.
13. Schwartz DA, Nair S, Hershey B, et al.: Vertebral arch hemangioma producing spinal cord compression in pregnancy: diagnosis by magnetic resonance imaging. Spine 14:888, 1989.
14. Bergstrand A, Hook O, Lidvall H: Vertebral hemangiomas compressing the spinal cord. Acta Neurol Scand 39:59, 1963.
15. Ghormley RK, Adson AW: Hemangioma of vertebrae. J Bone Joint Surg 23:887, 1941.
16. Gutierrez R, Spjut J: Skeletal angiomatosis: report of 3 cases and review of the literature. Clin Orthop 85:82, 1972.
17. Mirra JM, Arnold WD: Skeletal hemangiomatosis in association with hereditary hemorrhagic telangiectasia. J Bone Joint Surg 55A:850, 1973.
18. Govender S, Charles RW, Kelman IE: Vertebral haemangiomas: a report of 2 cases. S Afr Med J 72:640, 1987.
19. Lozman J, Holmblad J: Cavernous hemangiomas associated with scoliosis and a localized consumptive coagulopathy: a case report. J Bone Joint Surg 58A:1021, 1976.
20. Brower TD: Case records of the Massachusetts General Hospital. N Engl J Med 320:854, 1989.
21. Sherman RS, Wilner D: The roentgen diagnosis of hemangioma of bone. AJR 86:1146, 1961.
22. Banna M: Clinical Radiology of the Spine and the Spinal Cord. Rockville, Maryland: Aspen Systems Corp, 1985, pp 341–345.
23. McAllister VL, Kendall BE, Bull JW: Symptomatic vertebral hemangiomas. Brain 98:71, 1975.
24. Laredo J, Reizine D, Bard M, Merland J: Vertebral hemangions: radiologic evaluation. Radiology 161:183, 1986.
25. Gerard PS, Wilck E: Spinal hemangioma: an unusual photopenic presentation on bone scan. Spine 17:607, 1992.
26. Schnyder P, Frankhauser H, Mansouri B: Computed tomography in spinal hemangioma with cord compression. Report of two cases. Skeletal Radiol 15:372, 1986.
27. Laredo J, Assouline E, Gelbert F, et al.: Vertebral hemangiomas: fat content as a sign of aggressiveness. Radiology 177:467, 1990.
28. Reilly BJ, Davison JW, Bain H: Lymphangiectasis of the skeleton: a case report. Radiology 103:385, 1972.
29. Hambach R, Pujman J, Maly V: Massive osteolysis due to hemangiomatosis. Report of a case of Gorham's disease with autopsy. Radiology 71:43, 1958.
30. Kuroda S, Abe H, Akino M, et al.: Infiltrating spinal angiolipoma causing myelopathy: case report. Neurosurgery 27:315, 1990.
31. Dagi TF, Schmidek HH: Vascular tumors of the spine. In: Sundaresan N, Schmidek HH, Schiller AL, Rosenthal DI (eds): Tumors of the Spine: Diagnosis and Clinical Management. Philadelphia: WB Saunders, 1990, pp 181–191.
32. Manning JH: Symptomatic hemangioma of the spine. Radiology 56:58, 1951.
33. Kapur P, Banna M: Spinous osseous angioma: Gelfoam embolization. J Can Assoc Radiol 31:271, 1980.
34. Djindijian M, Nguyen J, Gaston A, et al.: Multiple vertebral hemangiomas with neurological signs: case report. J Neurosurg 76:1025, 1992.
35. Bednar DA, Esses SI: Double hemangioma of the spine with paraparesis: a case report. Spine 15:1377, 1990.

Eosinophilic Granuloma

Capsule Summary

Frequency of back pain—common
Location of back pain—lumbar spine
Quality of back pain—localized aching
Symptoms and signs—nontender swelling
Laboratory and x-ray tests—occasional peripheral eosinophilia; osteolysis without sclerosis in a vertebral body on plain roentgenogram; epidural extension of granuloma on MR
Treatment—curettage

PREVALENCE AND PATHOGENESIS

Eosinophilic granuloma occurs in solitary and multifocal forms and is characterized by the infiltration of bone with histiocytes, mononuclear phagocytic cells, and eosinophils. Eosinophilic granuloma, Hand-Schüller-Christian disease, and Letterer-Siwe disease are thought to have the same pathogenesis and are referred to collectively as histiocytosis X. Eosinophilic granuloma is the mildest form and Letterer-Siwe disease the most aggressive form of histiocytosis X.

Eosinophilic granuloma is a rare lesion occurring in less than 1% of primary infiltrative lesions of bone examined by biopsy.[1] It occurs most commonly in children and adolescents, with approximately 10% of patients being 20 years of age or older.[2] It has a higher incidence in males at a 2:1 ratio and is more frequent in Caucasians than in blacks. Approximately 1200 new cases of eosinophilic granuloma are reported yearly in the United States.[3]

The first reference to the term eosinophilic granuloma was made by Jaffe and Lichtenstein in 1944.[4] In the past, this lesion has gone by many different names, including pseudotuberculous granuloma, Taratynov's disease, traumatic myeloma, and histiocytic granuloma.

The pathogenesis of eosinophilic granuloma is not known. This disease belongs to the nonlipid histiocytoses, which are characterized by proliferation of histiocytes without a demonstrable disorder of lipid metabolism. These histiocytes accumulate cytoplasmic lipid, but, unlike true lipid metabolic disorders (Gaucher's disease), these lipids develop as a consequence of the ingestion of necrotic debris rather than an inborn error of metabolism. The cause of this lipid accumulation is unknown. Some investigators have suggested that eosinophilic granuloma may be the result of a viral infection, but this hypothesis remains unproven.[5] Immunologic alterations have been demonstrated in association with eosinophilic granuloma. Autoimmune complexes have been implicated as a possible cause of this disorder suggesting an immunologic origin for the disease.[6]

Approximately 10% of patients with unifocal eosinophilic granuloma have lesions in the spine. They are equally dispersed through the lumbar, thoracic, and cervical spine.[1] Unifocal (solitary) bone presentation is twice as common as multifocal osseous involvement. Eosinophilic granuloma may affect multiple spinal levels.[7]

CLINICAL HISTORY

The symptoms of spinal eosinophilic granuloma vary with the location and severity of the lesion. Back pain that is constant is the most common complaint. The pain is not relieved with rest or aspirin. The lesion may cause restricted motion and muscle spasm. A palpable mass may be noted if a lesion is close to the skin. Symptoms of spinal cord compression are uncommon but may occur secondary to vertebral body collapse or dislocation. Patients with eosinophilic granuloma may have neurologic symptoms including radicular pain and paresthesias.[8]

PHYSICAL EXAMINATION

A palpable mass may be present over the affected bone, but it is neither tender nor associated with redness or heat. A low-grade fever is present in few patients.[1] Spinal cord and nerve root compression secondary to vertebral body collapse results in corresponding abnormalities on neurologic examination.

LABORATORY DATA

Eosinophilic granuloma is associated with peripheral eosinophilia in 6% to 10% of patients. There is also an occasional patient with an elevated ESR. Bone marrow examination from an uninvolved area of bone will yield increased numbers of eosinophils even with normal differential counts.[9]

Examination of gross pathologic specimens usually reveals a soft reddish-brown tissue with hemorrhage and cysts. The histologic appearance of eosinophilic granuloma is characterized by collections of eosinophils and histiocytes without the formation of local, distinct granulomas (Fig. 13–18). The characteristic cell of eosinophilic granuloma is similar to the Langerhans' cell of the epidermis. On elec-

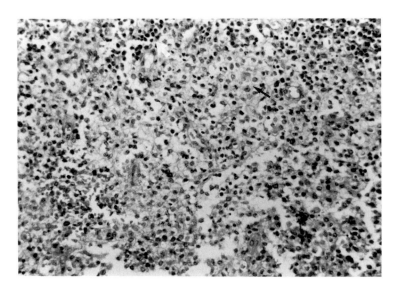

Figure 13–18. Eosinophilic granuloma. Histologic appearance of an eosinophilic granuloma with histiocytes containing large vesicular nuclei *(arrow)*. Other components of the polymorphous infiltrate include eosinophilic granulocytes and occasional lymphocytes. (Courtesy of Arnold Schwartz, M.D.)

tron microscopy, Langerhans' cells contain Birbeck bodies, which are granules shaped like tennis rackets. These pentalaminar, cytoplasmic inclusions are thought to be formed by the invagination of the cell membranes of Langerhans' cells. Birbeck granules are found in cells from eosinophilic granuloma lesions. Special stains also may be used to detect S-100 nuclear positive, dendritic system histiocytes, lysozyme, and esterase positive and S-100 negative macrophage system histiocytes.[1] S-100 protein cells are ubiquitous and may be found in a variety of neoplastic and benign conditions. Peanut agglutinin (PNA) is a more specific histiocyte marker. The paranuclear and surface pattern of PNA binding helps define Langerhans histiocytes.[10] The histiocytes have striking phagocytic activity. Some foci contain multinucleated giant cells with areas of hemorrhage and necrosis. The cytoplasm of the phagocytic cells often exhibits double refractile, neutral fat deposition. In areas where eosinophilic leukocytes are undergoing fragmentation, Charcot-Leyden crystals are noted. As the eosinophilic granuloma heals, eosinophils markedly diminish in number and are replaced by large histiocytes and fibrous tissue.[11, 12]

The pleomorphic appearance of the histiocytes may superficially resemble malignant cells of Hodgkin's disease. Histiocytes of eosinophilic granuloma are benign. With time, they may form giant cells and take on the appearance of foam cells after they have ingested necrotic tissue and converted it into cytoplasmic lipids. The presence of lipid in eosinophilic granuloma is a secondary phenomenon and is not of pathogenetic importance as it is in Gaucher's disease.

RADIOGRAPHIC EVALUATION

Eosinophilic granuloma in the spine is associated with a spectrum of radiographic abnormalities. The features of early lesions are those of a destructive, radiolucent oval area of bone lysis without peripheral sclerosis. Progressive destruction in a vertebral body results in a flattened vertebral body, termed vertebra plana (Fig. 13–19), first described by Calvé.[13] The degree of compression may be symmetric or asymmetric with preservation of the intervertebral disc. The body of the vertebra is affected with sparing of the posterior elements.[14] The compressed vertebra may project anteriorly and, in extreme circumstances, cause spinal dislocation. The association of vertebra plana and eosinophilic granuloma has been verified by biopsy.[15] Eosinophilic granuloma is the most common cause of vertebra plana in children. It may erode the posterior elements of a vertebral body and spare the vertebral body. One pedicle, a lamina, or one of the lateral masses may be affected. These lesions are not associated with vertebral collapse.[16] Rarely, eosinophilic granuloma can produce expansile lesions with extensive destruction of multiple vertebrae and paraspinal extension.[17] The vertebral height may be restored spontaneously or after treatment with the affected vertebra reverting to an almost normal configuration.[18]

Other radiographic techniques may be useful in the determination of bone involvement and the extent of soft tissue extension of lesions in the spinal canal. Bone scintigraphy may detect lesions in complex bones, but roentgenograms may be superior in the detection of early lesions.[19] CT is particularly helpful

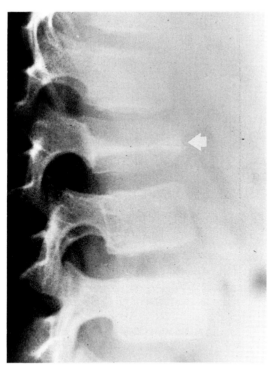

Figure 13–19. Eosinophilic granuloma involving a vertebral body *(arrow)* associated with some flattening of the vertebral body (vertebra plana) and preservation of disc spaces. (Courtesy of Anne Brower, M.D.)

in confirming periosteal reaction and cortical invasion. MR is very useful in the determination of epidural extension of extraosseous eosinophilic granulomas associated with neurologic compromise.[8]

DIFFERENTIAL DIAGNOSIS

The diagnosis of eosinophilic granuloma is made from the close inspection of biopsy material. Laboratory and radiographic features are too nonspecific to assure an accurate diagnosis. The careful inspection of biopsy material is essential to making the correct diagnosis. There are many pitfalls that may cause misinterpretation of biopsy specimens. The characteristic cells associated with this tumor are eosinophils and monocytoid histiocytes. Improperly stained eosinophils may be mistaken for neutrophils. The large number of "neutrophils" might be mistaken for osteomyelitis caused by bacterial, tuberculous, or fungal organisms. Histiocytes associated with eosinophilic granuloma may have single or multiple nuclei that are round, oval, or lobulated in shape. The pleomorphism of histiocytes can lead to the erroneous impression of a reticulum cell sarcoma or Hodgkin's disease.

Histiocytes in these malignant diseases have greater nuclear pleomorphism and more irregular nucleoli.

During the healing phase of eosinophilic granuloma, masses of multinucleate giant cells are seen in areas of the tumor that are being revascularized. The presence of these giant cells may result in an inappropriate diagnosis of giant cell tumor. The clinical, radiologic, and histologic features should prevent an erroneous diagnosis.

TREATMENT

Spontaneous healing of eosinophilic granuloma is manifested by partial restoration of vertebral body height. Restoration of vertebral height occurs most commonly in younger patients.[7] Therefore, surgical treatment or radiotherapy may not be indicated unless specific indications such as neurologic complications are present. In patients with biopsy evidence of the neoplasm and intractable symptoms, the treatment of choice for eosinophilic granuloma is curettage, with or without packing of the lesion with bone chips. Inaccessible lesions in the spine that may lead to pathologic fractures are best treated with low dosage radiation therapy of 300 to 600 rads. Lumbar braces are not usually required while affected vertebral bodies heal.[20] Healing may occur over months to years. Corticosteroids have been used in pediatric patients and have been effective in reversing bone lesions.[21] Steroids have been chosen in patients with lesions in a difficult operative location.[22] Diphosphonates have been utilized in a small number of patients to decrease bone pain and prevent the progression of bone lesions. Clodronate given in a dose of 1.6 gm per day for a 6 month period allowed for healing of bone lesions in two adult patients. The remission lasted for 3 years in one patient and 5 years in another.[23]

PROGNOSIS

Eosinophilic granuloma is a benign lesion, and the prognosis is good. Patients with vertebra plana may heal in time with partial reconstitution of the affected vertebral body. The prognosis of patients with multifocal eosinophilic granuloma may not be as good if their illness progresses to the diffuse involvement associated with other components of histiocytosis X. This is more of a concern for younger patients than for adults. If a patient has only a single lesion for 6 months, the chances are that the lesion will remain unifocal.[1]

References

EOSINOPHILIC GRANULOMA

1. Mirra JM: Bone Tumors: Clinical, Radiologic, and Pathologic Correlations. Philadelphia: Lea & Febiger, 1989, pp 1023–1045.
2. Cheyne C: Histiocytosis X. J Bone Joint Surg 53B:366, 1971.
3. Lavin PT, Osband ME: Evaluating the role of therapy in histiocytosis X. Hematol Oncol Clin North Am 1:35, 1987.
4. Jaffe HL, Lichtenstein L: Eosinophilic granuloma of bone: a condition affecting one, several or many bones, but apparently limited to the skeleton and representing the mildest clinical expression of the peculiar inflammatory histiocytosis also underlying Letterer-Siwe disease and Schüller-Christian disease. Arch Pathol 37:99, 1944.
5. Schajowicz F, Slullitel J: Eosinophilic granuloma and its relationship to Hand-Schüller-Christian and Lettere-Siwe syndromes. J Bone Joint Surg 55B:545, 1973.
6. Osband ME: Histiocytosis X: Langerhans' cell histiocytosis. Hematol Oncol Clin North Am 1:737, 1987.
7. Tomita T: Special considerations in surgery of pediatric spine tumors. In: Sundaresan N, Schmidek HH, Schiller AL, Rosenthal DI (eds): Tumors of the Spine: Diagnosis and Management. Philadelphia: WB Saunders, 1990, pp 258–271.
8. Kantererewicz E, Condom E, Canete JD, Del Olmo JA: Spinal cord compression by a unifocal eosinophilic granuloma: a case report of an adult with unusual roentgenological features. Neurosurgery 23:666, 1988.
9. Marcove RC: Bone marrow eosinophilia with solitary eosinophilic granuloma of bone: a report of two cases. J Bone Joint Surg 41A:1521, 1959.
10. Ree HJ, Kadin ME: Peanut agglutinin: a useful marker for histiocytosis-X and interdigitating reticulum cells. Cancer 57:282, 1986.
11. Huvos AG: Bone Tumors: Diagnosis, Treatment, and Prognosis, 2nd ed. Philadelphia: WB Saunders, 1991, pp 695–711.
12. Green WT, Farber S: "Eosinophilic or solitary granuloma" of bone. J Bone Joint Surg 24:499, 1942.
13. Calve, JA: Localized affection of spine suggesting osteochondritis of vertebral body, with clinical aspects of Pott's disease. J Bone Joint Surg 7:41, 1925.
14. David R, Oria RA, Kumar R, et al.: Radiologic features of eosinophilic granuloma of bone. AJR 153:1021, 1989.
15. Kieffer SA, Nesbit ME, D'Angio GJ: Vertebra plana due to histiocytosis X: serial studies. Acta Radiol [Diagn] (Stockh) 8:241, 1969.
16. Kaye JJ, Freiberger RH: Eosinophilic granuloma of the spine without vertebra plana: a report of two unusual cases. Radiology 92:1188, 1969.
17. Ferris RA, Pettrone FA, McKelvie AM, et al.: Eosinophilic granuloma of the spine: an unusual radiographic presentation. Clin Orthop 99:57, 1974.
18. Nesbit ME, Kieffer S, D'Angio GJ: Reconstitution of vertebral height in histiocytosis X: a long-term follow-up. J Bone Joint Surg 51:1360, 1969.
19. Kumar R, Balachandran S: Relative roles of radionuclide scanning and radiographic imaging in eosinophilic granuloma. Clin Nucl Med 5:538, 1980.
20. Ippolito E, Farsetti P, Tudisoc C: Vertebra plana. J Bone Joint Surg 66A:1364, 1984.
21. Avioli LV, Lasersohn JT, Lopresti JM: Histiocytosis X (Schüller-Christian disease): A clinicopathological survey, review of ten patients and the results of prednisone therapy. Medicine 42:119, 1963.
22. Carmago OPD, Oliveira NRBD, Andrade JS, et al.: Eosinophilic granuloma of the ischium: long-term evaluation of a patient treated with steroids. J Bone Joint Surg 74A:445, 1992.
23. Elomaa I, Blomqvist C, Porkka L, Holmstrom T: Experiences of clodronate treatment of multifocal eosinophilic granuloma of bone. J Intern Med 225:59, 1989.

Gaucher's Disease

Capsule Summary

Frequency of back pain—common
Location of back pain—lumbar spine
Quality of back pain—persistent ache
Symptoms and signs—generalized fatigue, abdominal distention, bleeding
Laboratory and x-ray tests—pancytopenia, increased nonprostatic acid phosphatase, decreased leukocyte acid beta-glucocerebrosidase, Gaucher's cells on bone marrow; vertebra plana on plain roentgenogram
Treatment—Alglucerase, gene therapy

PREVALENCE AND PATHOGENESIS

Gaucher's disease is a lipid metabolism disorder associated with the accumulation of ceramide glucoside in histiocytes. The massive accumulation of this lipid in cells of the reticuloendothelial system results in an enlarged spleen, destruction of bone, and abnormalities of the bone marrow.

Gaucher's disease is an uncommon illness that can become manifest at any time of life. However, the manifestations of the illness become more prominent as the affected individual ages. Ashkenazi Jews are at greatest risk to develop this illness, although Caucasians, blacks, and Orientals can also be affected.[1, 2] Of the three forms of the disease, type 1 is the most common with involvement limited to the spleen, liver, and skeletal system.[3] Type 1 is the most common form in Ashkenazi Jews. Type 2 and 3 are associated with neurologic involvement and differs from type 1. The age at the appearance of first symptoms is 25. Men and women are equally affected. The first reference to the disease was made by Gaucher in 1882.[4]

The pathogenesis of the disease is related to an inborn error of metabolism that causes the accumulation of complex lipids within histiocytes. In the past, the etiology of Gaucher's disease was thought to be excessive production of a lipid ceramide glucoside. More recently, the abnormality has been traced to a defective enzyme, beta-glucosidase, which is unable to degrade accumulating lipid.[5] Glucose is not cleaved from the lipid portion of sphingo-lipids. The accumulation of this material in cells throughout the body results in the manifestations of Gaucher's disease. The autosomal recessive inheritance of the disease suggests that a single biochemical defect does account for the abnormalities associated with this illness. Recently investigators have identified a gene mutation that causes a single base substitution (leucine to proline) that accounts for the loss of enzymatic activity.[6]

The gene that encodes the glucocerebrosidase enzyme is located on chromosome 1. A number of mutations have been identified with the various forms of Gaucher's disease. In the Jewish population, a mutation that results in the substitution of serine for asparagine at amino acid 370 of the processed protein accounts for most of the abnormalities of the Ashkenazi Jewish population. In the non-Jewish population, a larger variety of mutations is associated with Gaucher's disease.[7] This is the reason for the different clinical manifestations in non-Jewish Gaucher's patients.

In adults, the axial skeleton is frequently involved. Gaucher's disease causes vertebral body osteolysis, compression fractures, and spinal deformities. Any portion of the axial skeleton may be affected.

CLINICAL HISTORY

Clinical symptoms depend on the organ involved and the degree of involvement. Adult patients have abdominal distention secondary to hepatosplenomegaly. This may result in pancytopenia in association with episodes of bleeding and infections. Constitutional symptoms of generalized fatigue and weakness are common. Patients with skeletal disease have persistent bone pain, tenderness, difficulty walking, back pain, and loss of height. Symptoms relating to the skeletal system have been reported in up to 86% of patients.[8] Up to 37% of type 1 Gaucher patients develop acute bone crisis, including the lumbar spine and pelvis.[9] Pain is severe and resistant to narcotics. The involved bone is warm, swollen, and tender with systemic fever. Later in the course of the illness, bone pain becomes the major cause of morbidity. Neurologic symptoms are usually reserved for children with more severe disease. These manifestations include strabismus, seizures, tremors, clonus, mental retardation,

and loss of sensation. Neurologic symptoms, including radicular pain, occurs in rare circumstances in the setting of spinal cord compression. Cord compression occurs in later stages of the disease secondary to vertebral pathologic fractures.[10, 11]

PHYSICAL EXAMINATION

Patients with Gaucher's disease have massive splenomegaly, moderate hepatomegaly, and minimal lymphadenopathy. Deposits of lipid in the dermis give exposed skin a tan color, while deposits in the sclerae of the eye cause tan pingueculae to appear. Patient may complain of bone tenderness on palpation. This may be particularly prominent in patients who develop acute vertebral compression fractures. These individuals have percussion tenderness over the lumbar spine.

LABORATORY DATA

Anemia, leukopenia, and thrombocytopenia, which is associated with occasional episodes of bleeding, result from replacement of bone marrow cells with lipid-filled histiocytes. The abnormal blood counts are related to the status of the individual's spleen. Splenectomized patients are more likely to normalize blood counts than nonsplenectomized patients.[3] Serum acid phosphatase of nonprostatic origin is elevated.[12, 13] Other abnormalities include abnormal liver function tests, prolonged prothrombin and partial thromboplastin times, elevated serum ferritin levels, and angiotensin-converting enzyme activities. In one study, 15 of 23 (65%) patients with Gaucher's disease had elevated IgG levels, while a smaller percentage (43%) had diffuse hypergammaglobulinemia.[14]

Bone marrow aspirate is usually adequate in obtaining tissue that reveals characteristic Gaucher's cells. Gaucher's cells have two round-to-oval eccentric nuclei with striated cytoplasm, which readily stains with periodic acid-Schiff reagent (Fig. 13–20). In affected bones, the histiocytic cells form small nests that coalesce into large masses.[15] Gaucher's cells may be found in other body tissues, including the intervertebral discs.[16]

RADIOGRAPHIC EVALUATION

The infiltration of marrow with Gaucher's cells results in characteristic radiographic abnormalities. In the spine, cellular infiltrates result in increased radiolucency of vertebral bod-

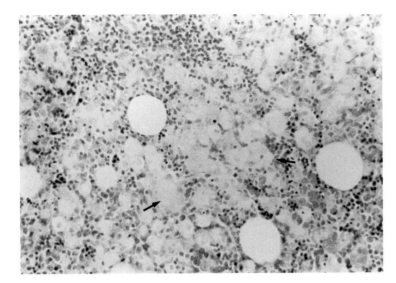

Figure 13–20. Gaucher's disease. Bone marrow specimen exhibiting large, lipid-filled histiocytes (Gaucher's cells) *(arrows)* that have replaced most of the other bone marrow elements. (Courtesy of Arnold Schwartz, M.D.)

ies, accentuation of vertical trabeculae, and compression fractures (Fig. 13–21).[17] Fractures may cause complete flattening of a vertebral body (vertebra plana) or the development of depressions in the superior and inferior margins of a vertebral body, referred to as an "H vertebra" (Fig. 13–22).[18] These lesions occur secondary to occlusion of vessels that are distributed to the chondro-osseous junction in the middle of the endplate. Disc spaces are usually spared. In an occasional patient, widespread disc degeneration with vertebral body overgrowth occurs.[19] Gaucher's disease is also associated with aseptic necrosis of bone, usually at the ends of long bones, but it has also been described near the sacroiliac joint. This process results in apparent obliteration of the articulation, simulating changes associated with ankylosing spondylitis.[18, 20]

Bone scan abnormalities include increased uptake surrounding the large joints of the extremities. On occasion, increased bone scan activity precedes roentgenographic abnormalities.[3] Bone scan abnormalities associated with Gaucher's disease identified by scintigraphy include aseptic necrosis, bone infarction, pathologic fractures, and osteomyelitis.[21]

CT is useful in quantifying the extent of skeletal involvement as well as delineating the degree of bone marrow replacement. The progression of disease reflects the infiltration of the marrow with Gaucher's cells moving from the axial to the appendicular skeleton. A combination of CT and technetium-99m sulfur colloid bone marrow scan offers assessment of gradations of increasing severity of bone disease.[22] The combination of these two tests show some patients with minimal to moderate

roentgenographic evidence of bone disease to have extensive skeletal involvement. Quantitative CT, a method for measuring bone calcium, is a useful method to measure the pro-

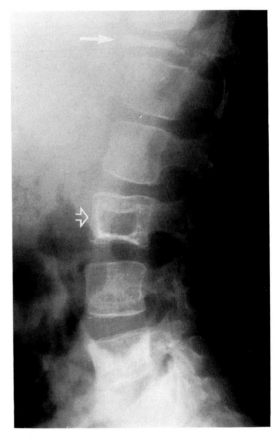

Figure 13–21. Gaucher's disease of the lumbar spine manifested by a vertebra plana *(arrow)* and rectangular lytic lesion in a vertebral body *(open arrow)*. (Courtesy of Anne Brower, M.D.)

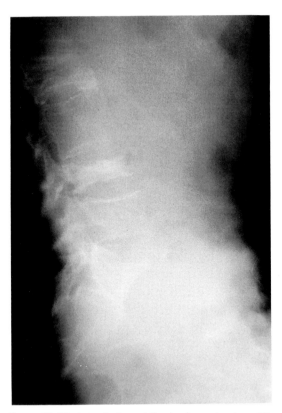

Figure 13–22. Lateral view of the lumbar spine in a 58-year-old woman with a 2-year history of intermittent low and mid back pain. The patient had a marked thoracic kyphosis. Mild anemia, thrombocytopenia, and elevated acid phosphatase were noted. Bone marrow aspiration revealed Gaucher's cells. The roentgenogram reveals generalized osteopenia and multiple compression fractures. (Courtesy of Peter Levitin, M.D.)

gression of disease as reflected by replacement of bone calcium.[23]

MR of patients with Gaucher's disease is useful in detecting the extent of organ replacement with Gaucher's cells. Replacement of normal fat with Gaucher's cells results in a characteristic hyposignal of bone marrow in T_1- and T_2-weighted sequences. Liver and spleen enlargement is readily visible with MR. MR detects increased fluid in bone associated with episodes of acute avascular necrosis. MR is useful in the orthopedic evaluation of the patient with the acute onset of skeletal pain.[24, 25] It is able to document sacroiliac joint involvement, including bone infarcts, effusions, and hematomas in surrounding muscle.[26]

DIFFERENTIAL DIAGNOSIS

The diagnosis of Gaucher's disease is confirmed by the presence of characteristic cells obtained by biopsy of affected tissues. Since the presence of pseudo-Gaucher's cells may occur in bone marrow specimens, the enzymatic assay of leukocyte acid beta-glucosidase is a more specific test.[3] In the future, DNA analysis for Gaucher's disease mutations will become the best method for diagnosis. The radiographic findings have considerable overlap with other disorders that produce osteoporosis and aseptic necrosis. Metabolic disorders associated with axial skeletal osteopenia include osteoporosis, osteomalacia, and hyperparathyroidism. Sickle cell anemia and thalassemia may cause similar radiographic findings. Tumors, including myeloma and metastatic lesions or leukemia, may cause loss of bone calcium, localized lucent areas, and cystic lesions, which are also seen in Gaucher's disease.

Osteosclerosis is not specific for Gaucher's disease. This radiographic finding occurs in Hodgkin's disease, myelofibrosis, mastocytosis, metastatic lesions, and tuberous sclerosis.

Patients with Gaucher's disease are at greater risk for developing infections, including osteomyelitis.[27] This diagnosis should be considered in a patient with Gaucher's disease who develops increased bone pain with an associated fever.

TREATMENT

Splenectomy is a surgical procedure utilized in patients with cytopenias and abdominal discomfort from splenomegaly. The procedure is most helpful for improving the rate of growth in children or adolescents. The effects of splenectomy on the progression of disease in other organs is questionable. In a study of the relationship between splenectomy and bone disease, an equal incidence of bone disease in splenectomized and nonsplenectomized patients was noted.[3] Splenectomy has no effect on the progression of skeletal disease.[28]

New treatments have been developed for Gaucher's disease. Alglucerase is a mannose-terminated form of human placental glucocerebrosidase developed to treat Gaucher's patients.[29] Primary therapy of Gaucher's disease focuses on the removal of the lipid metabolite that causes organ failure. Alglucerase is taken up by Gaucher's cells in the liver, spleen, and bone marrow where accumulated lipid is broken down. The drug is given intravenously (60U/kg) over 1 to 2 hours, usually every 2 weeks. The treatment must be continued indefinitely. In one study, 12 patients treated with infusions of alglucerase for 9 to 12 months showed an increase in hemoglobin concentration, platelet count, and a decrease in organ size.[30] Skeletal improvement also was noted in a quarter of patients. The cost of this enzyme is prohibitive and is estimated to be $382,200 per year. More effective methods to deliver the enzyme to macrophages are being investigated. A retroviral vector with the normal human DNA for the glucocerebrosidase gene has transduced bone marrow cells in long-term cultures. This method may prove useful to replace enzyme in patients. Bone marrow transplant is curative for the disease but is associated with the higher risks of the procedure. Transplantation is usually considered only for young patients with severe disease.[7, 31]

Patients with multiple bone fractures may benefit from treatment with bisphosphonates. Pamidronate (aminohydroxypropylidene bisphosphonate) has been associated with the reduction of bone resorption, increased calcium absorption, improved calcium balance, and improvement in bone density in the axial and appendicular skeleton in Gaucher's disease patients. Decreased bone pain was a result of the therapy.[32]

PROGNOSIS

Gaucher's disease has a protracted course punctuated with periods of increased symptoms. Compression fractures of the spine, aseptic necrosis of bone, and pathologic fractures in long bones can cause severe morbidity. Adult patients usually die of infection, bleeding, anemia, or severe weight loss.

The younger the age at clinical presentation, the more severe the disease. Patients with type 2 disease may die at birth.[31] A more closely linked factor with disease severity is the genotype of the patient. Certain genotypes are associated with milder disease (1226G/1226G), while others are associated with neuropathic disease and a poor prognosis (1226G/1448C).[3]

Gaucher's disease is commonly regarded as a progressive disorder leading to death. Recent studies have suggested that the disease is most progressive up to young adulthood with stabilization thereafter. Patients with long-standing disease are at risk of developing progressive skeletal disease involving the hip joints and the vertebral column. Skeletal disease, including compression fractures of the spine, aseptic necrosis of bone, and pathologic fractures in long bones, has the potential to become a source of morbidity in later life. Adult patients remain at risk for bleeding, anemia, and infection.

References

GAUCHER'S DISEASE

1. Greenfield GB: Miscellaneous diseases related to the hematologic system. Semin Roentgenol 9:241, 1974.
2. Novy SB, Naletson E, Stuart L, Whittock G: Gaucher's disease in a black adult. AJR 133:947, 1979.
3. Zimran A, Kay A, Gelbart T, et al.: Gaucher disease: clinical, laboratory, radiologic, and genetic features of 53 patients. Medicine 71:337, 1992.
4. Gaucher P: De l'epithelioma primitif de la rate, hypertrophie idiopathique de la rate sans l'eucemie. These de Paris, 1882.
5. Volk BW, Adachi M, Schneck L: The pathology of the sphingolipidoses. Semin Hematol 9:317, 1972.
6. Tsuji S, Choudary PV, Martin BM, et al.: A mutation in the human glucocerebrosidase gene in neuronopathic Gaucher's disease. N Engl J Med 316:570, 1987.
7. Beutler E: Gaucher disease: new molecular approaches to diagnosis and treatment. Science 256:794, 1992.
8. Goldblatt J, Sacks S, Beighton P: The orthopedic aspects of Gaucher's disease. Clin Orthop 137:208, 1978.
9. Yosipovitch Z, Katz K: Bone crisis in Gaucher's disease: an update. Isr J Med Sci 26:593, 1990.
10. Goldblatt J, Keet P, Dall D: Spinal cord decompression for Gaucher's disease. Neurosurgery 21:227, 1987.
11. Hermann G, Wagner LD, Gendal ES, et al.: Spinal cord compression in type I Gaucher disease. Radiology 170:147, 1989.
12. Tuchman LR, Swick M: High acid phosphatase level indicating Gaucher's disease in patients with prostatism. JAMA 164:2034, 1957.
13. Tuchman LR, Suna H, Carr JJ: Elevation of serum acid phosphatase in Gaucher's disease. J Mt Sinai Hosp 23:227, 1956.
14. Marti GE, Ryan ET, Papadopoulos NM, et al.: Polyclonal B-cell lymphocytosis and hypergammaglobulinemia in patients with Gaucher disease. Am J Hematol 29:189, 1988.
15. Mirra JM: Bone Tumors: Clinical, Radiologic, and Pathologic Correlations. Philadelphia: Lea & Febiger, 1989, pp 1060–1074.
16. Sack GH Jr: Clinical diversity in Gaucher's disease. Johns Hopkins Med J 146:166, 1980.
17. Greenfield GB: Bone changes in chronic adult Gaucher's disease. AJR 110:800, 1970.
18. Schwarz AM, Homer MJ, McCauley RGK: "Step off" vertebral body. Gaucher's disease vs. sickle cell hemoglobinopathy. AJR 132:81, 1979.
19. Colhoun EN, Cassar-Pullicino V, McCall IW, David MW: Unusual discovertebral changes in Gaucher's disease. Br J Radiol 60:925, 1987.
20. Kulowski J: Gaucher's disease in bone. AJR 63:840, 1950.
21. Israel O, Jerushalmi J, Front D: Scintigraphic findings in Gaucher's disease. J Nucl Med 27:1557, 1986.
22. Hermann G, Goldblatt J, Levy RN, et al.: Gaucher's disease type 1: assessment of bone involvement by CT and scintigraphy. AJR 147:943, 1986.
23. Rosenthal DI, Mayo-Smith W, Goodsitt MM, et al.: Bone and bone marrow changes in Gaucher disease: evaluation with quantitative CT. Radiology 170:143, 1989.
24. Lanir A, Hadar H, Cohen I, et al.: Gaucher disease: Assessment with MR imaging. Radiology 161:239, 1986.
25. Cremin BJ, Davey H, Goldblatt J: Skeletal complica-

tions of type I Gaucher disease: the magnetic resonance features. Clin Radiol 41:244, 1990.

26. Bisagni-Faure A, Dupont A, Chazerain P, et al.: Magnetic resonance imaging assessment of sacroiliac joint involvement in Gaucher's disease. J Rheumatol 19:1984, 1992.

27. Noyes FR, Smith WS: Bone crisis and chronic osteomyelitis in Gaucher's disease. Clin Orthop 79:132, 1971.

28. Stowens DW, Teitelbaum SL, Kahn AJ, Barranger JA: Skeletal complications of Gaucher disease. Medicine 64:310, 1985.

29. Whittington R, Goa KL: Alglucerase: A review of its therapeutic use in Gaucher's disease. Drugs 44:72, 1992.

30. Barton NW, Brady RO, Dambrosia JM, et al.: Replacement therapy for inherited enzyme deficiency—macrophage-targeted glucocerebrosidase for Gaucher's disease. N Engl J Med 324:1464, 1991.

31. Erikson A, Groth CG, Mansson JE, et al.: Clinical and biochemical outcome of marrow transplantation for Gaucher disease of the Norrbottnian type. Acta Paediatr Scand 79:680, 1990.

32. Ostlere L, Warner T, Meunier PJ, et al.: Treatment of type I Gaucher's disease affecting bone with aminohydroxypropylidene bisphosphonate (Pamidronate). Quar J Med 79:503, 1991.

33. Beutler E: Gaucher's disease. N Engl J Med 325:1354, 1991.

Sacroiliac Lipoma

Capsule Summary

Frequency of back pain—common
Location of back pain—sacroiliac junction
Quality of back pain—intermittent ache
Symptoms and signs—pain increased with sleeping, point tenderness
Laboratory and x-ray tests—none
Treatment—local injection, surgical excision

PREVALENCE AND PATHOGENESIS

Sacroiliac lipomas are fatty tumors located over the sacroiliac joints. They herniate through weak areas in the overlying fascia and become painful when they are strangulated by the fascia. The pain associated with herniation of these fatty tumors may be severe, may radiate into the buttock and thigh, and may be associated with limitation of flexion of the lumbosacral spine.

The prevalence of sacroiliac lipoma in the general population is unknown. Studies reporting on patients with sacroiliac lipomas suggest that the incidence is relatively high.[1, 2] Approximately 10% to 26% of the population may have these nodules, but the lipomas are symptomatic in only a small fraction of individuals.[3, 4] They become symptomatic most frequently when the patient is in the fifth decade. The male to female ratio is 1:4. Ries in

1939 was the first to describe the presence of sacroiliac lipomas and the clinical syndrome associated with them.[5]

The pathogenesis of sacroiliac lipomas is related to weaknesses in the fascia that runs from the cervical to the lumbosacral spine. The lipoma may herniate through a weakened area where there are deficiencies in fascia fibers or through one of the foramina where the lateral branches of the posterior primary division of the first, second, and third lumbar nerves pass.[6] The three types of herniations are pedunculated, nonpedunculated, and foraminal. With certain motions the fascia strangulates the herniated fatty tumor, compressing its blood supply and nerves, and this results in local pain with possible radiation in the distribution of the cutaneous nerves.

CLINICAL HISTORY

The typical patient is a middle-aged, obese female with unilateral low back pain radiating to the buttock or anterior thigh. Most symptomatic patients will have local pain or pain radiating to the thigh.[7] Patients with pain radiating to the calf or foot without other causes of radicular pain have been reported but are rare.[8] Flexion of the lumbosacral spine increases the pain, as does activity. The pain has an aching quality and occasionally may be bilateral. Compressing the area at night while sleeping may cause severe distress. There are no constitutional symptoms such as fatigue, weight loss, fever, or anorexia associated with the lesion.

PHYSICAL EXAMINATION

Physical examination demonstrates a tender nodule near the dimples in the sacroiliac area. The sacroiliac lipomas are very tender to palpation. Direct pressure on the nodule may recreate pain in the referral pattern of the sclerotome of the affected nerve.[8] Forward flexion causes pain, and that motion can be limited. The nodules may occur singly or in clusters. Neurologic examination, including straight leg raising tests, is normal.

LABORATORY DATA

Laboratory tests, including hematologic, chemical, and immunologic studies, are normal in patients with sacroiliac lipomas. The gross pathologic findings demonstrate rounded cylindric bodies, which measure from 1 to 5 cm in diameter. Microscopically, the lipomas consist of normal adipose tissue with little interposed connective tissue and a fibrous capsule. Nerve fibers are detected in some specimens.[9] Signs of edema and hemorrhage may be seen in some portions of the specimens.[10]

RADIOGRAPHIC EVALUATION

Sacroiliac lipomas are not associated with any radiographic abnormalities. MR may develop to a sufficient degree to identify the presence of these soft tissue tumors. At present, no MR studies have been completed systematically imaging the lumbar soft tissues for the presence of these soft tissue nodules.

DIFFERENTIAL DIAGNOSIS

The diagnosis of sacroiliac lipoma is not made unless physicians are aware of the existence of this entity as a cause of low back pain. Frequently, patients undergo extensive examinations before the correct diagnosis is made. Patients who have a history of pain that is increased by rolling over in bed and can be recreated by palpation of a tender nodule may have sacroiliac lipoma as the cause of their symptoms.

TREATMENT

The initial treatment for sacroiliac lipoma is injection of the nodules with local anesthetic such as xylocaine. These injections frequently produce relief from pain. Patients may notice relief for extended periods of time even from single injections.[1] Pain also may be relieved by dry needling of the lesion. The pathogenesis of pain may be pressure distension of the nodule. Multiple punctures of the nodule relieve this distension, which may be the mechanism of pain relief. Symptoms may increase for a few hours after the procedure. Surgical removal of the painful sacral lipoma is beneficial if injections do not relieve symptoms.[11]

PROGNOSIS

Since patients with sacral lipomas may experience severe pain and limitation of motion of the lumbosacral spine, they frequently undergo extensive evaluations including a variety of radiographic studies that are consistently normal. When no specific abnormality is discovered, these patients are thought to have psychogenic rheumatism and are referred for psychiatric evaluation. Some have had symptoms for as long as 7 years before the correct diagnosis was made.[6] The prognosis is excellent with the correct diagnosis and appropriate therapy. These patients suffer no functional impairment once they respond to therapy.

References

SACROILIAC LIPOMA

1. Singewald ML: Sacroiliac lipomata: an often unrecognized cause of low back pain. Bull Johns Hopkins Hosp 118:492, 1966.
2. Hucherson DC, Gandy JR: Herniation of fascial fat: a cause of low back pain. Am J Surg 76:605, 1948.
3. Copeman WSC, Ackerman WL: Edema or herniation of fat lobules as a cause of lumbar and gluteal "fibrositis." Arch Intern Med 79:22, 1947.
4. Swezey RI: Non-fibrositic lumbar subcutaneous nodules: prevalence and clinical significance. Br J Rheumatol 30:376, 1991.
5. Ries E: Episacroiliac lipoma. Am J Obstet Gynecol 34:490, 1937.
6. Copeman WSC: Fibro-fatty tissue and its relation to certain "rheumatic" syndromes. Br Med J 2:191, 1949.
7. Wollgast GF, Afeman CE: Sacroiliac (episacral) lipomas. Arch Surg 83:147, 1961.
8. Curtis P: In search of the "back mouse." J Fam Prac 36:657, 1993.
9. Hittner VJ: Episacroiliac lipomas. Am J Surg 78:382, 1949.
10. Herz R: Herniation of fascial fat as a cause of low back pain. JAMA 128:921, 1945.
11. Bonner CD, Kasdon SC: Herniation of fat through lumbosacral fascia as a cause of low-back pain. N Engl J Med 251:1102, 1954.

MALIGNANT TUMORS

Multiple Myeloma

Capsule Summary

Frequency of back pain—common
Location of back pain—lumbar spine
Quality of back pain—ache of increasing intensity
Symptoms and signs—generalized fatigue, bone pain, fever
Laboratory and x-ray tests—pancytopenia, hypergammaglobulinemia; diffuse osteolysis without reactive sclerosis on plain roentgenograms
Treatment—chemotherapy for general disease, radiotherapy for cord compression

PREVALENCE AND PATHOGENESIS

Multiple myeloma is a malignant tumor of plasma cells. Plasma cells produce immunoglobulins and antibodies and are located throughout the bone marrow. The multiplication of these cells in the bone marrow is associated with diffuse bone destruction characterized by bone pain, pathologic fractures, and increases in serum calcium. Multiple myeloma is the most common primary malignancy of bone in adults, accounting for 27% of bone tumors examined for biopsy and 45% of all malignant bone tumors.[1, 2] The incidence is 3 cases per 100,000 people in the United States.[3] The patients are usually in an older age group ranging between 50 and 70.[4] Multiple myeloma is rare in a patient younger than age 40.[5] There is a slight increase in the male to female ratio, but the ratio may be increased further for solitary plasmacytomas.[6]

Three physicians, Bence-Jones, Dalrymple, and Macintyre, first identified the bone lesion and urinary protein in the 1840s.[7–9] Von Rustizky in 1873 was the first to call the disease multiple myeloma.[10]

The pathogenesis of this plasma cell tumor is unknown. Viral infections, chronic inflammation, and myeloproliferative diseases have been suggested as possible initiating factors. Although the symptoms of a fracture associated with trauma are frequently the reason for a patient's initial evaluation by a physician, trauma is not a factor in the etiology of multiple myeloma. The lesions tend to occur in the bones with the greatest hematopoietic activity such as the spine, pelvis, ribs, skull, and proximal ends of the femora and humeri. A majority of patients with multiple myeloma have lesions in the axial skeleton. The thoracic spine is involved in 59% of patients, lumbosacral spine in 31%, and cervical spine in 10%. The spine is affected in 30% to 50% of patients with solitary plasmacytomas.[1]

The term *plasmacytoma* is used when one bone is involved by the disease. *Multiple myeloma* denotes the involvement of several bones throughout the skeleton. *Myelomatosis* refers to disseminated disease throughout the hematopoietic system including extraosseous locations. *Extramedullary plasmacytoma* refers to lesions in soft tissues independent of bone.[11]

CLINICAL HISTORY

Pain is the most common initial complaint of patients with multiple myeloma occurring in 75% of patients.[3] Low back pain is the presenting symptom in 35% of patients. The pain is mild, aching, and intermittent at the onset and is aggravated by weightbearing and relieved by bed rest. Pain when lying down is one of the symptoms that should raise the possibility of a spinal tumor, including multiple myeloma.[12] Some patients have radicular symptoms and are diagnosed as having herniated intervertebral discs, sciatica, or arthritis.[13–15] Approximately 20% of patients give a history of insignificant trauma that causes pathologic fractures of vertebral bodies and results in acute, severe localized pain. Paraplegia more often occurs with solitary plasmacytoma than with multiple myeloma.[16] Spinal cord or cauda equina compression also occurs in myeloma patients.[17, 18] Approximately 10% of patients with multiple myeloma may first present with a solitary lesion.[19] Monoclonal antibodies will develop as a sign of progression of isolated plasmacytoma to multiple myeloma.[20] Involvement of the ribs, sternum, and thoracic spine may result in kyphosis and loss in height. In this illness, pain is not confined to the back alone since bone pain may be found in any part of the skeleton and may be secondary to bone marrow expansion or microfractures.[21]

As a consequence of widespread bone destruction, abnormal immunoglobulin production, and infiltration of bone marrow, patients with multiple myeloma develop a broad range of clinical symptoms. Hypercalcemia due to bone destruction is associated with bone weakness, easy fatiguability, anorexia, nausea, vomiting, mental status changes (including coma), and kidney stones. Increased abnormal immunoglobulin concentrations cause progressive renal insufficiency, increased susceptibility to infection, and amyloidosis. Amyloid is a protein that forms from portions of abnormal myeloma immunoglobulins. This protein infiltrates certain structures including bone, muscle, perivascular connective tissue, kidney, and bladder.[22] Primary amyloidosis in the absence of multiple myeloma may infiltrate bone marrow and lead to radiographic changes in the vertebral column that are similar to those of multiple myeloma.[23] Infiltration of bone marrow is associated with anemia, bleeding secondary to a deficiency of platelets, thrombocytopenia, and generalized weakness. Most patients have symptoms for less than 6 months before seeking medical attention. Patients who are subsequently diagnosed with solitary lesions may have had symptoms for several years.

PHYSICAL EXAMINATION

In the early stages of the illness, the physical examination may be unremarkable. As the duration of illness increases and bone marrow infiltration progresses, diffuse bone tenderness, fever, pallor, and purpura become prominent findings on examination. Fever is usually a manifestation of a complicating infection. Fever associated with myeloma alone is not common.[24] Rib cage and spine deformities are common in later stages of the illness. Neurologic examination may demonstrate signs of compression of the spinal cord or nerve roots if vertebral collapse has progressed to a significant degree.[25]

LABORATORY DATA

Laboratory examination may reveal many abnormalities, including normochromic, normocytic anemia; rouleau formation on blood smear; elevated leukocyte count; thrombocytopenia; or positive Coomb's test; and an elevated erythrocyte sedimentation rate. Abnormal serum chemistries include hypercalcemia, hyperuricemia, and elevated creatinine.[26] Impaired coagulation is mediated through inhibitors of clotting factors, clearance of clotting factors, and platelet function abnormalities.[27]

Serum alkaline phosphatase is normal in most patients with multiple myeloma. A normal leukocyte alkaline phosphatase is associated with benign paraproteinemias, but an elevated level does not necessarily indicate a malignant condition.[28] Characteristic serum protein abnormalities occur in the vast majority of patients with multiple myeloma. The total serum protein concentrations are increased secondary to an increase in the globulin fraction. The increase in globulins is due to the presence of abnormal immunoglobulins of the G, A, D, E, or M classes. Immunoglobulins are composed of light and heavy chains. Multiple myeloma, instead of having a multitude of an-

tibodies, has one single antibody composed of a light and a heavy chain, an M-protein. It is produced to the exclusion of others. The balance between light and heavy chains may also be disturbed with excess light chain production resulting in Bence-Jones protein in the urine or excess heavy chain production resulting in heavy chain disease. Serum protein electrophoresis demonstrates the elevation in globulin levels, while quantitative immunoglobulin determination detects the class of immunoglobulin that is present in increased concentration. Serum protein electrophoresis demonstrates a spike in 76% of patients, hypogammaglobulinemia in 9%, and no abnormality in 15%.[4] Urine protein electrophoresis will detect the presence of Bence-Jones proteinuria. Other findings associated with abnormal immunoglobulins include increased serum viscosity, which results in the blockage of blood vessels, and a positive test for rheumatoid factor.

Examination of a bone marrow aspirate and biopsy show characteristic changes of multiple myeloma. Bone marrow aspirate demonstrates increased numbers of plasma cells at levels greater than 30%. Bone marrow biopsy demonstrates diffuse infiltration of bone marrow with plasma cells (Fig. 13–23). Plasma cells may be classified into three histologic grades: well differentiated, moderately differentiated, and poorly differentiated.[29] The well-differentiated plasma cells look much like normal plasma cells. Anaplastic myeloma cells may mimic undifferentiated carcinomas or small cell sarcomas. Differentiating myeloma cells from non-neoplastic plasma cells is difficult. Subtle abnormalities in the size of the nucleus, nucleocytoplasmic disproportion, and the ab-

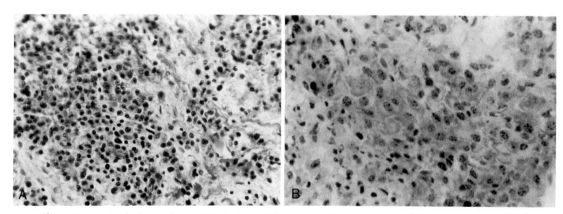

Figure 13–23. Multiple myeloma. Histologic sections of multiple myeloma exhibiting numerous atypical plasma cells. (Courtesy of Arnold Schwartz, M.D.)

sence of inclusions are a few of the many factors that may help to differentiate normal from malignant cells.[3]

Gross pathologic examination of bone shows a soft, gray, friable tumor in bone. The tumor frequently expands beyond the confines of the bone into the soft tissue. In the spine, pathologic fractures are commonly identified.

Bone lesions are frequently associated with myeloma lesions. Most patients have lytic abnormalities associated with unbalanced bone remodeling, leading to reduced bone mass and bone destruction.[30] Patients with sclerotic bone lesions had increased osteoblastic activity in the setting of increased bone resorption. These patients had a lambda subtype IgG myeloma, an immunoglobulin subtype associated with sclerotic myeloma.[31] An early manifestation of myeloma is enhancement of osteoblastic recruitment with increased generation of new osteoclasts that cause increased bone resorption. The early stimulation of osteoblasts results in increased amounts of interleukin 6, a potent myeloma growth factor and a cytokine for the formation of osteoclasts in bone marrow.[32]

RADIOGRAPHIC EVALUATION

The predominant radiographic abnormality of multiple myeloma is osteolysis (Fig. 13–24). Diffuse osteolysis of the axial skeleton resembles osteoporosis.[33] A characteristic finding is the absence of reactive sclerosis surrounding lytic lesions in the spine. Preferential destruction of vertebral bodies with sparing of posterior elements helps in differentiating multiple myeloma from osteolytic metastasis, which affects the vertebral pedicle and body (Fig. 13–25).[34] Paraspinous and extradural extension of tumor is seen in patients with multiple myeloma.

Benign solitary plasmacytoma may occur almost anywhere in the body, including bone and kidney. Bone plasmacytomas are most common in the vertebral column, pelvis, and long bones, in that order of decreasing frequency.[35] Solitary plasmacytomas, when located in the spine, have variable radiographic features. A purely osteolytic area without expansion or an expansile lesion with thickened trabeculae may be observed. An involved vertebral body may fracture and disappear completely, or the lesion may extend across the intervertebral disc to invade an adjacent vertebral body simulating the appearance of an infection.[16] The lesion may have coarse trabecu-

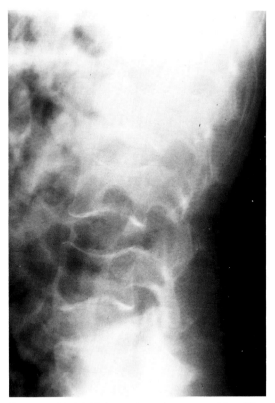

Figure 13–24. Multiple myeloma demonstrated by diffuse osteopenia. Diffuse osteopenia may be the sole radiographic abnormality in a majority of patients with this entity. (Courtesy of Anne Brower, M.D.)

lae with vertical striations simulating vertebral angioma or Paget's disease.[36] Occasionally, osteoblastic lesions have been reported in patients with multiple myeloma and plasmacytoma.[37, 38]

While bone scans are used in the early detection of metastatic lesions, they are not helpful in multiple myeloma because the osteolytic lesions, which lack bone forming (blastic) activity, will not be positive.[39, 40] In the unusual patient with a positive scintiscan, regression of tumor activity may be characterized by the disappearance of scan abnormalities with treatment.[11]

CT may demonstrate vertebral body involvement before plain radiographs. This is due to the fact that radiographs detect abnormalities in bone calcium only after 30% of the calcium is lost.[41] CT is useful in demonstrating the extent of tumor, delineating the soft tissue component of an osseous lesion, or detecting an extramedullary plasmacytoma. CT can be used to detect early bone or extraosseous lesions in areas of the spine that are difficult to image with simple radiographic techniques.[42]

MR detects abnormalities in bone marrow

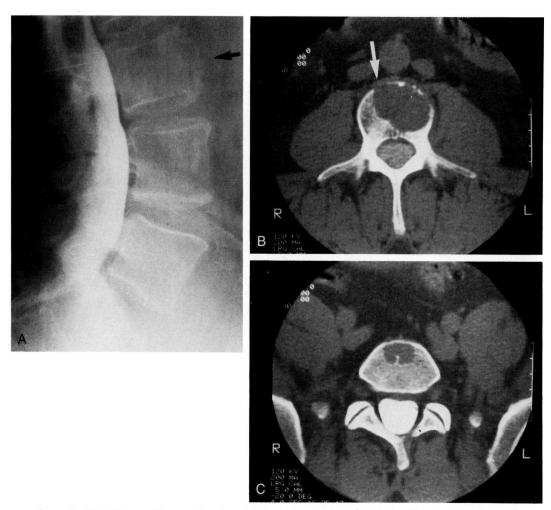

Figure 13–25. A 48-year-old man with a 6-week history of acute-onset back pain with radiation to the pelvis and right thigh associated with left leg weakness. Tenderness was demonstrated over the L3 vertebral body and there was decreased sensation in a left L2 dermatome and decreased strength in the left iliopsoas muscle. *A,* Myelogram revealing an expansile lesion of L3 *(arrow).* The spinal cord is normal. *B,* CT scan of L3 vertebral body demonstrating a sharply marginated hypodense area occupying the greater part of L3 associated with interruption of the anterior cortex *(arrow). C,* CT scan of L5 vertebral body revealing a similar, smaller lesion. A bone biopsy of the L3 vertebral body revealed collections of plasma cells consistent with multiple myeloma. Subsequently, lesions in the thoracic spine were noted and a monoclonal IgG kappa protein was identified. A diagnosis of multiple myeloma was made, and the patient was started on chemotherapy along with radiation therapy to the spine.

that are not readily visualized by other techniques. On T_1- and T_2-weighted images, myeloma will appear as decreased or increased signal intensity, respectively. Alterations in signal may occur with fatty infiltration of marrow. Foci of tumor are better visualized with T_2-weighted images (Fig. 13–26). MR appearance does not correlate with laboratory or bone marrow findings.[43]

DIFFERENTIAL DIAGNOSIS

The diagnosis of multiple myeloma requires the inclusion of clinical, radiographic, and laboratory data along with the presence of abnormal plasma cells on histologic examination. A combination of major and minor criteria for establishing the diagnosis of myeloma has been developed by the Southwest Oncology Group.[44] The major criteria include a plasmacytoma demonstrated on biopsy, bone marrow plasmacytosis with more than a 30% content of plasma cells, and a monoclonal spike of more than 3.5 gm for IgG, 2.0 gm per 100 ml for IgA, or 1.0 gm per 24 hours for urinary light chains. Minor criteria include bone marrow plasmacytosis, a monoclonal spike with small globulin concentrations, a lytic bone le-

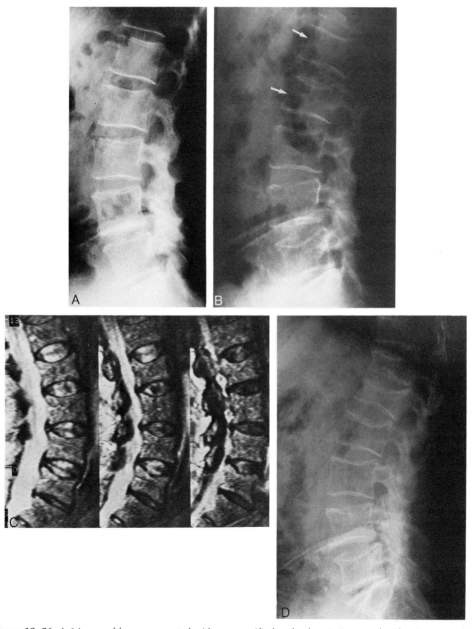

Figure 13–26. A 64-year-old man presented with nonspecific low back pain increased with spine extension. *A,* Lateral plain roentgenogram on 9/30/88 revealed disc degeneration at the L5-S1 intervertebral space. *B,* The pain increased over the ensuing 8 weeks. Lateral plain roentgenogram on 12/5/88 revealed a marked increase in generalized osteopenia with evidence of vertebral fractures (white arrows). *C,* MR scan, T_2-weighted image, of the lumbar spine revealed increased signal found diffusely in the vertebral bone marrow. A diagnosis of multiple myeloma was confirmed, and the patient received prednisone and melphalan. *D,* Lateral plain roentgenogram on 12/12/90 revealed increased generalized osteopenia with additional compression fractures. The patient's myeloma was in remission, and he had little back pain. (From Borenstein DG: Low back pain. In Klippel J, Dieppe P (eds): Rheumatology. St. Louis, CV Mosby, 1994. Sec 5, 4.10 and 4.16.)

sion, and serum immunoglobulin values less than 50 mg for IgM, 100 mg for IgA, and 600 mg per 100 ml for IgG. The presence of characteristic abnormalities, Bence-Jones protein and M-protein, on electrophoresis makes the diagnosis an easy one, but the diagnosis is more difficult in the patient who presents with diffuse osteoporosis and no detectable myeloma protein.[45] Low back pain in the middle-aged to elderly patient with osteoporosis on radiographs must be evaluated thoroughly for possible myeloma.[24]

Solitary plasmacytoma is also a difficult entity to diagnose. The diagnosis may be assumed if the character of the lesion is established by biopsy, if a bone survey is negative, if a bone marrow specimen is free of plasma cells, if hypergammaglobulinemia and Bence-Jones proteinuria are absent, and if the patient has been followed closely for years.

The list of other diseases that must be considered in the differential diagnosis of multiple myeloma is quite broad. Metastatic tumors and malignant lymphoma must be considered. Focal osteolysis on roentgenogram may be associated with a hemangioma. Infections, pyogenic and tuberculous, are associated with similar roentgenographic findings. Hyperparathyroidism may be associated with generalized bone lesions and hypercalcemia. Appropriate evaluation of blood tests and biopsy material should allow the treating physician the information to make the appropriate diagnosis.

A differential diagnosis of monoclonal gammopathy must also be considered in the patient with elevated globulins.[46] Some of the gammopathies have elevated globulin levels but do not cause bone lesions to the same degree as multiple myeloma. Examples of these gammopathies include benign monoclonal gammopathy, Waldenstrom's macroglobulinemia, IgE myeloma, and alpha heavy chain disease.[27]

TREATMENT

Clinically active multiple myeloma usually requires systemic therapy with melphalan and prednisone over an extended course.[47] Approximately 70% of patients respond to this therapy and have a reduction in bone destruction and pain, decreased concentration of abnormal proteins, and a normalization of hematocrit, urea nitrogen, creatinine, and calcium. Some patients have responded well to high-dose dexamethasone alone without the toxicities associated with other therapies.[48] Patients with more aggressive disease may benefit

by the M-2 drug program, combining vincristine, melphalan, cyclophosphamide, prednisone, and BCNU.[49] Other treatments include high-dose melphalan, autologous bone marrow transplantation, interferon, and cytokines.[50] In patients with cord compression secondary to multiple myeloma, decompressing laminectomy and/or local radiotherapy are indicated.[51] Radiotherapy is also indicated for a solitary plasmacytoma.

Bisphosphonates inhibit calcium release from bone and prevent bone resorption through inhibition of osteoclastic activity. These drugs are most effective in patients with idiopathic osteoporosis. Daily etidronate is not effective in reversing the osteopenia associated with myeloma.[52]

PROGNOSIS

The usual course of multiple myeloma is one of gradual progression. Therapy may have effects on clinical symptoms and amounts of myeloma protein, but the average survival remains about 5 years. Patients with D and G myeloma have poorer prognoses than A myeloma patients.[53, 54] Many patients may have more extensive disease than is clinically apparent. Over 50% of patients may have compression fractures at autopsy.[55] In addition, the effects of myeloma may extend beyond the involvement of bone alone. Even in the absence of a marrow packed with plasma cells, erythropoiesis may be depressed by an effect of the disease on progenitor cells.[56] Male patients with plasmacytosis, hypoalbuminemia, elevated alkaline phosphatase, hyperuricemia, or renal insufficiency are predictors of poor outcome at 2 years.[57] In a study of 130 Japanese patients, only 9 (6.9%) patients were alive at 10 years. Prognostic factors for survival included a younger age at diagnosis, low tumor mass, chemotherapy with cyclophosphamide, disappearance of myeloma protein, and a positive response to retreatment.[58]

Patients with solitary plasmacytomas have a better prognosis than those patients who initially have multiple lesions.[16] However, it is important to remember that some patients with solitary lesions may go on to develop disseminated disease, in some cases 20 years or more after their initial diagnosis.[59]

References

MULTIPLE MYELOMA

1. Mirra JM: Bone Tumors: Diagnosis and Treatment. Philadelphia: JB Lippincott Co, 1980, pp 398–406.

2. Dahlin DC, Unni KK: Bone Tumors: General Aspects and Data on 8,542 Cases, 4th ed. Springfield, Illinois: Charles C Thomas, 1986, pp 193–207.

3. Huvos AG: Bone Tumors: Diagnosis, Treatment and Prognosis, 2nd ed. Philadelphia: WB Saunders, 1991, pp 653–676.

4. Kyle RA: Multiple myeloma: review of 869 cases. Mayo Clin Proc 50:29, 1975.

5. Hewell GM, Alexanian R: Multiple myeloma in young persons. Ann Intern Med 84:441, 1976.

6. Todd IDH: Treatment of solitary plasmacytoma. Clin Radiol 16:395, 1965.

7. Bence-Jones H: On a new substance occurring in the urine of a patient with mollities ossium. Philos Trans R Soc Lond (Biol) 1:55, 1848.

8. Dalrymple J: On the microscopical character of mollities ossium. Dublin Q J Med Sci 2:85, 1846.

9. Macintyre W: Case of mollities and fragilitas ossium accompanied with urine strongly charged with animal matter. Med Chir Soc Trans 33:211, 1850.

10. Von Rustizky J: Multiples myelom. Dtsch Z Chir 3:162, 1873.

11. Bataille R, Chevalier J, Rossi M, Sany J: Bone scintigraphy in plasma cell myeloma. A prospective study of 70 patients. Radiology 145:801, 1982.

12. Nicholas JJ, Christy WC: Spinal pain made worse by recumbency: a clue to spinal cord tumors. Arch Phys Med Rehabil 67:598, 1986.

13. Lichtenstein L, Jaffee HL: Multiple myeloma: a survey based on 35 cases, 18 of which came to autopsy. Arch Pathol Lab Med 44:207, 1947.

14. Bayrd ED, Heck FJ: Multiple myeloma: a review of 83 proven cases. JAMA 133:147, 1947.

15. Lehmann O: Problems of pathological fractures. Bull Hosp Joint Dis 12:90, 1951.

16. Valderrama JAF, Bullough PG: Solitary myeloma of the spine. J Bone Joint Surg 50B:82, 1968.

17. Jacobs P, King HS, Le Roux I, Handler L: Extradural spinal myeloma and emergency neurosurgery. S Afr Med J 77:316, 1990.

18. Sinoff CL: Spinal cord compression due to myeloma. S Afr Med J 78:434, 1990.

19. Osserman EF: Plasma-cell myeloma. II. Clinical aspects. N Engl J Med 261:952, 1959.

20. Otto S, Vegh Z, Hindy I, Peter I: Multiple myeloma arising from solitary plasmacytoma of bone. Oncology 47:84, 1990.

21. Charkes ND, Durant J, Barry WE: Bone pain in multiple myeloma: studies with radioactive 87m Sr. Arch Intern Med 130:53, 1972.

22. Klein LA: Case Record 7–1986. N Engl J Med 314:500, 1986.

23. Axelsson U, Hallen A, Rausing A: Amyloidosis of bone: Report of two cases. J Bone Joint Surg 52B:717, 1970.

24. Duffy TP: The many pitfalls in the diagnosis of myeloma. N Engl J Med 326:394, 1992.

25. Davison C, Balser BH: Myeloma and its neural complications. Arch Surg 35:913, 1937.

26. Paredes JM, Mitchell BS: Multiple myeloma: current concepts in diagnosis and management. Med Clin North Am 64:729, 1980.

27. Kempin S, Sundaresan N: Disorders of the spine related to plasma cell dyscrasias. In Sundaresan N, Schmidek HH, Schiller AL, Rosenthal DI (eds). Tumors of the Spine: Diagnosis and Clinical Management. Philadelphia: WB Saunders, 1990, pp 214–225.

28. Majumdar G, Hunt M, Singh AK: Use of leukocyte alkaline phosphatase (LAP) score in differentiating malignant from benign paraproteinaemias. J Clin Pathol 44:606, 1991.

29. Bayrd ED: The bone marrow on sternal aspiration in multiple myeloma. Blood 3:987, 1948.

30. Bataille R, Chappard D, Marcelli C, et al.: Mechanisms of bone destruction in multiple myeloma: the importance of an unbalanced process in determining the severity of lytic bone disease. J Clin Oncol 7:1909, 1989.

31. Bataille R, Chappard D, Marcelli C, et al.: Osteoblast stimulation in multiple myeloma lacking lytic bone lesions. Br J Haematol 76:484, 1990.

32. Bataille R, Chappard D, Marcelli C, et al.: Recruitment of new osteoblasts and osteoclasts is the earliest critical event in the pathogensis of human multiple myeloma. J Clin Invest 88:62, 1991.

33. Carson CP, Ackerman LV, Maltby JD: Plasma cell myeloma: A clinical, pathologic and roentgenologic review of 90 cases. Am J Clin Pathol 25:849, 1955.

34. Jacobsen HG, Poppel MH, Shapiro JH, Grossberger S: The vertebral pedicle sign: a roentgen finding to differentiate metastatic carcinoma from multiple myeloma. AJR 80:817, 1958.

35. Eichner ER: The plasma cell dyscrasias: diverse presentations, pathophysiology and management. Postgrad Med 67:44, 1980.

36. Loftus CM, Micheisen CB, Rapoport F, Antunes JL: Management of plasmacytomas of the spine. Neurosurgery 13:30, 1983.

37. Brown TS, Paterson CR: Osteosclerosis in myeloma. J Bone Joint Surg 55B:621, 1973.

38. Roberts M, Rianudo PA, Vilinskas J, Owens G: Solitary sclerosing plasma-cell myeloma of the spine: case report. J Neurosurg 40:125, 1974.

39. Wooltenden JM, Pitt MJ, Durie BGM, Moon TE: Comparison of bone scintography and radiography in multiple myeloma. Radiology 134:723, 1980.

40. Wahner HW, Kyle RA, Beabout JW: Scintigraphic evaluation of the skeleton in multiple myeloma. Mayo Clin Proc 55:739, 1980.

41. Helms CA, Genant HK: Computed tomography in the early detection of skeletal involvement with multiple myeloma. JAMA 248:2886, 1982.

42. Solomon A, Rahamani R, Seligsohn U, Ben-Artzi F: Multiple myeloma: early vertebral involvement assessed by computerized tomography. Skel Radiol 11:258, 1984.

43. Libshitz HI, Malthouse SR, Cunningham D, et al.: Multiple myeloma: appearance at MR imaging. Radiology 182:833, 1992.

44. Durie BGM, Salmon SE: A clinical staging system for multiple myeloma: correlation of measured myeloma cell mass with presenting clinical features response to treatment and survival. Cancer 36:842, 1975.

45. Arend WP, Adamson JW: Nonsecretory myeloma: immunoflourescent demonstration of paraprotein within bone marrow plasma cells. Cancer 33:721, 1974.

46. Gandara DR, Mackenzie MR: Differential diagnosis of monoclonal gammopathy. Med Clin North Am 72:1155, 1988.

47. Costa G, Engle RL Jr, Schilling A, et al.: Melphalan and prednisone—an effective combination for the treatment of multiple myeloma. Am J Med 54:589, 1973.

48. Alexanian R, Dimopoulos MA, Delasalle, Barlogie B: Primary dexamethasone treatment of multiple myeloma. Blood 80:887, 1992.

49. Case DC Jr, Lee BJ III, Clarkson BD: Improved survival

times in multiple myeloma treated with melphalan, prednisone, cyclophosphamide, vincristine and BCNU–M-2 protocol. Am J Med 63:897, 1977.

50. Camba L, Durie BGM: Multiple myeloma: new treatment options. Drugs 44:170, 1992.

51. Gilbert RW, Kim JH, Posner JB: Epidural spinal cord compression from metastatic tumor: diagnosis and treatment. Ann Neurol 3:40, 1978.

52. Belch AR, Bergsagel DE, Wilson K, et al.: Effect of daily etidronate on the osteolysis of multiple myeloma. J Clin Oncol 9:1397, 1991.

53. Gompels BM, Votaw ML, Martel W: Correlation of radiological manifestations of multiple myeloma with immunoglobulin abnormalities and prognosis. Radiology 104:509, 1972.

54. Pruzanski W, Rother I: IgD plasma cell neoplasia: clinical manifestations and characteristic features. Can Med Assoc J 102:1061, 1970.

55. Kapadia SB: Multiple myeloma: a cliniopathologic study of 62 consecutively autopsied cases. Medicine 59:380, 1980.

56. Oken MM: Multiple myeloma: symposium on hematology and hematologic malignancies. Med Clin North Am 68:757, 1984.

57. Cherng NC, Asal NR, Kuebler JP, et al.: Prognostic factors in multiple myeloma. Cancer 67:3150, 1991.

58. Murakami H, Nemoto K, Miyawaki S, et al.: Ten-year survivors with multiple myeloma. J Intern Med 231:129, 1992.

59. Woodruff RK, Malpas JS, White FE: Solitary plasmacytoma II. Solitary plasmacytoma of bone. Cancer 43:2344, 1979.

Chondrosarcoma

Capsule Summary

Frequency of back pain—uncommon

Location of back pain—lumbar spine or sacrum

Quality of back pain—mild ache

Symptoms and signs—painless mass

Laboratory and x-ray tests—expansile, calcified mass on plain roentgenograms

Treatment—en-bloc resection

PREVALENCE AND PATHOGENESIS

Chondrosarcoma is a malignant tumor that forms cartilaginous tissue. It is frequently located in the pelvis, sacrum, or lumbar spine. Since the tumor has extremely slow growth and lesions are usually painless, chondrosarcoma of the pelvis and spine may be present for a long period of time before it is discovered. Chondrosarcoma makes up 11% to 22% of primary bone tumors examined by biopsy.[1, 2] Among malignant tumors, chondrosarcoma is the third most common neoplasm, following multiple myeloma and osteogenic sarcoma. The usual age of onset is between 40 and 60 years of age, and the ratio of men to women is 3:2.[3]

Chondrosarcoma has been known by many different names. These have included chondroblastic sarcoma, malignant chondroblastoma, myxoid chondrosarcoma, and clear cell chondrosarcoma, among others.

The pathogenesis of chondrosarcoma is unknown. Primary chondrosarcomas arise de novo from previously normal bone, while secondary chondrosarcomas develop from other cartilaginous tumors, such as an osteochondroma or enchondroma. Chondrosarcoma may be induced by irradiation, accounting for 9% of radiation-induced bone sarcoma.[4] It also develops in a small number of patients with Paget's disease, fibrous dysplasia, or Maffucci's syndrome (enchondromas with soft tissue hemangiomas).[5–7]

Approximately 9% of patients with chondrosarcoma have lesions involving the spine. A review of 553 chondrosarcoma patients documented spinal involvement in 6% of individuals.[8] The lumbosacral spine is the site of the tumor in 50% of patients, with 32% in the thoracic spine and 18% in the cervical spine.

CLINICAL HISTORY

Chondrosarcoma may be symptomless or may present with only mild discomfort and palpable swelling. Tumors in the pelvis are detected when they are palpable through the abdominal wall or cause nerve compression with radicular pain, mimicking symptoms of a herniated disc.[1, 9, 10] Pain, when it occurs, is strongly suggestive of an actively growing tumor. This is particularly important in a patient who has had an osteochondroma for decades that suddenly becomes painful. This is a very slow-growing tumor, so a history of symptoms for several years before the patient seeks medical evaluation is usual. Patients commonly complain of nocturnal pain with exacerbation on recumbency.[11, 12] Almost 50% of patients have neurologic symptoms at the time of diagnosis. With increased tumor growth, the pain becomes more severe and persistent.[13]

PHYSICAL EXAMINATION

Physical examination may demonstrate a painless tumor mass or one that is mildly painful on palpation. Range of motion of the spine is decreased secondary to pain and muscle spasm. Rectal examination may be helpful in detecting a mass originating in the pelvis or sacrum. Neurologic examination may be abnormal if neural elements are compressed by the tumor. With progression of compression, increasing weakness is noted. Lesions in the lumbar spine produce lower motor neuron weakness with flaccidity of muscles and loss of reflexes. Corresponding sensory deficits also are present.

LABORATORY DATA

Laboratory findings may not be abnormal until late in the course of the tumor. Abnormalities may correlate with tumor size and extent of metastasis. Useful data to obtain include blood counts, serum chemistries, and sedimentation rates. As many as 75% of patients with chondrosarcomas demonstrate an abnormal glucose tolerance curve and high insulin levels. Insulin and insulin growth factor are documented stimulators of cartilage metabolism.[11] The relationship of insulin to the development of abnormal cartilage growth is unknown.[11]

Gross pathologic inspection of chondrosarcomas reveal a pearly, translucent tissue that is lobulated. Areas of calcification within the lesions are represented by yellow-white areas of speckling. The extent and exact boundaries of the lesion are difficult to identify.[14] More reactive new bone is seen with slow-growing tumors than with high-grade anaplastic chondrosarcomas.[15] Peripheral chondrosarcomas may grow to very large sizes, particularly when they are situated in the pelvis.[16]

The microscopic appearance of chondrosarcoma is graded by the degree of abnormality in the nuclei of the cells. Grade 1 is the most benign form of chondrosarcoma and does not have any associated cellular atypia. Some lesions have double nuclei and abundant hyalin matrix. Microscopically, a grade 1 chondrosarcoma differs only slightly from a benign enchondroma. The malignant lesion is more cellular with larger cells that are binucleate. These changes may be present in only parts of the tumor necessitating review of many sections of a biopsy specimen to confirm the diagnosis (Fig. 13–27).[17] Grades 2 and 3 are increasingly malignant and are associated with higher degrees of cellularity, nuclear size, and mitoses (Fig. 13–28).[18] Grade 2 lesions have increased atypia, are more densely cellular, have multiple nuclei and foci of necrosis. Grade 3 lesions have marked atypia, mitotic figures, multinucleate cells, little matrix, and numerous areas of necrosis. In a study of 152 pelvic chondrosarcomas, 56 were Grade 1, 53 were Grade 2, and 43 were Grade 3.[1] Rare types of chondrosarcomas include clear cell, mesenchymal (characterized by a calcified soft tissue mass), myxoid, and periosteal. Dedifferentiation refers to the appearance of a more anaplastic connective tissue tumor in a Grade 1 chondrosarcoma.[19]

RADIOGRAPHIC EVALUATION

The characteristic radiographic findings of chondrosarcoma include a well-defined lesion with expansile contours (Fig. 13–29). The interior of the lesion may demonstrate lobular or fluffy calcification with scalloping of the interior cortex of bone. Periosteal and endosteal reactive bone formation leads to a thickened cortex of bone, which is typical of a slow-growing tumor.[20] Cortical destruction and soft tissue invasion are indicative of more aggressive lesions. In the spine, the vertebral body or pos-

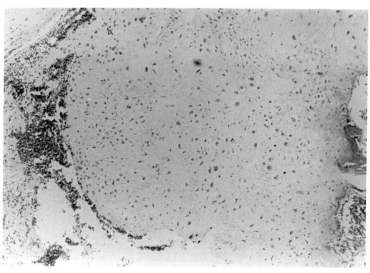

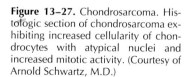

Figure 13–27. Chondrosarcoma. Histologic section of chondrosarcoma exhibiting increased cellularity of chondrocytes with atypical nuclei and increased mitotic activity. (Courtesy of Arnold Schwartz, M.D.)

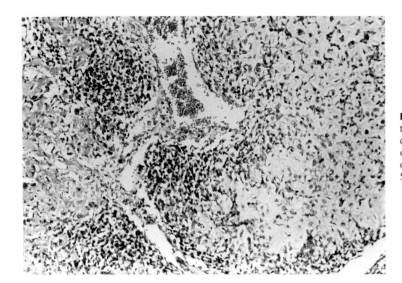

Figure 13–28. Chondrosarcoma. Histologic section of a high-grade chondrosarcoma with marked atypia, with clumps of chondroid matrix in a disorganized pattern. (Courtesy of Arnold Schwartz, M.D.)

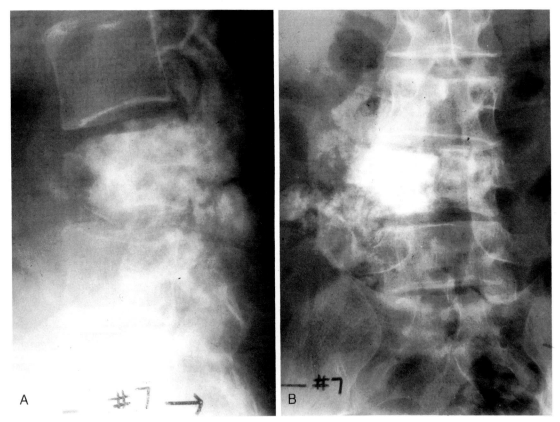

Figure 13–29. Chondrosarcoma. Lateral *(A)* and anterior *(B)* views of a vertebral body with soft tissue extension of the tumor associated with disorganized chondroid matrix calcification. Lateral view shows relative sparing of the disc spaces. (Courtesy of Anne Brower, M.D.)

terior elements may be the site of origin. Plain radiographs are useful in detecting tumors that have calcified. However, soft tissue extension may not be appreciated on these radiographs. A chondrosarcoma may develop in the cartilagenous cap of an osteochondroma. Malignancy should be suspected if the cap of the benign lesion becomes thicker than 1 cm, especially after skeletal maturity, and has the appearance of irregular calcification.[19] Plain roentgenograms are the most effective means for establishing the diagnosis of a cartilageous tumor. This technique detects calcifications, ossifications, and periosteal reaction more readily than CT or MR.[19]

For the evaluation of extraosseous extension of a tumor, CT and MR are essential. Both CT and MR can determine the presence or absence of soft tissue invasion by the tumor. CT depicts calcification in tumor matrix and cortical destruction that may be missed on MR.[17] Recent studies with gadolinium contrast-enhanced MR has detected scalloped margins and curvilinear septa of chondrosarcomas that correspond to fibrovascular bundles surrounding hyaline cartilage lobules.[21] Neither CT or MR are specific enough to establish a precise diagnosis before biopsy of the lesion. Particularly with MR, benign and malignant chondrogenic lesions have similar MR characteristics that do not allow for accurate differentiation of tumors.[27]

Arteriography may be useful in determining the extent of extraosseous involvement associated with a chondrosarcoma, and defining the major feeding blood vessels to the tumor.[22] Bone scintigraphy is helpful in detecting remote skeletal lesions and local intraosseous metastases.[17]

DIFFERENTIAL DIAGNOSIS

The diagnosis of Grade 1 chondrosarcoma must be based on clinical, radiographic, and pathologic findings. For the histopathologist, the chondrosarcoma is the most difficult of the malignant bone tumors to diagnose. The histologic appearance of a low-grade chondrosarcoma may be similar to that of a cellular enchondroma, a benign lesion. Malignant tumors with similar histologic appearances may have different aggressive properties. The findings of pain, rapid growth, cortical destruction, soft tissue extension, and anaplastic cells on biopsy are characteristic of higher-grade, more malignant chondrosarcoma.[3]

A wide range of benign and malignant processes may mimic the characteristics of chon-

drosarcoma. Those processes that may cause lesions of the lumbar spine include giant cell tumor, chordoma, and osteogenic sarcoma. Careful attention to the clinical symptoms of the patient along with a thorough review of biopsy material should give the pathologist adequate information to make the appropriate diagnosis.

TREATMENT

Surgery is the treatment of choice for chondrosarcoma. En-bloc resection of the tumor with a margin of normal tissue so that malignant cells are not implanted in the surgical wound offers the best chance of long-term survival. The 5-year survival rates for Grades 1, 2, and 3 pelvic chondrosarcoma after excisional surgery were 47%, 38%, and 15%, respectively.[9] Tumors that are partially resected frequently recur with increased cytologic malignancy.[23] Chondrosarcomas are radioresistant, and radiotherapy is reserved for tumors that are inaccessible to excision. Chemotherapy may play an adjunctive role in these difficult situations. A combination of surgical removal, radiation, and chemotherapy has been associated with prolonged survival.[24]

PROGNOSIS

The patients with chondrosarcoma who present with pain frequently have more malignant tumors.[25] Those with low-grade, well-differentiated chondrosarcoma have a longer survival rate and longer interval between treatment and recurrence than those with higher-grade tumors. These facts hold true for chondrosarcoma of the pelvis, spine, and sacrum. Chondrosarcoma with a low degree of malignancy grows slowly, recurs locally, and metastasizes late. High-grade tumors grow rapidly and metastasize early. The patients with the best outcome are those with low-grade tumors and successful en-bloc excision. Patients without en-bloc excision have progression of disease and are more likely to die from their tumor. In one study, 50% of patients with contaminated marginal excisions died after a local recurrence.[8] Patients with high-grade pelvic chondrosarcomas have a poor outcome, with a 5-year survival rate of only 20%.[26]

References

CHONDROSARCOMA

1. Huvos AG: Bone Tumors: Diagnosis, Treatment and Prognosis, 2nd ed. Philadelphia: WB Saunders, 1991, pp 343–381.

2. Dahlin DC, Unni KK: Bone Tumors: General Aspects and Data on 8,542 Cases, 4th ed. Springfield, Illinois: Charles C Thomas, 1986, pp 227–259.

3. Mirra JM: Bone Tumors: Diagnosis and Treatment. Philadelphia: JB Lippincott Co, 1980, pp 178–218.

4. Fitzwater JE, Caboud HE, Farr GH: Irradiation-induced chondrosarcoma: a case report. J Bone Joint Surg 58A:1037, 1976.

5. Feintuch TA: Chondrosarcoma arising in a cartilagenous area of previously irradiated fibrious dysplasia. Cancer 31:877, 1973.

6. Lewis RJ, Ketcham AS: Maffucci's syndrome: functional and neoplastic significance—case report and review of the literature. J Bone Joint Surg 55A:1465, 1973.

7. Thomson AD, Turner-Warwick RT: Skeletal sarcomata and giant cell tumor. J Bone Joint Surg 37B:266, 1955.

8. Shives TC, McLeod RA, Unni KK, Schray MF: Chondrosarcoma of the spine. J Bone J Surg 71A:1158, 1989.

9. Marcove RC, Mike V, Hutter RVP, et al.: Chondrosarcoma of the pelvis and upper end of the femur: an analysis of factors influencing survival time in 113 cases. J Bone Joint Surg 54A:561, 1972.

10. Smith FW, Nandi SC, Mills K: Spinal chondrosarcoma demonstrated by Tc-99m-MDP bone scan. Clin Nucl Med 7:111, 1982.

11. Cammisa FP Jr, Glasser DB, Lane JM: Chondrosarcoma of the spine: Memorial Sloan-Kettering Cancer Center experience. In: Sundaresan N, Schmidek, Schiller AL, Rosenthal DI (eds): Tumors of the Spine: Diagnosis and Clinical Management. Philadelphia: WB Saunders, 1990, pp 149–154.

12. Nicholas JJ, Christy WC: Spinal pain made worse by recumbency: a clue to spinal cord tumors. Arch Phys Med Rehabil 67:598, 1986.

13. Sim FH, Frassica FJ, Wold LE, McLeod RA: Chondrosarcoma of the spine: Mayo Clinic experience. In: Sundaresan N, Schmidek HH, Schiller AL, Rosenthal DI (eds): Tumors of the Spine: Diagnosis and Clinical Management. Philadelphia: WB Saunders, 1990, pp 155–162.

14. Goldenbeg RR: Chondrosarcoma. Bull Hosp Joint Dis 25:30, 1964.

15. Gilmer WS Jr, Kilgore W, Smith H: Central cartilage tumors of bone. Clin Orthop 26:81, 1963.

16. Norman A, Sissons HA: Radiographic hallmarks of peripheral chondrosarcoma. Radiology 151:589, 1984.

17. Greenspan A: Tumors of cartilage origin. Orthop Clin North Am 20:347, 1989.

18. Lichtenstein L, Jaffe HL: Chondrosarcoma of bone. Am J Pathol 19:553, 1943.

19. Ghelman B: Radiology of bone tumors. Orthop Clin North Am 20:287, 1989.

20. Barnes R, Catto M: Chondrosarcoma of bone. J Bone Joint Surg 48B:729, 1966.

21. Aoki J, Sone S, Fujioka F, et al.: MR of enchindroma and chondrosarcoma: rings and arcs of Gd-DTPA enhancement. J Comput Assist Tomogr 15:1011, 1991.

22. Kenney PJ, Gilola LA, Murphy WA: The use of computed tomography to distinguish osteochondroma and chondrosarcoma. Radiology 139:129, 1981.

23. Dahlin DC, Henderson ED: Chondrosarcoma: a surgical and pathological problem—review of 212 cases. J Bone Joint Surg 38B:1025, 1956.

24. Di Lorenzo N, Palatinsky E, Artico M, Palma L: Dural mesenchymal chondrosarcoma of the lumbar spine: case report. Surg Neurol 31:470, 1989.

25. Kaufman JH, Douglass HO Jr, Blake W, et al.: The importance of initial presentation and treatment upon the survival of patients with chondrosarcoma. Surg Gynecol Obstet 145:357, 1977.

26. Henderson ED, Dahlin DC: Chondrosarcoma of bone: a study of 280 cases. J Bone Joint Surg 45A:1450, 1963.

27. Petterson H, Sloane RM, Spanier S, et al.: Primary musculoskeletal tumors: Examination with MR imaging compared with conventional modalities. Radiology 164:237, 1987.

Chordoma

Capsule Summary

Frequency of back pain—common

Location of back pain—lumbar spine and sacrum

Quality of back pain—ache

Symptoms and signs—painless mass

Laboratory and x-ray tests—anemia, vertebral osteolysis with calcific soft tissue mass on plain roentgenograms

Treatment—en-bloc resection, radiotherapy

PREVALENCE AND PATHOGENESIS

Chordoma is a malignant tumor that originates from the remnants of embryonic tissue, the notochord. The notochord is the structure that develops into a portion of the vertebral bodies of the spine in the embryo. Chordomas are located exclusively in the axial skeleton. These tumors are slow-growing and may be present for an extended period of time before symptoms secondary to the compression of vital structures bring the patient to a physician.

Chordomas account for 3% of primary bone tumors.[1, 2] The tumors usually become evident between the ages of 40 and 70, and the tumor is rarely reported in patients 30 years of age or younger. The ratio of men to women with sacrococcygeal chordomas is 3:1, while the ratio is 1:1 for chordomas in other locations in the spine.[3] A Mayo Clinic study of 40 patients with chordomas, exclusive of the sacrum, reported the ratio of men to women to be 2:1.[4] A study of 88 chordoma patients, including those with sacral tumors, had a similar 2:1 ratio of men to women.[5] The mean age of sacral tumor patients was 56, while 47 was the mean age of those with tumors in the mobile spine.

Virchow in 1857 was the first to suggest the persistence of cells from the notochord in skeletal structures. Horwitz in 1941 proposed that chordomas arise from abnormal chordal remnants in vertebral bones.[6]

The etiology of the factors that initiate the regrowth of notochordal vestigial cells in the spine is unknown although trauma has been suggested as a possible initiating factor.[7] At Memorial Hospital in New York, 15% of patients with sacrococcygeal chordoma gave a history of previous trauma to the low back of a degree significant enough to require medical attention. The frequency of a history of trauma to the lower back requiring medical evaluation in patients with sacral chordoma may be as high as 50%.[8] Whether trauma is a causative factor or a chance event in the pathogenesis of the lesion remains conjectural at this time.

All chordomas are located in the axial skeleton, ranging from the spheno-occipital area in the skull to the tip of the coccyx. The most common location for chordoma is the sacrum, which is the site of 50% of the lesions. The skull is the location for 38% of the tumors. The cervical, lumbar, and thoracic spine are unusual locations for this neoplasm, accounting for 6%, 4%, and 2% of lesions, respectively.[8] Occasionally, chordomas may be present in other areas of the spine, such as the transverse process, and extraosseous locations, including the epidural space.[9–11]

CLINICAL HISTORY

The symptoms are dependent on the location and extent of the tumor. Patients with sacrococcygeal chordoma present with nondescript lower back pain. The pain may be characterized as dull or sharp and intermittent or constant and is localized in the sacrum. It may be of long duration, since the patient may not have thought it to be a significant problem.[12] Some patients present with severe constipation, urinary frequency or hesitancy, dysuria, incontinence, or muscular weakness.[12] These symptoms are secondary to direct pressure on pelvic structures or compression of neural elements. Patients with chordomas of the lumbar spine may experience pain in the hip, knee, groin, or sacroiliac region. This pattern of referred pain to the lower extremities may be confusing and may delay the discovery of the true location of the spinal tumor. Pain is not relieved by lying down and night pains are characteristic symptoms.[9]

PHYSICAL EXAMINATION

The rectal and neurologic examinations are helpful in detecting the presence of chordomas in the sacrum and spine. Chordomas of the sacrum extend anteriorly into the pelvis, and the presacral extension of a chordoma is detected on rectal examination. The tumor is a firm, roundish mass that is palpable through the posterior wall of the rectum. The examining finger glides easily over the tumor since the rectal mucosa and muscularis are rarely affected by the tumor. Neurologic examination may demonstrate flaccidity, while lesions higher in the axial skeleton are associated with muscle spasticity.

LABORATORY DATA

Laboratory findings may be unremarkable early in the course of this tumor. Abnormalities in hematologic and chemical parameters may appear late, after the tumor has grown extensively or has metastasized.

Gross examination of the tumor reveals a soft, lobulated, grayish mass that is usually well encapsulated except in the region of bony invasion. Sacral chordomas have a presacral extension that is covered by periosteum. In the vertebral column, it originates in the vertebral body and spreads either along the posterior longitudinal ligament or through the intervertebral disc.

Histologically, chordomas are characterized by cells of notochordal origin, physaliphorous cells (Fig. 13–30). These cells contain a large, clear area of cytoplasm with an eccentric, flattened nucleus and form columns that are interspersed in fibrous tissue.[13] The tumor is also characterized by the production of large amounts of mucin, and this histologic appearance bears a close resemblance to that of an adenocarcinoma. The nuclear size of tumor cells may vary greatly. Mitotic figures are rare. The tumor may show a wide range in its histologic appearance, including physaliphorous cells along with cells in arrangements that mimic spindle cell sarcomas or epithlial tumors.[14] The differentiation of chordomas from cartilage tumors and adenocarcinomas may be made by using special stain. Chordomas are positive for keratin and S-100 protein, while cartilage tumors are keratin negative and adenocarcinomas are S-100 negative.[5] Chordomas that contain chondroid components are usually limited to the sphenooccipital region of the spine. However, chondroid chordomas of the lumbosacral region have been reported. The distinction of conventional from chondroid chordomas is important since the later have a longer survival.[15]

RADIOGRAPHIC EVALUATION

Sacrococcygeal and vertebral chordomas produce lytic bone destruction with calcific foci and a soft tissue mass (Fig. 13–31).[16] The

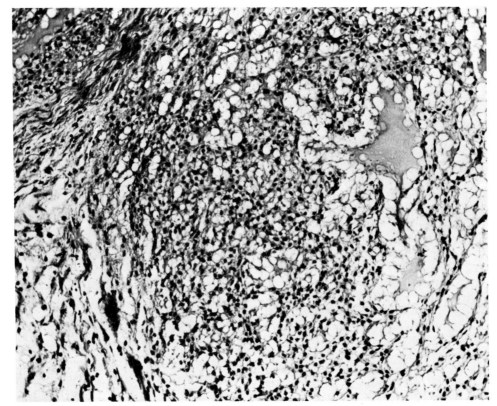

Figure 13–30. Chordoma. Histologic view of chordoma showing mucin-producing physaliphorous cells. The lesion must be differentiated from chondrosarcoma and metastatic carcinoma. (From Bogumill GP, Schwamm HA: Orthopaedic Pathology: A Synopsis with Clinical and Radiographic Correlation. Philadelphia: WB Saunders Co, 1984.)

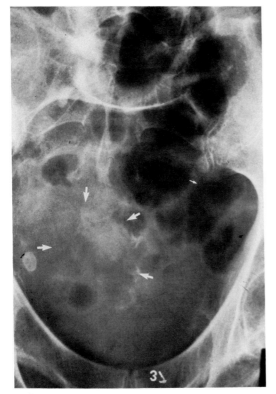

Figure 13–31. Chordoma of the sacrococcygeal spine associated with extensive bone destruction *(arrows)* with no associated calcification. (Courtesy of Anne Brower, M.D.)

tumor originates in a single vertebral body in the mobile spine. The lesion is osteosclerotic in most circumstances.[17] The soft tissue may extend superiorly to the tumor with amorphous, peripheral calcification. Sacral chordomas produce destruction of several sacral segments with a presacral soft tissue mass. Lesions may be difficult to identify because of the angle of the sacrum and overlying bowel gas. Soft tissue extension may be determined best by evaluation with intravenous pyelography, ultrasound, arteriography, venography, or CT (Fig. 13–32).[18, 19] Vertebral chordoma initially causes destruction of a vertebral body without intervertebral disc involvement. Subsequently, intervertebral discs become narrowed and opposing vertebral endplates are eroded.[20] Myelography is helpful in determining extradural extension of the tumor even in the absence of neurologic symptoms. However, it is important to remember that the sacral canal ends at the first or second sacral vertebra. Myelography may miss the intraspinal extension of tumor distal to the thecal sac.[21]

Bone scintigraphy may not detect sacral chordomas because of increased tracer accumulation in the bladder. Lateral scans may be needed to evaluate the sacrum. Reduced uptake in the sacrum, "cold spot," should raise the possibility of a chordoma.[22]

CT is superior to plain roentgenograms for the evaluation of chordomas. The total extent of the tumor mass and soft tissue component can be determined with CT without the need for angiography or myelography. CT detects calcific debris not apparent with plain roentgenograms.[23]

MR allows for imaging of the sacral region in three planes. MR detects the presence of bone pathology and is particularly helpful in determining the extent of the soft tissue mass accompanying the chordoma.[24] MR characteristics of chordomas include signal intensity similar to muscle on T_1-weighted images and increased intensity on T_2-weighted images.[25, 26] It is the best method to identify local recurrence after patients have received treatment for their tumors.[9]

DIFFERENTIAL DIAGNOSIS

The diagnosis of chordoma is suggested by its location and radiographic features, but the definitive diagnosis is dependent on the examination of a biopsy specimen. Needle biopsy of a vertebral chordoma is usually adequate. Fine-needle aspiration biopsy of chordomas produces adequate specimens for diagnosis. Specimens may be examined by microscopic, histochemical, and immunocytochemical examination, including tests for cytokeratin, epithelial membrane antigen, vimentin, carcinoembryonic antigen, and S-100. The use of these methods allows for differentiation of chondrogenic and metastatic adenocarcinomas from chordomas.[8, 27] Open biopsy is frequently required for sacral chordoma because of the tumor location.

A number of lesions need to be considered in the differential diagnosis of a chordoma. Giant cell tumor of bone frequently involves the sacrum. Other lesions include osteochondroma, chondrosarcoma, metastases, multiple myeloma, osteosarcoma, osteoblastoma, aneurysmal bone cyst, and intrasacral cysts. Undifferentiated sarcomas also may involve the sacrum.[28] Neurofibromas also may cause lytic lesions of the sacrum.[29]

Teratomas are benign or malignant tumors that occur in the sacrum and may be confused

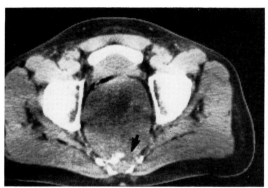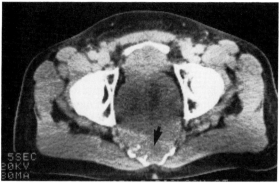

Figure 13–32. A 60-year-old man with minimal back discomfort with a mass detected on rectal examination. CT scan reveals a large mass anterior to the sacrum. The sacrum contains lytic lesions with destruction of the bony cortex *(arrows)*. A biopsy of this lesion revealed a chordoma.

with chordoma. Most teratomas are recognized at birth. However, a number have remained undiagnosed in adults for extended periods.[30] The symptoms of these tumors, such as rectal dysfunction, may be very similar to those seen with chordoma.[31] These tumors probably arise from Hensen's node near the coccyx.

TREATMENT

The definitive treatment for chordoma is en-bloc excision. Unfortunately, because of the size of the tumor at the time of diagnosis and the approximation of the tumor to vital structures, partial resection may be the only surgical option. Staging of the tumor before surgery with radiographic techniques and percutaneous biopsy help determine the possible surgical options for tumor removal.[32] Sacrococcygeal tumors are best treated by surgical excision, if the superior portion of the sacrum is uninvolved, followed by irradiation.[33] Postoperative radiation therapy results in reasonable local control of tumor without significant toxicity.[34] In patients with inaccessible sacral chordomas, radical radiation therapy may slow tumor growth.[35] Vertebral chordomas are treated by decompression laminectomy with excision of accessible tumor located in bone, soft tissues, and the extradural space. Aggressive surgical techniques have been developed that provide the ability to remove an entire vertebra or the sacrum with little residual dysfunction.[32, 36] Chemotherapy is usually ineffective.[37]

PROGNOSIS

Chordomas are slowly growing tumors which metastasize in 10% of patients late in the course of the illness.[38] The common locations for metastatic lesions are lung, bone, and lymph nodes.[39] Patients who undergo total resection of the tumor have a better survival rate than those with partial resection.[40, 41] The 5-year survival rates for sacrococcygeal tumors and vertebral tumors are 66% and 50%, respectively. The 10-year survival ranges between 10% and 40%.[18] A few patients have survived with a chordoma for 20 years. These data support the impression that chordoma is a tumor with a wide spectrum of behavior, from slow and indolent to rapidly progressive destructive growth. The prognosis of each patient must be determined by taking into account the location, pathologic characteristics, and invasiveness of the tumor. With the advent of more sensitive radiographic techniques, smaller tumors are identified with an improved opportunity for total removal of the tumor. This has resulted in a larger number of patients being disease free.[42]

References

CHORDOMA

1. Mirra JM: Bone Tumors: Clinical, Radiologic, and Pathologic Correlation. Philadelphia: Lea & Febiger, 1989, pp 648–690.
2. Dahlin DC, Unni KK: Bone Tumors: General Aspects and Data on 8,542 cases, 4th ed. Springfield, Illinois: Charles C Thomas, 1986, pp 379–393.
3. Mindell ER: Chordoma. J Bone Joint Surg 63A:501, 1981.
4. Bjornsson J, Wold LE, Ebersold MJ, Laws ER: Chordoma of the mobile spine: a clinicopathologic analysis of 40 patients. Cancer 71:735, 1993.
5. Sundaresan N, Rosenthal DI, Schiller AL, Krol G: Chordomas. In: Sundaresan N, Schmidek HH, Schiller AL, Rosenthal DI (eds): Tumors of the Spine: Diagnosis and Clinical Management. Philadelphia: WB Saunders, 1990, pp 192–213.
6. Horwitz T: Chordal ectopia and its possible relationship to chordoma. Arch Pathol 31:354, 1941.
7. Peyron A, Mellissinos J: Chordome, tumeur tramatique. Ann Med Legale 15:478, 1935.
8. Huvos AG: Bone Tumors: Diagnosis, Treatment and Prognosis, 2nd ed. Philadelphia: WB Saunders, 1991, pp 599–624.
9. Healey JH, Lane JM: Chordoma: A critical review of diagnosis and treatment. Orthop Clin North Am 20:417, 1989.
10. Tomlinson FH, Scheithauer BW, Miller GM, Onofrio BM: Extraosseous spinal chordoma. J Neurosurg 75:980, 1991.
11. Sebag G, Dubois J, Benianinovitz A, Lelouch-Tubiana A, Brunelle F: Extraosseous spinal chordoma: radiographic appearance. AJNR 14:205, 1993.
12. Hudson TM, Galceran M: Radiology of sacrococcygeal chordoma: difficulties in detecting soft tissue extension. Clin Orthop 175:237, 1983.
13. Congdon CC: Benign and malignant chordomas: A clinicoanatomical study of twenty-two cases. Am J Pathol 28:793, 1952.
14. Volpe R, Mazabrund A: A clinicopathologic review of 25 cases of chordoma: a pleomorphic and metastatic neoplasm. Am J Surg Pathol 7:161, 1983.
15. Hruban RH, May M, Marcove RC, Huvos AG: Lumbosacral chordoma with high-grade malignant cartilaginous and spincle cell components. Am J Surg Pathol 14:384, 1990.
16. Higinbotham NL, Phillips RF, Farr HW, Husty HO: Chordoma: thirty-five-year study at Memorial Hospital. Cancer 20:1841, 1967.
17. Bruine FTD, Kroon HM: Spinal chordoma: radiologic features in 14 cases. AJR 150:861, 1987.
18. Sundaresan N, Galicich JH, Chu FCH, Huvos AG: Spinal chordomas. J Neurosurg 50:312, 1979.

19. Krol G, Sundaresan N, Deck M: Computed tomography of axial chordomas. J Comput Assist Tomogr 7:286, 1983.

20. Pinto RS, Lin JP, Firooznia H, LeFleur RS: The osseous and angiographic manifestations of vertebral chordomas. Neuroradiology, 9:231, 1975.

21. Banna M: Clinical Radiology of the Spine and the Spinal Cord. Rockville, Maryland: Aspen Systems Corp, 1985, pp 353–357.

22. Rossleigh MA, Smith J, Yeh SD: Scintigraphic features of primary sacral tumors. J Nucl Med 27:627, 1986.

23. Smith J, Ludwig RL, Marcove RC: Sacrococcygeal chordoma. A clinicoradiological study of 60 patients. Skeletal Radiol 16:37, 1987.

24. Wetzel LH, Levine E: MR imaging of sacral and presacral lesions. AJR 154:771, 1990.

25. Yuh WTC, Flickinger FW, Barloon TJ, Montgomery WJ: MR imaging of unusual chordomas. J Comput Assist Tomogr 12:30, 1988.

26. Yuh WTC, Lozano RL, Flickinger FW, et al.: Lumbar epidural chordoma: MR findings. J Comput Assist Tomogr 13:508, 1989.

27. Walaas L, Kindblom L: Fine-needle aspiration biopsy in the preoperative diagnosis of chordoma: a study of 17 cases with application of electron microscopic, histochemical, and immunocytochemical examination. Hum Pathol 22:22, 1991.

28. Uppal GS, Kollmer CE, Rhodes A, et al.: Unique sacral sarcoma. Spine 16:594, 1991.

29. Whelan MA, Hila SK, Gold RP, et al.: Computed tomography of the sacrum 2. Pathology. AJR 139:1191, 1982.

30. Hunt PT, Davidson KC, Ashcraft KW, Holder TM: Radiography of hereditary presacral teratoma. Radiology 122:187, 1977.

31. Graham DF, McKenzie WE: Adult pre-sacral teratoma. Postgrad Med J 55:52, 1979.

32. Stener B: Complete removal of vertebrae for extirpation of tumors: a 20-year experience. Clin Orthop 245:72, 1989.

33. Dahlin DC, MacCarthy CS: Chordoma: a study of fifty-nine cases. Cancer 5:1170, 1952.

34. Schoenthaler R, Castro JR, Petti PL, et al.: Charged particle irradiation of sacral chordomas. Int J Radiation Oncology Biol Phys 26:291, 1993.

35. Pearlman AW, Friedman M: Radical radiation therapy of chordoma. 108:333, 1970.

36. Tomita K, Tsuchiya H: Total sacrectomy and reconstruction for huge sacral tumors. Spine 15:12, 1990.

37. Kamrin RP, Potanos JN, Pool JL: An evaluation of the diagnosis and treatment of chordoma. J Neurol Neurosurg Psychiatry, 27:157, 1964.

38. Wang CC, James AE Jr: Chordoma: brief review of the literature and report of a case with widespread metastases. Cancer, 22:162, 1968.

39. Hertzanu Y, Glass RBJ, Mendelsohn DC: Sacrococcygeal chordoma in young adults. Clin Radiol 34:327, 1983.

40. Bethke KP, Neifeld JP, Lawrence W Jr: Diagnosis and management of sacrococcygeal chordoma. J Surg Oncol 48:232, 1991.

41. Chetty R, Levin CV, Kalan MR: Chordoma: a 20-year clinicopathologic review of the experience of Groote Schuur hospital, Cape Town. J Surg Oncol 46:261, 1991.

42. Sundaresan N, Huvos AG, Krol G, et al.: Surgical treatment of spinal chordomas. Arch Surg 122:1479, 1987.

Lymphoma

Capsule Summary

Frequency of back pain—uncommon

Location of back pain—lumbar spine and sacrum

Quality of back pain—persistent ache

Symptoms and signs—pain that increases with recumbency, generalized fatigue, localized tenderness

Laboratory and x-ray tests—anemia; osteolytic lesion with compression fracture on plain roentgenogram

Treatment—chemotherapy and/or radiotherapy

PREVALENCE AND PATHOGENESIS

Lymphomas are malignant disease of lymphoreticular origin. They usually arise in lymph nodes, rarely initially in bone, and are classified into two major groups: Hodgkin's and non-Hodgkin's lymphoma. Hodgkin's lymphoma occasionally, and non-Hodgkin's lymphoma rarely, may present as back pain in an adult patient.

The incidence of Hodgkin's and non-Hodgkin's lymphomas is approximately 40 to 60 cases per million persons per year. Primary Hodgkin's and non-Hodgkin's disease of bone unassociated with lymph node involvement are rare tumors occurring in 1% to 7% of tumors examined by biopsy.[1, 2] Most bone involvement is secondary to hematogenous spread or direct extension of the tumor.[3] Approximately 30% of malignant lymphomas involve the skeletal system during the course of the illness.[4] A majority of patients who develop lymphomas are between the ages of 20 and 60, and the male to female ratio is approximately 2:1. The disease occurs with increasing frequency in each successive decade from the second to the eighth when the frequency declines.[5]

The pathogenesis of lymphomas remains unknown. Although viral infections have been implicated as the etiologic agents that result in lymphomas, the exact pathogenetic factors causing lymphoreticular malignancy remain to be identified.

Fourteen per cent of lymphomas affect the axial skeleton. The lumbosacral spine is the location of 55% of axial lesions, the thoracic spine 34%, and the cervical spine 11%.[2] In a study of 25 patients with primary lymphoma of bone, 24% of lesions occurred in the axial skeleton.[6] A similar percentage was noted in a larger, retrospective study of 246 patients with primary lymphoma of bone.[7]

CLINICAL HISTORY

Patients with primary Hodgkin's or non-Hodgkin's lymphoma of bone develop persistent pain over the affected bone. Bone pain may increase when the patient goes to bed. The pain often precedes the radiographic changes of lymphoma by months. A peculiar clinical finding relates to an increase of bone pain after the consumption of alcohol.[8] The duration of pain is usually measured in months before patients seek medical evaluation. Most patients with solitary lesions have no constitutional symptoms. Constitutional symptoms are more closely associated with multiple lesions of bone. Patients with spinal epidural lymphoma may complain of symptoms compatible with spinal stenosis.[9]

PHYSICAL EXAMINATION

The bone affected by primary lymphoma is tender to palpation. Soft tissue swelling may be associated with bony tenderness. Patients with axial skeletal disease may demonstrate neurologic deficits. Patients with primary disease of bone may have no peripheral signs of their tumor. Patients with generalized disease, of which bone infiltration is a part, may demonstrate lymphadenopathy and splenomegaly.

LABORATORY DATA

The patient with primary disease of bone will not demonstrate hematologic, chemical, or immunologic abnormalities associated with disseminated disease. The appearance of anemia, elevated sedimentation rate, and increased serum proteins in a patient with bone disease suggests either that the disease has extended to other tissue or that the bone lesion was secondary to disseminated disease and occurred late in its development.

Gross pathologic examination of affected bone reveals a main tumor mass in bone with variable amount of soft tissue extension.[10] The architecture of the bone is destroyed to a variable extent, and areas of necrosis are noted. The margins of the tumor and the involved bone are indistinct. The histologic picture of Hodgkin's disease includes typical Reed-Sternberg cells, atypical mononuclear cells, and an inflammatory component composed of lymphocytes, plasma cells, and scattered eosinophils. The reactive histiocytes and eosinophils

look superficially like eosinophilic granuloma. In an older adult, a lesion that resembles eosinophilic granuloma may be Hodgkin's disease.[11] Non-Hodgkin's lymphomas may exhibit marked histologic variation.[12] These lesions lack Reed-Sternberg cells and demonstrate different combinations of abnormal lymphocytes and supporting cells. New staining techniques may better characterize cells that cause the various kinds of lymphoma.[13] In a study of 34 Japanese patients with primary non-Hodgkin's lymphoma of bone, Ueda identified T-cell markers in 10% of tumors.[14] The frequency of T-cell lymphomas may be related to the increased frequency of retroviral associated lymphoma that is common in Japan. In a series from the United States, a B-lineage large cell lymphoma was the cause of primary bone neoplasms.[15]

RADIOGRAPHIC EVALUATION

Both primary Hodgkin's and non-Hodgkin's lymphoma have a predilection for the axial skeleton.[16] The bone changes of Hodgkin's disease may include lytic (75%), sclerotic (15%), mixed (5%), or periosteal (5%) lesions.[17] In the axial skeleton, Hodgkin's disease most frequently involves a vertebral body, and involvement of posterior elements of a vertebral body is much less common (Fig. 13–33). Occasionally, an osteoblastic lesion, an "ivory" vertebra, may be seen with Hodgkin's disease.[18] Hodgkin's involvement of the axial skeleton may result in compression fractures that spare the vertebral discs. Non-Hodgkin's lymphoma of bone has similar features characterized by lytic and blastic areas, with cortical destruction and little reactive new bone.

The degree and type of bony lesions may vary with the histologic classification of lymphoma. In a study of 179 patients with primary lymphoma of bone, 33% had two or more bones involved.[19] Skeletal lesions are more frequent and destructive in the more aggressive tumors. Sclerotic lesions are more common in less aggressive forms. Only 11% of patients with less aggressive tumors had bone lesions, in contrast to 64% of those with more malignant disease.[20]

CT and MR are helpful techniques for the determination of extraosseous, paravertebral extension of the neoplasm. CT reveals sequestra in 11% of patients with primary lymphoma of bone.[7] Sequestra are not only indicative of primary lymphoma but may also be associated with osteomyelitis, multiple myeloma, metastases, and bone sarcomas. CT scan is helpful

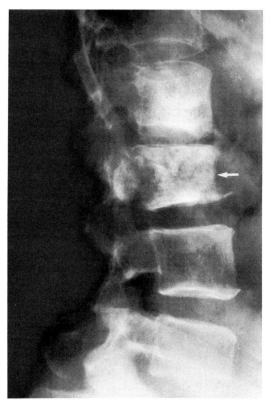

Figure 13–33. Lymphoma of the spine characterized by patchy sclerosis and lucency of two vertebral bodies with loss of body height. There is erosion of the anterior portion of one of the vertebral bodies *(arrow)* secondary to adjacent lymph node involvement. (Courtesy of Anne Brower, M.D.)

in staging lymphomas, differentiating primary lymphoma of bone (stage I) from bone lesions associated with disease in other sites (stage IV).[21] MR evaluation demonstrates low intensity signal on T_1-weighted images and high intensity signal on T_2-weighted images. Lymph gland enlargment can be identified with MR, but is unable to differentiate lymphadenopathy secondary to Hodgkin's disease, non-Hodgkin's disease, infection, or metastatic disease.[22]

DIFFERENTIAL DIAGNOSIS

The diagnosis of the lymphoma is based on the careful examination of adequate biopsy material. Even with adequate histologic material, however, the diagnosis of specific lymphoma is a difficult one to make because of the pleomorphic forms of the disease. The differential diagnosis of a single osteoblastic vertebral body must include Paget's disease and carcinoma of the breast or prostate. In younger patients with vertebra plana, the pos-

sibility of eosinophilic granuloma must be investigated. Careful review of all the clinical and pathologic data should render enough information for the treating physician to make the appropriate diagnosis.

TREATMENT

The treatment of lymphomas is based on the extent of the illness. All patients must be staged before treatment is initiated. Staging of lymphomas continues to be modified as additional information related to prognosis is gathered. A new predictive model for aggressive non-Hodgkin's lymphoma includes extranodal sites as one of the factors determining outcome.[23] Once the stage of disease is known, the patient should receive appropriate therapy for that degree of involvement. Treatment may include radiation therapy and/or chemotherapy.[24-26]

PROGNOSIS

The therapy for lymphoma has become more effective in the control of the disease, and patients have the potential for cure if the disease is not too extensive. In many circumstances, they are able to live productive lives for extended periods of time. Five-year survival rates of 40% to 50% have been reported. Recent studies have continued to report 50% survival for patients with lymphoma of bone.[27] Patients with solitary bone lesions have a better prognosis compared to the 42%, 5-year survival for patients with multiple lesions.[5] Prognosis may also be related to the pattern of cell associated with the tumor. Favorable patterns include noncleaved and multilobated cells. Unfavorable patterns are associated with cleaved cells and immunoblasts. The 5-year survival is 67% for cleaved cells and 21% for uncleaved cells.[28] Young patients who develop neural compression should receive aggressive radiotherapy and chemotherapy. Decompression is reserved for young patients with rapidly progressive paralysis. The results of decompression in the elderly is poor.[29] Patients with disease in the pelvis have the same survival rates as patients with bone involvement in other parts of the skeleton.[2]

References

LYMPHOMA

1. Mirra JM: Bone Tumors: Clinical, Radiologic, and Pathologic Correlation. Philadelphia: Lea & Febiger 1989, pp 1119–1185.

2. Dahlin DC, Unni KK: Bone Tumors: General Aspects and Data on 8,542 cases, 4th ed. Springfield, Illinois: Charles C Thomas, 1986, pp 206–226.
3. Steiner PE: Hodgkin's disease: the incidence, distribution, nature and possible significance of lymphogranulomatous lesions in bone marrow; review with original data. Arch Pathol 36:627, 1943.
4. Coles WC, Schulz MD: Bone involvement in malignant lymphoma. Radiology 50:458, 1948.
5. Aisenberg AC: Malignant Lymphoma: Biology, Natural History, and Treatment. Philadelphia: Lea & Febiger, 1991, pp 288–290.
6. Desai S, Jambhekar NA, Soman CS, Advani SH: Primary lymphoma of bone: a clinicopathologic study of 25 cases reported over 10 years. J Surg Oncol 46:265, 1991.
7. Mulligan ME, Kransdorf MJ: Sequestra in primary lymphoma of bone: prevalence and radiologic features. AJR 160:1245, 1993.
8. Conn HO: Alcohol-induced pain as a manifestation of Hodgkin's disease. Arch Intern Med 100:241, 1957.
9. Travlos J, du Toit G: Primary spinal epidural lymphoma mimicking lumbar spinal stenosis: a case report. Spine 16:377, 1991.
10. Huvos AG: Bone Tumors: Diagnosis, Treatment and Prognosis, 2nd ed. Philadelphia: WB Saunders, 1991, pp 625–637.
11. Jaffe HL: Metabolic, Degenerative and Inflammatory Diseases of Bones and Joints. Philadelphia: Lea and Febiger, 1972, p 887.
12. Reimer RR, Chabner BA, Young RC, et al.: Lymphoma presenting in bone: results of histopathology, staging, and therapy. Ann Intern Med 87:50, 1977.
13. Warnke RA, Gotter KC, Falini B, et al.: Diagnosis of human lymphoma with monoclonal antileukocyte antibodies. N Engl J Med 309:1275, 1983.
14. Ueda T, Aozasa K, Ohasawa M, et al.: Malignant lymphomas of bone in Japan. Cancer 64:2387, 1989.
15. Pettit CK, Zukerberg LR, Gray MH, et al.: Primary lymphoma of bone. A B-cell neoplasm with a high frequency of multilobated cells. Am J Surg Pathol 14:329, 1990.
16. Perttala Y, Kijanen I: Roentgenologic bone lesions in lymphogranulomatosis maligna: analysis of 453 cases. Ann Chir Gynaecol Fenn, 54:414, 1965.
17. Granger W, Whitaker R: Hodgkin's disease in bone, with special reference to periosteal reaction. Br J Radiol 40:939, 1967.
18. Dennis JM: The solitary dense vertebral body. Radiology, 77:618, 1961.
19. Ostrowski ML, Unni KK, Banks PM, et al.: Malignant lymphoma of bone. Cancer 58:2646, 1986.
20. Braunstein EM: Hodgkin disease of bone: radiographic correlation with the histological classification. Radiology 137:643, 1980.
21. Malloy PC, Fishman EK, Magid D: Lymphoma of bone, muscle, and skin: CT findings. AJR 159:805, 1992.
22. Holtas SL, Kido DK, Simon JH: MR imaging of spinal lymphoma. J Comput Assist Tomogr 10:111, 1986.
23. The International Non-Hodgkin's lymphoma prognostic factors project: A predictive model for aggressive non-Hodgkin's lymphoma. N Engl J Med 329:987, 1993.
24. Leslie NT, Mauch PM, Hellman S: Stage IA to IIB supradiaphragmatic Hodgkin's disease: long-term survival and relapse frequency. Cancer 55:2072, 1985.
25. Canellos GP, Come SE, Skarin AT: Chemotherapy in the treatment of Hodgkin's disease. Semin Hematol 20:1, 1983.
26. Dosoretz DE, Murphy GF, Raymond AK, et al.: Radiation Therapy for primary lymphoma of bone. Cancer 51:44, 1983.
27. Edeiken-Monroe B, Ediken J, Kim EE: Radiologic concepts of lymphoma of bone. Radiol Clin North Am 28:841, 1990.
28. Clayton F, Butler JJ, Ayala AG, et al.: Non-Hodgkin's lymphoma of bone: pathologic and radiologic features with clinical correlates. Cancer 60:2492, 1987.
29. Laing RJ, Jakubowski J, Kunkler IH, Hancock BW: Primary spinal presentation of non-Hodgkin's lymphoma: a reappraisal of management and prognosis. Spine 17:117, 1992.

Skeletal Metastases

Capsule Summary

Frequency of back pain—very common
Location of back pain—lumbar spine and sacrum
Quality of back pain—ache of increasing intensity
Symptoms and signs—increased pain with recumbency, prior malignancy
Laboratory and x-ray tests—anemia, bone biopsy may or may not show characteristics of primary tumor; bone scintigraphy most sensitive test
Treatment—palliative with radiotherapy, corticosteroids, decompressive laminectomy for neural compression

PREVALENCE AND PATHOGENESIS

A principal characteristic of malignant neoplastic lesions is the growth of tumor cells distant from the primary lesion. These distant lesions are referred to as metastases and are found commonly in the skeletal system. Skeletal lesions result either from dissemination through the blood stream or by direct extension. The axial skeleton and pelvis are common sites of metastatic disease.

Metastatic lesions in the skeleton are much more common than primary tumors of bone, with the overall ratio being 25:1.[1, 2] In a study of 1971 patients with neoplasms, only 29 (1.5%) had primary neoplasms of the lumbar spine.[3] The 18 primary lesions that occurred in adults were malignant. The prevalence of metastases increases with increasing age. This follows from the increasing numbers of tumors in a population of individuals as they grow older. Patients who are 50 years old or older are at greatest risk of developing metastatic disease. The ratio of men and women who develop metastases varies for each type of malignancy. Considering all neoplasms with the potential to metastasize, men and women are equally at risk of developing metastatic lesions.

Each tumor has a different propensity for metastasizing to bone. The true incidence of skeletal metastases from each tumor is difficult to ascertain. Complete examination of the skeleton can not be done with the same degree of care as evaluating other body organs. Therefore, great variability may be reported for the incidence of metastases from the same type of tumor. Neoplasms that are frequently associated with skeletal metastasis include tumors of the prostate, breast, lung, kidney, thyroid, and colon (Table 13–3).[4] Data from autopsy material suggest that up to 70% of patients with a primary neoplasm will develop pathologic evidence of metastasis to vertebral bodies in the thoracolumbar spine.[5] In an autopsy study of 832 individuals with malignant neoplasms, 36% had evidence of metastases to the spine. Occult metastases visible on autopsy but not detected by plain radiographs were present in 78 of 300 cases (26%).[6]

Metastases occur more commonly in the axial skeleton than in the appendicular skeleton. The axial skeleton is the third most common site of metastases after lung and liver.[7] In the axial skeleton, the thoracic and lumbar spine are most frequently affected. The lumbar and thoracic spine are affected in approximately 46% to 49% of cases, with the cervical spine involved to a lesser degree (6%).[8]

The propensity of bone, and the axial skeleton in particular, to be the site of metastases may be explained in part by the presence of Batson's plexus around the vertebral column and of bone marrow inside bone (Fig. 13–34). Batson's plexus is a network of veins located in the epidural space between the bony spinal column and the dura mater covering the spinal cord. It is connected to the major veins that return blood to the heart and the inferior and superior vena cava. This plexus of veins is unique in that there are no valves to control blood flow, and therefore any increased pressure in the vena caval system results in increased flow into Batson's plexus. Metastatic cells may enter this plexus and be deposited in the venous and sinusoidal systems of bones that are connected to Batson's plexus.[9] Supporting data for the importance of Batson's plexus in the distribution of skeletal metastasis are the frequency of axial skeleton metastases and the predilection of metastasis to the lumbar spine.[10, 11] The red bone marrow, located inside vertebral bodies, long bones, and flat bones, has a rich sinusoidal system. Sinusoidal vessels are usually under low hemodynamic pressure, allowing for pooling of blood. The pooling of blood, along with other factors such as fibrin deposits and thrombosis, may encourage tumor growth.

The incidence of skeletal metastases also may be related to the ability of tumor cell emboli to develop into secondary tumors. This is a property of each form of tumor. The effects of tumor cells on bone also vary for each type of neoplasm. Tumor cells may cause bone destruction or bone formation. Osteoclasts may be stimulated by products of tumor cells (in myeloma, for example) resulting in osteolysis.[12] On the other hand, osteoblasts may also be directly stimulated by tumor cell factors (as in prostatic carcinoma) that stimulate bone formation or may produce bone in reaction to increased bone destruction.[13–17] The effects of these processes of tumor cells on bone result in osteolysis or osteosclerosis that is discernible by radiographic techniques.

A number of chemical factors related to metastases have an effect on bone mineralization. These factors include parathyroid hormone, osteoclast-activating factor, prostaglandins (PGE_2), and transforming growth factor.[7, 18] Tumors associated with osteoblastic activity (prostate cancer), release factors that stimulate osteoblasts that produce bone.[19]

CLINICAL HISTORY

A high index of suspicion for the presence of metastasis is important in the evaluation of the patient with a prior history of malignancy or the adult over 50 years of age with back pain that is not associated with trauma. In a study of 1975 patients with low back pain, 13 individuals (0.66%) had cancer.[20] The patients with cancer were over 50 years of age, had a

TABLE 13–3. INCIDENCE OF SKELETAL METASTASES

TUMOR ORIGIN	INCIDENCE (%)	
	High	Low
Breast	85	47
Prostate	85	33
Thyroid	60	28
Kidney	64	30
Esophagus	7	5
Intestine	11	3
Rectum	61	8
Bladder	42	
Uterine cervix	56	50
Ovary	9	
Liver	16	
Melanoma	7	

Modified from Galasko CSB: Skeletal Metastases. Boston: Butterworths, 1986.

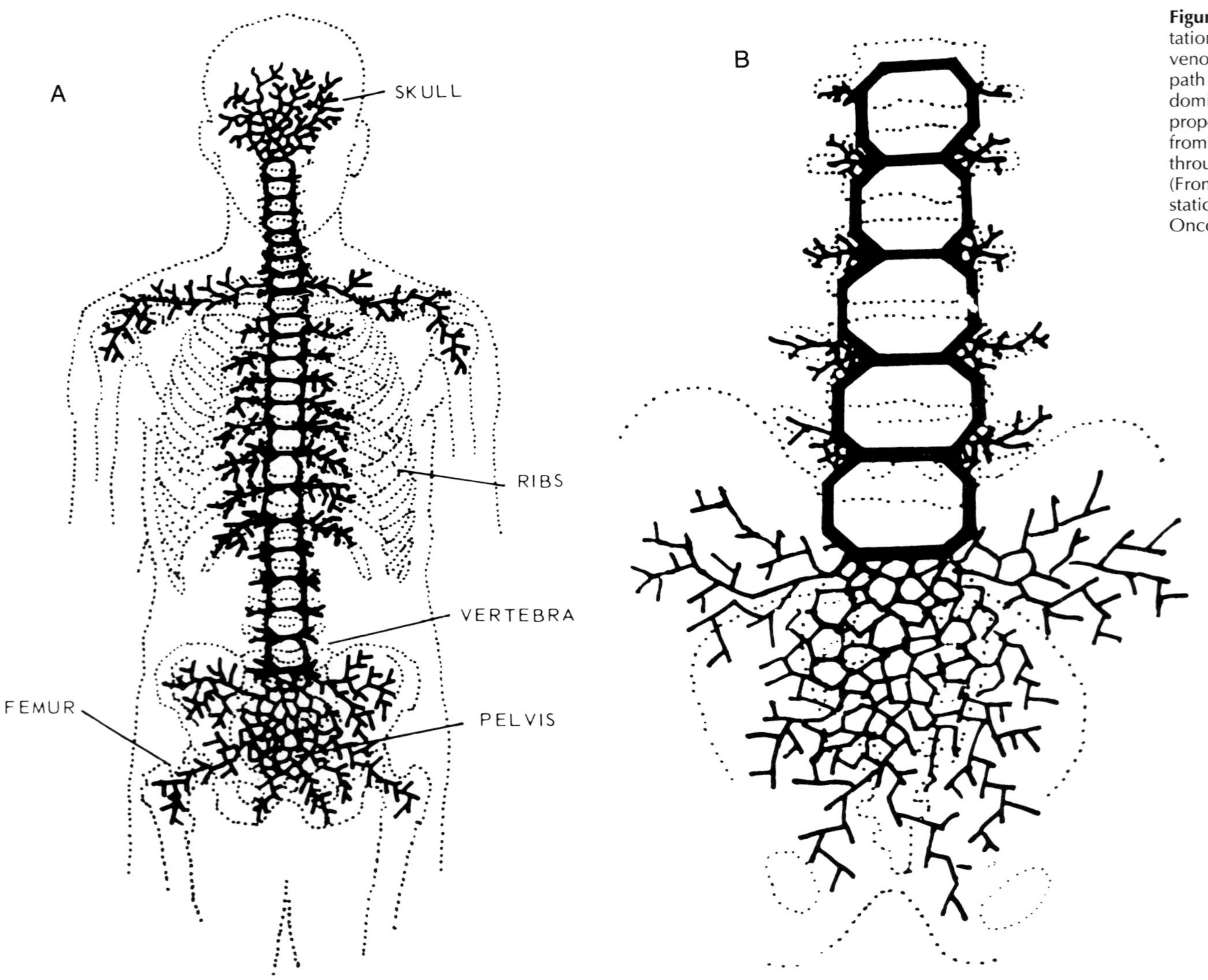

Figure 13-34. Diagrammatic representation of the vertebral vein system. This venous network is a common two-way path of metastatic spread of pelvic, abdominal, and thoracic tumors. A large proportion of bony metastases result from dissemination of neoplastic cells through the vertebral venous system. (From del Regato, JA: Pathways of metastatic spread of malignant tumors. Semin Oncol 4:33, 1977.)

SKULL

RIBS

VERTEBRA

PELVIS

FEMUR

A

B

previous history of cancer, had pain for over one month, and failed to respond to conservative therapy. Pain has a gradual onset and increases in intensity over time. It tends to be localized initially but may radiate in a radicular pattern over time. Pain in the lumbar spine is commonly increased with motion, cough, or strain. Radicular pain may increase at night as the spine lengthens with recumbency. Pain with recumbency is a symptom frequently associated with spinal tumors.[21]

Not all patients with skeletal metastases will have pain. In a review of 86 patients with breast cancer with radiographic evidence of skeletal metastases, only 65% complained of pain. Similar results have been reported by other investigators.[8, 16] Patients with spinal cord or nerve root compression secondary to bony or epidural lesions develop neurologic dysfunction that correlates with the location of the lesion. Neurologic symptoms may include numbness, tingling, unsteadiness of gait, weakness, bladder or bowel incontinence, or sexual dysfunction.[17, 22]

Three patterns of progression of neurologic symptoms may be noted. In 30% of patients, symptoms occur acutely, with progression to maximal neurologic deficit in 48 hours. Subacute deterioration over 7 to 10 days is noted in 60%. The remaining 10% of individuals develop symptoms over 4 to 6 months.[23]

PHYSICAL EXAMINATION

Physical examination may demonstrate pain on palpation over the affected bone. Muscle spasm and limitation of motion are associated findings. Careful attention to neurologic deficits (hyperesthesia, segmental muscular weakness, asymmetric reflexes, sphincter dysfunction) may help locate the lesion in the axial skeleton. Lesions that affect the T12 or L1 vertebrae may compress the conus medullaris, which contains the S3 through coccygeal nerve segments. Nerves originating from these segments innervate the urinary bladder, the bladder and rectal sphincter, and the sensory fibers of the perineal (saddle) region. Lesions that affect the conus may cause sphincter dysfunction and saddle anesthesia without neurologic abnormalities in the lower extremities. In contrast, lesions below L1 affect the nerve roots that are part of the cauda equina. Lesions of the cauda equina cause lower motor neuron abnormalities associated with motor and sensory loss and hyporeflexia.[24]

Frankel's classification is used to grade degrees of neurologic deficits. Grade A is associated with complete motor and sensory loss, while Grade E has normal motor and sensory function.[7]

LABORATORY DATA

Early in the course of lesions, laboratory parameters may be unremarkable. However, subsequent evaluation may demonstrate anemia, elevated ESR, abnormal urinalysis, or abnormal chemistries including increased serum alkaline phosphatase concentrations and increased prostatic acid phosphatase in metastatic prostate carcinoma. Therefore, initial negative laboratory data should not dissuade a physician from pursuing further diagnostic evaluation in an older patient with recent onset of back pain.

Biochemical tests are not always positive in patients. Bishop found false negative alkaline (18%) and acid phosphatase (36%) levels in patients with skeletal metastases from prostatic carcinoma.[25] In another study, only 30% of patients with positive scintiscan for metastatic disease had elevated alkaline phosphatase.[26]

In patients without a known primary tumor, bone biopsy may provide the first evidence of a malignancy. Occasionally, the histologic features of the biopsy specimen may suggest the source of the lesion, such as colloid material with thyroid adenocarcinoma, clear cells with renal cell carcinoma, or melanin with melanoma. On many occasions, the histologic features, squamous cells or mucin cells, may be associated with primary lesions in various organs (Figs. 13–35 and 13–36). Some lesions may be so undifferentiated that the pathologic findings offer no clue to the possible source of the tumor.[2] Radiologic identification of lesions may help localize the area for biopsy.[27]

RADIOGRAPHIC EVALUATION

Radiographic abnormalities associated with the axial skeleton include osteolytic, osteoblastic, or mixed lytic and blastic lesions.[28] Osteolytic lesions that affect a vertebral body or a posterior element such as a pedicle are associated with carcinomas of the lung, kidney, breast, and thyroid. Multiple osteoblastic lesions are associated with prostatic, breast, and colon carcinomas and bronchial carcinoid (Figs. 13–37 and 13–38). A single blastic vertebral body may be seen with prostatic carcinoma but is more closely associated with Hodgkin's disease or Paget's disease. Vertebral lesions that contain both lytic and blastic metastases are associated with carcinoma of the

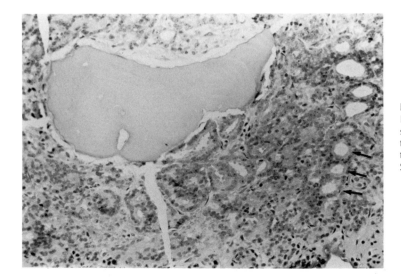

Figure 13–35. Metastatic carcinoma. Histologic section exhibiting metastatic prostatic carcinoma with collections of cells with glandular organization *(arrows)*. (Courtesy of Arnold Schwartz, M.D.)

Figure 13–36. Metastatic carcinoma. Histologic section of metastatic breast carcinoma exhibiting a lytic area of bone containing desmoplastic stroma with islands of malignant cells *(arrows)*. (Courtesy of Arnold Schwartz, M.D.)

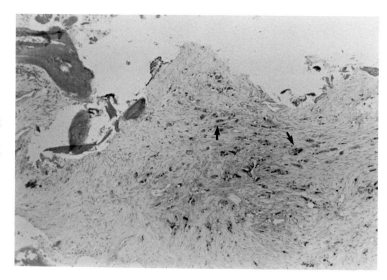

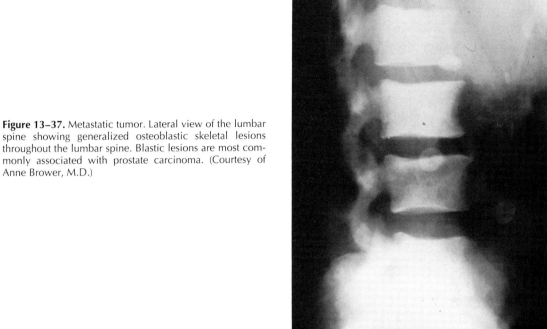

Figure 13–37. Metastatic tumor. Lateral view of the lumbar spine showing generalized osteoblastic skeletal lesions throughout the lumbar spine. Blastic lesions are most commonly associated with prostate carcinoma. (Courtesy of Anne Brower, M.D.)

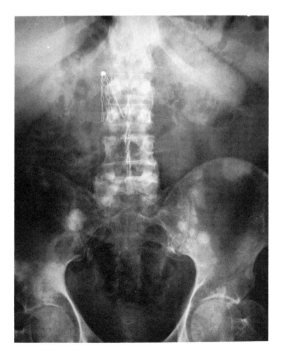

Figure 13–38. AP view of the lumbosacral spine and pelvis in a 66-year-old man with a 3-month history of back pain reveals multiple, discrete osteoblastic lesions, which proved to be metastatic prostatic carcinoma on biopsy.

breast, lung, prostate, or bladder. Because of their usual slow growth, kidney and thyroid carcinoma may cause an expansile lesion from periosteal growth without destruction. Osteolytic lesions are more frequently associated with vertebral body collapse than are osteoblastic lesions (Fig. 13–39). Vertebral body destruction is not associated with changes in the intervertebral disc, so the presence of vertebral body destruction and loss of intervertebral disc space suggests infection. However, radiographic and pathologic studies suggest that intervertebral discs may degenerate more rapidly, indent weakened vertebral bone, and form a Schmorl's node. Rarely it may be invaded by tumor, resulting in loss of disc integrity.[29, 30] Some metastases of tumors in the pelvis will affect the left side of the vertebral column more than the right; this is related to the proximity of lymph nodes to the axial skeleton.[31]

Early in the course of a metastatic lesion, plain roentgenographic examination will be unremarkable, since between 30% and 50% of bone must be destroyed before a lesion is evident on plain radiographs (Fig. 13–40).[32] However, scintigraphic examination with bone scan makes it possible to detect areas of symptomatic and asymptomatic bone involvement in up to 85% of patients with metastases (Figs. 13–41 and 13–42).[22, 33] A bone scan also may suggest the presence of tumor in patients with coincident degenerative disease or osteoporosis. In one study, bone scan was the single most useful diagnostic test in differentiating pain caused by metastatic disease from pain due to a benign lesion.[34] It is important to remember that there are reasons for false neg-

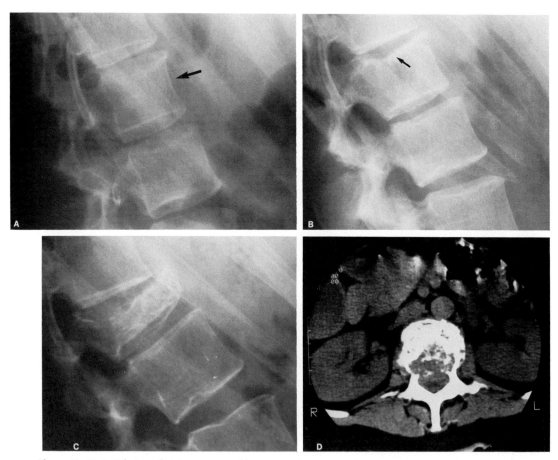

Figure 13–39. Serial view of L1 in a 43-year-old woman with metastatic breast cancer. *A,* 10/3/85. This patient developed radicular symptoms associated with an acute herniated lumbar disc. Her back pain resolved with conservative management. Calcification of bone is normal in L1 *(arrow). B,* 2/9/87. This patient developed acute-onset, localized back pain over the L1 vertebra. The lateral view reveals sclerosis of the superior endplate of L1 associated with a mild loss of vertebral body height. *C,* 4/17/87. The patient's pain persisted. Repeat roentgenogram demonstrates marked destruction of the L1 vertebral body. *D,* CT scan of L1 revealing marked destruction of the vertebral body and beginning encroachment of the tumor into the spinal canal.

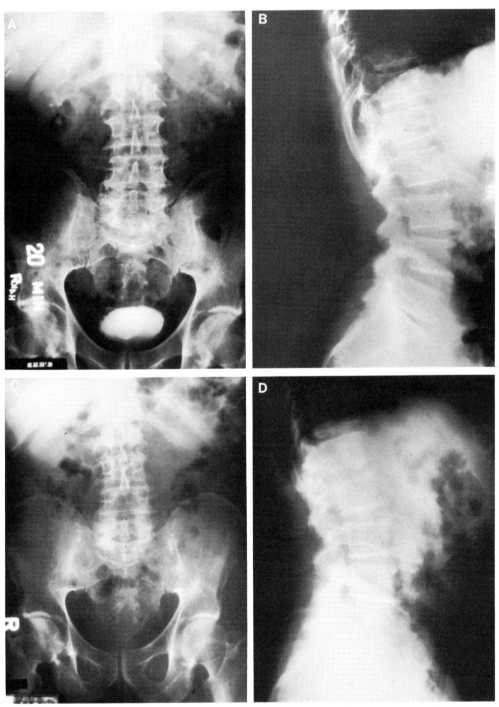

Figure 13–40. A 64-year-old man presented with diffuse low back pain. Evaluation included an intravenous pyelogram, which showed no abnormalities. The AP *(A)* and lateral *(B)* views reveal osteoarthritic changes associated with degenerative disc disease. The patient returned 6 months later with severe pain over the L4 vertebra. The AP *(C)* and lateral *(D)* views are presented. What is wrong with these pictures? (See repeat of Figures *C* and *D* and legend on next page.)

Illustration continued on following page

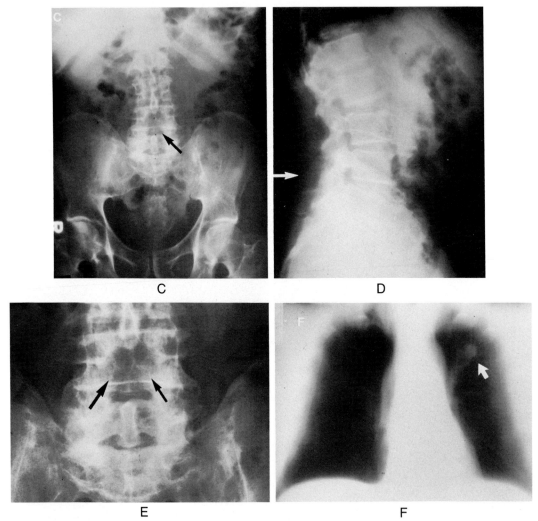

C

D

E

F

Figure 13–40 *Continued.* AP view *(C)* and lateral view *(D)* reveal loss of the spinous process of L4 *(arrows)*. Close-up *(E)* shows osteolysis of the process *(arrows)*. Tomogram *(F)* of the lung revealed the primary source of tumor in the upper lobe of the left lung *(arrow)*.

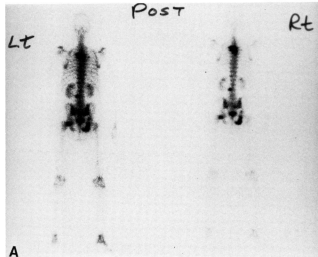

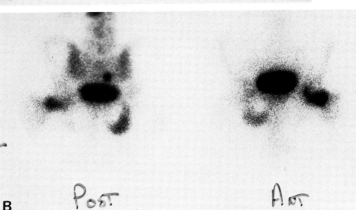

Figure 13–41. A 60-year-old man with a hard nodule in the prostate gland and bone pain. *A*, ^{99m}Tc MDP bone scan reveals uptake in the midthoracic spine, upper lumbar spine, left femoral neck, right ischium, and sacrum. *B*, Spot view reveals focal uptake in the same areas.

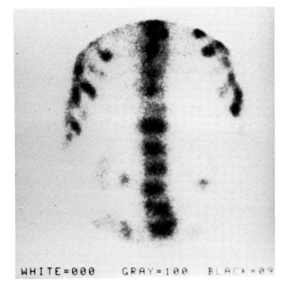

Figure 13–42. Bone scan of a 70-year-old man with metastatic prostatic carcinoma. Most of these "hot spots" on the scan were asymptomatic.

ative and false positive scintiscans (Table 13–4).[4] One of the most important of these to remember is the "superscan." In these scans, markedly increased, symmetric, generalized uptake by diffuse metastases may be interpreted as normal. The reduction of tracer in kidneys and urine should alert the radiologist to this possibility (Fig. 13–43).[35] The bone

TABLE 13–4. BONE SCAN

FALSE NEGATIVE	FALSE POSITIVE
1. Tumor lacks osteoblastic response (myeloma)	1. Site of injection (elbow)
2. Small deposits	2. Urinary incontinence
3. Lesions of sacrum and ischium masked by bladder	3. Abnormal bladder collections (diverticulum)
4. Generalized increased uptake ("superscan")	4. Incomplete isotope
	5. Superimposition of uptake

Modified from Galasko CSB: Skeletal Metastases. Boston: Butterworths, 1986.

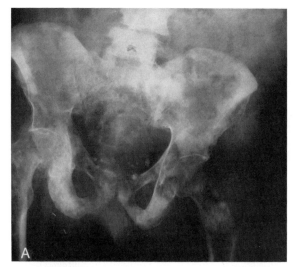

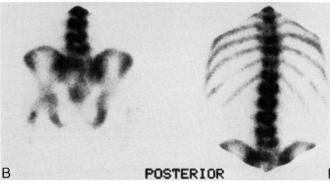

Figure 13–43. *A,* Posteroanterior view of pelvis of middle-aged man with metastatic prostate cancer (8/2/90). *B,* Bone scintiscan (9/26/90) with marked increase in uptake over axial skeleton without tracer in the kidney or bladder. (From Borenstein DG: Low back pain. In Klippel J, Dieppe P (eds): Rheumatology. St Louis: CV Mosby, 1994, Sec 5, 4.8 and 4.16.)

scintiscan is the most sensitive and economic test for detecting bone metastases.[35a]

CT may also be useful in localizing lesions that are difficult to identify on plain radiographs.[36] CT is normally reserved for assessment of patients with positive isotope scans but with negative radiographs. It enables differentiation among bony metastases, benign lesions, and no abnormality.[37, 38] With CT, differentiation can be made between metastases and degenerative joint disease when both coexisted in apophyseal articulations.[37] CT also may be useful in detecting the presence and extent of pelvic metastases, an area inadequately evaluated by scintiscan.[39] CT scan is particularly useful in demonstrating small areas of bone destruction and of bone and tumor impingement on the spinal canal.[40] It should not be used as a screening technique, since the exposure to radiation is great.

Myelography was the definitive diagnostic procedure for any patient with a metastatic lesion and spinal cord or nerve root compression. Injections of dye in two locations, lumbar and cisterna magna (cervical spine), was necessary to locate all potential areas of neural compression, since lesions in the lumbar spine were accompanied by "silent" lesions in the proximal spine.[41] Myelography may be used to identify whether the lesion is in extradural or intradural space.

The role of MR in the evaluation of patients with metastases continues to evolve as the technique becomes more sensitive in detecting neoplasms that replace normal tissues in the spine. Some studies have shown MR to be better at showing the extent of tumor inside the cord, the size of extraosseous extension, and bone marrow invasion, while CT is better at showing cortical bone destruction and degree of bone mineralization.[42, 43] MR is able to identify compression fractures secondary to osteopenia from replacement of bone marrow with malignant cells.[44] MR detects lesions that are not identified by roentgenograms or scintiscan.[45] A study of 40 patients with metastatic disease revealed patients with breast, kidney, prostate cancer, and multiple myeloma that was abnormal on MR but normal with other radiographic techniques including CT and scintiscan (Fig. 13–44).[46] MR also is sensitive to lesions in the pelvis that are not detected by

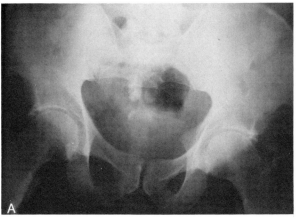
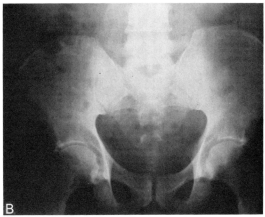
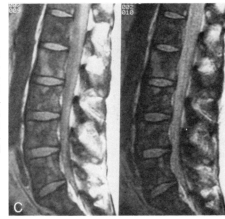

Figure 13–44. A 52-year-old man presented with right-sided low back and buttock pain. Plain roentgenogram *(A)* taken on 4/1/91 was unremarkable. He did not respond to conservative management and complained of increasing pain. Repeat roentgenogram *(B)* taken on 5/1/91 was suggestive of increased sclerosis in the pelvis. Serum acid phosphatase was elevated. *C*, MR of the lumbar spine (5/3/91) revealed on proton density (left) and T_2-weighted sequence (right) demonstrating decreased signal intensity in multiple vertebral bodies indicative of marrow replacement. Biopsy of prostate revealed adenocarcinoma. The patient expired from extensive metastatic disease in 6/93.

other radiographic techniques.[47] The importance of MR as a diagnostic tool has been further advanced by the availability of gadolinium-diethylenetriaminepentaacetic acid as a paramagnetic contrast agent. MR with contrast demonstrates the size, location, configuration, and characteristics of spinal tumors.[48] MR is the first procedure to be used for patients with spinal cord compression. It is a noninvasive technique that is sensitive in detecting extradural masses.[49] MR should be obtained of the entire spinal cord if compression is suspected since 10% of patients have multiple levels of impingement.[50] CT and myelography should be reserved for patients in whom MR is not feasible or does not satisfactorily explain neurologic findings.

DIFFERENTIAL DIAGNOSIS

In the patient with a known primary tumor who develops low back pain, a destructive spinal lesion is associated with the primary neoplasm in the vast majority of cases. These patients may not require a biopsy of the spinal lesion for diagnosis; however, patients with no known primary neoplasm who develop de-

structive lesions of the spine require a biopsy for tissue diagnosis. Closed needle biopsy of lesions in the lumbar spine can safely yield useful information.[51]

Other conditions may cause bony changes on radiographs and "hot spots" on scintiscans. Elevated alkaline phosphatase may be seen in osteomalacia, Paget's disease, hyperparathyroidism, and sarcoidosis. Only with careful review of all the data can the various diagnoses be eliminated. In some circumstances, tissue biopsy is the only sure way to obtain the data needed to make an accurate diagnosis.

TREATMENT

Treatment of metastatic disease of the spine is directed toward palliation of pain. A cure is rarely possible, since most solitary metastatic lesions are accompanied by a number of "silent" deposits that become evident only over time. The pain of the metastatic lesion of the spine may be secondary to bony destruction or pathologic fracture.[52] Therapy directed specifically at vertebral and cauda equina lesions may include radiation therapy, corticosteroids, or decompression. Radiotherapy may be used alone as primary treatment to decrease pain and slow growth or as adjunctive therapy after surgical decompression.[53, 54] If instability develops, patients may require the placement of rods to control their pain.[55] Metastatic lesions from breast, thyroid, and lymphomatoid tumors are most sensitive to radiotherapy. Corticosteroids may help reduce edema and alleviate symptoms in patients with spinal cord compression.[56] Decompression of the neural elements is usually of little help in returning function to patients with long-standing paraplegia, but it is recommended for those who have recently developed neurologic symptoms.[57] A number of new surgical procedures have been developed for spine stabilization in patients with an unstable vertebral column.[7] Patients with breast and prostate carcinoma who undergo laminectomy improve to a greater degree than those with lung or kidney carcinoma.[11] Surgery should be considered when the diagnosis of the spinal lesion is in doubt, in those with neurologic deterioration owing to metastatic epidural compression at a previously irradiated level, in those with progressive neurologic deterioration during radiotherapy despite large doses of corticosteroids, and in those with symptomatic spinal instability or bone compression of neural structures.[58]

PROGNOSIS

The course of each patient with skeletal metastasis is dependent on a number of factors: the type of tumor, extent of involvement, sensitivity to therapy, and degree of neurologic symptoms; but, in general, the prognosis is poor. In one study, 20% of patients with vertebral metastases developed cord compression.[24] Unless decompression is accomplished quickly, the return of function is minimal and the outcome debilitating. Metastatic disease of unknown primary is uncommon but particularly aggressive. The survival time of these patients is extremely short, with a 6-month-survival rate of 6%.[59]

References

SKELETAL METASTASES

1. Francis KC, Hutter RVP: Neoplasms of the spine in the aged. Clin Orthop 26:54, 1963.
2. Mirra JM: Bone Tumors: Clinical, Radiologic, and Pathologic Correlation. Philadelphia: Lea & Febiger, 1989, pp 1495–1517.
3. Delmarter RB, Sachs BL, Thompson GH, et al.: Primary neoplasms of the thoracic and lumbar spine: an analysis of 29 consecutive cases. Clin Orthop 256:87, 1990.
4. Galasko CSB: Skeletal Metastases. Boston: Butterworths, 1986.
5. Fornasier VL, Horne JG: Metastases to the vertebral column. Cancer 36:590, 1975.
6. Wong DA, Fornasier VL, MacNab I: Spinal metastases: the obvious, the occult, and the impostors. Spine 15:1, 1990.
7. Sundaresan N, Krol G, Digiacinto GV, Hughes JEO: Metastatic tumors of the spine. In: Sundaresan N, Schmidek HH, Schiller AL, Rosenthal DI (eds): Tumors of the Spine: Diagnosis and Clinical Management. Philadelphia: WB Saunders, 1990, pp 279–304.
8. Schaberg J, Gainor BJ: A profile of metastatic carcinoma of the spine. Spine 10:19, 1985.
9. Batson OV: The function of the vertebral veins and their role in the spread of metastasis. Ann Surg 112:138, 1940.
10. Galasko CSB, Doyle FH: The detection of skeletal metastases from mammary cancer. A regional comparison between radiology and scintigraphy. Clin Radiol 23:295, 1972.
11. Lenz M, Fried JR: Metastasis to skeleton, brain, and spinal cord from cancer of the breast and effects of radiotherapy. Ann Surg 93:278, 1931.
12. Mundy GR, Raisz LG, Cooper RA, et al.: Evidence for the secretion of an osteoclast activating factor in myeloma. N Engl J Med 291:1041, 1974.
13. Jacobs SC, Pikna D, Lawson RK: Prostate osteoblastic factor. Invest Urol 17:195, 1979.
14. Galasko CSB: The pathological basis for skeletal scintigraphy. J Bone Joint Surg 57B:353, 1975.
15. Galasko CSB: Skeletal metastases and mammary cancer. Ann Roy Coll Surg Engl 50:3, 1972.
16. Front D, Schenck SO, Frankel A, Robinson E: Bone metastases and bone pain in breast cancer. Are they closely associated? JAMA 242:1747, 1979.
17. Rodriguez M, Dinapoli RP: Spinal cord compression with special reference to metastatic epidural tumors. Mayo Clinic Proc 55:442, 1980.
18. Frassica FJ, Sim FH: Pathophysiology. In: Sim FH (ed): Diagnosis and Management of Metastatic Bone Disease: A Multidisciplinary Approach. New York: Raven Press, 1988, pp 7–14.
19. Rubens RD, Fogelman I: Bone Metastases: Diagnosis and Treatment. New York: Springer-Verlag, 1991, pp 1–247.
20. Deyo RA, Diehk AK: Cancer as cause of back pain: frequency, clinical presentation, and diagnostic strategies. J Gen Intern Med 3:230, 1988.
21. Nicholas JJ, Christy WC: Spinal pain made worse by recumbency: a clue to spinal cord tumors. Arch Phys Med Rehabil 67:598, 1986.
22. Fager CA: Management of malignant intraspinal disease. Surg Clin North Am 47:743, 1967.
23. Constans JP, De Divitiis E, Donzelli R, et al.: Spinal metastases with neurological manifestations: review of 600 cases. J Neurosurg 59:111, 1983.
24. Emsellem HA: Metastatic disease of the spine: diagnosis and management. South Med J 76:1405, 1986.
25. Bishop MC, Hardy JG, Taylor MC, et al.: Bone imaging and serum phosphatase in prostatic carcinoma. Br J Urol 57:317, 1985.
26. Cowan RJ, Young KA: Evaluation of serum alkaline phosphatase determination in patients with positive bone scans. Cancer 32:887, 1973.
27. Gatenby RA, Mulhern CB Jr, Moldofsky PJ: Computed tomography guided thin needle biopsy of small lytic bone lesions. Skeletal Radiol 11:289, 1984.
28. Young JM, Fung FJ Jr: Incidence of tumor metastasis

to the lumbar spine: a comparative study or roent-genographic changes and gross lesions. J Bone Joint Surg 35A:55, 1953.

29. Hubbard DD, Gunn DR: Secondary carcinoma of the spine with destruction of the intervertebral disc. Clin Orthop 88:86, 1972.

30. Resnick D, Niwayama G: Intervertebral disc abnormalities associated with vertebral metastasis: observations in patients and cadavers with prostatic cancer. Invest Radio 13:182, 1978.

31. Fisher MS: Lumbar spine metastasis in cervical carcinoma: a characteristic pattern. Radiology 134:631, 1980.

32. Edelstyn GA, Gillespie PG, Grebbel FS: The radiological demonstration of skeletal metastases: experimental observations. Clin Radiol 18:158, 1967.

33. Craig FS: Metastatic and primary lesions of bone. Clin Orthop 73:33, 1970.

34. Galasko CSB, Sylvester BS: Back pain in patients treated for malignant tumors. Clin Oncol 4:273, 1978.

35. Sy WM, Patel D, Faunce H: Significance of absent or faint kidney sign on bone scan. J Nucl Med 16:454, 1975.

35a. McNeil BJ: Value of bone scanning in neoplastic disease. Semin Nucl Med 4:277, 1984.

36. Wilson JS, Korobkin M, Genant HK, Bovill EG: Computed tomography of musculoskeletal disorders. AJR 13:55, 1978.

37. Redmond J, Spring DB, Munderloh SH, et al.: Spinal computed tomography scanning in the evaluation of metastatic disease. Cancer 54:253, 1984.

38. Muindi J, Coombes RC, Golding S, et al.: The role of computed tomography in the detection of bone metastases in breast cancer patients. Br J Radiol 56:233, 1983.

39. Cranston PE, Patel RB, Harrison RB: Computed tomography for metastatic lesions of the osseous pelvis. South Med J 76:1503, 1983.

40. Weissman DE, Gilbert M, Wang H, Grossman SA: The use of computed tomography of the spine to identify patients at high risk for epidural metastases. J Clin Oncol 3:1541, 1985.

41. Gilbert RW, Kim JH, Posner JB: Epidural spinal cord compression from metastatic tumor: diagnosis and treatment. Ann Neurol 3:340, 1978.

42. Zimmer WD, Berquist TH, McLeod RA, et al.: Bone tumors: magnetic resonance imaging versus computed tomography. Radiology 155:709, 1985.

43. Maravilla KR, Lesh P, Weinre JC, et al.: Magnetic resonance imaging of the lumbar spine with CT correlation. AJNR 6:237, 1985.

44. Yuh WT, Zachar CK, Barloon TJ, et al.: Vertebral compression fractures: distinction between benign and malignant causes with MR imaging. Radiology 172:215, 1989.

45. Khurana JS, Rosenthal DI, Rosenberg A, Mankin HJ: Skeletal metastases in liposarcoma detectable only by magnetic resonance imaging. Clin Orthop 243:204, 1989.

46. Avrahami E, Tadmor R, Dally O, Hadar H: Early MR demonstration of spinal metastases in patients with normal radiographs and CT and radionuclide bone scans. J Comput Assist Tomogr 13:598, 1989.

47. Beatrous TE, Choyke PL, Frank JA: Diagnostic evaluation of cancer patients with pelvic pain: comparison of scintigraphy, CT, and MR imaging. AJR 155:85, 1990.

48. Sze G, Stimac GK, Bartlett C, et al.: Multicenter study of gadopentetate dimeglumine as an MR contrast agent: evaluation in patients with spinal tumors. AJNR 11:967, 1990.

49. Carmody RF, Yang PJ, Seeley GW, et al.: Spinal cord compression due to metastatic disease: diagnosis with MR imaging versus myelography. Radiology 173:225, 1989.

50. Bonner JA, Lichter AS: A caution about the use of MRI to diagnose spinal cord compression. N Engl J Med 322:556, 1990.

51. Craig FS: Vertebral body biopsy. J Bone Joint Surg 38A:93, 1956.

52. Bhalla SK: Metastatic disease of the spine. Clin Orthop 73:52, 1970.

53. Bruckman JE, Bloomer WD: Management of spinal cord compression. Semin Oncol 5:135, 1978.

54. Khan FR, Glickman AS, Chu FCH, Nickson JJ: Treatment by radiotherapy of spinal cord compression due to extradural metastases. Radiology 89:495, 1967.

55. Dewald RL, Bridwell KH, Prodromas C, Rodts MF: Reconstructive spinal surgery as palliation for metastatic malignancies of the spine. Spine 10:21, 1985.

56. Clark PRR, Saunders M. Steroid-induced remission in spinal canal reticulum cell sarcoma: report of two cases. J Neurosurg 42:346–348, 1975.

57. Vieth RG, Odom GL: Extradural spinal metastases and their neurosurgical treatment. J Neurosurg 23:501, 1965.

58. Byrne TN: Spinal cord compression from epidural metastases. N Engl J Med 327:614, 1992.

59. Saengnipanthkul S, Jirarattanaphochai K, Rojviroj S, et al.: Metastatic adenocarcinoma of the spine. Spine 17:427, 1992.

Intraspinal Neoplasms

Capsule Summary

E = Extradural
IE = Intradural-Extramedullary
I = Intramedullary

Frequency of back pain
  E: very common
  IE: common
  I: rare
Location of back pain
  E: lumbar spine
  IE: low back and leg
  I: low back and leg
Quality of back pain
  E: increasing local ache
  IE: referred pain
  I: radicular
Laboratory and x-ray tests
  E: MR
  IE: MR
  I: MR
Treatment
  E: radiotherapy, corticosteroids, laminectomy
  IE: surgical excision
  I: surgical excision

PREVALENCE AND PATHOGENESIS

While bone is the tissue in the axial skeleton most frequently affected by primary and metastatic tumors, less commonly tissues inside the spinal column may be affected by neoplastic processes. These intraspinal neoplasms may be extradural, between bone and the covering of the spinal cord, the dura; intradural-extramedullary, between the dura and the spinal cord; and intramedullary, in the spinal cord proper (Fig. 13–45). Extradural tumors are most commonly metastatic in origin. Intradural-extramedullary tumors are predominantly meningiomas, neurofibromas, or lipomas. Intramedullary tumors are ependymomas and gliomas (Table 13–5).

Tumors of the spinal cord and its coverings are uncommon, constituting 10% of central nervous system neoplasms. A study in Norway revealed the annual incidence of primary intraspinal neoplasms as 5 per million for females and 3 per million for males.[1] They occur in individuals between the ages of 20 and 60 and have equal distribution in men and women.

Extradural tumors are metastatic lesions that have invaded the intraspinal space from contiguous structures. These are the most common tumors of the spinal canal. Of the intradural lesions, extramedullary neoplasms occur more commonly than intramedullary

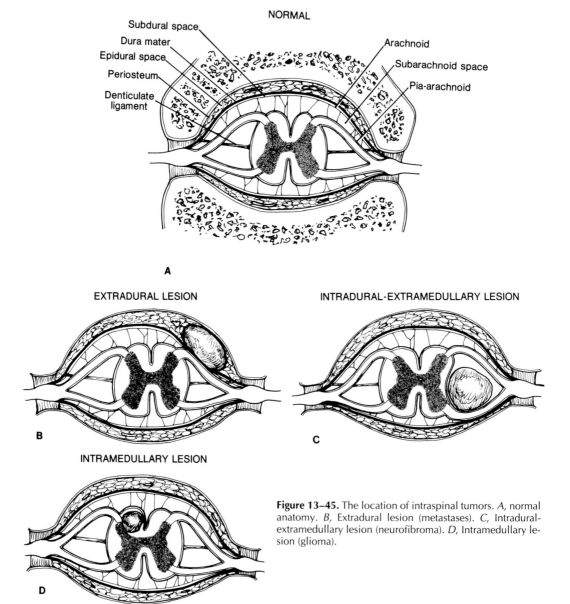

Figure 13–45. The location of intraspinal tumors. *A,* normal anatomy. *B,* Extradural lesion (metastases). *C,* Intradural-extramedullary lesion (neurofibroma). *D,* Intramedullary lesion (glioma).

TABLE 13–5. INTRASPINAL MASSES

EXTRADURAL (50%–60%)
Metastases
   Lung
   Prostate
   Breast
Lymphoma
Chordoma
Meningioma
Fibroma
Lipoma/Lipomatosis
Vascular malformation with bleeding
Abscess

INTRADURAL-EXTRAMEDULLARY (30%–35%)
Neurofibroma
Neurilemoma
Meningioma
Neurinoma
Lipoma
Arachnoid cyst
Leptomeningeal metastasis
Vascular abnormalities

INTRAMEDULLARY (10%–20%)
Glioma
   Ependymoma
   Astrocytoma
Arteriovenous malformation
Syringomyelia

neoplasms. Intraspinal neoplasms occur in adults, with a predominance in patients between 30 and 50 years of age.[2]

The extradural, or epidural, space is the predominant site for intraspinal malignant tumors. Metastatic tumors in the spinal canal are extradural in location because the dura is resistant to invasion from lesions that extend from foci in vertebral bone. The extradural space is also the location of Batson's plexus, which is a site for hematogenous spread of tumor.[3] Major structures in the intradural-extramedullary space are meninges and spinal nerve roots. Meningiomas and neurofibromas arise from these structures. Depending on the population of patients being studied, meningiomas may cause a quarter of intraspinal neoplasms. Intramedullary tumors arise in the spinal cord itself and are composed of cells that make up the support structure of the cord, ependymal and glial cells. Metastatic lesions to the spinal cord are extremely rare.[4] Gliomas of the spinal cord occur less frequently than neurofibromas or meningiomas. Gliomas affect men more commonly than women.

CLINICAL HISTORY

Intraspinal tumors may demonstrate a wide variety of clinical symptoms. Patients with extradural metastatic disease have pain as their initial complaint. Pain may localize to the affected area in the spine or may radiate to the lower extremities if neural elements are compressed. The pain characteristically increases in intensity and is unrelenting. The pain is increased at night with recumbency owing to lengthening of the spine. Pain with recumbency may occur with extradural or intradural-extramedullary lesions such as multiple myeloma, meningioma, or neurilemoma.[5] Activity also may exacerbate the discomfort. The pain is unresponsive to mild analgesics and requires narcotics for control. Not uncommonly, neurologic dysfunction rapidly follows axial pain. Neurologic symptoms include weakness, loss of sensation, and incontinence.

Intradural-extramedullary tumors grow in proximity to nerve roots and are associated with radicular pain or axial skeletal pain. Meningiomas and neurofibromas are slow-growing tumors, and this corresponds to slow evolution of symptoms in patients. Nocturnal symptoms are increased in these patients. Activity during the day may not be associated with symptoms. Neurologic symptoms are slower to develop than in patients with metastatic disease. Symptoms may persist and increase to the degree of complaints associated with a herniated lumbar disc. The slow, insidious onset of pain, without intermittency, may be helpful in identifying these patients but is not of great enough specificity to distinguish patients with neurofibroma from those with disc disease.[6] It is also important to remember that these tumors affect the nerves that travel to the lower extremities. Patients may present with dysesthesias in the buttock and lower leg, without back pain. This circumstance may occur with generalized neurofibromatosis (von Recklinghausen's disease), solitary neurofibroma, or other intramedullary-extradural neoplasms (such as lipoma).[7]

Intramedullary tumors are frequently painless owing to their location within the spinal cord proper, which disrupts the normal transmission of pain impulses. However, not all of these neoplasms are painless. Some patients may develop radicular or girdle type of pain as an early and persistent symptom. The onset may be insidious and the progression unrelenting. Not infrequently, weakness, spasticity, and sensory deficits below the level of the lesion develop. Conus medullaris tumors may cause stress incontinence as an early complaint associated with bladder dysfunction.[8] Some authors have described dysesthesias, "electricity-like" sensations, in patients with intramedullary tumors.[9]

The pain associated with intraspinal tumors is different from the pain associated with mechanical disease of the spine. Patients with intraspinal tumors will often tell of sleeping sitting up in a chair because of a marked increase in severity of pain when trying to sleep in a normal position. In contrast, in mechanical spinal disease the sitting position increases pressure on the anatomic structures of the lumbosacral spine and increases pain. The presence of this one part of the history should lead to a thorough evaluation for an intraspinal tumor.[10]

The motor and sensory features of compression are dependent on the extent and pattern of cord and nerve root distribution. Pure intramedullary tumors do not disturb nerve roots but ependymomas may involve the lower sacral cord and involve the corresponding roots. Extramedullary tumors between T11 and L2 compress cord and roots. Lesions below the cord cause cauda equina symptoms. Distinguishing conus (S2–S5) lesions from tumors in the cauda equina is difficult.[11]

PHYSICAL EXAMINATION

Examination of patients with extradural tumors may demonstrate pain on palpation with associated muscle spasm and limitation of motion. Neurologic findings correspond to the level and extent of compression on the spinal roots and cord. Patients with intradural-extramedullary tumors demonstrate slowly changing neurologic abnormalities, including gait disturbance, sensory changes, and urinary or rectal incontinence. They also may demonstrate lower extremity muscle atrophy. Patients with multiple neurofibromas may demonstrate spinal angulation, scoliosis, and/or kyphosis.[12] Those with von Recklinghausen's disease progress to develop paraplegia.[13] Patients with intramedullary tumors may have specific sensory changes that correlate with the location of these tumors in the center of the cord. Light touch and position sensation are normal, while pain and temperature sensation are lost. Hyperreflexia is a result of pressure on the pyramidal tracts. This finding helps differentiate patients with intramedullary tumors from those with herniated disc, in whom hyperreflexia is a distinctly unusual finding.[14] Hyperreflexia also may be associated with spasticity.

In addition to the neurologic examination, careful inspection of other organ systems may discover abnormalities that will suggest possible diagnoses. Examination of the skin may reveal café-au-lait patches or axillary freckles associated with neurofibromatosis. The presence of a tuft of hair, pigmented nevus, skin dimple indicates the presence of spina bifida or tumor such as lipomas, dermoid, or epidermoid cysts. Kyphosis may be related to wedge collapse of a vertebral body secondary to extradural tumor extension.

LABORATORY DATA

Abnormal laboratory values are most closely associated with extradural metastatic lesions. The location, degree of spread, and histologic type of tumor will have an effect on the pattern of laboratory abnormalities. Intradural tumors do not metastasize outside the spinal canal and are not associated with abnormal hematologic or chemical factors. Evaluation of cerebrospinal fluid obtained by lumbar puncture may demonstrate marked elevation in spinal fluid protein in all of these tumors. The fluid is usually obtained during myelographic study in a patient with suspected intraspinal tumor.

Histologic findings depend on the cell of origin of the tumor. The most common primary tumor causing extradural metastases in women is carcinoma of the breast, while carcinoma of the lung is most common in men.[15–17] Meningiomas are encapsulated, nodular soft tumors with a wide range of histologic patterns, including meningothelial, fibroblastic, and psammomatous types.[18] The most common forms of cord meningiomas, in decreasing incidence, are psammomatous, angioblastic, fibrous, and anaplastic. The lumbosacral spine is a relatively infrequent location for these tumors compared to the thoracic area.[10] Neurofibroma may appear as a fusiform swelling of a nerve root or as a pedunculated mass. Intraspinal neurofibromas may take on a dumbbell form with a central mass inside the vertebral canal connected by a shaft of tumor passing through the intervertebral foramen, forming a peripheral mass.[19] Histologic patterns of neurofibromas may vary but usually contain fibrous tissue in an interlacing configuration.

Ependymomas arise from cells that line the central ventricular system of the spinal cord. Gliomas arise from glial cells, which are the supporting cells for the nerve cells of the nervous system. Gliomas may be peripherally or centrally located in the spinal cord. Ependymomas and gliomas are associated with a variety of histologic forms. In adults, the forms most often encountered are ependymomas

(60%), astrocytomas (20%), glioblastomas (7%), and oligodendrogliomas (4%).[10, 20]

RADIOGRAPHIC EVALUATION

Radiographic evaluation of the patient with an intraspinal tumor can be very helpful in determining the exact location of tumor in the caudal-rostral orientation and its position in the extradural, intradural-extramedullary, or intramedullary space. Abnormalities noted on plain roentgenograms, CT scans, or MR can pinpoint the location of lesions and help determine their potential source (Fig. 13–46).

Radiographic abnormalities on plain roentgenograms of extradural tumors are characterized by destruction of bone in proximity to the growing lesion. Malignant tumors are associated with rapid destruction of bone with loss of posterior elements of vertebral body or vertebral body collapse. On lateral roentgeno-

grams, intraspinal lesions may be associated with posterior scalloping of the vertebral bodies, a consequence of their location and slow growth (Table 13–6).[21] Neurofibromas may grow through intervertebral foramina, which results in uniform dilatation of affected as compared with adjacent foramina. Intramedullary tumors rarely cause anatomic alterations that are discernible on plain roentgenograms.

Myelographic studies are very useful in determining the exact location of an intraspinal tumor.[22, 23] Extradural tumors frequently cause a complete block of the myelographic dye at the point of spinal cord compression. The block has irregular edges and varying radiographic densities, and displaces the spinal contents.

The myelographic features may be divided into four basic forms:

1. A lesion may be peripherally situated, displacing the dura and cord. This results in wid-

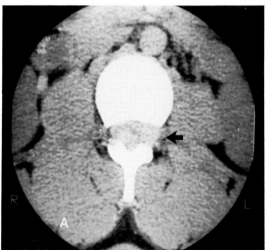

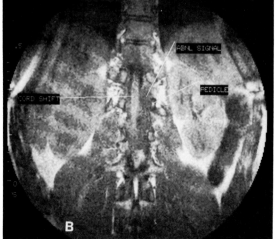

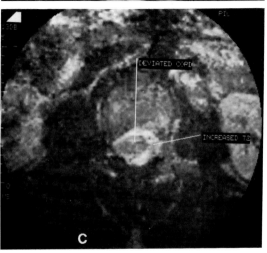

Figure 13–46. An 18-year-old man developed three episodes of midback pain that radiated to the right and left groin. *A,* A CT scan suggests a mass increasing the size of the L1 neural foramen *(arrow)*. *B,* MR revealed abnormal signal from T12 to L2 on the left. *C,* MR cross-sectional view demonstrated a mass pushing the spinal cord to the right. Hemilaminectomy of T12 to L2 revealed an intradural cyst filled with clear fluid extending from L2 to T11. Postoperatively, the patient had resolution of his pain.

TABLE 13–6. POSTERIOR VERTEBRAL SCALLOPING

1. Increased intraspinal pressure
   A. Generalized—communicating hydrocephalus
   B. Localized—syringomyelia, intraspinal cysts, intradural neoplasms
2. Bone resorption
   A. Acromegaly
3. Congenital disorders
   A. Idiopathic
   B. Neurofibromatosis
   C. Marfan's syndrome
   D. Ehlers-Danlos syndrome
   E. Mucopolysaccharidosis IV (Morquio's disease)
   F. Dysostosis multiplex (Hurler's disease)
   G. Osteogenesis imperfecta
4. Small spinal canal
   A. Achondroplasia
5. Normal variant
   A. Physiologic scalloping

Modified from Mitchell GH, Lourie H, Berne AS. The various cases of scalloped vertebrae with notes on their pathogenesis. Radiology 89:87, 1967.

ening of the space between the dye column and the pedicle on the side with the tumor and narrowing contralaterally.

2. An anterior or posterior tumor may cause flattening of the cord. This finding may simulate that associated with intramedullary tumors.

3. A shallow filling defect without cord displacement may be seen.

4. A lesion that encircles the cord causes constriction of the subarachnoid space without cord displacement.

Intradural-extramedullary lesions produce a sharp, smooth, concave outline, since the tumor is in direct contact with the dye. The spinal cord may be displaced to one side, and spinal nerve roots may be stretched over the lesion.

Intramedullary tumors arise in the spinal cord. The myelogram demonstrates fusiform enlargement of the spinal cord with tapering of the column of dye superiorly and inferiorly. Not all fusiform swellings of the cord are secondary to intramedullary tumors. Extradural tumors may flatten the contralateral aspect of the cord. Therefore, films must be taken at 90° angles so that intramedullary lesions are not confused with extradural lesions.

The addition of gadolinium contrast to the technique of MR has helped increase the sensitivity of this method in the detection of intraspinal tumors. In one study of intraspinal tumors, gadolinium enhancement detected ependymomas (intense, homogeneous, sharply margined lesions), and astrocytomas (patchy,

ill-defined lesions).[25] The differences in appearance of the two lesions was not adequate to allow MR to be useful in differentiating the histology of these intraspinal tumors. However, enhancement with gadolinium helps define the location, size, configuration, and character of the lesion.[26] Extramedullary-intradural tumors also are enhanced by gadolinium-contrast MR. The mechanism of enhancement is not the breakdown of the blood-brain barrier, but the highly vascular characteristics of the tumors, such as meningiomas and neurinomas. Gadolinium is helpful in the detection of leptomeningeal spread of a metastatic tumor, and in differentiating cystic lesions (syringomyelia) from intramedullary tumors that have similar radiographic characteristics on unenhanced MR. In patients with unexpected neurologic signs, contrast-enhanced MR may detect metastases to the pial membrane secondary to lymphoma, leukemia, adenocarcinoma of the lung, prostate carcinoma, malignant melanoma, or other tumors.[27]

DIFFERENTIAL DIAGNOSIS

The diagnosis of an intraspinal tumor is suggested by the presence of back pain that is persistent and increased by recumbency, neurologic dysfunction, and myelographic abnormalities. The definitive diagnosis requires histologic confirmation. A high level of suspicion is necessary to make this diagnosis. Patients with intradural tumor may present with lower extremity symptoms of long duration. This association must be kept in mind or the correct diagnosis may be missed.[7]

Extradural Lesions

The differential diagnosis of extradural lesions includes neoplastic and non-neoplastic lesions. Metastatic lesions from lung, prostate, or breast are frequent causes of epidural lesions. Primary tumors—lymphoma, chordoma, meningioma, fibroma, or lipoma—also may cause epidural lesions.

Angiolipomas make up approximately 2.2% of extradural tumors of the spine.[28] Angiolipomas occur more commonly in the thoracic spine, with occasional lumbar involvement. Lumbar lesions cause radicular symptoms with leg weakness. MR evaluation of these lesions reveals a homogeneous mass with T_1- and T_2-weighted images with signal close to that of subcutaneous fat. Gadolinium contrast increased uptake reveals the vascular nature of this benign tumor.[29] Angiolipoma is more common than lipoma and liposarcoma as a tumor of the epidural fat. The tumor is amenable to surgical excision. Careful review of CT scan and myelographic views are helpful in differentiating herniated discs from metastatic tumors.[30]

Epidural Abscess. A potentially diastrous non-neoplastic epidural lesion associated with delayed diagnosis is epidural abscess. These patients present with acute-onset, severe back pain with progressive neurologic dysfunction, which can progress to complete paraplegia in 2 hours.[31] These patients usually have evidence of a bacterial infection elsewhere, are acutely ill with fever, are disoriented, and exhibit signs of a parameningeal infection on cerebrospinal fluid examination. On myelogram, the extradural defect may extend over several vertebral levels.[52] MR has increased the opportunity to make the correct diagnosis of extradural abscess without the need for invasive procedures, such as myelograms (see Chapter 12, p 310).[33]

Epidural Hematoma. Spontaneous epidural hematoma may mimic the time course and symptoms of epidural abscess.[34] The bleeding may be associated with a small extradural vascular malformation or occur spontaneously without any specific anatomic abnormality. Most reported epidural hematomas are spontaneous and acute. The decreasing order of frequency of axial involvement is cervical, thoracic, and lumbar spine.[35] Most hematomas extend two or more segments and are located in a posterolateral position. Chronic epidural hematomas are rare and occur in the lumbar spine. In this location, the spinal canal is larger than in the cervial and thoracic spine, and the cauda equina is better able to tolerate pressure than the spinal cord. Patients with extradural caverous hemangiomas and bleeding have developed symptoms of sciatica secondary to nerve root compression.[36] Epidural hematomas have been associated with neurogenic claudication suggestive of lumbar spinal stenosis.[37] Epidural hematomas have been reported as complications of invasive procedures including surgery and myelograms and may occur in patients who are normotensive with normal blood coaguability (Fig. 13–47).[38, 39] Bleeding also may occur in individual on anticoagulants.[40] A hematoma may be a complication of patients with a bleeding diathesis secondary to a connective tissue disease (Fig. 13–48). The diagnosis is corroborated by a mass with a T_1-weighted increased signal intensity and T_2-weighted decreased signal intensity on MR. Epidural hematomas may be treated conservatively without surgery. However, surgical intervention is required if neurologic dysfunction does not resolve.

Epidural Lipomatosis. High-dose corticosteroid therapy may cause the accumulation of fat in an epidural location. Patients who have renal transplants, asthma, rheumatoid arthritis, radiation pneumonitis, polyarteritis nodosa, Cushing's disease, and morbid obesity develop epidural lipomatosis.[41] Corticosteroids in doses ranging from 5 to 180 mg/day have been associated with lipomatosis. The onset of lipomatosis may occur in 6 months to 13 years after starting therapy. Epidural lipomatosis can

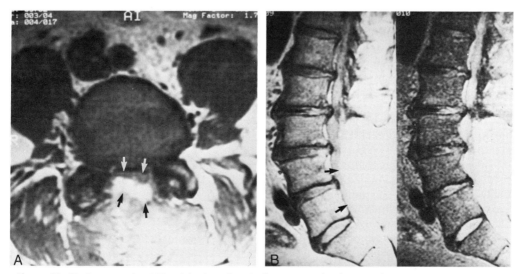

Figure 13–47. Postoperative MR axial *(A)* and sagittal *(B)* T₁-weighted image demonstrating a high signal intensity collection of fluid *(black arrows)* compressing the cauda equina *(white arrows)*. This collection was an epidural hematoma that required surgical evacuation. (From Borenstein DG: Low back pain. In Klippel J, Dieppe P (eds): Rheumatology. St. Louis: CV Mosby, 1994, Sec 5, 4.9.)

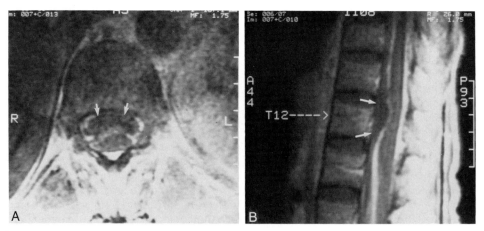

Figure 13–48. MR axial *(A)* and sagittal *(B)* T$_1$-weighted image of the T12 level demonstrating extradural and intradural fluid collection *(white arrows)* compressing the spinal cord. The signal in the subarachnoid space is compatible with blood. These lesions in this systemic lupus erythematosus patient resulted in paraparesis. She subsequently expired from extension of the hematoma and overwhelming sepsis.

cause neurologic symptoms of lower extremity weakness and loss of sensation. Symptoms associated with epidural lipomatosis include back pain, radicular pain, loss of sensation, burning dysesthesia, and lower extremity weakness. Upper motor neuron signs (Babinski sign, hyperreflexia) or lower motor neuron signs (hyporeflexia) have been reported depending on the location of epidural compression of the spinal cord or cauda equina, respectively. Additional signs include weakness, decreased proprioception, decreased pain sensation, positive straight leg raising test, and sphincter dysfunction. Transaxial CT scan reveals abundant soft tissue surrounding the thecal sac. T$_1$-weighted MR reveals increased signal intensity in the lipid mass. Fat has almost a pathognomonic appearance on MR (increased T$_1$-weighted signal and intermediate T$_2$-weighted signal intensity). MR is an ideal technique to identify extradural fat.[42] The treatment for this condition may be surgical or medical. Multilevel laminectomy may improve symptoms and signs but also is associated with significant mortality in patients requiring high-dose steroid treatment.[41] However, with cessation of steroid therapy, the epidural fat deposits may disappear with resolution of symptoms.[43]

Spinal Synovial Cyst. Intraspinal synovial cysts arise from the joint lining of the apophyseal joint and have been reported in the lumbar spine. The cysts occur most frequently at the L4-L5 level.[44] These lesions are associated with degenerative joint disease, trauma, and rheumatoid arthritis.[45, 46] These extradural lesions may be asymptomatic or may cause radicular symptoms associated with sensory and mo-

tor dysfunction. Spinal synovial cysts may appear and cause symptoms in less than 1 year.[47] CT appearance of lumbar intraspinal synovial cysts is characterized by a cystic mass with a broad base extending from the apophyseal joint. Hemorrhage into the cyst causes increased CT attenuation. Calcification of the cyst may occur in a chronic stage after hemorrhage. The presence of an attachment between the apophyseal joint and the synovial cyst can be proven by injecting contrast material into the joint and its subsequent dispersal throughout the cyst.[48] MR evaluation of cysts is difficult since the contents of the cyst have a significant effect on varying signal intensities. Cysts may recede spontaneously and do not require surgery. However, cysts that cause nerve root compression or neurogenic claudication require surgical decompression.[44]

Intradural-Extramedullary Lesions

Intradural-extramedullary lesions in adults are predominantly neurofibromas, neurilemomas (Schwannomas), and meningiomas. Neurofibromas arise from proliferating nerve fibers, fibroblasts, and Schwann cells. A neurilemoma consists of Schwann cells and collagen fibers. Meningiomas arise from the meninges, which support the spinal cord. The arachnoid may also be a source of lesions as well as vessel abnormalities.

Neurofibroma. Neurofibromatosis type-1 (peripheral neurofibromatosis) is the most common hereditary syndrome predisposing to neoplasms at a rate of 1/3000 live births in the United States.[49] Neurofibromatosis type-2 is associated with bilateral acoustic neuromas.

These entities are genetically separate: type-1 is associated with a locus on chromosome 17 and type-2 with a deletion on the long arm of chromosome 22.[50] Neurofibromas, like neurilemomas, contain Schwann cells but can be differentiated by histologic examination, since they have a more disorganized, plexiform appearance. Primary neurofibromas of the spinal cord occur most commonly in the cauda equina. They may involve sensory or motor roots or the entire nerve. Neurofibromas may occur singly or multiply (Von Recklinghausen's disease). The autosomal dominant illness with variable penetrance may be easily recognized when the cutaneous manifestations (café-au-lait spots, axillary freckling, and cutaneous neurofibromas) are present. The disease may become manifest when the patient is a child or as an adult with kyphoscoliosis, vertebral scalloping, and intervertebral foramen widening.[51] Malignant deterioration of neurofibromas occurs in 3% of cases and is more likely to occur in patients with multiple tumors as opposed to solitary lesions.[52] Neurofibromatosis also may be associated with malignant bone tumors, but rarely.[53] On occasion, tumors of the peripheral sciatic nerve must be differentiated from tumors in the central nervous system.[54] In patients with type-1 and type-2, the MR findings include multiple masses in both extramedullary and intradural locations.[55] Skeletal abnormalities include dural ectasias and posterior scalloping. Scoliosis occurred in 17% of individuals in a study of 47 neurofibromatosis patients.[56] A rare abnormality is spondyloptosis with verticalization of the sacrum.[57] A minority of patients will have no spinal abnormalities.

Neurilemoma. Neurilemomas are common cord tumors constituting 30% to 35% of all primary intraspinal neoplasms, occurring most often in adults between 30 to 40 years of age. Approximately 30% of these tumors occur in the lumbar area of which 70% are in an intradural-extramedullary position. These tumors are considered benign and slow growing and cause symptoms by exerting pressure on adjacent structures.[10] Neurilemoma is one of the extraosseous spinal lesions mimicking disc disease.[58] Patients with intraspinal tumors have painless neurologic deficits, pain with recumbency, pain disproportionate to that expected with lumbar disc disease, no improvement with disc surgery, and elevated spinal fluid protein. Neurilemoma is not limited to the lumbar spine but also may appear in the sacrum.[59] Lesions may become very large in the sacrum with minimal symptoms. MR of the lumbar spine is a noninvasive means to scan the conus and cauda equina for the presence of these tumors.

Meningioma. Meningiomas are benign, well-circumscribed tumors, which constitute about 25% of all primary intraspinal neoplasms. They occur in adults 40 to 70 years of age and more commonly in women. As opposed to neurofibromas, meningiomas tend to remain intradural. They are more common in the thoracic spine but occasionally occur at the lumbosacral level.[60] Only 2% occur in the lumbar spine.[11] Meningiomas differ from neurofibroma by occurring in older individuals, are located commonly in a lateral position, have a dumbbell shape only on occasion, calcify more often, and have more prominent sensory abnormalities than motor symptoms. Midline back pain is the most common early complaint with spinal meningiomas. The average duration of symptoms before diagnosis is 2 years but about 50% come to surgery within a year of onset. The ideal treatment is surgical excision of the tumor and its dural attachment.

Intradural Lipoma. Intradural lipomas may occur in the presence or absence of spina bifida. They are located most commonly in the lower thoracic and upper lumbar spine. The incidence of spinal lipoma with spina bifida varies from 40% to 78%. This lesion usually becomes manifest during childhood. Without spina bifida, intraspinal lipoma is a rare tumor that rarely affects the conus medullaris.[23]

Arachnoid Cyst. Cysts may arise from the arachnoid and are known by the terms arachnoid cyst or diverticulum.[61] These lesions occur in young adults most commonly in the thoracic spine and occasionally in the lumbar area. Patients may have fluctuating back and leg pain, sphincter malfunction, scoliosis, and paraparesis. The presence of posterior scalloping of a vertebral body helps raise the possibility of this lesion in a patient with neurologic symptoms. Perineural cysts in the sacral region (Tarlov cysts) are associated with perineal pain.[62] Atypical sciatic pain radiating to the groin may be present without difficulty in voiding. Neurologic examination may reveal decreased sensation in the perineal area or may be normal. MR of these patients is superior to CT with myelography in identifying the presence of sacral perineural cysts. In a study of 17 patients with perineal pain without urologic, gynecologic, or anorectal abnormalities, MR detected sacral cysts in 13 (76%) patients.[63] Surgical removal of the cysts is associated with resolution of perineal pain in a majority of patients with Tarlov cysts.

Arachnoiditis. Arachnoiditis is a nonspecific inflammatory process causing fibrosis of arachnoid membrane. The pathogenesis of arachnoiditis involves the development of a mild, inflammatory cellular exudate similar to the inflammatory response necessary to repair serous membranes like the peritoneum.[64] A fibrous exudate covers the nerve roots, causing them to adhere to one another and the thecal sac. Proliferating fibrocytes form dense collagenous adhesions around the roots. Arachnoiditis evolves from a stage of inflammation of the pia-arachnoid with hyperemia and swelling of the nerve roots, followed by arachnoditis and fibroblast proliferation and adhesion. The final stage of arachnoiditis causes complete encapsulation of the structure with hypoxia and atrophy of the nerve root.[65]

Inflammatory changes of the arachnoid space (arachnoiditis) may cause changes on myelogram which should not be confused with an arachnoid cyst. Cysts cause localized lesions. Arachnoiditis causes loculations of contrast dye, partial or complete obstruction of dye flow, and obliteration of nerve root sleeves (Fig. 13–49).

Causes of arachnoiditis are listed in Table 13–7.[66, 67, 68] A frequently implicated agent in

TABLE 13–7. CAUSES OF ARACHNOIDITIS

Surgery
  Extradural
    Discectomy
    Laminectomy
    Lumbar spine fusion
  Intradural
    Closure of spinal fistula
    Nerve root severed
Injected agents
  Contrast media
  Anesthetic agents
  Intradural steroids
Space-occupying lesion
  Neurofibroma
Infection
Intrathecal hemorrhage

the development of arachnoiditis is the oily contrast agent, iophendylate, when it is not removed from the spinal canal after myelography. A study of 98 patients who underwent iophendylate ventriculography did not develop arachnoiditis in a remote location in the lumbar spine despite a followup period of up to 28 years.[69] Oily contrast agents have been replaced with a water-soluble contrast agent not associated with the development of arachnoiditis. Other exogenous causes of arachnoiditis include infection (tuberculosis),[70] intrathecal medications and anesthetic agents such as bupivacaine.[71, 72] Arachnoiditis may be the cause of unsuccessful back surgery in more than 11% of individuals.[73, 74] Retained swab debris may be the source of the inflammatory response.[75]

The clinical symptoms associated with arachnoidits include diffuse constant back pain, radicular pain, paresthesias, dyesthesias, causalgia, motor weakness, and sphincter dysfunction. Physical signs include back tenderness, muscular spasm, atrophy, scoliosis, limited straight leg raising, hyporeflexia, and urinary sphincter dysfunction.

MR is the best radiographic technique to evaluate arachnoiditis. The three MR patterns of arachnoiditis are conglomerations of adherent nerve roots residing centrally within the thecal sac, nerve roots adherent to the meninges, and a soft tissue mass replacing the subarachnoid space (Fig. 13–50).[76, 77] Arachnoiditis that fills the subarachnoid space may have MR characteristics that mirror those of a spinal cord tumor.[78] Gadolinium enhanced MR does not increase the signal intensity of arachnoiditis, and the absence of enhancement helps differentiate neoplastic lesions from arachnoiditis.[76]

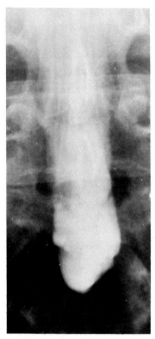

Figure 13–49. Arachnoiditis in patient who had undergone multiple back operations. Metrizamide was used; but because of scar tissue, it looks as if Pantopaque was employed. (From Wiesel SW, Bernini P, Rothman RH: The Aging Lumbar Spine. Philadelphia, WB Saunders Co, 1982.)

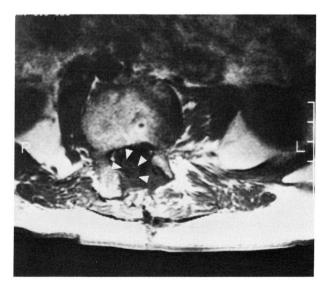

Figure 13–50. An 80-year-old woman had persistent burning leg pain after multiple surgical lumbar spine procedures. MR T₁-weighted axial view revealed a clumped mass of nerve roots *(white arrows)* in the dural sac characteristic of arachnoiditis.

The disability associated with arachnoiditis is the severe pain. The physical impairments change relatively little during the course of the illness. Urinary symptoms characterized by urgency, frequency, and incontinence develop late in the course of the illness. These patients have a poor prognosis since no therapy has been developed, which consistently decreases inflammation or diminishes their symptoms.

Arteriovenous Malformations (AVM). Vascular malformations may be located in the lumbar area of the spinal column. Lesions may be arterial, capillary, cavernous or arteriovenous. Vascular lesions affect the cervical and thoracic spinal cord more commonly than the cauda equina. Increased pressure in vessels causes structural alterations that result in vessel enlargement. Dysfunction of the spinal cord may occur secondary to impingement by the vessel mass or impairment of normal venous drainage secondary to abnormally high pressure in spinal cord capillaries. The majority of adults with AVM are over 30 years of age and male. The clinical course is one of progressive symptoms of back and radicular pain, dysesthesias, and painful claudication. Episodes of vessel thrombosis may accentuate the symptoms and signs. The clinical course of these patients may be hours to weeks. A cavernous angioma of the cauda equina may present with a subarachnoid hemorrhage.[79] Low back pain and sciatica also may be associated with a cavernoma of the cauda equina.[80] Electrophysiologic signs associated with AVM of the spinal cord include scattered, multiple, bilateral thoracolumbosacral radiculopathies consistent with axonal or neuronal destruction, associated with paraspinal fibrillations, or abnormal activation of motor unit potentials. The presence of these abnormalities depended on the caudal extension of the AVM, its arterial supply, and the duration of symptoms.[81] These lesions are best localized by spinal angiography.[82] AVM may not always be visualized by MR.[83] However, MR is a useful technique for the study of AVMs and is able to detect myelomalacia, edema, and reversible scalloping of the spinal cord; thrombosis and thickening of blood vessels; new bleeding versus old hematoma; and documents the alterations associated with angiographic or surgical correction of the lesion.[84, 85]

Vascular malformations also may be identified in an intramedullary location. These intramedullary vascular lesions are located in the cervical and thoracic spine. Lesions in the cervical spine are associated with arm and leg dysfunction, while thoracic cord lesions are associated with lower extremity motor or sensory abnormalities.[86, 87] Once identified, these lesions may be left alone, embolized, or surgically treated.[88] Clinical improvement is common in patients who have had operative resection or angiographic ablation.[89, 90] Patients with neurogenic claudication may undergo surgery for suspected spinal stenosis but may have an AVM as the cause of their symptoms. Relief of venous hypertension in both conditions may be one of the mechanisms by which surgical or angiographic intervention improves symptoms of neurogenic claudication.[91]

Leptomeningeal Metastases. Leptomeningeal spread of tumor is relatively rare, since the dura is a barrier to the spread of malignant tumors. In adults, this form of metastasis occurs with lymphoma, oat cell carcinoma, and breast cancer. In one study, 5% of patients with breast cancer had leptomeningeal involvement.[92] Lung carcinoma is the second most common primary tumor causing leptomeningeal disease, followed by melanoma.[93] Patients with widespread metastatic disease develop this problem, although it is occasionally the cause of initial symptoms of back pain in an individual patient. The clinical hallmark of this lesion is the involvement of the nervous system at more than one location. This may include extremity weakness, paresthesias, back or radicular pain, sphincter dysfunction, or all the symptoms of cauda equina compression. On physical examination, patients have focal weakness, asymmetric reflexes, and spotty sensory loss. The diagnosis is confirmed by cerebrospinal fluid cytologic examination. Patients may be treated with irradiation or intrathecal therapy. The prognosis is usually poor.

Intramedullary Lesions

Intramedullary lesions are primarily gliomas, vascular malformations, syringomyelia, lipoma, lymphoma, and melanoma. These lesions may occur with neurologic dysfunction without pain.

Syringomyelia. Syringomyelia is a fluid-filled cyst lined with benign glial cells that is located in the central portion of the spinal cord. Syringomyelia is associated with congenital abnormalities (Chiari malformations), trauma, infections (meningitis), or inflammatory processes (arachnoiditis).[94, 95] Arachnoiditis may cause syrinx formation by obliterating the spinal vasculature causing ischemia of the cord. Syringomyelia, by its growth laterally and longitudinally through the spinal cord, first causes loss of pain sensation, then abnormalities of motor function with weakness in the extremities and scoliosis in the axial skeleton, long tract signs (Babinski reflex), and autonomic dysfunction of the bladder and rectum. This lesion is found most commonly in the cervical spine and only occasionally in the lumbar spine.[96] In the past, diagnosis was made by myelography or CT.[97] MR has become the technique of choice to localize syringomyelias.[98] The treatment of syringomyelia is surgical removal of the fluid in the cystic cavity by needle aspiration or myelotomy.[99] The surgical treatment of syringomyelia must be approached with consideration of the pathogenesis of the specific lesion. Different shunting procedures are required depending on the location of the le-

sion.[100] Without effective therapeutic intervention to halt the progressive growth of the lesion, patients with syringomyelia suffer marked disability with spastic paraplegia, arthropathy, and infectious complications.

Neoplasms. Intramedullary tumors, mostly ependymomas and astrocytomas, grow slowly and insidiously in adults with few symptoms for many years. The symptomatology of both are similar. Patients may or may not have back pain with a sensory deficit to pinprick as their initial neurologic abnormality. The symptoms are of gradual onset and progress slowly. The average duration of symptoms before diagnosis is 3 years. Sudden bleeding into the tumor causes the onset of acute sciatic pain (Fincher's syndrome).[101] More than 50% of intraspinal ependymomas arise from the filum terminale, with the lumbar spine being the next most commonly affected structure. The tumor originates from the ependymal lining of the central canal or filum terminale and has very little capacity to invade the spinal cord. The tumor frequently grows posteriorly separating the proprioceptive columns. The tumors around the conus and cauda equina are of the myxopapillary variety.[11] Myxopapillary ependymomas may cause slow growing tumors in the sacrococcygeal region as well.[102] In adults, ependymomas comprise the majority of intramedullary tumors, accounting for nearly 65% of lesions.[11] Ependymoma is the most common primary tumor in the region of the conus and cauda equina. Astroytomas cause 20% to 25% of primary intraspinal neoplasms but affect the lumbar spine in only 20% of the time. Benign astrocytomas are slow-growing tumors associated with slowly progressive clinical symptoms. Astrocytomas cause enlargement of the cord, are relatively avascular, and may not have an identifiable plane of separation from the cord.

Radiographic evaluation demonstrates a fusiform expansion of the spinal cord. Ependymomas of the filum may cause marked deformity of vertebral bodies without producing symptoms.[10] Some conus intramedullary ependymomas have an exophytic extramedullary component extending into the lumbosacral canal. Contrast-enhanced MR is particularly effective for identifying the presence of intramedullary tumors, including those in the cauda equina. In one study of 32 spinal tumors, 30 neoplasms were enhanced. Ependymomas and astrocytomas were located with enhanced MR.[103] Enhanced MR has advantages over other radiographic techniques in differentiating solid tumor component from syrinx and from cysts. Also differentiated is recurrent or residual tumor from scar tissue in postoperative patients.

The treatment of these lesions is microsurgical removal of accessible lesions. Resection is completed to the extent consistent with preservation of neurologic function. Postoperative irradiation is helpful for those patients who have not had complete resection of the lesion. Presence of urinary difficulties at the time of diagnosis is a poor prognostic sign.[104] The 10-year survival of patients is up to 80% and is correlated with the use of irradiation after surgery in patients with incomplete resection of ependymoma.[105, 106]

Primary tumors such as lipomas, lymphomas, and melanomas are very rare causes of intramedullary tumor. For example, lipomas are 2% of intramedullary tumors.[11] Compared to extradural metastases, intramedullary metastatic lesions are very uncommon.[4] Some patients with intramedullary metastases may develop symptoms over a 6-month period. The common sources for metastases to the cord are lung, breast, lymphoma, colorectal, head and neck, and renal cell, in descending order. The prognosis is poor with a 20% survival rate at 3 months in one study.[107]

Vasculitis/Infarction. In the region below T8, the spinal cord is supplied anteriorly by the anterior spinal artery that arises from a single large vessel, the artery of Adamkiewicz, that arises from a segmental vessel between T9 and L2 on the left side. This artery is the largest vessel to reach the spinal cord and supplies 25% of the cord in 50% of individuals.[108] Branches of the anterior and posterior spinal arteries form a plexus around the cord that supplies the white matter and posterior horns of grey matter. The largest branches of the anterior spinal artery form a central artery that supplies the anterior grey matter and the innermost white matter.[109] Radicular arteries supply individual nerve roots.

In rare circumstances, connective tissue disorders that cause vasculitis may affect blood vessels, which supply blood to the spinal cord and cauda equina. Isolated granulomatous angiitis of the central nervous system is a form of vasculitis more commonly associated with cerebral vasculitis. Patients with isolated angiitis may develop spinal cord symptoms with or without cerebral involvement.[110, 111] These patients describe lower extremity weakness accompanied by sensory abnormalities including loss of pain proprioception and vibratory sense. Patients also develop incontinence. The prognosis for return of function is poor, although patients may survive for a number of years after

therapy with corticosteroids and radiation. Polyarteritis nodosa may cause neurologic dysfunction by affecting spinal cord arteries or by compression secondary to subarachnoid hemorrhage.[112, 113]

Infarction of the conus medullaris or cauda equina may occur by mechanisms other than inflammation of blood vessels, occlusion of the abdominal aorta during surgery, or by atheroma. Occlusion of the artery of Adamkiewicz results in paraplegia with relative sparing of the sacral roots. Blockage of this artery usually leads to watershed ischemia in its peripheral extension. Infarction of the conus may simulate the appearance of a spinal cord tumor on MR.[114] A severe prolapse of an intervertebral disc at the T12-L1 level may compress the anterior spinal artery and result in secondary ischemia. A very rare cause of infarction is embolization of disc material to spinal arteries causing infarction.[115] Patients with severe atherosclerosis, emboli, and sustained hypotension may be associated with cord infarction.[116] Patients with conus infarction have a poor prognosis unless definite improvement occurs within the first 48 hours after the onset of symptoms.

TREATMENT

Therapy directed at extradural metastatic lesions may include radiation therapy, corticosteroids, or spinal decompression.[117–119] The treatment of intradural-extramedullary tumors is complete surgical removal. Intramedullary tumors accessible to surgical excision should be removed.[120, 121] Some physicians suggest postsurgical radiation therapy of the spinal cord.

PROGNOSIS

In general, extradural and intramedullary tumors are malignant, while intradural-extramedullary tumors are benign. The course and prognosis of these tumors correspond to their invasiveness, rapidity of growth, and location. Extradural and intramedullary tumors have poor prognoses, while intradural-extramedullary tumors may be cured with surgical removal.

References

INTRASPINAL NEOPLASMS

1. Helseth A, Mork SJ: Primary intraspinal neoplasms in Norway 1955 to 1986: a population based survey of 467 patients. J Neurosurg 71:842, 1989.

2. Elsberg CA: Diagnosis and Treatment of Surgical Diseases of the Spinal Cord and Its Membranes, 2nd ed. Philadelphia: WB Saunders Co, 1941.

3. Batson OV: The function of vertebral veins and their role in the spread of metastases. Ann Surg 112:138, 1940.

4. Edelson RN, Deck MDF, Posner JB: Intramedullary spinal cord metastases: clinical and radiographic findings in nine cases. Neurology 22:1222, 1972.

5. Nicholas JJ, Christy WC: Spinal pain made worse by recumbency: a clue to spinal cord tumors. Arch Phys Med Rehabil 67:598, 1986.

6. Wiesel SW, Ignatius P, Marvel JP, Rothman RH: Intradural neurofibroma simulating lumbar disc disease. J Bone Joint Surg 58A:1040, 1976.

7. Robinson SC, Sweeney JP: Cauda equina lipoma presenting as acute neuropathic arthropathy of the knee. A case report. Clin Orthop 178:210, 1983.

8. Stein BM: Intramedullary spinal cord tumors. Clin Neurosurg 30:717, 1983.

9. Austin GM: The significance and nature of pain in tumors of the spinal cord. Surg Forum 10:782, 1959.

10. Davidoff RA: Handbook of the Spinal Cord. Vol 4 and 5. Congenital Disorders, Trauma, Infections, and Cancer. New York: Marcel Dekker, 1987.

11. Gurusinghe NT: Spinal cord compression and spinal cord tumours. In: Critchley E, Eisen A (eds): Diseases of the Spinal Cord. New York: Springer-Verlag, 1992, pp 351–408.

12. Winter RB, Moe JH, Bradford DS, et al.: Spine deformity in neurofibromatosis: a review of 102 patients. J Bone Joint Surg 61A:677, 1979.

13. Curtis BH, Fisher RL, Butterfield WL, Sauders FP: Neurofibromatosis in paraplegia. J Bone Joint Surg 51A:843, 1969.

14. McKraig W, Svien HJ, Dodge HW Jr, Camp JD: Intraspinal lesions masquerading as protruded lumbar intervertebral discs. JAMA 149:250, 1952.

15. Barron KD, Hirano A, Araki S, Terry RD: Experiences with metastatic neoplasms involving the spinal cord. Neurology 9:91, 1959.

16. Vieth RG, Odom GL: Extradural spinal metastases and their neurosurgical treatment. J Neurosurg 23:501, 1965.

17. Schaberg J, Gainor BJ: A profile of metastatic carcinoma of the spine. Spine 10:19, 1985.

18. Love JG, Dodge HW: Dumbbell (hourglass) neurofibromas affecting the spinal cord. Surg Obstet Gynecol 94:161, 1952.

19. Levy WJ, Bay J, Dohn D: Spinal cord meningioma. J Neurosurg 57:804, 1982.

20. Heshmat MY, Kovi J, Simpson C, et al.: Neoplasms of the central nervous system. Cancer 38:2135, 1976.

21. Mitchell GE, Lourie H, Berne AS: The various causes of scalloped vertebrae with notes on their pathogenesis. Radiology 89:67, 1967.

22. Resnick D, Niwayama G: Diagnosis of Bone and Joint Disorders. Philadelphia: WB Saunders Co, 1981, pp 432–445.

23. Banna M: Clinical Radiology of the Spine and the Spinal Cord. Rockville, Maryland: Aspen Systems Corporation, 1985.

24. Modic MT, Masaryk T, Paushter D: Magnetic resonance imaging of the spine. Radiol Clin North Am 24:229, 1986.

25. Parizel PM, Baleriaux D, Rodesch G, et al.: Gd-DTPA enhanced MR imaging of spinal tumors. AJNR 10:249, 1989.

26. Sze G, Stimac GK, Bartlett C, et al.: Multicenter study of gadopentetate dimeglumine as a MR contrast agent: evaluation in patients with spinal tumors. AJNR 11:967, 1990.

27. Lim V, Sobel DF, Zyroff J: Spinal cord pial metastases: MR imaging with gadopentetate dimeglumine. AJNR 11:975, 1990.

28. Haddad FS, Abla A, Allam CK: Extradural spinal angiolipoma. Surg Neurol 26:473, 1986.

29. Weill A, del Carpio-O'Donovan R, Tampieri D, et al.: Spinal angiolipomas: CT and MR aspects. J Comput Assist Tomogr 15:83, 1991.

30. Le May M, Jackson DM: Intervertebral disc protrusion masquerading as an intramedullary tumor. Br J Radiol 37:463, 1964.

31. Phillips GE, Jefferson A: Acute spinal epidural abscess: observations from fourteen cases. Postgrad Med J 55:712, 1979.

32. Baker AS, Ojemann RG, Swartz MN, Richardson EP Jr: Spinal epidural abscess. N Engl J Med 293:463, 1975.

33. Darouiche RO, Hamill RJ, Greenberg SB, et al.: Bacterial spinal epidural abscess: review of 43 cases and literature survey. Medicine 71:369, 1992.

34. Markham JW, Lynge HN, Stahlman GEB. The syndrome of spontaneous spinal epidural hematoma. Report of three cases. J Neurosurg 26:334, 1967.

35. Levitan LH, Wiens CW: Chronic lumbar extradural haematoma: CT findings. Radiology 148:707, 1983.

36. Hillman J, Bynke O: Solitary extradural caverous hemangiomas in the spinal canal: report of five cases. Surg Neurol 36:19, 1991.

37. Nakagami W, Yokota S, Ohishi Y, et al.: Chronic spontaneous lumbar spinal epidural hematoma. Spine 17:1509, 1992.

38. Stevens JM, Kendall BE, Gedroyc W: Acute epidural haematoma complicating myelography in a normotensive patient with normal blood coagulability. Br J Radiol 64:860, 1991.

39. DiLauro L, Poli R, Bortoluzzi M: Paresthesia after lumbar disc removal and their relationship to epidural haematoma. J Neurosurg 57:135, 1982.

40. Vinters HV, Barnett HJM, Kaufmann JCE: Subdural hematoma of the spinal cord and widespread subarachnoid hemorrhage complicating anticoagulant therapy. Stroke 11:459, 1980.

41. Fessler RG, Johnson DL, Brown FD, et al.: Epidural lipomatosis in steroid-treated patients. Spine 17:183, 1992.

42. Quint DJ, Boulos RS, Sanders WP, et al.: Epidural lipomatosis. Radiology 169:485, 1988.

43. Butcher DL, Sahn SA: Epidural lipomatosis: a complication of corticosteroid therapy. Ann Intern Med 90:60, 1979.

44. Lemish W, Apsimon T, Chakera T: Lumbar intraspinal synovial cysts: recognition and CT diagnosis. Spine 14:1378, 1989.

45. Pendleton B, Carl B, Pollay M: Spinal extradural benign synovial or ganglion cyst: case report and review of the literature. Neurosurgery 13:322, 1983.

46. Franck JI, King RB, Petro GR, Kanzer MD: A posttraumatic lumbar spinal synovial cyst. case report. J Neurosurg 68:293, 1987.

47. Cameron SE, Hanscom DA: Rapid development of a spinal synovial cyst. A case report. Spine 17:1528, 1992.

48. Bjokengren AG, Kurz LT, Resnick D, et al.: Symptomatic intraspinal synovial cysts: Opacification and treatment by percutaneous injection. AJR 149:105, 1987.

49. Skuse GR, Kosciolek BA, Rowley PT: The neurofi-

broma in von Recklinghausen neurofibromatosis has a unicellular origin. Am J Hum Genet 49:600, 1991.

50. Wertelecki W, Rouleau G, Superneau D, et al.: Neurofibromatosis: clinical and DNA linkage studies at a large kindred. N Engl J Med 319:278, 1988.

51. Wander JV, Das Gupta TK: Neurofibromatosis. Curr Probl Surg 14:1, 1977.

52. Thomeer RT, Bots GTAM, Van Dulken H, et al.: Neurofibrosarcoma of the cauda equina. Case report. J Neurosurg 54:409, 1981.

53. Ducatman BS, Scheithauer BW, Dahlin DC: Malignant bone tumors associated with neurofibromatosis. Mayo Clin Proc 58:578, 1983.

54. Thomas JE, Piepgras DG, Scheithauer B, et al.: Neurogenic tumors of the sciatic nerve. A clinicopathologic study of 35 cases. Mayo Clin Proc 58:640, 1983.

55. Egelhoff JC, Bates DJ, Ross JS, et al.: Spinal MR findings in neurofibromatosis types 1 and 2. AJNR 13:1071, 1992.

56. Disimone RE, Berman AT, Schwentker EP: The orthopedic manifestation of neurofibromatosis: a clinical experience and review of the literature. Clin Orthop 230:277, 1988.

57. Wong-Chung J, Gillespie R: Lumbosacral spondyloptosis with neurofibromatosis: case report. Spine 16:986, 1991.

58. Guyer RD, Collier RR, Ohnmeiss DD, et al.: Extraosseous spinal lesions mimicking disc disease. Spine 13:328, 1988.

59. Turk PS, Peters N, Libbey P, Wanebo HJ: Diagnosis and management of giant intrasacral schwannoma. Cancer 70:2650, 1992.

60. Davis RA, Washburn PL: Spinal cord meningiomas. Surg Gynecol Obstet 131:15, 1970.

61. Cillufo JM, Gomez MR, Reese DF, et al.: Idiopathic congenital spinal arachnoid diverticula: clinical diagnosis and surgical results. Mayo Clin Proc 56:93, 1981.

62. Nabors MW, Pait TG, Byrd E, et al.: Updated assessment and current classification of spinal meningeal cysts. J Neurosurg 68:366, 1988.

63. Van de Kelft E, Van Vyve M: Chronic perineal pain related to sacral meningeal cysts. Neurosurgery 29:223, 1991.

64. Delamarter RB, Ross JS, Masaryk TJ, et al.: Diagnosis of lumbar arachnoiditis by magnetic resonance imaging. Spine 15:304, 1990.

65. Burton CV: Lumbosacral arachnoiditis. Spine 3:24, 1978.

66. Shaw MDM, Russel JA, Grossart KW: The changing pattern of spinal arachnoiditis. J Neurol Neurosurg Psychiatry 41:97, 1978.

67. Bourne IHJ: Lumbo-sacral adhesive arachnoiditis: a review. J Roy Soc Med 83:262, 1990.

68. Quiles M, Marchisello PJ, Tsairis P: Lumbar adhesive arachnoiditis: etiologic and pathologic aspects. Spine 3:45, 1978.

69. Hughes DG, Isherwood I: How frequent is chronic lumbar arachnoiditis following intrathecal Myodil? Br J Radiol 65:758, 1992.

70. Freilick D, Swash M: Diagnosis and management of tuberculosis paraplegia with special reference to tuberculosis radiculomyelitis. J Neurol Neurosurg Psychiatry 42:12, 1979.

71. Sghirlanzoni A, Marazzi R, Pareyson D, et al.: Epidural anaethesia and spinal arachnoiditis. Anaesthesia 44:317, 1989.

72. Sklar EML, Quencer RM, Green BA, et al.: Complications of epidural anesthesia: MR appearance of abnormalities. Radiology 181:549, 1991.

73. Burton CV: Causes of failure of surgery on the lumbar spine: ten-year follow-up. Mt Sinai J Med 58:183, 1991.

74. Benoist M, Ficat C, Baraf P, Cauchoix J: Postoperative lumbar epiduro-arachnoiditis: Diagnosis and therapeutic aspects. Spine 5:432, 1980.

75. Hoyland JA, Freemont AJ, Denton J, et al.: Retained surgical swab debris in post-laminectomy arachnoiditis and peridural fibrosis. J Bone Joint Surg 70B:659, 1988.

76. Johnson CE, Sze G: Benign lumbar arachnoiditis: MR imaging with gadopentetate dimeglumine. AJR 155:873, 1990.

77. Ross JS, Masaryk TJ, Modic MT, et al.: MR imaging of lumbar arachnoiditis. AJR 149:1025, 1987.

78. Vloeberghs M, Herregodts P, Stadnik T, et al.: Spinal arachnoiditis mimicking a spinal cord tumor: a case report and review of the literature. Surg Neurol 37:211, 1992.

79. Ueda S, Saito A, Inomori S, Kim I: Cavernous angioma of the cauda equina producing subarachnoid hemorrhage: case report. J Neurosurg 66:134, 1987.

80. Pagni CA, Canavero S, Forni M: Report of a cavernoma of the cauda equina and review of the literature. Surg Neurol 33:124, 1990.

81. Armon C, Daube JR: Electrophysiological signs of arteriovenous malformations of the spinal cord. J Neurol Neurosurg Psychiatry 52:1176, 1989.

82. Djindjian R: Arteriography of the spinal cord. AJR 107:461, 1969.

83. Rosenblum DS, Myers SJ: Dural spinal cord arteriovenous malformation. Arch Phys Med Rehabil 72:233, 1991.

84. Minami S, Sagoh T, Nishimura K, et al.: Spinal arteriovenous malformations: MR imaging. Radiology 169:109, 1988.

85. Isu T, Iwasaki Y, Akino M, et al.: Magnetic resonance imaging in cases of spinal dural arteriovenous malformation. Neurosurgery 24:919, 1989.

86. Ogilvy CS, Louis DN, Ojemann RG: Intramedullary cavernous angiomas of the spinal cord: clinical presentation, pathological features, and surgical management. Neurosurgery 31:219, 1992.

87. Fontaine S, Melanson D, Cosgrove R, Bertrand G: Cavernous hemangiomas of the spinal cord: MR imaging. Radiology 166:839, 1988.

88. Logue V: Angiomas of the spinal cord: review of the pathogenesis, clinical features, and results of surgery. J Neurol Neurosurg Psychiatry 42:1, 1979.

89. McCormick PC, Michelsen WJ, Post KD, et al.: Cavernous malformations of the spinal cord. Neurosurgery 23:459, 1988.

90. Lundqvist C, Berthelsen B, Sullivan M, et al.: Spinal arteriovenous malformations: neurological aspects and results of embolization. Acta Neurol Scand 82:51, 1990.

91. Madsen JR, Heros RC: Spinal arteriovenous malformations and neurogenic claudication: report of two cases. J Neurosurg 68:793, 1988.

92. Yap HY, Yap BS, Tashima CK, et al.: Meningeal carcinomatosis in breast cancer. Cancer 42:283, 1978.

93. Wasserstrom WR, Glass JP, Posner JB: Diagnosis and treatment of leptomeningeal metastases from solid tumors: experience with 90 patients. Cancer 49:759, 1982.

94. Batzdorf U (ed): Syringomyelia: Current Concepts in

Diagnosis and Treatment. Baltimore: Williams & Wilkins, 1991, p. 208.

95. Caplan LR, Norohna AB, Amico LL: Syringomyelia and arachnoiditis. J Neurol Neurosurg Psychiatry 53:106, 1990.

96. McIlory WJ, Richardson JC: Syringomyelia: a clinical review of 75 cases. Can Med Assoc J 93:731, 1965.

97. Aubin ML, Vignaud J, Jardin C, Bar D: Computed tomography in 75 clinical cases of syringomyelia. Am J Neuroradiol 2:199, 1981.

98. Yeates A, Brant-Zawadzki M, Norman D, et al.: Nuclear magnetic resonance of syringomyelia. AJNR 4:234, 1983.

99. Gardner WJ, Bell HS, Poolos PN, et al.: Terminal ventriculostomy for syringomyelia. J Neurosurg 46:609, 1977.

100. Milhorat TH, Johnson WD, Miller JI, et al.: Surgical treatment of syringomyelia based on magnetic resonance imaging criteria. Neurosurgery 31:231, 1992.

101. Shen WC, Ho YJ, Lee SK, Lee KR: Ependymoma of the cauda equina presenting with subarachnoid hemorrhage. AJNR 14:399, 1993.

102. Domingues RC, Mikulis D, Swearingen B, et al.: Subcutaneous sacrococcygeal myxopapillary ependymoma: CT and MR. AJNR 12:171, 1991.

103. Parizel PM. Baleriaux D, Rodesch G, et al.: Gd-DTPA-enhanced MR imaging of spinal tumors. AJR 152:1087, 1989.

104. Schweitzer JS, Batzdorf U: Ependymoma of the cauda equina region: diagnosis, treatment, and outcome in 15 patients. Neurosurgery 30:202, 1992.

105. Clover LL, Hazuke MB, Kinzie JJ: Spinal cord ependymomas treated with surgery and radiation therapy. A review of 11 cases. Am J Clin Oncol 16:350, 1993.

106. Whitaker SJ, Bessell EM, Ashley SE, et al.: Postoperative radiotherapy in the management of spinal cord ependymoma. J Neurosurg 74:720, 1991.

107. Grem JL, Burgess J, Trump DL: Clinical features and natural history of intramedullary spinal cord metastasis. Cancer 56:2305, 1985.

108. Sliwa JA, Maclean IC: Ischemic myelopathy: a review of spinal vasculature and related clinical syndromes. Arch Phys Med Rehabil 73:365, 1992.

109. Aminoff MJ: Spinal vascular disease. In: Critchley E, Eisen A (eds): Disease of the Spinal Cord. New York: Springer-Verlag, 1992, pp 281–299.

110. Caccamo DV, Garcia JH, Ho K: Isolated granulomatous angiitis of the spinal cord. Ann Neurol 32:580, 1992.

111. Inwards DJ, Piepgras DG, Lie JT, et al.: Granulomatous angiitis of the spinal cord associated with Hodgkin's disease. Cancer 68:1318, 1991.

112. Ojeda VJ: Polyarteritis affecting the spinal cord arteries. Aust N Z J Med 13:287, 1983.

113. Rodgers H, Veale D, Smith P, Corris P: Spinal cord compression in polyarteritis nodosa. Ann Neurol 32:580, 1992.

114. Andrews BT, Kwei U, Greco C, Miller RG: Infarct of the conus medullaris simulating a spinal cord tumor: Case report. Surg Neurol 35:139, 1991.

115. Kestle JRW, Resch L, Tator CH, Kucharczyk W: Intervertebral disc embolization resulting in spinal cord infarction: case report. J Neurosurg 71:938, 1989.

116. Sandson TA, Friedman JH: Spinal cord infarction: report of 8 cases and review of the literature. Medicine 68:282, 1989.

117. Bruckmas JE, Bloomer WD: Management of spinal cord compression. Semin Oncol 5:135, 1978.

118. Clark PRR, Saunders M: Steroid-induced remission in spinal canal reticulum cell sarcoma. Report of two cases. J Neurosurg 42:346, 1975.

119. Khan FR, Glickman AS, Chu FCH, Nickson JJ: Treatment by radiotherapy of spinal cord compression due to extradural metastases. Radiology 89:495, 1967.

120. Greenwood J: Surgical removal of intramedullary tumors. J Neurosurg 26:275, 1967.

121. Vijayakumar S, Estes M, Hardy RW Jr, et al.: Ependymoma of the spinal cord and cauda equina: a review. Cleve Clin J Med 55:163, 1988.

14

Endocrinologic and Metabolic Disorders of the Lumbosacral Spine

Endocrinologic and metabolic disorders are systemic illnesses that can affect components of the musculoskeletal system throughout the body. Those endocrinologic and metabolic illnesses that produce symptoms of low back pain and characteristic laboratory and radiologic abnormalities include osteoporosis, osteomalacia, parathyroid disease, ochronosis, acromegaly, and microcrystalline disorders. Patients with these systemic diseases may present to a physician with low back pain as their initial or primary complaint, and a minor traumatic event is frequently thought to be the cause of the back discomfort. Evaluation by the physician, however, demonstrates compression fractures of the vertebral bodies secondary to inadequate bone stock, extensive degenerative disease of the spine, or accumulation of crystals, amino acids, or mucopolysaccharides in bone. A characteristic finding of endocrinologic and metabolic disorders is that, although symptoms may be limited to the axial skeleton, these illnesses cause bone changes in many locations. The bone abnormalities may be subtle but can be discovered if looked for carefully.

The history of back pain in patients with endocrinologic and metabolic diseases is usually nonspecific. Back pain is located predominantly in the lumbosacral spine, with occasional radiation into the lower extremities. Pain may be insidious in onset or acute, associated with a vertebral body compression fracture or acute gouty arthritis of the sacroiliac joint. Patients frequently have symptoms of bone or joint pain in other locations. In addition, the systemic manifestations of the endocrinologic or metabolic bone disorder may include symptoms of muscle weakness, renal stones, gastrointestinal malabsorption, or change in facial configuration. Physical examination may demonstrate the systemic quality of the underlying disorder. Not only will patients have back pain with percussion over the spine, loss of height, and dorsal kyphosis, they may also demonstrate muscle weakness, peripheral joint inflammation, tetany, pigmentation of cartilage, enlargement of the hands and jaw, or tophaceous deposits. Laboratory evaluation may be very helpful in making a specific diagnosis of the underlying disorder.

Abnormalities of calcium and phosphorus may raise the suspicion of osteomalacia or hyperparathyroidism. Bone biopsy confirms the diagnosis of osteoporosis or osteomalacia. Measurement of parathormone confirms the diagnosis of hyper- or hypoparathyroidism. Nonsuppressibility of growth hormone during a glucose tolerance test is characteristic of acromegaly. Detection of homogentisic acid in urine is diagnostic of ochronosis. Detection of urate or calcium pyrophosphate dihydrate crystals is essential for the diagnosis of gout or pseudogout, respectively. Prominent radiographic findings may indicate decreased bone stock, periosteal resorption, disc calcification, widened joint space, or bone erosions, but they are nonspecific. Although radiologic evaluation is not diagnostic, it is important in documenting the global involvement of the skeletal system with these diseases.

Therapy is tailored for each endocrinologic or metabolic illness. Calcium and vitamin D supplements are useful in patients with osteoporosis or osteomalacia. Surgical ablation of parathyroid or pituitary tumors is the therapy of choice for hyperparathyroidism or acromegaly, respectively. Patients with episodes of acute microcrystalline arthritis are benefitted by courses of nonsteroidal anti-inflammatory drugs.

OSTEOPOROSIS

Capsule Summary

Frequency of back pain—uncommon
Location of back pain—lumbar spine
Quality of back pain—chronic dull ache; acute, sharp with fracture
Symptoms and signs—back pain increases with motion, marked percussion tenderness over spine
Laboratory and x-ray tests—anemia, elevated sedimentation rate with secondary forms; diffuse vertebral involvement, compression fractures on plain roentgenograms; bone densitometry: dual energy x-ray absorptiometry (DEXA) or quantitated computed tomography (QCT)
Treatment—calcium, vitamin D, estrogens, calcitonin, etidronate

Prevalence and Pathogenesis

Osteoporosis, a metabolic bone disease related to several different disorders, is associated with loss of bone mass per unit volume even though the ratio of bone mineral content and bone matrix remains normal. The reduction of bone mass occurs predominantly in the axial skeleton, femoral neck, and pelvis. Loss of bone mass in the axial skeleton predisposes vertebral bodies to fracture, which results in back pain and deformity. Patients with osteoporosis may sustain multiple vertebral fractures over the years, with persistent mechanical pain and limitation of work potential. The diagnosis of osteoporosis is usually made on clinical grounds in a patient with a history of back pain and radiographic findings consistent with the disease. Other significant causes of osteoporosis, including tumors, hematologic disease, endocrinologic disorders, and drugs, must be considered in patients whose history,

physical examination, or laboratory findings are not consistent with idiopathic osteoporosis.

The absolute prevalence of osteoporosis is unknown. Patients who are symptomatic or who have radiographic changes of osteoporosis are easily recognized; however, many osteoporotic individuals are asymptomatic and have not come to medical attention. By radiographic criteria, 29% of women and 18% of men between 45 and 79 years of age have osteoporosis.[1] By a more sensitive method for determining vertebral bone mineral density, however, 50% of women past age 65 may be found to have asymptomatic osteoporosis.[2] Bone resorption increases with age, with bone loss normally beginning after age 40. In general, males have more bone mass than females, and blacks have more than whites. These facts correlate with the clinical finding of osteoporosis being more common in Caucasian women, particularly those of Northern European extraction. In at least 3% of patients with osteoporosis the disease is progressive, disabling, and an impediment to the activities of daily living.[3] During the course of their lifetime, women lose 50% of cancellous bone and 30% of cortical bone, while men lose 30% and 20%, respectively. The number of fractures related to osteoporosis is estimated to be 1.5 million with a cost in the United States of $10 billion.[4]

The cause of increased bone resorption on the endosteal (inner) surfaces of bone with inadequate compensatory bone formation, osteoporosis, is not well understood. Bone is living tissue which is constantly undergoing remodeling. Before adulthood, during growth, bone formation is greater than bone resorption. In the adult skeleton, up to the age of 30, the deposition and resorption of bone are equal and bone mass in both men and women is maximum at this age. Soon after, men start losing 0.3% of their skeletal bone calcium per year. In women, the rate is initially the same as in men but at menopause it increases to 3% per year.[5, 6] Patients with osteoporosis are individuals who either mature with a decreased skeletal mass or have an accelerated rate of bone loss after achieving peak bone density.

The causes of osteoporosis are listed in Table 14–1.[7] Primary osteoporosis includes postmenopausal or senile osteoporosis and idiopathic, adult or juvenile, osteoporosis. Senile osteoporosis is found in aging men and women, while postmenopausal osteoporosis occurs in women after menopause (Table 14–2).[8] Postmenopausal osteoporosis is the most common form of this illness. Juvenile idio-

TABLE 14–1. CAUSES OF OSTEOPOROSIS

PRIMARY
  Involutional (postmenopausal or senile)
  Idiopathic (juvenile or adult)

SECONDARY
Endocrine
  Hypogonadism
  Adrenocortical hormone excess (primary or iatrogenic)
  Hyperthyroidism
  Hyperparathyroidism
  Diabetes mellitus
  Growth hormone deficiency
Nutritional
  Calcium deficiency
  Phosphate deficiency
  Phosphate excess
  Vitamin D deficiency
  Protein deficiency
  Vitamin C deficiency
  Intestinal malabsorption
Drug
  Heparin
  Anticonvulsants
  Ethanol
  Methotrexate
Genetic
  Osteogenesis imperfecta
  Homocystinuria
Miscellaneous
  Rheumatoid arthritis
  Chronic liver disease
  Chronic renal disease
  Immobilization
  Malignancy (multiple myeloma)
  Metabolic acidosis
  Cigarette smoking

pathic osteoporosis occurs in early adolescence and is manifested by fragility in the axial skeleton. The disease may be severe and may cause vertebral fractures, kyphosis, and loss of height. Remissions can occur spontaneously, but the patients seldom achieve normal adult bone mass.

Idiopathic adult osteoporosis is found in men under 50 years of age.[9] This illness is often associated with idiopathic hypercalcemia, and the axial skeleton is the area most severely affected.

Secondary forms of osteoporosis may be caused by specific abnormalities, such as a hormonal imbalance that affects bone metabolism. Endocrine abnormalities that can cause osteoporosis should be investigated in any young or middle-aged person with decreased skeletal mass. Hypogonadism with decreased sex hormones can cause bone loss in both men and women, and this also plays a role in postmenopausal osteoporosis, particularly in women who undergo oophorectomy at an early age.[10] Amenorrhea may also play a role

in women who exercise excessively.[11] Adrenocortical hormone excess leads to decreased bone mass.[12] Glucocorticoids reduce bone calcium by decreasing intestinal absorption of calcium, by stimulating parathormone so as to increase bone resorption, and by exerting a direct inhibitory effect on bone metabolism and bone formation. This dual effect may explain the rapid bone loss associated with steroid therapy. The glucocorticoids from endogenous (Cushing's syndrome) or exogenous (cortisone) sources can cause osteoporosis.[13] Hyperthyroidism, by increasing general metabolic levels, increases bone turnover and remodeling. Parathormone exerts a direct effect on bone that causes an increase in resorption. Osteoporosis in hyperparathyroidism may develop because of parathyroid tumors or from illnesses that result in parathyroid gland hypertrophy. Whether or not diabetes contributes to the loss of bone mass is controversial, but studies suggest that bone density is decreased in patients with this illness.[14] Growth hormone is important for skeletal growth and maturation, and deficiencies are associated with decreased bone formation and mass.

The mineralization of bone is a complicated process involving a balance between calcium, phosphate, pH levels, hormones, and other factors. A nutritional deficiency of bone minerals or excess of any one of them may have a profound effect on bone mineralization. Low calcium consumption and decreased bone density are typical in women over 45 years of age.[15] The ratio of calcium to phosphorus or phosphate is altered by fluctuations in phosphorus concentration in nutritional sources, which may lead to bone resorption.[16] Vitamin

TABLE 14–2. TYPES OF INVOLUTIONAL OSTEOPOROSIS

	TYPE I (Postmenopausal)	TYPE 2 (Senile)
Age (yr)	50–75	Over 70
Sex ratio (M/F)	1:6	1:2
Type of bone loss	Trabecular	Trabecular and cortical
Fracture site	Vertebrae (crush), distal radius	Vertebrae (multiple wedge), hip
Main causes	Menopause	Aging
Calcium absorption	Decreased	Decreased
1,25-$(OH)_2$-vitamin D synthesis from 25-(OH) vitamin D	Secondary decrease	Primary
Parathyroid function	Decreased	Increased

Modified from Riggs BL, Melton LJ III: Involutional osteoporosis. N Engl J Med *314*:1676, 1986.

D in its activated form, 1,25-dihydroxyvitamin D$_3$, helps maintain serum calcium and phosphate levels by increasing both absorption of these substances from the intestine and their resorption from bone. Sources of vitamin D include fortified milk and fish along with the endogenous sources created by exposure of skin to the ultraviolet rays in sunlight. Osteoporosis may also be caused by deficiencies of protein and ascorbic acid (vitamin C) as well as by disorders such as celiac disease that result in intestinal malabsorption.

With extended use, certain drugs can lead to osteoporosis but the mechanisms are unknown. They include the anticoagulant heparin, anticonvulsants, like phenytoin, and methotrexate, an antimetabolite used in cancer chemotherapy. Chronic alcoholism is a common cause of bone loss in young men. Osteoporosis in alcoholics is probably related to poor dietary habits and decreased intestinal absorption. In addition, alcohol impairs vitamin D metabolism, has toxic effects on bone tissue, and decreases body mass resulting in decreased forces on skeletal structures.[17]

Genetic causes of osteoporosis are rare. Osteogenesis imperfecta is a severely deforming congenital disease occurring in children and to a lesser extent in adults and characterized by skeletal fragility, fractures, blue sclerae, and deafness. Specific disorders of collagen metabolism also result in weakened bones. Homocystinuria, a very rare heritable disorder related to a deficiency in the enzyme cystathionine beta-synthetase, causes mental retardation, tall stature, scoliosis, dislocated lens, and skeletal fragility.

A number of unrelated disorders may also cause osteoporosis. Increased blood flow related to synovial inflammation in rheumatoid arthritis causes osteoporosis that is periarticular in location. Immobilization results in osteoporosis. Mechanical stress increases bone mass and is necessary for maintenance of normal bone architecture.[16] Prolonged immobilization causes a proportionate loss of bone matrix and mineral. Focal loss occurs in bones that have been fractured and have been placed in casts. Generalized bone loss occurs in elderly patients who are chronically ill and are placed in bed.[18] Malignancies, particularly multiple myeloma and other hematologic neoplasms, cause local or general osteoporosis. Acidosis causes increased calcium resorption and if present on a chronic basis, results in osteoporosis. Women who smoke cigarettes may also be at risk of developing osteoporosis.[19]

Bone loss results from a disturbance of bone remodeling. Bone remodeling replaces old bone matrix with new matrix with an annual turnover rate of 25% in cancellous bone and 3% in cortical bone.[20] In adults, remodeling is the only important mechanism by which new bone is formed. Remodeling occurs in units of bone. A bone remodeling unit is comprised of a group of cells removing and replacing bone. These cells include osteoclasts, reversal cells, and osteoblasts.

The process of remodeling is initiated by denuding the bone surface of lining cells derived from osteoblasts. The retraction of these cells allows mononucleated osteoclasts to coalesce into multinucleated, mature osteoclasts in the area vacated by the surface lining cells. The activated osteoclasts resorb a predetermined volume of bone over 1 to 2 weeks. Osteoclasts then disappear from the surface and are replaced by mononucleated cells that prepare the surface for new bone formation by osteoblasts. During the reversal phase, a factor is released that signals the change from resorption to formation. Likely candidates for this factor are insulin-like growth factor (IGF) II or transforming growth factor (TGF-B), examples of osteoblast mitogens.[21] The recruitment of osteoblasts results in the filling in of the cavity made by the osteoclasts. The filling in process progresses and is concluded by mineralization of the osteoid manufactured by these cells after a 25- to 35-day delay. Disruption of the process results in an imbalance of resorption and formation, causing a loss of bone mineral. Increased activity of osteoclasts results in larger lacunae. Lack of the reversing factor may stall formation. Osteoblasts may have inadequate amounts of factors, such as calcium, phosphate, and vitamin D, to mineralize bone fully (osteomalacia).

As mentioned previously, parathormone (PTH), 1,25-dihydroxyvitamin D, and calcitonin are important in the maintenance of serum calcium levels. With increasing age, calcium intestinal absorption declines and renal function falls, limiting the amount of activated vitamin D manufactured. The increase in PTH levels is a secondary response to the lower calcium levels. Increased PTH causes activation of more remodeling units and greater loss of bone.

In postmenopausal women, the loss of estrogens results in the activation of increased numbers of remodeling units. The increased calcium levels inhibit the release of PTH and decrease the intestinal absorption of calcium. Estrogens may also have effects on a number of factors that affect bone metabolism including calcitonin, interleukins (IL) 1 and 6, TGF-B, prostaglandin E_2, tumor necrosis factor, and IGF.[22, 23] Increased levels of IL-1 and IL-6 recruit osteoclasts resulting in increased bone resorption. Estrogen treatment reverses the increased production of IL-1 in menopausal women.[24]

Local factors that have effects on bone metabolism may also play a role in the development of osteoporosis. Prostaglandins, osteoclast-activating factors, and bone-derived growth factors are a few of the substances that are the targets of studies researching the overall pathogenesis of osteoporosis.[25]

CLINICAL HISTORY

Certain risk factors predispose particular patients to osteoporosis, especially of the involutional (senile or postmenopausal) variety. Risk factors for osteoporosis include: (1) female gender, (2) age 20 years postmenopausal, (3) Caucasian or Oriental race, (4) positive family history, (5) premature menopause, (6) inactivity, (7) associated diseases (bowel resection, thyrotoxicosis, hyperparathyroidism), and (8) drugs (corticosteroids, anticonvulsants, ethanol, smoking).

Patients with vertebral osteoporosis may be asymptomatic, with the diagnosis being made on radiographs taken for other purposes. Symptomatic osteoporosis presents as midline back pain localized over the thoracic or lumbar spine, the most common location for fractures. Most vertebral body fractures occur after some mechanical stress such as slipping on a stair, lifting, or jumping. The patient with an acute fracture has severe pain localized over the affected vertebral body.

Occasionally the pain radiates into the flanks, upper portion of the posterior thighs, or abdomen. Spasm of the paraspinous muscles contributes to the back pain. Back motion aggravates the discomfort, and many patients attempt to reduce the pain by remaining motionless in bed, frequently lying on their side. Prolonged sitting, standing, and the Valsalva maneuver intensify the pain. Severe pain usually lasts 3 to 4 months and then resolves. However, some patients are left with persistent, nagging, dull spinal pain after vertebral body fracture secondary to osteoporosis, and this pain may persist even in the absence of new fractures on radiographs. The source of this pain may be microfractures too small to be detected by radiographs or biomechanical effects of the deformity on the lumbar spine below. Recurrent pain, increased deformity,

and loss of height suggest new fractures. Most patients do not have constant, sharp pain in the interval between fractures. Vertebral fractures of the dorsal spine result in anterior compression of the vertebral body. This kyphotic deformity (dowager's or widow's hump) can cause a compensatory flattening of the lumbar lordosis and low back pain. Multiple compression fractures may also cause persistent pain due to mechanical stress on ligaments, muscles, and apophyseal joints. They also result in a loss in height, and this is one of the parameters used to follow the progression of the disease. Since the disease affects only the anterior components of the vertebral bodies, neural compression is not associated with vertebral osteoporosis. Neurologic or radicular symptoms distant from an area of fracture are unusual, and if they are present, other pathologic conditions must be considered.

PHYSICAL EXAMINATION

Physical findings commonly include pain over the spinous process of the fractured vertebral body on percussion and associated spasm of surrounding paraspinous muscles. Patients with multiple fractures may demonstrate a loss of height and kyphoscoliosis. Neurologic examination is normal. On abdominal examination, patients with severe pain secondary to acute fracture may demonstrate a loss of bowel sounds, ileus, or bladder distention secondary to acute urinary retention.

LABORATORY DATA

Laboratory parameters in primary osteoporosis, such as serum calcium, phosphate, and alkaline phosphatase, are normal. Although urinary concentrations of calcium are normal, the amount of urinary calcium is high in relation to oral intake. Urinary hydroxyproline, an indicator of collagen breakdown, is normal. The presence of anemia, elevated ESR, rheumatoid factor, elevated serum proteins, or increased serum calcium suggests a secondary form of osteoporosis and requires further investigation. If there is a concern that osteomalacia may be playing a role in osteopenia, vitamin D levels should be measured. Thyroid hormone determinations along with any additional tests to eliminate renal, liver, parathyroid and gastrointestinal disorders may be indicated in the setting of the appropriate history.

New methods have been developed to detect bone resorption based upon the measurement

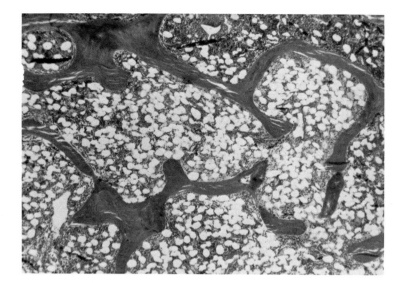

Figure 14–1. Osteoporosis. Histologic section demonstrating decreased bone and no osteoid. (Courtesy of Arnold Schwartz, M.D.)

of the breakdown products of collagen. Pyridinoline (Pyr) and deoxypyridinoline (D-Pyr) are nonreducible cross-links that stabilize the collagen chains in extracellular matrix. Pyr and D-Pyr are released from bone matrix during its degradation by osteoclasts.[26] These nonreducible cross-links are excreted in the urine in free form and can be measured by fluorimetry after high pressure liquid chromatography (HPLC) extraction of hydrolized urine. Elevated levels of D-Pyr are associated with patients with vertebral osteoporosis.[27] Currently, the test has assay variability with no synthetic standard. The amount excreted also varies with time of day and menstrual cycle. The development of radioimmunoassay for Pyr and D-Pyr should increase the availability of these tests and should allow validation of the measurement of these cross-links as an important measure of bone turnover and potential risk for osteoporosis.

Biopsy of osteoporotic bone reveals a reduction of thickness of cortical bone. In trabecular bone, the trabeculae within the medullary cavity are markedly thin and reduced in number. The biopsy contains no osteoid (Fig. 14–1).

RADIOGRAPHIC EVALUATION

Radiographic evaluation of osteopenia is best made from the lateral projection of the spine. Radiographic abnormalities of vertebral osteoporosis include changes in radiolucency, trabecular pattern, and shape of vertebral bone (Fig. 14–2).[28] Early osteoporosis may not be demonstrated on radiographs until 30% of bone mass has been lost.[29] An early finding is

the accentuation of the mineral density of the vertebral endplates since osteoporosis causes increasing lucency of the central portion of the vertebral body; however, the outer dimensions of the body remain the same, with sharply defined margins.[30] Horizontal trabecu-

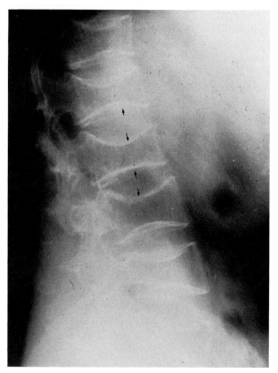

Figure 14–2. Osteoporosis. Radiograph shows generalized loss of bone mineral in multiple vertebral bodies along with thin cortical endplates in a 60-year-old woman with diffuse midline back pain. Disc expansion into vertebral bodies is associated with weakened bone structures *(arrows)*. (Courtesy of Anne Brower, M.D.)

lae are thinned, accentuating the vertical trabeculae that remain. This pattern is similar to that seen with hemangiomas. Prominent vertical trabeculae are limited to one vertebral body with a hemangioma, while multiple vertebrae are affected with osteoporosis. Osteoporosis may progress to the point where vertebral body contours may be affected, and "fish" or "codfish" vertebrae occur when intervertebral discs expand into weakened vertebral bone, causing an exaggerated biconcavity. "Fish" vertebrae are particularly common in the lower thoracic and upper lumbar spine. This deformity is more likely to be seen in young adults with osteopenia.

An anterior wedge compression fracture is manifested by a decrease in anterior height, usually 4 mm or greater, compared with the vertical height of the posterior body. A transverse compression fracture results in equal loss of both anterior and posterior heights. Many patients will demonstrate radiographic changes of "fish," anterior wedging, and compression vertebrae in the thoracic and lumbar

spine. The changes in osteoporotic vertebrae are unevenly distributed along the spine,[31] with no two affected exactly alike (Fig. 14–3). "Fish" vertebrae may occur asymptomatically. Anterior wedging and compression in osteoporosis indicate a fracture of the vertebral body and are associated with sudden, severe episodes of incapacitating back pain in most circumstances (Fig. 14–4).

For the most part, bone scintigraphy is not useful in differentiating the various forms of metabolic bone disease.[32] Bone scan is more helpful in detecting increased focal bone formation associated with acute spinal compression fractures. However, old fractures may remain "hot" on bone scan for months and may make identifying the most recent fracture site difficult. A number of radiographic techniques exist to measure bone calcium. They include radiographic photodensitometry, photon absorptiometry (single and dual), neutron activation, and CT.[28, 33] Controversy surrounds the utility of these radiographic techniques in predicting those individuals at risk for vertebral

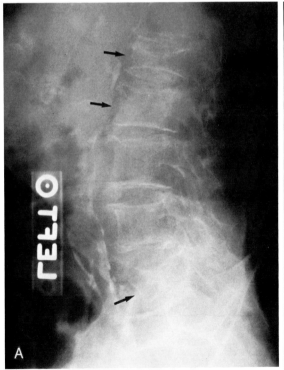
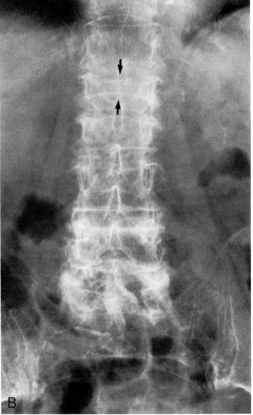

Figure 14–3. An 83-year-old woman presents with a history of acute low back pain localized to the thoracolumbar junction. *A,* Lateral view reveals generalized osteoporosis with diminished height of L1, L2, and L5 *(arrows). B,* AP view reveals marked loss of height of the L1 vertebral body *(arrows).*

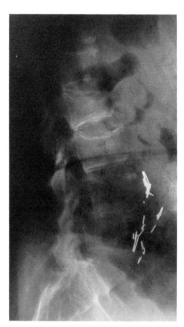

Figure 14–4. Osteoporosis. Lateral roentgenogram demonstrates vertebral compression fractures in vertebral bodies L1, L2, L3, and L4. Disc degeneration is noted at the L4-L5 with complete obliteration of the disc space with degenerative spondylolisthesis. (From Borenstein DG: Low back pain. In Kippel J, Duppe P (eds): Rheumatology. St Louis: CV Mosby, 1994, Sec 5, p 4.18.)

fractures. Two editorials in respected journals suggest that these techniques are not indicated in the common office setting.[34, 35] Since these editorials were written, greater sophistication has developed in the measurement of bone mineral calcium.[36] The major questions that concern bone densitometry are the accuracy and reproducibility of calcium measurement and associated risk of fracture. Characteristics of the more commonly utilized densitometry methods are listed in Table 14–3.[37] Plain radiographs may be helpful at estimating bone loss but are relatively inaccurate.[38] Physicians have been divided into two major camps in regard to the utility of vertebral bone densitometry. Some physicians believe that clinical risk factors should be used to identify women needing preventive therapy and that vertebral fractures are a better way to measure outcome than densitometry. Others believe that not all women with clinical risk factors should receive treatment because of toxicities of therapy, and treatment should be restricted to those whose bone mass is one to two standard deviations below age-matched controls.[39]

The two techniques most commonly thought to be accurate for the determination of vertebral bone density are dual energy x-ray absorptiometry (DEXA) and quantitated computed tomography (QCT).[40, 41] Both methods have their advantages and disadvantages. QCT is better able to separate the contribution of cortical and cancellous bone to bone density. It has somewhat better predictive value for spine fractures than DEXA. DEXA has better approximation of bone mineral with the use of lateral images that remove osteophytes and calcified ligaments from the measurement. This change in method has improved its accuracy. DEXA has 1/100 the x-ray exposure of QCT in the measurement of bone mineral. This difference in exposure is important when screening postmenopausal healthy women for the use of replacement estrogen.[42] The role of bone densitometry continues to evolve. The use of bone densitometry in general clinical practice will be decided on scientific and financial (reimbursement) concerns. Currently,

TABLE 14–3. BONE DENSITOMETRY METHODS FOR THE SPINE*

TECHNIQUE	RADIATION	PRECISION/ ACCURACY (%)†	SCAN TIME (MIN)	COMMENTS
Plain x-ray	400–1000 mrem	—	—	Available; insensitive
Dual photon absorptiometry (DPA)	5 mrem	2–4/4–6	20–30	Density correlates with risk for fracture; repositioning problem for sequential studies
Dual energy x-ray absorptiometry (DEXA)	5 mrem	1–2/2–6	7	Sequential studies are reliable; spurs increase bone density
Quantitative computed tomography (QCT)	400–1000 mrem	3–5/2–10	20	Density correlates with risk for spine fracture; expensive; low reading for extra marrow fat

*Modified from White PH: Osteopenic disorders of the spine. Semin Spine Surg 2:121, 1990.
†Precision: reproducibility of test; Accuracy: correct amount measured against standards.

screening is recommended only for individuals at high risk, particularly those who wish help in deciding about hormone replacement therapy.

DIFFERENTIAL DIAGNOSIS

In most patients with diffuse osteoporosis of the axial skeleton, vertebral compression fractures, and no abnormalities on laboratory evaluation, the diagnosis of osteoporosis is made on clinical grounds alone. Suspicion for the diagnosis is also heightened if the patient has any risk factors that are associated with osteoporosis, such as sedentary lifestyle; low calcium intake; early menopause or oophorectomy; cigarette smoking; excessive consumption of alcohol, protein, or caffeine; slender build; or a family history of osteoporosis.[43] Low levels of estrogen in the blood stream of menstruating women may also be a risk factor for decreased bone mass.[44]

Secondary causes of osteoporosis as listed in Table 14–1 should be considered in patients with abnormal laboratory findings such as anemia, elevated ESR, abnormal serum proteins, or hypovitaminosis D. Osteoporosis may be complicated by osteomalacia in 8% of postmenopausal women. Osteomalacia is a metabolic bone disease characterized by decreased bone mineralization with normal bone matrix, usually secondary to inadequate vitamin D. Osteomalacia is usually associated with normal or low concentrations of serum calcium, decreased concentration of phosphorus, and increased levels of alkaline phosphatase. Osteoporosis and osteomalacia may be indistinguishable by clinical and radiologic criteria. Bone biopsy is useful in detecting the presence of osteomalacia complicating osteoporosis and is indicated when the diagnoses are in doubt, since specific therapy is available for osteomalacia. Other methods for measuring bone calcium include dual photon absorptiometry (DPA), neutron activation analysis, and QCT; however, the significance of the measurement results remains to be determined. Therefore, these methods should not be utilized to predict patients at risk for osteoporosis in the usual clinical setting.

The differential diagnosis of abnormalities in vertebral body shape depends on the configuration of the alteration and its focal or generalized distribution. Biconcave ("fish") vertebrae occur with osteomalacia, Paget's disease, and hyperparathyroidism. Schmorl's nodes occur with Scheuermann's disease, trauma, and hyperparathyroidism. Flattened vertebrae occur with eosinophilic granuloma.

Trauma to the spine can cause vertebral fractures. Patients with such injuries experience acute pain over the area traumatized. Not only are the bones of the vertebral column affected, but the bony pelvis may be traumatized and cause back pain (Fig. 14–5).

Insufficiency fractures of the sacrum may oc-

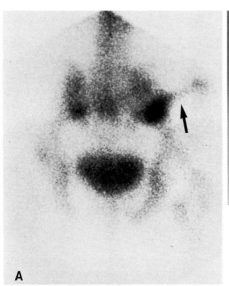
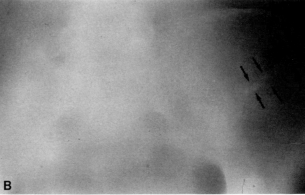

Figure 14–5. A 69-year-old woman was receiving nonsteroidal drugs and prednisone for an asymmetric polyarthritis. After a number of months on therapy, she developed excruciating low back pain without antecedent trauma. *A,* Bone scan reveals linear uptake in the left ilium *(arrow). B,* Tomogram of left ilium reveals healing fracture that resulted from osteoporosis *(arrows).* (Courtesy of David Caldwell, M.D.)

cur independent of trauma to the pelvis (Fig. 14–6). Patients with metabolic bone disease, pelvic irradiation, or corticosteroid therapy may be at increased risk of fracture.[45] Patients experience acute onset of back pain with radiation into the buttock or leg with no antecedent history of trauma. Subtle alterations in bone architecture seen on plain roentgenograms are frequently missed on initial readings (Fig. 14–6A). Bone scintiscan or computed tomography scans are useful to detect the presence of fractures. Most patients improve with resolution of pain and healing of fractures with an extended period of bed rest.

One other entity associated with vertebral collapse is Kümmell's disease or osteonecrosis of a vertebral body.[46] Not infrequently these patients are receiving long-term corticosteroid therapy and develop pain localized over a vertebral body (Fig. 14–7).[47] Plain roentgenograms demonstrate vertebral collapse with intravertebral body gas (Fig. 14–8). CT scan demonstrates the gas in the cortical margins of the vertebral body. The presence of gas in the body is distinctive. Metastatic lesions and fractures do not exhibit an intravertebral vacuum sign. Although it has not been reported in the spine, intraosseous gas accumulation does occur in osteomyelitis.[48] This possibility must be considered in the patient taking corticosteroids who develops intraosseous gas and collapse of a vertebral body. In these patients, MR examination may be useful in identifying spinal cord or nerve root compression associated with vertebral body collapse.[49] With MR, a distinction can be made between malignant compression fractures and those caused by benign processes.[50]

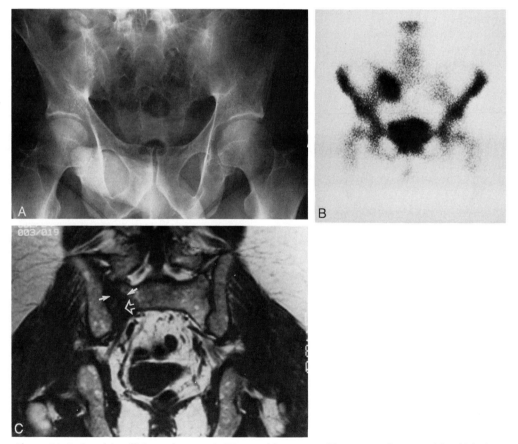

Figure 14–6. Sacral insufficiency fracture. A 57-year-old woman with severe asthma requiring high-dose corticosteroids for many years developed spontaneous right sided low back pain with radiation into the right buttock. *A,* Plain roentgenogram of the pelvis. No specific abnormality was noted. Persistent pain continued despite maximum medical therapy. *B,* Bone ⁹⁹ᵐTC MDP scintiscan. Marked increase in tracer uptake was noted over the right sacrum. *C,* MR of the pelvis. The coronal section of this T₁-weighted image reveals abnormal signal in the right sacrum. The changes are compatible with inflammation surrounding a fracture *(white arrows).* The fracture is noted in the lateral aspect of the sacrum *(open arrow).* This MR was originally misread as being normal. The patient improved with 6 weeks of controlled physical activity and crutch walking.

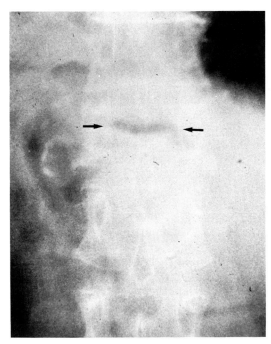

Figure 14–7. Osteonecrosis. AP view of the lumbar spine of a patient on long-term corticosteroid therapy who developed acute-onset low back pain. Osteonecrosis has resulted in an intravertebral vacuum sign *(arrows)*. (Courtesy of David Caldwell, M.D.)

TREATMENT

The treatment of osteoporosis should be primarily directed at young adult women at risk to help prevent the disease. Preventive factors include a high calcium intake, at least 1000 mg/day, regular exercise, and avoidance of excessive protein, alcohol, smoking, and caffeine.[51] In postmenopausal women, preventive measures may also be helpful in slowing bone calcium loss. These measures include increased calcium intake, administration of estrogens, and regular exercise against gravity, which must be performed at least 3 hours per week.[52, 53]

Combinations of these various therapies have been associated with varying degrees of slowing or preventing bone loss. Calcium and exercise is effective at slowing bone loss.[54] Calcium alone may be more helpful at slowing bone loss at the radius and hip than at the spine, and calcium citrate malate is more effective than supplementation with calcium carbonate according to a study.[55]

Patients who sustain an acute compression fracture experience severe pain and require bed rest for relief of the discomfort associated with physical activity. The period of bed rest, however, should be kept to a minimum, since immobilization speeds bone resorption. Bed rest is usually kept to about a week. Analgesics in the form of salicylates or other nonsteroidal anti-inflammatory drugs are useful in controlling pain. Pain from paravertebral muscle spasm is responsive to muscle relaxants. Lumbosacral corsets increase intraabdominal pressure and provide comfort but are usually poorly tolerated and tend to weaken abdominal muscles. The back pain usually resolves spontaneously over 3 to 4 months, and patients are encouraged to participate in non–weight-bearing exercises (such as swimming initially) and resume normal weight-bearing activity (walking, for example) as soon as possible.

The long-term goal in patients with osteoporotic fractures is to slow the rate of bone resorption, thereby reducing the possibility of additional fractures and progressive deformity. Medical therapies are directed at increasing calcium absorption and improving bone mineralization. No one regimen has been shown to be effective for all patients with osteoporosis

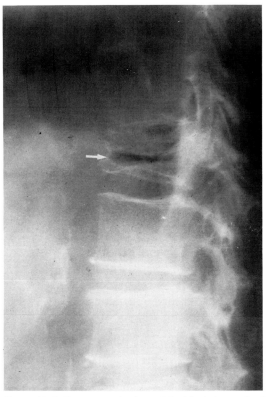

Figure 14–8. Osteonecrosis of a vertebral body in a patient with systemic lupus erythematosus receiving corticosteroids, demonstrated by linear lucency of the vertebral body *(arrow)*, vertebral body collapse, and relative preservation of intervertebral disc spaces. (Courtesy of Anne Brower, M.D.)

(Table 14–4). Calcium supplements alone have been shown to decrease the vertebral fracture rate in osteoporosis in some studies.[56] The daily requirement of calcium in perimenopausal women is approximately 1.3 to 1.5 gm/day.[57] In a more recent double blind, controlled study, it was shown that calcium supplements alone are not as effective as estrogen for the prevention of trabecular bone loss associated with postmenopausal osteoporosis.[58] It is important to remember that urinary calcium increases by about 6% of any increase in dietary intake of calcium. Therefore, an increase of 1000 mg of calcium will increase urinary calcium about 60 mg in 24 hours.

A study has tested the absorption of calcium from calcium salt preparations (calcium gluconate or calcium carbonate, for example) and milk. Approximately a third of the available calcium was absorbed from the calcium salts and milk. The applicability of the findings of the study to the absorption of calcium from over-the-counter calcium preparations is not clear, since the study used analytic grade preparations of the salts in capsules. In addition, the subjects used for the study were normal men. The application of the study findings to women and older individuals remains to be determined.[59]

Vitamin D helps increase calcium absorption from the gut. The improvement in bone mineralization after the institution of vitamin D therapy may be related to the presence of osteomalacia in some elderly patients with osteoporosis.[60] The principal effect of calcium supplements and vitamin D therapy may be to decrease bone turnover and increase intestinal absorption. Vitamin D does not increase bone mass or decrease fracture rates.[61] Doses of 50,000 units of vitamin D once a week are usually well tolerated; however, complications of vitamin D therapy given in more frequent doses include hypercalcemia, nephrocalcinosis, and/or nephrolithiases (renal stones). Measurement of 24-hour urinary calcium excretion every 4 to 6 months is indicated to detect the presence of hypercalciuria, a condition associated with the formation of calcium-containing renal stones.

Estrogens, female sex hormones, tend to decrease bone resorption and enhance bone mass by slowing the rate at which bone loss occurs.[62] A beneficial effect of estrogens in combination with calcium in preventing the progression of osteoporosis has been reported.[63] Estrogens are effective at decreasing the risk of fractures.[64] The effects of estrogens seem to be maximal when treatment is initiated early in the postmenopausal period. Patients are usually treated for a minimum of 5 to 10 years. Estrogens also are helpful in patients with well established osteoporosis.[65] These hormones are given daily for 3 weeks, and then withheld for 5 to 7 days to allow withdrawal bleeding and endometrial shedding. Estrogens also may be given by transdermal patches. This form of estrogen therapy is associated with decreased bone loss.[66] The use of low-dose progesterone may limit side effects of estrogen in postmenopausal women. Estrogens are not used routinely in patients with osteoporosis because of side effects, which include vaginal bleeding and breast engorgement. Another significant potential complication of estrogen therapy is the increase in risk of endometrial cancer.[67] The use of progesterone decreases this risk. In contrast, estrogen use was associated with no increased risk of breast cancer in a study of 1369 women with breast cancer and 1645 female controls.[68] Estrogens have other beneficial effects. Estrogens may not only improve bone status but may also reduce the risk for coronary artery disease.[69] Estrogens have beneficial effects on lipoproteins including decreasing LDL and increasing HDL levels.[70] In overall balance, estrogens have a beneficial effect on postmenopausal women and are indicated in women at risk for vertebral crush fractures secondary to osteoporosis as long as the patient is monitored carefully for toxicities. The effects of estrogen last only as long as the patient takes the hormone replacement. Rapid bone loss occurs once the estrogen is stopped.[71] Patients taking these replacement female hormones need to be followed closely by a gynecologist. Although additional study would be helpful, enough data are available to suggest that the risk:benefit ratio of estrogens in osteoporosis is on the side of benefit.[72]

Bisphosphonates are analogues of pyrophosphate that inhibit bone resorption. Etidronate is effective at decreasing bone fractures associated with osteoporosis.[73] The effect of this drug is similar to the effect of estrogen and calcitonin on bone.[74] The recommended dosage for etidronate is 400 mg daily for 2 weeks followed by 12 weeks off the drug. This cycle is continued for a 2-year period. Etridonate must be given on an empty stomach. Food should not be consumed 4 hours before and after taking the tablet. The time frame free of the drug is important in order to decrease the risk of osteomalacia, allowing bone to remineralize.

Sodium fluoride increases skeletal mass by

TABLE 14–4. THERAPY OF OSTEOPOROSIS

1. Encourage gravity exercises, including back extension exercises and balance exercises, strengthening abdominal muscles; acute fracture—analgesics, braces
2. Experimental therapy:

DRUG	POSITIVE EFFECTS	NEGATIVE EFFECTS	RECOMMENDED DOSES AND DURATION
Calcium	Prevents further bone loss Overcomes malabsorption	Rare Constipation	1000–1500 mg minimal daily requirement Milk 3–4 8 oz glasses Calcium citrate most easily absorbed
Vitamin D 1 alpha OH D_3 25-OH D_3 1,25-$(OH)_2$ D_3	Overcomes CA^{++} malabsorption of advancing age	Hyercalciuria Hypercalcemia	50,000 units 2 times weekly or 25-OH D 50 μg MWF in patients with 24-hour urine calcium <150 mg Do not allow urine calcium to exceed 300 mg/24 hours
Estrogens	Reduces bone resorption ? Risk of arteriosclerotic cardiovascular disease diminished	Bone formation rates will decrease after several months Cancer of uterus ? Breast cancer ? Vascular clotting ? Hypertension	Consider conjugated estrogen therapy in most women with early menopause and without a history of breast carcinoma Calcium supplements in most women with surgical oophorectomy before age 50 Starting dose 0.625 mg conjugated equine estrogen or 0.05 transdermal estrogen following blood test. Add progesterone if uterus intact. FDA approved
Calcitonin	Reduces bone resorption Best effect in high turnover osteoporosis fracture pain reduction	Allergic reactions Hypocalcemia	25–100 MRC units SQ daily or every other day. Need rest period off drug every 12–18 mo. FDA approved
Thiazides	Decreases urinary excretion of calcium	Hypokalemia Efficacy unproven	≥25 mg daily?
Bisphosphonates (etidronate)	Reduces bone resorption	Continuous use can result in osteomalacia Occasional GI upset	Cyclic therapy 400 mg daily for 2 wk, repeat every 3 mo Poor absorption with calcium (no calcium for 4 hr before or after taking etidronate)
Sodium fluoride	Stimulates osteoid formation Reduces bone resorption Replaces CA^{++} in hydroxyapatite: crystal is denser	Osteomalacia may occur Bone crystal may be brittle and cortical fractures increased GI discomfort Acne Arthralgias/arthritis Periostosis	NaF is available as Luride 2.2 mg tabs. Begin 4 three times a day with meals, increase slowly to attain doses between 50 and 75 mg/day

Courtesy of Patience White, M.D. Modified 1994.

boosting osteoblastic activity. Calcium supplements must be given with fluoride to ensure adequate bone mineralization. Sodium fluoride is given in daily doses of 40 to 65 mg in conjunction with calcium (1.5 gm daily) and vitamin D (50,000 units once or twice weekly). Fluoride dose may need to be increased to 75 mg daily. Fluoride therapy is associated with a number of potential toxicities. Although fluoridic bone may appear more dense on radiographic examination, it may be less elastic and more prone to fracture. Preliminary data suggest, however, that patients treated with fluoride for osteoporosis may have a decreased incidence of fracture.[75, 76] Other adverse side effects of fluorides include synovitis, gastric irritation, plantar fasciitis of the feet, and anemia. Most patients with vertebral osteoporotic fractures will heal spontaneously and will not require therapy other than the usual calcium and vitamin D. In patients with progressive bone loss, recurrent fractures, and deformity, sodium fluoride may be a useful drug to prevent progressive osteoporosis. Additional prospective studies investigating the fracture rate of postmenopausal women with osteoporosis using fluoride have been completed. Fluoride therapy increases cancellous bone but decreases cortical bone mineral density and increases skeletal fragility.[77] Fluoride is not effective at decreasing osteoporotic fractures.

Calcitonin, a hormone produced by C cells in the thyroid gland that suppresses bone resorption, is increased when postmenopausal women receive exogenous estrogen therapy. Intramuscular calcitonin injections along with calcium supplements may retard the rate of bone loss in osteoporotic women.[78] A recent study has reported the prevention of early postmenopausal bone loss in 30 women who used intranasal calcitonin (50 IU/day) and calcium 500 mg/day in comparison to 30 women who received calcium 500 mg/day alone.[79] Further studies are required to determine the efficacy of calcitonin to decrease fractures. Intranasal calcitonin is easier to administer than the intramuscular form and is effective at decreasing bone loss.[79] Calcitonin also may prove beneficial by controlling pain of fractures in osteoporotic patients through the release of endogenous analgesics, like beta-endorphin.

Thiazide diuretics block renal excretion of calcium. Studies have shown that bone mineral is increased in patients taking thiazides as compared with age-matched controls. The therapeutic effect of thiazides on osteopenia remains to be determined.[80] Another drug that may decrease bone loss is tamoxifen.[81] Tamoxifen is a synthetic anti-estrogen that is effective as an adjuvant therapy for invasive breast cancer. Tamoxifen is not a pure anti-estrogen. It has agonist estrogen effects. Tamoxifen decreases levels of cholesterol and increases sex hormone binding globulin. It might have either an agonist or antagonist effect on bone loss. Recent studies of bone mineral density in postmenopausal women with breast cancer demonstrated preservation of bone mineral. The effect on risk for fracture remains to be determined.

The therapy of symptomatic individuals with osteoporosis in whom urinary calcium is less than 100 mg/24 hours should include calcium 1000 to 1500 mg/day and vitamin D 50,000 units twice a week. Urinary calcium should be kept under 300 mg for 24 hours and should be monitored every 4 months. If the patients' urine contains greater than 100 mg of urinary calcium, calcium, vitamin D, and estrogen 0.625 mg every day to be cycled monthly should be considered. If new fractures occur within 6 to 12 months, the addition of calcitonin or fluoride should be considered.

Patients who receive corticosteroids are at risk of developing symptomatic osteoporosis, including vertebral fractures. Patients who take steroids should be considered for treatment with drugs that prevent osteoporosis including calcium, vitamin D, thiazide diuretics, and hormonal replacement. In patients with fractures, calcitonin and bisphosphonates may be helpful in decreasing symptoms.[82]

PROGNOSIS

Vertebral compression fractures occur episodically and are usually self-limited. Patients will usually have more than one fracture and a recurrence usually occurs within a few years of the first incident. Back pain may resolve within months of a fracture or may persist if increasing deformity causes a mechanical strain in the lumbar spine. The course of osteoporosis is variable, and it is impossible to predict the severity and frequency of fractures. Patients with osteoarthritis in conjunction with osteoporosis may be at less risk of bone fracture. Patients with both disorders are older, with a longer period of menopause, and are physically smaller in stature and body weight than those with the individual disorders.[83]

Patients with osteoporosis who continue to work are at risk of repeated fractures, and they should not be required to lift or carry heavy objects. They should refrain from work activities that jar the spine. Measures such as structured exercise and drug therapy may be helpful at slowing the progression of the disease. Individuals with strong back extensor muscles may have greater bone mineral density than individuals with weaker muscles.[84] Maintenance of muscle strength is worthwhile in a treatment program.

Osteoporosis and associated vertebral fractures cause significant morbidity in patients. Patients with fractures have decreased spinal motion and have difficulty walking. Psychologic perceptions of illness are also increased in the group with fractures. Osteoporosis is a significant medical disorder with physical and psychiatric impairments.[85] Long-term benefits may be found with the prolonged use of etidronate. A 4-year study demonstrated a decreased number of vertebral fractures in patients treated with cyclic etidronate therapy.[86]

References

OSTEOPOROSIS

1. Avioli LV: The osteoporosis problem. Curr Concepts Nutr 5:99, 1977.
2. Riggs BL, Wahner HW, Dunn WL, et al.: Differential changes in bone mineral density of appendicular and axial skeleton with aging. J Clin Invest 67:328, 1981.
3. Urist MP, Gurvey MS, Fareed DO: Long term observations on aged women with pathologic osteoporosis. In Barzel US (ed): Osteoporosis. New York: Grune and Stratton, 1970, pp 3–37.
4. Riggs BL, Melton LJ III: The prevention and treatment of osteoporosis. N Engl J Med 327:620, 1992.
5. Cohn SH, Vaswani A, Zanzi I, Ellis KJ: Effect of aging on bone mass in adult women. Am J Physiol 230:140, 1976.
6. Heaney RP, Recker RR, Saville PD: Calcium balance and calcium requirements in middle-aged women. Am J Clin Nutr 30:1603, 1977.
7. Lukert BP: Osteoporosis: a review and update. Arch Phys Med Rehab 63:480, 1982.
8. Riggs BL, Melton LJ III: Involutional osteoporosis. N Engl J Med 314:1676, 1986.
9. Jackson WPU: Osteoporosis of unknown cause in younger people. J Bone Joint Surg 40B:420, 1958.
10. Cann CE, Genant HK, Ettinger B, Gordon GS: Spinal mineral loss in oophorectomized women: determination by quantitative computed tomography. JAMA 244:2056, 1980.
11. Jones KP, Raunikar VA, Tulchinsky D, Schiff I: Comparison of bone density in amenorrheic women due to athletics, weight loss, and premature menopause. Obstet Gynecol 66:5, 1985.
12. Cushing H: The basophil adenomas of the pituitary body and their clinical manifestations. Bull Johns Hopkins Hosp 50:137, 1932.
13. Adinoff AD, Hollister JR: Steroid induced fractures and bone loss in patients with asthma. N Engl J Med 309:265, 1983.
14. McNair P, Madsbad S, Christiansen C, et al.: Osteopenia in insulin treated diabetes mellitus: its relation to age at onset, sex, and duration of disease. Diabetologia 15:87, 1978.
15. Albanese AA, Edelson AH, Lorenze EJ Jr, et al.: Problems of bone health in elderly. NY State J Med 75:326, 1975.
16. Lutwak L, Singer FR, Urist MR: Current concepts of bone metabolism. Ann Intern Med 80:630, 1974.
17. Schapira D: Alcohol abuse and osteoporosis. Semin Arthritis Rheum 19:371, 1990.
18. Smith EL, Reddon W: Physical activity: a modality for bone accretion in the aged. AJR 126:1297, 1976.
19. Cummings SR, Kelsey JL, Hevitt MC, O'Dowd KJ: Epidemiology of osteoporosis and osteoporotic fractures. Epidemiol Rev 7:178, 1985.
20. Dempster DW, Lindsay R: Pathogenesis of osteoporosis. Lancet 341:797, 1993.
21. Mohan S, Baylink D: Bone growth factors. Clin Orthop 263:30, 1992.
22. Jilja R, Hangoc G, Girasole G, et al.: Increased osteoclast development after estrogen loss: mediation by interleukin-6. Science 257:88, 1992.
23. Ralston SH, Rusell RGG, Gowen M: Estrogen inhibits release of tumor necrosis factor from peripheral blood mononuclear cells in postmenopausal women. J Bone Miner Res 5:983, 1990.
24. Pacific R, Brown C, Puscheck E, et al.: The effect of surgical menopause and estrogen replacement on cytokine release from human blood monocytes. Proc Natl Acad Sci USA 88:5134, 1991.
25. Raisz LG: Local and systemic factors in the pathogenesis of osteoporosis. N Engl J Med 318:818, 1988.
26. Delmas PD: Markers of bone formation and resorption. In Favus MJ (ed): Primer on the Metabolic Bone Disease and Disorders of Mineral Metabolism, 2nd ed. New York: Raven Press, 1993, pp 108–112.
27. Delmas PD, Schlemmer A, Gineyts E, et al.: Urinary excretion of pyridinoline crosslinks correlates with bone turnover measured on iliac crest biopsy in patients with vertebral osteoporosis. J Bone Miner Res 6:639, 1991.
28. Parfitt AM, Duncan H: Metabolic bone disease affecting the spine. In Rothman RH, Simeone FA (eds): The Spine, 2nd ed. Philadelphia: W B Saunders Co, 1982, pp 775–905.
29. Ardan GM: Bone destruction not demonstrable by radiography. Br J Radiol 24:107, 1951.
30. Thomson DL, Frame B: Involutional osteopenia: current concepts. Ann Intern Med 85:789, 1976.
31. Barnett E, Nordin BEC: The radiologic diagnosis of osteoporosis. A new approach. Clin Radiol 11:166, 1960.
32. Wahner HW: Assessment of metabolic bone disease: review of new nuclear medicine procedures. Mayo Clin Proc 60:827, 1985.
33. Genant HK, Cann CE, Ettinger B, Gordon GS: Quantitative computed tomography of vertebral spongiosa: a sensitive method for detecting early bone loss after oophorectomy. Ann Intern Med 97:699, 1982.
34. Ott S: Should women get screening bone mass measurements? (Editorial.) Ann Intern Med 104:874, 1986.
35. Hall FM, Davis MA, Baran DT: Bone mineral screening for osteoporosis. (Editorial.) N Engl J Med 316:212, 1987.
36. Lang P, Steiger P, Faulkner K, et al.: Osteoporosis: current techniques and recent developments in quantitative bone densitometry. Radiol Clin North Am 29:49, 1991.

37. White PH: Osteopenic disorders of the spine. Semin Spine Surg 2:121, 1990.
38. Michel BA, Lane NE, Jones HH, et al.: Plain radiographs can be useful in estimating lumbar bone density. J Rheumatol 17:528, 1990.
39. Mazess RB, Barden HS, Ettinger M: Radial and spinal bone mineral density in a patient population. Arthritis Rheum 31:891, 1988.
40. Pacifici R, Rupich R, Griffin M, et al.: Dual energy radiography versus quantitative computer tomography for the diagnosis of osteoporosis. J Clin Endocrinol Metab 70:705, 1990.
41. Haddaway MJ, Davie MWJ, McCall IW: Bone mineral density in healthy normal women and reproducibility of measurements in spine and hip using dual-energy x-ray absorptiometry. Br J Radiol 65:213, 1991.
42. Kellie SE: DEXA (letter). JAMA 268:475, 1992.
43. Heaney RP: Prevention of age-related osteoporosis in women. In Avioli LV (ed): The Osteoporotic Syndrome. New York: Grune and Stratton, 1983, pp 123–144.
44. Johnston CC Jr, Hui SL, Witt RM, et al.: Early menopausal changes in bone mass and sex steroids. J Clin Endocrinol Metab 61:905, 1985.
45. Crayton HE, Bell CL, De Smet AA: Sacral insufficiency fractures. Semin Arthritis Rheum 20:378, 1991.
46. Brower AC, Downey EF: Kümmell disease: report of a case with serial radiographs. Radiology 141:363, 1981.
47. Golimbu C, Firooznia H, Rafi M: The intravertebral vacuum sign. Spine 11:1040, 1986.
48. Ram PC, Martinez S, Korobkin M, et al.: CT detection of intraosseous gas. A new sign of osteomyelitis. AJR 137:721, 1981.
49. Chevalier X, Wrona N, Avouac B, et al.: Thigh pain and multiple vertebral osteonecroses: value of magnetic resonance imaging. J Rheumatol 18:1627, 1991.
50. Yuh WT, Zachar CK, Barloon TJ, et al.: Vertebral compression fractures: distinction between benign and malignant causes with MR imaging. Radiology 172:215, 1989.
51. Aloia JF, Vaswani AN, Yeh JK, Cohn SH: Premenopausal bone mass is related to physical activity. Arch Intern Med 148:121, 1988.
52. Chow R, Harrison JE, Notarius C: Effect of two randomised exercise programmes on bone mass of healthy postmenopausal women. Br Med J 295:1441, 1987.
53. Consensus Conference: Osteoporosis. JAMA 252:799, 1984.
54. Prince RL, Smith M, Dick IM, et al.: Prevention of postmenopausal osteoporosis: a comparative study of exercise, calcium supplementation, and hormone-replacement therapy. N Engl J Med 325:1189, 1991.
55. Dawson-Hughes B, Dallal GE, Krall EA, et al.: A controlled trial of the effect of calcium supplementation on bone density in postmenopausal women. N Engl J Med 323:878, 1990.
56. Riggs BL, Seeman E, Hodgson SF, et al.: Effect of the fluoride/calcium regimen on vertebral fracture occurrence in postmenopausal osteoporosis: comparison with conventional therapy. N Engl J Med 306:446, 1982.
57. Recker RR, Saville PD, Heaney RP: Effect of estrogens and calcium carbonate on bone loss in postmenopausal women. Ann Intern Med 87:649, 1977.
58. Riis B, Thomsen K, Christiansen C: Does calcium supplementation prevent postmenopausal bone loss? N Engl J Med 316:173, 1987.
59. Sheikh MS, Santa Ana CA, Nicar MJ, et al.: Gastrointestinal absorption of calcium from milk and calcium salts. N Engl J Med 317:532, 1987.
60. Lund B, Kjaer I, Friis T, et al.: Treatment of osteoporosis of aging with 1-hydroxycholecalciferol. Lancet 2:1168, 1975.
61. Riggs BL, Jowsey J, Kelley PJ, et al.: Effects of oral therapy with calcium and vitamin D in primary osteoporosis. J Clin Endocrinol Metab 42:1139, 1976.
62. Christiansen C, Christensen MS, Tansbol I: Bone mass in post-menopausal women after withdrawal of oestrogen/gestagen replacement therapy. Lancet 1:459, 1981.
63. Ettinger B, Genant HK, Cann CE: Postmenopausal bone loss is prevented by treatment with low-dosage estrogen with calcium. Ann Intern Med 106:40, 1987.
64. Lindsay R: Prevention and treatment of osteoporosis. Lancet 341:801, 1993.
65. Lindsay R, Tohme J: Estrogen treatment of patients with established postmenopausal osteoporosis. Obstet Gynecol 76:1, 1990.
66. Ribot C, Tremollieres F, Pouilles JM, et al.: Preventive effects of transdermal administration of 17B-estradiol on postmenopausal bone loss: a 2-year prospective study. Obstet Gynecol 75(suppl 4):43S, 1990.
67. Antunes CMF, Stolley PD, Rosenshein NB, et al.: Endometrial cancer and estrogen use: report of a large case-controlled study. N Engl J Med 300:9, 1979.
68. Wingo PA, Layde PM, Lee NC, et al.: The risk of breast cancer in postmenopausal women who have used estrogen replacement therapy. JAMA 257:209, 1987.
69. Stampfer MJ, Willet WC, Colditz GA, et al.: A prospective study of postmenopausal estrogen therapy and coronary heart disease. N Engl J Med 313:1044, 1985.
70. Walsh BW, Schiff I, Rosner B, et al.: Effects of postmenopausal estrogen replacement on the concentrations of metabolism of plasma lipoproteins. N Engl J Med 325:1196, 1991.
71. Lindsay R, Hart DM, MacLean A, et al.: Bone response to termination of estrogen treatment. Lancet 1:1325, 1978.
72. Goldman L, Tosteson ANA: Uncertainty about postmenopausal estrogen: time for action, not debate (editorial). N Engl J Med 325:800, 1991.
73. Storm T, Thamsborg G, Steiniche T, et al.: Effect of intermittent cyclical etidronate therapy on bone mass and fracture rate in women with postmenopausal osteoporosis. N Engl J Med 322:1265, 1990.
74. Watts NB, Harris ST, Genant HK, et al.: Intermittent cyclical etidronate treatment of postmenopausal osteoporosis. N Engl J Med 323:73, 1990.
75. Riggs BL, Hodgson SF, Hoffman DL, et al.: Treatment of primary osteoporosis with fluoride and calcium: clinical tolerance and fracture occurrence. JAMA 243:446, 1980.
76. Riggs BL, Seeman E, Hodgson SF, et al.: Effect of the fluoride/calcium regimen on vertebral fracture occurrence in postmenopausal osteoporosis. Comparison with conventional therapy. N Engl J Med 306:446, 1982.
77. Riggs BL, Hodgson SF, O'Fallon WM, et al.: Effect of fluoride treatment on the fracture rate in postmenopausal women with osteoporosis. N Engl J Med 322:802, 1990.
78. Gruber HE, Ivey JL, Baylink DJ, et al.: Long-term cal-

citonin therapy in postmenopausal osteoporosis. Metabolism 33:295, 1984.

79. Reginster JY, Denis D, Albert A, et al.: One-year controlled randomised trial of prevention of early postmenopausal bone loss by intranasal calcitonin. Lancet 2:1481, 1987.

80. Wasnich RD, Benfante RJ, Yano K, et al.: Thiazide effect on the mineral content of bone. N Engl J Med 309:344, 1983.

81. Love RR, Mazess RB, Barden HS, et al.: Effects of tamoxifen on bone mineral density in postmenopausal women with breast cancer. N Engl J Med 326:852, 1992.

82. Lukert BP, Raisz LG: Glucocorticoid-induced osteoporosis: pathogenesis and management. Ann Intern Med 112:352, 1990.

83. Verstraeten A, Van Ermen H, Haghebaert G, et al.: Osteoarthrosis retards the development of osteoporosis. Clin Orthop 264:169, 1991.

84. Sinaki M, McPhee MC, Hodgson SF, et al.: Relationship between bone mineral density of spine and nutritional strength of back extensors in healthy postmenopausal women. Mayo Clin Proc 61:116, 1986.

85. Lyles KW, Gold DT, Shipp KM, et al.: Association of osteoporotic vertebral compression fractures with impaired functional status. Am J Med 94:595, 1993.

86. Harris ST, Watts NB, Jackson RD, et al.: Four-year study of intermittent cyclic etidronate treatment of postmenopausal osteoporosis: three years of blinded therapy followed by one year of open therapy. Am J Med 95:557, 1993.

OSTEOMALACIA

Capsule Summary

Frequency of back pain—very common
Location of back pain—lumbar spine
Quality of back pain—acute, sharp (with fracture); chronic, dull ache
Symptoms and signs—pain increases with activity and standing
Laboratory and x-ray tests—decreased serum calcium, phosphate, vitamin D; increased alkaline phosphatase; decreased urinary calcium; increased parathormone; "codfish" vertebrae on plain roentgenograms; multiple Looser's zones on bone scan
Treatment—vitamin D, calcium, phosphate

PREVALENCE AND PATHOGENESIS

Osteomalacia is a metabolic bone disease associated with loss of bone mass per unit volume and a decrease in the ratio of bone mineral content to bone matrix. In essence, it is an abnormality in the mineralization of bone. Any disorder that affects calcium or phosphorus concentrations or alters the physiologic conditions needed for the formation of hydroxyapatite crystals may result in osteomala-

cia. It may occur in any of the long bones, pelvis, scapula, ribs, or axial skeleton. Loss of bone mineralization weakens the bone, which makes it vulnerable to fracture. Osteomalacia in the axial skeleton is associated with back pain, vertebral body weakening, fracture, and progressive kyphoscoliosis. It should be suspected in a patient with bone pain, radiographic evidence of decreased bone mass (osteopenia), and depressed levels of serum calcium and inorganic phosphate. The definitive diagnosis of osteomalacia is made based on the presence of a widened osteoid seam and decreased mineralization found in an undemineralized bone section. Osteomalacia may be caused by vitamin D deficiency, intestinal disorders, drugs, metabolic acidosis (usually associated with renal disorders, including tubular defects), phosphate deficiencies, and mineralization defects, both primary and secondary.

Evaluation of a patient with osteomalacia is directed at identifying the underlying disease process that results in the decreased bone mineralization. Treatment is directed toward the specific illness causing the osteomalacia and may include vitamin D supplements, pancreatic enzyme supplements, dietary modifications to increase intake of calcium and phosphorus, reduction of metabolic acidosis, and the discontinuation of drugs associated with osteomalacia.

The prevalence of osteomalacia is unknown. The number of illnesses associated with osteomalacia prohibits the computation of prevalence from all sources (Table 14–5).[1] Osteomalacia in children, rickets, is common outside the United States in areas of the world with malnutrition. Up to 9% of young children may demonstrate radiographic findings of rickets in impoverished urban areas.[2] Osteomalacia has been reported in 3% to 5% of acutely ill elderly patients.[3] Before the 1930s, vitamin D-sensitive osteomalacia was the most common form of osteomalacia. With the addition of vitamin D to the diet, the frequency of nutritional vitamin D osteomalacia has decreased. In the 1990s, some variant of vitamin D-resistant osteomalacia is a more commonly recognized form of disease.[4]

Osteomalacia includes a group of disorders with similar clinical symptoms and signs but with diverse etiologies. The most frequent abnormality associated with osteomalacia is vitamin D deficiency. Vitamin D in its activated form increases intestinal calcium absorption, renal tubular resorption of calcium and phosphate, and promotion of bone mineralization.[5]

TABLE 14–5. DISEASES ASSOCIATED WITH OSTEOMALACIA

DISORDER	METABOLIC DEFECT
Vitamin D	
Deficiency	Decreased generation of vitamin D_3
Dietary	
Ultraviolet light exposure	
Malabsorption	Decreased absorption of vitamins D_2 and D_3
Small intestine	
Inadequate bile salts	
Pancreatic insufficiency	
Abnormal metabolism	
Hereditary enzyme deficiency vitamin D-dependent rickets Type I	Decreased 1 alpha-hydroxylation of 25-(OH)-vitamin D
Chronic renal failure	Decreased 25-hydroxylation of vitamin D
Mesenchymal tumors	?P450 enzyme alteration of 25-hydroxyvitamin D
Systemic acidosis	conversion vs. decreased sunlight exposure
Hepatic failure	
Anticonvulsant drugs	
Peripheral resistance	Absent or abnormal $1.25\text{-}(OH)_2$-vitamin D
Vitamin D-dependent rickets (Type II)	receptors
Phosphate depletion	
Dietary	
Malnutrition (rare)?	Inadequate bone mineralization secondary to low
Aluminum hydroxide ingestion	serum concentrations
Renal tubular wasting	
Hereditary	Decreased serum phosphate concentrations
X-linked hypophosphatemic osteomalacia	
Acquired	
Hypophosphatemic osteomalacia	
Renal disorders	
Fanconi's syndrome	
Mesenchymal tumors	
Fibrous dysplasia	
Mineralization defects	
Hereditary	Abnormal alkaline phosphatase activity
Hypophosphatasia	
Acquired	
Sodium fluoride	Inhibition of bone mineralization
Disodium etidronate	
Miscellaneous	
Osteopetrosis	Abnormal osteoclast activity
Fibrogenesis imperfecta	Unknown
Axial osteomalacia	Unknown
Calcium deficiency	Inadequate bone mineralization secondary to low serum calcium concentration

The sources of vitamin D are exogenous (fortified dairy products) and endogenous (exposure of skin to ultraviolet rays in sunlight). Dairy products are fortified with vitamin D_2 (ergocalciferol, irradiation product of plant sterols) or vitamin D_3 (cholecalciferol). Adequate gastrointestinal absorption of dietary vitamin D requires an intact and functioning mucosal surface of the small intestine as well as an intact biliary system with adequate concentrations of bile salts. A more important source of vitamin D_3 is endogenous production generated by the exposure of 7-dehydrocholesterol in the skin to ultraviolet light.

Vitamin D (either D_2 or D_3) is transported to the liver by a carrier protein. Hepatic enzymes hydroxylate the precursor vitamin at the 25 position to form 25-hydroxyvitamin D. The 25-hydroxyvitamin D is then transported to the kidney, where hydroxylation at the 24 position will form 24,25-dihydroxyvitamin D, an active form of vitamin D. This form of vitamin D may contribute to mineralization of bone and modulation of parathyroid function, but it is less potent than the 1,25-dihydroxy form of vitamin D. Increased activity of 1-hydroxylase, the enzyme that controls hydroxylation at the 1 position, is mediated by decreased dietary intake of calcium, increased parathyroid hormone secretion, and hypophosphatemia.[5] Both inadequate intake of vitamin D-supplemented nutrition and an avoidance of the sun must occur to cause deficiency severe enough to result in osteomalacia.

Normal vitamin D absorption in the gut requires an intact intestinal mucosa, normal hepatobiliary circulation of bile salts, and, to a lesser degree, exocrine pancreatic function. Osteomalacia may occur despite adequate production of vitamin D_3 in the skin since the hepatic product 25-hydroxyvitamin D undergoes enterohepatic circulation like bile salts.[6] Most vitamin D is absorbed in the mid-jejunum, while a smaller component is absorbed in the terminal ileum.[7] Diseases associated with small bowel malabsorption, such as sprue, celiac disease, Crohn's disease, scleroderma, and jejunal diverticula, and bowel bypass surgery may all be complicated by osteomalacia.[8] Postgastrectomy patients are also prone to develop osteomalacia. Patients with hepatocellular disorders (cirrhosis, alcoholic hepatitis, or chronic active hepatitis) and those with biliary system disease (primary biliary cirrhosis) are unable to absorb vitamin D and develop osteomalacia.[9, 10] Malabsorption associated with pancreatic insufficiency may cause osteomalacia not only by decreasing levels of 25-hydroxyvitamin D but also by decreasing calcium absorption.[11] Osteomalacia may be the only symptom in some patients with gluten-sensitive enteropathy.[12]

$1,25\text{-}(OH)_2D_3$ is responsible for calcium and phosphorus homeostasis and maintenance of bone mineralization.[13] In the intestine, vitamin D increases the absorption of calcium and phosphorus. Parathyroid hormone binds to receptors on intestinal cells activating adenyl cyclase and cyclic adenosine monophosphate to allow calcium to enter the cell. Activated $1,23\text{-}(OH)_2$ vitamin D acts to enhance the message to synthesize cholecalcin or calbindin, binding proteins, that transport calcium across the cell membrane into the extracellular space.[14] The vitamin also affects skeletal tissues by mobilizing calcium and phosphorus from old bone and promotes mineralization in newly formed organic bone matrix.[4] 1,25-dihydroxyvitamin D also has effects on osteocalcin production, osteoclastic resorption, monocytic maturation, myelocytic resorption, skin growth, and insulin secretion.[15, 16]

The regulation of 1,25-dihydroxyvitamin D is determined by the interaction of serum calcium, serum phosphorus, and parathyroid hormone. Decreased serum calcium levels cause secretion of parathyroid hormone that stimulates 1,25 production. The result is an increase in absorption and mobilization of bone calcium and phosphorus. The increased phosphorus is excreted by the kidney resulting in increased serum calcium. In the setting of decreased vitamin D, gastrointestinal absorption of calcium is decreased resulting in decreased serum calcium concentration. This change in calcium results in secondary hyperparathyroidism causing a mobilization of bone calcium along with a phosphate diuresis. The chemical results of these changes are low serum calcium, diminished serum phosphate, decreased urinary calcium, reduced tubular resorption of phosphate, and increased alkaline phosphatase. The levels of vitamin D are decreased and parathormone is increased. The metabolic effects on bone are secondary to reduced mineral and secondary hyperparathyroidism.

Abnormalities, hereditary or acquired, in the metabolism necessary for the formation of 1,25-dihydroxyvitamin D result in rickets or osteomalacia. Patients with an autosomal recessive genetic condition of an absence of the renal 25-hydroxyl-1-hydroxylase are incapable of manufacturing adequate concentrations of 1,25-dihydroxyvitamin D. These patients develop vitamin D-dependent rickets.[17] Patients with chronic parenchymal liver disease are unable to form 25-hydroxyvitamin D.[18] Renal osteodystrophy is the bone disease associated with chronic renal failure. Osteomalacia, osteoporosis, osteosclerosis (particularly in the axial skeleton), and secondary hyperparathyroidism are all potential complications of renal disease. Osteomalacia in renal osteodystrophy occurs secondary to the impaired conversion of 25-hydroxyvitamin D to 1,25-dihydroxyvitamin D due to a decrease in kidney cell mass.[19] Hyperphosphatemia and systemic acidosis, complications of chronic renal failure, also may contribute to the deficiency of the renal metabolite.[20] Anticonvulsant drugs, phenytoin (Dilantin) and phenobarbital, induce hepatic hydroxylase enzymes that alter 25-hydroxyvitamin D, producing inactive metabolites.[21] Phenytoin also may decrease calcium absorption from the gut.[22] A rare cause of abnormal vitamin D metabolism is mesenchymal soft tissue tumors associated with low levels of 1,25-hydroxyvitamin D.[23] A study of 72 patients with tumor-associated osteomalacia and low levels of 1,25-dihydroxyvitamin D included about a third of tumors of vascular origin, such as hemangiopericytomas. Other common tumors included nonossifying fibromas, mesenchymal tumors, and giant cell tumors.

Only 10 of the 72 tumors were malignant.[24] Patients with hypophosphatemia and mesenchymal tumors may have clinical and radiologic findings in the sacroiliac joints that may resemble those of ankylosing spondylitis.[25] Patients may develop osteomalacia in the face of normal concentrations of 1,25-dihydroxyvitamin D when impaired end organ (gut and bone) responsiveness to the renal metabolite exists. This may occur with chronic renal failure or use of anticonvulsant drugs.[26] When no other etiology is evident, peripheral resistance to vitamin D associated with hypocalcemia, osteomalacia, and secondary hyperparathyroidism is referred to as vitamin D-dependent rickets Type II.[27]

Phosphate, as well as calcium, in the appropriate concentration is essential for normal bone mineralization and muscle function. Any disorder that causes phosphate deficiency will result in osteomalacia. Phosphorus is present in most foodstuffs. Therefore, phosphate deficiency on the basis of malnutrition is rare. Patients who ingest large quantities of phosphate-binding aluminum antacids for ulcer or renal disease are at risk of developing osteomalacia.[28] Aluminum may cause phosphate malabsorption by precipitation of aluminum phosphates in the gut. The result is decreased serum phosphate, normal serum calcium, and elevated alkaline phosphatase.[29] The most common cause of hypophosphatemia is related to hereditary or acquired renal tubular wasting of phosphate. A hereditary form of phosphate depletion is X-linked (male) hypophosphatemic osteomalacia. Phosphate reabsorption in the kidney is modulated predominantly by parathyroid hormone and, to a lesser degree, by serum calcium concentration.[30] Patients with X-linked hypophosphatemic osteomalacia (or familial vitamin D-resistant rickets) have complete absence of the parathyroid hormone-sensitive component of phosphate reabsorption. The disease is transmitted as a dominant trait in men, has onset in childhood, and results in short stature and bowing of legs in adults.[31] The disease may have an onset in adulthood (hypophosphatemic osteomalacia) in patients with no evidence of rachitic deformities.[32] Patients with familial vitamin D-resistant rickets develop increases in bone density in the axial skeleton along with ectopic calcification, which resembles ankylosing spondylitis.[33] Enthesopathy is a universal finding in adults with hypophosphatemic osteomalacia.[34] Many of these individuals are disabled secondary to degenerative joint disease in the lower extremities. A new form of hypophosphatemic osteomalacia is associated with hypercalciuria and increased levels of 1,25-dihydroxyvitamin D. The differentiation of these patients from those with other forms of hypophosphatemic osteomalacia is that the use of phosphate reverses osteomalacia and the use of vitamin D exacerbates the condition.[35]

Fanconi syndrome comprises a heterogeneous group of disorders that cause dysfunction in the renal tubules.[36] The syndromes have been classified by Mankin into proximal, distal, or combination of proximal and distal tubular diseases.[31] Tubular disorders may result in phosphate wasting, glycosuria, aminoaciduria, renal tubular acidosis, hypokalemia, or polyurias. A number of disorders, including cystinosis, Lowe's syndrome (oculocerebrorenal syndrome), Wilson's disease, tyrosinemia, nephrotic syndrome, and multiple myeloma may cause tubular dysfunction resulting in osteomalacia. Tumors, both benign and malignant, that inhibit renal phosphate absorption may cause osteomalacia.[37] Tumors associated with osteomalacia include giant cell tumor, nonossifying fibroma, osteoblastoma, and angiosarcoma.[38] These tumors may be producing a factor that is an antagonist to vitamin D.[39] Evidence for this proposal is the report of two patients who did not respond to increasing doses of vitamin D but became responsive to normal doses of vitamin D with removal of the tumors.[40] Neurofibromatosis also is associated with hypophosphatemia and osteomalacia.[41] The mechanism of phosphate wasting is of renal origin. These patients may improve with increased doses of vitamin D. Fibrous dysplasia, a disorder of unknown etiology that causes bone lesions with a ground-glass appearance in combination with precocious puberty and skin pigmentation, has been associated with osteomalacia.[42]

Alkaline phosphatase is an enzyme required for the normal mineralization of bone. Patients with hypophosphatasia have a deficiency in this enzyme resulting in elevated levels of plasma and urinary inorganic pyrophosphate, phosphorylethanolamine, and osteomalacia.[43] Adults with the disease have osteomalacia with axial skeletal ligamentous and tendinous calcification and develop marked limitation of motion in the lumbosacral spine.[44] Fluoride in increased concentrations causes inhibition of bone mineralization. Patients in areas where fluorosis is endemic or those who received sodium fluoride for osteoporosis are at risk of developing osteomalacia.[45] Diphosphonates, synthetic analogues of pyrophosphate, are inhibitors of bone formation and are used in the therapy of patients with Paget's disease. Patients receiving diphosphonates at increased doses for extended periods may develop inadequate mineralization of bone and pathologic fractures.[46] Aluminum causes osteomalacia by interfering with bone mineralization at the mineralization front in bone.[47]

A number of miscellaneous disorders may be associated with osteomalacia. Axial osteomalacia is a disease occurring in adult men who develop typical osteomalacic changes in bone limited to the axial skeleton, including the cervical and lumbar spine.[48] Some of these patients have features on radiographs that are similar to those of ankylosing spondylitis.[49] Fibrogenesis imperfecta ossium is a rare lesion in men over 50 who develop increased bone density, pseudofractures, and bone pain.[50] Osteopetrosis, also called marble bone or Albers-Schönberg disease, is a rare inherited disorder associated with increased osteosclerosis.[51] The benign form, autosomal dominant in inheritance, is associated with bone pain, fracture, osteomyelitis, and cranial nerve palsies due to bone overgrowth. The pathogenesis of the illness is related to the absence of osteoclastic activity in resorbing bone.

CLINICAL HISTORY

Patients with osteomalacia may present with a wide variety of symptoms depending on the underlying cause of their bone disease. The major complaint relating to their bone disease is bone pain. In nutritional osteomalacia, backache along with spine tenderness is present in over 90% of cases.[52] It is maximal in the lower extremities and axial skeleton and is worsened by activity. Lumbar pain increases with standing as opposed to the sudden and severe pain associated with osteoporosis. Back pain starts in the lumbar area and hips and then spreads to the upper portion of the spine and extremities.[53] Fractures of the spine causing sudden changes in height do not occur with osteomalacia unless the patient has concomitant osteoporosis.[54] The pain of osteomalacia tends to be more diffuse and less intense, but of longer duration. Muscle weakness and tenderness, along with episodes of muscle spasm, particularly in the proximal muscles in the lower extremities, may occur with hypocalcemia or hypophosphatemia. Movement of the spine is not necessarily painful. Patients with osteomalacia with long-standing disease may also have a history of fractures in appendicular bones. In rare circumstances, patients with X-linked hypophosphatemic osteomalacia may develop

symptoms of spinal stenosis associated with lower leg weakness. The level of stenosis is frequently the lower thoracic spine and is secondary to ossification of the ligamentum flavum.[55]

PHYSICAL EXAMINATION

Physical findings are sparse in osteomalacia. The affected bones are tender on palpation, and proximal muscles may be tender as well. Muscle weakness, exemplified by inability to climb stairs or to rise from a seated position, also may be present. The patient has a waddling gait similar to that associated with inflammatory proximal myopathies. Kyphoscoliosis of the thoracic and lumbar spine is prominent if osteomalacia of the axial skeleton is long-standing. Adult patients with a history of rickets may have short stature, bowing of the lower extremities, and enlargement of the costochondral junctions (rachitic rosary).

LABORATORY DATA

Laboratory abnormalities are frequent in patients with osteomalacia, which is in marked distinction to the normal values found in patients with osteoporosis.[1] Patients with abnormalities in vitamin D concentration or metabolism have low serum calcium and phosphate concentration, elevated serum alkaline phosphatase, a reduced renal phosphate threshold, generalized aminoaciduria, reduced urinary calcium excretion, increased parathyroid hormone (hyperparathyroidism secondary to hypocalcemia), and decreased serum concentrations of vitamin D (Table 14–6). The forms of vitamin D that are assayed are 25-hydroxyvitamin D and 1,25-dihydroxyvitamin D. These tests have assay variation and cross-react with materials that may not be vitamin constituents. Therefore, vitamin D assay results must be viewed critically and in light of other independent data (calcium, phosphate, and parathormone levels).[56] Urinary calcium excretion is less than 75 mg/day in 95% of patients with osteomalacia, and this measurement is a useful screening test.[57] Laboratory abnormalities associated with phosphate wasting include low serum phosphate, normal serum calcium, elevated serum alkaline phosphatase concentration, a reduced renal phosphate threshold, normal amino acid excretion, reduced urinary calcium excretion, increased parathyroid hormone concentration with therapy, and normal vitamin D concentrations. Additional laboratory abnormalities may be present depending

TABLE 14–6. LABORATORY FINDINGS IN SELECTED OSTEOMALACIC DISORDERS

	SERUM CALCIUM	SERUM PHOSPHORUS	SERUM ALKALINE PHOSPHATASE	SERUM BICARBONATE	URINARY CALCIUM EXCRETION	SERUM 25-(OH)- VITAMIN D	SERUM 1,25(OH)$_2$ VITAMIN D	SERUM PARATHORMONE	OTHER
Vitamin D deficiency	N, L	L	H	N, L	L	L	L, N	H	
Intestinal malabsorption	N, L	L	H	N, L	L	L	L, N	H	Malabsorption tests positive
Chronic renal failure	L, N	H	H	L	L	N	L	H	Abnormal kidney function
Phosphate depletion (antacids)	N	L	N, L	N	N, H	N	N, H	N	Urinary phosphate low
Phosphate depletion (renal wasting)	N, L	L	H	L	N, H	N	N	N	Urinary phosphate high
Phosphate depletion (tumor-related)	N	L	H	N	N	L	N	N	Tumor interference with renal tubular phosphate reabsorption
Axial osteomalacia	N	N	N	N	N	N	N	N	

N = normal; H = high; L = low.

on the underlying disease causing osteomalacia. Examples of these abnormalities might include decreased serum carotene, increased fecal fat in gastrointestinal malabsorption, increased urea nitrogen and creatinine in renal failure, and anemia and elevated ESR with a tumor. Patients with osteomalacia secondary to gastrectomy may not demonstrate typical laboratory abnormalities. These patients may have normal serum calcium and alkaline phosphatase concentrations. In some patients, 25-hydroxyvitamin D was normal but bone biopsy revealed osteomalacia.[58] Osteocalcin is a marker of osteoblast function. In patients with osteomalacia, osteocalcin is elevated along with serum alkaline phosphatase. The increase in osteocalcin is related to increased osteoid synthesis but not the mineralization defect.[59]

The definitive diagnosis of osteomalacia must be made by biopsy of undemineralized sections of a bone (Fig. 14–9). Tetracycline, which will fix to newly forming mineralized bone, is given to patients before the biopsy sample is taken. The extent of tetracycline fluorescence in bone is used to measure the decrease in the mineralization front. There is also an increase in osteoid thickness (more than 20 μ) and an increase in osteoid seams covering cortical and trabecular bone associated with osteomalacia.

RADIOGRAPHIC EVALUATION

The radiographic findings of osteomalacia are osteopenia and loss of bone mass, and they mimic the changes of osteoporosis. The generalized loss of bone density in osteomalacia is indistinguishable from bone loss in osteoporosis. In osteomalacia, the remaining trabeculae are thickened between radiolucent areas blurring the trabecular pattern. One of the major radiologic findings in osteomalacia is pseudofractures (Looser's zones, Milkman's fractures).[60] They occur in long or flat bones, usually oriented at right angles to the cortex, and incompletely span the diameter of the bone. Pseudofractures, which usually occur symmetrically, may or may not be associated with pain. Radiographic findings in the spine may include expansion of the intervertebral discs with "codfish" vertebrae and scoliosis if osteomalacia occurs during periods of growth. In contrast to osteoporosis, most vertebral bodies are involved to a similar degree (Figs. 14–10 and 14–11). Pseudofractures may occur in the ribs, pelvis, femoral neck, ulna, radius, scapula, clavicles, and phalanges. With long-standing disease and minimal trauma, patients with weakened areas of bone secondary to pseudofractures develop true fractures.

Patients with hypophosphatemic osteomalacia may develop radiographic enthesopathic changes in the axial skeleton that may mimic ankylosing spondylitis. The changes in the sacroiliac joints included mild widening, symmetric intra-articular and anterior para-articular bony bridging, and enthesopathic calcification. These changes may occur without marked changes of osteomalacia in other areas of the skeleton.[61]

Patients with renal osteodystrophy will have changes of osteomalacia but also will have findings associated with secondary hyperparathyroidism, which are predominant. These patients have areas of osteosclerosis in the spine (49% in one study), bone cysts, and erosion of

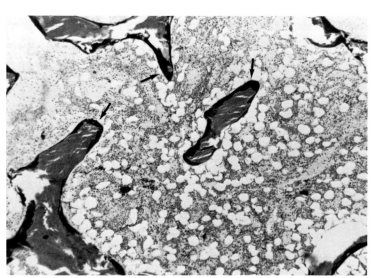

Figure 14–9. Osteomalacia. Histologic section exhibiting increased surface osteoid and increased osteoid thickness *(arrows)*. (Courtesy of Arnold Schwartz, M.D.)

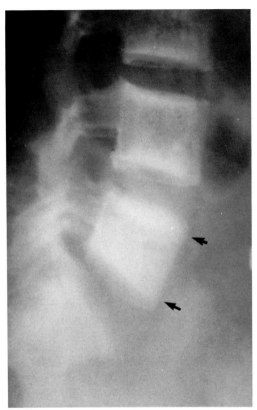

Figure 14–10. Osteomalacia. "Rugger jersey" spine of osteomalacia characterized by smudgy increased density of vertebral endplates *(arrows)* and osteopenia of the midportion of vertebral bodies with indistinct trabeculae. (Courtesy of Anne Brower, M.D.)

bone which may be noted around the sacroiliac joints.[62, 63]

Some investigators have suggested that bone scintigraphy is useful in the evaluation of metabolic bone decrease. Increased uptake of tracer is noted in areas of active bone metabolism. Although helpful, quantitative results from a number of conditions overlap, making the differentiation of these disorders by bone scintigraphy difficult.[64]

DIFFERENTIAL DIAGNOSIS

The diagnosis of osteomalacia can be suspected in a patient with bone pain and deformity, muscle weakness and tenderness, abnormal laboratory data consistent with disordered bone metabolism, and radiographic evidence of inadequate bone mineralization; and it can be confirmed, if necessary, by bone biopsy. A recent study reviewed the significance of clinical, radiographic, and biochemical abnormalities in the diagnosis of osteomalacia.[65] Patients

with osteomalacia had at least two of the following abnormalities: low serum calcium, low serum phosphate, elevated serum alkaline phosphatase, or radiographic evidence of pseudofractures. Tests that were not helpful included parathormone levels, 1,25-dihydroxyvitamin D, and decreased urinary calcium excretion. Histologic examination of a bone biopsy specimen is a useful test for patients in whom the diagnosis of osteomalacia remains in question after noninvasive screening tests are performed. Osteomalacia, like acute pain, is a sign of an underlying disease process that requires additional evaluation. The possibility that a patient has one of the diseases associated with osteomalacia listed in Table 14–5 would need to be investigated. In addition to osteoporosis, diffuse carcinomatosis of bone, polymyositis, or rhabdomyolysis would also have to be considered in a patient with bone pain or muscle weakness. The acute onset of pain, with pain-free intervals, and normal calcium and phosphate concentrations help differentiate patients with osteoporosis from those with osteomalacia. It should be remembered that vitamin D deficiency is not uncommon in the elderly, many of whom are not exposed to the sun and do not drink milk. These individuals may have a combination of metabolic bone diseases, osteomalacia, and osteoporosis.[66] Anemia and abnormal serum proteins are associated with diffuse carcinomatosis (multiple myeloma). Elevated muscle enzyme levels identify patients with primary muscle diseases.

Osteomalacia may occur in the setting of another illness that causes abnormalities of the skeleton. A notable prevalence of unrecognized osteomalacia was present in hospitalized patients with rheumatoid arthritis.[67] In these patients, 12.9% had unrecognized osteomalacia. They were elderly, had a poor diet, and were housebound. Osteomalacia should be considered in patients with other reasons for musculoskeletal pain who are at risk for vitamin D deficiency.

TREATMENT

The treatment of osteomalacia must be directed at the underlying abnormality that results in abnormal bone mineralization. The recommended daily intake of vitamin D is 400 IU for children and 100 IU for adults. This amount of vitamin D is adequate to heal bone lesions secondary to vitamin D nutritional deficiency, although higher doses can be given to speed healing.[53] Vitamin D comes in many

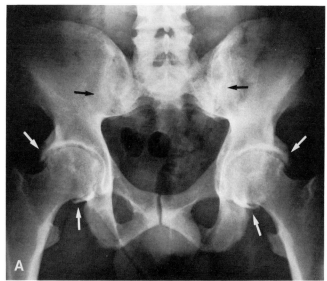

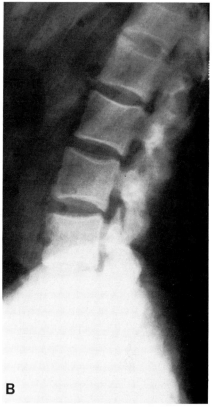

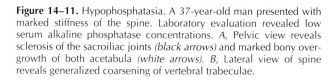

Figure 14–11. Hypophosphatasia. A 37-year-old man presented with marked stiffness of the spine. Laboratory evaluation revealed low serum alkaline phosphatase concentrations. *A,* Pelvic view reveals sclerosis of the sacroiliac joints *(black arrows)* and marked bony overgrowth of both acetabula *(white arrows). B,* Lateral view of spine reveals generalized coarsening of vertebral trabeculae.

different forms. These include vitamin D_2 (calciferol), dihydrotachysterol, 25-hydroxyvitamin D_3 (calcifediol, Calderol), and 1,25-dihydroxyvitamin D_3 (calcitriol, Rocaltrol).[68] Adequate calcium and phosphate intake are also required to assure normal mineralization of bone. Therapy for patients with osteomalacia secondary to gastrointestinal disorders should be directed at the underlying gut disease. For instance, a gluten-free diet may in itself correct osteomalacia in a patient with celiac disease. Patients with refractory gastrointestinal disease may benefit from pharmacologic doses of vitamin D (1 to 10 mg/day). Oral pancreatic enzymes may improve vitamin D absorption in pancreatic insufficiency. Increased oral intake of vitamin D (1 to 2 mg/day), along with correction of acidosis or removal of a tumor, will improve bone mineralization in patients with abnormal vitamin D metabolism. Patients with chronic renal failure may benefit from replacement with physiologic doses of 1,25-dihydroxyvitamin D_3. Discontinuing anti-epileptic drugs may be helpful in improving calcium absorption, decreasing osteomalacia, and improving musculoskeletal pain.[69]

Patients with phosphate-wasting forms of osteomalacia require phosphate supplementa-tion and vitamin D to reduce the possibility of decreased serum ionized calcium concentrations and secondary hyperparathyroidism. Some patients may also require alkali therapy to control renal tubular acidosis. Patients with osteomalacia secondary to hypophosphatemia associated with mesenchymal tumors improve with removal of the neoplasm.[70]

Mineralization defects caused by fluoride may be prevented if calcium supplements are administered. The pathologic fractures associated with disodium etidronate used in therapy of Paget's disease may be prevented by using doses of 5 mg/kg along with an alternating monthly schedule of giving and not giving the drug. Medical therapy of adult hypophosphatasia is ineffective. Treatment of aluminum-associated osteomalacia has a number of options. Discontinuing aluminum-containing medications is helpful. Desferrioxamine has been utilized to allow mineralization of bone despite the presence of aluminum. The proposed mechanism of action is relief of the inhibitory action of aluminum on parathyroid cells and osteoblasts.[71] Others have suggested that iron in patients with chronic renal failure may be the cause of osteomalacia.[72] Desferrioxamine may be helpful by removing iron from these patients allowing for improved bone metabolism.

PROGNOSIS

The prognosis of osteomalacia is based not only on the time of onset of the illness (rickets) and the extent of the bone disease, but also on the underlying disease and its reversibility with therapy. Many forms of osteomalacia are reversible with adequate vitamin D, calcium, and phosphorus supplementation. Pseudofractures heal and bone can be restored to normal mineralization and strength. Deformities secondary to bone weakening, lower extremity bowing, and kyphoscoliosis remain but do not progress. Patients with these reversible forms of osteomalacia are able to resume normal work activities without increased risk of fracture. Patients with hereditary abnormalities tend to be less responsive to therapy and areas of bone may continue to be osteomalacic in these patients despite therapy. Patients with chronic renal failure and those on chronic dialysis may continue to have osteomalacia despite efforts at maintaining calcium and phosphorus concentrations close to normal and correcting acidosis. Secondary hyperparathyroidism, which complicates renal osteodystrophy, may necessitate the removal of hypertrophied parathyroid tissue to prevent additional bone destruction. Patients with tumors and osteomalacia will have a prognosis that corresponds to the characteristics of the neoplasms. With so many diseases associated with osteomalacia, the prognosis for that disease must be evaluated on an individual basis, taking into account all factors that deal with the underlying disease process, extent of bone disease, and potential response to therapy.

References

OSTEOMALACIA

1. Dent CE, Stamp TCB: Vitamin D, rickets, and osteomalacia. In Avioli LV, and Krane SM (eds): Metabolic Bone Disease. New York: Academic Press, 1977, pp 237–305.
2. Richards IDG, Sweet EM, Arneil GC: Infantile rickets persists in Glasgow. Lancet 1:803, 1968.
3. Campbell GA: Osteomalacia: diagnosis and management. Br J Hosp Med 44:332, 1990.
4. Pitt MJ: Rickets and osteomalacia are still around. Radiol Clin North Am 29:97, 1991.
5. Haussler MR, McCain TA: Basic and clinical concepts related to vitamin D metabolism and action. N Engl J Med 297:974, 1977.
6. Arnaud SB, Goldsmith RS, Lambert PN, Go VLW: 25-hydroxyvitamin D_3: evidence of an enterohepatic circulation in man. Proc Exp Biol Med 149:570, 1975.
7. Schachter D, Finkelstein JD, Kowarski S: Metabolism of vitamin D. Part I. Preparation of radioactive vitamin D and its intestinal absorption in the rat. J Clin Invest 43:787, 1964.
8. Sitrin M, Meredith S, Rosenberg IH: Vitamin D deficiency and bone disease in gastrointestinal disorders. Arch Intern Med 138:886, 1978.
9. Compston JE, Thompson RPH: Intestinal absorption of 25-hydroxyvitamin D and osteomalacia in primary biliary cirrhosis. Lancet 1:721, 1977.
10. Long RG, Skinner RK, Willes MR, Sherlock S: Serum 25-hydroxyvitamin D in untreated parenchymal and cholestatic liver disease. Lancet 2:650, 1976.
11. Hahn TJ, Squires AE, Halstead LR, Strominger DB: Reduced serum 25-hydroxyvitamin D concentration and disordered mineral metabolism in patients with cystic fibrosis. J Pediatr 94:38, 1979.
12. De Boer WA, Tytgat GN: A patient with osteomalacia as single presenting symptom of gluten-sensitive enteropathy. J Intern Med 232:81, 1992.
13. Mankin HJ: Rickets, osteomalacia, and renal osteodystrophy: an update. Orthop Clin North Am 21:81, 1990.
14. Bronner F: Intestinal calcium absorption: mechanisms and applications. J Nutr 117:1347, 1987.
15. DeLuca HF: The vitamin D story: a collaborative effort of basic science and clinical medicine. FASEB J 2:224, 1988.
16. Reichel H, Koeffler P, Norman AW: The role of vitamin D endocrine system in health and disease. N Engl J Med 320:980, 1989.
17. Fraser D, Kooh SW, Kind HP, et al.: Pathogenesis of hereditary vitamin D-dependent rickets: an inborn error of vitamin D metabolism involving defective conversion of 25-hydroxyvitamin D to 1,25-dihydroxyvitamin D. N Engl J Med 289:817, 1973.
18. Imawari M, Akanuma Y, Itakura H, et al.: The effects of diseases of the liver on serum 25-hydroxyvitamin D and on the serum binding protein for vitamin D and its metabolites. J Lab Clin Med 93:171, 1979.
19. Avioli LV: Controversies regarding uremia and acquired defects in vitamin D_3 metabolism. Kidney Int 13(Suppl 8):36, 1978.
20. Lee SW, Russell J, Avioli LV: 25-dihydroxycholecalciferol to 1,25-dihydroxycholecalciferol: conversion impaired by systemic metabolic acidosis. Science 195:994, 1977.
21. Hahn TJ, Birge SJ, Scharp CR, Avioli LV: Phenobarbital-induced alterations in vitamin D metabolism. J Clin Invest 51:741, 1972.
22. Villareale ME, Chiroff RT, Bergstron WH, et al.: Bone changes induced by diphenylhydantoin in chicks on a controlled vitamin D intake. J Bone Joint Surg 60A:911, 1978.
23. Drezner MK, Feinglos MN: Osteomalacia due to 1,25-dihydroxycholecalciferol deficiency: association with a giant cell tumor of bone. J Clin Invest 60:1046, 1977.
24. Nuovo MA, Dorfman HD, Sun CC, Chalew SA: Tumor-induced osteomalacia and rickets. Am J Surg Pathol 13:588, 1989.
25. Moser CR, Fessel WJ: Rheumatic manifestations of hypophosphatemia. Arch Intern Med 134:674, 1974.
26. Brickman AS, Coburn JW, Massey SG: 1,25-dihydroxyvitamin D_3 in normal man and patients with renal failure. Ann Intern Med 80:161, 1974.
27. Brooks MD, Bell NH, Love L, et al.: Vitamin D-dependent rickets type II: resistance of target organs to

1,25-dihydroxyvitamin D. N Engl J Med 298:996, 1978.

28. Dent CE, Winter CS: Osteomalacia due to phosphate depletion from excessive aluminum hydroxide ingestion. Br Med J 1:551, 1974.

29. Kassem M, Eriksen EF, Melsen F, Mosekilde L: Antacid-induced osteomalacia: a case report with a histomorphometric analysis. J Intern Med 229:275, 1991.

30. Glorieux FH, Scriver CR: Loss of a parathyroid hormone-sensitive component of phosphate transport in X-linked hypophosphatemia. Science 175:997, 1972.

31. Mankin HJ: Rickets, osteomalacia and renal osteodystrophy. Part II. J Bone Joint Surg 56A:352, 1974.

32. Frymoyer JW, Hodgkin W: Adult-onset vitamin D-resistant hypophosphatemic osteomalacia. A possible variant of vitamin D-resistant rickets. J Bone Joint Surg 59A:101, 1977.

33. Steinbach HL, Kolb FO, Crane JT: Unusual roentgen manifestations of osteomalacia. AJR 82:875, 1959.

34. Reid IR, Hardy DC, Murphy WA, et al.: X-linked hypophosphatemia: a clinical, biochemical, and histopathologic assessment of morbidity in adults. Medicine 68:336, 1989.

35. Tieder M, Arie R, Bab I, et al.: A new kindred with hereditary hypophosphatemic rickets with hypercalciuria: implications for correct diagnosis and treatment. Nephron 62:176, 1992.

36. Dent CE: Rickets (and osteomalacia), nutritional and metabolic (1919–1969). Proc R Soc Med 63:401, 1970.

37. Harrison HE: Oncogenous rickets. Possible elaboration by a tumor of a humeral substance inhibiting tubular reabsorption of phosphate. Pediatrics 52:432, 1973.

38. Goldring SR, Krane SM: Disorders of calcification: Osteomalacia and rickets. In De Groot L (ed): Endocrinology, Vol. 2. New York: Grune and Stratton, 1979, pp 853–871.

39. Siris ES, Clemens TL, Dempster DW, et al.: Tumor-induced osteomalacia. Kinetics of calcium, phosphorus, and vitamin D metabolism and characteristics of bone histomorphometry. Am J Med 82:307, 1987.

40. Sparagana M: Tumor-induced osteomalacia: long-term follow-up of two patients cured by removal of their tumors. J Surg Oncol 36:198, 1987.

41. Konishi K, Nakamura M, Yamakawa H, et al.: Hypophosphatemic osteomalacia in von Recklinghausen neurofibromatosis. Am J Med Sci 301:322, 1991.

42. Dent CE, Gertner JM: Hypophosphatemic osteomalacia in fibrous dysplasia. Q J Med 45:411, 1976.

43. Jardon OM, Burney DW, Fink RL: Hypophosphatasia in an adult. J Bone Joint Surg 52A:1477, 1970.

44. Anderton JM: Orthopedic problems in adult hypophosphatasia. J Bone Joint Surg 61B:82, 1979.

45. Teotia SPS, Teotia M: Secondary hyperparathyroidism in patients with endemic skeletal fluorosis. Br Med J 1:637, 1973.

46. Kantrowitz FG, Byrne MH, Krane SM: Clinical and metabolic effects of the diphosphonate in Paget's disease of bone. Clin Res 23:445A, 1975.

47. Boyce BF, Byars J, McWilliams S, et al.: Histological and electron microprobe studies of mineralization in aluminum-related osteomalacia. J Clin Pathol 45:502, 1992.

48. Frame B, Frost HM, Ormond RS, Hunter RB: Atypical osteomalacia involving the axial skeleton. Ann Intern Med 55:632, 1961.

49. Nelson AM, Riggs BL, Jowsey JO: Atypical axial osteomalacia: report of four cases with two having features of ankylosing spondylitis. Arthritis Rheum 21:715, 1978.

50. Frame B, Frost HM, Pac CYC, et al.: Fibrogenesis imperfecta ossium: a collagen defect causing osteomalacia. N Engl J Med 285:769, 1971.

51. Johnston CC Jr, Lavy N, Lord T, et al.: Osteopetrosis: a clinical genetic, metabolic, and morphologic study of the dominantly inherited, benign form. Medicine 47:149, 1968.

52. Parfitt AM, Duncan H: Metabolic bone disease affecting the spine. In Rothman RH, Simeone FA (eds): The Spine, 2nd ed. Philadelphia: W B Saunders Co, 1982, pp 775–905.

53. Frame B, Parfitt AM: Osteomalacia: current concepts. Ann Intern Med 89:966, 1978.

54. Dent CE, Watson L: Osteoporosis. Postgrad Med J (Suppl) 42:582, 1966.

55. Adams JE, Davies M: Intra-spinal new bone formation and spinal cord compression in familial hypophosphataemic vitamin D resistant osteomalacia. Q J Med 236:1117, 1986.

56. Audran M, Kumar R: The physiology and pathophysiology of vitamin D. Mayo Clin Proc 60:851, 1985.

57. Nordin BEC, Hodgkinson A, Peacock M: The measurement and the meaning of urinary calcium. Clin Orthop 52:293, 1967.

58. Bisballe S, Eriksen EF, Melsen F, et al.: Osteopenia and osteomalacia after gastrectomy: interrelations between biochemical markers of bone remodelling, vitamin D metabolites, and bone histomorphometry. Gut 32:1303, 1991.

59. Demiaux B, Arlot ME, Chapuy MC, et al.: Serum osteocalcin is increased in patients with osteomalacia: correlations with biochemical and histomorphometric findings. J Clin Endocrinol Metab 74:1146, 1992.

60. Steinbach HL, Noetzli M: Roentgen appearance of the skeleton in osteomalacia and rickets. AJR 92:955, 1964.

61. Burnstein MI, Lawson JP, Kottamasu SR, et al.: The enthesopathic changes of hypophosphatemic osteomalacia in adults: radiologic findings. AJR 153:785, 1989.

62. Chan Y, Furlong TJ, Cornish CJ, Posen S: Dialysis osteodystrophy. A study involving 94 patients. Medicine 64:296, 1985.

63. Rubin LA, Fam AG, Rubenstein J, et al.: Erosive azotemic osteoarthropathy. Arthritis Rheum 27:1086, 1984.

64. Wahner HW: Assessment of metabolic bone disease: review of new nuclear medicine procedures. Mayo Clin Proc 60:827, 1985.

65. Bingham CT, Fitzpatrick LA: Noninvasive testing in the diagnosis of osteomalacia. Am J Med 95:519, 1993.

66. Barzel US: Vitamin deficiency: a risk factor for osteomalacia in the aged. J Am Geriatr Soc 31:598, 1983.

67. Ralson SH, Willocks L, Pitkeathly DA, et al.: High prevalence of unrecognized osteomalacia in hospital patients with rheumatoid arthritis. Br J Rheumatol 27:202, 1988.

68. Kumar R, Riggs BL: Vitamin D in the therapy of disorders of calcium and phosphorus metabolism. Mayo Clin Proc 56:327, 1981.

69. Ronin DI, Wu YC, Sahgal V, MacLean IC: Intractable muscle pain syndrome, osteomalacia, and axonopathy in long-term use of phenytoin. Arch Phys Med Rehabil 72:755, 1991.

70. McGuire MH, Merenda JT, Etzkorn JR, Sundaram M: Oncogenic osteomalacia: a case report. Clin Orthop 244:305, 1989.

71. Rapoport J, Chaimovitz C, Abulfil A, et al.: Aluminum-related osteomalacia: clinical and histological improvement following treatment with desferrioxamine. Isr J Med Sci 23:1242, 1987.
72. Phelps KR, Vigorita VJ, Bansal M, Einhorn TA: Histochemical demonstration of iron but not aluminum in a case of dialysis-associated osteomalacia. Am J Med 84:775, 1988.

PARATHYROID DISEASE

Capsule Summary

Frequency of back pain—rare
Location of back pain—lumbar spine
Quality of back pain—diffuse ache, severe localized (hyper); stiffness (hypo)
Symptoms and signs—ulcers, renal stones, bone pain with percussion (hyper); muscle spasm, tetany, decreased motion (hypo)
Laboratory and x-ray tests—hypercalcemia, hypophosphatemia, increased serum parathormone, "rugger-jersey" spine (hyper); hypocalcemia, hyperphosphatemia, decreased serum parathormone, calcified spinal ligaments (hypo)
Treatment—surgical (hyper); vitamin D, calcium (hypo)

PREVALENCE AND PATHOGENESIS

Parathyroid hormone is the dominant factor in the maintenance of serum calcium in a normal range. Hyperparathyroidism results in excess concentrations of parathyroid hormone in the blood stream and elevated serum calcium levels. Primary hyperparathyroidism is caused by abnormal growth of the parathyroid glands. Secondary hyperparathyroidism results from the secretion of parathyroid hormone in response to persistently low serum concentrations of calcium. Hyperparathyroidism, regardless of type, leads to bone disease and abnormal physiology in a number of organ systems that are dependent on calcium for normal function (nervous, genitourinary, and gastrointestinal). The loss of calcium from bone results in pain, weakening, and fracture. Untreated disease causes marked osteopenia of the vertebral column with progressive vertebral body fractures and spinal deformity.

Hypoparathyroidism, an illness associated with deficient activity of parathyroid hormone, causes hypocalcemia with associated soft tissue calcification and bony overgrowth. Paravertebral calcification of ligamentous structures in the lumbar spine leads to progressive stiffness and limitation of motion.

The absolute prevalence of parathyroid disease is unknown, although an incidence of 1 per 1000 patients was reported from data obtained at a diagnostic clinic.[1] The ratio of men to women affected is 1:3. After age 50, the incidence is 1 per 1000 males and 2 to 3 per 1000 females.[2] Rarely, hyperparathyroidism occurs in two familial syndromes associated with multiple endocrine neoplasms. Type I with pituitary and pancreatic tumors, and Type II with medullary thyroid carcinoma and pheochromocytoma.[3, 4]

Parathyroid hormone (PTH) maintains serum calcium levels by stimulating intestinal calcium absorption, activating osteoclasts for bone resorption, and stimulating renal tubular calcium reabsorption, phosphate excretion, and enzyme synthesis of the active form of vitamin D.[5] The concentration of serum calcium perfusing the four parathyroid glands located posterior to the thyroid gland is the dominant factor in the control of secretion of PTH. PTH is secreted in response to low serum calcium concentrations.

The hormone is released in an inactive form and is broken into at least two fragments (amino-terminal, short half-life, active component; and carboxyl-terminal, long half-life, inactive component) by the liver and kidney.[6] PTH exerts its effects through activation of membrane-bound adenylate cyclase generating cyclic adenosine monophosphate.

Primary hyperparathyroidism is a disease process within the parathyroid glands. In approximately 90% of cases, the abnormality is a neoplasm, usually the overgrowth of one gland forming an adenoma. Less often, the abnormality consists of multiple adenomas (2%), diffuse hyperplasia (6%), or a carcinoma of the parathyroids (2%).[7] Secondary hyperparathyroidism is the increased secretion of PTH in response to low serum calcium levels caused by abnormalities in other organ systems, such as the kidney, or when there is inadequate vitamin D metabolism. Alterations in calcium metabolism and relevant hormones occur with aging. The mean serum parathormone level is 20% to 40% higher in persons older than 70 years.[8] Calcitriol, the active form of vitamin D, is lower in older individuals.[9] Calcitonin levels are lower in older women. Tertiary hyperparathyroidism occurs when parathormone is irrepressible in patients with normal or low serum calcium levels.[10]

Hypoparathyroidism also occurs in primary and secondary forms. Primary or idiopathic hypoparathyroidism associated with cessation of function of the four parathyroid glands is uncommon and occurs more frequently in female children. The usual form of hypoparathyroidism is secondary and is caused by damage to or accidental removal of the parathyroid glands during thyroid gland surgery.[11]

CLINICAL HISTORY

The vast array of symptoms associated with hyperparathyroidism is related to direct effects of PTH and hypercalcemia. The patient with the florid syndrome of hyperparathyroidism is unusual, since many patients are discovered with hypercalcemia by multiphasic blood screening at an early stage of disease. Many individuals are asymptomatic when mild hypercalcemia is first discovered.[12] They complain of bone pain and may present with a history of back pain from vertebral compression fractures.[13] Dull back pain also may be related to renal colic secondary to nephrolithiasis. Other renal manifestations include polyuria and polydipsia. Gastrointestinal symptoms associated with hypercalcemia include anorexia, nausea, vomiting, constipation, and abdominal pain secondary to peptic ulcer disease or pancreatitis.[14] Markedly elevated serum levels of calcium may affect mental status and cause muscle weakness, hypotonia, and coma. Band keratopathy occurs in the eye. Musculoskeletal abnormalities may include generalized arthralgias and microcrystalline diseases.[15] The frequency of clinical symptoms is 40% for fatigue, 20% for musculoskeletal complaints, 20% for gastrointestinal complaints, 15% for renal failure, 10% for renal stones, and 10% for hypertension.[2]

The most prominent symptom of hypoparathyroidism is tetany. Tetany is tonic muscle spasm that occurs secondary to abnormally low concentrations of calcium. Persistent hypocalcemia may cause irritability, depression, and decrease in mental activity.

PHYSICAL EXAMINATION

Patients with hyperparathyroidism show muscle weakness on examination. Examination of the back may demonstrate percussion tenderness over a recently fractured vertebral body. Kyphosis occurs with wedging of vertebral bodies. Musculoskeletal examination may show joint inflammation (swelling, heat, redness, pain, loss of motion) in patients with acute gout or pseudogout. Both illnesses are commonly found in patients with hyperparathyroidism.[16, 17] Acute pseudogout occurs

in about 3.8% of patients with hyperparathyroidism.[18]

Patients with hypoparathyroidism may show signs of tetany when stressed with percussion over the facial nerve (Chvostek's sign) or carpal spasm with reduced blood flow from a blood pressure cuff (Trousseau's sign). They also may have limitation of motion of the lumbosacral spine secondary to soft tissue calcification.[19] These patients do not have spinal or pelvic tenderness on palpation but complain of pain with motion.

LABORATORY DATA

The laboratory parameter of greatest importance in the evaluation of a patient with suspected hyperparathyroidism is serum calcium. Serum calcium is elevated in over 96% of patients with primary hyperparathyroidism.[20] Mild disease can be associated with intermittent elevations, so repeated determinations are indicated if suspicion is great and the initial calcium value is normal. Other chemical tests are useful but not diagnostic. Findings associated with hyperparathyroidism include low serum phosphorus, elevated serum chloride, elevated serum alkaline phosphatase, and elevated urinary calcium excretion.[21] Measurement of parathormone by radioimmunoassay will become more helpful for the diagnosis of hyperparathyroidism once the specificities of the antibody for active PTH are improved and the normal range of values is determined.[22, 23] The antibody tests for intact parathormone have improved to a significant degree. In a study of 101 patients with a variety of disorders of calcium homeostasis including hyperparathyroidism, hypoparathyroidism, hypercalcemia of malignancy, or chronic renal failure, intact parathormone assay was superior to midregion/C-terminal parathormone assay in reflecting parathyroid function.[24]

Hypoparathyroidism is associated with low serum calcium, elevated serum phosphorus, and normal alkaline phosphatase. Secondary hyperparathyroidism, usually associated with chronic renal failure, seldom produces hypercalcemia but is associated with elevated phosphorus concentrations. The electrocardiogram may demonstrate a shortened Q-T interval with hyperparathyroidism and a prolonged interval with hypoparathyroidism.

Patients with hyperparathyroidism have little evidence of clinical bone disease at presentation, and bone biopsy is rarely performed. When it is, it usually demonstrates the effects of PTH on bone. Characteristic findings include an increased number of osteoclasts resorbing bone, osteoblasts repairing bone that is being resorbed, and numerous fibroblasts producing dense fibrous tissue. Bone resorption may result in bone cyst formation, and bleeding into the cysts results in brown discoloration of the fibrous tissue and is referred to as a brown tumor. Osteitis fibrosa cystica is the term used in reference to the bone disease of hyperparathyroidism (Fig. 14–12).

RADIOGRAPHIC EVALUATION

A variety of radiographic lesions are associated with hyperparathyroidism, including subperiosteal bone resorption, particularly on the radial aspects of the middle phalanges, resorption of the terminal tufts of the phalanges, "salt and pepper" appearance of the skull, and cystic lesions of the long bones.[25]

The axial skeleton is also involved in hyperparathyroidism. Most severely affected are the sacroiliac joints. Subchondral resorption affects the iliac side of the joint more than the sacrum, mimicking the "pseudowidening," sclerotic articular margins and bilateral symmetric distribution associated with ankylosing spondylitis. Resorption may also occur in the symphysis pubis (Fig. 14–13). Axial skeletal changes include osteopenia with wedging of vertebral bodies. Marked kyphosis may also be present. Sclerosis may develop at the superior and inferior margins of vertebral bodies, resulting in a "rugger-jersey" spine. This form of vertebral bony sclerosis may be associated with vertebrae of normal configuration or those that have undergone fracture and collapse. In one study, 20% of patients who

underwent parathyroidectomy for primary hyperparathyroidism had evidence of vertebral body fractures, compared with 13% in an age-matched control group. The difference in fracture rates was statistically significant.[26] Subchondral resorption at the discovertebral junction results in bone weakening and Schmorl's nodes. Other axial skeleton and joint manifestations of hyperparathyroidism include instability of the sacroiliac joints, calcium pyrophosphate dihydrate deposition disease, and gout.[27, 28] Hyperparathyroidism secondary to renal failure causes renal osteodystrophy and has radiologic similarities to primary hyperparathyroidism. Osteosclerosis with soft tissue and arterial calcification occurs more commonly with secondary hyperparathyroidism than with the primary disease.[29] Osteomalacia is also more frequently associated with renal osteodystrophy.

Brown tumors of bone are large cystic areas containing fibrous tissue. Brown tumors are most commonly found in the appendicular skeleton in hyperparathyroidism. Occasionally, brown tumors may involve the vertebral column and may be associated with vertebral collapse and spinal cord compression presenting as paraplegia.[30, 31] Brown tumors will appear as large cystic areas in bone.

The methods for identifying the location of hyperfunctioning parathyroid tissue utilizes thallium 201-technetium-99M parathyroid scan. The accuracy of these scans to identify parathyroid tissue is 87%.[10] The test was associated with false-positives, particularly with patients with concomitant thyroid disease. Ultrasound and CT also may be helpful to localize enlarged glands. In patients with an enlarged

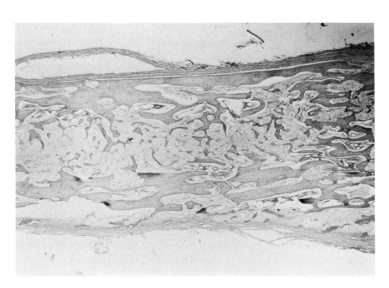

Figure 14–12. Secondary hyperparathyroidism associated with renal osteodystrophy. Histologic section exhibiting a combination of osteoporosis and osteomalacia. Bone matrix is decreased. Cortical osteoclastic activity is increased in association with bone resorption. (Courtesy of Arnold Schwartz, M.D.)

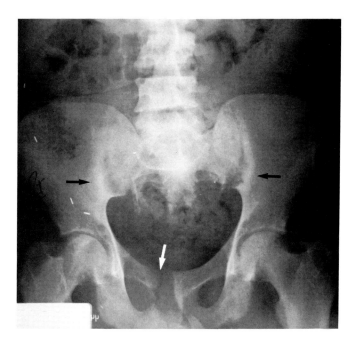

Figure 14–13. A 42-year-old man on hemo-dialysis after a failed kidney transplant with secondary hyperparathyroidism. AP view of pelvis reveals "pseudowidening" of both sa-croiliac joints with sclerosis most prominent in the ilium *(black arrows)*. Bone resorption of the symphysis pubis is noted *(white arrow).*

adenoma, CT scan may be the most effective test for localizing the malfunctioning parathyroid gland.[32]

Hypoparathyroidism is most commonly associated with osteosclerosis. Subcutaneous calcification and calcification of the longitudinal ligaments of the spine are the most common axial skeletal abnormalities.[19] The calcifications may become prominent to the same degree as those associated with ankylosing spondylitis.[33] In contrast to spondylitis, the sacroiliac joints are generally spared in hypoparathyroidism.

DIFFERENTIAL DIAGNOSIS

The diagnosis of hyperparathyroidism can be suspected in a patient who presents with hypercalcemia. The symptoms and signs of the more severe, classic disease are seldom observed. Evaluation of corroborating chemical and radiographic parameters help firm up the diagnosis, which can be definitively made by the surgical removal of abnormal parathyroid tissue.

A number of illnesses cause hypercalcemia and must be considered in the differential diagnosis of hyperparathyroidism.[34] The major categories to consider in the patient with back pain, vertebral fracture, and hypercalcemia include malignancies, secondary hyperparathyroidism, and granulomatous disorders such as sarcoidosis. Careful examination for the presence of a malignancy, urinalysis, chemical test-ing for renal function, and chest radiographs should help differentiate these illnesses from primary hyperparathyroidism.

The diagnosis of hypoparathyroidism is made based on the presence of decreased serum calcium in a patient who has undergone parathyroid surgery. Other diseases that cause generalized osteosclerosis (osteoblastic metastases, myelofibrosis, Paget's disease, fluorosis, and mastocytosis) rarely cause hypocalcemia.

TREATMENT

The treatment of hyperparathyroidism is the surgical removal of the malfunctioning parathyroid tissue in symptomatic patients. There is no effective medical therapy to control the effects of excessive parathyroid hormone. MR evaluation of the parathyroid glands identifies the size of the glands, and by the signal intensity of the lesions, the histologic characteristics of the adenomas.[35] Most patients have a single parathyroid adenoma, and its removal brings the hyperparathyroidism under control without recurrence.[36] In a smaller group of patients with diffuse hyperplasia of all the glands, total removal of all but a small portion of a single parathyroid gland is required.[37] Occasionally reoperation is needed for patients who have recurrence of the tumor or hyperplasia.[38] Patients with hypercalcemia who have clinically severe bone disease may require postoperative therapy with supplemental calcium, phosphorus, vitamin D, and magnesium. This is necessary to mineralize bone that has been chronically resorbed.[39] Most patients do not require this therapy unless tetany ensues after surgery. Therapy for patients with secondary hyperparathyroidism is directed toward control of the underlying disease process. For example, renal transplantation may slow down the bone regression of secondary hyperparathyroidism.[40]

Patients with back pain from hyperparathyroidism are treated for their underlying disease. Patients with compression fractures receive symptomatic therapy, analgesics, anti-inflammatory drugs, and braces while their skeletal lesions heal, but there may be residual deformity of the spine despite bone healing.

The logical replacement therapy for hypoparathyroidism would be PTH, but hormone replacement is not practical for clinical use. Vitamin D provides a satisfactory alternative since it has actions similar to those of PTH. Acute hypocalcemia requires intravenous calcium gluconate. Vitamin D, 25,000 to 50,000 units/day, is needed to maintain serum calcium concentrations at 8.5 mg/dl. Urine calcium needs to be checked for concentrations greater than 250 mg/day, which require increased fluid intake to prevent renal stone formation.

PROGNOSIS

Patients who have mildly elevated calcium concentrations and are asymptomatic may be followed closely without surgical intervention. In one 4-year study, 20% of 141 patients with hypercalcemia required surgical intervention.[41] Many patients may be followed by testing serum calcium, alkaline phosphatase, and renal function twice a year. Patients who become symptomatic require surgical intervention. Surgery is effective at controlling the disease, although an occasional patient may require reoperation. Bone lesions heal after the source of excess parathyroid hormone is removed. Brown tumors usually heal, but large cysts may not heal and carry a risk of pathologic fractures through areas of weakened bone. Lesions in the spine may heal, but areas of fracture and angular deformity are not reversible. Hypoparathyroidism is treated with calcium and vitamin D supplements.

References

PARATHYROID DISEASE

1. Boonstra CE, Jackson CE: Serum calcium survey for hyperparathyroidism. Results in 50,000 clinic patients. Am J Clin Pathol 55:523, 1971.

2. Petti GH Jr: Hyperparathyroidism. Otolaryngol Clin North Am 23:339, 1990.

3. Yamaguchi K, Kameya T, Abe K: Multiple endocrine neoplasm type I. Clin Endocrinol Metab 9:261, 1980.

4. Melvin KEW, Miller HH, Tashjian AH Jr: Early diagnosis of medullary carcinoma of the thyroid gland by means of calcitonin assay. N Engl J Med 285:115, 1971.

5. Raisz LG, Kream BE: Regulation of bone formation. N Engl J Med 309:29, 83, 1983.

6. Rosenblatt M: Pre-proparathyroid hormone: intracellular transport and processing. Mineral Electrolyte Metab 8:118, 1982.

7. Pyrah LN, Hodgkinson A, Anderson CK: Primary hyperparathyroidism. Br J Surg 53:234, 316, 1966.

8. Endres DB, Morgan CH, Garry PJ, et al.: Age-related changes in serum immunoreactive parathyroid hormone and its biological action in healthy men and women. J Clin Endocrinol Metab 65:724, 1987.

9. Clemens TL, Zhou XY, Myles M, et al.: Serum vitamin D2 and vitamin D3 metabolite concentrations and absorption of vitamin D2 in elderly subjects. J Clin Endocrinol Metab 63:656, 1986.

10. Voorman GS, Petti GH Jr, Schulz E, et al.: The pitfalls of technetium Tc 99 mm/thallium 201 parathyroid scanning. Arch Otolaryngol Head Neck Surg 114:993, 1988.

11. Nusynowitz ML, Frame B, Kolb FO: The spectrum of the hypoparathyroid states: a classification based on physiologic principles. Medicine 55:105, 1976.

12. Potts JT Jr: Management of asymptomatic hyperparathyroidism. J Clin Endocrinol Metab 70:1489, 1990.

13. Dauphine RT, Riggs BL, Scholz DA: Back pain and vertebral crush fractures: an unemphasized mode of presentation for primary hyperparathyroidism. Ann Intern Med 83:365, 1975.

14. Lockwood K, Bruun E, Tansbol I: Disease of the parathyroid glands. Adv Surg 9:177, 1975.

15. Hamilton EBD: The arthritis of hyperparathyroidism, haemochromatosis, and Wilson's disease. Clin Rheum Dis 1:109, 1975.

16. Scott JT, Dixon ASJ, Bywaters EGL: Association of hyperuricemia and gout with hyperparathyroidism. Br Med J 1:1070, 1964.

17. Bywaters EGL: Discussion of simulations of rheumatic disorders by metabolic bone disease. Ann Rheum Dis 18:64, 1959.

18. Geelhoed GW, Kelly TR: Pseudogout as a clue and complication in primary hyperparathyroidism. Surgery 106:1036, 1989.

19. Jimenea CV, Frame B, Chaykin LB, Sigler JW: Spondylitis of hypoparathyroidism. Clin Orthop 74:84, 1971.

20. Hect A, Gershberg H, St Paul H: Primary hyperparathyroidism: laboratory and clinical data in 73 cases. JAMA 233:519, 1975.

21. O'Riordan JLH, Adami S: Pathophysiology of hyperparathyroidism. Horm Res 20:38, 1984.

22. Posen S, Clifton-Bligh P, Mason RS: Testing for disorders of calcium metabolism. (Editorial.) Pathology 12:511, 1980.

23. Kao PC: Parathyroid hormone assay. Mayo Clin Proc 57:596, 1982.

24. Rudnicki M, McNair P, Tansbol I, Lindgren P: Diagnostic applicability of intact and midregion/C-terminal parathyroid hormone assays in calcium metabolic disorders. J Intern Med 228:465, 1990.

25. Genant HK, Heck LL, Lanzi LH, et al.: Primary hyperparathyroidism: a comprehensive study of clinical, biochemical, and radiographic manifestations. Radiology 109:513, 1973.

26. Kochersberger G, Buckley NJ, Leight GS, et al.: What is the clinical significance of bone loss in primary hyperparathyroidism? Arch Intern Med 147:1951, 1987.

27. Resnick D, Niwayama G: Subchondral resorption of bone in renal osteodystrophy. Radiology 118:315, 1976.

28. Pritchard MH, Jessop JD: Chondrocalcinosis in primary hyperparathyroidism: influence of age, metabolic bone disease, and parathyroidectomy. Ann Rheum Dis 36:146, 1977.

29. Greenfield GB: Roentgen appearance of bone and soft tissue changes in chronic renal diseases. AJR 116:749, 1972.

30. Shaw MT, Davies M: Primary hyperparathyroidism presenting as a spinal cord compression. Br Med J 4:230, 1968.

31. Sundarim M, Scholz C: Primary hyperparathyroidism presenting with acute paraplegia. AJR 128:674, 1977.

32. Carmalt HL, Gillett DJ, Chan J, et al.: Perspective comparison of radionuclide, ultrasound and computed tomography and the preoperative localization of parathyroid glands. World J Surg 12:830, 1988.

33. Chaykin LB, Frame B, Sigler JW: Spondylitis: a clue to hypoparathyroidism. Ann Intern Med 70:955, 1970.

34. Goldsmith RS: Differential diagnosis of hypercalcemia. N Engl J Med 274:674, 1966.

35. Auffermann W, Guis M, Tavares NJ, et al.: MR signal intensity of parathyroid adenomas: correlation with histopathology. AJR 153:873, 1989.

36. Attie JN, Wise L, Mir R, Ackerman LV: The rationale against routine subtotal parathyroidectomy for primary hyperparathyroidism. Am J Surg 136:437, 1978.

37. Block MA, Frame B, Jackson CE, Horn RC Jr: The extent of operation for primary hyperparathyroidism. Arch Surg 109:798, 1974.

38. Sayle AW, Brennan MF: Strategy and technique of reoperative parathyroid surgery. Surgery 89:417, 1981.

39. Gonzales-Villapando C, Porath A, Berelowitz M, et al.: Vitamin D metabolism during recovery from severe osteitis fibrosa cystica of primary hyperparathyroidism. J Clin Endocrinol Metab 51:1180, 1980.

40. David DS, Sakai S, Brennan L, et al.: Hypercalcemia after renal transplantation: long-term follow-up data. N Engl J Med 289:298, 1973.

41. Purnell DC, Scholz DA, Smith LH, et al.: Treatment of primary hyperparathyroidism. Am J Med 56:800, 1974.

PITUITARY DISEASE

Capsule Summary

Frequency of back pain—common

Location of back pain—lumbar spine

Quality of back pain—ache

Signs and symptoms—headache, visual disturbance, muscle weakness, normal range of spine motion, coarsened facial features

Laboratory and x-ray tests—increased growth hormone and somatomedin-C, posterior scalloping vertebral bodies, increased disc space on plain roentgenograms

Treatment—surgical ablation of pituitary tumor

PREVALENCE AND PATHOGENESIS

Excessive growth hormone (GH) secretion from tumors in the anterior pituitary gland causes gigantism in growing children and acromegaly in adults. A number of morphologic and physiologic abnormalities occur secondary to hypersecretion of GH, including increased growth of bone, cartilage, and visceral organs; hypermetabolism resulting in impaired glucose tolerance; and osteoporosis. Low back pain is a prominent symptom of patients with acromegaly, although the range of motion of the lumbosacral spine remains normal.

The prevalence and incidence of pituitary tumors are unknown. In one study, 13% of patients had small pituitary tumors that were asymptomatic and were only discovered at autopsy.[1] In symptomatic disease, recent epidemiologic studies have indicated an incidence rate of 3.3/million/year and a prevalence rate of 66/million.[2] The disease usually begins insidiously 30 to 50 years of age and affects men and women equally.

Growth hormone has multiple actions, including maintenance of serum glucose levels, protein synthesis, calcium absorption from the gut, renal tubular absorption of phosphate, epiphyseal periosteal bone growth, production of connective tissue, and collagen synthesis. Growth hormone secretion is stimulated primarily by hypoglycemia, and to a lesser degree by exercise, sleep, and stress. Overproduction of GH while the growth plates are still open causes a marked overgrowth of bone, resulting in extreme height, which is referred to as hyperpituitary gigantism. In the adult with closed growth plates, new bone formation is endochondral, with periosteal growth resulting in widening bones and excess cartilage formation. The newly formed cartilage is friable and is easily damaged, causing fissuring and ulceration of the articular surface. Degeneration of the cartilage initiates increased cartilage and bone repair, and secondary osteoarthritis. Acromegaly is the disease associated with excessive GH production in the adult.[3] The source of GH is usually an acidophilic or chromophobic adenoma of the anterior lobe of the pituitary gland, which is located in the center of the skull in the sella turcica.

CLINICAL FINDINGS

The symptoms associated with acromegaly are related to the growth of the tumor intracranially as well as to the effect of GH on the musculoskeletal system and other viscera.

Headaches and visual disturbances are directly related to the growth of a tumor in the sella turcica. Rheumatic disease symptoms of carpal tunnel syndrome, backache, limb pain, muscle weakness, and Raynaud's phenomenon are common.[4] Arthropathy is the mode of presentation of acromegaly in a small minority of patients.[5] Spinal stenosis and disc herniation are unusual complications of acromegaly but have been more frequently recognized as a complication of this illness.[6, 7] Back pain is a symptom in 50% of patients. The pain is localized to the lumbosacral spine in most circumstances but may radiate into the lower extremities when there is secondary cauda equina compression from spinal stenosis.[8] Pain in the lumbar area is insidious in onset and slowly progressive. In general, acromegalic patients with longer duration disease have more severe musculoskeletal symptoms and signs.[9, 10] In the axial skeleton, the lumbosacral region is most often affected, the next most often is the cervical spine, and rarely the thoracic spine.[3, 11] A patient may also notice a gradual enlargement of facial features, deepening of the voice, thickening of the tongue, enlargement of the extremities, particularly the fingers, and diminished libido.

PHYSICAL EXAMINATION

Facial characteristics of the patient with acromegaly usually are prominent and alert the physician to the potential diagnosis. The jaw is large, and the skin over the face is thickened and coarse. A broad based nose is usual, and the forehead is bossed. The musculoskeletal examination is characterized by joint swelling due to periarticular thickening and noninflammatory synovial hypertrophy. Coarse crepitation with motion is common. The hands become "spade-like" and broad, with blunted fingers. Compression of the median nerve in the carpal tunnel elicits paresthesias in the sensory distribution of the nerve, and there is a positive Phalen's test (wrist flexion test).

Lumbar spine examination may be unremarkable even in the 50% of acromegalic patients with back pain. Examination of the back may demonstrate percussion tenderness over the spine. The range of motion of the lumbar spine remains normal. This preservation of motion may be related to thickened intervertebral discs that retain their turgor. However, with progressive disease, painful kyphosis of the axial skeleton may occur. Long tract signs indicative of spinal cord compression also may be found in some patients.[12] Secondary osteoarthritic changes may appear in the knees, hips, and shoulders. Rarely, an acute episode of joint inflammation may be seen secondary to crystal-induced synovitis from calcium pyrophosphate dihydrate deposition.[13]

LABORATORY DATA

Abnormal laboratory parameters include elevated GH levels, excessive somatomedin-C/insulin-like growth factor I, elevated serum glucose levels indicative of glucose intolerance, and elevated levels of serum phosphorus and alkaline phosphatase in proportion to skeletal growth.[14] Basal GH levels are elevated and are nonsuppressible during a standard glucose tolerance test. Glucose tolerance is impaired and is relatively resistant to insulin therapy. Growth hormone levels may be measured 2 hours after a patient ingests 75 to 100 gm of glucose. A value greater than 5 ng/ml should initiate definitive testing for acromegaly.[15]

The activity of acromegaly and the pathologic effects of the disease on cartilage may be more closely correlated with a hepatic protein, somatomedin-C, than with GH itself.[16] Increased somatomedin-C concentrations may be an indication of acromegaly in those individuals with the disease and equivocally elevated GH levels.[17]

RADIOGRAPHIC EVALUATION

Radiographic findings in the axial skeleton are prominent in patients with acromegaly. Anterior and lateral osteophytes of the lumbar and thoracic vertebral bodies are very prominent and may resemble diffuse idiopathic skeletal hyperostosis (DISH). Posterior osteophytes are less prominent. Posteriorly, the vertebral bodies are scalloped as a result of bone resorption.[18, 19] Disc spaces are well maintained and may be increased in size (Figs. 14–14 and 14–15). Anterior intervertebral disc calcification, thought to be secondary to calcium pyrophosphate deposition, also may be seen. Other characteristic radiographic findings of acromegaly include increased heel pad thickness and widening of joint spaces secondary to growth of cartilage.[20]

Bone mineral density varies in the skeleton depending on the effects of excess GH and the hypogonadism resulting from the inhibition of gonadotropin production by the pituitary tumor. Peripheral bone densities are increased in the forearm secondary to increased GH, while vertebral values are decreased secondary to hypogonadism.[21]

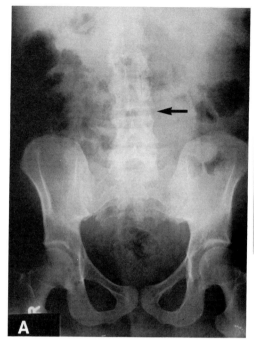

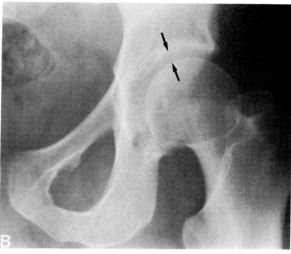

Figure 14–14. Acromegaly in a 34-year-old man. *A,* AP view of the lumbosacral spine demonstrating well maintained disc spaces *(arrow). B,* Left hip joint with increased joint space *(arrows).*

DIFFERENTIAL DIAGNOSIS

The diagnosis of acromegaly can be suspected in a patient with the clinical symptoms and signs previously described and confirmed by measurement of GH in basal and suppressible states. Once abnormalities of GH are determined, evaluation of the sella turcica by CT scan or MR is essential.[22]

The differential diagnosis of a patient with symptoms and signs of headaches, head and extremity enlargement, and glucose intolerance is essentially limited to acromegaly. The radiographic changes of acromegaly with increased articular space and increased bone surface are easily differentiated from those of other disease processes. The later stages of joint disease of acromegaly are similar to those of primary osteoarthritis and are difficult to differentiate from this disorder. Unusual locations for osteophytes (metacarpophalangeal joints) and the lack of subchondral erosions have been suggested as factors differentiating acromegaly from secondary osteoarthritis.[23] Scalloped vertebral bodies, while associated with acromegaly, also may be seen as other disease processes associated with increased intraspinal pressure, weakness of the dural sac, or genetic abnormalities with tissue accumulation of mucopolysaccharides.[24] Lesions associated with increased intraspinal pressure include intraspinal tumors and cysts, syringomyelia, and communicating hydrocephalus.

Disorders of connective tissue that result in weakness in the covering of the spinal cord dura predispose vertebral bodies to scalloping. These disorders, which occasionally cause low back pain, include Marfan and Ehlers-Danlos

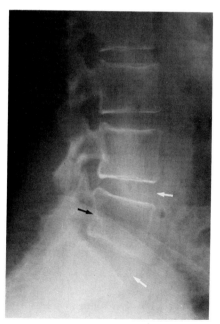

Figure 14–15. Acromegaly in a 46-year-old woman with a 5-year history of clinical symptoms of the disease. Lateral view of the lumbosacral spine reveals large intervertebral disc spaces *(white arrows)* and early scalloping of the L5 vertebral body *(black arrow).*

syndromes. Tumors of spinal nerves, neurofibromas, also may cause vertebral body indentation. The mucopolysaccharidoses, a heterogeneous group of genetic abnormalities that result in the excessive accumulation of mucopolysaccharides in various organs, may cause skeletal abnormalities. Hurler's and Morquio's syndromes are most closely associated with posterior skeletal abnormalities.[25] The physical appearance of these patients helps differentiate them from patients with acromegaly.

TREATMENT

The goals of therapy to cure acromegaly include the total elimination of the pituitary tumor and its mass effects, along with complete restoration of normal GH physiology.[26] Surgery is the preferred means to obtain the goals of therapy.[17] A transsphenoidal approach is adequate to remove the pituitary tumor unless massive suprasellar extension requires a craniotomy. The mortality rate is 1%. GH levels are reduced to 10 ng/ml or less in 70% of patients.[26] Surgical hypopituitarism occurs in 10% to 18% of patients. Patients who suffer from spinal stenosis may benefit from surgical decompression to relieve nerve compression.[27]

Radiation therapy may normalize GH levels but may require 2 to 4 years to achieve this goal. Between 10% and 15% of patients may continue with elevated levels of GH despite 10 years of radiation therapy. The toxicity of radiation therapy is the risk of multihormonal pituitary insufficiency in between 15% and 50% of irradiated patients.

Medical therapy may include bromocriptine or GH inhibitory factor. Although 70% of acromegaly patients experience clinical improvement when treated with bromocriptine, GH levels are only reduced to 5 ng/ml in 20% of patients. Bromocriptine is taken orally every 8 to 12 hours. The side effects include malaise, nausea, vomiting, postural hypotension, nasal congestion, and depression. The somatostatin analog, octreotide acetate, inhibits the secretion of GH. Octreotide treatment results in a significant reduction in GH levels in up to 94% of patients.[28] The drug is injected subcutaneously 2 to 3 times/day. The most common toxicities include loose acholic stools, abdominal discomfort, and gallstones.

Unfortunately, therapeutic measures that are effective in controlling the pituitary lesion have little effect on the progression of acromegalic arthropathy in the axial skeleton or peripheral joints once the joint disease has developed. These patients develop progressive degenerative joint disease and are treated in a similar fashion with nonsteroidal anti-inflammatory drugs, physical therapy, and orthopedic surgery.

PROGNOSIS

Articular symptoms of acromegaly may range from mild joint pain to severe disabling arthritis of the peripheral joints and axial skeleton. Degenerative changes may be progressive, causing marked joint destruction that requires joint replacement of the hip or knee. Bony or disc enlargement in the spine may cause compressive symptoms requiring decompression procedures. The usual course of the illness, in general, is one of benign chronicity; however, some patients have a premature demise from congestive heart failure, complications of diabetes, or unrecognized hypopituitarism.

References

PITUITARY DISEASE

1. Kovacs K, Bryan N, Horvath E, et al.: Pituitary adenomas in old age. J Gerontol 35:16, 1980.
2. Bengtsson BA, Eden S, Ernest I, et al.: Epidemiology and long-term survival in acromegaly. A study of 166 cases diagnosed between 1955 and 1984. Acta Med Scand 223:327, 1988.
3. Ney RL: The anterior pituitary gland. In Bondy PK, Rosenberg LE (eds): Duncan's Diseases of Metabolism, 7th ed, Vol II Endocrinology. Philadelphia: WB Saunders Co., 1974, p 966.
4. Bluestone R, Bywaters EGL, Hartog M, et al.: Acromegalic arthropathy. Ann Rheum Dis 30:243, 1971.
5. Molitch ME: Clinical manifestations of acromegaly. Endocrinol Metab Clin North Am 21:597, 1992.
6. Parikh M, Iyer K, Elias AN, Gwinup G: Spinal stenosis in acromegaly. Spine 12:627, 1987.
7. Cheng CL, Chow SP: Lumbar disc protrusion in an acromegalic patient. Spine 15:50, 1990.
8. Gelman MI: Cauda equina compression in acromegaly. Radiology 112:357, 1974.
9. Lieberman SA, Bjorkengren AG, Hoffman AR: Rheumatologic and skeletal changes in acromegaly. Endocrinol Metab Clin North Am 21:615, 1992.
10. Layton MW, Fudman EJ, Barkan A, et al.: Acromegalic arthropathy: characteristics and response to therapy. Arthritis Rheum 31:1022, 1988.
11. Podgorski M, Robinson B, Weissberger A, et al.: Articular manifestations of acromegaly. Aust N Z J Med 1828, 1988.
12. Hornstein S, Hambrook G, Eyerman E: Spinal cord compression by vertebral acromegaly. Trans Am Neurol Assoc 96:254, 1971.
13. Silcox DC, McCarty DJ: Measurement of inorganic pyrophosphate in biologic fluids: elevated levels in some patients with osteoarthritis, pseudogout, acromegaly, and uremia. J Clin Invest 52:1836, 1973.
14. Chang-DeMoranville BM, Jackson IMD: Diagnosis and endocrine testing in acromegaly. Endocrinol Metab Clin North Am 21:649, 1992.
15. Thorner MO, Vance ML, Horvath E, Kovacs K: The anterior pituitary. In Wilson JD, Foster DW (eds):

Textbook of Endocrinology, 8th ed. Philadelphia: W B Saunders, 1992, pp 221–310.

16. Clemmons DR, Van Wyk JJ, Ridgway EC, et al.: Evaluation of acromegaly by radioimmunoassay of somatomedin-C. N Engl J Med 301:1138, 1979.

17. Thomas JP: Treatment of acromegaly. Br Med J 286:330, 1983.

18. Stuber JL, Palacios E: Vertebral scalloping in acromegaly. AJR 112:397, 1971.

19. Lang EK, Bessler WT: The roentgenologic features of acromegaly. AJR 86:321, 1961.

20. Steinbach HL, Russell W: Measurement of the heel pad as an aid to diagnosis of acromegaly. Radiology 82:418, 1964.

21. Diamond T, Nery L, Posen S: Spinal and peripheral bone mineral densities in acromegaly: the effects of excess growth hormone and hypogonadism. Ann Intern Med 111:567, 1989.

22. Daughaday WH: New criteria for evaluation of acromegaly. (Editorial.) N Engl J Med 301:1175, 1979.

23. Tornero J, Castaneda S, Vidal J, Herrero-Beaumont G: Differences between radiographic abnormalities of acromegalic arthropathy and those of osteoarthritis. Arthritis Rheum 33:455, 1988.

24. Mitchell GE, Lourie H, Berne AS: The various causes of scalloped vertebrae with notes on their pathogenesis. Radiology 89:67, 1967.

25. McKusick VA, Kaplan D, Wise D, et al.: The genetic mucopolysaccharidoses. Medicine 44:445, 1965.

26. Frohman LA: Therapeutic options in acromegaly. J Clin Endocrin Metab 72:1175, 1991.

27. Kaufman HH, Ommaya AK, Dopman JL, Roth JA: Hypertrophy of the ligamentum flavum: secondary cord syndrome in an acromegalic. Arch Neurol 25:256, 1971.

28. Vance ML, Harris AG: Long-term treatment of 189 acromegalic patients with the somatostatin analog octreotide: results of the International Multicenter Acromegaly Study Group. Arch Intern Med 151:1573, 1991.

MICROCRYSTALLINE DISEASE

Capsule Summary

Frequency of back pain—rare

Location of back pain—sacroiliac joints (gout), lumbar spine (CPPD)

Quality of back pain—acute and sharp, chronic ache

Signs and symptoms—generalized microcrystalline disease, straightened lumbosacral spine

Laboratory and x-ray tests—monosodium urate or calcium pyrophosphate dihydrate crystals; joint erosions, disc calcification on plain roentgenograms

Treatment—nonsteroidal anti-inflammatory drugs, colchicine

PREVALENCE AND PATHOGENESIS

Microcrystalline disease, gout, and calcium pyrophosphate dihydrate disease (CPPD) are commonly associated with peripheral joint arthritis. Occasionally, patients with gouty axial skeletal disease may develop episodes of acute low back pain secondary to spinal or sacroiliac joint involvement. CPPD is associated with radiographic findings of disc calcification, and degenerative changes of the discs and vertebral bodies. Symptoms of back pain may develop secondary to these degenerative changes.

The actual prevalence of gout and CPPD is not known. In one study approximately 5% of a large adult population had hyperuricemia,[1] while in another report 6% of an elderly population had CPPD in a joint.[2] Men develop gout during the fourth or fifth decade; women develop it after menopause. Prevalence increases with age in both sexes and is higher among males at all ages.[3] In North America, gout develops at rates of 1.7 and 0.2 cases/1000 person-years among men and women respectively, aged 30 and older.[4] A similar rate was found in a cohort of male physicians who were enrolled in a study at Johns Hopkins.[5] The etiology is related to the inability of the body to eliminate uric acid. This may occur secondary to underexcretion of uric acid through the kidney or to overproduction during protein metabolism. Uric acid accumulates in tissues throughout the body. The presence of crystals in joints, soft tissues, and other areas may initiate the inflammatory response that results in acute symptoms. Uric acid may accumulate into large collections, tophi, which may be located in superficial structures such as the olecranon bursae, as well as in deep areas such as the kidney, heart, and sacroiliac joints.[6] Risk factors for the development of acute gout include hyperuricemia, primarily, obesity, hypertension, alcohol consumption, lead exposure, and renal insufficiency.[7]

CPPD causes symptomatic disease in about half the number of patients affected by gouty arthritis.[8] CPPD occurs in 5% to 10% of all adults. CPPD shows a marked increase with age, with a prevalence as high as 30% in those older than 75.[9] Like gout, CPPD affects men more than women. The disease becomes symptomatic in patients in the sixth or seventh decade. Calcium pyrophosphate dihydrate is the crystal in CPPD that initiates the inflammatory response, but the factors that facilitate the deposition of these crystals in cartilage and surrounding articular structures are poorly understood. Inorganic pyrophosphate (PP) is a byproduct in the formation of cyclic adenosine monophosphate. PP is normally hydrolyzed by an inorganic pyrophosphatase resulting in very low tissue concentrations of PP.

Elevated levels of PP are noted in individuals who develop CPPD.[10] PP levels are increased 5- to 8-fold in individuals with CPPD compared to those with other arthropathies. Pyrophosphatase is inhibited by the presence of divalent cations including iron, calcium, and copper. This may be reflected in the illnesses that are associated with CPPD. The disease may be associated with a number of metabolic conditions, including hyperparathyroidism, hemochromatosis, hypothyroidism, Wilson's disease, and ochronosis. The disorders that are currently believed to be associated with chondrocalcinosis and pseudogout include hypophosphatasia, hypomagnesemia, hyperparathyroidism, and hypothyroidism. Chronic arthropathy of CPPD is associated with hemochromatosis, acromegaly, and ochronosis.[11]

CLINICAL FINDINGS

Back pain secondary to gout is a rare occurrence. Those patients who present with back pain secondary to gout have a long history of peripheral gouty arthritis, are mostly men over 50 years of age, and have nonradiating low back pain due to chronic gouty arthritis.[12] Occasionally they may have a sudden onset of low back pain associated with an acute gouty attack in the sacroiliac joints. These patients may experience pain-limiting back motion to a severe degree.[13] Tophaceous deposits may affect the spine and spinal cord to the point of the development of radicular symptoms or paraparesis.[14, 15] Patients with spinal cord compression from tophi frequently have chronic polyarthritis.[16]

Patients with CPPD of the spine may also have symptoms of low back pain associated with straightening and stiffening of the spine.[17] Rarely do they have neurologic symptoms. Back pain associated with CPPD is an uncommon symptom. In one study, only 7% of patients had back pain as part of their symptom complex.[18] In rare circumstances, patients with CPPD may develop symptoms of spinal stenosis secondary to calcification in the spinal canal.[19]

PHYSICAL EXAMINATION

Physical findings in the lumbosacral spine in the patient with gout may demonstrate spinal stiffness, loss of motion, and muscle spasm with pain on motion. Patients with acute gout of the lumbosacral spine may be febrile on initial presentation.[13] Examination of extensor surfaces (elbows, Achilles tendons) and ears may demonstrate tophaceous deposits. Peripheral joints may be affected at the same time as the lumbar spine. However, even in patients with polyarticular gout, involvement of the lumbar spine is unusual.[20]

Patients with CPPD disease may have restricted motion as a result of associated degenerative disease of the spine. Neurologic signs with CPPD are rare.[21] Patients with CPPD may also develop prolonged fever and elevated ESR.[22]

LABORATORY DATA

Hyperuricemia is a prerequisite for the diagnosis of gout and many patients will have an elevated level of uric acid during an acute attack. However, a normal level does not eliminate the possibility of gout since uric acid concentrations fluctuate, particularly with anti-inflammatory medications. The presence of arthritis and elevated uric acid concentration does not equate with a diagnosis of gout. Hyperuricemia may occur without acute gout. The diagnosis of gout is established definitively by the demonstration of characteristic crystals of monosodium urate monohydrate in synovial fluid or from aspirates of tophaceous deposits. These crystals are negatively birefringent. Other synovial fluid characteristics of gout include a fair mucin clot test, elevated white blood cell count, and increased protein concentration. In a patient with gouty nephropathy, renal function as measured by blood urea nitrogen and creatinine may be impaired, and red blood cells may be present in the urine of the patient with uric acid renal stones.

Blood studies in CPPD are of no use except to detect associated diseases such as hemochromatosis or hyperparathyroidism. Synovial fluid aspiration of acute effusions will demonstrate calcium pyrophosphate dihydrate crystals in the vast majority of patients. A careful examination for these crystals is necessary since they are less numerous than uric acid crystals in an inflamed joint and they polarize light weakly in contrast to urate crystals. White blood cell count and protein concentration in synovial fluid will be elevated, at levels similar to those occurring in gout.

RADIOGRAPHIC EVALUATION

Radiographic abnormalities in the sacroiliac joint and axial skeleton are unusual in gout, but the disease may cause joint margin sclerosis with cystic areas of erosion in the ilium and sacrum.[23] Gout also may cause erosions of endplates of vertebral bodies, disc space narrow-

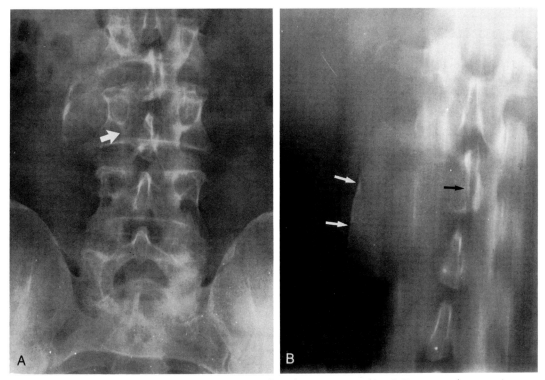

Figure 14–16. Gout. *A,* Huge tophus of gout eroding the R lamina *(arrow)* of L2. *B,* Tomogram shows erosion of the posterior spinous process *(black arrow).* There is a rim of expanding cortex present *(white arrows).* (Courtesy of Anne Brower, M.D.)

ing, and vertebral subluxation (Fig. 14–16).[24] The changes associated with gout in the intervertebral disc may be confused with infectious discitis. Biopsy material from suspected areas should be placed in absolute alcohol and not formalin so that crystals will not be leached out from the specimen.[25] Occasionally, extradural deposits of urate may cause nerve compression and can be detected by myelographic examination.[26] Pathologic fractures in posterior elements of vertebral bodies are also found in patients with extensive gouty involvement.[27] Indium-111–labeled leukocyte scintigraphy will identify accumulation of tracer in involved joints during an acute attack. This type of scan has been utilized in patients with appendicular arthritis. The utility of this type of scan with axial involvement with gout is not known.[28] Repeat scan will demonstrate decreased uptake after therapy corresponding to the patient's course.

Radiographic manifestations of CPPD in the spine include intervertebral disc calcifications, primarily in the annulus fibrosus. The nucleus pulposus is not involved.[29, 30] Calcification also may be present in the symphysis pubis and the sacroiliac joint.[10] The ligamentum flavum may be calcified.[21] Calcifications of the ligamentum flavum may be better visualized by CT scan or MR. Patients with spinal stenosis secondary to ligamentum flavum calcification frequently have evidence of CPPD in peripheral joints.[31] Disc space narrowing associated with vertebral osteophyte formation may occur and is a common finding in the spine.[32] Vertebral body destruction may become severe enough to cause degenerative spondylolisthesis.[18, 33]

DIFFERENTIAL DIAGNOSIS

The diagnosis of microcrystalline disease is confirmed by the detection of the specific crystal in a clinical specimen. Patients with back pain secondary to microcrystalline disease usually have extensive disease in other locations, so that aspiration of the facet or sacroiliac joints is not necessary. Careful monitoring of response to therapy will show rapid improvement if the diagnosis is correct.

Infection must always be considered if the patient has extreme pain, fever, and an elevated peripheral white blood count. Patients with septic sacroiliac joints or osteomyelitis will not improve with anti-gout therapy and they will require further evaluation with blood cultures and joint aspiration to rule out infection.

Hemochromatosis

Hemochromatosis, a disease associated with increased body stores of iron, is an important illness to consider in the differential diagnosis of CPPD.[34] The pathologic processes associated with iron deposition do occur in the spine in patients with hemochromatosis. Radiographic changes are seen in the lumbosacral spine in 15% of patients, but patients rarely have symptoms in the axial skeleton associated with these changes.[35] Most patients with symptomatic hemochromatosis are men between the ages of 40 and 60 years. Arthritis occurs in 20% to 50% of patients and is a late manifestation of the disease. The arthritis may have characteristics of chronic disease similar to that of osteoarthritis or symptoms of acute disease similar to those of CPPD. Radiographic features associated with hemochromatosis include axial skeleton osteoporosis associated with "fish vertebrae"; chondrocalcinosis affecting the symphysis pubis, intervertebral discs and sacroiliac joints; joint space narrowing; and osteophytosis (Fig. 14–17).[21] These spinal abnormalities may lead to fracture and vertebral collapse, back pain, and deformity.[36] The diagnosis of hemochromatosis is suspected because of the presence of bronze skin, diabetes, cirrhosis, and elevated levels of iron and the iron-binding complex, ferritin. The diagnosis is confirmed by the presence of excessive amounts of iron on liver biopsy. MR is a noninvasive method of confirming excess iron deposition in the liver. MR is able to detect excess iron of 400 μg/gram of tissue. Liver biopsy is not always required. The therapy for hemochromatosis is the removal of iron through phlebotomy. Unfortunately, the changes of arthritis are progressive despite control of iron concentrations.

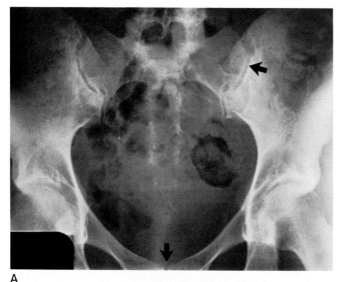

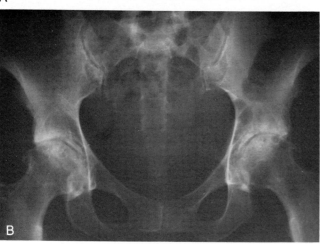

Figure 14–17. Hemochromatosis. *A,* A 53-year-old woman with occasional low back pain with an elevated level of serum ferritin. AP of pelvis reveals chondrocalcinosis of the left sacroiliac joint and symphysis pubis *(arrows).* Degenerative disease of the right hip is noted. *B,* A roentgenogram of the same patient at age 63 demonstrating progressive degenerative disease of both hips. The patient's primary clinical complaint was hip pain. The chondrocalcinosis in the symphysis pubis and sacroiliac joint was no longer visible. The patient was treated with phlebotomy with normalization of serum ferritin.

TREATMENT

Therapy for gout requires the immediate control of inflammation during the acute attack and the chronic control of hyperuricemia to prevent tophaceous deposits.[37] An acute gouty attack may be controlled with intravenous colchicine or nonsteroidal anti-inflammatory drugs, particularly indomethacin or phenylbutazone. The nonsteroidal drug (indomethacin, 150 mg/day, or phenylbutazone, 300 mg/day) is continued for 7 to 10 days or until the attack is alleviated. In patients where nonsteroidal drugs or colchicine is contraindicated, corticotrophin in the form of an intramuscular injection of 40 to 80 IU is used. Corticosteroids given by either oral or intravenous route may also be effective. The corticosteroids are gradually tapered over a 2 to 3 week period as the attack subsides. A maximum dose of intravenous colchicine for the treatment of an acute attack of gout should not exceed 2 mg. The use of a maximum dose less than 4 mg per attack may prevent potential toxicities of cytopenias and renal failure.[38] Once the acute inflammation has subsided, uric acid concentrations may be controlled by increasing uric acid excretion with probenecid or sulfinpyrazone or by inhibiting uric acid production with the xanthine oxidase inhibitor allopurinol, along with colchicine prophylaxis.[39, 40]

Therapy for CPPD is primarily directed toward control of inflammation with nonsteroidal anti-inflammatory drugs. Occasionally, aspiration of a joint to remove crystals is helpful in controlling joint symptoms, but this is not practical for axial skeletal involvement. Oral colchicine is not as effective in preventing attacks in CPPD as it is in gout. Controlling diseases associated with CPPD may help to arrest its progression, but the calcium pyrophosphate deposits are not resorbed.[40]

PROGNOSIS

Acute attacks of gout and CPPD do not occur with any specific intervals between episodes. Some patients have only one attack, while others have frequent, painful bouts of inflammatory arthritis. Both the acute and chronic manifestations of gout can be well controlled with available therapy; if diagnosed early enough, patients should have limited dysfunction from the disease. Those with CPPD also have a variable period between attacks, but anti-inflammatory therapy is usually effective at controlling the associated inflammation. There is, however, no effective therapy to either control or reverse the calcification of tissues or the secondary degenerative changes associated with crystal deposition. Patients with severe disease may develop progressive axial skeletal involvement with limited function. Fortunately, these circumstances are rare.

References

MICROCRYSTALLINE DISEASE

1. Hall AP, Barry PE, Dawber TR, McNamara PM: Epidemiology of gout and hyperuricemia: a long-term population study. Am J Med 42:27, 1967.
2. McCarty DJ, Hogan JM, Gatter RA, Grossman M: Studies on pathological calcifications in human cartilage. Part I. Prevalence and types of crystal deposits in the menisci of 215 cadavers. J Bone Joint Surg 48A:309, 1966.
3. Star VL, Hochberg MC: Prevention and management of gout. Drugs 45:212, 1993.
4. Abbott RD, Brand FN, Kannel WB, Castelli WP: Gout and coronary heart disease: the Framingham study. J Clin Epidemiol 41:237, 1988.
5. Roubenoff R, Klag MJ, Mead LA, et al.: Incidence and risk factors for gout in white men. JAMA 266:3004, 1991.
6. Lichtenstein L, Scott HW, Levin MH: Pathologic changes in gout: survey of eleven necropsied cases. Am J Pathol 32:871, 1956.
7. Campion EW, Glynn RJ, DeLabry LO: Asymptomatic hyperuricemia: risks and consequences in the Normative Aging Study. Am J Med 82:421, 1987.
8. O'Duffy JD: Clinical studies of acute pseudogout attacks: comments on prevalence, predispositions and treatment. Arthritis Rheum 19:349, 1976.
9. Felson DT, Anderson JJ, Naimark A, et al.: The prevalence of chondrocalcinosis in the elderly and its association with knee osteoarthritis: the Framingham study. J Rheumatol 16:1241, 1989.
10. Jensen PS: Chondrocalcinosis and other calcifications. Radiol Clin North Am 26:1315, 1988.
11. Jones AC, Chuck AJ, Arie EA, et al.: Diseases associated with calcium pyrophosphate deposition disease. Semin Arthritis Rheum 22:188, 1992.
12. Malawista SE, Seegmiller JE, Hathaway BE, Sokoloff L: Sacroiliac gout. JAMA 194:954, 1965.
13. Leventhal LJ, Levin RW, Bomalaski JS: Peripheral arthrocentesis in the work-up of acute low back pain. Arch Phys Med Rehabil 71:253, 1990.
14. Reynolds AF, Wyler AR, Norris HT: Paraparesis secondary to sodium urate deposits in the ligamentous flavum. Arch Neurol 33:795, 1976.
15. Varga J, Giampaolo C, Goldenberg DL: Tophaceous gout of the spine in a patient with no peripheral tophi: case report and review of the literature. Arthritis Rheum 28:1312, 1985.
16. Magid SK, Gray GE, Arand A: Spinal cord compression by tophi in a patient with chronic polyarthritis: case report and literature review. Arthritis Rheum 24:1431, 1984.
17. Reginato A, Valenzuela F, Martinez V, et al.: Polyarticular and familial chondrocalcinosis. Arthritis Rheum 13:197, 1970.

18. Resnick D, Niwayama G, Goergen TG, et al.: Clinical, radiographic, and pathologic abnormalities in calcium pyrophosphate dihydrate deposition disease (CPPD): pseudogout. Radiology 122:1, 1977.

19. Delamarter RB, Sherman JE, Carr J: Lumbar spinal stenosis secondary to calcium pyrophosphate crystal deposition (pseudogout). Clin Orthop 289:127, 1993.

20. Lawry GV, Fan PT, Bluestone R: Polyarticular versus monoarticular gout: a prospective, comparative analysis of clinical features. Medicine 67:335, 1988.

21. Ellman MH, Vazquez T, Ferguson L, Mandel N: Calcium pyrophosphate deposition in ligamentum flavum. Arthritis Rheum 21:611, 1978.

22. Berger RG, Levitin PM: Febrile presentation of calcium pyrophosphate dihydrate deposition disease. J Rheumatol 15:642, 1988.

23. Alarcon-Segovia D, Cetina JA, Diza-Jouanen E: Sacroiliac joints in primary gout. Clinical and roentgenographic study of 143 patients. AJR 118:438, 1973.

24. Hall MC, Selin G: Spinal involvement in gout. J Bone Joint Surg 42A:341, 1960.

25. De AD: Intervertebral disc involvement in gout: brief report. J Bone Joint Surg 70B:671, 1988.

26. Litvak J, Briney W: Extradural spinal depositions of urates producing paraplegia: case report. J Neurosurg 39:656, 1973.

27. Burnham J, Fraker J, Steinbach H: Pathologic fracture in an unusual case of gout. AJR 129:116, 1977.

28. Palestro CJ, Vega A, Kim CK, et al.: Appearance of acute gouty arthritis on indium-111-labeled leukocyte scintigraphy. J Nucl Med 31:682, 1990.

29. McCarty DJ Jr, Haskin ME: The roentgenographic aspects of pseudogout (articular chondrocalcinosis): an analysis of 20 cases. AJR 90:1248, 1963.

30. Bundens WD Jr, Brighton CT, Weitzman G: Primary articular cartilage calcification with arthritis (pseudogout syndrome). J Bone Joint Surg 47A:111, 1965.

31. Brown TR, Quinn SF, D'Agostino AN: Deposition of calcium pyrophosphate dihydrate crystals in the ligamentum flavum: evaluation with MR imaging and CT: Radiology 178:871, 1991.

32. Webb J, Deodhar S, Lee P: Chronic destructive polyarthritis due to pyrophosphate crystal arthritis ("pseudogout" syndrome). Med J Aust 2:206, 1974.

33. Richards AJ, Hamilton EBD: Spinal changes in idiopathic chondrocalcinosis articularis. Rheumatol Rehabil 15:138, 1976.

34. Hamilton E, Williams R, Barlow KA, Smith PM: The arthropathy of idiopathic haemochromatosis. Q J Med 37:171, 1968.

35. Bywaters EGH, Hamilton CBP, Williams R: The spine in idiopathic haemochromatosis. Ann Rheum Dis 30:453, 1971.

36. Hirsch JH, Killien C, Troupin RH: The arthropathy of hemochromatosis. Radiology 118:591, 1976.

37. Yu TF, Gutman AB: Principles of current management of primary gout. Am J Med Sci 254:893, 1967.

38. Roberts WN, Liang MH, Stern SH: Colchicine in acute gout: reassessment of risks and benefits. JAMA 257:1920, 1987.

39. Klinenberg JR, Goldfinger S, Seegmiller JE: The effectiveness of the xanthine oxidase inhibitor allopurinol in the treatment of gout. Ann Intern Med 62:639, 1965.

40. McCarty DJ: Calcium pyrophosphate dihydrate crystal deposition disease (pseudogout syndrome)—clinical aspects. Clin Rheum Dis 3:61, 1977.

OCHRONOSIS

Capsule Summary

Frequency of back pain—very common
Location of back pain—lumbar spine
Quality of back pain—ache
Signs and symptoms—decreased back motion, pigmentation of sclerae, ears, nose
Laboratory and x-ray tests—homogentisic acid in urine; extensive disc calcifications on plain roentgenograms
Treatment—nonsteroidal anti-inflammatory drugs

PREVALENCE AND PATHOGENESIS

Ochronosis is a rare metabolic disorder associated with the deposition of homogentisic acid in connective tissue throughout the body. The accumulation of homogentisic acid results in darkened pigmentation and progressive degeneration of connective tissue. Ochronotic arthropathy develops in the fourth decade of life and is associated with progressive low back pain, stiffness, and obliteration of the normal lumbar lordosis. Peripheral joint disease also may occur in the hips, knees, and shoulders.

The prevalence of ochronosis is approximately 1 in 10 million.[1] The illness has a wide geographic distribution, although most large series have been reported from Central European countries.[2] Men are slightly more commonly affected than women.

The cause of this illness is the congenital absence of the enzyme homogentisic acid oxidase.[3] Without the enzyme there is an accumulation of homogentisic acid. Alkaptonuria is the disease associated with the excretion of homogentisic acid in the urine. Ochronosis, which is caused by the same enzyme deficiency, is the discoloration of connective tissue from the deposition of a black pigment that is thought to be a polymer of homogentisic acid.[4] The pigment affects the integrity of cartilage matrix and chondrocytes and results in cartilage damage and degeneration.[5] The inheritance of the disorder is autosomal recessive.[2]

CLINICAL HISTORY

Alkaptonuria is usually unrecognized during childhood, although occasionally discoloration of urine is detected before adulthood. Symptoms of ochronosis first appear in the fourth decade of life. Low back pain and stiffness are frequently the initial symptoms of the illness.[6] Herniation of an intervertebral disc, particularly in men, can be the initial symptom of disease in some patients.[7] This is associated with severe sharp pain.[8–10] Peripheral joint involvement may cause loss of motion and pain in the hips, knees, and shoulders. Pain in some patients is most intense in the morning. Some also describe episodes of acutely swollen, inflamed joints, particularly the knees. This symptom is related to the association of calcium pyrophosphate dihydrate deposition (CPPD) disease and ochronosis.[11] Ochronotic deposition in other organs may cause prostatic enlargement with calculi, renal calculi with renal failure, and myocardial infarction.

PHYSICAL EXAMINATION

Physical examination demonstrates limited motion of the lumbar spine and localized tenderness with percussion. Muscle spasm is usually absent. With advanced disease, there is rigidity of the axial skeleton. Chest wall expansion is also limited. Kyphosis may be prominent and is associated with a loss in height. Dark pigmentation may be discovered in the nose, ears, sclerae, and fingernails.

LABORATORY DATA

The characteristic laboratory finding is the presence of homogentisic acid in urine. Alkalinization of a urine specimen will cause darkening, which is indicative of the presence of homogentisic acid.[5] Synovial fluid analysis may demonstrate a "ground-pepper" appearance of the fluid or pyrophosphate crystals.[11, 12]

Pathologic examination demonstrates pigment deposition in connective tissue, including articular cartilage, tendons, and ligaments. Pathologic changes in the axial skeleton first occur in the lumbar spine. Pigment is located in the nucleus pulposus and annulus fibrosus. The discs become brittle.[13, 14] The ligaments may also become calcified. Transmission electron microscopy has demonstrated the binding of ochronotic pigment to collagen fibrils in the presence of mucopolysaccharide ground substance.[15] The presence of mucopolysaccharide ground substance may be the factor located in tissues that attracts deposition of ochronotic pigment.

RADIOGRAPHIC FINDINGS

Radiographic examination of the lumbar spine in ochronosis demonstrates marked disc

space narrowing, osteophyte formation, and disc calcification (Fig. 14–18). "Vacuum" phenomena may be seen in an intervertebral disc and are suggestive of the diagnosis of ochronosis when it occurs at multiple levels. Disease of long duration may be associated with total obliteration of disc spaces, bony fusion, and loss of lumbar lordosis, and may be confused with the axial skeletal changes of ankylosing spondylitis (Fig. 14–19).[16] Osteoporosis of the vertebral bodies is common and accentuates the prominence of disc calcification.

Bone scintigraphy may demonstrate a "whisker sign" in the axial skeleton in patients with ochronosis.[17] The increased uptake near the axial skeleton is a result of intervertebral discs accumulating radioactivity allowing spread of the uptake bilaterally beyond the confines of the vertebral column.

DIFFERENTIAL DIAGNOSIS

A diagnosis of ochronosis is based on the characteristic clinical symptoms and radiographic findings along with the presence of homogentisic acid in urine. Other diseases, such as CPPD, hemochromatosis, hyperparathyroidism, and acromegaly, may involve intervertebral disc calcification and must be considered in the differential diagnosis (Table 14–7).[18] Patients with ankylosing spondylitis may have symptoms and signs similar to those of ochronosis but will not have skin pigmentation or disc calcification. The coexistence of ochronosis and ankylosing spondylitis in patients has been recently reported.[19–21] These patients have characteristic evidence of ochronosis, including increased urinary homogentisic acid, along with bilateral sacroiliac joint fusion. Interestingly, HLA-B27 is positive in only 1 of 3 patients with both illnesses.

Patients with generalized degenerative disc disease (intervertebral osteochondrosis) will have loss of disc space, vacuum phenomena, traction osteophytes, and marginal sclerosis. The absence of widespread disc calcification should help differentiate these diseases.[22]

TREATMENT

Specific treatment for this disease, replacement of homogentisic acid oxidase, is not available. Treatment is symptomatic and includes rest, exercise, analgesics, and anti-inflammatory drugs. Low tyrosine–low phenylalanine diets lower homogentisic acid levels but

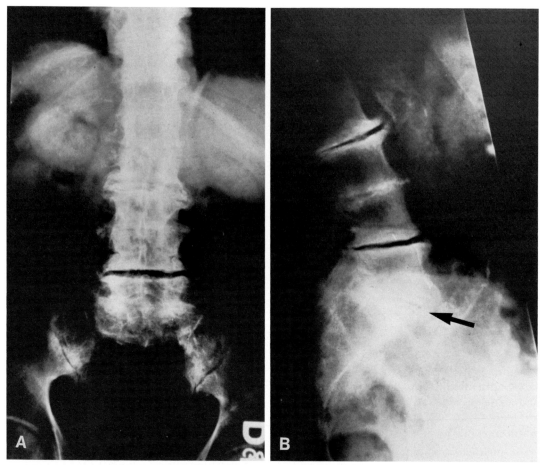

Figure 14–18. Ochronosis. *A,* AP view reveals disc space narrowing and marked osteophyte formation of the vertebral bodies and sacroiliac joints. *B,* Lateral view shows disc space calcification *(arrow).* (Courtesy of Randall Lewis, M.D.)

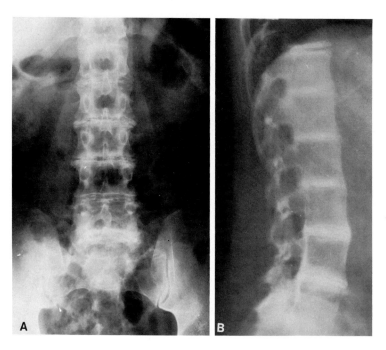

Figure 14–19. Ochronosis. *A,* AP view demonstrating generalized disc space narrowing and diffuse disc calcification. *B,* Lateral view of lumbar spine simulating ankylosing spondylitis. Notice multiple disc calcifications, which are not characteristic of ankylosing spondylitis. (Courtesy of Anne Brower, M.D.)

TABLE 14–7. DISC CALCIFICATION

DISEASE	CHARACTER OF DISC	DIAGNOSIS
Ochronosis	Diffuse distribution, "wafer-like" configuration Broad outer band-like osteophytes	Homogentisic acid in urine
Ankylosing spondylitis	Perservation of disc space Central calcification Vertically-oriented thin syndesmophytes	Radiographic distribution Clinical history (iritis)
Calcium pyrophosphate dihydrate disease (Hemochromatosis, hyperparathyroidsm)	Outer portion of the annulus fibrosus Disc narrowing	Presence of crystals
Acromegaly	Anterior portion of disc Increased disc height	Increased growth hormone

do not seem to produce major benefits in regard to the course of the illness.[5]

PROGNOSIS

The course of ochronosis is progressive and disabling. Ochronosis is a generalized disease that affects the appendicular and axial skeleton with destructive disease. The disease may progress to the degree that patients have severely limited function because of musculoskeletal disease. The osteoporotic spine of the ochronotic patient is at risk for fracture from minimal injury.[23]

References

OCHRONOSIS

1. Seradge H, Anderson MG: Alkaptonuria and ochronosis. Historical review and update. Orthop Rev 7:41, 1978.
2. Srsen S: Alkaptonuria. Johns Hopkins Med J 145:217, 1979.
3. LaDu BN, Zannoni VG, Laster L, Seegmiller JE: The nature of the defect in tyrosine metabolism in alkaptonuria. J Biol Chem 230:251, 1985.
4. Milch RA: Biochemical studies on the pathogenesis of collagen tissue changes in alkaptonuria. Clin Orthop 24:213, 1962.
5. Schumacher HR, Holdsworth DE: Ochronotic arthropathy. Part I. Clinicopathologic studies. Semin Arthritis Rheum 6:207, 1977.
6. McCollum DE, Odom GL: Alkaptonuria, ochronosis, and low back pain: a case report. J Bone Joint Surg 47A:1389, 1965.
7. O'Brien WM, LaDu BN, Bunim JJ: Biochemical, pathologic, and clinical aspects of alkaptonuria, ochronosis, and ochronotic arthropathy. Am J Med 34:813, 1963.
8. Acosta C, Watts CC, Simpson CW: Ochronosis and degenerative lumbar disc disease. A case report. J Neurosurg 28:488, 1968.
9. Feild JR, Higley GB, Disaussare RL Jr: Case report. Ochronosis with ruptured lumbar disc. J Neurosurg 20:348, 1963.
10. Ortiz AC, Neal EG: Alkaptonuria and ochronotic arthritis. A general review and report of two cases. Clin Orthop 25:147, 1962.
11. Rynes RI, Sosman JL, Holdsworth DE: Pseudogout in ochronosis. Report of a case. Arthritis Rheum 18:21, 1975.
12. Hunter T, Gordon DA, Ogryzlo MA: The ground pepper sign of synovial fluid. A new diagnostic feature of ochronosis. J Rheumatol 1:45, 1974.
13. Bywaters EGL, Dorling J, Sutor J: Ochronotic densification. Ann Rheum Dis 29:563, 1970.
14. Lagier R, Sitaj S: Vertebral changes in ochronosis. Anatomical and radiological study of one case. Ann Rheum Dis 33:86, 1974.
15. Gaines JJ: The pathology of alkaptonuric ochronosis. Hum Pathol 20:40, 1989.
16. Simon G, Zorab PA: The radiological changes in alkaptonuric arthritis: a report of 3 cases (one an Egyptian mummy). Br J Radiol 34:384, 1961.
17. Paul R, Ylinen S: The "whisker sign" as an indicator of ochronosis in skeletal scintigraphy. Eur J Nucl Med 18:222, 1991.
18. Weinberger A, Myers AR: Intervertebral disc calcification in adults. A review. Semin Arthritis Rheum 8:69, 1978.
19. Zanetakis E, Khan MA, Yagan R, Kushner I: Ochronotic arthropathy, post-traumatic spinal pseudoarthrosis and HLA-B27. J Orthop Rheumatol 2:48, 1989.
20. Gemignani G, Olivieri I, Semeria R, et al.: Coexistence of ochronosis and ankylosing spondylitis. J Rheumatol 17:1707, 1990.
21. Weinberger KA: The coexistence of ochronosis and ankylosing spondylitis. J Rheumatol 18:1948, 1991.
22. Resnick D, Niwayama G: Radiographic and pathologic features of spinal involvement in diffuse idiopathic skeletal hyperostosis (DISH). Radiology 119:559, 1976.
23. Millea TP, Segal LS, Liss RG, Stauffer ES. Spine fracture in ochronosis. Report of a case. Clin Orthop 281:208, 1992.

FLUOROSIS

Capsule Summary

Frequency of back pain—rare
Location of back pain—lumbar spine
Quality of back pain—ache
Symptoms and signs—bone pain, decreased spine motion, discolored teeth

Laboratory and x-ray tests—increased urinary fluoride, increased alkaline phosphatase; osteosclerosis and osteophytes on plain roentgenograms

Treatment—limit exposure to fluoride

PREVALENCE AND PATHOGENESIS

Fluorine is an element that is found extensively throughout the environment since, like silicon and phosphorus, it is a common constituent of the earth's crust. Fluorine serves as a trace element in the human body. At optimal concentrations, fluoride compounds stabilize the crystalline structure of teeth and bone. At high concentrations, fluoride is a cell poison. Between optimum (1 mg/day) and toxic (100 mg/day) intake levels, fluoride ingestion causes alterations primarily of bone.

Fluoride poisoning occurs in three circumstances:

1. Endemic fluorosis occurs in regions of the world where drinking water contains fluoride in concentrations greater than 4 parts/million (ppm).[1] Endemic fluorosis occurs in parts of India, Africa, and South America where water supplies are contaminated with fluorine compounds. Fluoride is added to water in developed countries to help reduce the incidence of dental caries. The concentration of fluoride in water in developed countries is 1 ppm and causes no harm to man.

2. Industrial fluorosis occurs in industrial workers exposed to fluoride compounds (aluminum mining, phosphate fertilizer industries), in laboratory workers who inhale fluorine fumes, or with exposure to insecticides. This form of fluorosis occurs with exposure over many years.[2]

3. Iatrogenic fluorosis occurs in patients treated with sodium fluoride for osteoporosis, or with other medications or liquids that contain increased concentrations of fluoride.[3–5]

The prevalence of fluorosis in the United States is unknown. For the most part, it is a very rare illness outside of endemic areas. In endemic areas, fluoride intoxication of bone is the most common form of bone disease. The effects of fluoride on the skeleton are related to the interaction of fluoride ions with bone and the parathyroid glands. Fluoride ions enter the surface of bone from the extracellular fluid. Fluoride ions, because of their similarity to hydroxyl ions, substitute for hydroxyl groups in the hydroxyapatite lattice structure of bone. The new crystals, hydroxyfluoroapatite, are harder and more resistant to dissolution and growth and to the actions of parathyroid hormone.[6, 7] Fluoride causes simultaneous increases in bone formation and bone resorption.[8] These findings are reflected in the osteoblastic appearance of bone and the increased plasma levels of alkaline phosphatase.[7] The new bone that is formed is osteomalacic secondary to inadequate mineralization.

CLINICAL HISTORY

In the initial stages of exposure, the patients have no specific complaints. As the skeletal disease advances, patients complain of vague pains in the small joints of hands and feet. As the spine becomes involved, patients complain of back stiffness and loss of motion. With severe disease, patients complain of inability to flex the fingers, rigidity of the spine, flexion deformities of the appendicular skeleton, and shortness of breath secondary to decreased chest expansion.

PHYSICAL EXAMINATION

Physical examination may demonstrate abnormalities of the teeth. Tooth enamel is weakened by high concentrations of fluoride. The enamel becomes mottled, with discoloration and pitting. Examination of the musculoskeletal system reveals decreased range of motion of the spine along with percussion tenderness. Appendicular joints also have decreased motion. In advanced disease, kyphosis and spinal angulation occur, which may result in neurologic signs including sensory disturbance, muscle weakness, and atrophy proceeding to paralysis.[9]

LABORATORY DATA

Laboratory evaluation of patients with fluorosis reflects the increased bone and PTH activity. Plasma levels of alkaline phosphatase are extremely high. In the urine, increased phosphate clearance in association with decreased tubular reabsorption of phosphate is noted along with decreased concentrations of calcium. Urinary fluoride concentrations are elevated.[7]

RADIOGRAPHIC EVALUATION

Involvement of the axial skeleton, including the spine and pelvis, is commonplace in patients with fluorosis.[10, 11] Osteosclerosis is the predominant finding in adults who have ingested fluoride for many years. Osteoblastic activity occurs along trabecular surfaces, leading to thickening of trabeculae and loss of detail in bony architecture. Osteophytes are numerous and large and may encroach on the spinal canal. Encroachment on the spinal canal may result in compromise of nerve function resulting in myelopathy or neuropathy.[12] Calcification of supporting ligaments also is common. In severe cases, osteophytosis may resemble a "bamboo spine" and corresponds to the symptom of spinal rigidity.

DIFFERENTIAL DIAGNOSIS

In the United States, the diagnosis of fluorosis should be considered in an individual with an industrial exposure to the chemical or someone who is ingesting sodium fluoride as part of a therapeutic regimen for osteoporosis.[13] Workers in the manufacture of aluminum, nickel, copper, gold, glass-works, and pesticides are at risk. Fluorosis also has occurred in communities neighboring fluoride-polluting industries.[14] Fluorosis should also be considered in individuals whose primary source of drinking water are ground wells.[15] Acute fluoride poisoning has also been reported from excess fluoridation of water from a public water system in Alaska.[16] The diagnosis is confirmed by the presence of increased fluoride concentration in the urine. The combination of generalized axial skeletal sclerosis, osteophytosis, and ligamentous calcification is almost diagnostic of the illness.

Osteosclerosis alone may be noted in patients with bone metastases, hematologic disorders (myelofibrosis), renal osteodystrophy, and Paget's disease. Vertebral osteophytosis is found in patients with DISH, spondyloarthropathy, neuroarthropathy, and ochronosis. Ligamentous calcifications are also associated with DISH. It is the combination of all three findings in a single patient that helps differentiate fluorosis from these other more common illnesses.

TREATMENT

The most important aspect of therapy for patients with fluorosis is to limit any additional exposure to the chemical. Excess body stores of fluoride trapped in bone crystals are released only when bone resorption occurs and some of the liberated fluoride is redeposited at sites of new bone formation. If intake is minimized, urinary excretion of the chemical will gradually decrease.

PROGNOSIS

Questions remain concerning the strength of fluorotic bone and whether it is at greater risk for fracture than normal bone. Evans has suggested that fluorotic bone is weaker and prone to fracture.[17] In contrast, Franke observed increased strength of fluorotic bone.[18] Clinically, fluoride in combination with calcium may improve bone strength and decrease bone fracture.[19] Additional studies are needed to determine the effect of fluorine on bone.

References

FLUOROSIS

1. Singh A, Jolly SS, Bansal BC, Mathur CC: Endemic fluorosis. Epidemiological, clinical, and biochemical study of chronic fluorine intoxication in the Punjab (India). Medicine 42:229, 1963.
2. Boillat MA, Garcia J, Velebit L: Radiological criteria of industrial fluorosis. Skel Radiol 5:161, 1980.
3. O'Duffy JD, Wahner HW, O'Fallon WM, et al.: Mechanism of acute lower extremity pain syndrome in fluoride-treated osteoporotic patients. Am J Med 80:561, 1986.
4. Meunier PJ, Courpron P, Smoller JS, Briancon D: Niflumic acid-induced skeletal fluorosis. Iatrogenic disease or therapeutic perspective for osteoporosis? Clin Orthop 148:304, 1980.
5. Johnson FF, Fischer LL: Report on fluorine in urine. Am J Pharm 107:512, 1939.
6. Faccini JM, Teotia SPS: Histopathological assessment of endemic skeletal fluorosis. Calcif Tissue Res 16:45, 1974.
7. Teotia SPS, Teotia M: Secondary hyperparathyroidism in patients with endemic skeletal fluorosis. Br Med J 1:637, 1973.
8. Aggarwal ND: Structure of human fluorotic bone. J Bone Joint Surg 55A:331, 1973.
9. Singh A, Jolly SS, Bansal BC: Skeletal fluorosis and its neurological complications. Lancet 1:197, 1961.
10. Stevenson CA, Watson AR: Fluoride osteosclerosis. AJR 78:13, 1957.
11. Largent EJ, Bovard PG, Heyroth FF: Roentgenographic changes and urinary fluoride excretion among workmen engaged in the manufacture of inorganic fluorides. AJR 65:42, 1951.
12. Fisher RL, Medcalf TW, Henderson MC: Endemic fluorosis with spinal cord compression: a case report and review. Arch Intern Med 149:697, 1989.
13. Riggs BL, Hodgson SF, Hoffman DL, et al.: Treatment of primary osteoporosis with fluoride and calcium. JAMA 243:446, 1980.
14. Nemeth L, Zsogon E: Occupational skeletal fluorosis. Clin Rheumatol 3:81, 1989.
15. Felsenfeld AJ, Roberts MA: A report of fluorosis in the United States secondary to drinking well water. JAMA 265:486, 1991.
16. Gessner BD, Beller M, Middaugh JP, et al.: Acute fluoride poisoning from a public water system. N Engl J Med 330:95, 1994.
17. Evans FG, Wood JL: Mechanical properties and density of bone in a case of severe endemic fluorosis. Acta Orthop Scand 47:489, 1976.

18. Franke J, Runge H, Grau P, et al.: Physical properties of fluorosis bone. Acta Orthop Scand 47:20, 1976.
19. Riggs BL, Seeman E, Hodgson SF, et al.: Effect of the fluoride/calcium regimen on vertebral fracture occurrence in postmenopausal osteoporosis. N Engl J Med 306:446, 1982.

HERITABLE GENETIC DISORDERS

Capsule Summary

Frequency of back pain—common
Location of back pain—lumbar spine
Quality of back pain—chronic ache
Symptoms and signs—abnormalities noticeable early in life; structural alterations—kyphoscoliosis, short stature
Laboratory and x-ray tests—specific for each illness
Treatment—symptomatic bracing

This section will review a number of heritable disorders of connective tissue that are associated with back pain (Table 14–8). For the most part, these diseases are rare. Many of the patients with these disorders are not evaluated by internists, since many of these patients do not live to adulthood.

Within the major categories of heritable disorders of connective tissue, impairment of the back and spine is common. However, not all of the entities included in a single disorder (Ehlers-Danlos syndrome, for example) have associated back pain. Those subclasses of these disorders associated with back pain will be identified and the clinical characteristics of each group listed. The disorders of connective tissue may involve fibrous connective tissue elements (collagen or elastin), ground substance (mucopolysaccharide), cartilage, or bone.[1, 2]

Marfan Syndrome

Marfan syndrome is a connective tissue disorder associated with arachnodactyly, myopia, and aortic disease.[3] The musculoskeletal abnormalities associated with this syndrome include loose-jointedness, scoliosis, and prominent ribs. Marfan syndrome is a familial disorder that is inherited as an autosomal dominant trait. Both sexes are equally affected. The etiology of this disease is related to an abnormality in the fibrillin gene on chromosome 15.[4] Fibrillin is a large glycoprotein that is one of the structural components of

TABLE 14–8. HERITABLE DISORDERS ASSOCIATED WITH BACK PAIN

DISORDER	SPINAL MANIFESTATIONS
Marfan syndrome	Kyphoscoliosis
	Vertebral body—posterior scalloping, increased height
Homocystinuria	Kyphoscoliosis
	Vertebral body—posterior scalloping, compression fractures
Ehlers-Danlos syndrome	Kyphoscoliosis
	Vertebral body—posterior scalloping, anterior wedging
	Spondylolysis
	Spondylolisthesis
Achondroplasia	Kyphoscoliosis
	Lumbar lordosis, small spinal canal
	Vertebral body—decreased height, posterior scalloping
	Pedicles short and thick
Osteogenesis imperfecta	Kyphoscoliosis
	Fractures
	Osteoporosis
	Vertebral body—flattening, "fish" vertebrae, anterior wedging
Mucopolysaccharidoses	
Hunter syndrome	Vertebral bodies—ovoid, hypoplastic
	Kyphoscoliosis
	Osteoporosis
Morquio syndrome	Vertebral bodies—flattening, central beaking
	Kyphoscoliosis
Maroteaux-Lamy	Vertebral bodies—central beaking, hypoplasia
Tuberous sclerosis	Osteosclerosis of sacroiliac joints and vertebrae
Spondyloepiphyseal dysplasia	Vertebral bodies—flattened irregular endplates
	Intervertebral disc space narrowing

microfibrils. Microfibrils are components of a number of tissues in the body that are abnormal in Marfan syndrome including the suspensory ligament of the lens, periosteum of bone, and the media of the aorta.[5] A variety of mutations on chromosome 15 result in alterations in fibrillin polypeptides that result in the phenotypic expression of Marfan syndrome.[6]

Clinically, these patients are tall and thin with disproportionately long arms in comparison to the trunk (dolichostenomelia). The thoracic kyphosis is lost (straight back) with scoliosis at multiple levels. Joint laxity is prominent. Radiographic evaluation reveals a high proportion of patients with scoliosis of the thoracolumbar spine, which is similar in configuration to that seen with idiopathic scoliosis. However, scoliosis associated with Marfan syndrome starts at an earlier age and does not have a female predominance. Other roentgenographic findings include posterior scalloping of the vertebral bodies and increased vertebral height. Dural ectasia, a result of hydraulic forces of pulsatile cerebrospinal fluid on weakened connective tissue, may be noted in 63% of Marfan patients.[7] Dural ectasia results in Tarlov, or perineural, cysts, arachnoid cysts, or pelvic meningoceles that are associated with neurologic signs including sensory deficits.[8] The spinal deformity is progressive and potentially painful.[9] Sinclair reported that 7 of 40 patients with Marfan syndrome had associated back pain.[10]

The diagnosis of Marfan syndrome is a clinical one, since most patients have only some of the characteristic manifestations of disease.[11] In one study, arachnodactyly occurred in 89%, aortic murmurs in 62%, and ectopia lentis in 57%.[12] Schlesinger has suggested the possibility of Marfan syndrome in patients with refractory low back syndrome, dural ectasia, and protracted pain after lumbar puncture with a marfanoid habitus.[13]

Homocystinuria is the disease that must be differentiated from Marfan syndrome. Homocystinuric patients are long-limbed and tall but have restricted movements as opposed to lax ones. In addition, homocystinuria is associated with nervous system disorders including mental retardation and seizures. Between 25% and 60% of homocystinuric patients have skeletal abnormalities, including scoliosis, posterior scalloping, and osteoporosis with compression fractures.[14, 15] Unlike in Marfan syndrome, a specific biochemical abnormality is detectable in homocystinuric patients. Levels of homocysteine, homocystine, and methionine are elevated. Cystathionine B-synthetase deficiency is the most common cause of homocystinuria.[16]

The treatment of Marfan syndrome starts early in life with bracing to decrease abnormal spinal curvature. Surgical stabilization is needed if scoliosis progresses to too great a degree. Surgical intervention also may be required to control the growth of arachnoid cysts.[17]

Ehlers-Danlos Syndrome (EDS)

Ehlers-Danlos syndrome (EDS) comprises a group of disorders characterized by skin hyperelasticity and fragility, loose-jointedness, and decreased tensile strength of elastic tissues. Eleven different forms of EDS have been reclassified into nine entities that have been separated on the basis of clinical or biochemi-

cal differences.[18, 19] Types I (Gravis), II (Mitis), and III (Hypermobile) account for 80% of all cases of EDS. The phenotypic heterogeneity within the EDS syndrome results from mutations in collagen genes that affect Type I procollagen, Type III procollagen, or enzymes that modify collagens.[20]

In general, EDS patients have hyperelastic skin that tears with minimal trauma. Patients experience easy bruisability. Loose-jointedness ("India rubber man") is characteristic of the disorder. Hypermobility results in back pain in 6% of patients, with radiographic evidence of spinal deformity appearing in 23%.[21] Spinal deformity is noted in patients with Type I, VI (ocular-scoliotic), and, most commonly, VII (arthrochalasis multiplex congenita). Radiographically, EDS patients present with kyphoscoliosis at the thoracolumbar junction in association with anterior wedging and posterior scalloping of the vertebral bodies.[22] Patients may also develop spondylolysis and spondylolisthesis secondary to tissue laxity. EDS is associated with vascular fragility, bleeding, compartment syndromes, and sciatic neuropathy.[23] The treatment for EDS is nonsurgical. Bracing and muscle strengthening exercises are used to prevent deformities. Bracing of the spine may be worthwhile early in the course of the illness before scoliosis appears.

Achondroplasia

Achondroplasia is a skeletal defect associated with a quantitative decrease in endochondral bone growth. The etiology of the disease is unknown, and no biochemical abnormality has been identified. The disease is transmitted as a autosomal dominant trait, but only 10% have an affected parent. Spontaneous mutations occur in 90%.[24]

The diagnosis of achondroplasia is made at birth. Patients have short limbs, prominent forehead, kyphoscoliosis, and prominent buttocks associated with accentuated lumbar lordosis. Patients have normal intelligence and no visceral lesions.

Achondroplasts have increasing back pain as they become adults, which is associated with their hyperlordosis and small spinal canal.[25] Patients develop facet joint hypertrophy, which further narrows the canal. Achondroplasts have severe and persistent sciatica secondary to disc disease in the lower lumbar canal, which often requires surgery.[26] These patients also develop cord or cauda equina compression at the thoracic or upper lumbar level.[27]

Radiographically, the height of vertebral bodies is reduced with flaring of the upper and lower endplates resulting in posterior scalloping. The pedicles are short and thick. The interpediculate distances become progressively smaller from L1 to L5.[28] Increased disc spaces are also noted. Hyperlordosis is marked, with the sacrum directed sharply posterior.[29] The spinal canal is very narrow. (Fig. 14–20).[30]

Treatment for neurologic complications is surgical, including extensive laminectomy.[31] Leg lengthening also has been proposed as a means to decrease lumbar hyperlordosis in achondroplastic dwarfs.[32] Physiotherapy, nonsteroidal anti-inflammatory drugs, and injections are useful for back pain. Some patients may benefit from bracing.[9, 33]

Osteogenesis Imperfecta

Osteogenesis imperfecta (OI) is an inherited disorder of connective tissue affecting bones, ligaments, skin, sclerae, and teeth. In all its forms, OI affects between 1/5000 to 1/10,000 individuals of all racial and ethnic backgrounds.[34] The primary abnormality of OI is abnormal maturation of collagen. Significant progress has been made in determining the exact mutations resulting in alterations of collagen production. The principal collagen genes, COL1A1 for the alpha 1 chain on chromosome 17 and COL1A2 for the alpha 2 chain on chromosome 7, code for the formation of procollagen.[35] Collagen is a heterotrimer consisting of 2 alpha 1 and 1 alpha 2 chains. A number of defects, including decreased rate of collagen synthesis, abnormal aldehyde cross-linkages, and alterations in the usual proportions of Type I and Type II collagen have been reported.[36–39] OI has several phenotypically distinct entities with different inheritance patterns.[40] Type I OI, the most common variety, has an autosomal dominant pattern of inheritance with variable penetrance and is associated with short stature, blue sclerae, hearing loss, and variable bone fragility.[41] Type II OI has autosomal dominant inheritance and is the lethal form with in utero fractures associated with rearrangements of the COL1A1 and COL1A2 genes and substitution of bulkier amino acids for glycine in the alpha 1 chain.[35] Type III OI has autosomal recessive inheritance and a variable phenotypic appearance with marked deformity, scoliosis, joint laxity, and variable scleral color associated with a deletion in alpha 2 chains. Type IV has autosomal dominant inheritance with point mutations in the alpha 2 chain and is like Type I with normal sclerae. The diagnosis of OI is confirmed by the presence of two of three criteria: (1) abnormal fragility of the skeleton, (2) blue sclerae, and (3) dentinogenesis imperfecta. Other features of OI include premature otosclerosis, ligamentous laxity, episodic diaphoresis, easy bruisability, constipation, and premature vascular calcification.[42]

Skeletal manifestations of OI include short stature secondary to multiple fractures, kyphoscoliosis, and bowing of the long bones. Fractures are very numerous before puberty. Back pain may be present secondary to fractures or

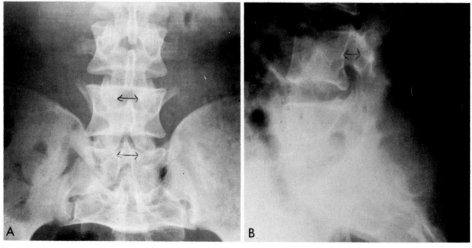

Figure 14–20. AP (A) and lateral (B) views of an achondroplast showing decreased spinal canal size and posterior scalloping of the vertebral bodies. (From Wiesel SW, Bernini P, Rothman RH [eds]: The Aging Lumbar Spine. Philadelphia: W B Saunders Co, 1982, p 12.)

chronic muscle strain resulting from scoliosis. Facial features, including temporal bulging, micrognathia, and blue sclerae, are common. The teeth are frequently discolored. Hearing loss secondary to otosclerosis is common.

Roentgenographic features of OI include diffuse osteopenia of the axial and appendicular skeleton. Spine studies reveal flattening of vertebral bodies, "fish" vertebrae, and anterior wedge deformity. Severe kyphoscoliosis results from ligamentous laxity, fractures, and osteopenia (Fig. 14–21).[43]

Therapy of OI is essentially symptomatic. Fractures are casted. Sofield procedures (intramedullary rodding) may be needed to add support to bones that are chronically fractured. Hanscom has reported the natural history of radiographic changes in six defined groups of patients with OI.[44] Patients with mild disease (Type A), that maintained the contours of vertebral bodies, had a halt to progression of spinal curvature with spinal fusion. More severely affected patients with OI (Types B–F) had a less successful response to bracing and surgery. Nonsteroidal anti-inflammatory and analgesic drugs are necessary to diminish pain associated with skeletal fractures. The use of sodium fluoride and anabolic steroids has not decreased fracture rates and is not recommended.[45]

Mucopolysaccharidoses

The diseases in this class of inborn errors of metabolism result in deposition of mucopolysaccharides in various tissues. The distinct types of mucopolysaccharidosis are distinguished on the basis of combined clinical, genetic, biochemical, and allelic subtypes.[46] Many of the patients with mucopolysaccharidoses do not live into adulthood. The forms of

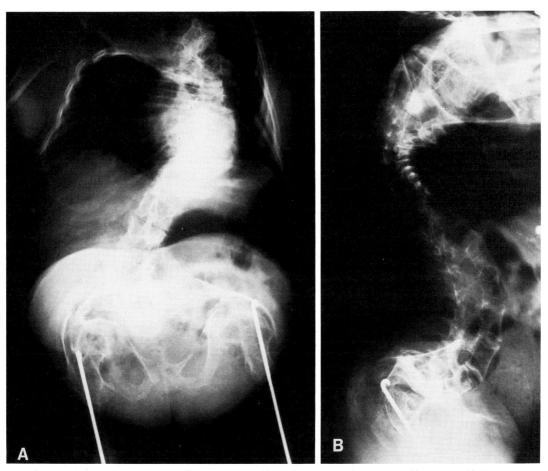

Figure 14–21. Osteogenesis imperfecta. AP *(A)* and lateral *(B)* views of a 24-year-old woman with Type III osteogenesis imperfecta who has sustained over 100 fractures. Severe kyphoscoliosis is noted associated with generalized osteoporosis and flattening of the vertebral bodies. Sofield procedures have been performed in the femoral bones for added support to decrease fractures.

mucopolysaccharidoses that may be seen by an internist include: Type II, Hunter syndrome; Type IV, Morquio syndrome; and Type VI, Maroteaux-Lamy syndrome.

Hunter syndrome (Type II) is an X-linked syndrome with a deficiency of iduronate sulfatase resulting in accumulation of dermatan sulfate and heparan sulfate. The patients are men with mild mental retardation and mild hearing loss. The roentgenographic abnormalities include ovoid vertebral bodies with hypoplasia of vertebrae near the thoracolumbar junction resulting in kyphosis and osteoporosis.[47]

Morquio syndrome (Type IV) is an autosomal recessive disorder with abnormalities in galactosamine-6-sulfate sulfatase (Type A) or beta-galactosidase (Type B) resulting in ineffective keratan sulfate catabolism and keratan sulfaturia. Clinical manifestations of Morquio syndrome include dwarfism, facial deformity, corneal opacification, deafness, pectus carinatum, ligamentous laxity, hepatomegaly, and normal intelligence. The spinal roentgenograms of Morquio's patients reveal platyspondyly with central beaking of vertebral bodies, atlantoaxial subluxation, and kyphoscoliosis.[48] Patients who have symptomatic back pain may benefit from analgesics and anti-inflammatory drugs.[9] The use of a Milwaukee corset can prevent the appearance of medullary compressions of the spinal cord.[49]

Maroteaux-Lamy syndrome (Type VI) is an autosomal recessive syndrome with arylsulfatase B deficiency which results in accumulation of dermatan sulfate. Clinical manifestations of the syndrome include kyphoscoliosis, pectus carinatum, genu valgum, hepatosplenomegaly, and joint contractures.[40] Variations in the severity of clinical manifestations of the illness may be related to the heterogeneity of genetic mutations that result in corresponding alterations in the activity or amounts of the arylsulfatase B enzyme.[50] Roentgenograms of the lumbar spine may demonstrate beaked vertebral bodies, hypoplasia of vertebral bodies, and abnormal ossification of ring epiphyses.

TUBEROUS SCLEROSIS

Tuberous sclerosis is a phakomatosis, a disorder of neuroectodermal tissues. The illness is also termed Bourneville's disease. Tuberous sclerosis is a rare disorder with a variable pattern of inheritance and an estimated incidence of 1 to 2/100,000 population.[51] A more recent study suggests the point prevalence of tuberous sclerosis in Olmstead County, Minnesota to be 6.9/100,000 persons. The higher

rate of diagnosis is related to the use of CT and MR to detect cerebral lesions.[52] The classic diagnostic triad consists of facial adenoma sebaceum, mental retardation, and epilepsy. Depigmented nevi, café-au-lait spots, and shagreen patches are other associated cutaneous manifestations. The cause of these abnormalities is considered to be hamartomas of the skin, brain, and other body organs. Although some of the manifestations of tuberous sclerosis are present at birth, some do not appear until adulthood.[53, 54] Therefore, it is possible for the diagnosis to be overlooked.

Skull films will demonstrate calcification in up to 80% of patients. The calcifications are usually multiple and are located in the basal ganglia and paraventricular areas.[55, 56]

In the axial skeleton, osteoblastic lesions are common and have multiple discrete shapes (round and ovoid). Patchy areas of increased density are also noted. The sacroiliac joints, vertebral bodies, and posterior elements are also involved (Fig. 14–22). These areas may have a mottled appearance. The lesions do not expand the bone.[57] These lesions are usually

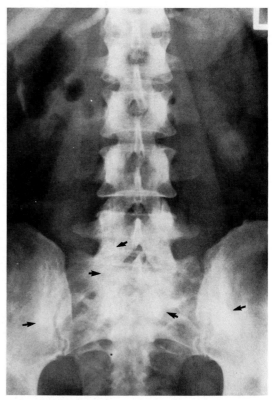

Figure 14–22. Tuberous sclerosis. AP view of a 50-year-old woman with adenoma sebaceum and episodes of middle back pain. Pain was worse with bending or rotation. Irregular areas of osteosclerosis are noted in the ilium, sacrum, and vertebral bodies (arrows). (Courtesy of Eric Gall, M.D.)

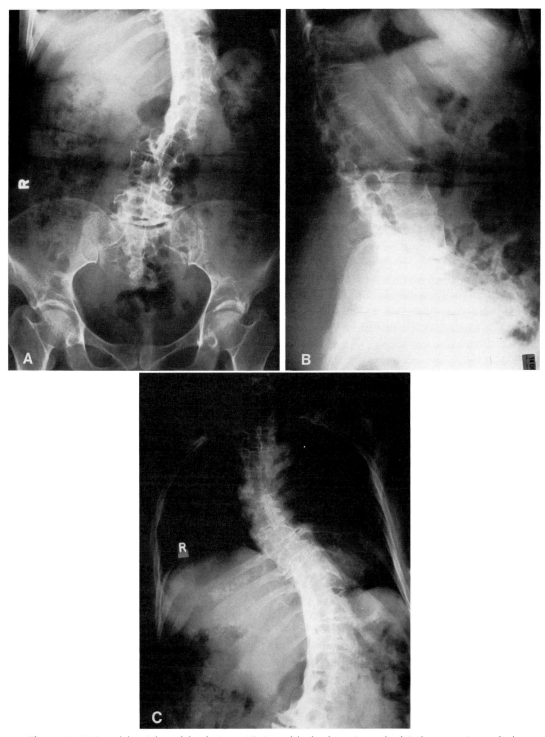

Figure 14–23. Spondyloepiphyseal dysplasia. *A,* AP view of the lumbar spine and pelvis demonstrating marked scoliosis and hypoplastic ilia. *B,* Lateral view reveals generalized osteopenia associated with flattening of the vertebrae (platyspondyly) and irregularity of the contour of the vertebral bodies. *C,* AP view of the thoracolumbar spine shows postsurgical fusion from T9 to L2. This 64-year-old woman had progressive kyphoscoliosis as a young adult and had surgery to prevent additional deformity. She experienced diffuse low back pain with occasional episodes of L5 radiculopathy manifested by weakness in her foot. Electromyography documented radiculopathy. Her symptoms responded to a 6-day course of oral corticosteroid therapy. In 1991, progressive leg pain and motor weakness in the left foot associated with calf atrophy was noted. Laminectomy was undertaken to decompress the L5 and S1 nerve roots. Surgery was successful in decreasing pain. In 1993, the patient's weakness was slowly progressive. An ankle brace was being considered to improve ambulation.

asymptomatic. Other areas of the skeleton that frequently have abnormalities include the hands and feet. Skeletal involvement is present in approximately 50% of patients with tuberous sclerosis.[58]

Tuberous sclerosis is a generalized disease and affects other organ systems in addition to the musculoskeletal and neurologic systems. Hamartomas affect the kidneys, heart, liver, lungs, and gastrointestinal tract. There is no specific therapy for the disorder. Therapy is directed at symptomatic relief of clinical complaints.

SPONDYLOEPIPHYSEAL DYSPLASIA

The epiphyseal dysplasias have been defined by Spranger as a group of heterogeneous disorders characterized by defective or excessive bone formation in the secondary ossification centers of tubular bones and vertebrae.[59] Since there is no known biochemical abnormality to differentiate these disorders, they have been divided into two large categories based on skeletal disease: (1) spondyloepiphyseal dysplasias (SD) with vertebral beaking and (2) multiple epiphyseal dysplasia without spinal involvement.[60] Abnormalities in Type II collagen have been identified in some of the forms of SD.[61] One abnormality is associated with a higher ratio of hydroxylysine to lysine than in normal collagen.[62] The spectrum of clinical severity of SD may be related to the extent of alteration and proximity of defects to the carboxyl terminus of the collagen molecule.

The disease has an autosomal dominant inheritance. Spinal involvement in multiple epiphyseal dysplasia, if it occurs, is mild compared with the marked alterations that occur in the appendicular skeleton. Most forms of the illness affect the phalanges, shoulders, hips, or elbow and knee joints. The vertebral changes mimic those of Scheuermann's disease. The vertebral bodies are wedge-shaped, with mild platyspondyly and scoliosis. The spine is also osteoporotic.[63] This disorder is occasionally confused with Morquio syndrome. Patients with SD of Maroteaux also mimic Morquio syndrome but have no abnormality at birth and have no biochemical abnormality.[64] Morquio syndrome is not manifest at birth and results in increased mucopolysaccharide in the urine.[65]

SD is recognized to have two primary forms, congenita and tarda. The spine and some appendicular bones are involved in the congenita form. The vertebrae are flattened with an irregular aspect to the superior and inferior endplates along with a bulging configuration to the posterior portion of the vertebral body (Fig. 14–23).[66]

The tarda form of SD is a male sex-linked recessive disorder that becomes manifest in late childhood as short stature with spinal abnormalities, pectus carinatum, and a broad thorax.[67] Roentgenograms of patients with this form of dysplasia reveal generalized flattening of vertebral bodies with irregular endplates, intervertebral disc space narrowing, and small iliac bones. The appendicular skeleton is minimally affected (Fig. 14–24).

A review of 30 patients with epiphyseal dysplasia reported by Kahn determined that 13% had lumbar stiffness and pain suggestive of ankylosing spondylitis.[68] Six patients with the tarda form of disease had disc narrowing to a severe degree. Fusion of the disc space occurred in these patients and has been reported previously.

One other rare form of dysplasia is spondylometaphyseal dysplasia, reported by Kozlowski.[69] These patients are dwarfs with a waddling gait, kyphoscoliosis, and decreased joint motion. As opposed to the abnormalities in the dysplasias described above, the epiphyses are normal in this disorder, and the metaphys-

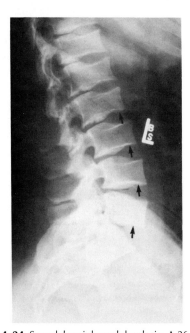

Figure 14–24. Spondyloepiphyseal dysplasia. A 26-year-old man with progressive scoliosis and broadening of the thorax. Lateral view of the lumbar spine demonstrating elongation of vertebral bodies at all levels (black arrows). (From Borenstein DG: Low Back Pain. In Klippel JH, Dieppe P (eds): Rheumatology. St Louis, CV Mosby, 1994, Sec 5, p 4.8.)

eal areas of bone are the primary locations of the bony abnormalities.[70]

References

HERITABLE GENETIC DISORDERS

1. Pyeritz RE: Heritable and development disorders of connective tissue and bone. In McCarty DJ, Koopman WJ (eds): Arthritis and Allied Conditions, 12th ed. Philadelphia: Lea & Febiger, 1993, pp 1483–1509.
2. Beighton P (ed): McKusick's Heritable Disorders of Connective Tissue, 5th ed. St. Louis: CV Mosby, 1993, pp 748.
3. Pyeritz RE, McKusick VA: The Marfan syndrome: diagnosis and management. N Engl J Med 300:772, 1979.
4. Tsipouras P, Del Mastro R, Sarfarazi M, et al.: Genetic linkage of the Marfan Syndrome, ectopia lentis, and congenital contractural arachnodactyly to the fibrillin genes on chromosomes 15 and 5. N Engl J Med 326:905, 1992.
5. Maddox BK, Sakai LY, Keene DR, Glanville RW: Connective tissue microfibrils. J Biol Chem 264:21381, 1989.
6. Kainulainen K, Sakai LY, Child A, et al.: Two mutations in Marfan syndrome resulting in truncated fibrillin polypeptides. Proc Natl Acad Sci 89:5917, 1992.
7. Magid D, Pyeritz RE, Fishman EK: Musculoskeletal manifestations of the Marfan syndrome: radiologic features. AJR 155:99, 1990.
8. Stern WE: Dural ectasia and the Marfan syndrome. J Neurosurg 69:221, 1988.
9. Kahn MF, De Sese S: Rheumatic manifestations of heritable disorders of connective tissue. Clin Rheum Dis 1:3, 1975.
10. Sinclair RJG: The Marfan syndrome. Bull Rheum Dis 8:153, 1958.
11. Pyeritz RE: The Marfan syndrome. In Royce PM, Steinmann B (eds): Connective Tissue and Its Heritable Disorders: Molecular, Genetic, and Medical Aspects. New York: Wiley-Liss, 1993, pp 437–468.
12. Robins PR, Moe JH, Winter RB: Scoliosis in Marfan syndrome. Its characteristics and results of treatment in thirty-five patients. J Bone Joint Surg 57A:358, 1975.
13. Schlesinger EB: The significance of genetic contributions and markers in disorders of spinal structure. Neurosurgery 26:944, 1990.
14. Brenton DP, Dow CJ, James JIP, et al.: Homocystinuria and Marfan's syndrome. A comparison. J Bone Joint Surg 54B:277, 1972.
15. Brill PW, Mitty HA, Gaull GE: Homocystinuria due to cystathionine synthetase deficiency: Clinical roentgenologic correlation. AJR 121:45, 1974.
16. Skovby F: The homocystinurias. In Royce PM, Steinmann B (eds): Connective Tissue and Its Heritable Disorders: Molecular, Genetic, and Medical Aspects. New York: Wiley-Liss, 1993, pp 469–486.
17. Raftopoulos C, Pierard GE, Retif C, et al.: Endoscopic cure of a giant sacral meningocele associated with Marfan's syndrome: case report. Neurosurgery 130:765, 1992.
18. Beighton P. The Ehlers-Danlos syndromes. In Beighton P (ed): McKusick's Heritable Disorders of Connective Tissue, 5th ed. St. Louis: CV Mosby, 1993, pp 189–251.
19. McKusick VA, Scott CI: A nomenclature for constitutional disorders of bone. J Bone Joint Surg 53A:978, 1971.
20. Byers PH: Inherited disorders of collagen gene structure and expression. Am J Med Gen 34:72, 1989.
21. Beighton P, Horan F: Orthopaedic aspects of the Ehlers-Danlos syndrome. J Bone Joint Surg 51B:444, 1969.
22. Goldman AB: Collagen diseases, epiphyseal dysplasias, and related conditions. In Resnick D, Niwayama G (eds): Diagnosis of Bone and Joint Disorders, 2nd ed. Philadelphia: WB Saunders, 1988, pp 3374–3441.
23. Schmalzried TP, Eckardt JJ: Spontaneous gluteal artery rupture resulting in compartment syndrome and sciatic neuropathy: report of a case in Ehlers-Danlos syndrome. Clin Orthop 275:253, 1992.
24. Horton WA, Hecht JT: The chondrodysplasias. In Royce PM, Steinmann B (eds): Connective Tissue and its Heritable Disorders: Molecular, Genetic, and Medical Aspects. New York: Wiley-Liss, 1993, pp 641–675.
25. Pyeritz RE, Sack GH Jr, Udvarhelyi GB: Cervical and lumbar laminectomy for spinal stenosis in achondroplasia. Johns Hopkins Med J 146:203, 1980.
26. Bailey JA: Orthopaedic aspects of achondroplasia. J Bone Joint Surg 52A:1285, 1970.
27. Epstein JA, Malis LI: Compression of spinal cord and cauda equina in achondroplastic dwarfs. Neurology 5:875, 1955.
28. Alexander E Jr: Significance of the small lumbar spinal canal: cauda equina compression syndromes due to spondylosis. Part 5. Achondroplasia. J Neurosurg 31:513, 1969.
29. Langer LO Jr, Baumann PA, Gorlin RJ: Achondroplasia. AJR 100:12, 1967.
30. Caffey J: Achondroplasia of pelvis and lumbosacral spine: some roentgenographic features. AJR 80:449, 1958.
31. Shikata J, Yamamuro T, Iida H, et al.: Surgical treatment of achondroplastic dwarfs with paraplegia. Surg Neurol 29:125, 1988.
32. Vilarrubias JM, Ginebreda I, Jimeno E: Lengthening of the lower limbs and correction of lumbar hyperlordosis in achondroplasia. Clin Orthop 250:143, 1990.
33. Siebens AA, Hungerford DS, Kirby NA: Achondroplasia: effectiveness of an orthosis in reducing deformity of the spine. Arch Phys Med Rehabil 68:384, 1987.
34. Byers PH, Steiner RD: Osteogenesis imperfecta. Ann Rev Med 43:269, 1992.
35. Gertner JM, Root L: Osteogenesis imperfecta. Orthop Clin North Am 21:151, 1990.
36. Prockop DJ, Constantinou CD, Dombrowski KE, et al.: Type I procollagen: the gene-protein system that harbors most of the mutations causing osteogenesis imperfecta and probably more common heritable disorders of connective tissue. Am J Med Gen 34:60, 1989.
37. Fugi K, Tanzer ML: Osteogenesis imperfecta: biochemical studies of bone collagen. Clin Orthop 124:271, 1977.
38. Sykes B, Francis MJO, Smith R: Altered relation of two collagen types in osteogenesis imperfecta. N Engl J Med 296:1200, 1977.
39. Uitto J, Murray LW, Blumberg B, Shamban A: Biochemistry of collagen in diseases. Ann Intern Med 105:740, 1976.
40. Levin LS, Salinas CF, Jogenson RJ: Classification of

osteogenesis imperfecta by dental characteristics. Lancet 1:332, 1978.

41. Sillence DO, Senn A, Danks DM: Genetic heterogeneity in osteogenesis imperfecta. J Med Genet 16:101, 1979.

42. Falvo KA, Root L, Bullought PG: Osteogenesis imperfecta: clinical evaluation and management. J Bone Joint Surg 56A:783, 1974.

43. King JD, Bobechko WP: Osteogenesis imperfecta: an orthopaedic description and surgical review. J Bone Joint Surg 53B:72, 1971.

44. Hanscom DA, Winter RB, Luther L, et al.: Osteogenesis imperfecta: radiographic classification, natural history, and treatment of spinal deformities. J Bone Joint Surg 74:598, 1992.

45. Shoenfeld Y, Fried A, Ehrenfeld NE: Osteogenesis imperfecta: review of the literature with presentation of 29 cases. Am J Dis Child 129:679, 1975.

46. Whitley CB: The mucopolysaccharidoses. In Beighton P (ed): McKusick's Heritable Disorders of Connective Tissue. St. Louis: CV Mosby, 1993, pp 367–499.

47. Hunter C: A rare disease in two brothers. Proc R Soc Med 10:104, 1971.

48. McAlister WH: Osteochondrodysplasias, dysostoses, chromosomal aberrations, mucopolysaccharidoses, and mucolipidoses. In Resnick D, Niwayama G (eds): Diagnosis of Bone and Joint Disorders, 2nd ed. Philadelphia: WB Saunders, 1988, pp 3442–3515.

49. Blaw ME, Langer LO: Spinal cord compression in Morquio-Brailsford disease. J Pediatr 74:593, 1969.

50. Jin W, Jackson CE, Desnick RJ, Schuchman EH: Mucopolysaccharidosis type IV: identification of three mutations in the arylsulfatase B gene of patients with the severe and mild phenotypes provides molecular evidence for genetic heterogeneity. Am J Hum Genet 50:795, 1992.

51. Critchley M, Earl CJC: Tuberose sclerosis and allied conditions. Brain 55:311, 1932.

52. Shepherd CW, Beard CM, Gomez MR, et al.: Tuberous sclerosis complex in Olmstead County, Minnesota, 1950–1989. Arch Neurol 48:400, 1991.

53. Medley BE, McLeod RA, Houser OW: Tuberous sclerosis. Semin Roentgenol 11:35, 1976.

54. Rosenberg S, Mendez MF: Tuberous sclerosis in the elderly. J Am Geriatr Soc 37:1058, 1989.

55. Lagos JC, Holman CB, Gomez MR: Tuberous sclerosis. Neuroroentgenologic observations. AJR 104:171, 1968.

56. Fitz CR, Harwood-Nash DCF, Thompson JR: Neurobiology of tuberous sclerosis in children. Radiology 110:635, 1974.

57. Komar NN, Gabrielsen TO, Holt JF: Roentgenographic appearance of lumbosacral spine and pelvis in tuberous sclerosis. Radiology 89:701, 1967.

58. Bell DG, King BF, Hattery RR, et al.: Imaging characteristics of tuberous sclerosis. AJR 156:1081, 1991.

59. Spranger J: The epiphyseal dysplasias. Clin Orthop 114:46, 1976.

60. Rubin P: Dynamic Classification of Bone Dysplasias. Chicago, Year Book Medical Publishers, 1964, p 120.

61. Rimoin DL, Lachman RS: Genetic disorders of the osseous skeleton. In Beighton P (ed): McKusick's Heritable Disorders of Connective Tissue. St Louis: CV Mosby, 1993, pp 557–689.

62. Murray LW, Baustista J, James PL, Rimoin DL: Type II collagen defects in the chondrodysplasias. 1. Spondyloepiphyseal dysplasias. Am J Hum Genet 45:5, 1989.

63. Hulvey JT, Keats T: Multiple epiphyseal dysplasia. A contribution to the problem of spinal involvement. AJR 106:170, 1969.

64. Doman AN, Maroteaux P, Lyne ED: Spondyloepiphyseal dysplasia of Maroteaux. J Bone Joint Surg 72A:1364, 1990.

65. Saldino RM: Radiographic diagnosis of neonatal short-linked dwarfism. Med Radiogr Photogr 48:61, 1973.

66. Spranger JW, Langer LO Jr: Spondyloepiphyseal dysplasia congenita. Radiology 94:313, 1970.

67. Langer LO Jr: Spondyloepiphyseal dysplasia tarda. Hereditary chondrodysplasia with characteristic vertebral configuration in the adult. Radiology 82:833, 1964.

68. Kahn MF, Corvol MT, Jarmand SH, et al.: Le rhumatisme chondrodysplastique. Rev Rheum 37:825, 1970.

69. Kozlowski K, Beighton P: Radiographic features of spondyloepimetaphyseal dysplasia with joint laxity and progressive kyphoscoliosis. Fortschr Roentgenstr 141:337, 1984.

70. Thomas PS, Nevin NC: Spondylometaphyseal dysplasia. AJR 128:89, 1977.

15

Hematologic Disorders of the Lumbosacral Spine

Disorders of the hematologic system may involve any area of the body where bone marrow is located. Since the axial skeleton contains a significant proportion of an adult's bone marrow, disorders that cause hyperplasia of bone marrow or the replacement of normal bone marrow cells with abnormal ones may be associated with low back pain. A characteristic of hematopoietic disorders is that although symptoms may be localized to various areas of the skeleton, these illnesses are systemic in origin and cause significant abnormalities in a number of other organ systems. The hematologic disorders that produce symptoms of low back pain include the hemoglobinopathies, myelofibrosis, and mastocytosis.

The symptoms of back pain in a patient with a hemoglobinopathy (sickle cell anemia) occur at the height of a vaso-occlusive crisis. These crises occur secondary to the blockage of small vessels and the infarction of tissue by sickled cells. Back pain is acute in onset and has a duration of 4 to 5 days. Patients frequently have bone pain in the extremities as well. Patients with myelofibrosis have an insidious onset of low back pain secondary to the fibrosis and osteosclerosis that occurs as the bone marrow is replaced with fibrous tissue. Patients with mastocytosis may also have insidious onset of back pain in the setting of a systemic illness characterized by skin eruptions, flushing, weight loss, and diarrhea.

Physical examination of a patient with a hemoglobinopathy will demonstrate a chronically ill individual in acute distress during a crisis. Abnormal findings may include fever, tachycardia, and tenderness to palpation over the back and extremities with associated muscle spasm. The patient with myelofibrosis will have pallor, splenomegaly, and bone tenderness on palpation. The patient with mastocytosis has skin rash, hepatosplenomegaly, and bone tenderness.

Laboratory evaluation of these patients is very helpful in making a specific diagnosis of the underlying disorder. Patients with hemoglobinopathies have characteristic abnormalities on blood smear, including sickle and target cells. The specific hemoglobin abnormality is identified by hemoglobin electrophoresis. The blood smear in myelofibrosis contains abnormal red blood cell forms, mature and immature white blood cell forms, and variable numbers of platelets. The diagnosis of myelofibrosis is confirmed by bone marrow biopsy, which characteristically reveals marrow fibrosis, an increased number of megakaryocytes, and osteosclerosis. Findings in mastocytosis include increased urinary histamine, increased fibrosis, and mast cells, which may be confused with granulomatous cells on bone marrow biopsy.

Radiographic findings associated with hemoglobinopathies include evidence of marrow expansion secondary to hyperplasia, characterized by loss of trabeculae and cortical thinning, distinctive cup-like depression in vertebral bodies ("H" vertebrae), sclerosis, and fractures compatible with aseptic necrosis of bone. Radiographic findings of myelofibrosis include diffuse osteosclerosis in the axial skeleton and proximal long bones. Mastocytosis may cause osteosclerosis, osteoporosis, or a mixed picture on plain radiographs. Bone scintiscan may show diffusely increased uptake.

Therapy for these hematopoietic disorders is essentially symptomatic. Patients with sickle cell anemia are educated to avoid circumstances that may precipitate a painful crisis. They are treated with hydration and analgesics during vaso-occlusive crises. Transfusions are reserved for life-threatening complications such as a cerebrovascular accident. There is no effective therapy that alters the course of myelofibrosis. Antihistamines are the cornerstone of therapy for mastocytosis. These drugs counteract the effects of the chemical mediators released by mast cells. The prognosis of patients with hematologic disorders is related to the severity of the illness in sickle cell disease and the possibility of malignant degeneration in myelofibrosis and mastocytosis. Hemoglobinopathies are systemic illnesses that affect the musculoskeletal, pulmonary, cardiovascular, renal, and nervous systems. Patients with severe sickle cell anemia die prematurely from cardiac failure or infection.

Patients with myelofibrosis are at risk of developing acute leukemia. Many patients die from leukemia within 5 years of the diagnosis of their illness.

Mastocytosis is associated with a broad spectrum of diseases, including urticaria pigmentosa with or without systemic disease. The patients with the worst prognosis are those with marked systemic involvement who develop mast cell leukemia.

HEMOGLOBINOPATHIES

Capsule Summary

Frequency of back pain—common
Location of back pain—lumbar spine
Quality of back pain—ache, boring
Symptoms and signs—intermittent episodes of pain with crises, bone tenderness
Laboratory and x-ray tests—anemia, abnormal blood smear; coarsened trabeculae with "fish" vertebrae on plain roentgenograms
Treatment—hydration, analgesics

PREVALENCE AND PATHOGENESIS

Hemoglobinopathies are a clinical group of disorders associated with defects in the physi-

cal properties or manufacture of the polypeptide chains that are the protein parts of hemoglobin. The presence of abnormal hemoglobin in red blood cells causes continuous premature destruction of these cells and chronic hemolytic anemia. Abnormal hemoglobins also change the shape of red cells, causing sickling and obstruction of the vascular microcirculation. Vascular obstruction leads to deoxygenation, tissue necrosis, and pain, and this condition is referred to as a vaso-occlusive or thrombotic crisis. In adults with hemoglobinopathies, particularly sickle cell anemia, acute back pain and extremity pain are the most common symptoms of vascular crises. Persistent bone destruction secondary to vaso-occlusion and hyperplasia of bone marrow in the axial skeleton results in compression fractures, accentuated dorsal kyphosis, and lumbar lordosis.

Herrick in 1910 was the first to describe the sickle-shaped erythrocytes of sickle cell anemia.[1] Cooley and Lee in 1925 used the Greek word for "the sea" to propose thalassemia as the name for the severe anemia associated with splenomegaly in patients of Mediterranean origin.[2]

The most common clinically significant hemoglobinopathies include sickle cell anemia (hemoglobin SS), sickle cell hemoglobin C disease (hemoglobin SC), and sickle cell beta-thalassemia. Human adult hemoglobin consists of two pairs of coiled polypeptide chains, alpha and beta, and is referred to as hemoglobin A. Substitution of gamma or delta chains for beta chains results in hemoglobin F (fetal) or hemoglobin A_2. Patients with hemoglobin S have normal alpha chains but have glutamic acid replaced with valine at the sixth amino acid position in the beta chain. Chromosome 16 is the location for the gene that produces the alpha chain and chromosome 11 the beta chain.[3] Hemoglobin C has lysine substituted in the sixth position of the beta chain.

Sickle cell anemia (hemoglobin SS) is a relatively common disorder, present in 1 of 625 black Americans.[4] Hemoglobin SC affects 1 in 833 black Americans. Hemoglobin S beta-thalassemia occurs in 1 in 1667. Sickle cell trait (hemoglobin having only one abnormal beta chain with valine) occurs in 8% of black Americans. Sickle cell trait may also be seen infrequently in persons from the eastern Mediterranean, India, or Saudi Arabia.

The function of hemoglobin is to carry oxygen in red blood cells to cells throughout the body. When hemoglobin S is oxygenated, it has normal solubility. However, upon deoxygenation, hemoglobin S has decreased solubility and polymerizes into rigid, elongated rods that alter the biconcave shape of red cells into a sickle form.[5]

The change in morphology results in two major clinical features of sickle cell disease: chronic hemolysis with anemia and acute vaso-occlusive crises associated with pain, organ necrosis, and significant morbidity and mortality. Red blood cells that are sickled are irreversibly deformed. They are removed by the reticulo-endothelial system at an earlier stage in their life span than normal red blood cells. Marrow hyperplasia is unable to produce an adequate supply to replace those prematurely removed from the blood stream. Chronic anemia is the result.

Sickle cell crises occur when acute sickling of red blood cells causes a rise in blood viscosity, decreased blood flow, and vessel obstructions. Vessel blockage leads to ischemia, increased concentrations of deoxygenated hemoglobin, and a progression to sickle crises. Some of the initiating factors that may result in sickle crises include infections, acidosis, fever, and dehydration.[6] These factors play a role as manifestations of systemic infection. The most important factor is the degree of deoxygenation. Sickle cell trait cells will sickle at oxygen tensions of about 15 mm Hg, while sickle anemia cells will sickle at about 40 mm Hg. Low temperatures causing vasoconstriction also may predispose to crises. Acidosis shifts the oxygen dissociation curve to the right, favoring the deoxy conformation of hemoglobin resulting in polymerization of hemoglobin S. Increases of mean corpuscular hemoglobin concentration secondary to dehydration promote sickling. The vascular endothelium of patients with severe disease has increased propensity to cause red cell adherence.[7] The severity of crises varies from patient to patient and may be related to the concentration of S and other hemoglobins in red blood cells. The frequency of painful crises cannot be predicted.

Sickle cell crises occur most commonly in patients with hemoglobin SS. Patients with sickle trait usually do not have sufficient hemoglobin S in their red blood cells to cause sickling. Patients with hemoglobin SC have equal amounts of hemoglobin S and C and very small quantities of hemoglobin F and A_2 in each red blood cell. Hemoglobin SC causes milder diseases and relatively infrequent crises.[8] The degree of anemia is less in SC disease partly because of the red cell survival for 29 days versus 17 days for erythrocytes from sickle cell disease patients.[9] Crises may occur when patients are stressed during surgery or medical emergencies.[10] In addition, patients with hemoglobin SC have a higher frequency of aseptic necrosis of bone.[11]

Thalassemia is a defect in the production of an entire polypeptide chain of hemoglobin. Patients with beta-thalassemia produce normal alpha chains but no beta chains in the homozygous state. Patients with thalassemia minor are usually heterozygous for a beta globin mutation and have either mild or no anemia. Patients with alpha-thalassemia have abnormalities in the production of the A chains and accumulate beta chains. The imbalance in chain production causes accumulation of unpaired chains in developing erythroblasts, which eventually causes death of the cell, giving rise to changes in the bone marrow that result in ineffective erythropoiesis.[12] In sickle cell–beta-thalassemia, the beta-thalassemia defect is combined with sickle trait to produce a disease similar to sickle cell anemia.

The severity of sickle cell–beta-thalassemia is related to the amount of normal hemoglobin that is produced.[13] Patients with sickle cell–β^0-thalassemia produce no normal beta chains and have a disease very similar to sickle cell anemia. Patients with β^+-thalassemia produce hemoglobin A but in reduced amounts. These patients have milder disease. Beta-thalassemia is associated with four clinical syndromes corresponding to the concentrations of hemoglobin produced. These syndromes include thalassemia major, thalassemia intermedia, thalassemia trait, and silent carrier. Bone and joint pathology is noted most frequently in thalassemia major and intermedia patients who have not received sufficient blood transfusions. Normalizing hemoglobin levels suppresses ineffective erythropoiesis that result in bone pathology.[14] Alpha-thalassemia also may be found in patients with hemoglobin SS. The decreased levels of alpha chains results in decreased amounts of sickle hemoglobin per cell and prolonged red cell survival. However, the persistence of cells with sickle hemoglobin promotes vaso-occlusive events by blocking microvasculature that might otherwise be able to accommodate more rigid cells at a lower hematocrit. The end result is that patients with alpha-thalassemia and sickle hemoglobin are less anemic but experience frequent vaso-occlusive episodes, including an increased incidence and severity of aseptic necrosis of bone.[15]

CLINICAL HISTORY

Patients with sickle cell anemia usually present with a painful vaso-occlusive crisis during childhood. The hand-foot syndrome may be the first manifestation of their disease. Diffuse swelling of the hands and feet occurs along with associated warmth and pain. Infarction of bone marrow, which is present in bones of the hands and feet in children, is the cause of this syndrome.[16]

In adults, the most common manifestation of vaso-occlusive crises is back and extremity pain. Back pain may be most severe over the axial skeleton but frequently radiates to the flanks. Muscle spasm may also contribute to the severity of pain in the lumbosacral area. In the extremities, pain is usually asymmetric and unassociated with soft tissue swelling. The duration of symptoms is 4 to 5 days. The patient may be left with no residual pain and resolution of the crisis. Sickle cell crises may also present as severe abdominal pain, which may mimic an acute surgical abdomen. The presence of bowel sounds and the absence of peritoneal signs in sickle cell crisis help differentiate it from the acute abdomen. The use of pain drawings has been useful in detecting an amplification of pain symptoms during crises. Patients with pain amplifications have pain drawings with sites inconsistent with expected sickle cell disease pain patterns. These patients may benefit from specific psychologic evaluation for improved pain control.[17] Other forms of acute crises include the splenic sequestration, aplastic, and hyperhemolytic crises.[18] Patients with hemoglobin SC and sickle cell–β^{+}-thalassemia have milder disease and as adults may present with occasional bone pain along with a history of abdominal or bone pain in childhood.

Tissue infarction secondary to chronic vaso-occlusion is associated with abnormalities in a number of organ systems in patients with sickle cell anemia. In the musculoskeletal system, sickle cell anemia causes bone infarctions, joint effusions, hemarthroses, septic arthritis, and osteomyelitis.[11] Cholelithiasis from chronic hemolysis and hepatitis from congestive, viral, or intrahepatic cholestasia are complications in the gastrointestinal system.[19] Pneumonia and pulmonary infarction are frequently the cause of hospitalization of sickle cell patients.[20] Renal function may be impaired by glomerular sclerosis, papillary necrosis, and a renal concentrating defect.[21] Stroke and subarachnoid hemorrhage are potentially life-threatening complications of the CNS in sickle cell anemia.[22] Osteomyelitis is a serious complication of sickle cell anemia. In a study of 15 sickle cell patients, Epps described two individuals who had osteomyelitis in the ilium and lumbar vertebrae.[23] These patients were infected with *Salmonella* and *Proteus mirabilis*. Although *Salmonella* has been more frequently associated with bone infection in sickle cell patients, *Staphylococcus aureus* was a more frequent cause of osteomyelitis in the individuals in this study.[3, 23]

Patients with thalassemia major become symptomatic by the first 2 years of life. The anemia is severe and requires transfusion. Hyperplasia of the bone marrow causes organomegaly, including splenomegaly, and skeletal abnormalities, including osteopenia, which is associated with fractures.[24] Patients with thalassemia may rarely develop neurologic symptoms secondary to spinal cord compression resulting from extramedullary hematopoiesis.[25]

PHYSICAL FINDINGS

Physical findings demonstrate obvious distress when the patient is in sickle crisis. The affected areas (back, extremities) are tender to palpation. The patient is febrile, often with tachycardia, systolic hypertension, and tachypnea. Other physical signs found in painful crises include a tender, rigid abdomen and normal bowel sounds. Abnormal breath sounds and signs of pleural disease are present in the patient with pneumonia or pulmonary infarction.

Patients with thalassemia have hyperpigmented skin. Abdominal examination reveals hepatosplenomegaly. Marrow hyperplasia may cause bone expansion manifested by frontal bossing and maxillary prominence. Patients with vertebral compression fractures have percussion tenderness over the affected vertebrae.

LABORATORY DATA

Laboratory test results demonstrating abnormalities in the hematologic system are universal in patients with sickle cell anemia. Hematocrit values are in a range of 16% to 36% with hemoglobin of 5 to 12 gm/100 ml.[18] Leukocyte counts are usually elevated in the 20,000/mm range, with increased reticulocytosis to levels of 33%. In general, hemoglobin, hematocrit, and reticulocyte counts remain unchanged during a crisis. A leukocytosis and mild thrombocytopenia may occur.[7]

Blood smear will show the presence of sickled cells and erythrocytes with Howell-Jolly bodies. Howell-Jolly bodies are cytoplasmic

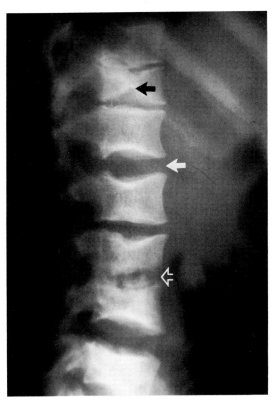

Figure 15–1. Sickle cell anemia. "Fish vertebrae" with widening of the intervertebral disc space *(white arrow)* are associated with sickle cell anemia. Also demonstrated is an "H" shape vertebral body *(black arrow)* and a chronic disc space infection *(open arrow)*. (Courtesy of Anne Brower, M.D.)

remnants of nuclear chromatin that are normally removed by the spleen.

The inability to concentrate urine is manifested by a low urine specific gravity. Evidence of persistent hemolysis is reflected in increased serum bilirubin and lactic dehydrogenase concentrations.

Thalassemia also causes anemia. The anemia is hypochromic and microcytic on smear. Nucleated red blood cells, reticulocytes, and "target" cells are seen in increased number.

RADIOGRAPHIC EVALUATION

The radiographic abnormalities of sickle cell anemia are not unique but are distinctive and are diagnostic when detected in multiple sites.[26] In the spine, marrow hyperplasia causes loss of bone trabeculae and cortical thinning. This results in osteoporosis and coarsening of the remaining trabeculae in the axial skeleton. Vertebral bodies develop a distinctive cup-like depression on the superior and inferior endplates ("fish vertebrae") (Figs. 15–1 and 15–

2).[27] Central depression of the vertebral endplate with "squared off" edges may be caused by a growth abnormality of the subchondral bone, and the resulting deformity is referred to as an "H" vertebra (Fig. 15–3).[28] "H" vertebrae may be seen in other conditions as well (Table 15–1). Irregular sclerosis of the sacroiliac joints secondary to bone infarctions may mimic the radiologic abnormalities of ankylosing spondylitis.[29] Infarction or osteomyelitis may result in bony ridging in the axial skeleton and hip.[30]

Beta-thalassemia causes osteopenia of the vertebrae, which is most evident in the vertebral bodies. Reduction of trabeculae, thinning of vertebral endplates, and biconcave deformities are common. "H" vertebrae occur more rarely in thalassemia major than they do in sickle cell anemia.[31]

Bone scintigraphic abnormalities are frequent in sickle cell patients who experience osseous and bone marrow infarctions. Abnormal uptake also may be noted in patients with osteomyelitis. Expansion of the bone marrow space, in the absence of infarction, may be associated with increased uptake on scinti-

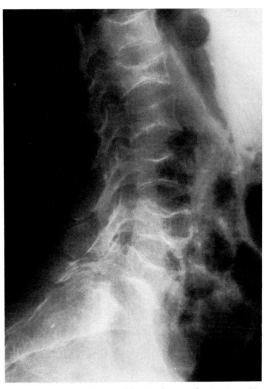

Figure 15–2. Lateral view of the lumbosacral spine in a 30-year-old woman with severe sickle cell anemia manifested by frequent, painful crises. The roentgenogram reveals diffuse osteopenia and multiple "fish vertebrae."

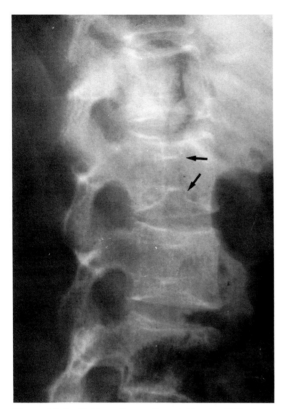

Figure 15–3. Sickle cell anemia resulting in "H" shape vertebral bodies. There is a square indentation of the endplates *(arrows)*. The indented area corresponds to areas of ischemia beneath the cartilaginous endplates, which result in abnormalities of bone growth. (Courtesy of Anne Brower, M.D.)

TABLE 15–1. DISEASE ASSOCIATED WITH "H" VERTEBRAE

Sickle cell anemia
Sickle cell–hemoglobin C disease
Sickle cell–thalassemia disease
Thalassemia
Gaucher's disease
Congenital hereditary spherocytosis
Osteoporosis

MR is also an excellent method to determine the extent of extramedullary hematopoiesis near the vertebral column. Thalassemia patients with neurologic dysfunction can be studied with MR to determine the location and extent of spinal cord or nerve root impingement.[37]

DIFFERENTIAL DIAGNOSIS

The diagnosis of sickle cell anemia is suspected in a child or young adult black patient with diffuse back, bone, or abdominal pain with anemia. A blood smear shows sickled cells and red blood cells with Howell-Jolly bodies, which are usually removed by a normally functioning spleen. A "sickle prep" helps confirm the diagnosis. Red blood cells are circulated with 2% sodium metabisulfite for 1 hour, which causes sickling. The exact proportion of normal and abnormal hemoglobins is determined by the separation of the individual hemoglobins on hemoglobin electrophoresis.

The diagnosis of sickle cell anemia is not in doubt when a patient demonstrates the symptoms and signs of crisis and has abnormal hemoglobin on electrophoresis. However, patients with sickle cell anemia are susceptible to infection and must be evaluated for that possibility when they present with a crisis. The spine may be infected occasionally with *Salmonella,* or more commonly with *Staphylococcus aureus.*[38]

The diagnosis of thalassemia major is usually made when the affected child has severe anemia. Hemoglobin electrophoresis measures increased concentrations of hemoglobin F and A_2, which occur secondary to the inadequate amounts of hemoglobin A.

TREATMENT

Medical management of sickle cell crises includes hydration, analgesics for pain, and antibiotic therapy in crises when there is an ongoing infection. Narcotic therapy for sickle cell patients can be a difficult problem for the

graphic scan. The differentiation of these abnormalities by scintigraphy may be difficult.[32] The use of gallium-67 and indium-111 leukocyte scans is helpful in differentiating infection from infarction.[33, 34]

MR may be very helpful in differentiating the disease processes that complicate the course of the sickle cell patients.[35] The expansion of bone marrow is noted by the replacement of fat signal. Osteonecrosis is readily identified in the femoral heads and other bony locations by MR. Acute infarction, characterized by areas of low signal intensity on T_1-weighted pulse sequences and high signal intensity on T_2-weighted pulse sequences may be determined in the spine by MR evaluation. Old infarction is associated with low signal with T_1 and T_2 images. Although the signal intensities of osteomyelitis and acute infarction are similar, the presence of defined cortical involvement, marrow edema beyond the infarcted zone, sinus tracts, and a soft tissue mass suggests the presence of osteomyelitis.[36]

treating physician. The patient complains of pain but may have no objective physical signs of an ongoing crisis. Ballas has reviewed some of the behavioral patterns used by patients during a vaso-occlusive crisis.[39] A better understanding of the patient's fears, a knowledge of the pharmacokinetics of the narcotic analgesics, and trust between the patient and physician are important in optimizing medical care for these individuals. Nonsteroidal anti-inflammatory drugs may be useful adjuncts to the narcotics for individuals with musculoskeletal pain. The use of alkali to reverse acidosis does not seem to be effective during acute crises. Oxygen is not needed if the patient has no ventilatory hypoxia. Oxygen therapy may be detrimental owing to a re-emergence of irreversible sickled cells appearing with oxygen cessation.[3] Standard red cell transfusions and exchange transfusions are reserved for patients with severe complications of sickle cell anemia such as strokes. Transfusions also may be useful preoperatively for patients who are undergoing surgery. Other forms of therapy are in the experimental stage. These therapies include hydroxyurea to increase fetal hemoglobin synthesis and bone marrow transplantation for thalassemia. The efficacy of these therapies for the usual patient with sickle cell disease awaits further study.[40–42]

Thalassemia is treated with transfusions maintaining a hemoglobin level of 12 gm/100 ml. Iron overload is limited as much as possible with deferoxamine. Occasionally, splenectomy is required to control hypersplenism. In patients with greater risk for infection, including pneumonia and osteomyelitis, pneumococcal vaccine is indicated.

PROGNOSIS

The course of sickle cell anemia is difficult to predict. Some patients with the disease have occasional crises, once every year or two, and have little in the way of organ dysfunction from their disease. On the other end of the spectrum are patients who are in almost continuous crises and are frequently hospitalized. These patients commonly show evidence of generalized disease affecting many organ systems. Patients must avoid situations that predispose to sickle crisis (dehydration) and receive comprehensive medical care. Immunization with pneumococcal vaccine, good nutrition, vitamins, and psychologic support have improved their long-term outlook. However, until the time comes when the genetic defect

of sickle hemoglobin is corrected, patients with sickle cell anemia will be at risk for the complications of their disease and can expect a decreased work potential as well as a shortened life span.

Thalassemia major is also a cause of shortened life span. Either the results of the chronic anemia or the complications of chronic transfusion therapy are detrimental. As with sickle cell anemia, correction of the underlying genetic defect is the most appropriate therapy for this illness.

References

HEMOGLOBINOPATHIES

1. Herrick JB: Peculiar elongated and sickle-shaped red blood corpuscles in a case of severe anemia. Arch Intern Med 6:517, 1910.
2. Cooley TB, Lee P: A series of cases of splenomegaly in children with anemia and peculiar bone changes. Trans Am Pediatr Soc 37:29, 1925.
3. Bunn HF, Forget BG (eds): Hemoglobin: Molecular, Genetic and Clinical Aspects. Philadelphia: WB Saunders Co, 1986.
4. Motulsky AG: Frequency of sickling disorders in U. S. blacks. N Engl J Med 288:31, 1973.
5. Dean J, Schechter AN: Sickle-cell anemia: molecular and cellular bases of therapeutic approaches. Parts 1, 2, and 3. N Engl J Med 299:752, 804, 863, 1978.
6. Diggs LW: Sickle cell crises. Am J Clin Pathol 44:1, 1965.
7. Steingart R: Management of patients with sickle cell disease. Med Clin North Am 76:669, 1992.
8. Neel JV, Kaplan E, Zuelzer WW: Further studies on hemoglobin C. I: A description of 3 additional families segregating for hemoglobin C and sickle cell hemoglobin. Blood 8:724, 1953.
9. Nagel RL, Lawrence C: The distinct pathobiology of sickle cell-hemoglobin C disease: therapeutic implications. Hematol Oncol Clin North Am 5:433, 1991.
10. Bannerman RM, Serjeant B, Seakins M, et al.: Determinants of hemoglobin level in sickle cell–hemoglobin C disease. Br J Haematol 43:39, 1979.
11. Schumacher HR: Rheumatological manifestations of sickle cell disease and other hereditary haemoglobinopathies. Clin Rheum Dis 1:37, 1975.
12. Canale V: Beta-thalassemia: A clinical review. Pediatr Ann 3:6, 1974.
13. Reynolds J, Pritchard JA, Ludders D, Mason RA: Roentgenographic and clinical appraisal of sickle cell beta-thalassemia. AJR 118:378, 1973.
14. Johanson NA: Musculoskeletal problems in hemoglobinopathy. Orthop Clin North Am 21:191, 1990.
15. Steinberg MH: The interactions of alpha-thalassemia with hemoglobinopathies. Hematol Oncol Clin North Am 5:453, 1991.
16. Pearson HA, Diamond LK: The critically ill child: sickle cell disease crises and their management. Pediatrics 48:629, 1971.
17. Gil KM, Phillips G, Abrams MR, Williams DA: Pain drawings and sickle cell disease pain. Clin J Pain 6:105, 1990.
18. Karayalcin G, Rosner F, Kim KY, et al.: Sickle cell ane-

mia: clinical manifestations in 100 patients and review of the literature. Am J Med Sci 269:51, 1975.

19. Cameron JL, Maddrey WC, Zuidema GD: Biliary tract disease in sickle cell anemia: surgical considerations. Ann Surg 174:702, 1971.

20. Barret-Connor E: Pneumonia and pulmonary infarction in sickle cell anemia. JAMA 224:997, 1973.

21. Buckalew VM Jr, Someren A: Renal manifestations of sickle cell disease. Arch Intern Med 133:660, 1974.

22. Powars D, Wilson B, Imbus C, et al.: The natural history of stroke in sickle cell disease. Am J Med 65:461, 1978.

23. Epps Ch, Bryant DD III, Coles MJM, Castro O: Osteomyelitis in patients who have sickle-cell disease. J Bone Joint Surg 73A:1281, 1991.

24. Finsterbush A, Farber I, Mogle P, Goldfarb A: Fracture patterns in thalassemia. Clin Orthop 192:132, 1985.

25. Abbassioun K, Amir-Jamshidi A: Curable paraplegia due to extradural hematopoietic tissue in thalassemia. Neurosurgery 11:804, 1982.

26. Reynolds J: Radiologic manifestations of sickle cell hemoglobinopathy. JAMA 238:247, 1977.

27. Reynolds J: A re-evaluation of the "fish vertebra" sign in sickle cell hemoglobinopathy. AJR 97:693, 1966.

28. Rohlfing BM: Vertebral end-plate depression: report of two patients with hemoglobinopathy. AJR 128:599, 1973.

29. Schumacher HR, Andrews R, McLaughlin G: Arthropathy in sickle cell disease. Ann Intern Med 78:203, 1978.

30. Diggs LW: Bone and joint lesions in sickle cell disease. Clin Orthop 52:119, 1967.

31. Cassady JR, Berdon WE, Baker DH: The "typical" spine changes of sickle cell anemia in a patient with thalassemia major (Cooley's anemia). Radiology 89:1065, 1967.

32. Glaser Am, Chen DCP, Siegel ME, et al.: An unusual scintigraphic pattern in sickle cell patients. Eur J Nucl Med 15:357, 1989.

33. Amundsen TR, Siegel MF, Siegel BA: Osteomyelitis and infarction in sickle cell hemoglobinopathies: differentiation by combined technetium and gallium scintigraphy. Radiology 153:807, 1984.

34. Rao VM, Sebes JI, Steiner RM, Ballas SK: Noninvasive diagnostic imaging in hemoglobinopathies. Hematol Onc Clin North Am 5:517, 1991.

35. Steiner Rm, Mitchell DG, Rao VM, et al.: Magnetic resonance imaging of bone marrow: diagnostic value in diffuse hematologic disorders. Mag Res Quart 6:17, 1990.

36. Modic MT, Pflanze W, Fieglin DH, Belhobek G: Magnetic resonance imaging of musculoskeletal infections. Radiol Clin North Am 24:247, 1986.

37. Hassoun H, Lawn-Tsao, Langevin R Jr, et al.: Spinal cord compression secondary to extremeduallry hematopoiesis: A noninvasive management based on MRI. Am J Hematol 37:201, 1991.

38. Specht CE: Hemoglobinopathic *Salmonella* osteomyelitis: orthopedic aspects. Clin Orthop 79:110, 1971.

39. Ballas SK: Treatment of pain in adults with sickle cell disease. Am J Hematol 34:49, 1990.

40. Charache S: Hydroxyurea as treatment for sickle cell anemia. Hematol Onc Clin North Am 5:571, 1991.

41. Stamatoyannopoulos JA, Nienhuis AW: Therapeutic approaches to hemoglobin switching in treatment of hemoglobinopathies. Annu Rev Med 43:497, 1992.

42. Lucarelli G, Galimberti M, Polchi P, et al.: Bone marrow transplantation in thalassemia. Hematol Onc Clin North Am 5:549, 1991.

MYELOFIBROSIS

Capsule Summary

Frequency of back pain—uncommon
Location of back pain—lumbar spine
Quality of back pain—ache or sharp
Symptoms and signs—weakness, weight loss, bone pain
Laboratory and x-ray tests—anemia, leukoerythroblastic smear; osteosclerosis on plain roentgenograms
Treatment—transfusions, chemotherapy, bone marrow transplant

PREVALENCE AND PATHOGENESIS

Myelofibrosis is a disease of the hematopoietic system characterized by fibrosis of bone marrow and myeloid metaplasia or the production of blood cells in nonmarrow-containing organs such as the liver and spleen. The disease is characterized by anemia, organomegaly, osteosclerosis, and extramedullary hematopoiesis. Bone and joint pain in the axial and peripheral skeleton is associated with myeloid metaplasia. Patients may develop localized masses of hematopoietic tissue near the spinal cord which can cause neurologic symptoms of weakness, hyperreflexia, and sensory deficit.

Myelofibrosis is a relatively uncommon disorder that appears in patients during the sixth decade of life.[1] Both sexes are equally afflicted. The pathogenesis of this disorder is unknown. While initially thought to be a compensatory mechanism for bone marrow failure, myelofibrosis is part of the spectrum of primary myeloproliferative disorders that affect blood stem cells, including erythrocytes, granulocytes, and platelets.[2] The marrow fibrosis that is characteristic of the illness is a secondary phenomenon. In the past the disease has been considered a primary bone disease, a reactive response to marrow necrosis, a leukemic variant, or a myeloproliferative disorder. The term myeloproliferative disorder was proposed by Dameshek, who noticed a spectrum of illnesses (polycythemia rubra vera, chronic myelocytic leukemia, essential thrombocythemia, and agnogenic myeloid metaplasia [myelofibrosis]) that were associated with marked marrow proliferation that evolved into an illness progressing to a blast crisis similar to acute myeloblastic leukemia.[3] More recently, the unity of these disorders under the concept of myeloproliferation has been challenged.[4] In the light of these proposed etiologies of myelofibrosis, it should not be surprising to find a number of terms used in the description of this illness. Starting in the 1870s, the disease has been known as leukocythemia, agnogenic myeloid metaplasia, aleukemic myelosis, leukoerythroblastic anemia, osteosclerosis, myelosclerosis, and myelofibrosis.[5, 6]

Myelofibrosis is probably mediated through a number of different pathologic processes.[7] It has been associated with toxin exposure to benzol, paint thinners, and thorium dioxide. Radiation exposure has been associated with myelofibrosis in survivors of the Hiroshima atomic bomb explosion. A number of karyotypic abnormalities (in approximately 50% of patients), including loss of the Y chromosome, trisomy 8, and trisomy 1q, along with familial predisposition, have been reported. The primary abnormality of myelofibrosis seems to reside in the bone marrow stem cells and not the bone marrow fibroblasts. All the bone marrow stem cells contain the same G6PD isoenzymes that are separate from the isoenzyme in the fibroblasts. This suggests the bone marrow fibrosis is mediated by non-malignant bone marrow fibroblasts in response to a malignant process.

CLINICAL HISTORY

Patients with myelofibrosis present with symptoms secondary to anemia (weakness, fatigue, weight loss) and abdominal pain associated with fullness or heaviness. The onset of symptoms is insidious, with a usual delay of 1 to 2 years before the diagnosis is made.[8] Patients may also experience a gradual progressive weight loss, acute gouty arthritis, nephrolithiasis, jaundice, edema, and lymphadenopathy. As many as 13% of patients may have an episode of acute gout before the diagnosis of myelofibrosis is recognized.[9] Bone pain in the extremities and axial skeleton may be mild to severe.[10] Neurologic symptoms of lower extremity weakness and sensory loss may be present with spinal cord compression.[11]

PHYSICAL EXAMINATION

Physical examination reveals a patient who appears chronically ill with pallor. Abdominal examination is remarkable with a markedly enlarged spleen. Hepatomegaly and ascites occur less frequently. Bones affected in the lumbar spine by myelofibrosis may be tender to palpation. Examination of the extremities demonstrates edema and purpura. Hyperreflexia and Babinski's signs are seen in the patients with spinal cord compression.

LABORATORY DATA

Myelofibrosis is associated with a number of hematologic abnormalities. Anemia is found in the vast majority of patients and is initially normochromic but becomes hypochromic with progression of the illness. Blood smears reveal an abnormal configuration of cells, polychromatic cells (reticulocytes), and increased numbers of white blood cells with both mature and immature forms. This blood smear is characteristic of leukoerythroblastic anemia.[12] Platelets may be present in high, normal, or low numbers. The bleeding time may be prolonged even with normal numbers of platelets, indicating a platelet functional disorder. The neutrophil alkaline phosphatase score is high.

Bone marrow in myelofibrosis is unobtainable by needle aspiration because of the fibrosis and hypocellularity. Bone marrow biopsy, which protects the positional integrity of bone and marrow elements, shows fibrosis, increased numbers of megakaryocytes, and osteosclerosis.[13]

Other laboratory features include an elevated serum or urinary uric acid concentration in most patients with myelofibrosis.[14] Secondary gout, with tophi and uric acid stones, occurs in an occasional patient.[15] An elevation in lactate dehydrogenase, a decrease in albumin, or prolongation in prothrombin time is noted in a majority of patients.[9] A number of autoimmune factors are abnormal in patients with myelofibrosis, including complement components indicative of activation, presence of excess immune complexes, elevated antinuclear antibodies, rheumatoid factor, positive direct Coomb's test, lupus anticoagulant, polyclonal increases in serum immunoglobulins, and platelet associated IgG and IgM.[7, 9]

The fibroblasts in the bone marrow produce a number of collagens, including I, III, IV, and V with a predominance of III. The procollagen III molecule is cleaved and the aminoterminal fragments are released into the serum. The serum level of fragments has been associated with the degree of marrow fibrosis associated with primary and secondary myelofibrosis.[16] Marrow fibrosis has also been associated with type IV collagen metabolites.[17] Hyaluronan is a polysaccharide that is a component of ground substance of connective tissues. This material is detected by a radioimmunoassay and has been found elevated in a variety of fibrosing conditions.[18] Although a differentiation between normals and individuals with myelofibrosis is not possible, serial samples of hyaluronan follow the response of patients to therapy for myelofibrosis.

RADIOGRAPHIC FINDINGS

The radiologic findings of myelofibrosis are those of osteosclerosis in the axial skeleton and proximal long bones.[19] Osteosclerosis is observed in 40% to 50% of patients.[20] In vertebral bodies the sclerosis is increased at the superior and inferior endplates. The sclerosis may be uniformly dense or disrupted by small areas of radiolucency (Fig. 15–4). In the spine, increased radiodensity or condensation of bone at the superior and inferior margins of the vertebral body may result in a "sandwich vertebrae".[21] Other bones that may show sclerosis include the pelvis, skull, ribs, proximal femur, and humerus. Paravertebral soft tissue masses may be identified in patients with spinal cord compression and neurologic abnormalities.[11, 22]

MR of patients with myelofibrosis can identify the extent of bone marrow replacement.[20] Through the use of spin-echo images, the degree of replacement of normal marrow with fat, fibrosis, and hemosiderosis secondary to transfusions is possible.[23] The location and extent of extramedullary hematopoiesis that causes spinal cord compression can be determined with MR.[24]

DIFFERENTIAL DIAGNOSIS

The diagnosis of myelofibrosis may be suspected in the patient with anemia, splenomegaly, and osteosclerosis and can be confirmed by identifying the characteristic abnormalities on bone marrow biopsy. However, splenomegaly and osteosclerosis are not found exclusively in myelofibrosis.

Disseminated carcinoma that involves the bone marrow may produce a leukoerythroblastic smear. It may also cause sclerosis of bone, particularly if the primary lesion is in the prostate.

Patients with chronic myelogenous leukemia (CML) have splenomegaly and abnormal blood smears. These patients also may present with back pain.[25] Leukocyte counts are higher with chronic myelogenous leukemia, and there is an increased proportion of immature cells. CML rarely produces a leukoerythroblastic smear. The Philadelphia chromosome is positive in 90% of CML patients. CML is associated with a low neutrophil alkaline phosphatase score. Radiographic abnormalities are uncommon.[26]

The differential diagnosis of osteosclerosis is quite broad. These entities include osteoblastic metastases, mastocytosis, lymphomas, Paget's disease, fluorosis, renal osteodystrophy, and axial osteomalacia. Careful review of blood tests and bone biopsy material should differentiate these entities from myelofibrosis (Table 15–2).[21]

TREATMENT

The treatment of myelofibrosis is mostly supportive. Anemia is helped by transfusions and, occasionally, by androgen therapy (oral oxymetholone, 150 mg/day). Patients with bone pain or spinal cord compression may benefit from local radiotherapy.[24] Chemotherapy with low doses of busulfan (2 to 4 mg/day) may decrease spleen size but may cause pancytopenia. Splenectomy is not always helpful in improving blood counts, and it may be associated with excessive bleeding postoperatively. Hyperuricemia may be controlled with allopurinol. Patients who develop aggressive disease with increasing organomegaly, peripheral blast cells, anemia, and thrombocytopenia are gen-

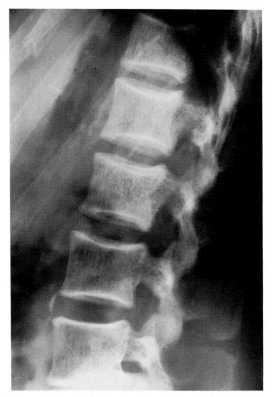

Figure 15–4. Myelofibrosis. Lateral view of the lumbar spine showing diffuse increased density of bone associated with a thickened trabecular pattern. (Courtesy of Anne Brower, M.D.)

TABLE 15–2. DIFFERENTIAL DIAGNOSIS OF OSTEOSCLEROSIS*

	SKELETAL METASTASIS	MASTO-CYTOSIS	MYELO-FIBROSIS	LYMPHOMAS	PAGET'S DISEASE	FLUOROSIS	RENAL OSTEO-DYSTROPHY	AXIAL OSTEO-MALACIA
Distribution	Axial > appendicular	Axial > appendicular	Axial > appendicular	Axial > appendicular	Axial > appendicular	Axial > appendicular	Axial > appendicular	Axial
Diffuse sclerosis	+	+	+	+	+	+	+	+
Focal sclerosis	+	+	–	+	+	–	–	–
Osteopenia or bone lysis	+	+	+	+	+	–	+	–
Bony enlargement	–	–	–	–	+	–	–	–
Osteophytosis, ligament ossification	–	–	–	–	–	+	–	–
Splenomegaly	–	+	+	+	–	–	–	–

* +, Common; –, uncommon or rare.
From Resnick D, Niwayama G (eds): Diagnosis of Bone and Joint Disorders, 2nd ed. Philadelphia: WB Saunders Co, 1988, p 2486.

erally resistant to therapeutic intervention.[27] Bone marrow transplantation has been utilized with patients with acute or secondary myelofibrosis. The degree of marrow fibrosis does not appear to limit the efficiency of engraftment.[7]

PROGNOSIS

Occasionally, the course of myelofibrosis is benign with a survival greater than 5 years after diagnosis.[1] Bone marrow fibrosis may be reversed through the use of alkylating agents, ^{32}P therapy, or splenectomy.[28] In the usual circumstance, the disease is progressive with a survival of only 2 to 3 years after diagnosis.[8] Many patients die from infections or thromboembolic events.[9] Bad prognostic factors include a short period of time between the first symptoms and diagnosis, anemia, significant leukocytosis, and the presence of immature granulocyte precursors in the peripheral blood.[29] Rarely, patients may have an acute myelofibrosis that is highly aggressive, with death occurring within a year. This is heralded by fever, weight loss, and increased anemia and thrombocytopenia in the absence of organomegaly and a hypercellular marrow with bone marrow biopsy. Approximately 20% of patients with myelofibrosis develop acute myelogenous leukemia and usually are resistant to therapeutic intervention.[30]

References

MYELOFIBROSIS

1. Silverstein MN, Gomes MR, ReMine WH, Elveback LR: Agnogenic myeloid metaplasia. Arch Intern Med 120:546, 1967.
2. Adamson JW, Fialkow PJ: The pathogenesis of myeloproliferative syndromes. Br J Haematol 38:229, 1978.
3. Dameshek W: Some speculations on myeloproliferative syndromes. Blood 6:372, 1951.
4. Ward HP, Vautrin E, Kurnick J: Presence of a myeloproliferative factor in patients with polycythemia vera and agnogenic myeloid metaplasia: I. Expansion of the erythropoietin responsive stem cell compartment. Proc Soc Exp Biol Med 147:305, 1974.
5. Wood HC: On relations of leukocythemia and pseudoleukemia. Am J Med Sci 62:373, 1871.
6. Leigh TF, Corley CC Jr, Huguley CM Jr, Rogers JV Jr: Myelofibrosis: the general and radiologic findings in 25 proven cases. AJR 82:183, 1959.
7. Smith RE, Chelmowski MK, Szabo EJ: Myelofibrosis: a concise review of clinical and pathologic features and treatment. Am J Hematol 29:174, 1988.
8. Bouruncle BA, Doan CA: Myelofibrosis: clinical, hematologic and pathologic study of 110 patients. Am J Med Sci 243:697, 1962.
9. Hasselbalch H: Idiopathic myelofibrosis: a clinical study of 80 patients. Am J Hematol 34:291, 1990.
10. Glew RH, Haese WH, McIntyre PA: Myeloid metaplasia with myelofibrosis: the clinical spectrum of extramedullary hematopoiesis and tumor formation. Johns Hopkins Med J 132:253, 1973.
11. Cromwell LD, Kerber C: Spinal cord compression by extramedullary hematopoiesis in agnogenic myeloid metaplasia. Radiology 128:118, 1978.
12. Vaugh JM: Leuco-erythroblastic anaemia. J Pathol 42:541, 1936.
13. Roberts BE, Miles DW, Woods CG: Polycythaemia vera and myelosclerosis: a bone marrow study. Br J Haematol 16:75, 1969.
14. Gilbert HS: The spectrum of myeloproliferative disorders. Med Clin North Am 57:355, 1973.
15. Yu TF: Secondary gout associated with myeloproliferative disorders. Arthritis Rheum 8:765, 1965.
16. Hochweiss S, Fruchtman S, Hahn EG, et al: Increased serum procollagen III aminoterminal peptide in myelofibrosis. Am J Hematol 15:343, 1983.
17. Hasselbalch H, Junker P, Lisse I, et al: Serum markers for type IV collagen and type III procollagen in the myelofibrosis-osteomyelosclerosis syndrome and other chronic myeloproliferative disorders. Am J Hematol 23:101, 1986.
18. Hasselbalch H, Junker P, Lisse I, et al: Circulating hyaluronan in the myelofibrosis/osteomyelosclerosis syndrome and other myeloproliferative disorders. Am J Hematol 36:1, 1991.
19. Pettigrew JD, Ward HP: Correlation of radiologic, histologic, and clinical findings in agnogenic myeloid metaplasia. Radiology 93:541, 1969.

20. Kaplan KR, Mitchell DG, Steiner RM, et al: Polycythemia vera and myelofibrosis: correlation of MR imaging, clinical, and laboratory findings. Radiology 183:331, 1992.

21. Resnick D, Niwayama G (eds): Diagnosis of Bone and Joint Disorders. Philadelphia: WB Saunders Co, 1981, p 2011.

22. Close AS, Taira Y, Cleveland DA: Spinal cord compression due to extramedullary hematopoiesis. Ann Intern Med 48:421, 1958.

23. Steiner RM, Mitchell DG, Rao VM, et al.: Magnetic resonance imaging of bone marrow: diagnostic value in diffuse hematologic disorders. Magn Reson Q 6:17, 1990.

24. Klippel ND, Dehou MF, Bourgain C, et al.: Progressive paraparesis due to thoracic extramedullary hematopoiesis in myelofibrosis. J Neurosurg 79:125, 1993.

25. Klier I, Santo M: Low back pain as a presenting symptom of chronic granulocytic leukemia. Orthop Rev 11:111, 1982.

26. Chabner BA, Haskell CM, Canellos GP: Destructive bone lesions in chronic granulocytic leukemia. Medicine 48:401, 1969.

27. Ward HP, Block MH: The natural history of agnogenic myeloid metaplasia (AMM) and a critical evaluation of its relationship with the myeloproliferative syndrome. Medicine 50:357, 1971.

28. Talarico L, Wolf BC, Kumar A, Weintraub LR: Reversal of bone marrow fibrosis and subsequent development of polycythemia in patients with myeloproliferative disorders. Am J Hematol 30:248, 1989.

29. Visani G, Finelli C, Castelli U, et al.: Myelofibrosis with myeloid metaplasia: clinical and haematological parameters predicting survival in a series of 133 patients. Br J Haematol 75:4, 1990.

30. Silverstein MN, Linman JW: Causes of death in agnogenic myeloid metaplasia. Mayo Clin Proc 44:36, 1969.

MASTOCYTOSIS

Capsule Summary

Frequency of back pain—uncommon

Location of back pain—lumbar spine

Quality of back pain—ache

Symptoms and signs—urticaria, diarrhea, flushing, bone tenderness, hepatosplenomegaly

Laboratory and x-ray tests—anemia, increased mast cells on bone marrow biopsy associated with increased fibrosis; lytic and/or sclerotic vertebral body lesions on plain roentgenograms

Treatment—H_1- and H_2-receptor blockers, oral chromolyn

PREVALENCE AND PATHOGENESIS

Systemic mastocytosis is a rare disorder associated with the proliferation of mast cells in skin, bone, liver, spleen, and lymph nodes.[1] Mast cells contain vasoactive compounds, such as histamine, which cause some of the clinical symptoms of the illness, including hives, flushing, diarrhea, and brownish skin lesions. Patients with mast cell proliferation in the axial skeleton may have back pain.

The prevalence of disease associated with mast cells is unknown. Approximately 1 in every 1000 to 8000 patients in dermatology clinics have mastocytosis.[2] However, an unknown number of patients may have disease without skin involvement.[3] The disease may start at any age. The disease usually becomes manifest after the age of 20. The age range is 25 to 80 years, with a median of 60 years. Men and women are equally affected.[4] A recent study of 58 cases revealed a male/female ratio was 1.33:1.[5]

The pathogenesis of mastocytosis is unknown. Mast cells originate from pluripotent bone marrow cells that are disseminated as precursors and then undergo proliferation and maturation in specific tissues.[6] Mast cells in the skin or in other organs start to proliferate. Mast cells in the skin, gastrointestinal tract, liver, spleen, lymph nodes, and bone produce chemical mediators that have effects on a number of these organ systems. The mediators include histamine, arachidonic acid metabolites (possibly including leukotrienes C_4 and B_4), and platelet activating factor.[7] Mast cells contain secretory granules and membrane-derived factors that are from three biologically active categories. These categories include: (1) histamine, a proteogylcan, and neutral proteinases; (2) cysteinyl and dihydroxyleukotrienes, prostaglandin D_2, and platelet activating factor; (3) interleukin-1, -3, -4, -5, -6, tumor necrosis factor alpha, granulocyte–macrophage colony stimulating factor, and interferon gamma.[6] These factors have potent effects on immune function, inflammation, blood vessels, and fibroblasts. The clinical manifestations of the disease can be directly correlated with the products released by mast cells.[8]

Nettleship in 1869 was the first to describe the cutaneous manifestations of the disease,[9] while Sangster in 1878 coined the term "urticaria pigmentosa."[10] In 1958, Ende was the first to report the occurrence of systemic mastocytosis in the absence of skin involvement.[11]

CLINICAL HISTORY

Systemic mastocytosis may manifest itself in a number of ways. The clinical manifestations may be divided into five distinct syndromes: (1) urticaria pigmentosa (95% to 99% of all mastocytoses), (2) cutaneous involvement with bone disease, (3) systemic mastocytoses with cutaneous and other internal organ involvement including bone, (4) systemic mastocytosis without urticaria pigmentosa, and (5) mast cell leukemia.[12-15] A recent consensus conference held in 1991 has classified mastocytosis into four forms: indolent, mastocytosis with hematologic disorders, aggressive mastocytosis, and mast cell leukemia (Table 15–3).[16]

The symptoms of patients with the illness depend on the extent and degree of mast cell organ involvement and physiologic response to histamine. Approximately 10% to 20% of patients with a systemic disease have bone pain, including back pain. Fractures may be present in 16%.[5] Patients have attacks that begin with a sensation of flushing, followed by palpitations and lightheadedness due to vasodilitation with associated hypotension.[17] Other common symptoms include generalized fatigue, night sweats, weakness, vomiting, diarrhea, and weight loss. Patients may also complain of cutaneous flushing, pruritus, dizziness, syncope, and various neuropsychiatric disorders including irritability and inability to concentrate.[2]

PHYSICAL EXAMINATION

Skin or mucous membrane lesions include confluent macules, papules, or nodules, which may become pigmented. Progressive disease will affect the oral, nasal, and rectal mucosa. Dermatographism is also a common finding. Cutaneous manifestations are the most prevalent abnormality on physical examination.[18] Other prominent findings in systemic disease include hepatosplenomegaly, generalized lymphadenopathy, and tenderness on palpation of affected bones in the vertebral column.

LABORATORY DATA

The infiltration of mast cells into the bone marrow, the release of mast cell products, and the associated fibrosis have marked effects on laboratory parameters. Anemia is seen in many patients in association with normal leukocyte counts. A minority of patients have leukopenia, while leukocytosis with eosinophilia occurs in 10% to 20% of patients.[7, 19] A minority of patients may be thrombocytopenic.[5] Patients with systemic mastocytosis with urticaria pigmentosa may have normal blood parameters. Patients with malignant mastocytosis have blood abnormalities involving the red blood cells, white blood cells, or platelets, invariably.[20] The ESR is elevated. The biochemical diagnosis of mastocytosis may be suspected even in the absence of histologic proof of the illness. In patients with episodes of systemic mastocytic activation, mast cell mediators will

TABLE 15–3. MASTOCYTOSIS CLASSIFICATION

1. Indolent mastocytosis	
A. Cutaneous disease	Major form
Urticaria pigmentosa (U.P.)	
Diffuse cutaneous mastocytosis	
B. Systemic disease	Unaltered life expectancy
Bone marrow	
Mast cell aggregates	
Gastrointestinal	
Ulcer disease	
Malabsorption	
Hepatosplenomegaly	
Skeletal disease	
Lymphadenopathy	
2. Mastocytosis with a hematologic disorder	
A. Myeloproliferative	Prognosis of hematologic disorder
Nonlymphatic leukemia	
Malignant lymphoma	
B. Myelodysplastic	
Chronic neutropenia	
3. Aggressive	
A. Lymphadenopathic mastocytosis with eosinophilia	Prognosis of extent of organ infiltration
4. Mast cell leukemia	Invariably fatal

be elevated during these episodes and will be normal at quiescent times. In contrast, patients with proliferative mast cell disease, such as leukemia, usually exhibit chronic overproduction of mast cell mediators.[21] Mast cell secretory products include heparin, histamine, PGD_2, and tryptase. Episodes of mast cell activation are short-lived, usually lasting up to 60 minutes. Blood samples should be obtained while a patient is experiencing an episode of mast cell activation.

Heparin from mast cells may cause a prolongation of the partial thromboplastin time (PTT). An abnormal PTT is encountered only during severe episodes of activation. The specificity of the abnormal PTT secondary to heparin may be increased by the presence of a normal protime that is less sensitive to heparin and the reversal of the abnormal PTT by the addition of protamine, a heparin antagonist. Measurement of urinary histamine and its metabolites will document increased concentrations along with increased prostaglandin D_2 metabolites.[22, 23] Many difficulties are associated with the quantification of histamine in plasma and urine. Mass spectrometric analysis is the most accurate but least available means to measure histamine.[21] Plasma histamine may be increased by basophils activated during phlebotomy. Bacteria add to the the levels of urinary histamine. Elevated levels of histamine during a period of mast cell activation with a return to normal may be more indicative of overproduction of histamine secondary to systemic mastocytosis. Prostaglandin D_2 metabolites are elevated but are difficult to quantify since mass spectrometric analysis is necessary. Tryptase is a neutral protease found in mast cell granules and not in basophil granules. Tryptase is more specific than histamine as a measure of mast cell activation.[24] Tryptase is measured by an ELISA assay. Samples may be obtained up to 2 or more hours after an attack of mast cell activation.[25] Elevated alkaline phosphatase may be seen in a minority of patients with significant bone involvement. Patients have also been described with abnormal lipoproteins, particularly prebetalipoprotein. These patients had accelerated coronary atherosclerosis.[26]

Bone marrow biopsy is the definitive diagnostic procedure for systemic mastocytosis. Bone marrow is hypercellular with increased reticulin and increased myeloid elements.[27] Superficially, the lesions have a granulomatous appearance, but there are no giant cells. The mast cells are present but may be difficult to recognize, since the mast cells of systemic mastocytosis are immature and contain fewer granules than mature mast cells.[28] Mast cells are paratrabecular and perivascular in location. The bone cells, osteoblasts and osteoclasts, are prominent in this disease. Both types of cells are enlarged. In certain areas, osteoclasts predominate and there is associated bone lysis. In other areas bone density is increased corresponding to increased osteoblastic activity. A study of 9 patients with mastocytosis investigated the pathologic changes associated with osteopenia and osteosclerosis.[29] Patients with osteopenia had active bone-forming surfaces that were outpaced by bone resorption by osteoclasts. In these patients, bone marrow infiltration by mast cells and fibrosis was not as extensive as that with osteosclerosis. Patients with osteosclerosis had extensive skin and visceral organ involvement. Bone marrow mast cells and fibrosis was significantly increased. Skin biopsy may also demonstrate increased numbers of mast cells.[8]

RADIOGRAPHIC EVALUATION

Although bone pain may be a symptom in a minority of patients, skeletal changes on radiographic evaluation occur in up to 70% of patients with mastocytosis. The abnormalities include either diffuse or localized osteoblastic or osteolytic lesions (Fig. 15–5). In the axial skeleton, diffuse lesions predominate. In a number of reviews, generalized osteosclerosis was the most common pattern (16% to 45%) (Fig. 15–6). Mixed osteosclerosis with focal osteolytic areas and generalized osteoporosis occur less commonly.[12, 13, 30–32] Patients with mastocytosis may present with compression fractures as a manifestation of osteopenia. Osteopenia may be the sole manifestation of mastocytosis independent of skin disease.[33] In the axial skeleton, the loss of delineation of the bony trabeculae results in a homogeneous, radiodense appearance of bone. Osteolytic areas are discrete (5 cm or less in diameter) with a thin rim of sclerotic bone.

Bone scan may also have a variable pattern. In one study, patients had a variety of scans ranging from normal to unifocal, multifocal, or diffuse increased uptake.[34] The finding of osteolytic and osteosclerotic bone abnormalities on plain roentgenograms and a diffuse increased uptake on bone scan should suggest the possibility of mast cell disease.[35] Mast cells absorb gallium. Gallium scans may identify the location of increased numbers of mast cells.[36] Dual photon absorptiometry has been used to document the increased amount of bone min-

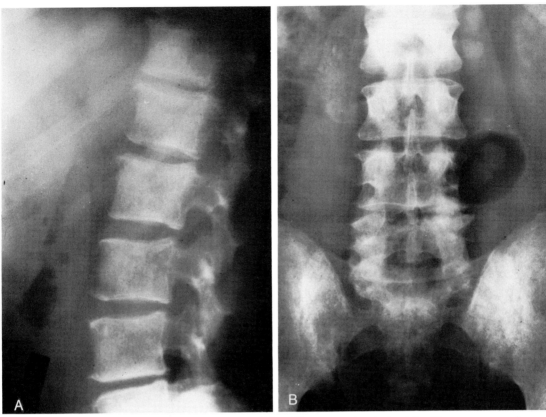

Figure 15-5. *A* and *B*, Mastocytosis demonstrated by diffuse osteosclerosis involving ilium, sacrum, and vertebral bodies. (Courtesy of Anne Brower, M.D.)

eral calcium in patients with systemic mastocytosis.[37]

DIFFERENTIAL DIAGNOSIS

The diagnosis of mastocytosis is not difficult in the patient with urticaria pigmentosa, positive Darier's sign (urticaria formation with gentle stroking of the skin), cutaneous flushing, hepatosplenomegaly, histaminuria, and osteosclerosis on plain films associated with back pain. A problem exists in making the diagnosis because mastocytosis has a broad spectrum of disease. Importantly, patients may present with systemic involvement without cutaneous lesions.[38] In these patients, biopsy of an involved area (bone marrow, liver, skin) should yield tissue with mast cells. The histologic demonstration of increased numbers of mast cells in the appropriate clinical setting is diagnostic.

The radiographic picture of mastocytosis may be confused with that of other diseases that cause osteosclerosis. These include myelofibrosis, fluorosis, sickle cell anemia, Paget's disease, and metastatic lesions, particularly prostatic carcinoma (see Table 15-2).[39] Each disease has laboratory or clinical parameters that differentiate it from mastocytosis.

TREATMENT

Treatment of mastocytosis is directed at counteracting the effects of mast cell products. A major part of therapy is antihistamines. Treatment may include histamine 1 receptor antagonists, such as chlorpheniramine 12 to 24 mg/day, and histamine 2 receptor antagonists, such as cimetidine 800 to 1200 mg/day or ranitidine 300 to 600 mg/day.[40] The H_1 antagonists inhibit flushing and pruritis, while the H_2 anatgonists limit gastrointestinal manifestations.

Oral cromolyn sodium (100 to 400 mg/day) may ameliorate pruritis, abdominal pain, and neuropsychiatric dysfunction.[44] The mechanism of action of this agent may be to block absorption of factors from the gut that stimulate mast cell discharge of active products. At 800 mg/day, oral cromolyn is significantly better than placebo for the gastrointestinal manifestations of mastocytosis.[42]

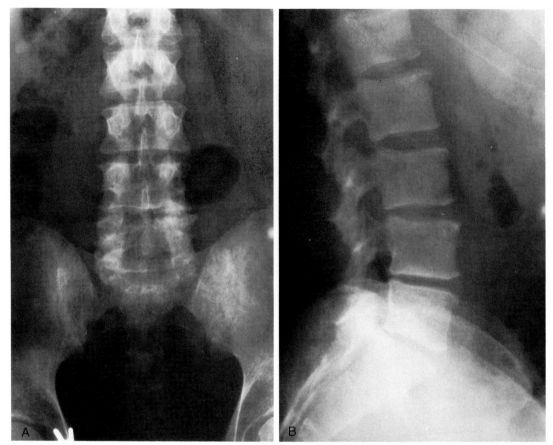

Figure 15–6. AP *(A)* and lateral *(B)* views of the lumbosacral spine of a 55-year-old man with systemic mastocytosis. The patient had urticaria pigmentosa. The patient had chronic low back pain since a fall as a child. In the past year, the pain had increased. The roentgenograms reveal advanced lower lumbar spondylosis. The bones reveal a granular quality consistent with early osteosclerosis, most evident in the pelvis.

The use of nonsteroidal anti-inflammatory agents is controversial. Some patients with mastocytosis are aspirin sensitive and develop bronchospasm with aspirin ingestion. Other patients have used nonsteroidals to block the production of prostaglandin D_2 by mast cells, thereby decreasing symptoms.[23] In patients with severe disease who have not responded to antihistamines, a trial of aspirin is warranted. Small doses of aspirin (60 to 120 mg) along with antihistamines should be given as tolerated. Small increments of aspirin are given as tolerated.

Radiotherapy has been utilized in patients with severe spinal involvement. Mast cell degranulation with increased histamine levels does not occur with radiation therapy.[43]

In patients who develop shock, emergency procedures are needed. These patients require intravenous fluids and dopamine or epinephrine. Transfusions may be indicated for patients who develop profound anemia.

PROGNOSIS

The prognosis in mastocytosis varies with two factors: age at onset and absence of systemic disease. Patients who are older at time of onset or have systemic manifestations have a worse prognosis. About 15% to 30% of adult patients with skin disease may progress to systemic mastocytosis. The patients at greatest risk of developing mast cell leukemia are those with no skin disease, marked splenomegaly, and severe myeloid hyperplasia.[27] In one study, 40% of 43 patients with mastocytosis developed leukemia. The leukemias included myelogenous, monocytic, and mast cell malignancies. This suggests that systemic mastocytosis may be part of a spectrum of myeloproliferative disorders that include polycythemia, chronic myelogenous leukemia, and essential thrombocythemia.

The prognosis of 58 patients with mast cell disease was evaluated by uni- and multivariate analysis.[5] Most of the deaths from mastocytosis occurred during the first 3 years after diagnosis. Older men with constitutional symptoms, anemia, thrombocytopenia, abnormal liver function tests, lobulated mast cell nuclei, and few cells in bone marrow biopsy were at greatest risk.

References

MASTOCYTOSIS

1. Mutter RD, Tannenbaum M, Ultmann JE: Systemic mast cell disease. Ann Intern Med 59:887, 1963.
2. Fine J: Mastocytosis. Int J Dermatol 19:117, 1980.
3. Turk J, Oates JA, Roberts LJ II: Intervention with epinephrine in hypotension associated with mastocytosis. J Allergy Clin Immunol 71:189, 1983.
4. Korenblat PE, Wedner HJ, Whyte MP: Systemic mastocytosis. Arch Intern Med 144:2249, 1984.
5. Travis WD, Li C, Bergstralh EJ, et al: Systemic mast cell disease: analysis of 58 cases and literature review. Medicine 67:345, 1988.
6. Austen KF: Systemic mastocytosis. (Editorial) N Engl J Med 326:639, 1992.
7. Lewis RA: Mastocytosis. J Allergy Clin Immunol 74:755, 1984.
8. Olafsson JH: Cutaneous and systemic mastocytosis in adults. A clinical, histopathological and immunological evaluation in relation to histamine metabolism. Acta Derm Venereol (Suppl) 115:1, 1985.
9. Nettleship E: Rare forms of urticaria. Br Med J 2:323, 1869.
10. Sangster A: An anomalous mottled rash, accompanied by pruritis, factitious urticaria, and pigmentation, urticaria pigmentosa? Trans Clin Soc Lond 11:161, 1878.
11. Ende W, Cherniss EL: Splenic mastocytosis. Blood 13:631, 1958.
12. Brunning RD, McKenna RW, Rosai J: Systemic mastocytosis: extracutaneous manifestations. Am J Surg Pathol 7:425, 1983.
13. Webb TA, Li CY, Yam LT: Systemic mast cell disease: a clinical and hematopathologic study of 26 cases. Cancer 49:927, 1982.
14. Hills E, Dunstan CR, Evans RA: Bone metabolism in systemic mastocytosis. J Bone Joint Surg 63A:665, 1981.
15. Travis WD, Li C, Hoagland HC, Travis LB, Banks PM: Mast cell leukemia: report of a case and review of the literature. Mayo Clin Proc 61:957, 1986.
16. Metcalfe DD: Classification and diagnosis of mastocytosis: current status. J Invest Dermatol 96:2S, 1991.
17. Kuter I: Case records of the Massachusetts General Hospital. N Engl J Med 326:472, 1992.
18. Austen KF, Horan RF: Systemic mastocytosis: retrospective review of a decade's clinical experience at the Brigham and Women's hospital. J Invest Dermatol 96:5S, 1991.
19. Yam LT, Yam CF, Li CY: Eosinophilia in systemic mastocytosis. Am J Clin Pathol 73:48, 1980.
20. Horny HP, Ruck M, Wehrmann M, Kaiserling E: Blood findings in generalized mastocytosis: evidence of frequent simultaneous occurrence of myeloproliferative disorders. Br J Heamatol 76:186, 1990.
21. Roberts LJ, Oates JA: Biochemical diagnosis of systemic mast cell disorders. J Invest Dermatol 96:19S, 1991.
22. Keyzer JJ, de Monchy JGR, Van Doormaal JJ, van Voorst Vader PC: Improved diagnosis of mastocytosis by measurement of urinary histamine metabolites. N Engl J Med 309:1603, 1983.
23. Roberts LJ II, Sweetman BJ, Lewis RA, et al.: Increased production of prostaglandin D2 in patients with systemic mastocytoses. N Engl J Med 303:1400, 1980.
24. Schwartz LB, Metcalfe DD, Miller JS, et al.: Tryptase levels as an indicator of mast cell activation in systemic anaphylaxis and mastocytosis. N Engl J Med 316:1622, 1987.
25. Schwartz LB, Yunginger JW, Miller J, et al.: Time course of appearance and disappearance of human mast cell tryptase in the circulation after anaphylaxis. J Clin Invest 83:1551, 1989.
26. Frieri M, Papadopoulos NM, Kaliner MA, Metcalfe DD: An abnormal prebeta lipoprotein in patients with systemic mastocytosis. Ann Intern Med 97:227, 1982.
27. Rudders RA: Case 38–1986. N Engl J Med 315:816, 1986.
28. Lennert K, Parwaresch MR: Mast cells and mast cell neoplasia: a review. Histopathology 3:349, 1979.
29. Gennes CD, Kuntz D, Vernejoul CD: Bone mastocytosis: a report of nine cases with a bone histomorphometric study. Clin Orthop 279:281, 1992.
30. Rafii M, Firooznia H, Golimbu C, Bathazar E: Pathologic fracture in systemic mastocytosis. Clin Orthop 180:260, 1983.
31. Sagher F, Cohen C, Schorr S: Concomitant bone changes in urticaria pigmentosa. J Invest Dermat 18:425, 1952.
32. Poppel MH, Gruber WF, Silber R, et al.: The roentgen manifestations of urticaria pigmentosa (mastocytosis). AJR 82:239, 1959.
33. Chines A, Pacifici R, Avioli LV, et al.: Systemic mastocytosis presenting as osteoporosis: a clinical and histomorphometric study. J Clin Endocrinol Metab 72:140, 1991.
34. Rosenbaum RC, Frieri M, Metcalfe D: Patterns of skeletal scintigraphy and their relationship to plasma and urinary histamine levels in systemic mastocytosis. J Nucl Med 25:859, 1984.
35. Gagnon JH, Kalz F, Kadri AM, Von Graefe I: Mastocytosis: unusual manifestations; clinical and radiologic changes. Can Med Assoc J 112:1329, 1975.
36. Ensslen RD, Jackson FI, Reid AM: Bone gallium scans in mastocytosis: correlation with count rates, radiography, and microscopy. J Nucl Med 24:568, 1983.
37. Arrington ER, Eisenberg B, Hartshorne MF, et al.: Nuclear medicine imaging of systemic mastocytosis. J Nucl Med 30:2046, 1989.
38. Duffy TP: Clinical problem solving. N Engl J Med 328:1333, 1993.
39. Tubiana JM, Dana A, Petit-Perrin D, Duperray B: Lymphographic patterns in systemic mastocytosis with diffuse bone involvement and hematological signs. Radiology 131:651, 1979.
40. Achord JL, Langford H: The effect of cimetidine and propantheline on the symptoms of a patient with systemic mastocytosis. Am J Med 69:610, 1980.
41. Soter NA, Austen KF, Wasserman SI: Oral disodium cromoglycate in the treatment of systemic mastocytosis. N Engl J Med 301:465, 1979.
42. Horan RF, Sheffer AL, Austen KF: Cromolyn sodium in the management of systemic mastocytosis. J Allergy Clin Immunol 85:852, 1990.
43. Janjan NA, Conway P, Lundberg J, Derfus G: Radiation therapy in a case of systemic mastocytosis: evaluation of histamine levels and mucosal effects. Am J Clin Oncol 15:337, 1992.

16

Neurologic and Psychiatric Disorders of the Lumbosacral Spine

Disorders of the neurologic system may be associated with systemic illnesses that alter nerve function or with local compression that causes isolated neurologic abnormalities. Charcot joint disease, which affects the spine, occurs in the setting of decreased sensation in the skeletal system and results in marked destruction of bony structures. Syphilis and diabetes remain the most common etiologies of this arthropathy of the spine.

In addition to systemic disorders, peripheral neuropathy may affect nerves that course through the lumbosacral spine. Abnormalities of these nerves may superficially resemble impingement of a nerve root by a herniated nucleus pulposus or spinal stenosis. However, careful history and physical examination should localize the lesion outside the central nervous system and should raise the possibility of a wide range of disorders that affect the structures embedded in the retroperitoneum (retroperitoneal bleeding or tumor, for example).

The diagnosis of neurologic disorders is made by the careful review of the findings discovered during the physical examination and data obtained from a limited number of electrophysiologic and radiographic tests.

The therapy of neurologic disorders associated with back pain must be directed at the underlying disorder causing nerve dysfunction. Most commonly, strict control of glucose metabolism in diabetes is necessary. When compression of a peripheral nerve is relieved, total return of function is possible.

Psychiatric disorders are also associated with back pain. A small minority of patients with psychiatric illness actually complain of low back pain. The hallucinations and other psychotic thoughts of these patients do not usually involve pain.

In contrast, those patients with chronic low back pain very frequently develop neurotic behavior. Neurosis increases with the duration of pain. Patients with chronic pain lose control over their lives and become depressed. The initial injury that caused the pain may have healed entirely, but the patient continues to exhibit pain behavior. The diagnosis of chronic pain syndrome is made in a patient who has no new organic disease, has had pain for 6 months or longer, and has experienced progressive physical and emotional deterioration. In patients with chronic pain, therapy must take a multidisciplinary form including drugs, physical therapy, psychiatric therapy, and vocational rehabilitation.

Malingerers are individuals who feign their symptoms and signs willfully to gain some advantage. The number of patients with back pain who are malingering is very small. A careful history and physical examination frequently reveal the inconsistencies between malingerers' symptoms and signs and those of patients with organic disease. If the patient is thought to be malingering, that fact should be corroborated by another physician. Extensive evaluations and prolonged courses of treatment are counterproductive in the patient with feigned illness.

NEUROLOGIC DISORDERS

Capsule Summary

Frequency of back pain—rare

Location of back pain—radicular distribution—thigh, lower leg

Quality of back pain—neuropathic—burning, stinging, radiating

Symptoms and signs—burning pain or painless, diabetes most common illness, loss of sensation, local muscle wasting

Laboratory and x-ray tests—glucose intolerance; neuroarthropathy—marked destruction and disorganization of vertebral bodies

Treatment—glucose control, antidepressants, anticonvulsants

Neuropathic Arthropathy (Charot Joints)

Neuropathic arthropathy is a joint disease that occurs secondary to a wide range of neurologic disorders with a common characteristic—diminished sensory function. Although Charcot described the relationship between joint disease and neurologic dysfunction with tabes dorsalis (syphilis), Charcot joint disease has become synonymous with any articular disorder associated with neurologic deficits.[1]

The pathogenesis of neuropathic joint disease, regardless of the anatomic site, is the result of a combination of factors, including an absence of normal pain sensation, preservation of motor strength, repeated trauma to the anesthetic part, and damage to afferent proprioceptive neurons, that lead to joint instability and destruction.[2] The deprivation of normal protective reactions results in repeated trauma to articular constituents (neurotropic mechanism). Severe cumulative injury damages the articular cartilage, fractures subchondral bone, and disorganizes the joint. Some patients undergo rapid destruction of a joint without bone repair. The rapid resorption of bone without accompanying bone repair has been proposed as evidence for a neurovascular mechanism in the pathogenesis of Charcot joint disease.[3] In this hypothesis, neurally initiated vascular reflex mediated through the sympathetic nerves leads to increased blood flow resulting in dissolution of bone and cartilage.[4] Proof supporting this theory is the development of Charcot joints in patients who have been immobilized with limited exposure to trauma.[5] Local microfractures lead to hyperemia and hyperactive resorption of bone. Hy-

peractive resorption of bone results in osteopenia. These weakened bones are then at greater risk from local fracture secondary to minor trauma. Fracturing and repair are a secondary phenomenon.

Other factors that predispose to joint destruction include chondrocalcinosis (CPPD neuropathic joints in absence of neurologic disturbance) and increased stress on subchondral bone that has stiffened as a result of healing of trabecular fractures. Increased bone stiffness may hasten articular cartilage dissolution and accelerate the breakdown of Charcot joints.[6–8]

The pathologic findings associated with Charcot joint disease includes fibrillation and erosion of articular cartilage, formation of loose bodies, and marginal osteophytes.[9] The marginal osteophytes are markedly larger than those ordinarily associated with osteoarthritis. Dense subchondral sclerosis is common. Subluxation in association with juxta-articular fractures, which may involve articular facet joints, results in formation of additional callus. Parts of osteophytes may fracture and become incorporated into the joint capsule and synovium.[10, 11] These pathologic abnormalities have also been reported in the axial skeleton.[12]

The pathology of acute neuropathic joint disease reveals an intact articular surface.[4] Most of the bone directly beneath the articular cartilage is replaced by a vascular connective tissue reticulum. Remaining bone trabeculae are surrounded by numerous dilated vascular channels and are being resorbed by numerous osteoclasts. The increase in vascular channels correlates with increased vascularity noted with neuropathic lesions of the lower extremity.[13]

Neurologic disorders that cause Charcot joints may be of central (upper motor neuron) or peripheral (lower motor neuron) origin (Table 16–1). In general, central lesions and those that spare the sympathetic nervous system result in hypertrophic joint changes, while peripheral lesions and those that affect the postganglionic sympathetic nerve fibers are more closely associated with destructive joint alterations.[14, 15]

John Kearsley Mitchell in 1831 was the first to describe vertebral column abnormalities with spinal cord disease.[16] Vertebral neuroarthropathy (Charcot spine) was first reported with syphilitic tabes dorsalis by Kronig in 1884.[17] In modern times, Charcot spine is more likely secondary to diabetes mellitus, most often, or syringomyelia.[18] Lumbar spine involvement is most commonly associated with tabes dorsalis and occasionally occurs in patients with diabetes and syringomyelia.[19–21]

TABLE 16–1. CHARCOT ARTHROPATHY[1]

Central (upper motor neuron)
  Trauma
  Syringomyelia
  Meningomyelocele
  Syphilis (tabetic)
  Multiple sclerosis
  Congenital vascular anomalies
  Charcot-Marie-Tooth syndrome[31]
  Cervical myelopathy (compression)
  Arachnoiditis
  Diabetes
  Tuberculosis
  Pernicious anemia
Peripheral (lower motor neuron)
  Diabetes[18]
  Alcoholism
  Infections (leprosy)
  Trauma
  Pernicious anemia[32]
  Corticosteroids
Unknown
  Congenital insensitivity to pain[33]
  Familial dysautonomia[34]

Vertebral neuroarthropathy accounts for up to 12% of all neuropathic joints.[12] In tabetic patients, the proportion may rise to 21%.[22] The patients are between 50 and 60 years of age and the male:female ratio is 3 to 1. In the axial skeleton, the thoracolumbar and lumbar spine are most frequently affected.[12] Up to 20% of patients with neuropathic joints may have no sign of neurologic dysfunction at time of presentation.[23]

In contrast to peripheral Charcot joints, axial involvement is frequently symptomatic. The patients have pain in the low back that may radiate to the lower extremities. The source of pain is posterior nerve root compression resulting from malalignment of vertebral bodies, disc protrusion, and facet joint hypertrophy.[2] Some patients are asymptomatic or are only slightly uncomfortable, and the diagnosis of these patients is made as an incidental finding on roentgenographic evaluation of the lumbosacral spine.[19]

Physical examination reveals kyphosis, scoliosis, sensory disturbances, and lack of local tenderness. Neurologic dysfunction is discovered in those patients with nerve impingement secondary to extradural compression of the spinal cord associated with marked destruction of the vertebral column.

Roentgenographic abnormalities may occur solely in the spine or in combination with peripheral lesions. Axial neuropathy is limited to one to three contiguous vertebral bodies and is characterized by either marked sclerosis or destruction (lysis). Associated with this appearance of the vertebrae is fragmentation of bone with compression of vertebral bodies and discs, bony debris in the paravertebral soft tissues, and subluxation. Kyphoscoliosis is associated with facet joint involvement. The atrophic, or resorbed, lesions of the spine are a diagnostic problem. These lesions may be mistaken for a rampant infection or an aggressive bone tumor. There is extensive bone resorption with no evidence of accompanying bone repair. There is a sharp zone of transition between the area of resorption and the remaining bone.

The more common roentgenographic abnormality is vertebral sclerosis. Sclerosis involves the vertebral bodies, facet joints, spinous processes, and laminae. Large osteophytes, out of proportion to disc space narrowing, are usual. Sclerosis is a result of bone reaction to fracture. Sclerosis occurs early in the course of the disease. Osteolysis is less common and is associated with rapidly progressive disease. The disc spaces and facet joints may narrow or dissolve (Fig. 16–1).[2] A mixed pattern containing areas of lysis and bone production may also be noted.

Nuclear imaging is often used to differentiate Charcot arthropathy from infection and tumor. The three phase bone scan [blood flow, blood pool (1 minute image), and delayed uptake (2 to 4 hour images)] of ^{99m}TC methylene diphosphonate in the bone and joint uniformly demonstrates abnormality of high turnover and increased uptake in the neuropathic lesion. This corresponds with the increased blood flow to the lesion.[4] A differentiation between Charcot joint and septic arthritis may be made by the initial increased blood flow in the area of interest versus the increase in the third phase of the scan in septic arthritis.[24] Gallium-67 citrate scan has been utilized for detection of infectious lesions but has been capable of detecting lesions in only 80% of chronic osteomyelitis patients.[4] Indium-111 white blood cell scan has differentiated infectious from noninfectious lesions in patients with diabetic neuroarthropathy.[25] However, subsequent evaluation of indium-111 scans reported a significant number of false-positive and false-negative results. The use of MR in this same study also resulted in a number of false-positive tests for infection. The conclusion of these studies suggests that a negative result with indium scan and MR makes a diagnosis of osteomyelitis unlikely.[26]

The discovery of vertebral neuroarthropathy requires the identification of the underlying neurologic disorder. An evaluation for patients

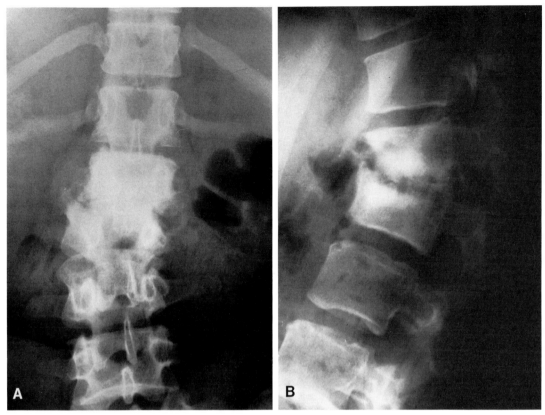

Figure 16–1. Neuropathic spine. AP *(A)* and lateral *(B)* view of the lumbar spine demonstrates total disintegration of the L1–L2 intervertebral disc space with associated extensive osteosclerosis. L1 appears to be "tumbling" into L2. This patient had congenital insensitivity to pain. (Courtesy of Anne Brower, M.D.)

with lumbar disease should include, at a minimum, a work-up for syphilis and diabetes. The differential diagnosis of sclerotic axial neuropathy includes spondylosis, vertebral osteomyelitis, and osteoblastic metastasis. Unlike degenerative spondylosis, neuropathic joint disease is rapidly progressive and is associated with florid osteophyte formation. In contrast to osteomyelitis, sclerosis of axial neuropathy parallels the vertebral endplates, involves the posterior arch, and is associated with paraspinal debris but not a soft tissue mass. Unlike blastic metastases, Charcot spine involves the disc spaces and preferentially affects the facet joints and vertebral bodies. Similar explanations could be given for the differential diagnosis of the lytic form of spinal neuroarthropathy. Bacterial infection must be considered in the patients with a progressive destructive lesion.[27] Tuberculosis and osteolytic metastases need to be considered in this form of the disease.[1]

Therapy for Charcot spine disease is directed at immobilization of the vertebral column by the use of a corset or brace.[28] Arthrodesis of Charcot joints is frequently unsuccessful. Infection and nonunion are frequent complications of the surgical procedure. Failures of surgery in the past were likely due to early mobilization and inadequate instrumentation. Staged procedures with anterior and posterior fusion, instrumentation, and prolonged immobilization have been associated with successful fusion of the unstable Charcot segment that is frequently located at the thoracolumbar junction.[29, 30] However, the same forces that led to spinal destruction and instability remain present. These patients are at risk of developing accelerated degenerative abnormalities at vertebral levels contiguous to the fusion.

Neuropathies

Neurologic disorders most commonly associated with the lumbosacral spine are radiculopathies associated with alterations of the lumbar disc (herniation) and the spinal canal (spinal stenosis). These entities are discussed in Chapter 10. Patients with herniated disc and spinal stenosis may have back pain as part of their symptom complex but more prominently have symptoms that affect the lower extremities. The involvement of the lower extremities follows a specific pattern that correlates with motor and sensory abnormalities associated with dysfunction of a specific nerve root.

Distal to the neural foramen, nerve roots from multiple levels form trunks that are incorporated into the lumbar and sacral plexuses. Because the structures are continuous, the lumbar and sacral plexuses can be considered as one unit, the lumbosacral plexus (see Fig. 5–8). A nerve distal to the spinal cord will have a distribution not as a single root but as a peripheral nerve with abnormalities in cutaneous or muscular structures innervated by multiple nerve root segments.

The lumbosacral plexus forms from the spinal roots of L1 through S5 and lies just lateral to both sides of the vertebral column in a retroperitoneal and posterior pelvic position. Any pathologic disease process that alters the anatomy of retroperitoneal or posterior pelvic areas may affect the plexus (tumor, fibrosis). Systemic disorders that affect the vasa nervorum may also have marked effects on plexus function (vasculitis).

Lumbosacral Plexus

Tumors. Tumors of the pelvic organs spread by direct or lymphatic extension to involve the lumbosacral plexus.[35] Tumors in the pelvis (cervix, prostate, bladder, and rectum) spread to pelvic lymph nodes that neighbor the sacral plexus. The nerves supplying the gluteal muscles, the posterior cutaneous nerve of the thigh, and the sciatic nerve are affected. Tumors that spread to abdominal lymph glands in the lower aortic chain (testicular, ovarian) involve the lumbar plexus and are more likely to affect obturator, femoral, and genitofemoral nerves along with the psoas muscle. Lymphoma involving the retroperitoneal nodes may invade the lumbar plexus. Lymph nodes near the pelvic brim may affect the femoral and obturator nerves. Primary retroperitoneal sarcomas may have a similar effect.[36] Nonmalignant processes that cause fibrosis of the retroperitoneum (retroperitoneal fibrosis) may also cause a similar clinical picture.[37]

The clinical symptom commonly associated with tumors affecting the lumbosacral plexus is constant, deep boring pain. The pain is predominantly in the hip and posterolateral thigh. With involvement of the motor neurons, atrophy of the gluteal and thigh muscles re-

sults in increasing hip instability and gait abnormalities. Radiographic evaluation of the retroperitoneum may demonstrate mass lesions or increased osteoblastic activity on scintigraphy. Radiation treatment of the affected area is used to decrease pain and halt progressive paralysis.[38]

Vasculitis. Systemic vasculitis can affect the blood vessels supplying nerves. When blood flow to a nerve is compromised, neurologic dysfunction in the form of motor and/or sensory loss occurs. Most often, mononeuritis multiplex is associated with this pathologic process.[39] Mononeuritis multiplex is associated with a variety of connective tissue disorders including polyarteritis nodosa (PAN), systemic lupus erythematosus (SLE), and rheumatoid arthritis (RA). However, in a review of 35 patients with mononeuritis, 15 had no identifiable rheumatic disease. Of the 14 patients with mononeuritis multiplex and a connective tissue disease, 5 had SLE.[39] A significant number of individuals may develop mononeuritis without an identifiable, associated connective tissue disorder.

Ischemic nerve lesions may be distributed along the entire length of the affected nerves, although the majority of lesions are located in the proximal nerve trunks.[40] These lesions occur only with extensive disease, because the peripheral nerves receive extensive collateral circulation. Multiple small vessels of the aorta must be occluded before limb nerve ischemia occurs. Chronic, severe peripheral arterial insufficiency is associated with neurologic deficits in the lower extremities. Up to 88% of individuals with chronic arterial disease may demonstrate sensory abnormalities in the lower extremities.[41] The vasculitides associated with these lesions are listed in Table 16–2. Connective tissue disorders include PAN, allergic granulomatosis, Wegener's granulomatosis, vasculitis associated with cryoglobulinemia, and RA.[42] Other vasculitides associated with peripheral neuropathy include SLE, Sjögren's syndrome, and temporal arteritis.[41] Peripheral nerve lesions in inflammatory vascular disorders occurs less frequently than with atherosclerotic vascular disease. A variety of peripheral neuropathic syndromes occur in 14% of patients with temporal arteritis.[43] Approximately 10% of SLE patients have a peripheral neuropathy.[44] The frequency of peripheral neuropathy associated with Sjögren's syndrome has been quantified at 30% of individuals with primary disease.[45]

The clinical symptoms associated with vasculitis of a plexus or major nerve branch is the

TABLE 16–2. RHEUMATIC DISORDERS ASSOCIATED WITH NEUROPATHY

DISORDER	PERCENT WITH NEUROPATHIES	REFERENCE
Polyarteritis nodosa	67%	46
Wegener's granulomatosis	20%	47
Rheumatoid vasculitis	42%	50
Systemic lupus erythematosus	10%	49
Sjögren's syndrome	30%	48
Temporal arteritis	14%	43
Scleroderma	1%	51, 55
Cryoglobulinemia/myeloma	13%	52, 53, 56, 57
Lyme disease	5%	54

sudden onset of profound weakness or paralysis of a group of muscles supplied by a major nerve and radiating, burning, aching, or shooting pain associated with dysesthesias or numbness in a matching cutaneous distribution. The onset may take hours to days but is maximal at the beginning of the insult to the nerve. The damage to the nerve can be profound, so that function does not return. If the damage is not complete, return of function may occur over months to a year or longer. Laboratory evaluation will reveal systemic factors associated with the specific form of vasculitis (rheumatoid factor—rheumatoid vasculitis; eosinophils—allergic granulomatosis) and nonspecific signs of generalized vessel inflammation (elevated ESR, thrombocytosis). CSF remains normal in most cases since the nerve lesions are extraspinal. Electromyogram reveals denervation in the affected muscle along with slowed conduction in the corresponding nerve on nerve conduction studies. The appearance of neurologic abnormalities in the setting of vasculitis is indicative of more aggressive, potentially life-threatening disease. These patients usually require large doses of corticosteroids and immunosuppressive drugs such as cyclophosphamide.[46, 58] Other manifestations of connective tissue diseases may also cause neurologic dysfunction similar to a radiculopathy or plexopathy. On rare occasions, rheumatoid arthritis causes a pachymeningitis of the cauda equina and lumbosacral meninges. These patients develop abnormal CSF leukocytosis and elevated protein. Cauda equina symptoms are associated with this meningeal inflammation and resolve after treatment with high-dose corticosteroids.[59]

Bradley reported an inflammatory lesion of the lumbosacral plexus associated with perivascular inflammation in epineural arterioles associated with markedly elevated sedimentation rates in six patients. All patients presented with buttock or thigh pain or with mononeuritis multiplex symptoms of the lower extremities. Involvement was characterized by asymmetric radicular involvement initially associated with weakness and pain in a sciatic nerve distribution. Subsequently the process became bilateral and was associated with progressive motor and sensory dysfunction. Sural nerve biopsies demonstrated axonal degeneration and epineural arteriolar inflammation. Patients who were treated with immunosuppressive drugs had resolution of their symptoms.[60]

Radiation Therapy. Radiation therapy to the pelvis has been reported to cause damage to the lumbosacral plexus.[61] Patients receiving 5900 to 6760 rads to the pelvis developed signs of neurologic injury 6 to 48 months after exposure. Asymmetric patchy involvement of the entire plexus was manifested by spotty sensory, motor, and reflex abnormalities in both lower extremities. The major difficulty for the clinician in this circumstance is to distinguish plexus abnormalities from recurrent tumor. Patients with radiation damage develop neurologic dysfunction secondary to fibrosis.[62] Fibrosis may also be a manifestation of recurrent tumor. Surgical exploration may be needed to differentiate the possible diagnoses.

Peripheral Nerve Syndromes

Peripheral nerves are the extension of the spinal nerve roots that comprise the lumbosacral plexus. These nerves supply sensory function alone or a combination of sensory and motor function. Pathologic processes that compress (tunnel syndromes) or decrease blood flow (diabetes) to peripheral nerves are associated with neurologic symptoms of dysesthesias and muscular weakness in the distribution of the corresponding nerve. Many of the rheumatic diseases that cause mononeuritis multiplex may also be associated with a peripheral polyneuropathy or a multifocal mononeuropathy.[63] A number of nerves are affected in different locations in the lower extremity.

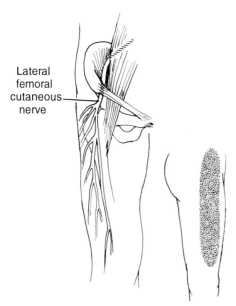

Figure 16–2. Meralgia paresthetica. The lateral femoral cutaneous nerve supplies the cutaneous structures of the lateral thigh. An area from the inguinal ligament to the knee may be affected.

Careful physical examination allows for the differentiation of spinal root from peripheral nerve lesions. Specific areas of sensory loss are characteristic of individual peripheral nerve lesions such as meralgia paresthetica and ilioinguinal syndrome (Figs. 16–2 and 16–3). A complete listing of lower extremity tunnel syndromes are listed in Table 16–3.

Femoral Neuropathy. The femoral nerve, the largest branch of the lumbar plexus, arises from the posterior divisions of the L2, L3, and L4 nerve roots (Fig. 16–4). The nerve emerges through the lower lateral border of the psoas muscle and descends along the line of junction of the psoas and iliacus muscles. The nerve supplies innervation to these muscles, runs with them under the inguinal ligament, and enters the femoral triangle, at which point it divides into superficial and deep branches. The superficial branch supplies cutaneous innervation to the anterior thigh and medial aspect of the lower leg. The deep branches innervate the rectus femoris, pectineus, vastus lateralis, vastus medialis, and vastus internus, and the knee joint and its medial ligament. In its course from the spine to the leg, the nerve is at greatest risk for compression in the iliac fossa, where it is included in a fascial compartment.

Patients with femoral neuropathy have deep pain that radiates into the flank, low back, and groin. Burning dysesthesias may also be felt in the cutaneous distribution of the nerve in the thigh and lower leg. Muscle weakness is manifested by weakness in hip flexion and loss of the patellar reflex. In pure femoral neuropathy, the patellar reflex is abolished while the adductor reflex is preserved. There are many etiologies for femoral neuropathy secondary to compression, traction, or direct injury to the nerve (Table 16–4). The most common cause of femoral neuropathy is diabetes.[64]

Femoral neuropathy may also be caused by bleeding disorders. In hemophilia, 75% to 80% of episodes of nerve compression are caused by bleeding into muscles.[65, 66] About 35% of hemophilic neuropathies involve the femoral nerve or lumbar plexus secondary to a psoas hematoma. Iatrogenic forms of bleeding secondary to anticoagulant therapy may also cause femoral neuropathy or lumbar plexus compression. Bleeding occurs in the iliopsoas.[67, 68] If bleeding occurs in the buttock, sciatica from sciatic nerve compression can occur.[69] A differentiation of the location of bleeding can be made in that bleeding into the psoas muscle causes hip muscle paralysis as well as quadriceps weakness. Sensory loss involves the anterior thigh, medial leg, medial upper thigh, and anterolateral thigh, corresponding to the femoral, saphenous, obturator, and lateral femoral cutaneous nerves, respectively.[68] Hemorrhage into the iliacus

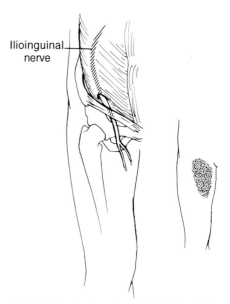

Figure 16–3. Ilioinguinal syndrome. The ilioinguinal nerve lies within the transversis abdominis and emerges below the inguinal ligament. An area near the medial thigh near the genitalia is affected.

TABLE 16–3. COMPRESSION NEUROPATHIES OF THE LOWER EXTREMITY

SYNDROME	NERVE	LOCATION OF COMPRESSION	CLINICAL MANIFESTATIONS
Lumbosacral tunnel	L5 nerve root	Iliolumbar ligament	L5 dysesthesias
Iliacus/femoral	Femoral nerve (L2, L3, L4)	Iliopectineal arch	Iliopsoas weakness (hip flexion); patellar reflex; dysesthesias: medial lower leg
Obturator	Obturator (L2, L3, L4)	Obturator tunnel	Dysesthesias: medial thigh, posterior knee; leg adductor weakness (partial)
Piriformis	Sciatic (L4–S3)	Sciatic notch	Sciatica; Freiberg's sign +; gluteal muscle atrophy, distal leg muscles
Meralgia paresthetica	L2, L3 nerve roots (lateral femoral cutaneous nerve)	Inguinal ligament, fascia lata	Dysesthesias: anterolateral thigh
Ilioinguinal	L1 nerve root	Transversis abdominus muscle	Dysesthesias: scrotum, labia, inguinal ligament
Saphenous	Femoral (cutaneous)	Adductor canal mid-thigh	Dysesthesias: medial lower leg
Common peroneal	Peroneal (L4–S2)	Fibular head	Dysesthesias: lateral lower leg, dorsal foot; foot weakness dorsiflexion
Superficial peroneal	Peroneal (L4–S1)	Crural fascia mid-lower leg	Dysesthesias: dorsal foot; foot weakness eversion
Deep peroneal	Peroneal (L5–S1)	Dorsal pedis fascia; anterior tarsal tunnel	Dysesthesias: dorsum great and 2nd toes; weakness great toe extension
Tarsal tunnel	Tibial (L5–S1)	Medial malleolus	Dysesthesias: medial plantar foot; weakness intrinsic foot flexors

muscle, which affects the femoral nerve alone, results in quadriceps weakness. Although some have suggested fasciotomy to relieve nerve compression, most allow healing to occur without surgical intervention.[65, 69, 70, 71] It is also important to remember that femoral neuropathy and psoas weakness may be a sign of a ruptured abdominal aneurysm (Fig. 16–5).[72]

Other causes of femoral neuropathy include retroperitoneal masses. These may be benign, such as appendiceal or renal abscesses, or malignant, such as retroperitoneal lymphoma or metastatic lesions.[73, 74] Femoral nerve palsies also occur secondary to leg traction during orthopedic procedures, to thermal injuries during hip replacement, or to bleeding from a bone biopsy site.[75, 76]

Hernias may also be associated with femoral neuropathy. This occurs more commonly with femoral hernias. The repair of hernias and other pelvic operations have been associated with postoperative femoral nerve palsies.[77–79]

Patients with femoral neuropathy must be evaluated for the possibility of a L3–4 disc herniation. This lesion is uncommon compared with lesions at the L4–5, and L5–S1 intervertebral disc interspaces. However, it is a lesion that is easily overlooked unless the possibility is kept in the differential diagnosis. Careful physical examination (hip and knee weakness or knee weakness alone) helps localize the area of compression. When there is doubt, CT scan of the retroperitoneum is very helpful in identifying anatomic abnormalities.

Piriformis Syndrome. The piriformis muscle arises from the pelvic surface of the second, third, and fourth sacral vertebrae. The muscle is directed toward the greater sciatic foramen and inserts into the upper border and medial side of the greater trochanter of the femur. The sciatic nerve, which arises from L4–S3 nerve roots, passes over the lower edge of the sciatic notch and lies just beneath the piriformis muscle and just above the obturator internus muscle (Fig. 16–6). Branches of the sciatic nerve that supply the gluteus medius and minimus and tensor fasciae latae separate from the nerve before the main branch travels beneath the piriformis muscle. The sciatic nerve continues down the leg to supply innervation to

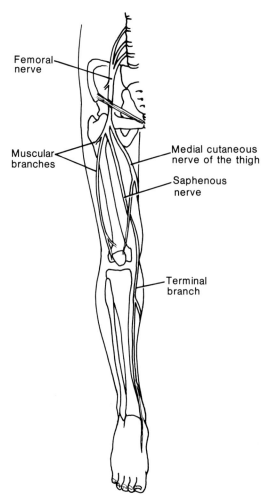

Figure 16–4. Femoral nerve. The nerve supplies hip flexors proximally and the cutaneous structures of the medial aspect of the lower leg distally.

(The piriformis is a lateral rotator of the hip.) Internal rotation puts stretch on the muscle and causes reflex pain and spasm. A more consistent positive finding is pain and weakness on resisted abduction and external rotation of the thigh. Rectal examination also may identify the increased tone in the affected muscles.

EMG of the upper sciatic muscles (gluteal, tensor fasciae latae) and paraspinous lumbosacral muscles will be normal, while those below the piriformis muscle may show mild denervation potentials. These findings are consistent with an entrapment neuropathy of the upper sciatic nerve. Abnormal H-reflex may be noted when forcible pressure is placed on the sciatic nerve with internal rotation of an affected limb in an adducted, flexed position.[83] CT scan or MR may identify soft tissue enlargement of the piriformis muscle on the lateral wall of the pelvis.[84]

Therapy for the piriformis syndrome is bed rest, analgesic medications, and anti-inflammatory drugs. Injection of the piriformis muscle is difficult to do and is rarely done. Caudal injection of an anesthetic and corticosteroids may be of value since the medication diffuses along the nerve root sleeves to the proximal portion of the sciatic nerve.[85] Section of the piriformis by surgical means is rarely indicated. However, sectioning of the piriformis muscle at its tendinous origin causes little functional loss and may relieve sciatic symptoms.[86]

Piriformis syndrome may complicate the symptoms of patients with other disease processes. Abnormalities of the inferior gluteal artery are associated with piriformis syndrome.[87] Disorders that cause inflammation of the sacroiliac joints may irritate the origin of the

the hamstring and muscles of the lower leg along with sensory innervation of the leg and foot. Any disease process that irritates the piriformis muscle will cause it to contract, compressing the sciatic nerve against the obturator internus and the sharp edge of the greater sciatic notch. Patients with piriformis syndrome have sciatic pain that radiates down the leg to the foot, following the course of the sciatic nerve but in no specific dermatome. Females may experience dyspareunia. Both sexes may develop a limp with dragging of the lower leg on the affected side.[80, 81] The pain associated with the piriformis syndrome is referred to as "pseudosciatica." The straight leg test is usually negative. The patient may have sciatic notch tenderness. The characteristic test that is positive in the patient with piriformis syndrome is re-creation of pain with internal rotation of the hip (Freiburg's sign).[82]

TABLE 16–4. ETIOLOGY OF FEMORAL NEUROPATHY

Diabetes mellitus
Bleeding disorders
  Inherited
    Hemophilia
  Iatrogenic
    Anticoagulants
  Acquired
    Ruptured aneurysm
Retroperitoneal tumors
  Benign
  Malignant
Surgical
  Leg traction
  Thermal injury
Femoral hernia
Postanesthetic
Idiopathic

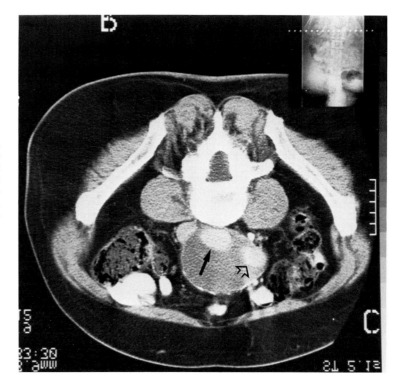

Figure 16–5. Abdominal aneurysm. CT scan with contrast dye reveals the aorta *(black arrow)* and left iliac artery *(open arrow)* involved with an expanding aneurysm. This is a patient at risk of developing rupture, retroperitoneal bleeding, and femoral neuropathy.

muscle and cause "psuedosciatica." Patients with spondyloarthropathy may be prone to the development of this disorder. The following case report illustrates the difficulty of diagnosing piriformis syndrome:

Case Study 16–1: A 26-year-old man with ankylosing spondylitis (AS) was referred for evaluation of persistent right leg pain. The diagnosis of AS was made on the basis of a history of sacroiliac (SI) joint pain, morning stiffness, and bilateral sacroiliitis on plain roentgenograms of the pelvis. The patient required indomethacin therapy at a dose of 75 mg/day on an intermittent basis. The patient stopped his medicine and within a few months developed bilateral low back pain, more severe on the right, with radiation of pain down the leg to the foot. His physical examination by his family physician revealed bilateral SI joint pain, a negative straight leg raising test, and no sensory or motor abnormalities. The patient underwent an evaluation for a herniated disc, including CT scan and myelogram, which were unrevealing for disc pathology. Evaluation by the rheumatologist at the time of his referral for continued back and leg pain revealed bilateral SI joint percussion tenderness, positive Faber tests, increased pain with internal rotation of the right hip, and increased pain with palpation of the right lateral wall of the rectum on rectal examination. A diagnosis of AS with piriformis syndrome was made and the patient started on indomethacin 75 mg slow-release capsules twice a day. Within 4 weeks, the leg pain resolved and the SI joint symptoms were remarkably improved.

Other Lower Extremity Peripheral Neuropathies

Obturator neuropathy occurs secondary to an obturator hernia or osteitis pubis. Patients develop groin pain that radiates to the thigh. Physical examination reveals weakness of the thigh adductors. Atrophy of the muscles is not seen, since the adductor magnus and longus may receive innervation from the sciatic and femoral nerves, respectively. Patients with adductor weakness will have an increased lateral swing to their gait associated with the unopposed action of the thigh abductors. If oral medications are ineffective, obturator nerve block may be performed.

Meralgia paresthetica is compression of the lateral femoral cutaneous nerve. Middle-aged, obese men are more commonly affected.[88] The nerve may be compressed near the inguinal ligament, the aponeurotic expansion of the sartorius muscle, or at its emergence from the iliac fascia. Physical examination reveals numbness in the distribution of the nerve (see Fig 16–2). Treatment in the form of weight reduction can be helpful. Most patients have resolution of the syndrome without the need for injection or decompression of the nerve. Surgical intervention is less successful if compression has been present longer than 18 months.[89]

Ilioinguinal syndrome is associated with pain

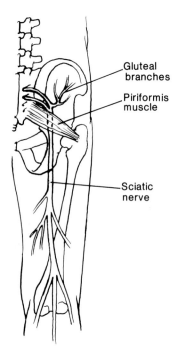

Gluteal
branches

Piriformis
muscle

Sciatic
nerve

Figure 16–6. Piriformis syndrome. The piriformis muscle originates from the sacrum and inserts on the medial side of the greater trochanter of the femur. Spasm of the piriformis muscle will affect motor and sensory supply to the lower extremity but will spare the proximal gluteal muscles.

in the inguinal region. The nerve is compressed in the transversis abdominis muscle. Patients may develop this syndrome after repair of an inguinal hernia or blunt abdominal trauma.[90] Injection of a trigger point medial and below the anterosuperior iliac spine is diagnostic and therapeutic for this syndrome.[91]

The saphenous nerve is a purely sensory nerve and is the longest cutaneous branch of the femoral nerve. *Entrapment of the saphenous nerve* causes pain along the medial aspect of the knee and lower leg. The nerve is frequently compressed in the adductor canal. Injection into the adductor canal provides improvement in 80% of patients with saphenous nerve compression.[92]

Lesions of the lower leg include involvement of the common peroneal nerve. *Compression of the common peroneal nerve* is associated with footdrop with weakness of ankle dorsiflexion or eversion. Involvement of the common peroneal nerve occurs more frequently than selective disease of the deep or superficial peroneal nerve. Parethesias may be noted over the dorsum of the foot if the common nerve is compressed in the fibular tunnel.[93] The similarities in clinical symptoms between L5 radiculopathy and common peroneal compression may be differentiated by EMG studies.

Diabetic neuropathy describes a heterogeneous and often overlapping group of neuropathic syndromes associated with diabetes mellitus. The absolute prevalence of neuropathy in diabetes is not known, but at time of diagnosis 8% of patients have signs of neurologic dysfunction and electrophysiologic abnormalities are encountered in 100% of patients.[94] The prevalence of physical signs of neurologic disease increase with longer duration of the disease.[95] The pathogenesis of diabetic mononeuropathies is ischemia of the nerve. Multiple infarctions of the femoral nerve and other peripheral nerves were demonstrated by Raff and Asbury.[96] Pathologic evaluation of the nerves demonstrated thickening and hyalinization of the arteriolar capillary walls, leading to luminal narrowing of nutrient vessels, with resultant discrete ischemic lesions. The pathogenesis of symmetric diabetic neuropathy is related to a deficiency of myoinositol, a sugar alcohol that has a myriad of biochemical effects on peripheral nerves resulting in decreased oxygen uptake, decreased high-energy phosphates, decreased glutathione, and increased oxygen-derived free radicals and membrane peroxidation. The end result of these biochemical abnormalities is slowed conduction.[97] Depletion of peripheral nerve myoinositol results in alterations of phosphoinositide metabolism that reduces protein kinase C–mediated Na^+/K^+–ATPase activity. The decrease in Na^+/K^+–ATPase activity results in impairment of nerve conduction velocity.[98] Therefore, myoinositol abnormalities in peripheral nerves seem to play a role in the pathogenesis of diabetic mononeuropathies. The nerves most commonly affected by mononeuropathy are those anatomically exposed to external mechanical compression. In patients with peripheral mononeuropathy, the nerve may be sensitized to the noxious effects of compression by the abnormality in carbohydrate metabolism. Most diabetic mononeuropathies are reversible over time with strict control of glucose metabolism, diminished compression of the nerve (removal of tight garments), and analgesics for pain.

Other forms of diabetic neuropathy that might be confused with femoral neuropathy include diabetic radiculopathy and diabetic amyotrophy. *Diabetic radiculopathy* is associated with the acute onset of radicular pain in an older patient, whose pain is worse at night. The trunk and areas supplied by the upper lumbar nerve roots are affected. The pain may be confused with pain of pulmonary, cardiac, or gastrointestinal origin. The relationship of pain with physical activities, such as Valsalva maneuver, is variable. Patients may have a history of weight loss of 15 to 40 pounds. The pain does not cross the midline. Physical examination reveals dysesthesia and a loss of muscle tone. Involvement may include the intercostal and abdominal muscles. The diagnosis is confirmed by nerve conduction and EMG studies. This form of neuropathy, like the mononeuropathy, resolves spontaneously. The period of time of resolution may be as long as 2 years.[99]

Diabetic amyotrophy, or proximal motor neuropathy, is a rare form of proximal muscle weakness that affects men between 50 and 60 years of age with new onset or mild diabetes.[100] Neurologic symptoms begin after a period of weight loss followed by severe thigh pain.[101] The pain is also experienced in the low back and hip. It is unilateral and radiates down the leg. The pain may be confused with that associated with a lumbar disc or hip disease. The pain has a burning, causalgic component with dysesthesias of the overlying skin. Simultaneously, the patient develops increasing weakness and wasting of the proximal muscles of one leg, then the other. Involvement of the quadriceps, iliopsoas, and adductors of the thigh is common.[99, 102] Walking becomes increasingly difficult. Physical examination reveals wasting and weakness of the proximal thigh muscle that does not conform to any one nerve root or peripheral nerve. Scapulohumeral and lumbar spinal muscles are affected rarely and to a lesser degree. The straight leg raising test is normal, and hip motion is unrestricted. Reflexes are reduced if the corresponding muscle is weak from the disease. Laboratory abnormalities include increased CSF protein and abnormal EMG findings consistent with denervation. The usual course of the illness is progressive over the first 6 months followed by a partial and variable recovery over the subsequent 2- to 3-year period. Strict glucose control is recommended, although proof that documents improvement of amyotrophy with glucose control is lacking.[103] The weakness and pain remit during the same time frame.[99] The pain associated with diabetic neuropathy and amyotrophy may improve with carbamazepine 300 mg 3 times a day.[104] Other therapies, which may be helpful but have not been tested in double-blind studies, include trazodone and doxepin.[105] Amitriptyline and fluphenazine were helpful in controlling pain associated with diabetic neuropathy in one study.[106] However, a more recent small double-blind study of the same drugs demonstrated no greater improvement from these drugs than from placebo.[107]

Aldose reductase inhibitors, drugs which limit the conversion of glucose to sorbitol in nerves, are a new class of agents that may improve nerve conduction velocities and diminish pain associated with diabetic neuropathy. The accumulation of sorbitol and its conversion to fructose is thought to play a role in the pathogenesis of diabetic neuropathy. Aldose reductase inhibitors (sorbinil, for example) have been reported to decrease neuropathic pain in diabetic patients.[108]

In patients with diabetic or other peripheral neuropathies (traumatic, compressive, postherpetic), the oral administration of mexiletine, a class IB antiarrhythmic agent, is helpful in decreasing neuropathic pain that is resistant to conventional therapies of glucose control, antidepressants, anticonvulsants, and nonsteroidal anti-inflammatory drugs. Mexiletine at doses between 150 to 900 mg in 2 or 3 divided doses per day is required. Congestive heart failure patients may have difficulty with this agent secondary to worsening of their cardiac condition.[109]

Miscellaneous Disorders

Other conditions that may on occasion be associated with back pain or cause symptoms that may be confused with sciatica include *coccydynia* (pain in the coccyx, usually secondary to fracture); *hip arthritis*, which usually radiates pain to the groin but on occasion radiates up to the buttock and lumbar region; and *iliopsoas bursitis* (pain in the inguinal area). The coccyx is usually protected by the buttocks and is not usually traumatized by a fall. However, a fall on a projecting object or a fall by a thin individual may damage the bone. The primary symptom is pain that is produced by sitting and relieved with standing or walking. Rectal examination recreates pain with palpation and movement of the coccyx. Therapy will include a circular cushion for sitting, nonsteroidal anti-inflammatory drugs, injection of anesthetics, and transcutaneous nerve stimulation. While surgery may be contemplated, it is not helpful in many patients since the patient may still have pain secondary to the surgical scar.

Hip arthritis may cause back pain on a referred basis (hip joint capsule is supplied by branches of nerves that innervate muscle and skin of the back) or by a change in gait that puts strain on the lumbar spine on a mechanical basis. The diagnosis is apparent after the patient is observed walking and examination of hip motion recreates hip pain. Most patients will have roentgenographic evidence of hip disease.

Iliopsoas bursitis occurs in individuals with inflammation of the bursa that complicates the course of degenerative or inflammatory arthropathy of the hip joint. The bursa is located between the iliopsoas muscle and the anterior capsule of the hip joint. Awareness of the syndrome as a cause of pain in the inguinal area has increased with the availability of radiographic methods that image the pelvis. The diagnosis should be suspected in patients presenting with anterior hip pain or an inguinal mass. Oral medications are usually effective in controlling the pain associated with bursitis. Injection therapy is limited to refractory cases.[110]

References

NEUROLOGIC DISORDERS

1. Goldman AB, Freiberger RH: Localized infections and neuropathic diseases. Semin Roentgenol 14:19, 1979.
2. Feldman F, Johnson AM, Walter JF: Acute axial neuropathy. Radiology 111:1, 1974.
3. Brower AC, Allman RM: Pathogenesis of the neurotropic joint: neurotraumatic vs neurovascular. Radiology 139:349, 1981.
4. Allman RM, Brower AC, Kotlyarov EB: Neuropathic bone and joint disease. Radiol Clin North Am 26:1373, 1988.
5. Norman A, Robbins H, Milgram JE: The acute neuropathic arthropathy—a rapid, severely disorganizing form of arthritis. Radiology 90:1159, 1968.
6. Jacobelli S, McCarty DJ, Silcox DS, Mall JC: Calcium pyrophosphate dihydrate crystal deposition in neuropathic joints: four cases of polyarticular involvement. Ann Intern Med 79:340, 1973.
7. Helms CA, Chapman GS, Wild JH: Charcot-like joints in calcium pyrophosphate dihydrate deposition disease. Skeletal Radiol 7:55, 1981.
8. Radin EL: Mechanical aspects of osteoarthrosis. Bull Rheum Dis 26:862, 1976.
9. Potts WJ: The pathology of Charcot joints. Ann Surg 86:596, 1927.
10. Horwitz T:Bone and cartilage debris in the synovial membrane. Its significance in the early diagnosis in neuroarthropathy. J Bone Joint Surg 30A:579, 1948.
11. Johnson JTH: Neuropathic fractures and joint injuries. Pathogenesis and rationale of prevention and treatment. J Bone Joint Surg 49A:1, 1967.
12. McNeel DP, Ehni G: Charcot joint of the lumbar spine. J Neurosurg 30:55, 1969.
13. Edelman SV, Kosofsky Em, Paul RA, Kozak GP: Neuroosteoarthropathy (Charcot's joint) in diabetes mellitus following revascularization surgery—three case reports and a review of the literature. Arch Intern Med 147:1504, 1987.
14. Resnick D: Neuroarthropathy. In Resnick D, Niwayama G. (eds): Diagnosis of Bone and Joint Disorders, 2nd ed. Philadelphia: WB Saunders Co, 1988, pp 3162–3185.
15. Wirth CR, Jacobs RL, Rolander SD: Neuropathic spinal arthropathy. A review of Charcot spine. Spine 5:558, 1980.
16. Mitchell JK: On a new practice in acute and chronic rheumatism. Am J Med Sci 8:55, 1831.
17. Campbell DJ, Doyle JO: Tabetic Charcot's spine. Br Med J 1:1018, 1954.
18. Zucker G, Marder MJ: Charcot spine due to diabetic neuropathy. Am J Med 12:118, 1952.
19. Ramani PS, Sengupta RP: Cauda equina compression due to tabetic arthropathy of the spine. J Neurol Neurosurg Psychiatry 32:260, 1973.
20. Harrision BR: Charcot joint: two new observations. AJR 128:807, 1977.
21. Briggs JR, Freehafer AA: Fusion of the Charcot spine: report of 3 cases. Clin Orthop 53:83, 1967.
22. Feldman MJ, Becher KL, Reefe WE, Longo A: Multiple neuropathic joints including the wrist in a patient with diabetes mellitus. JAMA 209:1690, 1969.
23. Katz I, Rabinowitz JG, Dziadiw R: Early changes in Charcot's joints. AJR 86:965, 1961.
24. Gandsman EJ, Deutsch SD, Kahn CB, Deutsch AM: Dynamic bone scanning in diabetic osteoarthropathy. J Nucl Med 24:664, 1987.
25. Knight D, Gray HW, McKillop JH, Bessent RG: Imaging for infection: caution required with the charcot joint. Eur J Nucl Med 13:523, 1988.
26. Seabold JE, Flickinger FW, Kao SCS, et al: Indium-111-leukocyte/technetium-99m-MDP bone and magnetic resonance imaging: difficulty of diagnosing osteomyelitis in patients with neuropathic osteoarthropathy. J Nucl Med 31:549, 1990.
27. Pritchard JC, Desoia MF: Infection of a Charcot spine: a case report. Spine 18:7674, 1993.
28. Hoppenfeld S, Gross M, Giangarra C: Nonoperative treatment of neuropathic spinal arthropathy. Spine 15:54, 1990.
29. Piazza MR, Bassett GS, Bunnell WP: Neuropathic spinal arthropathy in congenital insensitivity to pain. Clin Orthop 236:175, 1988.
30. Harrison MJ, Sacher M, Rosenblum BR, Rothman AS: Spinal Charcot arthropathy. Neurosurgery 29:273, 1991.
31. Bruckner FE, Kendal BE: Neuroarthropathy in Charcot–Marie–Tooth disease. Ann Rheum Dis 28:577, 1969.
32. Halonen PI, Jarvinen KAJ: On the occurrence of neuropathic arthropathies in pernicious anaemia. Ann Rheum Dis 7:152, 1948.
33. Thrush DG: Congenital insensitivity to pain. A clinical genetic, and neurophysiological study of four children from the same family. Brain 96:369, 1973.
34. Brunt PW: Unusual cause of Charcot joints in early adolescence (Riley–Day Syndrome). Br Med J 4:277, 1967.
35. McKinney AS: Neurologic findings in retroperitoneal mass lesions. South Med J 66:862, 1973.
36. Thomas MH, Chisholm GD: Retroperitoneal fibrosis associated with malignant disease. Br J Cancer 28:453, 1973.
37. Lepor H, Walsh P: Idiopathic retroperitoneal fibrosis. J Urol 122:1, 1979.
38. Layzer RB: Neuromuscular Manifestations of Systemic Disease. Philadelphia: FA Davis Co, 1985.
39. Hellmann DB, Laing TJ, Petri M, et al.: Mononeuritis multiplex: the yield of evaluations for occult rheumatic diseases. Medicine 67:145, 1988.
40. Dyck PJ, Conn DL, Okazaki H: Necrotizing angiopathic neuropathy. Three-dimensional morphol-

ogy of fiber degeneration related to sites of occluded vessels. Mayo Clin Proc 47:461, 1972.

41. Schaumburg HH, Berger AR, Thomas PK: Disorders of Peripheral Nerves, 2nd ed. Philadelphia: F A Davis Co, 1992, pp 130–135.

42. Fauci AS, Haynes BG, Katz P: The spectrum of vasculitis. Clinical, pathologic, immunologic and therapeutic consideration. Ann Intern Med 89:660, 1978.

43. Casseli RJ, Daube JR, Hunder GC, Whisnant JP: Peripheral neuropathic syndromes in giant cell (temporal) arteritis. Neurology 38:685, 1988.

44. McCombe PA, McLeod JG, Pollard JD, et al.: Peripheral sensorimotor and autonomic neuropathy associated with systemic lupus erythematosus. Brain 110:533, 1987.

45. Kennett R, Harding AE: Peripheral neuropathy associated with sicca syndrome. J Neurol Neurosurg Psychiatry 49:90, 1986.

46. Guillevin L, Du LTH, Godeau P, et al.: Clinical findings and prognosis of polyarteritis nodosa and Churg–Strauss angiitis: A study in 165 patients. Br J Rheumatol 27:258, 1988.

47. Fauci AS, Haynes BF, Katz P, Wolff SM: Wegener's granulomatosis: prospective and therapeutic experience with 85 patients for 21 years. Ann Intern Med 98:76, 1983.

48. Mellgren SI, Conn DL, Stevens JC, Dyck PJ: Peripheral neuropathy in primary Sjogren's syndrome. Neurology 39:390, 1989.

49. Feinglass EJ, Arnett FC, Dorsch CA, et al.: Neuropsychiatric manifestations of systemic lupus erythematosus: diagnosis, clinical spectrum, and relationship to other features of the disease. Medicine 55:323, 1976.

50. Scott DGI, Bacon PA, Tribe CR: Systemic rheumatoid vasculitis: a clinical and laboratory study of 50 cases. Medicine 60:288, 1981.

51. Lee P. Bruni J, Sukenik S: Neurological manifestations in systemic sclerosis (scleroderma). J Rheumatol 11:480, 1984.

52. Walsh JC: The neuropathy of multiple myeloma: an electrophysiological and histological study. Arch Neurol 25:404, 1971.

53. Vallat JM, Desproges-Gotteron R, Leboutet MJ, et al.: Cryoglobulinemic neuropathy: a pathological study. Ann Neurol 8:179, 1980.

54. Pachner AR, Steere AC: The triad of neurologic manifestations of Lyme disease: meningitis, cranial neuritis, and radiculoneuritis. Neurology 35:47, 1985.

55. Oddis CV, Eisenbeis CH Jr, Reidbord HE, et al.: Vasculitis in systemic sclerosis: association with Sjogren's syndrome and CREST syndrome variant. J Rheumatol 14:942, 1987.

56. Thomas FP, Lovelace RE, Ding XS, et al.: Vasculitic neuropathy in a patient with cryoglobulinemia and anti-MAG IgM monoclonal gammopathy. Muscle Nerve 15:891, 1992.

57. Gemignani F, Pavesi G, Fiocchi A, et al.: Peripheral neuropathy in essential mixed cryoglobulinaemia. J Neurol Neurosurg Psychiatry 55:116, 1992.

58. Moore PM, Fauci AS: Neurologic manifestations of systemic vasculitis. A retrospective and prospective study of the clinicopathologic features and response to therapy in 25 patients. Am J Med 71:517, 1981.

59. Markenson JA, McDougal JS, Tsairis P, et al.: Rheumatoid meningitis: a localized immune process. Ann Intern Med 90:786, 1979.

60. Bradley WG, Chad D, Verghese JP, et al.: Painful lumbosacral plexopathy with elevated erythrocyte sedimentation rate: a treatable inflammatory syndrome. Ann Neurol 15:457, 1984.

61. Ashenhurst EM, Quartey GRC, Starreveld A: Lumbosacral radiculopathy induced by radiation. Can J Neurol Sci 4:259, 1977.

62. Van der Kogel AJ, Barendsen GW: Late effects of spinal cord irradiation with 300 KV x-rays and 15 MeV neutrons. Br J Radiol 47:393, 1974.

63. Olney RK: AAEM minimonograph 38: neuropathies in connective tissue disease. Muscle Nerve 15:531, 1992.

64. Chopra JS, Hurwitz LJ: Femoral nerve conduction in diabetes and chronic occlusive disease. J Neurol Neurosurg Psychiatry 31:28, 1968.

65. Ehrmann L, Lechner K, Mamoli B, et al.: Peripheral nerve lesions in haemophilia. J Neurol 225:175, 1981.

66. Hoskinson J, Duthie RB: Management of musculoskeletal problems in hemophilias. Orthop Clin North Am 9:455, 1978.

67. Butterfield WC, Neiraser RJ, Robert MP: Femoral neuropathy and anticoagulants. Ann Surg 176:56, 1972.

68. Emery S, Ochoa J: Lumbar plexus neuropathy resulting from retroperitoneal hemorrhage. Muscle Nerve 1:330, 1978.

69. Parkes JD, Kidner PH: Peripheral nerve and root lesions developing as a result of hematoma formation during anticoagulation treatment. Postgrad Med J 46:146, 1970.

70. Young MR, Norris JW: Femoral neuropathy during anticoagulant therapy. Neurology 26:1173, 1976.

71. Niakan E, Carbone JE, Adams M, Schroeder FM: Anticoagulants, iliopsoas, hematoma and femoral nerve compression. Am Fam Physician 44:2100, 1991.

72. Owens ML: Psoas weakness and femoral neuropathy: neglected signs of retroperitoneal hemorrhage from ruptured aneurysm. Surgery 91:363, 1982.

73. Biedmond A: Femoral neuropathy. In Vinlen PJ, Bruyn BW (eds): Handbook of Clinical Neurology. Vol 1, Part II, Diseases of nerves. Amsterdam: North Holland Publishing, 1970, pp 303–310.

74. Nelson LM, Hewett WJ, Chu Ang JT: Neural manifestations of para-aortic node metastasis in carcinoma of the cervix. Obstet Gynecol 40:45, 1972.

75. Weber ER, Daube JR, Coventry MB: Peripheral neuropathies associated with total hip arthroplasty. J Bone Joint Surg 58A:66, 1976.

76. Walton RJ: Femoral palsy complicating iliac bone biopsy. Lancet 2:497, 1975.

77. Kline DG: Operative management of major nerve lesions of the lower extremity. Surg Clin North Am 52:1247, 1972.

78. Sinclair RH, Pratt JH: Femoral neuropathy after pelvic operation. Am J Obstet Gynecol 112:404, 1972.

79. McDaniel GC, Kukliy WH, Gilbert SC: Femoral nerve injury associated with the Pfannenstiel incision and abdominal retractors. Am J Obstet Gynecol 87:381, 1967.

80. Yoemans WE: The relation of arthritis of the sacroiliac joint to sciatica. Lancet 2:1119, 1928.

81. Pace JB, Nagle D: Piriformis syndrome. West J Med 124:435, 1976.

82. Freiburg AA, Vinke TA: Sciatica pain and its relief by operation on muscle and fascia. J Bone Joint Surg 16:126, 1934.

83. Fishman LM, Zybert PA: Electrophysiologic evidence of piriformis syndrome. Arch Phys Med Rehabil 73:359, 1992.

84. Jankiewicz JJ, Henrikus WL, Houkom JA: The appear-

ance of the piriformis muscle syndrome in computed tomography and magnetic resonance imaging. Clin Orthop 262:205, 1991.

85. Mullin V, de Rosayro M: Caudal steroid injection for treatment of piriformis syndrome. Anesth Analg 71:705, 1990.

86. Vandertop WP, Bosma NJ: The piriformis syndrome: a case report. J Bone Joint Surg 73A:1095, 1991.

87. Padopoulos SM, McGillicuddy JE, Albers JW: Unusual cause of "piriformis muscle syndrome." Arch Neurol 47:1144, 1990.

88. Stuart JD, Morgan RF, Persing JA: Nerve compression syndromes of the lower extremity. Am Fam Physician 40:101, 1989.

89. Macnicol MF, Thompson WJ: Idiopathic meralgia paresthetica. Clin Orthop 254:270, 1990.

90. Starling JR, Harms BA, Schroeder ME, Eichman PL: Diagnosis and treatment of genitofemoral and ilioinguinal entrapment neuralgia. Surgery 102:581, 1987.

91. Knockaert DC, O'Heygere FG, Bobbaers HJ: Ilioinguinal nerve entrapment: a little known cause of iliac fossa pain. Postgrad Med J 65:632, 1989.

92. Romanoff ME, Cory PC, Kalenak A, et al.: Saphenous nerve entrapment at the adductor canal. Am J Sports Med 17:478, 1989.

93. Donnell ST, Barrett DS: Entrapment neuropathies: 2. lower limb. Brit J Hosp Med 46:99, 1991.

94. Fraser DM, Campbell IW, Ewing DJ, et al.: Peripheral and autonomic nerve function in newly diagnosed diabetes mellitus. Diabetes 26:546, 1977.

95. Campbell IW, Fraser DM, Ewing DJ, et al.: Peripheral and autonomic nerve function in diabetic ketoacidosis. Lancet 2:167, 1976.

96. Raff MC, Asbury AK: Ischemic mononeuropathy and mononeuropathy multiplex in diabetes mellitus. N Engl J Med 279:17, 1968.

97. Green DA, Lattimer SA, Ulbrecht J, Carroll P: Glucose-induced alterations in nerve metabolism: current perspective on the pathogenesis of diabetic neuropathy and future directions for research and therapy. Diabetes Care 8:290, 1985.

98. Green DA, Lattimer SA: Altered myoinositol metabolism in diabetic nerve. In Dyck PJ, Thomas PK, Asbury AK, et al. (eds): Diabetic Neuropathy. Philadelphia: WB Saunders, 1987, pp 289–298.

99. Asbury AK: Focal and multifocal neuropathies of diabetes. In Dyck PJ, Thomas PK, Asbury AK, et al. (eds): Diabetic Neuropathy. Philadelphia: WB Saunders, 1987, pp 45–55.

100. Subramony SH, Wilbourn AJ: Diabetic proximal neuropathy. Clinical and electromyographic studies. J Neurol Sci 53:293, 1981.

101. Chokroverty S, Reyes MG, Rubino FA: The Bruns-Garland syndrome of diabetic amyotrophy. Trans Am Neurol Assoc 102:173, 1977.

102. Donovan WH, Sumi SM: Diabetic amyotrophy: a more diffuse process than clinically suspected. Arch Phys Med Rehabil 57:397, 1976.

103. Ellenberg M: Diabetic neuropathic cachexia. Diabetes 23:418, 1974.

104. Rull JA, Quibrera R, Gonzales-Millan H, Castaneda OL: Symptomatic treatment of peripheral diabetic neuropathy with carbamazepine. Double-blind crossover study. Diabetologia 5:215, 1969.

105. Kurana RC: Treatment of painful diabetic neuropathy with trazadone. JAMA 250:1392, 1983.

106. David JL, Lewis SB, Gerich JE, et al.: Peripheral diabetic neuropathy treated with amitriptyline and fluphenazine. JAMA 238:2291, 1977.

107. Mendel CM, Klein RF, Chappell DA, et al.: A trial of amitriptyline and fluphenazine in the treatment of painful diabetic neuropathy. JAMA 255:637, 1986.

108. Fagius J, Brattberg A, Jameson S, Berne C: Limited benefit of treatment of diabetic polyneuropathy with an aldose reductase inhibitor: a 24-week controlled trial. Diabetologia 28:323, 1985.

109. Dejgard A, Peterson P, Kastrup J: Mexiletine for treatment of chronic painful diabetic neuropathy. Lancet 1:9, 1988.

110. Toohey AK, LaSalle TL, Martinez S, Polisson RP: Iliopsoas bursitis: clinical features, radiographic findings, and disease associations. Semin Arthritis Rheum 20:41, 1990.

PSYCHIATRIC DISORDERS, CHRONIC PAIN, AND MALINGERING

Capsule Summary

P = psychiatric disorders
CP = chronic pain
M = malingering

Frequency of back pain
P — rare
CP — very common
M — very common

Location of back pain
P — low back
CP — low back
M — low back

Quality of back pain
P — unremitting, persistent, descriptive language (burning through my back)
CP — continuous with irregular fluctuations
M — unremitting, unresponsive to all therapies, disabling

Symptoms and signs
P — neurotic
CP — traumatic injury, loss of control over life
M — incapacitating pain, attempt to impress with severity of lesion, pain not consistent with anatomic findings, entire back, entire limb affected

Laboratory and x-ray tests
P — normal
CP — normal
M — normal

Therapy
P — antipsychotic drugs
CP — antidepressants, pain clinic
M — none

Psychiatric Disorders

Patients with psychiatric disorders may develop pain as part of the symptoms associated with their illness. The prevalence of pain as a symptom in psychiatric patients ranges from 22% to 66%, depending on the population studied (inpatient vs. outpatient, VA system vs. private clinic).[1-3] In many of these patients, pain is recognized as a result of their mental illness but is not a major complaint. However, in at least 25% of psychiatric patients, pain is severe.[3]

The pain that these patients experience is as "real" to the individuals with psychiatric illness as to those with a fractured femur. Pain is defined by the International Association for the Study of Pain as "an unpleasant sensory and emotional experience which we primarily associate with tissue damage or describe in terms of such damage, or both."[4] The definition of pain has two parts. One part deals with tissue damage or the threat of damage. It is necessary to experience an emotional response to that injury in order to experience pain. Therefore, those psychiatric patients who experience an emotional response to an event that they believe to be damaging have felt pain.

Walters was one of the first to report on pain in psychiatric patients.[5] In a study of 430 patients referred for evaluation of pain, 112 patients (26%) had low back pain. Other locations for pain included the head, chest, trunk, pelvis, and whole body. Pain was usually described dramatically. The most common diagnoses in these 430 patients was "other neuroses and situational states" in 336, conversion hysteria in 26, and psychoses in 68. Psychiatric patients with minor physical trauma had greater levels of pain than would have been expected.

Merskey reported his experience with 76 patients with mental illness and pain. Pain associated with neurosis was more common than pain associated with schizophrenia or endogenous depression.[6] Merskey discovered a relatively high association of neurosis, hysteria, and conversion symptoms with pain. Spear also found an increased number of neurotic patients with pain.[2] He found, as in the Mersky study, that the proportion of neurotic patients with pain to psychotic individuals with pain was similar.

Psychologic test studies yield comparable results. A number of researchers reported that the Minnesota Multiphasic Personality Inventory (MMPI) scores for hypochondrosis and conversion reaction were elevated compared with those for depression in psychiatric patients who complained of back pain.[7, 8] Sternbach has demonstrated that the conversion

pattern on the MMPI was found in patients who had pain that was chronic in duration. An unexpected finding was the relative absence of depression as a psychiatric diagnosis.[9] In a comparison between patients in chronic pain clinics and psychiatric patients with pain, depression was identified more commonly in the psychiatric population but only 10% of the psychiatric patients.[10, 11]

Merskey has suggested four reasons why psychologic illness causes the appearance or exacerbation of pain.[12] The first relates to a state of anxiety. Increased anxiety or worry about a lesion or experience heightens the intensity of pain. The mechanism of anxiety-associated pain remains speculative, but from a clinical standpoint alleviation of anxiety has a beneficial effect in the reduction of pain.

A second mechanism is associated with psychiatric hallucination. This mechanism is a rare cause of pain and is most closely associated with schizophrenic patients. Schizophrenic patients may experience hallucinatory damage to their person but infrequently associate that with pain.[13]

The third proposed mechanism concerns increased tension in muscles, which is associated with inadequate circulation and the accumulation of metabolic byproducts (lactic acid).[14] Individuals who use muscles in a new way may develop aching and discomfort in a body part. It is proposed that generalized muscle tension in those with chronic anxiety and stress similarly causes pain. In actuality, this hypothesis is not proven in fact. In a number of studies of pain, particularly headache, increased muscle tension accounted for only a small percentage of pain in patients with chronic pain. The pain was more closely related to a patient's personality disorder than to the level of muscle contraction.[15, 16]

The fourth mechanism of pain production in psychiatric patients is hysteria with conversion reactions. Conversion reaction or hysterical conversion is a mechanism for transforming anxiety or other emotions into a dysfunction of bodily structures or organs supplied by the voluntary portion of the nervous system. The symptoms lessen anxiety and symbolize the underlying mental conflict. The patient may gain benefits from his situation and may not be overly concerned about the dysfunction. The mental anguish associated with the patient's condition is not easily recognized by the people who surround him, but a somatic complaint, like back pain, is one that is readily accepted and understood.

Psychogenic rheumatism is a term that may

be used in patients who have musculoskeletal symptoms, like back pain, associated with a psychiatric disorder.[17] The criteria for this diagnosis include the absence of an organic disease or the insufficiency of disease that is present to account for the complaints, "functional" character of the complaints, and a positive diagnosis for a psychiatric illness. In one large population of rheumatology patients, approximately 7% had a diagnosis of psychogenic rheumatism. However, the separation of psychogenic rheumatism and organic disease was seldom distinct.

One specific form of psychiatric disorder associated with back pain is camptocormia.[18] Camptocormia is derived from the Greek words kamptein, to bend, and kormos, trunk. It is a special form of conversion hysteria occurring mainly in soldiers and industrial workers. The disease consists of assumption of a position in which the back is flexed acutely, the arms hang loosely, and the eyes are directed downward after a trivial trauma. The position disappears when the patient assumes a recumbent position. Many of these individuals are men whose parents have had back disorders. Therapy for the condition is separation of the individuals from the source of stress. Patients have had quick recoveries within days of receiving the news of discharge from the Armed Forces.[18]

Case Study 16–2: *A 23-year-old hotel maintenance man developed acute low back pain while lifting heavy sofa cushions at work. He had no response to conservative therapy and developed a severe headache and increased back pain after a myelogram. He described his pain as constant with radiation up his back to his neck and down to his feet. His pain was so severe that he was limited to walking 15 minutes/day. He was unable to shave or dress himself and relied on his wife for activities of daily living. His physical examination revealed an individual "stuck" in a forward flexed posture at 20°. The motion of the lumbar spine was severely limited. The patient was unable to raise his arms secondary to low back pain. He also reported back pain with movement of his wrists and hands. He had cogwheeling movements of his lower extremities and "no feeling" in his entire left leg. He had back pain with vertical loading over his skull. He also had facial grimacing, muscle tremors, cramps of his hands, sweating, and gagging during his examination. Although in the standing position he was unable to straighten his spine, he was able to lie flat on the examining table when assuming a supine position. During a functional capacity examination and work hardening program, he was unable to complete minimal tasks (lifting a 1 pound weight from waist to shoulder level) secondary to pain. This individual has a form of camptocormia in*
which his physical condition maintains his role as a patient for all the individuals with whom he interacts including his family and his employer. The possibility of return to work for these types of individuals is poor.

Rotes-Querol has suggested a list of symptoms and signs found in patients with psychogenic rheumatism.[17] These symptoms do not have diagnostic importance until the possibility of organic disease has been ruled out. The symptoms and signs include the following:

1. Dramatic urgency for an appointment not justified by the severity of disease.

2. A written list of complaints so that no fact is left out.

3. Multiple test results including EKG, EMG, EEG, barium enema, upper GI, CT scans, myelograms, MR.

4. The necessity to review the laboratory data first to determine the cause of the patient's symptoms. Any minor abnormalities are highlighted by the patient.

5. Preoccupation with future disability from minor physical changes.

6. Those who accompany the patient may be separated from the patient's condition or intensively supportive, highlighting every abnormality and frequently using the pronoun "we" during the description of tests or medications taken.

7. Inability to relax during the examination.

8. Marked theatrical responses to questions concerning pain.

9. Patient frequently holds on to the physician during the course of the examination as a gesture of seeking support.

The evaluation of the psychiatric patient must be complete. A thorough history is essential to remove the possibility of an organic cause of a patient's pain. This type of evaluation also gains the patient's confidence that the physician has been thorough and concerned about the problem. At a second session, the possibility of stress as a cause of the patient's pain is raised. Additional portions of the patient's history concerning job or family stresses or conflicts are asked. The patient may be willing to talk about the faults of others in the workplace but will remain reticent about sexual conflicts with spouses, or conflicts with parents or children, unless specifically asked about these interpersonal difficulties.

The patient must be told that the pain is of psychogenic origin. Statements by the physician denying the presence of an illness ("It is all in your own imagination") are inappropriate. The explanation of the fact that patients who are anxious, threatened, or stressed experience real pain is reassuring to the patient. These patients are referred to a mental health professional for care of their psychiatric disorders. While the patient is undergoing psychiatric therapy, the referring physician should encourage the patient to be as physically active as possible. Interaction with other people in an exercise class may be very useful.

Patients with low back pain frequently ask the question concerning the association of stress or anxiety with the onset or exacerbation of pain. Feuerstein studied the mood fluctuations of patients with recurrent low back pain with matched healthy controls. Patients with pain had higher levels of anxiety, tension, and fatigue and lower levels of vigor. No mood state was predictive of pain onset, but fatigue was more common after the onset of pain. No mood set predicted the severity of pain, but greater levels of pain were correlated with levels of fatigue. Although this study does not clearly demonstrate the correlation of anxiety and the initiation of pain, the control of established pain requires the reduction of anxiety and the improvement of functional endurance to counteract the fatigue factor associated with low back pain. A regular exercise program has the potential to decrease fatigue, relieve stress, and reduce pain.[19]

Despite careful evaluation and the institution of appropriate therapy, patients with psychogenic rheumatism may not improve. The following case study demonstrates the difficulties in the treatment of these patients:

Case Study 16–3: A 26-year-old woman was referred for evaluation of back pain. The patient had worked as a bookkeeper for her husband's company but was now unemployed. She had been divorced once and had two children by her first marriage. She had remarried but had become disenchanted with her marriage because of physical threats by her spouse. Eight months prior to her evaluation, she was pushed down by her husband, hitting her lower back on the ground. Subsequent to that event, the patient experienced severe back pain radiating down both legs, anterior and posterior aspects. The patient felt most comfortable standing, since sitting and lying increased her pain. An extensive work-up including a CT scan, myelogram, and MR revealed a minimal protrusion of a disc without nerve impingement. A multitude of therapeutic modalities, including nonsteroidals, physical therapy, and nerve blocks, were ineffective.

On examination, the patient had exquisite pain of the lumbar area with slight pressure on the skin over the low back. With palpation of the back, the patient would grimace and jump. She had low back pain with lateral bending of the neck and downward pressure on her head. Her muscle tests revealed cogwheeling and resisting movements.

The possibility of a psychiatric problem as a cause of the patient's pain was offered as one explanation of her symptoms. The patient's thought that an operation to remove a disc would "cure" her problem was discounted.

Attempts at involving the patient in psychiatric therapy were not successful. The patient remained at home with her husband. On subsequent visits, she offered the history that she was fearful and anxious and could not decide whether to leave her spouse or stay at home. Her back pain continued to be severe.

Despite the best of efforts, some patients with low back pain will not improve. Some patients with psychiatric disorders fit into this group. All the clinician can do is rule out the possibility of an organic cause of pain and discuss, in a frank but supportive fashion, the psychologic sources of the patient's symptoms. The care of these patients is time-consuming. Often a busy practitioner will not have the time to treat these patients. If that is the case, these patients should be referred to a psychiatrist, psychologist, or other mental health care professional for continued evaluation and therapy.

Psychiatric Illness Associated with Chronic Pain

Patients with acute injuries recognize the linkage between pain (nociception) and tissue injury. The pain serves a purpose to warn the host that injury has occurred and removal of the body part from the injurious stimulus is warranted. The pain that remains after the immediate injury results in decreased use of that body part during the healing process. That portion of the body is protected. Once the injury heals, the pain disappears.

The patient with chronic pain does not follow this scenario. Chronic pain is defined as pain that has been present for 6 months or longer.[20] The most significant factor differentiating chronic from acute pain is that the pain is no longer serving a useful biologic or survival function and has become a disease itself. The emotional state of patients, involving affective, vegetative, cognitive, and behavioral components of personality, is affected. This was noted during the Civil War by Mitchell, who described the development of dejection and anger in soldiers who developed chronic causalgia.[21] The patient undergoes a progressive physical and emotional deterioration caused by loss of appetite, insomnia, depression, anxiety, decreased physical activity, demoralization, and depressive symptoms of worthlessness, helplessness, and hopelessness. These patients have the clinical signs and symptoms of the chronic pain syndrome.[22]

The effects of the chronic pain syndrome will vary depending on the patient's ethnic background, coping skills, and self-image and the support system contributed by the patient's family and fellow workers. Understanding the patient's psychosocial dynamics has a profound effect on the prognosis and the choice of therapy. A psychosocial assessment of the patient with chronic pain can identify the strengths and weaknesses in the patient's personality structure that will influence the manifestations of the pain syndrome and identify those factors that may hinder compliance with the treatment regimen.

The psychologic assessment of the patient with chronic pain may include evaluation of the patient's personality and conceptualization of the pain, along with a rating scale for the severity of pain. The MMPI is the most widely used personality test.[23] The purpose of the test is to categorize psychiatric patients and to discriminate between psychiatric patients and normal patients through the answers to 566 true/false questions. The questions are divided into the following 10 clinical scales: hypochondriasis, depression, hysteria, psychopathic deviance, masculinity/femininity, paranoia, psychasthenia, schizophrenia, hypomania, and social introversion.

Patients with chronic pain indicate an elevation in neuroticism manifested by increases on the hypochondriasis, depression, and hysteria scales. The basic interpretation of this profile is that it reflects a preoccupation with physical symptoms, bodily functions, depression, negativism, hostility, and use of denial to cope with psychologic conflicts. The data record for patients who have less depression forms a "V" shape on the MMPI, which is referred to as a "conversion V" pattern. These patients somatosize their problems when under stress. Physical symptoms are easier for these patients to understand than psychologic conflicts.

The results of the MMPI taken by chronic pain patients have been reported by a number of investigators. Sternbach reported neurotic scale elevation in patients with chronic back pain as compared with those who have acute low back pain.[24] Neurosis was not a permanent part of the patient's personality as shown by a reduction in neurotic scales in patients who had pain relief after back surgery.[25] Fordyce has noted that the degree of neuroticism in MMPI studies is related more to the chronicity of the pain than to the physical lesion.[26]

Bradley has identified three homogeneous subgroups of low back pain patients based upon MMPI profiles.[27] The first group is normal patients who are functioning well in their job and family life with a minimum of disruption, despite back pain. The second, most common, group is composed of patients who are neurotic. The third group manifests a psychopathologic profile that shows elevations in all scales except the masculinity/femininity scale. These patient have significant psychiatric dysfunction diagnosed as schizophrenia, psychotic depression, or inadequate personality. Heaton also has used the MMPI to characterize chronic pain patients into seven groupings.[28] A report by Love and Peck suggests that the psychologic etiology of chronic low back pain and the response of individuals to specific therapy cannot be differentiated by the MMPI.[29]

MMPI has been used in the evaluation of industrial workers who report injury associated with chronic pain. In a prospective study of industrial workers, MMPI was used to predict the likelihood of reporting back injury.[30] MMPI scale 3 (lassitude/malaise) had the greatest predictive power of those who report back pain from an injury. However, job dissatisfaction is also a contributing factor since 75% of workers in this study had back pain but only 5% reported a painful injury.

The results of all the studies of MMPI suggest that the test is helpful in characterizing the psychologic profile of some patients with chronic low back. However, the test is cumbersome, does not predict all individuals who will develop pain, and does not define the appropriate and effective therapy for chronic pain patients.

The McGill pain questionnaire assesses how patients conceptualize their pain by using words to qualify and quantify it. There are a total of 78 pain descriptors in the questionnaire. In one study, psychiatric disturbance was associated with a greater total number of pain descriptors.[31] Patients may also use visual pain analogue scales to quantify their pain. A daily log of the patient's pain level, along with degree of physical activity, and medication usage can be used to assess the patient's functional status and monitor progress. Whether estimations of pain intensity are correlated with the clinical status and health care utilization of a patient has been challenged by Fordyce.[32] Patient self-reports of pain may not accurately describe their level of functioning. However, the ratings of pain by the patient do help in monitoring progress in treatment.

In addition to those tests already mentioned, a mental status examination and a social and work history are essential. These evaluations focus on the patient's thought processes and self-image. The work history is important to list the patient's work experiences and test those job skills the patient retains that may be used in vocational rehabilitation.

The classification of psychiatric diagnoses of pain patients is difficult. The Diagnostic and Statistical Manual of Mental Disorders, 3rd Edition (DSM-III) is the standard for the nomenclature of psychiatric diagnoses. In a study of 1801 patients seen by a psychiatric consultation service, 167 pain patients were compared with the remainder in regard to their DSM-III diagnosis. The pain patients had more serious medical problems, lack of improvement in medical condition, and decreased mobility. Nonpain patients had more serious psychiatric disorders. The psychiatric diagnoses of the pain patients were nonspecific for the problem of pain, including dysthymic disorder, and depressed mood. DSM does not provide specificity of the clinical state of pain including the separation of chronic and acute syndromes.[33]

A variety of DSM diagnoses, including depression, somatosensory conversion disorder, anxiety, and personality disorders, were used for the characterization of 283 chronic pain patients at a pain center. Diagnosis of schizophrenia and psychogenic disorders was rare. The authors of this study also agree that difficulties exist in characterizing patients with chronic pain with the current DSM classification.[34]

Treatment of patients with chronic pain must be directed at physical-structural abnormalities if they persist and, equally important, at pain behavior of the patient. The four most important factors determining successful outcome in rehabilitation of chronic pain patients are the following in order of importance: (1) motivation, (2) social support system, (3) chronicity, and (4) degree of tissue pathology.[35] Correction of tissue pathology is important but may not be adequate to alter pain behavior. If the condition has been chronic, patients may have altered their behavior because of the pain to the point where they have lost control over their lives.[36] These individuals, in response to the loss of control, develop reduced motivation to initiate responses to the environment, inability to learn new responses, depression, and anxiety disorders. Depression was noted in over 50% of patients with chronic low back

pain resistant to medical and surgical therapy.[37] The reality of being in pain and out of work can also contribute to psychologic dysfunction. Dependency becomes all-encompassing in a patient who is unemployed, is financially insecure, and is experiencing deteriorating interpersonal relationships with family members and social isolation. Therapy of these individuals must be directed at returning control of their lives back to each patient.

Patients with chronic, resistant back pain benefit from an evaluation by a pain center. Pain centers have the resources to deal with a patient's situation in a multidisciplinary fashion. Psychiatrists, psychologists, neurosurgeons, anesthesiologists, physical therapists, vocational rehabilitation counselors, and social workers are part of the treatment team. Through the concerted effort of all these health professionals and the motivation of the patient, improvement in the patient's condition can occur. A study of 38 patients with disabling chronic pain at an inpatient/outpatient pain center demonstrated an improvement in patient function at 3 weeks. Patients at the pain center had significant reduction in addictive medications, subjective pain ratings, the number of functional activities that caused pain, and the number of health professional visits.[38]

Malingering

Malingering, which may be defined as conscious misrepresentation of thoughts, feelings, and facts, is a condition in which symptoms and signs associated with back pain are entirely feigned for secondary gain.[39] Most commonly, malingering occurs in the setting of the workplace and workmen's compensation. However, the secondary gain associated with malingering may not be financial alone. Individuals may feign back symptoms to continue in a less strenuous job at work. They may receive a parking space closer to their place of employment. These individuals may feign symptoms to gain control over family members or fellow workers. The injured party may allow others to do work the patient would do ordinarily.

The actual percentage of chronic back pain patients who are malingering is undetermined. Obviously, the ascertainment of the inaccuracy of the patient's report of pain and disability is a difficult process. Each health care provider has an internalized standard of symptoms and signs by which those with chronic low back pain are judged. However, most physicians who see a large population of low back pain patients believe that the number of individuals who are true malingerers—those who totally feign injury and pain in a willful manner to collect workmen's compensation or disability payments— is a very small percentage of the individuals with low back pain. A survey of a total of 300 orthopedists and neurosurgeons quantified the percentage of malingerers among back pain patients to be 5% or less.[40]

The possibility of malingering should be raised in the mind of the treating physician when major discrepancies or inconsistencies appear in the patient's medical situation. Seventeen patients with chronic low back pain with inconsistencies in their statements or behaviors were compared to subjects assessed without inconsistencies. Inconsistent subjects were more likely to have pending litigation and were more focused on pain with more dramatized complaints, lower levels of medical findings, and less interest in treatment.[41]

These inconsistencies may involve the patient's history or physical examination. The following two case studies are examples of how patients who are malingering can be identified by history or physical examination.

Case Study 16–4: A 24-year-old woman slipped and fell while working at a restaurant. She experienced acute low back pain. Over the next year, the patient complained of continued pain that was unrelenting. The pain was so severe that the patient had decreased range of motion of the lumbar spine. The patient stated that the pain with motion was so severe that she was unable to bend her back. She had received courses of nonsteroidal anti-inflammatory drugs, muscle relaxants, physical therapy, and transcutaneous nerve stimulation. All these therapies had no effect on her pain. She could not go back to work because she could not bend or carry objects. Formal testing of the motion of her lumbar spine was markedly limited. No palpable muscle spasm was noted. During the physical examination, nail polish was noted on her fingers and toes. She was asked who applied the polish to her nails. She said she did her own nails. Her lack of motion was feigned. In the privacy of her home, she had full range of motion of her spine. Other distraction tests completed during the physical examination corroborated the fact that the patient was malingering.

The second case illustrates the suggestibility of the malingering patient. They are willing to agree with any of the statements of the examining physician. The patient believes that whatever the physician suggests as symptoms or signs of the disease must be correct.

Case Study 16–5: A 36-year-old man was working on a construction site when he developed back pain while lifting some lumber. The patient developed localized, right-sided lumbar pain. The patient was placed on bed rest and nonsteroidal anti-inflammatory drugs. He had no response to therapy. He was referred to our office and was evaluated. A suspicion of malingering was raised, but the patient was given another course of nonsteroidals to monitor his response. When he returned he reported no response to therapy. It was suggested to him that palpation of areas other than the lumbar spine may cause low back pain. The patient's nose was pressed and patient complained that the maneuver recreated his low back pain. We referred to this as "Rudolph, the Red-Nosed Reindeer" sign.

The assessment of malingering by the treating physician is very difficult. It is difficult to positively prove conscious misrepresentation of thoughts, feelings, and facts by the patient. However, the inconsistencies in history and physical examination are useful in documenting one's suspicions.

Two separate sets of criteria have been developed to document the likelihood of malingering.[42, 43] Although the Emory Pain Control Center "inconsistency profile" and Ellard's profile of inconsistency were developed independently, they are remarkably similar. The Emory profile is an amalgamation of those factors which would lead the examining physician to suspect malingering. The profile includes the following:

1. Discrepancy between a person's complaint of "terrible pain" and an attitude of calmness and well-being.

2. Complete negative work-up for organic disease by two or more physicians.

3. "Dramatized" complaints that are vague or have global implications ("It just hurts" or "I hurt bad").

4. Exaggeration of trivial pathology, embellished with medical terms learned from previous contacts with physicians ("My back spasms paralyze my legs").

5. Overemphasized gait or posture abnormalities that develop suddenly, persist, and cannot be substantiated objectively (the presence of a limp which is not confirmed by a specific pattern of wear of old shoes, the use of a cane, or a back brace that is said to be used on a daily basis but shows little wear).

6. Resistance to evaluation or rehabilitation when the stated goal of therapy is return to gainful employment.

7. Lack of motivation to learn new coping skills, despite verbal reports of compliance with treatment (no increase in back motion despite claims of completing range of motion exercise on a daily basis).

8. Missed appointments for studies that

measure function, motion, or vocational capabilities.

9. Unconventional response to treatment (no discrimination between saline and analgesic injection into affected areas; reports of increased symptoms with therapy that follow no anatomic or physiologic pattern—response to tranquilizers as stimulants and vice versa).

10. Resistance to treatment procedures, especially in presence of intense complaints of pain.

11. Absence of psychologic or emotional disturbances.

12. Inconsistent psychologic test profile with clinical presentations. For example, MMPI profile indicative of a psychotic disorder with no clinical signs of psychosis.

13. Discrepancies between reports of patient and spouse or other close relatives.

14. Unstable personal and occupational history.

15. A personal history that reflects a character disorder that might include drug and/or alcohol abuse, criminal behavior, erratic personal relationships, and violence.

As suggested by the inconsistency profile, physical examination of the malingerer is often helpful and revealing. The patient may refuse to cooperate with components of the examination.[44] Patients with low back pain may be better able to exaggerate symptoms than those individuals who are pain free when using pain questionnaires.[45] Gait abnormalities may not be present when the patient initially enters the office but are during the formal examination. A normal lumbar lordosis without paraspinous muscle spasm is unusual in the patient with persistent low back pain, in whom a decreased lordosis would be expected. Gently touching the skin over the back results in intense pain with reflex spasm. The area of tenderness may vary during the examination. It is worthwhile to retest the area of tenderness during the course of the physical examination. Not infrequently, the patient does not remember the exact location of the tenderness and an inconsistency is noted. Patients will be unable to bend forward more than 5° despite the absence of muscle spasm. (Patients without spasm should be able to rotate around the hips, resulting in flexion of the upper body despite lumbar spine disease.) Patients may have a limited straight leg raising test in the supine position, but normal motion without pain with the modified straight leg test in the seated position or the bilateral straight leg test. The Hoover test will document the patient's

effort to complete the requested physical test. The absence of muscle atrophy belies a history of chronic leg weakness.

Once all the data have been collected, the physician should make a determination of malingering by the patient. This is a difficult process which requires the diagnostic and detective skill of the physician. Very few things in medicine are black and white. The same can be said about malingering. Very few malingerers are totally without pain or the fear of being placed back in a job situation that may be perceived as harmful.

Some physicians prefer to remove themselves from the determination of malingering, and leave it to others, including lawyers, to make the determinations of impairment and disability. If the process is allowed to function without medical input, those who do not really deserve compensation or consideration will diminish the resources that rightfully belong to those who have organic difficulties and are attempting to function at their maximum capacity. If the physician believes the patient is a malingerer, he should terminate further treatment of the patient. The patient should be told that there is no anatomic abnormality that can explain the pain. If the patient has been evaluated only once, he should be referred to another physician for an additional opinion. If the first physician was in error, the second physician can initiate appropriate therapy. If the first physician was correct, no additional investigations are ordered, and therapy is discontinued.

References

PSYCHIATRIC DISORDERS, CHRONIC PAIN AND MALINGERING

1. Klee GD, Ozelis S, Greenberg I, Gallant LJ: Pain and other somatic complaints in a psychiatric clinic. Maryland St Med J 8:188, 1959.
2. Spear FG: Pain in psychiatric patients. J Psychosom Res 11:187, 1967.
3. Delaplaine R, Ifabumuyi OI, Mersky H, Zarfas J: Significance of pain in psychiatric hospital patients. Pain 4:361, 1978.
4. International Association for the Study of Pain (Subcommittee on Taxonomy): Pain terms: a list with definitions and notes on usage. Pain 6:249, 1979.
5. Walters A: Psychogenic regional pain alias hysterical pain. Brain 84:1, 1961.
6. Merskey H: The characteristics of persistent pain in psychological illness. J Psychosom Res 9:291, 1965.
7. Pilling LF, Brannick TL, Swenson WM: Psychological characteristics of patients having pain as a presenting symptom. Can Med Assoc J 97:387, 1967.
8. Hanvik LH: MMPI profiles in patients with low-back pain. J Consult Clin Psychol 15:350, 1956.

9. Sternbach RA: Pain Patients: Traits and Treatment. New York: Academic Press, 1974.

10. Pilowsky I, Chapman CR, Bonica JJ: Pain, depression, and illness behavior in a pain clinic population. Pain 4:183, 1977.

11. Pelz M, Merskey H: A description of the psychological effects of chronic painful lesions. Pain 14:293, 1982.

12. Merskey H: Pain and Psychological Medicine. In Wall PD, Melzack R (eds): Textbook of Pain. Edinburgh: Churchill Livingstone, 1984, pp 496–502.

13. Watson GD, Chandarana PC, Merskey H: Relationships between pain and schizophrenia. Br J Psychiatry 138:33, 1981.

14. Lewis T, Pickering GW, Rothschild P: Observations upon muscular pain in intermittent claudication. Heart 15:359, 1931.

15. Sainsbury P, Gibson JG: Symptoms of anxiety and tension and the accompanying physiological changes in the muscular system. Psychosom Med 17:216, 1954.

16. Harper RC, Steger JC: Psychological correlates of frontalis EMG and pain in tension headache. Headache 18:215, 1978.

17. Rotes-Querol J: The syndrome of psychogenic rheumatism. Clin Rheum Dis 5:797, 1979.

18. Rockwood CA Jr, Eilbert RE: Camptocormia, J Bone Joint Surg 51A: 553, 1969.

19. Feuerstein M, Carter RL, Papciak AS: A prospective analysis of stress and fatigue in recurrent low back pain. Pain 31:333, 1987.

20. Sternbach RA: Pain: A Psychophysiological Analysis. New York: Academic Press, 1968.

21. Mitchell SW, Moorehouse GR, Keen WW: Gunshot Wounds and Other Injuries of Nerves. Philadelphia: JB Lippincott Co, 1864.

22. Black RG: The chronic pain syndrome. Surg Clin North Am 4:999, 1975.

23. Dahlstrom WG, Welsh GS, Dahlstrom LE: An MMPI Handbook, Vol I and II. Minneapolis: University of Minnesota Press, 1972.

24. Sternbach RA, Wolf SR, Murphy RW, Akeson WH: Traits of pain patients: the low-back "loser." Psychosom 14:226, 1973.

25. Sternbach RA, Timmermans G: Personality changes associated with reduction of pain. Pain 1:177, 1975.

26. Fordyce WE: Behavioral methods in chronic pain and illness. St Louis: CV Mosby Co, 1976.

27. Bradley LA, Prokop CK, Margolis R, Gentry DD: Multivariate analysis of the MMPI profiles of low back pain patients. J Behav Med 1:253, 1978.

28. Heaton RK, Getto CJ, Lehman RAW, et al.: A standardized evaluation of psychosocial factors in chronic pain. Pain 12:165, 1982.

29. Love AW, Peck CL: The MMPI and psychological factors in chronic low back pain: a review. Pain 28:1, 1987.

30. Fordyce WE, Bigos SJ, Battie MC, Fisher LD: MMPI scale 3 as a predictor of back injury report: what does it tell us? Clin J Pain 8:222, 1992.

31. Kremer EF, Atkinson JH, Kremer AM: The language of pain: affective descriptors of pain are a better predictor of psychological disturbance than sensory and effective descriptors. Pain 16:185, 1983.

32. Fordyce WE, Lansky D, Calsyn DA, et al.: Pain measurement and pain behavior. Pain 18:53, 1984.

33. King SA, Strain JJ: The problem of psychiatric diagnosis for the pain patient in the general hospital. Clin J Pain 5:329, 1989.

34. Fishbain DA, Goldberg M, Meagher BR, et al.: Male and female chronic pain patients categorized by DSM-III psychiatric diagnostic criteria. Pain 26:181, 1986.

35. Ng LKY (ed): New Approaches to Treatment of Chronic Pain: A Review of Multidisciplinary Pain Clinics and Pain Centers. US Dept HEW, NIDA, Monograph Series 36, 1981.

36. Woodforde JM, Merskey H: Personality traits of patients with chronic pain. J Psychosom Res 16:167, 1972.

37. Maruta T, Swanson DW, Swenson WM: Low back pain in a psychiatric population. Mayo Clin Proc 51:57, 1976.

38. Smith GT, Hughes LB, Duvall RD, Rothman S: Treatment outcome of a multidisciplinary center for management of chronic pain: a long-term follow-up. Clin J Pain 4:47, 1988.

39. Finneson BE: Low Back Pain, 2nd ed. Philadelphia: JB Lippincott Co, 1981, pp 179–197.

40. Leavitt F, Sweet JJ: Characteristics and frequency of malingering among patients with low back pain. Pain 25:357, 1986.

41. Chapman SL, Brena SF: Patterns of conscious failure to provide accurate self-report data in patients with low back pain. Clin J Pain 6:178, 1990.

42. Ellard J: Psychological reactions to compensable injury. Med J Aust 8:349, 1970.

43. Brena SF, Chapman SL: Pain and litigation. In Wall PD, Melzack R (ed): Textbook of Pain. Edinburgh: Churchill Livingstone, 1984, pp 832–839.

44. Cunnien AJ: Psychiatric and medical syndromes associated with deception. In Rogers R (ed): Clinical Assessment of Malingering and Deception. New York: The Guilford Press, 1988, pp 13–33.

45. Leavitt F: Detection of simulation among persons instructed to exaggerate symptoms of low back pain. J Occup Med 29:229, 1987.

17

Referred Pain

Back pain occurs not only with diseases that affect the bones, joints, ligaments, tendons, and other component parts of the lumbosacral spine but also as a significant symptom of disorders of the vascular, genitourinary, and gastrointestinal systems. Some of the visceral organs of the abdomen and pelvis lie in proximity to the lumbosacral spine. Inflammation, infection, or hemorrhage that originates in the aorta, pancreas, or kidney may spread beyond the confines of these organs, stimulating sensory nerves within the lumbosacral spine. This direct stimulation of sensory nerves not only results in pain that is localized to the damaged area but also may be experienced in a location other than the one being stimulated. The pain occurs in superficial tissues supplied by the same segment of the spinal cord that sends afferent sensory fibers to the diseased area. This is called "referred pain."

Referred pain occurs as a result of the organization of the nervous system and the embryologic location of the visceral organs. Sensory impulses of somatic origin (skin and parietal peritoneum, for example) travel by somatic afferent neurons to the dorsal root ganglia and then into the posterior horn of the spinal cord. They synapse either with a second neuron that crosses to the opposite side of the cord and ascends to the cerebral cortex through the lateral spinothalamic tract or with motor neurons in the anterior horn of the spinal cord at the same level. Sensory impulses from visceral structures, such as the duodenum or pancreas, travel in visceral afferent nerve fibers that accompany fibers of the sympathetic nervous system through the rami communicantes and the posterior horn to join somatic sensory neurons in the posterior horn of the spinal cord. The visceral afferent fibers may travel cranially or caudally in the gray matter of the dorsal horn before synapsing with neurons of the spinothalamic tract.

Sensory impulses of visceral origin travel the same path to the brain as somatic afferent nerves. The radiation of visceral afferents to a number of spinal cord segments may explain the diffuse, poorly localized character of visceral pain. The organization of the spinal segment is further complicated by projections of neurons from higher centers in the brain that may intensify or diminish either visceral or somatic pain. Sensory stimulation of visceral origin may spill over in the dorsal horn to affect somatic sensory nerves and result in pain that is felt only in the corresponding segmental somatic distribution (a dermatome of skin). Sensory input may also stimulate motor fibers in the anterior horn, and their stimulation results in muscle contraction and spasm.

The segment of the spinal cord that supplies a visceral structure is dependent not on its anatomic location in the fully developed adult, but on its original location in the developing human embryo. Visceral organs migrate to their final location taking along their nerve and vascular supplies, and referred pain from these organs will be sensed in the somatic distribution of their embryologic origin. For example, since the twelfth thoracic and first lumbar nerves supply the visceral sensory input of the uterus, referred somatic pain originating from the uterus is felt in the groin area, which receives its somatic sensory input from the same L1 segment.

Patients with visceral disease in the abdomen may experience three types of pain. True visceral pain is felt at the site of primary stimulation and is dull and aching in character. It has a diffuse and deep location. This is particularly true of visceral structures that originate in the midline (small intestine) and have visceral sensory input from both sides of the spinal cord. Visceral pain from the kidney is more easily localized, since the sensory innervation to it is unilateral.

Deep somatic pain in the abdomen is related to stimulation of the parietal peritoneum. These impulses are transmitted by somatic pathways. The pain is localized, sharp, and intense in character. These pains are frequently associated with reflex abdominal wall muscle spasm.

Referred pain to the lumbosacral spine from lesions in the aorta or the genitourinary or gastrointestinal tract is characteristically sharp and relatively well localized to the skin. Hyperalgesia may be noted in the area of referred pain, and reflex muscle contraction also may be present. Although referred pain usually occurs in combination with visceral and somatic pain, occasionally it may exist in the absence of visceral pain or symptoms of an underlying disease.

In the setting of low back pain and no associated visceral symptoms, a complete history, physical examination, and laboratory evaluation are essential to discover the source of the visceral referred pain. Characteristically, back pain that is referred from visceral structures is not aggravated by activity or relieved by recumbency. Abdominal examination may uncover an asymptomatic pulsatile mass, indicative of an abdominal aortic aneurysm, or rectal examination may reveal blood in the stool, suggesting a hidden malignancy. Laboratory evaluation may show pyuria, indicative of urinary tract infection, or increased amylase, reflective of pancreatitis. Referred pain from a visceral structure must be considered as the cause of low back pain when mechanical, rheumatologic, infectious, metabolic, and neoplastic origins of the pain have been eliminated as possibilities.

VASCULAR DISEASES

Abdominal Aortic Disease

Capsule Summary

Frequency of back pain—rare to uncommon

Location of back pain—left lumbar paraspinous area

Quality of back pain—dull ache to sharp tearing

Symptoms and signs—epigastric pain, not affected by position; hypertension, smoking history, pulsatile mass, hypotension with rupture

Laboratory and x-ray tests—decreased hematocrit with rupture; curvilinear calcification on plain roentgenogram, aortic enlargement on sonogram or CT scan

Treatment—surgical excision with enlargement greater than 5 cm

ABDOMINAL ANEURYSM

Low back pain associated with disease of the abdominal aorta may occur secondary to aneurysmal dilatation, rupture, or obstruction of the vessel. The abdominal aorta is located in the retroperitoneum, just to the left of the midline. The abdominal aorta splits at the L4 vertebra to form the common iliac arteries, which supply the lower extremities. An arterial aneurysm is a localized or diffuse enlargement of an artery. One or all three layers (intima, media, and adventitia) of the aorta make up the wall of the aneurysm. A dissecting aneurysm is caused by the formation of a false channel in the wall of the aorta that splits apart the layers of the vessel. Saccular aneurysms are bulbous protrusions of all three layers on one side of the vessel. A fusiform aneurysm is a diffuse, circumferential expansion of a segment of the vessel.

Abdominal aneurysms occur most commonly in white men between the ages of 60 and 70[1]; however, they have been reported in patients as early as in the fourth decade of life and are quite common in people over the age of 50.[2] The aneurysms occur four times more often in men than in women. The incidence of abdominal aneurysm is increasing as the number of elderly people increases.[3] Between 10 and 40 per 1000 people over the age of 50 may have this abnormality. Abdominal aortic aneurysms were responsible for 14,982 deaths in the United States in 1988 among people 55 years of age or older.[4] In a Swedish study, the incidence among men increased rapidly after age 55, with a peak of 5.9% at age 80; among women, the increase occurred after age 70 with a peak of 4.5% at age 90.[5] The estimated financial loss for hospitals who have patients with ruptured aneurysms is $24,655 per individual.[6]

The aneurysms are fusiform in configuration and extend from an area just inferior to the renal arteries to the common iliac artery bifurcation. Only 5% have dilatation of the suprarenal aorta.[2] The inferior mesenteric artery frequently arises out of the aneurysm. The iliac arteries and common and superficial femoral arteries are occasionally affected. Patients with abdominal aneurysms may have aneurysms of other types (saccular) and location (thoracic, popliteal) in association with generalized arterial disease.

The pathogenesis of the aneurysm is related to atherosclerotic degeneration with structural weakening of the connective tissue (collagen) of the vessel wall. Patients with abdominal aneurysm are usually hypertensive and may demonstrate manifestations of generalized atherosclerosis, including angina, previous myocardial infarction, stroke, or peripheral vascular disease.[7] Trauma, in itself, is not an etiologic factor, although it may cause rupture of a pre-existent aneurysm.[8] A number of studies have also described a familial tendency (possible genetic predisposition) for the development of abdominal aneurysm.[9, 10] First-degree relatives are at significantly increased risk for development of aneurysmal degeneration. At a minimum, review of family history for aortic disease is warranted in patients with back pain. Noninvasive screening tests to detect early aortic disease may be indicated in patients with a strong family history of aneurysms. Family studies have demonstrated increased prevalence of aneurysms in brothers and sons of patients who died secondary to ruptured aneurysms.[11]

Two theories have been proposed as the cause of aneurysmal enlargement. The first cause is that a genetic linked deficit in the quantity and quality of collagen and elastin in the arterial wall causes generalized arteriomegaly. This would explain the fact that a number of vessels may be affected in a patient. A second cause is that plaque from atherosclerosis interferes with the blood supply of the arterial wall resulting in weakening of the wall.[12] Inflammatory mediators, such as interleukin-8 and monocyte chemoattractant protein-1, have been identified in aortic aneurysms. These factors are chemoattractant to leukocytes and recruit inflammatory cells to the arterial wall causing weakening of the wall.[13] Atherosclerosis may represent a secondary, nonspecific response to vessel-wall injury.

The risk of rupture has been associated with the size and expansion rate of the aneurysm. The average increase in size is 0.4 cm/year. Approximately 80% of small aneurysms increase in diameter, with 20% increasing more than 0.5 cm/year.[4] Aneurysms larger than 5 to 6 cm expand more rapidly. However, the rate of expansion in each patient is unpredictable. Some aneurysms remain stable for years and then expand rapidly. The risk for rupture is 2% in aortic aneurysms less than 4.0 cm in diameter.[14] The 5-year risk of rupture for aneurysms 5.0 cm or more is up to 41%.[15, 16]

Pain associated with abdominal aortic aneurysm occurs secondary to compression of surrounding structures by expansion or rupture of the aneurysm. Patients with stable or slowly enlarging aneurysms are asymptomatic, and this may be the case in a majority of those with an abdominal aneurysm.[1] The aneurysm may be noted as an incidental finding on a radiograph of the abdomen, or as a pulsatile abdominal mass at the level of the umbilicus, which is minimally tender if found on physical examination.

Extension of the aneurysm is associated with increased pain and clinical symptoms. Most frequently, patients experience abdominal pain that is dull, steady, and unrelated to activity or eating. Some patients notice or complain of a ''pounding'' sensation or palpitations in their abdomen. Back pain, when it occurs, is usually associated with epigastric discomfort and may radiate to the hips or thighs. Pressure of the aneurysm on lumbar nerves may give rise to this symptom. With increasing expansion, stretching of the mesenteric root or obstruction of the duodenum is associated with acute episodes of pain and gastrointestinal symptoms of nausea and vomiting. This may simulate gastrointestinal diseases such as pancreatitis or peptic ulcer disease.

Rupture of an abdominal aneurysm is associated with excruciating pain, circulatory shock from blood loss, and an expanding mass. The pain of rupture may be the first clinical sign in a previously asymptomatic patient with an aneurysm. An exacerbation of previously milder pain in a patient with an aneurysm is a harbinger of extension or impending rupture. Ruptures of the abdominal aorta are frequently located at the junction of the aortic attachment to the vertebral bodies and the portion that is unattached in the retroperitoneum. Blood from the ruptured aneurysm may be contained in the retroperitoneum or may pass into the peritoneal cavity or a hollow viscus. Rupture into the retroperitoneum is associated with the sudden onset of severe, tearing, or piercing pain that is continuous and increasing in intensity. The pain is present in the deep abdomen and is referred into the back, legs, and groin.[17] Extension into the lower extremities may be confused with radiculopathy. Patients with a ruptured aorta may present with a history of chronic back pain of a month or more.[12] The hematoma is confined to the retroperitoneal space.

The common physical finding in patients with uncomplicated abdominal aortic disease is the presence of a expansile, pulsatile mass that is located near the level of the umbilicus and frequently extends into the lower abdomen. Palpation of a normal aorta may cause discomfort. The normal aorta is pulsatile, expands in an anterior and lateral direction, and measures approximately 2.5 cm in diameter. As the individual ages, the aorta loses its elasticity and becomes tortuous. The aorta bulges anteriorly to the left or, less commonly, to the right. A tortuous aorta should be rolled under the examining hand to establish a true measure of its size. The ability to palpate an aneurysm in both planes separates true aneurysms from transmitted pulsations, which are palpable only in the anteroposterior direction. The size of the aneurysm, thickness of the abdominal wall, and relaxation of the abdominal wall will have a significant effect on the chances of palpating an aneurysm. The examination is best performed with the patient in the supine position, knees flexed. Pressure should be applied to the abdomen between respirations as the abdominal musculature relaxes.

The patient with an asymptomatic aneurysm may complain of pain with palpation of the abdomen. Tenderness may be more pronounced with impending rupture. Palpation should be gentle to avoid causing the patient discomfort or perturbing the aneurysm.

Physical examination of the patient with abdominal aortic rupture demonstrates hypotension, profuse sweating, and, rarely (because of surrounding hematoma, which camouflages vessel movement), a pulsatile abdominal mass that is tender. The classic triad of hypotension, back pain, and a pulsatile mass may be present in only 50% of patients with ruptured aneurysms.[18] Palpation of the aneurysm may elicit low back pain that radiates into the thigh or lower abdomen.[19] The abdominal wall is usually not rigid. Less frequently, patients have hemorrhagic discoloration of the skin in the back and flanks secondary to a retroperitoneal hematoma, or loss of sensation in the distribution of the femoral nerve along with weakness in the quadriceps musculature as a manifestation of rupture in the psoas region.[20, 21] The status of distal pulses in both lower extremities does not correlate with the presence or absence of an aneurysmal rupture. Neurologic signs, such as leg weakness, may be detected if expansion of the aneurysm compromises blood flow to the spinal cord. In rare circumstances, infarction of the spinal cord may occur.[22]

Laboratory tests may be normal in patients with asymptomatic aneurysm. Patients with ruptured aneurysms may have mild to profound anemia at the time of evaluation depending on the degree of extravascular blood loss. Thrombocytopenia may result from active thrombus deposition.

Ultrasonography and CT of the abdomen are noninvasive diagnostic methods used to identify the presence and extent of an aneurysm (Figs. 17–1 and 17–2). These methods are very reliable in identifying the location of the aneurysm in the abdomen.[23, 24]

Abdominal ultrasonography detects aneurysms with a sensitivity that approaches 100%.[25] The longitudinal and transverse diameters can be determined without radiation or contrast medium. The effectiveness of ultra-

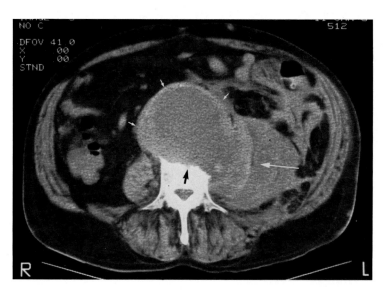

Figure 17–1. CT scan of ruptured abdominal aneurysm. A 72-year-old man presented with abdominal pain and left-sided back pain of acute onset that radiated to the left leg. The abdomen was distended with minimal pulsations of the aorta. Abdominal CT demonstrates old aneurysm (*small white arrows*) and new retroperitoneal bleed (*large white arrow*). An unusual finding is the remodeling of the vertebral body by the aneurysm (*black arrow*). (Courtesy of Joseph Giordano, M.D.)

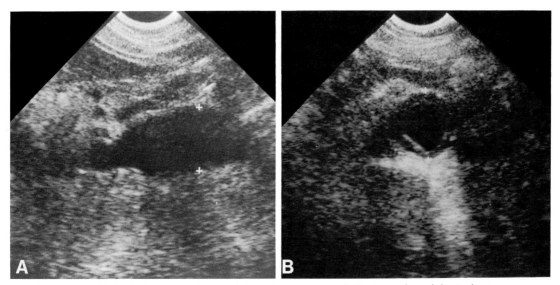

Figure 17–2. Abdominal ultrasound. Sagittal *(A)* and cross-sectional *(B)* views of an abdominal aneurysm. Increased signal in the vessel wall compatible with vascular calcification. (Courtesy of Michael Hill, M.D.)

sound is diminished by excessive bowel gas that obscures the infrarenal abdominal aorta and the pancreas that hides the suprarenal aorta. Therefore, ultrasound is a good screening tool but is not adequate for planning surgery.

CT is highly sensitive and specific for the identification of aneurysms. CT visualizes the suprarenal and infrarenal aorta and accurately determines the size and shape of the aneurysm to a greater degree than ultrasound. Unlike ultrasonography, CT visualizes aortic anomalies, horseshoe kidneys, inferior vena cava anomalies, and involvement of iliac and hypogastric arteries. CT identifies rupture or leaking into the retroperitoneal space. CT may be inaccurate in the evaluation of a tortuous aorta. The use of contrast media and exposure to ionizing radiation are the disadvantages of this radiographic method. Therefore, CT should not be used as a screening method for abdominal aneurysms. CT is most effective when the aneurysm has been identified and a resection is planned. CT scan may be the most useful test in the emergency room setting if surgery is contemplated. CT scan reveals the extent of the aneurysm and extravasation of blood which is important in the preoperative evaluation of the patient by the vascular surgeon.

Magnetic resonance (MR) is another very useful imaging technique and can be used to depict involvement of the renal and iliac arteries.[26] MR can identify vascular anatomy in three planes without the need for contrast dye

or radiation. However, MR is not as accurate as other methods for defining the caudal extension of aneurysms.[27] MR is also more expensive and less available than other radiographic techniques.

Aortography is done in patients with abdominal aneurysm to delineate vascular anatomy. The lack of time to complete the test in the compromised patient with an acute rupture occasionally results in surgery being performed without an angiogram.[28, 29] Aortography may not determine the true size of an aneurysm. Aneurysms commonly have thrombus lining the inner wall. Since the aortogram visualizes only the lumen, the thrombus obscures the true diameter of the aorta. Aortography may be useful in the patient with an aneurysm associated with occlusive disease and ischemic symptoms involving the lower extremities. It depicts the status of the iliac, femoral, and popliteal vessels of the lower extremity prior to operation in these patients (Fig. 17–3). Aortography is used selectively by vascular surgeons for the preoperative planning of aneurysmal resections.

Review of plain films of the abdomen is helpful in detecting abdominal aneurysms. Anteroposterior and lateral projections of the abdomen may demonstrate a curvilinear thin layer of calcification in the wall of the aorta in 70% of patients.[30] Vertebral body erosion is generally not found with an abdominal aneurysm.[31]

The spectrum of abdominal aortic disease is quite broad in regard to both the severity of

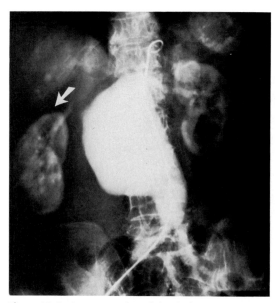

Figure 17–3. Aortogram of an abdominal aneurysm. A 70-year-old woman presented with acute low back pain and a history of a pulsatile aorta. The aortogram reveals an 8-cm aneurysm arising below the renal arteries. A right retroperitoneal mass (hematoma) has caused marked inferior displacement of the right kidney (arrow). (Courtesy of Edward Druy, M.D.)

arterial disease and the extent of organs affected by the expanding aneurysm (Table 17–1). The diagnosis should be considered in the elderly patient with nondescript back pain that does not improve with rest and is exacerbated with activity. Patients with impending rupture have more severe symptoms that may simulate a wide range of illnesses. Disorders that cause back pain that may be mimicked by an aneurysm include peptic ulcer disease, pancreatitis, biliary or renal colic, acute appendicitis, and a herniated intervertebral disc. A misdiagnosis may occur in 30% of patients, with the most common incorrect diagnoses of renal colic, diverticulitis, and gastrointestinal hemorrhage.[32] Careful evaluation of the abdomen with noninvasive methods should identify the presence of an aneurysm (Fig. 17–4). *Salmonella* infection may localize in an abdominal aortic aneurysm and cause progressive symptoms that may call for surgical intervention to repair the aneurysm.[33] Inflammation of the three layers of the aorta may result in narrowing and decreased blood flow. Takayasu's arteritis occurs most commonly in young women. Back pain is a symptom in up to 10% of patients with this disease.[34]

Therapy of abdominal aneurysms is surgical. The presence of an aneurysm 6 cm or more in external diameter is associated with an in-

creased mortality, and if there is no major contraindication, elective resection and bypass of the aneurysm should be considered.[35] Improved survival has been documented for patients who have undergone surgery for intact aneurysms.[36] The mortality from an elective procedure is 2% to 5%. Patients with evidence of a ruptured aneurysm require immediate surgical intervention, since up to 80% of patients with ruptured aneurysms live at least 6 hours after the onset of symptoms. Early operation is the most important factor influencing survival. Recent surgical data suggest that over 70% of patients with ruptured abdominal aneurysms can survive surgery.[37] Complications associated with surgery include shock, myocardial infarction, necrosis of viscera, and renal failure. Infection of the aneurysm may be a complicating factor both pre- and post-operatively.[37–39]

Patients for whom extensive surgery would present a high risk may be treated by alternate means. Induced thrombosis by ligature of both iliac arteries or ligature of the aorta above and below the aneurysm with an axillofemoral artery bypass graft has been utilized. These techniques should be considered only in patients who would not survive extensive surgery.[40, 41]

The prognosis for individuals identified before aortic rupture is good. Even in patients 80 years or older, the operative mortality rate is 3%.[42] The operative mortality for individuals 80 or older with ruptured aneurysms is 91%.[43] Reviewing data from many studies, operative mortality in all age groups of individuals with nonruptured aneurysms is 4% and ruptured aneurysms is 49%.[4] The quality of life is also different for individuals who undergo elective versus emergency surgery. Patients with ruptured aneurysms have a deterioration of quality of life even with a successful operation.[44]

TABLE 17–1.   SPECTRUM OF AORTIC DISEASE

Asymptomatic aneurysm
Symptomatic aneurysm
  Abdominal fullness or pulsation
  Pain—abdominal or lumbar
    Dull, gnawing
    Initially intermittent, then continuous
    Obstruction—ureter, duodenum, vena cava, lower aorta
      Peptic ulcer, renal colic, lower limb claudication
Dissection and/or rupture
  Sudden onset
    Severe pain radiating from abdomen or back into
      groin, buttocks, thighs
  Hypovolemic shock
  Gastrointestinal or retroperitoneal bleeding

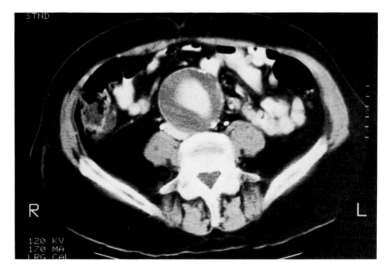

Figure 17–4. Abdominal CT scan with contrast dye. A 73-year-old man presented with very mild, diffuse back pain. CT scan demonstrates an abdominal aneurysm. Contrast dye (white) accentuates the surrounding intraluminal thrombus. (Courtesy of Joseph Giordano, M.D.)

Young patients with small aneurysms should consider resection even with a small risk of expansion.[45] Contraindications for elective reconstruction include myocardial infarction within 6 months, intractable congestive heart failure, severe pulmonary insufficiency, intractable angina pectoris, chronic renal insufficiency, stroke, or a life expectancy of less than 2 years.[5] In regard to screening, an abdominal examination is inexpensive but relatively insensitive for men 60 to 80 years old.[46] A single screen with abdominal ultrasound is of greater benefit but at added cost.[32]

AORTIC OCCLUSION

Obstruction of the abdominal aorta is associated with pain located in the muscles of the low back and gluteal areas. The pain may be of either acute or gradual onset. Patients who develop acute embolic obstruction of the terminal aorta develop acute claudication of the lower extremities and acute, severe low back pain.[47, 48] The source of the embolus is most frequently a mural thrombus from the left side of the heart, which may be generated by a myocardial infarction, cardiomyopathy, valvular disease, atrial fibrillation, or atrial myxoma.[48] The embolus lodges at the bifurcation of the aorta, blocking blood flow to the lower half of the body.[49] Patients experience pain in the thighs, low back, buttocks, and lower abdomen. Neurologic function is impaired, as evidenced by weakness, numbness, and paresthesias. Pulses are lost in the lower extremities, and the skin turns pale. Removal of the clot is required for the patient to survive. Embolectomy may be accomplished with the use of an intra-arterial balloon catheter.

Surgical intervention is usually necessary to restore blood flow. There is a 20% mortality among patients who have had a successful revascularization operation because of underlying cardiac disease.

Low back pain may also be a symptom in patients who develop gradual obstruction of the abdominal aorta.[50] Occasionally they will present with low back pain as their initial symptom, and this pain may occur without associated symptoms of claudication, neurologic dysfunction, or pallor. Back pain from arterial obstruction may be limited to repeated activity, with the pain subsiding with rest. Patients with aortic obstruction may develop Leriche syndrome associated with buttock or thigh claudication and impotence. Claudication occurs in the muscles of the lower extremity, most commonly in the calf and less commonly in the thigh and buttocks. Cramping occurs with exercise and is relieved by rest in 3 to 5 minutes. Rest pain is a symptom of more severe peripheral vascular disease. Rest pain occurs in the toes or forefoot and at night while the individual is recumbent. The supine position lessens the beneficial effect of gravity increasing blood flow to the most distal part of the lower extremity. The sleeping state also decreases cardiac output and blood pressure, further reducing flow. If individuals do not have pain in their feet while recumbent, they do not have rest pain.

Claudication occurs secondary to narrowing or occlusion of major arteries in the lower extremities. With exercise, the peripheral vascular bed dilates to increase blood flow. The arterial pressure does not change despite marked increases in blood flow. In the situation of the patient with claudication, the arterial pressure in arteries distal to the obstruction is reduced to levels below the pressure generated by contracting muscles. The arteries are closed off and symptoms of claudication occur.

Examination of patients with claudication reveals absent pulses and bruits over the iliac or femoral arteries. On occasion, distal pulses may remain palpable. Measurement of ankle arterial pressures is a means to differentiate neurogenic from vascular claudication. The presence of normal ankle pressures following exercise definitively rules out vascular disease as the cause of lower extremity pain.[12] The use of a treadmill and a stationary bicycle has been suggested as a means of differentiating patients with neurogenic and vascular claudication. Patients with neurogenic pain may cycle for long distances without pain, while patients with vascular disease develop pain. However, the treadmill test will not differentiate patients with neurogenic pain if they flex while walking.[51] The results of these exercise tests must be examined carefully to determine the cause of claudication. Vascular pressure measurements or Doppler tests may be required to establish vascular disease.

By-pass grafting is successful in controlling symptoms in 80% of patients undergoing such surgery. Mortality from the operation is greatest with those who have cardiac disease.[50]

References

VASCULAR DISEASES

1. Gore I, Hirst AE Jr: Arteriosclerotic aneurysms of the abdominal aorta: a review. Prog Cardiovasc Dis 16:113, 1973.
2. DeBakey ME, Crawford ES, Cooley DA, et al.: Aneurysm of abdominal aorta. Ann Surg 160:622, 1964.
3. Rob C: Surgical diseases of the iliac and mesenteric arteries. Arch Surg 93:21, 1966.
4. Ernst CB: Abdominal aortic aneurysm. N Engl J Med 328:1167, 1993.
5. Bengtsson H, Bergqvist D, Sternby NH: Increasing prevalence of abdominal aortic aneurysms: a necropsy study. Eur J Surg 158:19, 1992.
6. Breckwoldt WL, Mackey WC, O'Donnell TF Jr: The economic implications of high-risk abdominal aortic aneurysm. J Vasc Surg 13:798, 1991.
7. Spittell JA: Hypertension and arterial aneurysm. J Am Coll Cardiol 1:533, 1983.
8. Cannon JA, Van De Water J, Barker WF: Experience with surgical management of 100 consecutive cases of abdominal aneurysm. Am J Surg 106:128, 1963.
9. Tilson MD, Seashore MR: Fifty families with abdominal aortic aneurysms in two or more first order relatives. Am J Surg 147:551, 1984.
10. Johansen K, Koepsell T: Familial tendency for abdominal aortic aneurysms. JAMA 256:1934, 1986.
11. Bengtsson H, Sonesson B, Lanne T, et al.: Prevalence of abdominal aortic aneurysm in the offspring of patients dying from aneurysm rupture. Br J Surg 79:1142, 1992.
12. Giordano JM: Vascular versus spinal disease as a cause of back and lower extremity pain. Semin Spine Surg 2:136, 1990.
13. Koch AE, Kunkel SL, Pearce WH, et al.: Enhanced production of the chemotactic cytokines interleukin-8 and monocyte chemoattractant protein-1 in human abdominal aortic aneurysms. Am J Pathol 142:1423, 1993.
14. Ouriel K, Green RM, Donayre C, et al.: An evaluation of new methods of expressing aortic aneurysm size: relationship to rupture. J Vasc Surg 15:12, 1992.
15. Nevitt MP, Ballard DJ, Hallett JW Jr: Prognosis of abdominal aortic aneurysms: a population-based study. N Engl J Med 321:1009, 1989.
16. Limet R, Sakalihassan N, Albert A: Determination of the expansion rate and incidence of rupture of abdominal aortic aneurysms. J Vasc Surg 14:540, 1991.
17. Barratt-Boyes BG: Symptomatology and prognosis of abdominal aortic aneurysm. Lancet 2:716, 1957.
18. Rohrer MJ, Cutler BS, Wheeler HB: Long-term survival and quality of life following ruptured abdominal aortic aneurysm. Arch Surg 123:1213, 1988.
19. DeHoff JB, Finney GG: Sign of ruptured aneurysm of abdominal aorta. N Engl J Med 281:47, 1969.
20. Beebe RT, Powers SR Jr, Ginouves E: Early diagnosis of ruptured abdominal aneurysm. Ann Intern Med 48:834, 1958.
21. Owens ML: Psoas weakness and femoral neuropathy: neglected signs of retroperitoneal hemorrhage from ruptured aneurysm. Surgery 91:363, 1982.
22. Sandson TA, Friedman JH: Spinal cord infarction: report of 8 cases and review of the literature. Medicine 68:282, 1989.
23. Bluth EL: Ultrasound of the abdominal aorta. Arch Intern Med 144:377, 1984.
24. Gomes MN, Schellinger D: Abdominal aortic aneurysms: diagnostic review and new technique. Ann Thorac Surg 27:479, 1979.
25. LaRoy LL, Cormier PJ, Matalon TAS, et al.: Imaging of abdominal aortic aneurysms. AJR 152:785, 1989.
26. Amparo EG, Hoddick WK, Hricak H, et al.: Comparison of magnetic resonance imaging and ultrasonography in the evaluation of abdominal aortic aneurysms. Radiology 154:451, 1985.
27. Durham JR, Hackworth CA, Tober JC, et al.: Magnetic resonance angiography in the preoperative evaluation of abdominal aortic aneurysms. Am J Surg 166:173, 1993.
28. Wheeler WE, Beachley MC, Ranniger K: Angiography and ultrasonography: a comparative study of abdominal aortic aneurysms. AJR 126:95, 1976.
29. Nano IN, Collins GM, Bardin JA, Bernstein EF: Should aortography be used routinely in the elective management of abdominal aortic aneurysm? Am J Surg 144:53, 1982.
30. Janower ML: Ruptured arteriosclerotic aneurysms of the abdominal aorta. N Engl J Med 265:12, 1961.
31. Wheelock F, Shaw RS: Aneurysm of abdominal aorta and iliac arteries. N Engl J Med 255:72, 1956.
32. Marston WA, Ahlquist R, Johnson G Jr, Meyer AA: Misdiagnosis of ruptured abdominal aneurysms. J Vasc Surg 16:17, 1992.
33. Mendelowitz DS, Ramstedt R, Yao JST, Bergan JJ: Abdominal aortic salmonellosis. Surgery 85:514, 1979.
34. Ishikawa K: Patterns of symptoms and prognosis in occlusive thromboaortopathy (Takayasu's disease). J Am Coll Cardiol 8:1041, 1986.
35. Foster JH, Bolasny BL, Gobbel WG, Scott HW Jr: Comparative study of elective resection and expectant

treatment of abdominal aortic aneurysm. Surg Gynecol Obstet 129:1, 1969.

36. Crawford ES, Saleh SA, Babb JW III, et al.: Infrarenal abdominal aortic aneurysm. Ann Surg 193:699, 1981.

37. Diehl JT, Cali RF, Hertzer NR, Beven EG: Complications of abdominal aortic reconstruction: an analysis of perioperative risk factors in 557 patients. Ann Surg 197:49, 1983.

38. Bennett DE, Cherry JK: Bacterial infection of aortic aneurysms: a clinicopathologic study. Am J Surg 113:321, 1967.

39. Russinovich NAE, Karem GG, Luna RF: Radiology rounds: persistent lumbar pain and low-grade fever in a 62-year-old man. Ala J Med Sci 19:67, 1982.

40. Compion ML, Kreel L, Rothman MT, Pardy BJ: Induced thrombosis of abdominal aortic aneurysm. J Roy Soc Med 78:72, 1985.

41. Kwaan JHM, Khan RJ, Connally JE: Total exclusion technique for the management of abdominal aortic aneurysms. Am J Surg 146:93, 1983.

42. Paty PS, Lloyd WE, Chang BB, et al.: Aortic replacement for abdominal aortic aneurysm in elderly patients. Am J Surg 166:191, 1993.

43. Dean RH, Woody JD, Enarson CE, et al.: Operative treatment of abdominal aortic aneurysms in octagenarians. When is it too much too late? Ann Surg 217:721, 1993.

44. Magee TR, Scott DJ, Dunkley A, et al.: Quality of life following surgery for abdominal aortic aneurysm. Br J Surg 79:1014, 1992.

45. Katz DA, Littenberg B, Cronenwett JL: Management of small abdominal aneurysms . . . early surgery vs watchful waiting. JAMA 268:2678, 1992.

46. Frame PS, Fryback DG, Patterson C: Screening for abdominal aortic aneurysm in men ages 60 to 80 years. A cost-effectiveness analysis. Ann Intern Med 119:411, 1993.

47. Schalz IJ, Stanley JC: Saddle embolus of the aorta. JAMA 235:1262, 1976.

48. Filtzer DL, Bahnson HT: Low back pain due to arterial obstruction. J Bone Joint Surg 41B:244, 1959.

49. Danto LA, Fry WJ, Kraft RO: Acute aortic thrombosis. Arch Surg 104:569, 1972.

50. Crawford ES, Bomberger RA, Galeser DH, et al.: Aortoiliac occlusive disease: factors influencing survival and function following reconstruction operation over a twenty-five-year period. Surgery 90:1055, 1981.

51. Dong G, Porter RW: Walking and cycling tests in neurogenic and intermittent claudication. Spine 14:965, 1989.

GENITOURINARY DISEASES

Capsule Summary

Frequency of back pain—common
Location of back pain—flanks, sacrum
Quality of back pain—colicky or dull ache
Symptoms and signs—colicky flank and referred pain, tender costovertebral angle
Laboratory and x-ray tests—abnormal urinalysis, positive cultures; filling defects or masses with contrast studies or sonography, calcifications on plain roentgenograms
Treatment—surgical removal of mass, lysis or removal of stone, antibiotics

The organs that compose the genitourinary tract are located in the retroperitoneum and pelvis and lie close to the lumbosacral spine. Diseases that affect the genitourinary organs may be associated with both local pain and referred pain that radiates to the lumbosacral area. Primary renal disease causes flank pain. The flank is the region of the back bounded superiorly by the ribs, inferiorly by the iliac crests, medially by the spine, and laterally by the sides of the body. Stretching of the renal capsule causes pain in the distribution of T10–T12, the source of sensory innervation. Renal pain is not exacerbated by movement or increased by palpation or percussion except in the setting of pyelonephritis or renal infarcts.[1]

Processes that obstruct the outflow of urine will cause symptoms. Obstruction may be secondary to congenital narrowing, stones, and/or tumor. Tumors may also cause pain, but of a slow and insidious variety as opposed to the sharp pain associated with acute obstruction of the urinary tract. The blockage of blood flow and associated tissue necrosis (renal infarction) will also cause acute pain.

Acute inflammatory involvement of glomeruli may cause flank pain. Hereditary disorders associated with structural abnormalities of the kidney cause back pain. Blockage of vessel outflow in the form of renal vein thrombosis causes renal capsular swelling and low back pain.

Kidney

The kidneys are located at the level of the tenth through twelfth thoracic and first lumbar vertebrae. Pain from diseases that affect the kidneys is felt at the costovertebral angle just lateral to the paraspinous muscles at T12-L1. It often radiates around the flank toward the umbilicus and usually is dull and constant. The source of the pain is thought to be the sudden distention of the capsule of the kidney. Diseases that cause or are associated with acute kidney obstruction (stone, hemorrhage, hydronephrosis, or acute pyelonephritis) are painful. Disease processes that cause only gradual capsular distention are not associated with kidney pain (stone with partial obstruction, tumor, congenital obstruction).

KIDNEY STONES

Nephrolithiasis, urinary stones, may also be associated with back pain. Stones located in the pelvis of the kidney will cause dull flank pain if there is capsular distention, and colic if there is obstruction or spasm at the uretero-pelvic junction. Approximately 2% to 3% of people in the United States and Western Europe have an attack of renal colic during their lifetimes. The risk for recurrent attacks ranges from 20% to 50% over the subsequent 10 years.[2, 3] The major types of stones include calcium oxalate, struvite (magnesium ammonium phosphate, or stones of infection), calcium phosphate, uric acid, and cystine. Many of the factors that predispose to renal lithiasis are unknown. However, factors that either increase urinary concentration or decrease urinary solubility do promote stone formation in general. Other factors may predispose to the formation of specific stones. These include hypercalcemia, hyperoxaluria, and hyperuricosuria for calcium oxalate stones; urinary infection causing alkaline urine (urea-splitting organisms) for struvite stones; persistent alkaline urine from oral antacids, renal tubular acidosis, or primary hyperparathyroidism for calcium phosphate stones; acid urine for uric acid stones; and cystinuria for cystine stones.[4]

The clinical symptoms associated with a kidney stone are correlated with stone size and the duration, location, and degree of obstruction. Although kidney stones frequently produce symptoms of renal colic or acute urinary tract infection, some stones are discovered incidentally during an x-ray examination for another condition. Pain, when it occurs, is secondary to stretching of the collecting system or renal capsule and is not necessarily caused by increased peristalsis. Severity of pain correlates with the rate of distention rather than the degree of dilatation. Acute obstruction from a renal calculus causing sudden hydronephrosis of a mild degree may be very painful, while chronic obstruction of insidious onset may be painless. Patients with stones in the kidney or calyceal system may experience sharp, cramping pain or pain that is dull and persistent. Acute obstruction may be characterized by a steady crescendo of pain in the flank, which may radiate downward toward the groin and into the genitalia if the area near the ureter is affected.[5] The pain is steady and continuous in its onset and may have a duration as short as 30 minutes or as long as 24 hours. The patient may find that walking or other movement is preferred over lying still in bed. In general, the character of the pain is not changed with movement or position. The pain is associated with nausea and vomiting and may mimic an acute surgical abdomen. A history of chills and fever suggests a complicating infection.

Physical examination may demonstrate costovertebral angle tenderness with percussion. Some paraspinous muscle spasm may accompany the tenderness. Acute nonstructural scoliosis may occur in severe cases. Abdominal examination may elicit tenderness in the appropriate upper quadrant, particularly with an associated infection. Abdominal distention and paralytic ileus may accompany acute renal colic.

Examination of the urine is the most important part of the laboratory evaluation of the patient with a suspected stone. Hematuria may range from a few erythrocytes on microscopic evaluation to gross blood. Proteinuria is also present. If the pH of the urine is alkaline, the stone may be struvite in origin. A pH constantly in the 6.0 to 6.5 range may be associated with renal tubular acidosis. A low pH is associated with uric acid stones. Microscopic evaluation of urine for crystals is worthwhile, since the different crystals that cause stones have different shapes. Calcium oxalate and phosphate are rectangular, uric acid is rhomboidal, cystine is hexagonal, and struvite is a rectangle within a rectangle. A 24-hour urine collection along with samples collected individually over a 24-hour period aids in diagnosis. Hypercalciuria favors the formation of calcium oxalate stones. Hyperuricosuria favors calcium oxalate or uric acid stones.[6]

Blood tests may also be useful in detecting the potential source of stones. Hypercalcemia is associated with oxalate stones, while hyperuricemia is associated with oxalate and uric acid stones. Hyperchloremia suggests renal tubular acidosis, which is associated with phosphate stones.[7] Tests of serum creatinine and urea nitrogen are obtained to assess renal function and document the extent of renal disease that may be associated with nephrolithiasis.

Plain roentgenograms of the abdomen may be adequate to detect the presence of stones. Radiopaque stones contain calcium and are oxalate or phosphate (Fig. 17–5). Moderate size stones or staghorn calculi are frequently composed of struvite. Cystine stones are moderately radiopaque. Uric acid stones are radiolucent. Intravenous pyelography (IVP) is useful to localize a calcific shadow as long as the kidneys are functioning and are not acutely obstructed. Radiolucent stones may appear as holes in the column of dye.[8] Ultrasonography

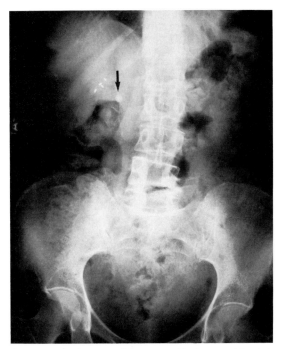

Figure 17–5. A 55-year-old woman with rheumatoid arthritis developed colicky right-sided back pain most noticeable in the flank. Plain roentgenogram of the abdomen revealed a radiopaque stone in the right kidney *(arrow)*. (Courtesy of Arnold Kwart, M.D.)

and/or CT can localize stones if the IVP proves inadequate.[9] MR visualizes the organs of the genitourinary system well, but does not identify stones. The usefulness of this technique is limited in these patients.[10]

The diagnosis of nephrolithiasis is suggested by the patient's history, physical examination, and urinalysis, and is confirmed by the presence of the stone on radiographic studies. Chemical analysis of passed stones specifies the type of stone that is at fault. Patients with other kidney conditions may have flank pain. Pyelonephritis may complicate nephrolithiasis as well as occur independently. Renal tumor with an obstructive blood clot may cause pain. Papillary necrosis with obstruction of the pelvis will cause pain. Infarction of the kidney will cause flank pain. Renal tubular acidosis (RTA), independent of nephrolithiasis, may cause back pain. In one study, 16% of patients with RTA had low back pain in the absence of a mechanical cause for pain.[7]

The patient with acute pain associated with nephrolithiasis is treated with increased fluid intake and analgesia. The patient may pass the stone without any other therapy. Between 80% and 90% of stones will pass spontaneously, especially if the stones are 1 to 5 mm in diame-

ter.[4] If a kidney is totally blocked for a few days, removal of the stone needs to be considered. In the past, open surgery may have been considered. The treatment of choice for upper tract stones (above the upper third of the ureter) is extracorporeal shock wave lithotripsy.[11] The stones are fragmented by shock waves and subsequently passed through the ureter into the bladder to be voided out. Even large stones may be fragmented by this method. Treatment has been reported to be successful in 70% of patients.[12] Two forms of percutaneous disintegration include ultrasonic lithotripsy and electrohydraulic disintegration. These procedures require endoscopic surgery.[13, 14] The ability of these procedures to remove renal stones continues to improve.[15]

If the other procedures are contraindicated or ineffective, open surgery is advised. This may be particularly true for staghorn calculi.[16]

The prognosis for patients with an episode of nephrolithiasis is that they will have a recurrence. Patients with stones should undergo a careful metabolic evaluation to identify the source of their stones. After appropriate evaluation, specific therapy in the form of phosphates, thiazides, allopurinol, penicillamine, or antibiotics may be given to reverse the underlying metabolic abnormality predisposing to stone formation.[17–19]

PYELONEPHRITIS

Acute pyelonephritis is a bacterial infection of the parenchyma of the kidney.[20] Bacteria are able to travel retrograde from the bladder to the kidney when there is an obstruction of vesicoureteral reflux in the genitourinary system, which allows access to the kidney parenchyma.

Urinary tract infection (UTI) is the most common of all the bacterial infections. Between the ages of 1 and 50, when prostate infection increases the prevalence of UTI in men, the ratio of men to women with UTI is 1:50. The yearly incidence in females older than 10 years of age is approximately 5%.[21] Most of the infections are of the bladder (cystitis). In individuals over 65 years of age, the male to female ratio is 1:10.

Over 95% of urinary tract infections occur via the ascending route from the urethra, bladder, and ureter to the kidney. Only 3% to 5% are of hematogenous origin.[4] Vesicoureteral reflux allows infected urine to reach the pelvicalyceal system. The urine gains access to the kidney parenchyma at the papillary tips and then spreads along the collecting tubules. The medullary portion of the kidney is predisposed to infection because of its chemical environment, characterized by high urea and ammonia concentrations and high osmolarity, which inhibits granulocyte function as well as complement activation.[22] The infection is focal, causing localized swelling with an inflammatory infiltrate composed of polymorphonuclear leukocytes initially, and lymphocytes subsequently. Persistent and/or repeated infections will cause scarring of the kidneys.

Patients with pyelonephritis complain of severe, constant, aching pain over one or both costovertebral angles that is not affected by position or movement. The pain may radiate to the lower abdominal quadrants. Patients have frequency, urgency, and burning on urination. Nausea and vomiting may be part of the symptom complex.

Patients with acute pyelonephritis are systemically ill with high fever, tachycardia, and chills. They exhibit exquisite percussion tenderness over the costovertebral angle with associated back muscle spasm. Abdominal signs may include muscle guarding of the abdominal wall and hypoactive bowel sounds.

Laboratory tests confirm the presence of pyuria and bacteria, and cultures of urine and blood will grow the offending organism. *Escherichia coli*, staphylococcal species, and *Streptococcus faecalis* are the most common pathogens. Urine will show many white blood cells on an unspun specimen. The presence of bacteria on a Gram stain of an unspun urine specimen is also suggestive of a significant infection.[23] The use of the antibody-coated bacteria assay has proved to be too nonspecific to separate upper tract from lower tract infection.[24] The response to single-dose antibiotic therapy is a more sensitive means of separating lower tract from upper tract disease. Other laboratory findings include elevated white blood cell counts to the level of 40,000 cells/ml. The ESR is also increased.

Radiographic evaluation, including IVP or ultrasonography, is indicated in a patient with pyelonephritis. Plain film of the abdomen may show some obliteration of the renal shadow secondary to edema of the kidney. The IVP or ultrasound is useful to survey the urinary tract for the presence of obstruction or vesicoureteral reflux. If the infection is severe, the involved kidney is enlarged and its nephrographic image is diminished in intensity. These investigations are most useful in patients who do not respond to antibiotic therapy. Gallium-67 can be used to localize the site of infection in the kidney. Although 86% ac-

curacy has been claimed, both false-positive and false-negative findings can occur.[25] This technique cannot differentiate acute pyelonephritis from renal abscess.

The differential diagnosis of patients with acute back pain not relieved by rest and associated with systemic signs includes pancreatitis, pneumonia, acute cholecystitis, acute appendicitis, and acute diverticulitis. Gastrointestinal problems are associated with normal urinalysis and changes in bowel habits. Pleuritic pain is associated with pneumonia. Herpes zoster, before vesicles appear, can simulate the pain of pyelonephritis if the T12 or L1 dermatomes are affected.

Treatment with appropriate intravenous antibiotics results in the control of the infection and resolution of the pain.[4] When the infection is resistant to cure because of structural abnormalities such as polycystic kidneys or vesicoureteral reflux, the patient may develop chronic pyelonephritis. This disorder may be clinically silent except in acute exacerbations of the chronic infection, when localized renal pain will be present.[26] The ideal duration of antibiotic therapy depends on the location of the infection in the upper or lower portion of the genitourinary tract. For upper tract infection, intravenous therapy is given until the patient is afebrile. Oral antibiotics, such as trimethoprim-sulfamethoxazole or quinolones, may be used to complete a 2 week course of therapy.[27, 28]

PERINEPHRIC ABSCESS

Infections that escape the confines of the renal capsule will lodge in the perinephric tissues and form a perinephric abscess. Frequently patients with these abscesses have a history of chronic renal disease from urinary tract infections, a urinary calculus with hydronephrosis, trauma, or hematogenous spread from a distant infected area. The site of pain associated with perinephric abscess is the costovertebral angle, and the pain is insidious in onset. Patients may be symptomatic for weeks before seeking medical attention. Patients may have symptoms of dysuria, hematuria, or urinary retention along with anorexia, fever, and weight loss. Patients may have mild to severe tenderness on palpation, as well as muscle spasm with a scoliotic posture. A mass may be palpated over the flank in 50% of patients. Laboratory evaluation reveals anemia, leukocytosis, elevated ESR, and abnormal urinalysis with positive urine culture for the infecting organism. Renal function is usually normal since the infection is unilateral. Urinalysis may be normal in 30% and urine culture sterile in 40% of cases. Blood cultures are positive in 40% of individuals. Radiologic findings in the abdomen include ptosis of a kidney and obliteration of the psoas shadow. Chest roentgenograms may demonstrate an elevated or fixed hemidiaphragm, pleural effusion, empyema, lung abscess, and lower lobe atelectasis. Excretory urography demonstrates poor vizualization of the kidney, displacement of the kidney, and obstruction. Gallium scan, sonogram, or CT may reveal an inflammatory mass. Of these techniques, CT scan demonstrates the full extent of the infection to the best degree.[29] MR may identify edema but may not be able to distinguish cysts from other inflammatory processes. Treatment includes appropriate antibiotics and percutaneous and/or open surgical drainage.[30]

URETEROPELVIC JUNCTION OBSTRUCTION

Abnormalities of the ureteropelvic junction are most commonly congenital malformations that cause stenosis or obstruction. The stricture elicits symptoms associated with urinary obstruction. Rarely, stenosis of the junction may occur in adults as one of the sequelae of renal injury. Extravasation of urine or blood results in fibrosis of the junction. A historical fact that helps localize the site of the lesion at the junction is the scenario of increased water intake exacerbating back pain.[31] The pain is intermittent. In acute circumstances, the pain may be sharp and colicky. Over time, the pain becomes dull and persistent. Tenderness at the costovertebral angle or flank is common. The diagnosis is confirmed by demonstration of hydronephrosis and enlargement of the renal pelvis as seen on IVP, sonogram, or renal scan (Fig. 17–6). Surgical repair of the stenosis is indicated. The goal of surgery is to relieve obstruction at the junction.[32] If the process of obstruction continues on a chronic basis, causing hydronephrosis and atrophy of the kidney with loss of renal function, nephrectomy may be required.

RENAL INFARCTION

Infarcts of the kidney are caused by arterial occlusion. The major causes of occlusion include thrombi in the atria or ventricles, secondary to myocardial infarction, myocarditis, or infective endocarditis, that embolize to the kidney (Fig. 17–7). Plaques associated with arteriosclerosis may also be a source of emboli.

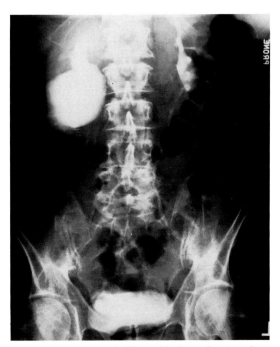

Figure 17–6. IVP reveals bilateral hydronephrosis and enlargement of both renal pelves in a patient with ureteropelvic junction obstruction. (Courtesy of Arnold Kwart, M.D.)

Primary vascular inflammation (e.g., polyarteritis nodosa) will cause vascular occlusion. Trauma to the blood vessels to the kidney will also interrupt blood flow. Aneurysms of the renal artery may also be a source of emboli (Fig. 17–8).

If the main renal artery is occluded, the entire kidney may become infarcted, becoming functionless and atrophic. This process is associated with sudden onset of severe, sharp costovertebral angle pain. Smaller areas of infarction may cause no symptoms. The development of symptoms is due in part to the acuteness of onset and the amount of kidney tissue affected.

Physical examination elicits pain over the paraspinal muscles on the affected side. The kidney is not enlarged on abdominal examination. Bowel sounds may be hypoactive. Urinalysis will usually contain erythrocytes. Repeated urinalyses are indicated if the first specimen is normal, since blood flow to the kidney is impaired and urine containing erythrocytes may take hours to appear. IVP may fail to visualize a portion of the kidney with a partial infarction. Total occlusion results in an absence of any radiographic image of the kidney.

The definitive diagnosis is made through the use of a renal scan or arteriogram. The

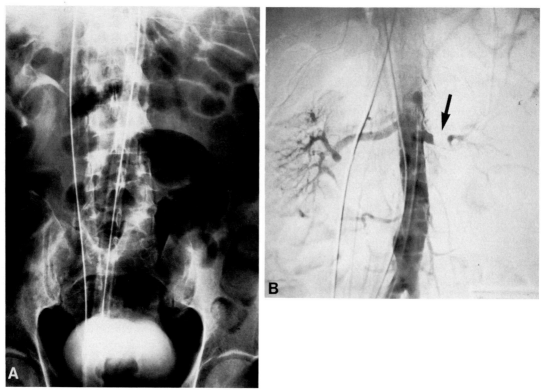

Figure 17–7. IVP *(A)* demonstrates no flow to the left kidney. Subtraction view *(B)* of renal arteriogram reveals an embolus in the left renal artery *(arrow)*. The patient had developed severe left-sided back pain while recovering from a coronary artery bypass graft operation. (Courtesy of Edward Druy, M.D.)

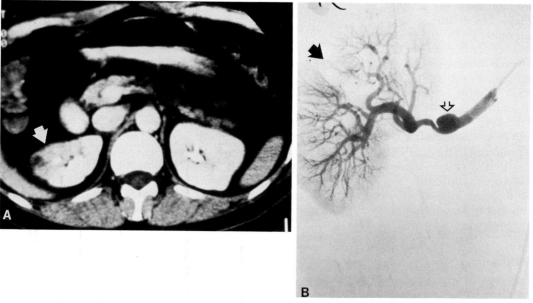

Figure 17–8. A 40-year-old man presented with acute-onset right-sided costovertebral angle pain. Urinalysis was initially normal. The patient continued with pain and became febrile. Microscopic hematuria appeared on the third day of hospitalization. *A,* CT scan of the abdomen showed an infarct of the upper outer aspect of the right kidney *(arrow)*. *B,* Renal angiogram (subtraction view) revealed a large renal artery aneurysm *(open arrow)* with area of decreased blood vessels corresponding to the area of infarction *(black arrow)*. Surgery was done to correct the aneurysm. (Courtesy of Edward Druy, M.D.)

arteriogram will identify the location and extent of vessel involvement. Possible sources of emboli should be investigated by the appropriate methods (echocardiogram, for example) if renal infarction is documented. Therapy of infarction, if the diagnosis is made promptly, is embolectomy by either medical or surgical means. Anticoagulants are useful to prevent progressive thrombosis and may improve renal function. If hypertension ensues from a partial occlusion of the renal artery that is not responsive to medical therapy, renal endarterectomy or nephrectomy may be required.[33] A more recent study has reported the successful use of intra-arterial streptokinase to dissolve clots causing renal infarcts.[34]

RENAL CANCER

Tumors of the kidney include renal cell carcinoma (85%), renal pelvis tumor (8%), Wilms' tumor (5%), and sarcoma (2%).[4] Of all the renal tumors, renal cell carcinoma is the most prevalent and, because of the diverse and nonrenal symptoms that are associated with the tumor, is the most difficult to diagnose. In the United States, the incidence is 19,000 new cases per year.[35] The ratio of men to women with renal cell tumor is 2:1. The peak age of incidence is 60 years. The most common site of origin of renal tumors is the proximal convoluted tubular epithelium. In light of this fact, the designation of kidney tumors as renal cell carcinoma as suggested by Mostofi is a more appropriate name than hypernephroma.[36]

Patients with renal cell carcinoma may present with a range of symptoms. They may be symptomless, have renal symptoms, or develop systemic complaints. The classic triad of hematuria, flank pain, and palpable renal mass occurs in 10% of patients. The most common finding is hematuria (63%), with flank or back pain occurring in 41%.[37, 38] The pain is usually a constant, dull ache in the back or abdomen. The dull ache occurs as the tumor extends beyond its capsule into retroperitoneal structures. Acute low back pain that is sharp or colicky will occur with clot formation that obstructs part of the calyceal system. As part of the systemic or paraneoplastic manifestations of renal cell carcinoma, patients will complain of fever, anorexia, weight loss, or neurologic symptoms.[39]

Physical examination will reveal fever in 20% of patients, and a palpable mass in a similar number.[40] The appearance of a left-sided varicocele is noted in up to 11% of male patients. This finding is secondary to blockage of the left gonadal vein at its point of entry into the left renal vein by a tumor thrombus.[41] Edema of the lower extremities may also occur in 11% of patients.

Laboratory tests may be very helpful in documenting the systemic nature of the patient's disease. The ESR is elevated in a majority of patients. Anemia, with normal white cell and platelet counts, is seen in 40%. Hypercalcemia, secondary to a hormone effect of a material released by the tumor, is noted in 15%. Urinalysis is positive for erythrocytes and protein. Pathologic evaluation of the tumor reveals adenocarcinoma in most circumstances. Those tumors with more mitotic figures or anaplasia are more invasive.

IVP will demonstrate a space-occupying lesion (Fig. 17–9). Renal ultrasonography shows a solid mass as opposed to a cyst, which lacks

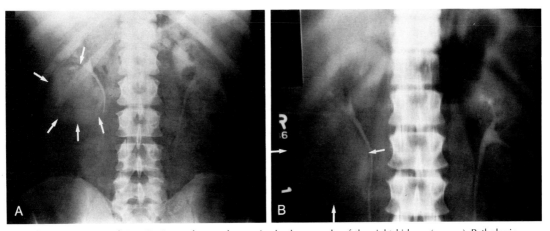

Figure 17–9. *A* and *B*, IVP views of a renal mass in the lower pole of the right kidney *(arrows)*. Pathologic examination revealed a renal cell carcinoma. (Courtesy of Arnold Kwart, M.D.)

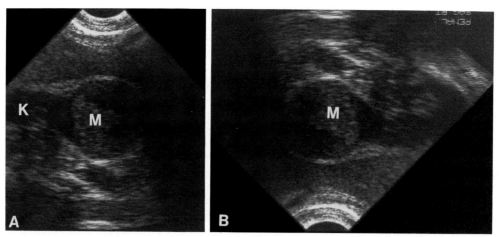

Figure 17–10. Ultrasound. *A,* Sagittal scan of the kidney (K) demonstrating a solid intrarenal mass (M) compatible with a renal cell carcinoma. *B,* Cross-sectional scan revealing solid intrarenal mass. (Courtesy of Michael Hill, M.D.)

internal echoes and has a smooth, sharp border (Fig. 17–10). If any doubt remains in regard to whether the mass is solid or cystic, a CT scan will demonstrate the status of the lesion along with the extension of the tumor within the vena cava.[42, 43] Arteriography may be necessary to document the vascular supply of the tumor in order to plan for operative intervention.[44] MR is able to identify the presence of a mass and is most helpful in staging the neoplasm. It determines the origin of the mass, vascular patency (renal vein or vena cava), the presence of lymph node metastases, and the direct tumor invasion to adjacent organs.[45]

The therapy for renal cell carcinoma is radical nephrectomy. This procedure includes the removal of regional lymph nodes.[43] The need for chemotherapy and/or radiotherapy is determined by the extension of the tumor locally and the number of metastases distally.[46] In general, chemotherapy and radiotherapy are ineffective in controlling tumor growth. The prognosis is best for patients with Stage I disease (tumor confined to kidney capsule), in whom the survival rate is 75% at 5 years. Patients with Stage IV disease (distant metastases) have a 5-year survival rate of 25%.[47]

MISCELLANEOUS KIDNEY DISORDERS

Glomerulonephritis is an inflammatory disorder of the kidney characterized by the abrupt onset of hematuria, proteinuria, decreased filtration rate, hypertension, and oliguria. Inflammation of the glomerulus may be caused by a variety of disorders including mul-

tisystem diseases such as systemic lupus erythematosus.[4] Patients may present with malaise and a dull persistent aching in the flanks bilaterally. Interstitial edema within the renal parenchyma and stretching of the renal capsule is the cause of flank pain. Physical examination reveals hypertension and evidence of fluid overload (rales, edema, dyspnea). Laboratory evaluation reveals red cell casts and proteinuria on urinalysis. Renal function tests may demonstrate a variable degree of dysfunction. Treatment is based on the underlying disease and may include corticosteroids or cytotoxic therapy.

Hereditary disorders causing structural damage to the kidney may be associated with back pain. Autosomal dominant polycystic kidney disease may present as back pain in 20% of all patients.[1] Between the ages of 20 to 24, up to 50% of affected females will present with back pain as the initial symptom. The flank pain is dull in quality and is associated with flank masses and gross hematuria. Patients may have renal insufficiency at initial presentation. Ultrasound of the kidney demonstrates multiple cysts. The disease inevitably progresses to renal failure.

Other disorders associated with flank pain include renal vein thrombosis and nephrotic syndrome. When the venous outflow from the kidney is obstructed, the associated swelling results in flank pain. Nephrotic syndrome is a result of excessive excretion of albumin. The resulting hypoalbuminemia causes interstitial edema of the kidney. Interstitial edema within the renal parenchyma causes stretching of the renal capsule. Patients with nephrotic syndrome often complain of dull bilateral fullness in the area of the costovertebral angles.

Ureter

The ureter is a thin tube composed of smooth muscle that connects the renal pelvis with the bladder. The ureter is anatomically narrowed at three locations. These include the ureteropelvic junction, a point crossing over the iliac vessels, and the ureterovesical junction. These are the three locations that are most frequently obstructed by urinary stones. Other inflammatory (retroperitoneal fibrosis) or neoplastic (transitional cell) processes may affect the ureter along its path from the kidney to the bladder.[48, 49] These processes may cause obstruction that occurs on a chronic basis (Fig. 17–11).

URETERAL STONE

Renal stones are initially formed in the proximal urinary tract and pass progressively into the calyces, renal pelvis, and ureter. In the ureter, specific locations that become obstructed are associated with specific symptoms. In the upper or proximal ureter, stones cause acute, sharp, spasmodic pain that is localized to the flank. If acute renal capsular distention occurs, pain may radiate along the course of

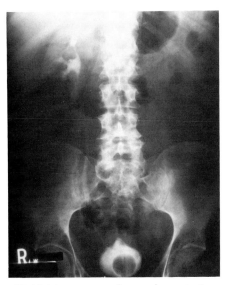

Figure 17–11. Intravenous pyelogram demonstrating an obstructive pattern involving the right kidney. An entire column of dye is visualized while the left kidney has emptied. This 56-year-old man had developed vague, right-sided flank pain. The cause of the obstruction was a ureteral transitional cell cancer.

the ureter into the ipsilateral testicle, since the nerve supply to the kidney and testis is the same. As the stone passes along the ureter, it may lodge at the level where the ureter passes over the iliac vessels. The pain remains sharp and intermittent, corresponding to peristalsis of the ureter. The pain radiates to the lateral flank and lower quadrant of the abdomen.

As the stone passes into the distal ureter, the pain remains intermittent and sharp, corresponding to the waves of ureteral peristalsis. In women, the pain will radiate into the genitalia, particularly the labia. In men, the pain radiates along the inguinal canal into the groin and scrotal wall. The stone in this location may give rise to excruciating pain, causing the patient to writhe about trying to find a comfortable position. This is in contrast to patients with abdominal disease, such as peritonitis, who lie quietly because motion increases discomfort.[50] When the stone approaches the bladder, urgency and frequency with burning on urination develop as a result of inflammation of the bladder wall around the ureteral orifice.

The sensory innervation of the kidneys and abdominal organs is similar. Ureteral disease may cause autonomic reflex symptoms in the gastrointestinal tract manifested by nausea, vomiting, and paralytic ileus. The differential diagnosis of a ureteral stone includes abdominal or pelvic processes (appendicitis, colitis, salpingitis, or cholecystitis).

Physical examination reveals a patient in significant distress, who is in constant motion, unable to find a comfortable position. Fever is present if the patient has an associated infection. The costovertebral angle is tender to percussion. Bowel sounds may be hypoactive on abdominal examination.

Urinalysis is an essential part of the evaluation. Hematuria, either gross or microscopic, is frequent.

Plain film of the abdomen may reveal the presence of a stone, since over 90% are radiopaque (Fig. 17–12). Oblique films will separate renal stones from other calcified structures such as gallstones, mesenteric lymph nodes, and pelvic phleboliths. IVP findings may include a delay in visualization of the collecting system on the affected side, followed by an intense nephrographic effect. The column of dye will end at the level of stone obstruction. Ultrasonography can identify hydronephrosis in patients who are allergic to intravenous dye or are anuric.

A majority of ureteral stones will pass through the urinary tract spontaneously.[51] Hy-

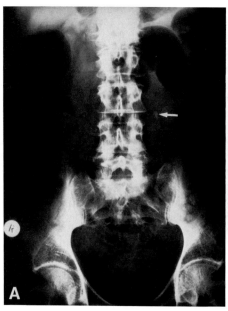
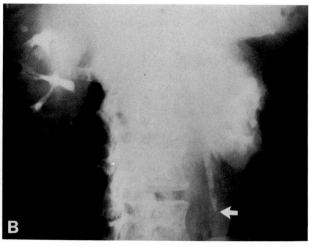

Figure 17–12. *A,* Plain roentgenogram reveals a radiopaque structure lateral to the L3–L4 intervertebral disc space *(arrow)* in a patient with left-sided back pain. *B,* IVP, oblique view, confirms the object as a ureteral stone that has obstructed the left ureter *(arrow).* (Courtesy of Arnold Kwart, M.D.)

dration and analgesics are generally useful in treating symptoms of stone obstruction. Stones in the lower tract pass spontaneously more often than those in the upper system. If fever develops, or if severe nausea and vomiting or complete obstruction occurs, manipulative or surgical therapy is needed. Manipulative therapy includes lithotripsy or stone removal by endourologic procedures.[52] Open surgical measures are infrequently used.

VESICOURETERAL REFLUX

The ureterovesical junction is a specialized structure that allows urine to enter the bladder but prevents urine from re-entering the ureter, particularly during voiding.[53] The kidney is protected from the high pressures developed in the bladder during excretion and limits infections to the bladder. If the valve becomes incompetent, on either a congenital (short intravesical ureter) or an environmental (infectious) basis, refluxed urine will reach the kidney and play a key role in the pathogenesis of infection. Hydronephrosis also may occur. About 8% of adults with bacteriuria have reflux.[54] Patients with reflux are usually asymptomatic. Occasionally they develop dull, unilateral or bilateral flank pain. On rare occasions, this may be associated with voiding. Patients may have episodes of acute pyelonephritis (particularly in females) or may have pyuria

without symptoms. The physical examination may be unremarkable. Laboratory evaluation may show bacteriuria without pyuria. Renal function tests (creatinine, BUN) are abnormal in a minority. Radiographic evaluation with IVP may be normal, but a dilated lower ureter, visualization of the entire length of the ureter, and healed pyelonephritis are clues to the presence of reflux. Cystography may directly visualize reflux. Therapy of vesicoureteral reflux in adult women is to control infection, if present in the urinary tract, with antibiotics, and if necessary, to administer chronic suppression treatment for 6 months or more. Surgical therapy is necessary if acute pyelonephritis recurs and is not preventable with antibiotics. Reimplantation of the ureter into the bladder may be necessary in these circumstances.[55] If reflux is not treated, the end result may be markedly diminished renal function.[56]

Bladder

Bladder pain is visceral in origin and is usually felt in a suprapubic or lower abdominal location. It is occasionally located in the sacral area.

BLADDER RETENTION

Patients who develop obstruction at the bladder neck develop urinary retention. In acute circumstances, the bladder fills rapidly, becomes distended, and causes suprapubic pain. Slowly developing obstruction, frequently from prostatic hypertrophy, causes pain of a dull variety that may be suprapubic or sacral in location. Patients are men over 60 years of age who have difficulty in maintaining a normal urinary stream. Examination of these patients demonstrates a lower abdominal midline mass frequently associated with prostatic hypertrophy discovered during rectal examination. Laboratory data are consistent with renal dysfunction in a minority. IVP demonstrates a post-void residual in the bladder with associated hydronephrosis. Sonography can be used to document bladder size if the patient is allergic to contrast media. Therapy for bladder retention is relief of the obstruction. Acute obstruction is relieved by catheterization. Special consideration must be made for individuals with massively distended bladder that become unobstructed acutely.[57] Rapid decompression is ill advised. Slow removal of fluid (100 to 300 ml/hr) will decrease the likelihood of gross hematuria. Prostatectomy is required for those men with outflow obstruction secondary to prostatic hypertrophy.

BLADDER INFECTION

Bladder infections (cystitis) are very common, particularly in women. The greater frequency of this infection in women can be directly related to the length of the urethra in each sex. Bacteria on the introitus can gain entry into the bladder with greater ease in women than in men.[58] Prostatic secretions contain bacteriostatic factors, which also may inhibit entry of bacterial organisms into the bladder in men. The bladder is able to clear infections spontaneously by voiding the organism in the urine. The urine also contains bacteriostatic substances, while the mucosa of the bladder has properties that inhibit bacterial invasion.[4] However, if these defense mechanisms are inadequate to clear the organisms, cystitis will occur. Patients with severe cystitis (local infection or inflammation of the bladder) may experience mild, diffuse low back pain that resolves with the resolution of the inflammation.

Patients with acute cystitis describe burning pain with urination, but little fever and no chills. Those with chronic cystitis who develop signs of obstruction, including cystoceles, may have persistent, low-grade sacral back pain. Some patients with symptoms of cystitis (nocturia, dysuria, frequency, and hematuria) may

have urethral irritation without bacteriuria.[13] Patients with cystitis are frequently sexually active women. On physical examination, the patient complains of pain with palpation over the lower abdomen, and tenderness of the bladder on palpation during pelvic examination. Positive laboratory tests are usually limited to urinalysis, which shows hematuria and pyuria with positive urine cultures. Therapy for uncomplicated cystitis is a single large dose of an effective antimicrobial agent—3 gm of oral amoxicillin, 2 double-strength trimethoprim-sulfamethoxazole tablets, or 2 gm of oral sulfisoxazole. Patients who have infections limited to the bladder will respond to single-dose therapy with eradication of bacteria and relief of symptoms.[59] If infection recurs after a several-week delay after the completion of therapy, the reappearance of symptoms is secondary to reinfection. If the same organism reappears in the first few days after completion of therapy, the infection is a relapse of the original infection and a hidden focus (pyelonephritis, bladder diverticulum) must be sought.[60] Cystoscopy, which allows direct visualization of the bladder wall, documents the extent of bladder inflammation and the obstruction in the patient with persistent symptoms.

Male Genital Organs

PROSTATE

The prostate gland is located in the pelvis at the base of the bladder in males. Diseases of the prostate are not usually associated with visceral pain from the gland itself. Instead, pain is localized to the perineal or rectal area and the sacral portion of the lumbosacral spine.

Prostatitis

Prostatitis may be defined as a disease state characterized by inflammation of the prostatic acini, which is frequently caused by bacterial infection. Bacteria gain entry into the bladder from the urethra. In a retrograde manner, bacteria travel past the urethra to the bladder, and gain entry into the prostate. Antegrade infection occurs less frequently from a source in the kidney.[61] Among male patients, prostatitis accounts for 25% of office visits for genitourinary tract complaints.[62] Acute prostatitis is characterized by severe urinary frequency, urgency, dysuria, and nocturia. Pain in the low back, perineum, or external genitalia may be noted. Symptoms of systemic infection are usual, including fever, diffuse myalgias, nausea, vomiting, and anorexia. Rectal examination reveals a very tender, enlarged, warm prostate that is firm to the examining finger. Laboratory evaluation reveals positive cultures of urine or prostatic fluids. The differential diagnosis of prostatitis includes other forms of prostatitis and infections of other parts of the urinary system (Table 17–2). Pain of acute pyelonephritis with bladder irritability is primarily lumbar in location, while prostatitis is sacral. The choice of therapy is limited because of the inability of most antibiotics to gain entry into the prostate. Trimethoprim-sulfamethoxazole enters the prostate gland and is the antibiotic of choice. Therapy of 6 to 12 weeks has had a significantly better cure rate than a conventional 2-week course of therapy.[63] After completion of successful therapy, the patient should undergo serial examinations with prostatic fluid cultures for a minimum of 4 months to ensure resolution of the infection.

Chronic prostatitis has the same pathogenesis as acute disease, but the symptoms and signs are milder. Patients may develop chronic prostatitis without any prior history of acute prostatitis. They may have symptoms of recurrent urinary tract infections. They may note an aching or "fullness" in the bladder area and a dull, aching pain in the low back. Pain with ejaculation may be a symptom. Rectal examination reveals a boggy, indurated prostate gland with areas of fibrosis. Massage of the gland is productive of an inflammatory fluid that contains numerous leukocytes and few organisms. Reports of increased incidence of sacroiliitis on plain roentgenograms with chronic prostatitis have not been substantiated.[64] Therapy includes long-term antibiotic therapy, particularly with trimethoprim-sulfamethoxazole.[65] Other antibiotics recommended for prolonged periods of 2 to 6 weeks include carbenicillin, erythromycin, minocycline, doxycycline, cephalexin, or fluoroquinolones (norfloxacin, ciprofloxacin, ofloxacin).[66] Sitz baths, twice daily, are prescribed for pain in the perineum, back, and rectum. Prostatic massage is useful to relieve symptoms of fullness and to reduce pain.

Prostatic Neoplasms

Neoplasms of the prostate are among the most common malignancies found in men.[35] Benign prostatic hypertrophy, a hyperplastic growth of the glandular tissue of the prostate, develops slowly and is not associated with low back pain. Flank pain may occur with benign prostatic hypertrophy if obstruction of the outflow tract causes hydronephrosis. Adenocarcinoma of the prostate does not cause back pain when the tumor is confined to the limits of the gland capsule; however, the cancer may spread through the pelvic lymph channels and through vertebral veins to bones in the pelvis and lumbosacral spine.[67] Many tumors are asymptomatic when first diagnosed by detection of a nodule or diffuse induration of the prostate on rectal examination. In other instances, symptoms of obstruction may be the initial presenting features. Symptoms of low back pain with radiation down one or both legs associated with symptoms of bladder obstruction in men, especially in those over 50 years of age, suggest metastases to the axial skeleton by prostatic cancer. Rectal examination documents a hard, fixed, nodular prostate.

Anemia, hematuria, decreased renal function, and elevated serum acid phosphatase may be present on initial laboratory examination. Serum prostate-specific antigen (PSA) is a serine protease produced only by prostatic epithelial cells. When PSA is more than 10 ng/ml, the test is 92% specific for prostate cancer.[68] However, when used as a screening test, PSA may identify individuals who do not have cancer and who receive therapy with an unfavorable effect.[69] Additional studies are necessary to determine the utility of PSA as a screening test for prostatic carcinoma. The test is most useful in detecting recurrence after radical prostatectomy.[70] Transrectal ultrasonography is an efficient radiographic technique for staging the local extent of disease. Malignant nodules appear hypoechoic when viewed sonographically.[71] However, the technique has a high false-positive rate with benign hypertrophy and does not identify hypertrophy of pelvic lymph nodes. MR and CT scans detect soft tissue involvement with lymph nodes but do not differentiate benign from malignant lesions limited to the prostate itself.[72] Osteoblastic lesions from metastases to bone are demonstrated on plain radiographs

TABLE 17–2. DIFFERENTIAL DIAGNOSIS OF PROSTATITIS

Acute bacterial prostatitis
Chronic bacterial prostatitis
Acute nonspecific granulomatous prostatitis—
    eosinophilia/vasculitis (Wegener's)
Nonbacterial prostatitis—?autoimmune
Prostatodynia—voiding dysfunction
Acute diverticulitis
Pyelonephritis with bladder irritability
Prostatic carcinoma

of the pelvis. Bone scintiscan may demonstrate multiple lesions throughout the axial skeleton (see Chapter 13). Quantitative bone scintigraphy may be used after therapy to document the response of skeletal lesions to treatment.[73] Diagnosis is confirmed by biopsy of the gland.[74] Most prostatic neoplasms are adenocarcinomas.[75] The lesions are evaluated by the Gleason grading system, which identifies well, moderately, and poorly differentiated tumors.[76] Poorly differentiated tumors are the ones that have more malignant characteristics and metastasize to a greater degree.[77] The anaplastic characteristics of the tumors also may be noted by the DNA status of the cells. Patients with diploidy have a better prognosis than patients with aneuploidy.[78] Once the diagnosis is established, staging of the tumor is necessary before appropriate therapy can be instituted.[79]

Great controversy exists regarding optimum therapy for prostatic carcinoma.[80] Involvement of pelvic lymph nodes limits therapy in that radical prostatectomy or radiotherapy will not be curative. About 80% of patients with lymph nodes develop metastatic disease in 5 years.[81] Therapy for prostatic cancer includes surgical, endocrine, and radiation modalities.[82] The basic premise for therapy of metastatic disease is to deprive the tumor of androgen. This may be achieved through surgical castration or administration of estrogen (diethylstilbestrol), analogues of luteinizing hormone releasing hormone (LHRH), or anti-androgens such as flutamide or cyproterone acetate. Aminoglutethimide and ketoconazole block steroid biosynthesis and may be useful in patients with advanced disease. Combination chemotherapy with cyclophosphamide, cisplatin, fluorouracil, and/or doxorubicin is reasonably effective in palliating pain from widespread bone metastases. Radiotherapy is used to decrease pain in isolated areas of metastatic disease.[83–85]

The therapy of prostatic carcinoma depends on the stage of the tumor. Stages A (limited to the gland with well-differentiated cells) and B (tumor confined to the gland in one or more lobes) may be treated with transurethral prostatectomy, radical prostatectomy, or radiation therapy.[86] Stages C (extension beyond capsule) and D (distant metastases) require radiotherapy and hormonal manipulation. A variety of treatment protocols are under study to determine the most effective means of controlling the growth of metastatic prostatic carcinoma.[87, 88]

The prognosis is good when prostate cancer is diagnosed early (stage A or B) with a 77%

to 80% 5-year survival rate.[89] In stage C disease, the survival rate is 58% and in stage D, 27%.[73] Rectal examination is a simple procedure but is relatively insensitive. Transrectal ultrasound and serum markers are more expensive and are not recommended for asymptomatic men. A positive PSA test is correlated with a tumor 30% of the time. A negative test does not eliminate prostatic cancer as a possibility. The therapy for prostatic cancer does not improve survival and has significant toxicities. The best screening mechanism to detect early cancers remains to be determined.[90]

TESTIS

The testicles are rarely affected by disease processes that are associated with back pain. However, malignancies of the testicles may metastasize locally to structures that will be associated with back pain. Testicular examination is frequently omitted from the evaluation of men with back pain. Failure to do a testicular examination in a young man may cause the scrotal mass that is indicative of testicular disease to be missed.

Testicular Carcinoma

Approximately 5000 cases of testicular cancer are diagnosed yearly in the United States. The peak age of incidence is 20 to 35 years. White men are more commonly affected than blacks. Men with maldescended testicles are at greater risk of developing the tumor. Back pain may be a presenting symptom in 10% to 21% of patients. Patients present with back pain in the absence of any testicular symptoms.[91, 92] The pain may be dull and insidious or persistent and sharp. The pain is localized over the bones of the lumbosacral spine and the para-aortic area. The source of the pain is metastatic disease to the para-aortic or caval nodes. The history of back pain that prevents sleep in a young man should raise the possibility of testicular cancer.[93] Physical examination will usually reveal a testicular mass. Diffuse induration without nodularity may be the initial finding. In rare circumstances, the testis may feel normal despite the presence of a tumor. Laboratory tests are obtained to identify tumor markers. Two useful markers are alpha-fetoprotein and human chorionic gonadotropin (HCG). These markers can also be used to follow the response to therapy.[94] The kinds of testicular tumors include seminoma (most benign), embryonal cell cancer, teratoma, and choriocarcinoma (most malignant).

Once the diagnosis is established, staging of

the lesion is necessary. Patients with back pain will have Stage II or more advanced disease. Therapy for patients with back pain will usually include orchiectomy along with chemotherapy including cisplatin and etoposide.[95, 96] The outcome is better if the disease is recognized at Stage I. The chance of diagnosis is improved if a testicular exam is added to the routine examination of the young adult man. Back pain may be the presenting symptom of recurrence of tumor before radiologic abnormalities are identified.[97]

Female Genital Organs

Females with disease in the pelvic organs may experience visceral, somatic, or referred pain.[98] Visceral pain from the uterus, fallopian tubes, or ovary is transmitted through nerves that travel with the sympathetic nervous system to spinal segments T11-12 and with the parasympathetic system to segments S2-4. The pain is deep, diffuse, and not well localized. Somatic nerves supply supporting tissues of the pelvis, including muscles, ligaments (e.g., uterosacral), peritoneum, and periosteum of bone. Irritation, traction, or pressure on these structures results in more localized, sharp pain that is felt in the suprapubic area or sacrum. Referred pain to the low back develops when sympathetic or parasympathetic nerves are stimulated by a disease process in the pelvic organs and causes sensory fibers in the dorsal horn of the corresponding spinal segment (T12, S2) to be activated. Back pain secondary to a gynecologic disorder is almost invariably associated with symptoms and signs of disease in the pelvic organs. A number of pathologic processes that affect the uterus, tubes, or ovaries may be associated with low back pain.

UTERUS

The uterus is an organ composed chiefly of smooth muscle lined by endometrium. New growths in the form of leiomyomas may be associated with back pain. Abnormal position of the uterus may put traction on ligamentous structures, which may cause pain. The lining of the uterus may escape the confines of that organ and implant on structures in the pelvis, which will result in cyclic pain. Pregnancy may cause pain on the basis of either the size of the uterus or the effects of hormones on musculoskeletal structures.

Leiomyomas

Leiomyomas are the most common form of uterine tumor.[99] One out of every 4 or 5 women over 35 years of age has uterine myomas. They are benign tumors composed of smooth muscle which arise in the wall of the uterus. Small myomas usually do not produce symptoms; however, these tumors may become quite large. Tumors occur and grow most commonly during the reproductive years and regress following menopause. Large tumors produce symptoms of heaviness in the pelvis and may produce back or lower extremity pain if they place pressure on nerves in the sacral portion of the bony pelvis. A dull aching soreness is usual. Myomas are palpable on physical examination of the pelvis. They are firm, irregular nodules arising from the pelvis and extending into the lower abdomen. The masses may be movable if they are pedunculated. The differential diagnosis may prove to be a problem. Symmetric enlargement of the uterus may be confused with pregnancy. The soft pregnant uterus and positive HCG test should help make the diagnosis of an intrauterine pregnancy. A pedunculated tumor may be confused with an ovarian tumor. Endometriosis can cause uterine scarring, which may be difficult to distinguish from subserous myomas. Ultrasonography may help differentiate among these possibilities (Fig. 17–13). Surgical removal is indicated for persistent symptoms of pain, uterine bleeding, infertility, size or position of the uterus preventing proper pelvic ex-

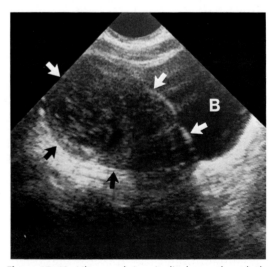

Figure 17–13. Ultrasound. Longitudinal scan through the pelvis demonstrating a large uterus *(arrows)* with multiple fibroid masses. (B = urinary bladder.) (Courtesy of Michael Hill, M.D.)

amination, or impingement on adjacent organs (such as the ureter).

Malposition

The uterus is normally directed forward in the pelvis.[100] In about a third of patients the uterus is retroverted or inclined posteriorly toward the sacrum and gently retroflexed. The most common simple displacement of the uterus is retroversion. Retroversion is congenital, acquired following a pregnancy, or a result of cul-de-sac pathology. The position of the uterus in itself is usually not associated with back pain. However, a retroverted uterus may be associated with chronic congestion of pelvic veins. Back pain may also occur as a result of permanent uterine retroversion. The pain is associated with the underlying condition (endometriosis, salpingitis). Pelvic pain, low back pain, abnormal menstrual bleeding, and infertility have been associated with retroversion of the uterus. Pelvic examination allows determination of the position of the uterus. Bimanual replacement of the uterus is inadequate to obtain appropriate positioning of the uterus. Use of a pessary is more successful at relieving symptoms.

Women who have had multiple births may experience weakening of the uterosacral and cardinal ligaments as well as of the pelvic musculature that supports the uterus.[101] In addition, patients who have a pelvic or presacral tumor or sacral nerve disorder may develop uterine prolapse. Uterine prolapse is the migration of the uterus down into the vagina. Patients with moderate prolapse will complain of a sensation of heaviness in the pelvis, lower abdominal pulling discomfort, and low back pain. Pelvic examination reveals descent of the cervix into the vagina. Therapy includes use of a pessary or surgical removal of the uterus.

Endometriosis

Endometriosis is a disease in which the presence of functioning tissue from the lining of the uterus (endometrium) occurs outside the uterine cavity. Adenomyosis is the presence of endometrial tissue within the uterine musculature. Endometrial tissue may be located most commonly on the ovaries or the dependent portion of the pelvic peritoneum. However, peritoneal surfaces as well as extraperitoneal sites have been remote locations for this tissue. Three theories proposed as the cause of endometriosis include metaplastic transformation of cells lining the pelvic peritoneum, transplantation of endometrium to ectopic locations, or induction of endometrial tissues

from mesenchymal tissues by factors released by shed endometrium.[102] Endometrial tissue outside the uterus undergoes the same monthly cycle of growth, shedding, and bleeding as the endometrial lining in the uterus, and symptoms of endometriosis are correlated with the site of the abnormal tissue. The disease may occur at any age after the onset of menses. Endometriosis is a familial disease with mothers, daughters, and sisters of patients more frequently affected than appropriate controls.[103] Older women who had endometriosis during their menses may develop recurrent disease if they receive estrogen replacement therapy. The estimated prevalence of endometriosis in women aged 15 to 50 is 2.5% to 3.3%.[104]

Implants in the rectovaginal septum, colon, and ureter are associated with low back pain, which may radiate to the rectum or to the medial or posterior portions of the thighs. The radiation of pain correlates with the innervation of the pelvic peritoneum by nerves from the lumbar and sacral spinal segments. The pain may be intermittent or persistent, but characteristically increases at the time of menstruation and persists throughout the entire period of bleeding. Other symptoms associated with endometriosis include dysmenorrhea, dyspareunia, infertility, and menorrhagia. About 20% of patients may be asymptomatic. Endometriosis causes sciatica with invasion of the sciatic nerve. Laparoscopy reveals a "pocket sign," an evagination of the pelvic peritoneum with endometriosis at its base on the sciatic nerve, in these patients.[105]

Physical examination reveals uterine tenderness and enlargement. Ovarian tenderness and enlargement also may be discovered. The uterus may be fixed in a retroverted position. Endometriosis may lodge within surgical scars. Inguinal endometriosis may mimic the signs of an incarcerated hernia.[102]

The diagnosis of endometriosis is frequently made at the time of a pelvic operative procedure. The diagnosis and extent of the disease in the pelvis can be adequately determined during laparoscopy or laparotomy.[103] MR is useful in the identification of endometriosis in women with adnexal masses.[106] The sensitivity and specificity for the identification by MR was 90% and 98%, respectively.[107] Endometriosis is frequently discovered in the pouch of Douglas, ureterosacral ligaments, ovaries, uterine surface, rectovaginal septum, fallopian tubes, bowel, or appendix. The urinary tract may be involved, as indicated by symptoms of obstruction. The intestinal tract also may be obstructed. Biopsy demonstrates endometrial glandular tissue. The most recently proposed classification system, from the work of the Brisbane series, is based on severity and extent of disease (Table 17–3).[103] The American Fertility Society also has published a classification system for endometriosis. The more advanced the stage of disease, the greater is the chance for the patient to experience symptoms of pain and infertility. Cytologic examination of peritoneal washings and ultrasonography are inadequate to make an accurate diagnosis of endometriosis.[108, 109]

Patients with endometriosis frequently experience dysmenorrhea. Painful menstruation and dysmenorrhea from all etiologies is the most common of all gynecologic complaints and is a leading cause of absenteeism of women from work. Dysmenorrhea may be primary or secondary. When primary, it is unassociated with any identifiable gynecologic disease. Secondary dysmenorrhea is caused by pelvic disease such as uterine malposition, cervical stenosis, salpingitis, or endometriosis. Painful menses occurs in ovulatory cycles and is associated with nausea, vomiting, and diarrhea. Dysmenorrheic pain occurs in the pelvis; is crampy, correlating with uterine contractions; and is frequently referred to the low back. In women with uterine retroversion, pain may be increased during menses; however, even those with normal uterine position may experience abdominal and back pain associated with their menses.

Pain starts just before the onset of bleeding and lasts 1 to 2 days after bleeding has stopped. Many patients with primary dysmenorrhea obtain relief with the use of nonsteroidal anti-inflammatory drugs or oral contraceptives.[110] Secondary dysmenorrhea may be associated with pelvic inflammatory disease and pelvic neoplasms. Other symptoms of endometriosis may mimic gastrointestinal, urologic, or neurologic disorders.

Laparoscopy or laparotomy is essential to make an appropriate diagnosis, since noninvasive tests are unreliable for making an accurate diagnosis of endometriosis. Therapy for endometriosis may include medications, including LHRH agonists (medical oophorectomy), oral contraceptives, danazol, nonsteroidal anti-inflammatory drugs, pregnancy, and surgery to remove foci of abnormal implants and lyse adhesions.[103] Danazol has been demonstrated to decrease pain even for an extended period of time after discontinuing the drug.[111]

Pregnancy

Pregnant women complain of low back pain with increasing size of the gravid uterus. Low back pain may be secondary to increasing tension in the uterosacral ligaments or to a marked increase in lumbar lordosis with concomitant muscle strain. Pain is experienced in the sacroiliac joints and the pubis and may radiate to the thighs. Low back pain in pregnancy may also be related to pelvic girdle relaxation. In the nonpregnant state there is practically no motion in the joints of the pelvis, symphysis, and sacroiliac joints. During pregnancy, women produce a hormone, relaxin, that allows increased motion in the pelvic joints, and this causes tension in the relaxed capsule and ligaments. Pain develops about the sacroiliac joints, the symphysis pubis, and the medial part of the thighs. It is increased by active movement such as climbing stairs. Most patients have resolution of their symptoms post partum. Rarely, they continue with symptoms of pelvic relaxation and require bracing or operative stabilization of joints in order to resolve their complaints.[112]

The frequency of back pain in pregnancy has been reported by Fast and associates. Caucasians had a statistically higher incidence of back pain as compared with other groups. Overall, 56% of mothers had pain. Pain radiated from the low back to the lower extremities in 45% of patients. The pain usually started during the fifth to seventh month of pregnancy.[113] In another study, Svensson reported back pain in 24% of the 1514 women who had been pregnant.[114]

TABLE 17–3. BRISBANE SERIES CLASSIFICATION OF ENDOMETRIOSIS

STAGE	EXTENT OF DISEASE
0	Minimal disease, no hemorrhage
1	Minimal disease, hemorrhage, no adhesions
2	Progression with hemorrhage, adhesions
3	Progression to organ destruction, dense adhesions
4	Total loss of reproductive function, extensive organ destruction, dense adhesions, progression to "frozen pelvis"

FALLOPIAN TUBES

The fallopian tubes are appendages of the uterus and convey ova from the ovary to the uterus. The problems that affect the fallopian tubes and cause back pain are pelvic inflammatory disease and ectopic pregnancy.

Pelvic Inflammatory Disease

The most common disorder that affects the fallopian tubes and is associated with low back pain is pelvic inflammatory disease.[115] Pelvic inflammatory disease is a term for acute or chronic infection of the tubes and ovary. Bacteria, particularly *Neisseria gonorrhoeae*, gain access to the tube by direct spread from the endometrial lining or lymphatic dissemination. Other organisms causing infection include *Chlamydia trachomatis* (most common pathogen), *Escherichia coli*, *Streptococcus viridans*, anaerobic cocci, and *Clostridium perfringens*. The infection may localize to the tube or spread to involve the ovary (tubo-ovarian abscess) or the pelvic peritoneum. The chief clinical symptom of a patient with acute salpingitis is lower abdominal and pelvic pain, which may be unilateral or bilateral. Patients have a feeling of pelvic pressure and may have radiation of low back pain into the thighs. Nausea also may be present. Physical examination finds an acutely ill patient with or without fever, hypoactive bowel sounds, lower quadrant abdominal tenderness, purulent cervical discharge, and exquisite tenderness on movement of the pelvic organs during pelvic examination. Laboratory examination of the discharge may show pathogenic organisms on Gram stain and on culture. Therapy for acutely ill patients is hospitalization for intravenous antibiotics and bed rest in the semi-Fowler's position.[116] Repeated infections or inadequate treatment of acute salpingitis can result in recurrent episodes of pelvic infection or tubo-ovarian or pelvic abscess. Complications of these very serious infections include infertility, peritonitis, intra-abdominal abscesses, bowel obstruction, or septic emboli. About 1 million American women (1% of sexually active females) will develop pelvic inflammatory disease. This group will experience ectopic pregnancy (5%), infertility (10%), pelvic pain (15%), and recurrent infection (25%).[117]

A number of conditions must be considered during the evaluation of a patient with pelvic pain. These include ectopic pregnancy, acute appendicitis, acute pylonephritis, adnexal torsion, endometriosis, ovarian cysts, renal stones, myomata, and psychogenic pain syndromes.

Ectopic Pregnancy

Ectopic pregnancy is a pregnancy that is implanted outside the uterine cavity. The most common site for ectopic pregnancy is the fallopian tube. The number of hospitalizations for ectopic pregnancies in the United States in 1989 was 88,400.[117a] The death rate is 1 in 1000 cases.[118] The major sources of disease and death with ectopic pregnancy are delay by patients in reporting early symptoms and delay by physicians in initiating appropriate treatment. One study showed delay in diagnosis in 50% or more of patients with ectopic pregnancy.[118] The problem for the examining physician is the fact that symptoms of ectopic pregnancy mimic those of other abdominal and pelvic problems. Ectopic pregnancy should remain on the list of possible diagnosis in all women between menarche and menopause.

Patients with structural abnormalities of the fallopian tubes are at risk of developing an ectopic pregnancy. Chronic pelvic inflammatory disease is a common cause of both problems. Approximately 5% of patients with pelvic inflammatory disease develop ectopic pregnancies. The chances for ectopic implantation are greater with increasing severity of salpingitis.[118a] Distorted tubal anatomy may be associated with a ruptured appendix or endometriosis. Patients who utilize an IUD as a contraceptive device also are at greater risk of developing ectopic pregnancy since pelvic inflammatory disease is a frequent result of their use.[119]

The first symptoms of ectopic pregnancy are missed period, nausea, and breast tenderness. The classic triad of pain, irregular uterine bleeding, and an adnexal mass on physical examination is found in a minority of patients when seen in an emergency room setting.[119a] Pain develops in the lower quadrant as rupture is imminent. As rupture occurs, blood collects in the inferior portion of the pelvis and abdomen. Pain in the sacral area may radiate to the thighs as the pelvic peritoneum is irritated. Nausea and vomiting may occur with rupture.

Physical examination reveals fever in less than 2% of patients.[118] Pulse rate is increased in patients hemorrhaging from a ruptured tubal pregnancy. Abdominal signs vary. Lower abdominal tenderness is common, with rebound tenderness and guarding occurring less often. Pelvic examination may be normal in a minority of patients. Usually tenderness is present along with an adnexal mass in about half. A mass in the cul-de-sac, when present, is due to collection of blood in the area.

Anemia is found in a minority along with leukocytosis. The pregnancy test is positive in 82% of patients with the radioimmunoassay for HCG.[120] A pregnancy may be detected by

HCG assay or maternal serum by day 7.[121] Culdocentesis is a valuable test for diagnosing rupture of an ectopic pregnancy. In a study of 300 surgically treated patients, culdocentesis revealed nonclotting blood in 95% of patients.[118]

The differential diagnosis of ectopic pregnancy includes a wide range of disorders including normal intrauterine pregnancy, ruptured corpus luteum cyst, acute appendicitis, salpingitis, acute pyelonephritis, degenerating fibroid, and incomplete abortion. Careful history, along with pregnancy tests, may help differentiate the nonpregnant from the pregnant state. Ultrasonography may help identify the location of the pregnancy.[122] The use of transvaginal ultrasonography is able to detect the presence of an adnexal mass that may be missed by transabdominal ultrasound (Fig. 17–14).[123]

The treatment of ectopic pregnancy has evolved over the past 7 years to include medical and surgical therapies. Early ectopic pregnancies may resolve spontaneously at a rate of 75% to 83%.[124] These patients are asymptomatic and have falling HCG levels. Methotrexate, given intramuscularly 1 mg/kg with leukovorin rescue, 0.1 mg/kg, has had a 96% success rate of resolving pregnancies with minimal toxicity. This therapy works best when HCG levels are less than 10,000 mU/ml.[125] Surgical intervention, in the form of laparoscopy, has been associated with preservation of fertility. This procedure is less costly than laparotomy and has equally good results.[126] At the time of laparoscopy, the diagnosis can be made and the appropriate fallopian tube can be preserved if at all feasible. The ovary is spared unless it is involved by an extensive hematoma arising from the tube.

OVARY

The ovaries have great potential of producing an unusual number of neoplasms of both epithelial and connective tissue origin. While ovarian neoplasms may occur at any age, they are most common during the reproductive years. Benign tumors occur most commonly during years of ovulation (age 30 to 40 years), while malignant tumors occur after ovulation has ceased (50 years and up).

Benign Tumors

Benign tumors of the ovary include a wide range of lesions which may include functional cysts (corpus luteum cysts) to new growths (serous cystadenoma, granulosa cell tumor, or dermal cyst). Functional cysts occur at times of pregnancy or ineffective ovulation. These growths are associated with symptoms if they grow to a large size or are complicated by torsion, rupture, or hemorrhage. Of the benign tumors, serous cystadenoma and mucinous cystadenoma are the most common, constituting 25% of all benign tumors.[100]

Back pain associated with benign ovarian tumors is rare. When back pain occurs, it is localized to the sacrum. The pain has a quality of pressure and aching. Most benign tumors are asymptomatic until they reach a large size. The symptoms these tumors cause are frequently related to pressure on neighboring structures (ureters, colon, veins, or lymphatics). Pain from benign lesions may be referred to the iliac or inguinal areas, the inner aspect of the upper thigh, or the vulva. A sudden change in symptoms may occur if there is hemorrhage, torsion, or rupture of a cyst. These complications of benign tumors result in abdominal symptoms.

Physical examination reveals a unilateral, freely movable, smooth mass. Ascites may be present. The uterus may be displaced if the tumor is large. Careful pelvic examination should be able to identify the location of the

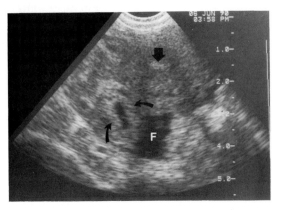

Figure 17–14. Transvaginal sonogram of a right tubal ectopic pregnancy. The uterine cavity *(large arrow)* is empty. An echogenic ring-like structure is present in the right adnexa *(curved arrows)* representing the ectopic gestational sac. A small amount of fluid (F) is present in the cul-de-sac. (Courtesy of Michael Hill, M.D.)

mass in relation to the ovary. Lesions of the colon, bladder, uterus, and fallopian tube must be differentiated. Ultrasonography does not replace the pelvic examination in determining the site of a lesion, but it may discriminate between uterine and adnexal masses and distinguish cystic from solid tumors (Fig. 17–15).[127]

The management of ovarian neoplasms may be medical for functional growths and surgical for benign tumors. For functional cysts, a course of oral contraceptives can accelerate involution of non-neoplastic ovarian enlargement. In one study, 72% of patients had resolution of ovarian enlargement after a 6-week trial of therapy.[128] Benign tumors larger than 5 cm and those that do not respond to hormonal therapy require an exploratory operation. The extent of surgery depends on the findings at operation, including the type of tumor and extent of the lesion. Benign tumors are usually removed. Removal of the opposite ovary and uterus depends on the age of the patient and the potential for developing the same lesion in the remaining tissue.

Malignant Tumors

Carcinoma of the ovary causes 6% of all cancer deaths in women in the United States. The annual incidence of cases is 22,000.[129] It is the most common cause of death among gynecologic cancers.[130] Women who are nulliparous and have a family history of ovarian cancer have an increased risk. The most important risk factor is heredity, having two first-degree relatives with the tumor.[131]

Like benign tumors, malignant tumors may be asymptomatic until the tumor reaches a large size. Abdominal distention and pain are very common complaints. Back pain occurs rarely. The pain may have an aching quality, with radiation from the paraspinous area and sacrum to the thighs. The pain may occur when the blood supply to the ovary is compromised. Patients also may develop back pain by direct extension of the tumor or spread through lymphatics.[132]

Physical examination, including pelvic examination, is very revealing, particularly in the postmenopausal patient. The ovaries are usually not palpable in postmenopausal women. Palpable ovaries in this group of women require additional evaluation. Cul-de-sac nodularity may be secondary to metastatic disease. Examination of inguinal and supraclavicular nodes may detect the spread of an unsuspected malignant ovarian tumor.

Transvaginal ultrasonography is more sensitive than CT scan for imaging the ovary and is predictive in detecting the presence of cancer.[133] This technique is able to differentiate simple cysts from complex cysts associated with malignancies.

Once an ovarian tumor is suspected, surgical staging is necessary for diagnosis and determination of the extent of disease. Areas of lymph drainage (iliac and para-aortic nodes) must be sampled along with the cul-de-sac, the abdominal gutters, and the diaphragm.[134] Determination of glycoprotein markers for ovarian cancer, CA 125 and DF 3, are useful for following the response to treatment and detecting early disease.[135] The CA 125 test is more useful for following diagnosed patients than in detecting the presence of an ovarian neoplasm. Elevated levels may be detected with other neoplasms and with other gynecologic conditions such as endometriosis and pregnancy.[136]

Therapy of early stage disease (I and II—limited to the ovary or true pelvis, respectively) is surgical. Disease with extension beyond the pelvis (III) and distant metastases (IV) requires chemotherapy. The benefit of therapy with a single drug versus combination therapy remains to be determined.[137, 138] Current chemotherapy that includes platinum has improved response rates and prolonged median survival. Taxol, a diterpene plant product isolated from the bark of the Pacific yew tree, has been effective as an adjunct to platinum in patients resistant to platinum and cyclophosphamide chemotherapy.[136]

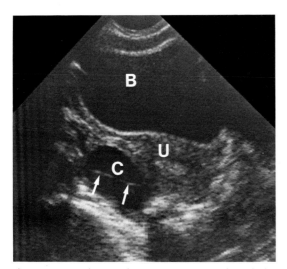

Figure 17–15. Ultrasound. Transverse section through the pelvis revealing a right ovarian cyst (C), which is septated *(arrows)*. (U = uterus; B = bladder.) (Courtesy of Michael Hill, M.D.)

References

GENITOURINARY DISEASES

1. Gibson SM, Kimmel PL: Genitourinary disease affecting the spine. Semin Spine Surg 2:145, 1990.
2. Johnson CM, Wilson DM, O'Fallan WM, et al.: Renal stone epidemiology: a 24-year study in Rochester, Minnesota. Kidney Int 16:624, 1979.
3. Recurrent renal calculi. (Editorial.) Br Med J 282:5, 1981.
4. Brenner BM, Rector FC Jr (eds): The Kidney, 3rd ed. Philadelphia: WB Saunders Co, 1986.
5. Risholm L: Studies on renal colic and its treatment by posterior splanchnic block. Acta Chir Scand (Suppl) 184:1, 1954.
6. Elliot JS: Urinary calculus disease. Surg Clin North Am 45:1393, 1965.
7. Harrington TM, Bunch TW, Van Den Berg CJ: Renal tubular acidosis: a new look at treatment of musculoskeletal and renal disease. Mayo Clin Proc 58:354, 1983.
8. Kaye AD, Pollack HM: Diagnostic imaging approach to the patient with obstructive uropathy. Semin Nephrol 2:55, 1982.
9. Brennan RE, Curtis JA, Kurtz AB, Dalton JR: Use of tomography and ultrasound in the diagnosis of non-opaque renal calculi. JAMA 244:594, 1980.
10. Spirnak JP, Resnick MI: Urinary stones. In Tanagho EA, McAninch JW (eds): General Urology, 13th ed. Norwalk, Connecticut: Appleton & Lange, 1992, pp 271–298.
11. Wickham JEA, Webb DR, Payne SR, et al.: Extracorporeal shock wave lithotripsy: the first 50 patients treated in Britain. Br Med J 290:1188, 1985.
12. Chaussy C, Schuller J, Schmiedt E, et al.: Extracorporeal shock-wave lithotripsy (ESWL) for treatment of urolithiasis. Urology 23:59, 1984.
13. Brannen GF, Bush WH, Correa RJ, et al.: Kidney stone removal, percutaneous versus surgical lithotomy. J Urol 133:6, 1985.
14. Clayman R: Techniques in percutaneous removal of renal calculi: mechanical extraction and electrohydraulic lithotripsy. Urology 25:11, 1984.
15. Segura JW: The role of percutaneous surgery in renal and ureteral stone removal. J Urol 141:780, 1989.
16. Maddern JP: Surgery of the staghorn calculus. Br J Urol 39:237, 1967.
17. Pak CYC, Peters P, Hurt G, et al.: Is selective therapy of recurrent nephrolithiasis possible? Am J Med 71:615, 1981.
18. Crawhall JC, Scowen EF, Watts RWE: Effect of penicillamine on cystinuria. Br Med J 1:588, 1963.
19. Silverman DE, Stamey TA: Management of infection stones: The Stanford experience. Medicine 62:44, 1983.
20. Sanford JP: Urinary tract symptoms and infections. Annu Rev Med 26:485, 1975.
21. Stamey TA: Pathogenesis and Treatment of Urinary Tract Infections. Baltimore: Williams & Wilkins Co, 1972.
22. Kaye D, Santoro J: Urinary tract infection. In Mandell GL, Douglas RG Jr, Bennett JE (eds): Principles and Practice of Infectious Disease. New York: John Wiley & Sons, Inc, 1979, p 537.
23. Latham RH, Wong ES, Larson A, et al.: Laboratory diagnosis of urinary tract infection in ambulatory women. JAMA 254:3333, 1985.
24. Rubin RH, Fang LST, Jones SR, et al.: Multicenter trial of single dose amoxicillin therapy of acute, uncomplicated urinary tract infection localized by the antibody-coated technique. JAMA 244:561, 1980.
25. Hurwitz SR, Kessler WO, Alazraki NP, Ashburn WL: Gallium-67 imaging to localize urinary-tract infections. Br J Radiol 49:156, 1976.
26. Smith JW, Jones SR, Reed WP, et al.: Recurrent urinary tract infections in men—characteristics and response to therapy. Ann Intern Med 92:544, 1979.
27. Stamm WE, McKevitt M, Counts GW: Acute renal infection in women: treatment with trimethoprim-sulfamethoxazole or ampicillin for two or six weeks. A randomized trial. Ann Intern Med 106:341, 1987.
28. Tolkoff-Rubin NE, Rubin RH: Ciprofloxacin in management of urinary tract infection. Urology 31:359, 1988.
29. Piccirillo M, Rigsby C, Rosenfield AT: Contemporary imaging of renal inflammatory disease. Infect Dis Clin North Am 1:927, 1987.
30. Thorley JD, Jones SR, Sanford JP: Perinephric abscess. Medicine 53:441, 1974.
31. Covington T Jr, Reeser W: Hydronephrosis associated with overhydration. J Urol 63:438, 1950.
32. Perlberg S, Pfau A: Management of ureteropelvic junction obstruction associated with lower polar vessels. Urology 23:13, 1984.
33. Tse RL, Leberman PR: Acute renal artery occlusion—etiology, diagnosis, and treatment. Report of a case with subsequent revascularization. J Urol 108:32, 1972.
34. Rudy DC, Seigel RS, Parker TW, Woodside JR: Segmental renal artery emboli treated with low-dose intra-arterial streptokinase. Urology 19:410, 1982.
35. Silverberg E: Cancer statistics. CA 35:19, 1985.
36. Mostofi FK: Pathology and Spread of Renal Cell Carcinoma. In King JS Jr (ed): Renal Neoplasia. Boston: Little, Brown and Co, 1967, p 41.
37. Skinner DG, Colvin RB, Vermillion CD, et al.: Diagnosis and management of renal cell carcinoma. A clinical and pathologic study of 309 cases. Cancer 28:1165, 1971.
38. Gibbons RP, Montie JE, Correa RJ Jr, Mason JT: Manifestations of renal cell carcinoma. Urology 8:201, 1976.
39. Chisholm GD, Roy RR: The systemic effects of malignant renal tumor. Br J Urol 43:687, 1971.
40. Berger L, Sinkoff MW: Systemic manifestations of hypernephroma: a review of 273 cases. Am J Med 22:791, 1957.
41. Pinals RS, Krane SK: Medical aspects of renal carcinoma. Postgrad Med J 38:507, 1982.
42. Weyman PJ, McCleannan BL, Stanley RJ, et al.: Comparison of computed tomography and angiography in the evaluation of renal cell carcinoma. Radiology 137:417, 1980.
43. Richie JP, Garnick MB, Seltzer S, Bettmann MA: Computerized tomography scan for diagnosis and staging of renal cell carcinoma. J Urol 129:114, 1983.
44. Watson RC, Fleming RJ, Evans JA: Arteriography in the diagnosis of renal carcinoma. Radiology 91:188, 1968.
45. Hricak H, Thoeni RF, Carroll PR, et al.: Detection and staging of renal neoplasms: a reassessment of MR imaging. Radiology 166:643, 1988.
46. Robson CJ, Churchill BM, Anderson W: The results of radical nephrectomy for renal cell carcinoma. Trans Am Assoc Genitourin Surg 60:122, 1968.
47. Waters WB, Richie JP: Aggressive surgical approach to renal cell carcinoma: review of 130 cases. J Urol 122:306, 1979.

48. Baker LR, Mallinson WJ, Gregory MC, et al.: Idiopathic retroperitoneal fibrosis: a retrospective analysis of 60 cases. Br J Urol 60:497, 1987.

49. Babian RJ, Johnson DE: Primary carcinoma of the ureter. J Urol 123:357, 1980.

50. Thomas WC Jr: Clinical concepts of renal calculus disease. J Urol 113:423, 1975.

51. Anderson EE: The management of ureteral calculi. Urol Clin North Am 1:357, 1974.

52. Drach GW: Stone manipulation. Urology 12:286, 1978.

53. Amar AD: Vesiculoureteral reflux in adults: a 12 year study of 122 patients. Urology 3:184, 1974.

54. Smith DR: Vesiculoureteral reflux and other abnormalities of the ureterovesical junction. In Campbell MF, Harrison JH (eds): Urology, 4th ed. Philadelphia: WB Saunders Co, 1978.

55. Ahmed S, Smith AJ: Results of ureteral reimplantation in patients with intrarenal reflux. J Urol 120:332, 1978.

56. Bakshandeh K, Lynne C, Carrion H: Vesicoureteral reflux and end stage renal disease. J Urol 116:557, 1976.

57. Martinez-Maldonado M, Kumjian DA: Acute renal failure due to urinary tract obstruction. Med Clin North Am 74:919, 1990.

58. Cox CE, Lacy SS, Hinman F Jr: The urethra and its relationships to urinary tract infections. II. The urethral flora of the female with recurrent urinary infection. J Urol 99:632, 1968.

59. Fang LST, Tolkoff-Rubin NE, Rubin RH: Efficacy of single-dose and conventional amoxicillin therapy in urinary tract infection localized by the antibody-coated bacteria technic. N Engl J Med 298:413, 1978.

60. Stamey TA: Urinary tract infections in the female: a perspective. In Remington JS, Swartz MW (eds): Current Clinical Topics in Infectious Diseases, Vol 2. New York: McGraw-Hill Book Co, 1981, p 31.

61. Meares EM Jr: Prostatitis syndromes: new perspectives about old woes. J Urol 123:141, 1980.

62. Lipsky BA: Urinary tract infections in men: epidemiology, pathophysiology, diagnosis, and treatment. Ann Intern Med 110:138, 1989.

63. Gleckman R, Crowley M, Natsios GA: Therapy of recurrent invasive urinary-tract infection of men. N Engl J Med 301:878, 1979.

64. Moller P, Vinje O, Fryjordet A: HLA antigens and sacroiliitis in chronic prostatitis. Scand J Rheumatol 9:138, 1980.

65. Drach GW: Prostatitis and prostatodynia: their relationship to benign prostatic hypertrophy. Urol Clin North Am 7:79, 1980.

66. Meares EM Jr: Acute and chronic prostatitis: diagnosis and treatment. Infect Dis Clin North Am 1:855, 1987.

67. Whitmore WF Jr: Natural history and staging of prostate cancer. Urol Clin North Am 11:205, 1984.

68. Catalona WJ, Smith DS, Ratliff TL, et al.: Measurement of prostate-specific antigen in serum as a screening test for prostate cancer. N Engl J Med 324:1156, 1991.

69. Kramer BS, Brown ML, Prorok PC, et al.: Prostate cancer screening: what we know and what we need to know. Ann Intern Med 119:914, 1993.

70. Lange PH, Ercole CJ, Lightner DJ, et al.: The value of serum prostate-specific antigen determinations before and after radical prostatectomy. J Urol 141:873, 1989.

71. Lee F, Torp-Pedersen ST, Siders DB, et al.: Transrectal ultrasound in the diagnosis and staging of prostatic carcinoma. Radiology 170:609, 1989.

72. Hricak H, Dooms GC, Jeffrey RB, et al.: Prostatic carcinoma: staging by clinical assessment, CT, and MR imaging. Radiology 162:331, 1987.

73. Sundkvist GMG, Ahlgren L, Mattsson S, et al.: Repeated quantitative bone scintigraphy in patients with prostatic carcinoma treated with orchiectomy. Eur J Nucl Med 14:203, 1966.

74. Kass LG, Woyke S, Schreiber K, et al.: Thin-needle aspiration biopsy of the prostate. Urol Clin North Am 11:237, 1984.

75. Klein LA: Prostatic carcinoma. N Engl J Med 300:824, 1979.

76. Gleason DF: The Veterans Administration Cooperative Urological Research Group: histologic grading and clinical staging of prostatic carcinoma. In Tannenbaum M (ed): Urologic Pathology. The Prostate. Philadelphia: Lea & Febiger, 1977, p 171.

77. McCullough DL, Prout GR Jr, Daly JJ: Carcinoma of the prostate and lymphatic metastases. J Urol 111:65, 1974.

78. McIntire TL, Murphy WM, Coon JS, et al.: The prognostic value of DNA ploidy combined with histologic substaging for incidental carcinoma of the prostate gland. Am J Clin Pathol 89:139, 1988.

79. McCullough DL: Diagnosis and staging of prostatic cancer. In Skinner DG, de Kemion JB (eds): Genitourinary Cancer. Philadelphia: WB Saunders Co, 1978, p 295.

80. Narayan P, Lange PH: Current controversies in the management of carcinoma of the prostate. Semin Oncol 7:460, 1960.

81. Barzell W, Bean MA, Hilaris BS, Whitmore WF Jr: Prostatic adenocarcinoma: relationship of grade and local extent to the pattern of metastases. J Urol 118:278, 1977.

82. Elder JS, Catalona WJ: Management of newly diagnosed metastatic carcinoma of the prostate. Urol Clin North Am 11:283, 1984.

83. Trachtenberg J: Ketoconazole therapy in advanced prostatic cancer. J Urol 132:61, 1984.

84. Labrie F, Dupont A, Belanger A: Complete androgen blockade for the treatment of prostate cancer. In Devita VT Jr, Hellman S, Rosenberg SA (eds): Important Advances in Oncology, 1985. Philadelphia: JB Lippincott Co, 1984, p 193.

85. Torti FM, Carter SK: The chemotherapy of prostatic adenocarcinoma. Ann Intern Med 92:681, 1980.

86. Consensus Conference: The management of clinically localized prostate cancer. JAMA 258:2727, 1987.

87. Crawford ED, Eisenberger MA, McLeod DG, et al.: A controlled trial of leuprolide with and without flutamide in prostatic carcinoma. N Engl J Med 321:419, 1989.

88. Peeling WB: Phase III studies to compare goserelin (Zoladex) with orchiectomy and with diethylstilbestrol in treatment of prostatic carcinoma. Urology 33(5 suppl):45, 1989.

89. Andriole GL, Catalona WJ: Early diagnosis of prostate cancer. Urol Clin North Am 14:657, 1987.

90. Dorr VJ, Williamson SK, Stephens RL: An evaluation of prostate-specific antigen as a screening test for prostate cancer. Arch Intern Med 153:2529, 1993.

91. Paulson DF, Einhorn L, Peckham M, Williams SD: Cancer of the testis. In De Vita VT, Hellman S, Rosenberg SA (eds): Cancer: Principles and Practice of Oncology. Philadelphia: JB Lippincott Co, 1982, pp 786–822.

92. Cantwell BMJ, Mann KA, Harris AL: Back pain—a presentation of metastatic testicular germ cell tumors. Lancet 1:262, 1987.

93. Smith DB, Newlands ES, Rustin GJ, et al.: Lumbar pain in stage 1 testicular germ cell tumors: a symptom preceding radiological abnormality. Br J Urol 64:302, 1989.

94. Lange PH, McIntire KR, Waldmann TA, et al.: Serum alpha fetoprotein and human chorionic gonadotropin in the diagnosis and management of non-seminomatous germ-cell testicular cancer. N Engl J Med 295:1237, 1976.

95. Garnick MB, Canellos GP, Richie JP: Treatment and surgical staging of testicular and primary extragonadal germ cell cancer. JAMA 250:1733, 1983.

96. Williams SD, Einhorn LH, Greco AF, et al.: VP-16-213 salvage therapy for refractory germinal neoplasms. Cancer 46:2154, 1980.

97. Woll PJ, Rankin EM: Persistent back pain due to malignant lymphadenopathy. Ann Rheum Dis 46:681, 1987.

98. Walde J: Obstetrical and gynecological back and pelvic pains, especially those contracted during pregnancy. Acta Obstet Gynecol Scand 41:11, 1962.

99. Stearns HC: Uterine myomas: clinical and pathologic aspects. Postgrad Med 51:165, 1972.

100. Danforth DN, Scot JR, DiSaia PJ, et al. (eds): Obstetrics and Gynecology. Philadelphia: JB Lippincott Co, 1986.

101. Te Linde RW: Prolapse of the uterus and allied conditions. Am J Obstet Gynecol 94:444, 1966.

102. Olive DL, Schwartz LB: Endometriosis. N Engl J Med 328:1759, 1993.

103. O'Connor DT: Endometriosis. New York: Churchill Livingstone, 1987.

104. Guzick DS: Clinical epidemiology of endometriosis and infertility. Obstet Gynecol Clin North Am 16:43, 1989.

105. Torkelson SJ, Lee RA, Hidahl DB: Endometriosis of the sciatic nerve: a report of two cases and a review of the literature. Obstet Gynecol 71:473, 1988.

106. Johnson IR, Symonds EM, Worthington BS, et al.: Imaging ovarian tumors by nuclear magnetic resonance. Br J Obstet Gynecol 91:260, 1984.

107. Togashi K, Nishimura K, Kimura I, et al.: Endometrial cysts: diagnosis with MR imaging. Radiology 180:73, 1991.

108. Protuondo JA, Herran C, Echanojaurgei AD, Riego AG: Peritoneal flushing and biopsy in laparoscopically diagnosed endometriosis. Fertil Steril 38:538, 1982.

109. Goldman SM, Minkin SI: Diagnosing endometriosis with ultrasound: accuracy and specificity. J Reprod Med 25:178, 1980.

110. Ylikorkala O, Dawood MY: New concepts in dysmenorrhea. Am J Obstet Gynecol 130:833, 1978.

111. Teloimaa S, Puolakka J, Ronnberg L, Kaupilla A: Placebo-controlled comparison of danazol and high-dose medroxyprogesterone acetate in the treatment of endometriosis. Gynecol Endocrinol 1:13, 1987.

112. Hagen R: Pelvic girdle relaxation from an orthopaedic point of view. Acta Orthop Scand 45:550, 1974.

113. Fast A, Shapiro D, Docommun EJ, et al.: Low-back pain in pregnancy. Spine 12:368, 1987.

114. Svensson H, Andersson GBJ, Hagstad A, Jansson P: The relationship of low-back pain to pregnancy and gynecologic factors. Spine 15:371, 1990.

115. Eschenbach DA, Holmes KK: Acute pelvic inflammatory disease: current concepts of pathogenesis, etiology, and management. Clin Obstet Gynecol 18:35, 1975.

116. Ansbacher R: Recognition and treatment of pelvic inflammatory disease. Modern Med 55:79, 1987.

117. Eschenbach DA: Acute pelvic inflammatory disease Urol Clin North Am 11:65, 1984.

117a. Ectopic pregnancy–United States. MMWR 41:591, 1992.

118. Brenner PF, Roy S, Mishell DR Jr: Ectopic pregnancy. A study of 300 consecutive surgically treated cases. JAMA 243:673, 1980.

118a. Joesoef MR, Westrom L, Reynolds G, et al.: Recurrence of ectopic pregnancy: the role of salpingitis. Am J Obstet Gynecol 165:46, 1991.

119. Burkman RT: Association between intrauterine device and pelvic inflammatory disease. The Women's Health Study. Obstet Gynecol 57:269, 1981.

119a. Stovall TG, Kellerman AL, Ling FW, Buster JE: Emergency department diagnosis of ectopic pregnancy. Ann Emerg Med 19:1098, 1990.

120. Barnes RB, Roy S, Yee B, et al.: Reliability of urinary pregnancy tests in the diagnosis of ectopic pregnancy. J Reprod Med 30:827, 1985.

121. Helsa JS, Rock JA: Emergent management of ectopic pregnancy. Infertil Reprod Med Clin North Am 3:775, 1992.

122. Lawson TL: Ectopic pregnancy: criteria and accuracy of ultrasonic diagnosis. AJR 131:153, 1978.

123. Shapiro BS, Cullen M, Taylor KJ, DeCherney AH: Transvaginal ultrasound for the diagnosis of ectopic pregnancy. Fertil Steril 50:425, 1988.

124. Leach RE, Ory SJ: Modern management of ectopic pregnancy. J Reprod Med 34:324, 1989.

125. Stoval TG, Ling FW, Gray LA, et al.: Methotrexate treatment of unruptured ectopic pregnancy: a report of 100 cases. Obstet Gynecol 77:749, 1991.

126. Zouves C, Urman B, Gomel V: Laparoscopic surgical treatment of tubal pregnancy: a safe, effective alternative to laparotomy. J Reprod Med 37:205, 1992.

127. O'Brien WS, Buck DR, Nash JD: Evaluation of sonography in the initial assessment of the gynecological patient. Am J Obstet Gynecol 149:598, 1984.

128. Spanos WJ: Preoperative hormonal therapy of cystic adrenal masses. Am J Obstet Gynecol 116:551, 1973.

129. Boring CC, Squires TS, Tong T: Cancer statistics, 1993. CA Cancer J Clin 43:7, 1993.

130. Richardson GS, Scully RE, Nikrui N, Nelson JH Jr: Common epithelial cancer of the ovary. N Engl J Med 312:415, 474, 1985.

131. Lynch HT, Lynch JF: Hereditary ovarian carcinoma. Hematol Oncol Clin North Am 6:783, 1992.

132. Julian CG, Goss J, Blanchard K, Woodruff JD: Biologic behavior of primary ovarian malignancy. Obstet Gynecol 44:873, 1974.

133. van Nagell JR Jr, Higgins RV, Donaldson ES, et al.: Transvaginal sonography as a screening method for ovarian cancer: a report on the first 1000 cases screened. Cancer 65:573, 1990.

134. Buchsbaum HJ, Lifshitz S: Staging and surgical evaluation of ovarian cancer. Semin Oncol 11:227, 1984.

135. Bast RC Jr, Knapp RC: Immunologic approaches to the management of ovarian carcinoma. Semin Oncol 11:264, 1984.

136. Cannistra SA: Cancer of the ovary. N Engl J Med 329:1550, 1993.

137. Parker LM, Griffiths CT, Yankee RA, et al.: Combination chemotherapy with adriamycin-cyclophosphamide for advanced ovarian carcinoma. Cancer 46:669, 1980.

138. Williams CJ, Mead GM, Macbeth FR, et al.: Cisplatin combination chemotherapy versus chlorambucil in advanced ovarian carcinoma: mature results of a randomized trial. J Clin Oncol 3:1455, 1985.

GASTROINTESTINAL DISEASES

Capsule Summary

Frequency of back pain—common
Location of back pain—lumbar spine
Quality of back pain—dull ache, colicky
Signs and symptoms—alteration of bowel habits, abdominal tenderness
Laboratory and x-ray tests—abnormal serum enzymes, bilirubin, WBC; abnormal filling defects on contrast radiographs
Treatment—surgical removal of mass or stones, antibiotics

The organs of the gastrointestinal tract associated with back pain are those in direct contact with the retroperitoneum or those with referred pain distribution to the back. Diseases of the pancreas, duodenum, gallbladder, and colon may be associated with low back pain of visceral, somatic, or referred origin. A common finding in the history of patients with back pain secondary to a gastrointestinal disorder is the relationship between pain and eating or bowel function such as defecation.[1]

Pancreas

The pancreas is located at the level of the first and second lumbar vertebrae in the retroperitoneum. Pain from diseases that affect the pancreas is felt deep in the midepigastrium secondary to somatic irritation and is referred to the back in the region of L1. Acute inflammatory diseases of the pancreas cause severe, persistent pain, which may be out of proportion to physical findings. Infiltrative diseases of the pancreas, such as pancreatic carcinoma, may not cause pain until the lesion has invaded peripancreatic nerves. Disease processes that affect the head of the pancreas cause pain to the right of the spine, while lesions of the body and tail are felt to the left of the spine.

ACUTE PANCREATITIS

Acute pancreatitis is an inflammatory disease of the pancreas in which the digestive enzymes produced by that organ act on pancreatic tissue.[2] Conditions that may precipitate episodes of pancreatitis include gallstones, ethanolism, drugs (azathioprine, oral contraceptives, tetracycline, furosemide), hyperlipidemia, trauma, hypercalcemia, and obstruction to the outflow of pancreatic enzymes. The incidence of acute pancreatitis is 28 per 100,000 population per year.[3] The median age is 53, and men and women are affected equally.[4]

Most often the presenting and most significant symptoms include steady, boring, severe epigastric pain, which radiates through to the upper lumbar spine and is increased in the supine position. The pain reaches peak intensity within an hour. Approximately 50% of patients have pain that radiates to the vertebral area. Pain gradually resolves over 3 to 7 days.[5]

Patients with pancreatitis are systemically ill with fever, tachycardia, hypotension (with severe disease), and abdominal tenderness without abdominal muscle guarding. They frequently assume a characteristic position, sitting with the trunk flexed, the knees drawn up, and arms folded across the abdomen so as to get relief. Bowel sounds are diminished. Nausea and vomiting occur in a majority of patients. Fever, tachycardia, and hypotension may be present. Two rare but dramatic signs of severe pancreatitis are Cullen's sign, faint blue discoloration about the umbilicus, and Turner's sign, discoloration of the flanks reflecting hemorrhage into the retroperitoneum. Laboratory tests reveal an elevated white cell count, between 10,000 and 30,000 cells/mm³, and elevated sedimentation rate. Elevated amylase and lipase concentrations on laboratory evaluation reflect pancreatic inflammation. However, increased amylase concentrations may arise from tissue other than the pancreas (salivary gland, intestine) or disease states (renal insufficiency, pancreatic carcinoma, ruptured ectopic pregnancy). Elevated lipase and trypsin levels should differentiate pancreatic disease from disorders of the salivary gland. Serum immunoreactive trypsinogen/trypsin is a specific and sensitive test for the diagnosis of acute pancreatitis.[6] If the increased amylase is more than 3 times normal in the presence of normal renal function, the diagnosis of pancreatitis is likely. If amylase remains elevated, a nonpancreatic source of amylase should be sought.

Radiographic findings in the abdomen may include the presence of a single, dilated loop of small bowel with edematous walls in the left upper quadrant (a "sentinel loop") or generalized ileus. The plain roentgenogram of the abdomen is also helpful to exclude other disorders that may complicate pancreatitis. Left-sided pleural effusions may be seen on chest films.

Ultrasonography and CT scan are accurate methods of delineating the extent of pancreatic inflammation but do not have a place in the initial diagnosis of acute pancreatitis.

Bowel gas may obscure the image of an abdominal sonogram, and CT scan may not detect inflammatory changes in a significant number of patients with mild pancreatitis. The techniques are better utilized to detect complications that predispose to pancreatitis (gallstones—ultrasonography) or exacerbate symptoms (pseudocyst—CT scan).[7] Ultrasonography has 93% sensitivity and 96% specificity for the diagnosis of cholelithiasis and acute cholecystitis.[8] The CT scan is useful in patients with severe disease, in which the technique detects the presence of a phlegmon or retroperitoneal necrosis. MR is no better and is more expensive than CT scan for the evaluation of acute pancreatitis.[9]

Treatment for acute pancreatitis includes general supportive measures with fluids, nasogastric suction, respiratory support if respiratory failure intervenes, surgical intervention for local complications (pseudocyst), and removal of precipitating factors that may provoke additional attacks (gallstones). In one study, 63% of patients who required surgery for acute pancreatitis had the disease as a result of biliary tract abnormalities.[10] Removal of stones by endoscopic retrograde cholangiopancreatographic technique is indicated in the treatment of acute pancreatitis.[11]

CHRONIC PANCREATITIS

Inflammation of the pancreas may result in chronic, irreversible damage to the organ. About 75% of adult patients with chronic pancreatitis have the disease on the basis of alcohol abuse. Men are more frequently affected than women, and the average age of onset is 38 years. Other cases of chronic pancreatitis are classified as idiopathic, traumatic, familial, hypercalcemic, and nutritional.

Chronic pancreatitis is associated with a variety of pain. It may cause intermittent, aching pain or boring, constant pain, which radiates from the epigastrium to the back in about 66% of patients.[12] Pain may last for up to 2 weeks and gradually diminish. If chronic pancreatitis is associated with severe exocrine insufficiency, patients may have pain along with anorexia, weight loss, malabsorption in the form of steatorrhea, and new-onset diabetes. Patients are usually thin, and physical examination occasionally reveals a palpable right quadrant mass (pseudocyst).

Serum analysis of patients with quiescent chronic pancreatitis may be normal. Serum enzymes may be normal even with acute exacerbations of pain. Decreased serum trypsinogen levels determined by radioimmunoassay strongly suggest pancreatic exocrine insufficiency. Trypsinogen levels are helpful in differentiating patients with chronic pancreatic insufficiency from those with other pancreatic disorders, such as acute pancreatitis, which is associated with an elevated concentration.[13] Low trypsinogen concentrations are associated with both chronic pancreatitis and carcinoma of the pancreas. In these circumstances, the presence of CA 19-9 antigen with pancreatic tumors will help differentiate patients with carcinoma from those with chronic pancreatitis.

Another useful test in the evaluation of a chronic pancreatitis is the bentiromide test. Bentiromide is a molecule with a terminal para-aminobenzoic acid (PABA) group. The enzymatic function of the pancreas is necessary for the PABA to be separated from the molecule. The orally ingested bentiromide is absorbed through the gut and PABA is excreted by the kidney, where it is collected over a 6-hour period. A collection of less than 50% of the ingested PABA associated with bentiromide is compatible with abnormal function.[14]

Plain films of the abdomen may demonstrate diffuse calcifications in 30% of patients with chronic pancreatitis. These calcifications are pathognomonic of the illness (Fig. 17–16). Other noninvasive tests that may prove useful in detecting calcifications and pseudocysts are ultrasonography and CT scan. CT scan is a better test than ultrasound for detecting cysts, but the lower cost and lack of radiation exposure make ultrasound a worthwhile initial test.[15]

Endoscopic retrograde cholangiopancreatography (ERCP) is an invasive test accom-

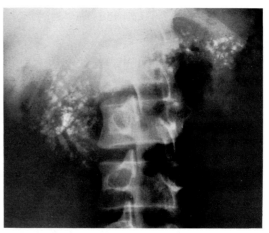

Figure 17–16. Plain roentgenogram of abdomen reveals diffuse calcification in a patient with chronic pancreatitis. (Courtesy of William Steinberg, M.D.)

plished by cannulating the pancreatic duct at its junction with the duodenum (papilla of Vater) and visualizing the system for ductal architecture. The demonstration of widespread duct abnormalities during ERCP is characteristic of chronic pancreatitis.[16] An evaluation for chronic pancreatitis would include serum amylase; Sudan stain for stool fat; flat plate of abdomen for calcification; sonography for dilated pancreatic ducts or pseudocysts; CT scans for calcifications not detected by plain film; ERCP for stricture and dilatation of ducts; and pancreatic secretory tests associated with decreased bicarbonate output after secretin stimulation and decreased trypsin with cholecystokinin stimulation, which is the most sensitive way to diagnose chronic pancreatitis.

Abstinence from alcohol once chronic pancreatitis has been established has no effect on the course of recurrent attacks. Patients with pancreatic insufficiency and malabsorption benefit by replacement of pancreatic enzyme preparations.[17] Complications associated with diabetes mellitus are treated with insulin. Surgical intervention is needed to bypass biliary tract obstruction and to drain pseudocysts if they become large.[18, 19] It should be noted that once calcifications and insufficiency appear, pain symptoms may decrease. After 5 years, many patients will have resolution of their back pain.

PANCREATIC TUMOR

Carcinoma of the pancreas occurs in 10 per 100,000 persons in the general population and 100 per 100,000 in the population over the age of 75.[20] Pancreatic carcinoma is the fourth most common cause of cancer deaths in men. The sex ratio, men to women, is 2:1. Blacks are more commonly affected than Caucasians. The disease occurs most commonly in the elderly. The etiology of this neoplasm is unknown, although cigarette smoking, ingestion of animal fats, juvenile-onset diabetes, and chronic pancreatitis have been implicated.

Pancreatic tumors are frequently asymptomatic until they have metastasized to surrounding abdominal viscera. Patients may present with a nondescript, dull, midepigastric pain that radiates to the back.[20] Pain that radiates to the back in patients with carcinoma implies direct invasion of adjacent retroperitoneal organs or splanchnic nerves.[21] Patients also may have symptoms of anorexia, weight loss, nausea, vomiting, and jaundice.[22] Physical findings include a hard abdominal mass, which may be associated with a distended,

nontender gallbladder, Courvoisier's sign. Commonly, abnormal laboratory tests include decreased hematocrit, elevated ESR, elevated serum alkaline phosphatase, and hyperbilirubinemia. Unfortunately these test results are nonspecific and do not allow for early diagnosis of the tumor. Tumor antigens, particularly carcinoembryonic antigen (CEA), have been reported to be elevated in over 70% of patients with pancreatic malignancy. Unfortunately, most patients had unresectable tumors at the time of diagnosis of their malignancy.[23] The CEA has low sensitivity and is associated with benign and malignant disorders.[24] A new antigen, CA 19-9, has been shown to have greater sensitivity and specificity than CEA. CA 19-9 was detectable in 79% of patients with resectable tumors.[25] However, CA 19-9 also may be present in the setting of other gastrointestinal tumors (bile duct and colon).[26] The antigen may also be negative in early stages of pancreatic cancer and is not suitable for screening.

A number of radiographic techniques, including upper gastrointestinal series, sonography, angiography, endoscopic retrograde cholangiopancreatography, and CT of the abdomen, may be useful in identifying the presence of a pancreatic tumor.[27] Ultrasonography and CT scan can detect pancreatic masses as small as 2 cm.[28] CT provides better definition of the tumor and surrounding structures.[29] MR is not significantly better than CT scan in differentiating pancreatic tumors from normal pancreatic tissue.[30]

Diagnosis of pancreatic tumor is confirmed by intraoperative biopsy or fine needle aspiration biopsy of the pancreas.[31] Pancreatic tumors must be differentiated from other retroperitoneal tumors, which also may cause back pain. Some of the lesions associated with retroperitoneal tumors include malignant fibrous histiocytoma, liposarcoma, leiomyosarcoma, fibrosarcoma, paraganglioma, and neurofibroma.[32]

Therapy for pancreatic carcinoma includes surgical removal of the pancreas and duodenum as well as surrounding lymph nodes. In most circumstances, only up to 22% have resectable tumors.[33]

Chemotherapy and radiation therapy are adjunctive methods of treatment. Unfortunately, cures of this neoplasm are very rare.[34] The prognosis of patients with pancreatic cancer was related to the presence of back pain in one study. Patients with back pain had a shorter survival than those who did not have back pain with their tumor. This outcome correlated with the extent of disseminated disease in those with back pain.[35] Pancreatic cancer has a very poor prognosis with a 20% survival rate at 1 year and 3% survival at 5 years.[28]

Gallbladder

The gallbladder receives its innervation from both greater splanchnic nerves (T5-9). The brain interprets biliary pain to be in the midline in relationship to the bilateral innervation of the gallbladder. When biliary pain is severe, the discomfort may radiate to the back in a T5-9 distribution. Occasionally patients may experience pain lower in the thoracic area that they consider to be low back pain.

ACUTE CHOLECYSTITIS

In certain patients, the bile that is stored in the gallbladder crystallizes to form gallstones (cholelithiasis). The presence of these stones may cause inflammation of the gallbladder, which results in chronic cholecystitis. Gallstones are a very common medical problem, with 5 million men and 15 million women affected in the United States.[36] Women younger than 30 years of age who have had more than three pregnancies are at greatest risk of developing stones.[37] A majority of stones are asymptomatic. When the cystic duct is obstructed by a stone, acute cholecystitis occurs. Bacterial infection and ischemia may play a role in the pathogenesis of acute cholecystitis. Lodging of a stone in the cystic duct or the common bile duct causes severe steady pain lasting 15 to 60 minutes. The pain typically occurs in the mid-epigastrium and moves to the right upper quadrant. Pain may radiate around the sides to the back or directly through to an area below the tip of the right scapula or occasionally in the dorsolumbar spine.[38] The pain is intense, begins abruptly, and subsides gradually. The quality of the pain varies from excruciating or lancinating to aching or cramping. Associated with the abdominal and back pain, patients may develop nausea, vomiting, and dyspepsia.

Physical examination demonstrates a positive Murphy's sign (inspiratory arrest with palpation in the right subcostal area), abdominal guarding, rebound tenderness, fever, and jaundice. The gallbladder is palpable in 30% of patients. Generalized rebound tenderness suggests the possibility of rupture. In a study of patients referred for gallstones, the most characteristic signs and symptoms were pain in the upper abdomen, radiation to the back, a steady quality, duration for 1 to 24 hours, and onset more than a hour after meals. These clinical findings required confirmation by radiographic imaging.[39]

Laboratory tests demonstrate an elevated white blood cell count, which may be as high as 15,000 cells/mm³. Increased alkaline phosphatase suggests a common bile duct stone. Elevated amylase also suggests pancreatic inflammation and a common bile duct stone.

The primary imaging modality for diagnosis of cholelithiasis is ultrasonography, with oral cholecystography playing a secondary role. These techniques have sensitivity and specificity in the 95% to 100% range.[40]

Cholescintigraphy is a reasonably specific test to confirm the diagnosis of acute cholecystitis.[41] Under normal circumstances, technetium-labeled iminodiacetic acid (IDA) is preferentially concentrated in the biliary tree and enters the gallbladder. In acute cholecystitis, radiolabeled material enters the common bile duct but does not enter the gallbladder. The scan may not be helpful in patients with severe hyperbilirubinemia. An alternative to scintigraphy is ultrasonography (Fig. 17–17). Sonography detects the presence of gallstones with 95% accuracy. However, the technique is unable to determine the extent of inflammation in the gallbladder.[42, 43] These tests have taken the place of oral cholecystography.

Treatment for acute cholecystitis is frequently surgical removal of the gallbladder. Patients who do not elect cholecystectomy may be at risk of perforation. Laparoscopic chole-

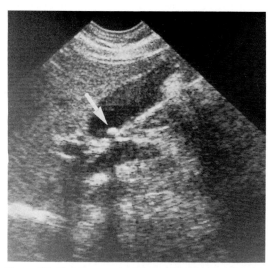

Figure 17–17. Ultrasound of the gallbladder demonstrates a large gallstone (arrow). (Courtesy of Michael Hill, M.D.)

cystectomy has become the surgical method of choice for removal of the gallbladder.[44]

For those who choose to forego surgery, symptoms may resolve in as little time as 48 hours or continue for weeks despite antibiotics. The back pain associated with cholecystitis will follow a similar course. Those who have had one attack of cholecystitis are at risk of developing another. Those patients with recurrent attacks should consider surgical removal of the gallbladder.

Hollow Viscus

The term hollow viscus refers to the stomach, duodenum, and small and large bowel. Most gastric ulcers tend to occur in the antrum of the stomach and are most commonly associated with epigastric pain. In very rare circumstances, gastric pain may be referred to the back at the L1 level. Gastric lesions cause back pain less often than duodenal lesions. When gastric pain is referred to the back, it may occur in the lumbar area but almost never is felt exclusively in the back.

The duodenum is located retroperitoneally at the level of the first lumbar vertebra. The primary disease of the duodenum that is associated with low back pain is peptic ulceration of its posterior wall.[45] Patients taking nonsteroidal anti-inflammatory drugs have decreased protection of the mucosa by altered production of bicarbonate and prostaglandins that maintain blood flow.[46] Patients taking these drugs on a regular basis are at risk of developing gastric and duodenal ulcerations. Bleeding and perforation occur less frequently than simple ulceration. Patients with *Helicobacter pylori* infection of the intestinal tract have an increased risk of developing ulcers.[47]

Patients with duodenal peptic ulcer generally present with burning, epigastric pain that occurs 1 to 3 hours after meals, awakens the patient from sleep, and is relieved with food.[48] A minority have pain that radiates to the back.[49] The pain is localized to the L1-2 vertebral body level and to the right of the midspinal line for up to 3 cm. The pain is episodic and has no relation to physical activity. The pain follows the same relationship to eating as anterior ulcer pain. Duodenal ulcers may cause pain that occurs only in the back. Physical examination may reveal little more than epigastric tenderness. When the pain is present in the back, the involved area may be tender on palpation. Laboratory evaluation is of little benefit unless a decreased hematocrit is present to suggest hemorrhage or an elevated serum amylase concentration indicates posterior penetration into the pancreas. Upper gastrointestinal radiography may outline the ulcer with barium, while endoscopy allows for direct visualization of the ulcer crater (Figs. 17–18 and 17–19).[50] Medical treatment of peptic ulcers, which includes antacids, histamine H_2-receptor antagonists, and sulcralfate, is successful in greater than 85% of patients. Eradication of *H. pylori* infection may also be helpful in healing ulcerations.[51] However, persistence or a change in symptoms suggests a complication of the disease. An increase in pain, the loss of relief with food, and the onset of radiation to the back suggests a posterior penetration through the wall of the duodenum into the underlying pancreas and acute pancreatitis, which is an unusual complication of this disease.[52] Back pain may occur in the absence of anterior abdominal pain and may become persistent. The complications of an untreated posterior penetrating ulcer include pancreatitis, obstruction, and giant duodenal ulcers.[53] In most circumstances, as the ulcer responds to therapy, back pain begins to resolve. Back pain should be absent once the ulcer has healed.

Colon

Of the portions of the colon, ascending, transverse, descending, sigmoid, and rectum, only the transverse and sigmoid colon are located outside the retroperitoneum. Pain of colonic origin that is related to distention is usually felt locally in the abdomen; however, disease processes that affect the rectum may be associated with midsacral back pain. The sigmoid colon and rectum are located just anterior to the sacrum and coccyx.

DIVERTICULITIS

Diverticulitis of the colon may be associated with low back pain. Diverticula are outpouchings of the wall of a portion of the gut and are found most commonly in the colon. The cleft made by the nutrient artery passing into the wall of the gut is their most frequent location. Autopsy studies show diverticula in 50% of all individuals over 60 years of age.[54] Diverticula in the gut are usually asymptomatic. However, diverticulitis, a disease associated with infection and inflammation of diverticula, causes constitutional symptoms such as fever.[55] Of those with diverticulosis, a small percentage

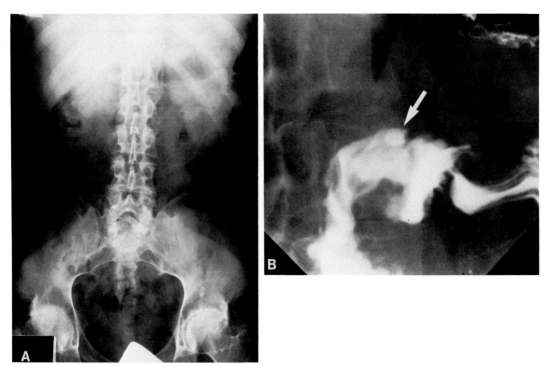

Figure 17–18. A 33-year-old man with Reiter's syndrome had three different types of back pain during a 1-month period. *A,* Plain roentgenogram of the abdomen reveals bilateral sacroiliitis and severe joint narrowing of both hips. The patient had continuous low back pain localized over the sacroiliac joints. The patient developed acute colicky flank pain associated with hematuria and later passed a stone. *B,* Within 1 month of passing the stone, the patient developed epigastric pain that radiated to the middle part of his spine. Upper gastrointestinal roentgenogram revealed an ulcer crater in the duodenum *(arrow).* The patient's symptoms resolved with anti-ulcer therapy.

will develop symptoms and signs of diverticulitis. The patients develop acute, persistent pain that localizes to the left lower quadrant and then radiates to the low back. The pain is often severe and gripping. The pain lasts from hours to days. Relief of pain may occur with a bowel

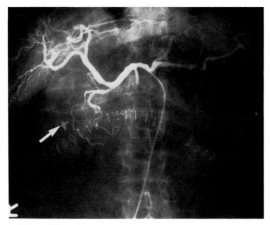

Figure 17–19. Arteriogram of a patient with an actively bleeding duodenal ulcer with dye extravasation *(arrow).* (Courtesy of Edward Druy, M.D.)

movement, while pain is increased with eating. The mechanism of pain is inflammation in the colonic wall. Patients frequently have fever and a change in bowel habits with diverticular disease. Dysuria will also be present if the bladder is involved. Physical examination demonstrates tenderness, which is more pronounced with palpation, a mass in the colon, and depressed bowel sounds.

Laboratory examination will show an elevation in white blood cells. Plain radiographs of the abdomen may show evidence of an ileus or intestinal obstruction. A barium enema must be performed with care during the acute stage of the disease for fear of potential perforation. CT scan is a useful technique for the diagnosis of acute diverticulitis.[56] CT scan identifies changes in the wall of the colon and pericolic fat that are altered with the inflammation of the diverticulum. It also identifies colonic abscesses without the need for contrast. The noninvasive character of the test makes it a technique of choice in these patients. However, CT scan is limited in that marked thickening of the colonic wall can not be differentiated from a neoplasm. Some patients may require contrast enema to exclude carcinoma and confirm the diagnosis of acute diverticulitis.[57] Ultrasonography may also play a useful role as a technique for identifying diverticulitis that is noninvasive and does not utilize ionizing radiation. Sonography was able to identify diverticulitis confirmed by other more invasive means, such as surgery or colonoscopy, in 46 of 54 (85%) patients with clinical signs of colonic disease.[58] Treatment of acute diverticulitis includes antibiotic therapy to control infection and prevent perforation. Surgical drainage of an abscess is necessary if the diverticular disease has perforated into the peritoneum. The damaged segment of bowel is removed and a colostomy may be needed. Back pain will resolve as the swelling and inflammation of diverticular disease resolves.

COLORECTAL CARCINOMA

Rectal adenocarcinoma is another colonic cause of low back pain.[59] The incidence of colorectal cancer has risen to 140,000 new cases per year.[60] Data from 1991 revealed 157,000 new cases in the United States with 61,000 related deaths, second only to lung cancer.[61] Patients are asymptomatic in the early stages of the illness except for a change in bowel habits. Subsequently, they may complain of fatigue, which is secondary to occult bleeding. Those who develop systemic symptoms of anorexia, weight loss, and weakness may have a tumor that has invaded through the wall and has metastasized. Patients with infiltration of the rectum with tumor experience deep pelvic and midsacral back pain, which may radiate to the lower extremities if local invasion irritates the sacral nerves. The patients with rectal carcinoma may have tenesmus and a reduction in stool diameter. Rectal examination may show a hard mass that is fixed and nontender. Carcinoma of the colon may present as a localized, walled-off perforation that simulates a local diverticular abscess. Patients may also have palpable masses anywhere along the length of the colon. Metastatic disease is associated with ascites, hepatomegaly, or lymphadenopathy. The diagnosis of rectal carcinoma may be made through the use of colonoscopy or barium enema. Biopsy and brush cytology specimens can be obtained from lesions at the time of endoscopy. Repeat rectal examination will provide information about the fixation of the rectum and the potential for removal of the tumor. A thorough search for metastatic lesions is essential in order to plan for appropriate therapy. Determination of increased carcinoembryonic antigen (CEA) and lactic dehydrogenase levels may be useful in detecting metastatic disease. In one study, median survival was 8 months when boths tests were elevated. CEA has low predictive value in asymptomatic individuals and is not useful as a screening test.[62] Curative resection for rectal cancer involves removal of the rectal lymph nodes and surrounding perineal structures.[63] Palliative surgery is offered to those patients with metastatic disease who are at risk of obstruction.[64] Radiation therapy may be helpful, but chemotherapy for rectal carcinoma has been disappointing. A number of treatment regimens have been developed with some improvement in survival. Surgical removal of the lesion remains the best chance for cure.[65] The chances for cure from surgery for patients with back pain associated with colon cancer is very small, since the presence of back symptoms is usually associated with locally invasive disease.

Miscellaneous

Other lesions of the abdominal viscera or thorax on very rare occasions may produce back pain. Subphrenic abscess, acute retrocecal appendicitis, and lower lobe pneumonia may all have a component of back pain.[66] An important consideration in differentiating these lesions from mechanical abnormalities of the lumbosacral spine is that the former also produce either anterior pain or additional symptoms in the organ system involved. Rarely is back pain the exclusive sensory symptom of visceral disease. Other examples might include femoral inguinal or obturator hernias, which may cause chronic aching pelvic and sacral pain associated with radiation into the anteromedial or inner thigh. Retroperitoneal bleeding from anticoagulant therapy may also cause back pain that is not associated with mechanical factors.

References

GASTROINTESTINAL DISEASES

1. Roberts I: Gastrointestinal disorders presenting with back pain. Semin Spine Surg 2:141, 1990.
2. Geokas MC, Van Lancker JL, Kadell BM, Machleder HI: Acute pancreatitis. Ann Intern Med 76:105, 1972.
3. The Copenhagen Pancreatitis Study Group: An interim report from a prospective epidemiological multicenter study. Scand J Gastroenterol 26:305, 1981.
4. O'Sullivan JW, Nobrega FT, Morlock CG, et al.: Acute

and chronic pancreatitis in Rochester, Minnesota, 1940–1969. Gastroenterology 62:373, 1972.

5. Scholhamer CF Jr, Spiro HM: The first attack of acute pancreatitis: a clinical study. J Clin Gastroenterol 1:325, 1979.

6. Werner M, Steinberg WM, Pauley C: Strategic use of individual and combined enzyme indicators for acute pancreatitis analyzed by receiver-operator characteristics. Clin Chem 35:967, 1989.

7. Mendez G Jr: CT of acute pancreatitis: interim assessment. AJR 135:463, 1980.

8. Carroll BA: Preferred imaging techniques for the diagnosis of cholecystitis and cholelithiasis. Ann Surg 21:1, 1989.

9. Stark DD, Moss AA, Goldberg HI, et al.: Magnetic resonance and CT of the normal and diseased pancreas. A comparative study. Radiology 250:153, 1984.

10. Martin JK Jr, van Heerden JA, Bess MA: Surgical management of acute pancreatitis. Mayo Clin Proc 59:259, 1984.

11. Fan ST, Lai EC, Mok FP, et al.: Early treatment of acute biliary pancreatitis by endoscopic papillotomy. N Engl J Med 329:1228, 1993.

12. Grendell JH, Cello JP: Chronic pancreatitis. In Sleisenger MH, Fordtran JS (eds): Gastrointestinal Disease: Pathophysiology, Diagnosis, and Management. Philadelphia, WB Saunders Co, 1983, pp 1485–1514.

13. Steinberg WM, Goldstein SS, Davis ND, et al.: Predictive value of low serum trypsinogen. Dig Dis Sci 30:547, 1985.

14. Toskes PP: Bentiromide as a test of exocrine pancreatic function in adult patients with pancreatic exocrine insufficiency. Determination of appropriate dose and urinary collection interval. Gastroenterology 85:565, 1983.

15. Foley WD, Stewart ET, Lawson TL, et al.: Computed tomography, ultrasonography, and endoscopic retrograde cholangiopancreatography in the diagnosis of pancreatic disease: a comparative study. Gastrointest Radiol 5:29, 1980.

16. Feller ER: Endoscopic retrograde cholangiopancreatography in the diagnosis of unexplained pancreatitis. Arch Int Med 144:1797, 1984.

17. Bank S: Chronic pancreatitis: clinical features and medical management. Am J Gastroenterol 81:153, 1986.

18. Prinz RA, Greelee HB: Pancreatic duct drainage in 100 patients with chronic pancreatitis. Ann Surg 194:313, 1981.

19. Shatney CH, Lillehei RC: Surgical treatment of pancreatic pseudocysts: analysis of 119 cases. Ann Surg 189:386, 1979.

20. Morgan RGH, Wormsley KG: Progress report—cancer of the pancreas. Gut 18:580, 1977.

21. Hermann RE, Cooperman AM: Current concepts in cancer: cancer of the pancreas. N Engl J Med 301:482, 1979.

22. Weingarten L, Gelb AM, Fischer MG: Dilemma of pancreatic ductal carcinoma. Am J Gastroenterol 71:473, 1979.

23. Mackie CR, Moosa AR, Go VLW, et al.: Prospective evaluation of some candidate tumor markers in the diagnosis of pancreatic cancer. Dig Dis Sci 25:161, 1980.

24. Fabris C, Del Favero G, Basso D, et al.: Serum markers and clinical data in diagnosing pancreatic cancer: a constrastive approach. Am J Gastroenterol 83:549, 1988.

25. Steinberg WM, Gelfand R, Anderson KK, et al.: Comparison of the sensitivity and specificity of the CA 19-9 and carcinoembryonic antigen assays in detecting cancer of the pancreas. Gastroenterology 90:343, 1986.

26. Steinberg W: The clinical utility of the CA 19-9 tumor-associated antigen. Am J Gastroenterol 85:350, 1990.

27. Simeone JF, Wittenberg H, Ferruci JT: Modern concepts of imaging of the pancreas. Invest Radiol 15:620, 1980.

28. Warshaw AL, Fernandez-del Castillo C: Pancreatic carcinoma. N Engl J Med 326:455, 1992.

29. Balthazar EJ, Chako AC: Computed tomography of pancreatic masses. Am J Gastroenterol 85:343, 1990.

30. Steiner E, Stark DD, Hahn PF, et al.: Imaging of pancreatic neoplasms: comparison of MR and CT. AJR 152:487, 1989.

31. Yamanaka T, Kimura K: Differential diagnosis of pancreatic mass lesion with percutaneous fine-needle aspiration biopsy under ultrasonic guidance. Dig Dis Sci 24:694, 1979.

32. Lane RH, Stephens DH, Reiman HM: Primary retroperitoneal neoplasms: CT findings in 90 cases with clinical and pathologic correlation. AJR 152:83, 1989.

33. Connolly MM, Dawsin PJ, Michelassi F, et al.: Survival in 1001 patients with carcinoma of the pancreas. Ann Surg 206:366, 1987.

34. Edis AJ, Kiernan PD, Taylor WF: Attempted curative resection of ductal carcinoma of the pancreas: review of Mayo Clinic experience, 1951–1975. Mayo Clin Proc 55:531, 1980.

35. Mannell A, van Heerden JA, Weiland LH, Istrup DM: Factors influencing survival after resection for ductal adenocarcinoma of the pancreas. Ann Surg 203:403, 1986.

36. Friedman GD, Kannel WB, Dawber TR: The epidemiology of gallbladder disease: observation in the Framingham study. J Chron Dis 19:273, 1966.

37. Maringhini A, Ciambra M, Baccelliere P, et al.: Sludge, stones, and pregnancy. Gastroenterology 95:1160, 1988.

38. French EG, Robb WAT: Biliary and renal colic. Br Med J 2:135, 1963.

39. Diehl AK, Sugarek NJ, Todd KH: Clinical evaluation for gallstone disease: usefulness of symtpoms and signs in diagnosis. Am J Med 69:29, 1990.

40. Marton KI, Doubilet P: How to image the gallbladder in suspected cholecystitis. Ann Intern Med 109:722, 1988.

41. Boucher IAD: Imaging procedures to diagnose gallbladder disease. Br Med J 288:1632, 1984.

42. Laing FC, Federle MP, Jeffrey RB, Brown TW: Ultrasonic evaluation of patients with acute right upper quadrant pain. Radiology 140:449, 1981.

43. Fink-Bennett D, Freitas JE, Ripley SD, Bree RL: The sensitivity of hepatobiliary imaging and real time ultrasonography in the detection of acute cholecystitis. Arch Surg 120:904, 1985.

44. The Southern Surgeons Club: A prospective analysis of 1518 laparoscopic cholecystectomies. N Engl J Med 324:1073, 1991.

45. Ross JR, Reave LE III: Syndrome of posterior penetrating peptic ulcer. Med Clin North Am 50:461, 1966.

46. Soll AH (moderator): Nonsteroidal anti-inflammatory drugs and peptic ulcer disease. Ann Intern Med 114:307, 1991.

47. Graham DY: *Campylobacter pylori* and peptic ulcer disease. Gastroenterology 96:615, 1989.

48. Earlam R: A computerized questionnaire analysis of duodenal ulcer symptoms. Gastroenterology 71:314, 1976.

49. Gibson SB: Back pain in peptic ulcer. NY State J Med 61:625, 1961.

50. Laufer I, Mullens JE, Hamilton J: The diagnostic accuracy of barium studies of the stomach and duodenum: correlation with endoscopy. Radiology 115:569, 1975.

51. Rauws EAJ, Tytgat GNJ: Cure of duodenal ulcer associated with eradication of *Helicobacter pylori*. Lancet 335:1233, 1990.

52. Norris JR, Haubrich WS: The incidence and clinical features of penetration in peptic ulceration. JAMA 178:386, 1961.

53. Mistilis SP, Wiot JF, Nedelman SH: Giant duodenal ulcer. Ann Intern Med 59:155, 1963.

54. Painter NS, Buckett DP: Diverticular disease of the colon, a 20th century problem. Clin Gastroenterol 4:3, 1975.

55. Asch MJ, Markowitz AM: Diverticulosis coli: A surgical appraisal. Surgery 62:239, 1967.

56. Morris J, Stellato TA, Haaga JR, Lieberman J: The utility of computed tomography in colonic diverticulitis. Ann Surg 204:128, 1986.

57. Balthazar EJ, Megibow A, Schinella RA, Gordon R: Limitations in the CT diagnosis of acute diverticulitis: comparison of CT, contrast enema, and pathologic findings in 16 patients. AJR 154:281, 1990.

58. Wilson SR, Toi A: The value of sonography in the diagnosis of acute diverticulitis of the colon. AJR 154:1199, 1990.

59. Falterman KW, Hill CB, Markey JC, et al.: Cancer of the colon, rectum and anus: a review of 2,313 cases. Cancer 34:951, 1974.

60. American Cancer Society: Cancer Facts and Figures. New York, American Cancer Society, 1982.

61. Boring CC, Squires TS, Tong T: Cancer statistics, 1991. CA Cancer J Clin 41:19, 1991.

62. Bates SE: Clinical applications of serum tumor markers. Ann Intern Med 115:623, 1991.

63. Kemeny N, Braun DE: Prognostic factors in advanced colorectal carcinoma: the importance of lactic dehydrogenase, performance status and white blood cell count. Am J Med 74:786, 1983.

64. Enker WE, Laffer UT, Block GE: Enhanced survival of patients with colon and rectal cancer is based upon wide anatomic resection. Ann Surg 190:350, 1979.

65. Bresalier RS, Kim YS: Malignant neoplasms of the large intestine. In Sleisenger MH, Fordtran JS (eds): Gastrointestinal Disease: Pathophysiology, Diagnosis, Management, 5th ed. Philadelphia: WB Saunders Co, 1993, Vol 2, pp 1449–1493.

66. Sullivan JE: Backache due to visceral lesions of the chest and abdomen. Clin Orthop 26:67, 1963.

18

Miscellaneous Diseases

PAGET'S DISEASE OF BONE

Capsule Summary

Frequency of back pain—uncommon
Location of back pain—lumbar spine
Quality of back pain—deep, boring, ache
Symptoms and signs—pain with walking, decreased spine motion
Laboratory and x-ray tests—increased alkaline phosphatase; lytic and sclerotic enlarged vertebrae on plain roentgenograms
Treatment—calcitonin, diphosphonates, nonsteroidal anti-inflammatory drugs

PREVALENCE AND PATHOGENESIS

Paget's disease of bone is a localized disorder of bone characterized by a remarkable degree of bone resorption and subsequent formation of disorganized and irregular new bone. The disease was first described by Sir James Paget in 1877.[1]

Paget's disease is a common disorder in certain areas of the world. It is more common in Western Europe, Australia, and New Zealand than in the United States. Most Americans with Paget's disease are of Western European or Mediterranean descent. Paget's disease is rare in blacks in Africa, but is reported in blacks in the United States.[2] It affects up to 3% of people over 40 years of age,[3] and increases to 10% in individuals 80 years or older.[4] The prevalence increases to 10% to 20% with a positive family history.[5] Men are slightly more commonly affected than women by a ratio of 1.3:1.[6] In New York State between 1980 to 1983, the rate for Paget's disease for hospitalized patients was 26 per 100,000 for the age group 65 to 74 years and 34 for the group 75 years and older. The average length of hospitalization for these groups was 9 and 11 days, respectively.[7]

The pathogenesis of Paget's disease is unknown. There is little evidence to support abnormalities in hormone secretion, vascular supply, or connective tissue metabolism as a cause of this illness. The primary abnormality resides in osteoclasts, cells that resorb bone. Histologic examination of pagetic bone reveals increased numbers of osteoclasts, with marked increases in size and number of nuclei in these cells. Pagetic osteoclasts in long-term marrow cultures have a 10 to 20 fold increase in number compared to normal marrow cultures, are larger in size, have more nuclei per cell, increased levels of tartrate-resistant acid phosphatase activity, and are hyperresponsive to $1,25(OH)_2$ vitamin D.[8] Levels of interleukin-6 (IL-6) are increased in long-term marrow cultures of Paget's disease bone cells. IL-6 is an important regulator of bone function, acting as a stimulator of osteoclast cell formation.[9] This change in the number of osteoclasts results in increased bone resorption and inadequate new bone formation. New pagetic bone is less compact, more vascular, and weaker than normal bone.[10]

Other investigators have suggested that the osteoblast is the source of the primary abnormality of Paget's disease.[11, 12] The evidence for this hypothesis is the focal nature of Paget's disease and the presence of viral genome in cells other than osteoclasts in bone, including the osteoblast. Osteoblasts are not distributed via the bloodstream. The osteoclasts are derived from progenitor cells in bone marrow and distributed through the peripheral circulation. If osteoclasts were the putative cause of Paget's disease, the illness should be systemic following the body-wide distribution of the osteoclasts. In addition, osteoblasts produce

562

large amounts of IL-6. Additional evidence has been reported suggesting the importance of deregulation of c-fos protooncogene expression in bone cells by the insertion of a paramyxovirus may be the primary lesion of Paget's disease.

Ultrastructural studies of pagetic bone have demonstrated the presence of nuclear and cytoplasmic inclusions that resemble portions of paramyxoviruses.[13] The characteristics of a slow virus infection—long latent period, single organ disease, and lack of inflammatory response—match closely those of Paget's disease. However, the infectious agent has not been isolated from cultured pagetic cells and the specific virus has not been identified. Polymerase chain reaction techniques have been utilized to screen for paramyxovirus sequences in ribonucleic acid extracted from bone from patients with Paget's disease. No evidence of viral products were identified in RNA extracts from 10 patients.[14] Therefore, any conclusion concerning the role of viruses as the etiologic agent of Paget's disease cannot be made at this time.

CLINICAL HISTORY

Most patients with Paget's disease are asymptomatic.[15] Frequently the possibility that a patient may have the disease is raised by the presence of an elevated serum alkaline phosphatase level on screening chemistry tests or by the discovery of an area of bony change on radiographs. When patients become symptomatic, however, they frequently develop rheumatologic complaints. Back pain is common, affecting 34% of 290 patients in one study and 43% in another.[6, 16] However, other investigators have reported prevalences as low as 11% and have suggested that Paget's disease has been inappropriately diagnosed as the cause of back pain in a large proportion of patients.[17, 18] A recent study has documented spine involvement in 35% of 248 patients with Paget's disease.[19] The problem arises that these patients may have osteoarthritis of the spine which may be the actual cause of back pain. A recent study investigating this specific point reported only 12% of patients (3 of 25) with Paget's disease having back pain directly related to their underlying illness. The remaining patients had back pain that could be related to Paget's disease and/or coexistent osteoarthritis.[20] A similar frequency (13%) of back pain related to Paget's disease alone was reported in the study of 248 patients, while

mechanical causes of back pain were present in 27%.[19]

Pain of Paget's disease is of a deep boring quality and is not increased at night. Pain secondary to Paget's disease uncomplicated by mechanical disorders is unrelated to activity, not relieved by rest, and is not significantly relieved with nonsteroidal anti-inflammatory drugs.[19] The pain may radiate with a radicular pattern in the gluteal region, thighs, legs, or feet. Cauda equina symptoms with saddle anesthesia, progressive weakness, and bladder or bowel incontinence are present in a small percentage of patients.[6, 21] The lumbosacral spine is the area of the axial skeleton most commonly symptomatic. The pelvis and sacrum are the most common primary sites of bone involvement with the polyostotic form of Paget's disease.[22]

The pain of Paget's disease involving the axial skeleton may be of bone, joint, or nerve origin. Vertebral bodies may fracture, facet joints may develop secondary osteoarthritis due to deformity, and neural elements may become compressed by new bone growth including extradural structures such as ligamentum flavum.[17, 23–26] Monostotic Paget's disease affecting a vertebral body may be associated with pain not related to fracture or compression of neural elements.[27] Pain also may be generated by compression of neural elements by intraspinal soft tissue, neural ischemia produced by arterial steal phenomenon, interference with blood supply to the cord by compression of expanding bone, or platybasia with compression of the medulla.[19] The increased vascularity associated with Paget's disease has been implicated as the cause of spontaneous spinal epidural hematomas associated with neurologic dysfunction, including cauda equina syndrome.[28, 29] Neurologic complications are relatively uncommon but may cause significant disability such as myelopathy, radiculopathy, and cranial nerve signs including optic atrophy, deafness, and cerebellar dysfunction.[30] Spinal cord compression occurs most commonly in the thoracic spine where vertebral width is narrowed.[31] Occasionally, cord compression develops suddenly as a result of a collapse of a vertebra.[32]

Other frequently affected sites are the skull, pelvis, femurs, and tibias. Patients may experience pain in weight-bearing bones with walking. Paget's disease may also cause deformities in bones and results in increased size of the skull, hip joint disease (osteoarthritis), and bowing of the legs. Bone softening may give rise to invagination of the base of the skull which may result in obstructive hydrocephalus.[2]

Other complications of Paget's disease include hyperuricemia with gout,[33] hypercalcemia in the immobilized patient, and high-output cardiac failure due to the increased blood flow to bones. Malignant degeneration develops in patients with polyostotic Paget's disease but is a rare occurrence. Less than 1% of Paget's disease patients develop osteosarcoma or fibrosarcoma.[34] Metastases also may involve Pagetic bone and may only be differentiated from sarcomas by tissue biopsy.[35]

PHYSICAL EXAMINATION

Physical examination may be entirely normal in the patient with asymptomatic Paget's disease. Increasing disease activity, manifested by rapid bone growth, may correspond to physical findings consistent with rapid bone metabolism, and the temperature over bones may be elevated from increased blood flow. Bone growth of the skull is manifested by increased skull circumference and dilated scalp veins. Angioid streaks are an occasional finding on funduscopic examination. Resting tachycardia is seen in patients with high cardiac output.

Musculoskeletal abnormalities may include a pagetic stature (dorsal kyphosis) and abnormal gait. In the weight-bearing bones, new bone formation leads to lateral bowing in the femur and anterior bowing in the tibia. Decreased motion may be demonstrated in the lumbar spine, and point tenderness may be elicited over vertebral bodies that have sustained fractures. The lumbar spine may be straightened, fixed, or reversed on examination. Scoliosis may be present. Straight leg raising may be reduced. Neurologic examination may be remarkable for cranial nerve, sensory, motor, or cerebellar dysfunction if bone growth has resulted in nerve compression.

LABORATORY DATA

The most characteristic laboratory abnormality is an elevation of the serum alkaline phosphatase, since this mirrors the extent of new bone, osteoblastic activity. A measure of bone resorption is 24-hour total urinary hydroxyproline. This amino acid is formed from collagen matrix during bone breakdown. Together the tests can provide an indication of bone disease, its progression, and its response to therapy. From a practical standpoint, measurement of serum alkaline phosphatase is used routinely, since 24-hour urine collections are difficult to obtain on a regular basis.

Serum levels of calcium and phosphorus are normal, since bone resorption and formation are closely linked. Elevations of calcium occur in pagetic patients who are immobilized, who have coexistent primary hyperparathyroidism, or who have metastatic disease to bone. In rare circumstances, hypercalcemia has been reported in monostotic Paget's disease unassociated with immobilization.[36] Serum uric acid concentrations may be increased in men with extensive disease. Serum osteocalcin is a vitamin K-dependent protein that has a high affinity for hydroxyapatite, binds calcium, and is produced by osteoblasts. Osteocalcin levels have lower sensitivity and specificity than other biochemical markers for activity of Paget's disease.[37] Histocompatibility testing of a small group of patients has demonstrated a greater frequency of HLA-DR2 compared to controls.[38] This test has no diagnostic significance at this time.

Pathologic abnormalities of early disease are characterized by an increased number of osteoclasts. Subsequently new bone is produced in a chaotic, mosaic pattern, and woven bone, as opposed to normal lamellar bone, is produced. The amount of minerals in pagetic new bone appears normal. Histologically, the bone contains irregular, broad trabeculae, with numerous osteoclasts and fibrous vascular tissue replacement of the bone marrow space (Fig. 18–1). Malignant tumors may arise in pagetoid lesions. The most common is osteosarcoma. Other neoplasms include fibrosarcoma and malignant giant cell tumor.[39]

RADIOGRAPHIC EVALUATION

Radiographic abnormalities vary with the stage of disease. The osteolytic phase corresponds to localized lytic lesions of bone. There is a well-demarcated area of lucency without associated bony reaction. These lesions are most commonly discovered in the skull and are referred to as osteoporosis circumscripta. Lytic lesions may be seen in long bones but are rarely seen in the spine.[40] Paget's disease is monostotic in 35% of cases (Fig. 18–2).[41]

The mixed phase consists of bone sclerosis combined with osseous demineralization. The bone increases in size with greatly thickened and widely spaced trabeculae, cortical thickening, and irregularly distributed zones of increased and reduced density. A "cotton wool" appearance is a term used to describe the patchy involvement.

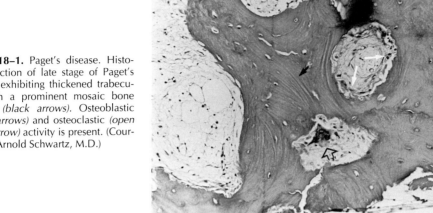

Figure 18–1. Paget's disease. Histologic section of late stage of Paget's disease exhibiting thickened trabeculae with a prominent mosaic bone pattern *(black arrows).* Osteoblastic *(white arrows)* and osteoclastic *(open black arrow)* activity is present. (Courtesy of Arnold Schwartz, M.D.)

The sclerotic phase of disease appears as areas of homogeneous increase in bone density. This form of disease may be too difficult to distinguish clearly from the mixed form of disease.

In the spine, mixed or sclerotic radiographic changes are usually demonstrated.[42] Vertebral bodies may develop coarse, parallel, vertical striations which may simulate the appearance of a hemangioma. Increased cortical thickening at the inferior and superior vertebral borders may result in a "picture frame" appearance (Fig. 18–3). Marked osteoblastic changes may result in a homogeneously sclerotic "ivory" vertebra (Fig. 18–4). The "ivory" vertebra is usually enlarged in Paget's disease, and this helps differentiate it from metastatic disease (Fig. 18–5).[43] Compression fractures and large osteophytes may also be seen. Paget's disease may invade soft tissue and cartilage structures such as intervertebral discs. This process, causing disc space narrowing, may be entirely asymptomatic.[44]

Bone scintiscans are sensitive in detecting increased bone activity even in locations where plain radiographs are normal. In a patient with localized disease and normal biochemical parameters, a bone scan may give the only objective indication of the presence and activity of disease.[45] In a patient with Paget's disease, a positive scan in a "normal" area of skeleton suggests involvement at that location.[46] Multiple areas of increased activity also may be associated with diffuse skeletal metastases. Roentgenographic evaluation of areas of increased scintiscan activity may be able to differentiate areas with Paget's disease from those with a maliganancy.[47] Response to treatment is characterized by radiographic changes in an area of normal activity on scan. Paget's disease may be noted on indium-111 white blood cell scintigraphy as "cold" areas. The cold bone defects are related to the loss of the bone marrow component in pagetic bone.[48]

CT generally is not required for the evaluation of uncomplicated Paget's disease.[49] CT demonstrates the coarsened trabeculae of Paget's disease (Fig. 18–6). It is most useful at identifying complications of Paget's disease in-

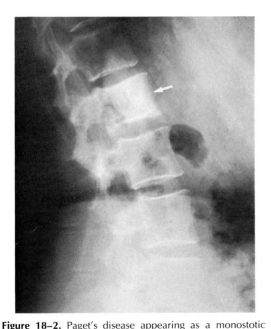

Figure 18–2. Paget's disease appearing as a monostotic lesion in the second lumbar vertebra *(arrow).* This early lesion has vertical striations simulating a hemangioma (see Fig. 13–14). This 51-year-old woman was asymptomatic and had a normal serum alkaline phosphatase. (From Borenstein DG: Low back pain. In Klippel JH, Dieppe P (eds): Rheumatology. St Louis: CV Mosby, 1994, Sec 5, p 4.18.)

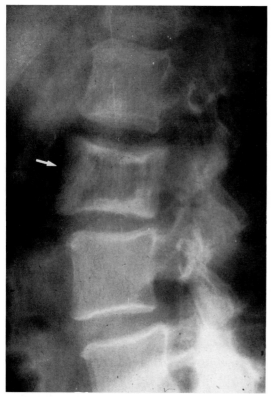

Figure 18–3. Paget's disease seen as a "picture-frame" vertebral body. Lateral view demonstrates generalized enlargement of the vertebral body associated with thickening of the vertebral endplates and the cortex. Also visible are the straightening of the convexity of the anterior surface of the body (arrow) and thickening of the trabecular pattern. (Courtesy of Anne Brower, M.D.)

cluding articular disease, neoplastic degeneration, and neurologic impingement secondary to vertebral involvement.[50]

MR also is not required for the diagnosis of Paget's disease. However, the frequent use of MR in a variety of skeletal conditions results in the identification of Paget's disease serendipitously. Complications of spinal stenosis secondary to Paget's disease are readily identified by MR.[51]

DIFFERENTIAL DIAGNOSIS

In the great majority of patients, the history, physical examination, and chemical, plain radiographic, and bone scan abnormalities are adequate to confirm the diagnosis of Paget's disease. In an occasional patient with unusual clinical or radiologic presentation, bone biopsy may be necessary to confirm the diagnosis.

The problem for the clinician may not be discovering the presence of Paget's disease in

the spine, but rather the association of the patient's back symptoms with the lumbar spine pagetoid lesion. Paget's disease causes alterations of the lumbar spine, many of which can cause back pain (Table 18–1). Altman has suggested that in order for a patient's symptoms to be directly related to Paget's disease and not another disorder (osteoarthritis) they should fulfill the following characteristics: (1) nonspecific low back pain without radiculopathy, (2) normal or minimal findings on examination, (3) roentgenographically demonstrated vertebral sclerosis (ivory vertebra) with facet sclerosis and normal disc space and facet joint, (4) bone scan revealing isolated vertebral Paget's disease, and (5) CT demonstrating an enlarged vertebra and neural arch but no facet joint arthritis or bony impingement.[20]

The differential diagnosis of Paget's disease is broad, since all lesions that may cause sclerosis of bone must be included. Diseases associated with sclerotic vertebral bodies, including metastatic tumor, lymphoma, myelofibrosis, fluorosis, mastocytosis, renal osteodys-

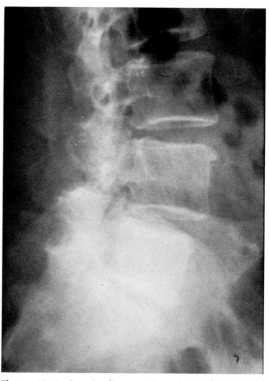

Figure 18–4. Paget's disease—"ivory" vertebra. Lateral view of the lumbar spine of a 72-year-old black women with a 3-year history of low back and right leg pain. Abnormal findings include narrowing of the L5–S1 disc space and dense sclerosis of the L5 vertebral body. Craig needle biopsy revealed Paget's disease. (Courtesy of Randall Lewis, M.D.)

trophy, tuberous sclerosis, axial osteomalacia, and fibrogenesis imperfecta ossium, may be confused with Paget's disease. Abnormalities on physical and radiologic examination, such as hepatosplenomegaly (myelofibrosis) or anemia (metastatic tumor), help differentiate these disorders from Paget's disease. A history of renal disease along with laboratory evidence of renal failure helps with the diagnosis of renal osteodystrophy. A history of urticaria pigmentosa is common in patients with mastocytosis. Fibrous dysplasia may also cause sclerosis of vertebral bodies. A careful history, physical examination, and review of laboratory data should help the clinician in making the appropriate diagnosis.

Fibrous Dysplasia

Fibrous dysplasia is a developmental anomaly of the bone-forming mesenchymal tissue of bone which may occur in a monostotic or polyostotic form. It was first described by Lichenstein in 1938.[52] It also may be associated with endocrine abnormalities (precocious female development) and cafe-au-lait spots, which is

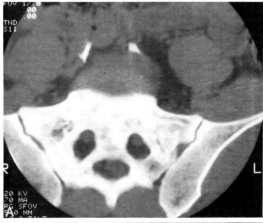

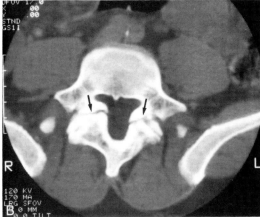

Figure 18–6. Paget's disease. CT scan of sacrum *(A)* and fifth lumbar vertebral body *(B)* of a 61-year-old Caucasian man with a history of parathyroid adenoma with hyperparathyroidism, prostatic hypertrophy, and right sacral and anterior thigh pain. Pelvic radiographs and bone scan were suggestive of Paget's disease. The axial view of the sacrum *(A)* demonstrated replacement of normal trabecular pattern with hyperdense bony pattern compatible with Paget's disease. At level L5 *(B)* a spondylolysis *(black arrows)* is surrounded by reactive sclerosis that is not Paget's disease. His back and leg pain was responsive to nonsteroidal anti-inflammatory therapy suggesting a mechanical source of his pain.

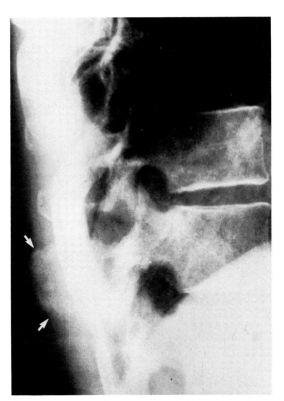

Figure 18–5. Paget's disease—expanded bone. Lateral view of the lumbar spine in a 60-year-old Caucasian man with an expanded spinous process of T12 *(white arrows)*. This isolated lesion was aymptomatic. (Courtesy of Randall Lewis, M.D.)

associated with Albright's syndrome and neurofibromatosis.[53] The diverse metabolic abnormalities arise from cells that respond to extracellular signals through the activation of the hormone-sensitive adenylyl cyclase system.[54] McCune-Albright syndrome may occur secondary to a mutation of the gene encoding a subunit of the stimulatory G protein of adenylyl cyclase.[55] Being a developmental abnormality, this illness is usually diagnosed in adolescents, particularly if they suffer from polyostotic lesions. Occasionally, patients with monostotic lesions are not discovered to have fibrous dysplasia until adulthood. In the skele-

TABLE 18–1. MANIFESTATIONS OF LUMBAR SPINE PAGET'S DISEASE

ANATOMIC PART	MECHANISM	CLINICAL CORRELATE
Vertebra	Total enlargement	Altered lordosis/scoliosis
	Posterior element enlargement	Spinal stenosis/paraplegia
	Uneven subchondral enlargement (disc fracture)	Degenerative disc
	Enlargement stressing ligamentous attachment	Osteophytes
	Spinal osteoporosis, fibrous replacement, bone weakening	Compression fractures (kyphosis)
	Hypervascularity	Paraplegia (spinal artery steal syndrome)
Neural arch	Medial facet enlargement	Lateral recess syndrome, stenosis, loss or reversal of lordosis
	Facet joint enlargement	Facet osteoarthritis
	Altered joint congruity	
Spinal ligaments	Ligamentous calcifications	
	Ankylosing hyperostosis form	Back pain?
	Ankylosing spondylitis form	Back pain?
Any bone	Sarcomatous degeneration	Severe pain
	Metastatic disease to hypervascular bone	Severe pain
Pelvis	Protrusion acetabulae with hip flexion contractures	Forward bend to trunk
Lower extremity	Tibial bowing	Forward or altered pelvic tilt, abnormal gait, muscle spasm

Modified from Altman R: Low back pain in Paget's disease of bone. Clin Orthop 217:152, 1987.

ton, the pelvis is involved in 80% of patients and the axial skeleton in 8% of patients with polyostotic disease.[56] Bone involvement may be associated with localized pain if the lesion is large or if a pathologic fracture occurs. Neurologic deficits, including paralysis, have been described in association with vertebral compression, osseous expansion, or fibrous tissue extending into the spinal canal.[57] Fibrous dysplasia causes the replacement of normal bone with a slow-growing mass of fibrous tissue and woven bone, which leads to expansion of bone that is structurally weak and results in marked deformity. A helpful test in differentiating fibrous dysplasia from Paget's disease is measurement of the alkaline phosphatase levels, which is minimally elevated in a minority of patients with fibrous dysplasia in contrast with the markedly elevated levels in Paget's disease. The radiographic features of fibrous dysplasia include a radiolucent, "ground-glass" appearance of the bone. These areas are bordered by a sclerotic rim (Fig. 18–7). The interior of the bone contains variable amounts of calcification and bony septa. Vertebral changes may show deformed vertebral bodies or posterior elements with variable areas of lucency and cysts (Fig. 18–8).[58] Monostotic fibrous dysplasia of the spine has been reported.[59, 60] The bone scan is not helpful in differentiating fibrous dysplasia from Paget's disease.[61] MR reveals an expanded bone contour, a decreased signal on T_1-weighted image, and variable signal on T_2-weighted images. MR is most helpful in determining the extent of fibrous dysplasia within an affected bone.[62] The age of the patient (under 30 in fibrous dysplasia versus over 30 in Paget's disease) and the radiographic and alkaline phosphatase differences should allow the differentiation of these diseases.

TREATMENT

Most patients with Paget's disease are asymptomatic and do not require therapy. Indications for treatment include disabling bone pain that is not relieved with nonsteroidal anti-inflammatory agents, progressive skeletal deformity with frequent fractures, vertebral compression, acetabular protrusion, neurologic complications, deafness, high-output congestive heart failure, or immobilization.

A number of new agents have been developed for the treatment of Paget's disease. Many of these agents are available in Europe but have not been released in the United States as of 1993 for use with Paget's disease.[63]

None of the three classes of agents used for Paget's disease to produce symptomatic improvement and better control of bone metabolism cures the illness. Calcitonin, a polypeptide hormone from the parafollicular cells of

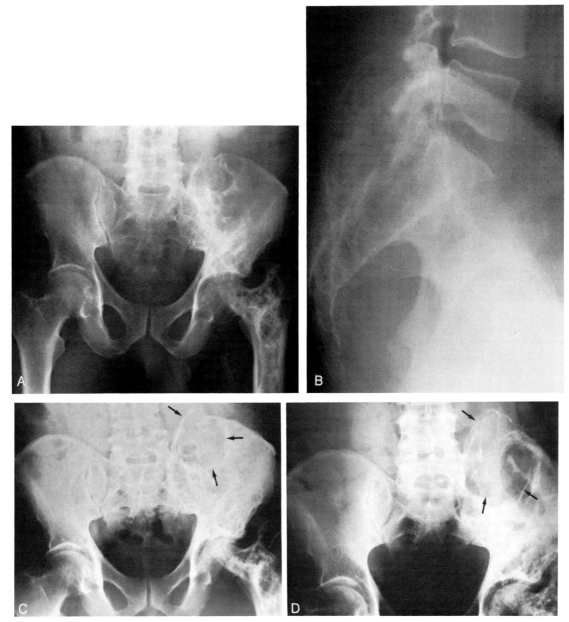

Figure 18–7. Fibrous dysplasia. AP *(A)* and lateral *(B)* views of the pelvis of a 56-year-old black man with left-sided back and leg pain. An expansile lesion with areas of sclerosis is present involving the left hemipelvis and left femur. The alkaline phosphatase of this patient was normal. The patient's symptoms improved with a heel lift for a leg length discrepancy and indomethacin 75 mg every evening. These radiographs were obtained in 1983. *C,* is an AP view of the pelvis taken in 1988. The left hemipelvis has increased in size. The superior rim of the left pelvis *(black arrows)* has expanded the cortex, which is compatible with an aneurysmal bone cyst. The patient complained of left buttock pain. *D,* is an AP view of the pelvis taken in 1991. The area of the aneurysmal bone cyst has expanded in size. The patient complained of an enlarging mass that was warm to the touch that expanded on an intermittent basis.

Illustration continued on following page

the thyroid gland, slows osteoclastic bone resorption. Injection of 50 to 100 units of calcitonin three or more times per week results in a gradual decrease in serum alkaline phosphatase to about half of the initial elevated con-

centrations and resolution of bone pain; however, patients may develop antibodies to calcitonin, which abrogates its beneficial effects.[64] Salmon calcitonin is the most commonly utilized form of calcitonin and the type

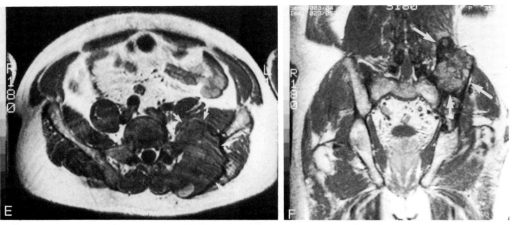

Figure 18–7 *Continued E,* MR exam of the pelvis, axial T₁-weighted image, demonstrates a huge expansile lesion in the left ilium *(white arrows). F,* MR coronal view of pelvis demonstrates extensive involvement of the left ilium with a mixed signal abnormality compatible with fibrous dysplasia *(white arrows).* As of 1993, the lesion is cool to touch on physical examination and had not expanded further. The patient's symptoms are controlled with indomethacin 75 mg twice a day.

most commonly associated with antibody production. Human calcitonin differs from salmon calcitonin at 16 of the 32 amino acid sites.[65] Anti-salmon calcitonin antibodies do not bind human calcitonin. Patients resistant to salmon calcitonin have responded to human calcitonin.[66] Intranasal salmon calcitonin is available in Europe for the treatment of Paget's disease.[67] Intranasal calcitonin is more convenient than parenteral calcitonin, but the efficacy relative to parenteral calcitonin remains to be determined. The absence of side effects is probably related to the 60% reduction in plasma levels obtained from intranasal

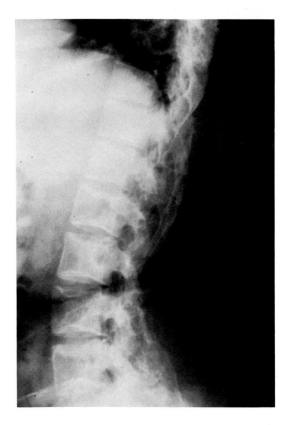

Figure 18–8. Fibrous dysplasia of the vertebral bodies and posterior elements. The bones have multiple lytic lesions caused by the fibrous replacement. (Courtesy of Anne Brower, M.D.)

installation compared to the same dose given by subcutaneous injection. Intranasal calcitonin produces a maximum reduction in bone turnover of 30% to 40% after 6 months of therapy.

Diphosphonates are structural analogues of pyrophosphate that, when ingested by osteoclasts, decrease the osteoclast's ability to resorb bone. In addition, to a variable extent, they interfere with the mineralization of normal bone, and this limits the dose and duration of a course of diphosphonate therapy. Diphosphonates are given at a dose of 5 mg/kg/day for 6 months of the year. Some physicians give a course for a 6-month period and discontinue therapy for 6 months, while others give therapy every other month for 6 months and then re-evaluate the response. Diphosphonates may increase the tendency of Paget's patients to develop pathologic fractures.[68] Editronate has been the most commonly utilized diphosphonate. Pamidronate, an aminohydroxypropilidene bisphosphonate, has been utilized in the United States for intravenous treatment of hypercalcemia associated with malignancy.[69] In Europe, pamidronate is used regularly for the control of Paget's disease. The drug may be used orally or intravenously. As opposed to other diphosphonates, pamidronate inhibits bone resorption without any significant detrimental effect on bone growth and mineralization.[70] Pamidronate decreases serum alkaline phosphatase to near normal values, almost completely relieves bone pain, and maintains the response for 6 months or longer after the cessation of therapy.[71] The dose range of pamidronate has been between 300 mg to 1200 mg/day. An oral dose of 600 mg/day has been associated with low back pain relief in 56% of 156 patients with Paget's disease.[72]

Diphosphonate therapy has been shown to cause improvement of symptoms in 60% or more of patients even in the presence of secondary osteoarthritis.[73] Diphosphonates may be helpful in patients with low back pain secondary to Paget's disease alone or to Paget's disease and associated osteoarthritis.[20]

Mithramycin is an antibiotic that binds to DNA and inhibits RNA synthesis. It has a cytotoxic effect on osteoclasts and is used as a treatment for hypercalcemia related to cancer. The drug is potent and rapidly effective but, since it is associated with toxicity, it cannot be used as a first-line agent.[74] It is administered intravenously to patients with progressive neurologic compression syndromes secondary to Paget's disease. Pamidronate may control hypercalcemia with less toxicity than mithramycin.

Other therapies utilized for Paget's disease have included gallium nitrate, oral tiludronate, and clodronic acid. These agents have been associated with a beneficial effect on the clinical symptoms and biochemical parameters of Paget's disease.[63, 75, 76]

Physicians usually use one agent at a time, following the patient's symptoms, serum alkaline phosphatase, and bone activity on bone scan. Many have remission of their disease after a course of therapy and may not need to resume the drug for an extended period. More complete biochemical suppression is associated with more prolonged clinical remission not requiring a resumption of therapy.[77] Patients with persistent neurologic syndromes may require a combination of agents for adequate control.[78]

PROGNOSIS

Most patients with Paget's disease have an asymptomatic illness. In others, more active disease can usually be controlled with nonsteroidal anti-inflammatory drugs and agents that modify bone metabolism. Patients with Paget's disease uncomplicated by osteoarthritis may respond to a combination of calcitonin and bisphosphonates or bisphosphonates alone.[27, 79] Improvement may be manifested by a decrease in bone scintiscan activity. However, complete resolution of increased activity is unusual.[80] The complications of Paget's disease that cause disability and mortality are rare. Occasionally patients develop neurologic symptoms from spinal cord compression. Increased drug therapy or laminectomy can be effective in controlling these complications. Malignant transformation of Paget's disease is associated with a very poor prognosis but is fortunately a very rare occurrence. In a series of 22 cases of sarcoma complicating Paget's disease, one patient had involvement of the sacrum and another, the thoracic spine.[81] Sarcoma occurred in areas of advanced disease and presented as a destructive lesion without periosteal reaction. The 5-year survival is 15% of patients.[82]

References

PAGET'S DISEASE OF BONE

1. Paget J: On a form of chronic inflammation of bones (osteitis deformans). Trans Roy Chir Soc London 60:37, 1877.
2. Siris ES, Jacobs TP, Canfield RE: Paget's disease of bone. Bull NY Acad Med 56:285, 1980.
3. Schmorl G: Ueber Osteitis deformans Paget. Virchows Arch Pathol Anat Physiol 283:694, 1932.

4. Barker DJ: The epidemiology of Paget's disease of bone. Metab Bone Dis 3:231, 1981.

5. Rosenthal MJ, Hartnell JM, Kaiser FE, et al.: Paget's disease of bone in older patients. Am J Ger Soc 37:639, 1989.

6. Altman RD: Musculoskeletal manifestations of Paget's disease of bone. Arthritis Rheum 23:1121, 1980.

7. Polednak AP: Rates of Paget's disease of bone among hospital discharges, by age and sex. J Am Ger Soc 35:550, 1987.

8. Kukita A, Chenu C, McManus LM, et al.: Atypical multinucleated cells form in long-term marrow cultures from patients with Paget's disease. J Clin Invest 85:1280, 1990.

9. Roodman GD, Kukihara N, Ohsaki Y, et al.: Interleukin 6: a potential autocrine/paracrine factor in Paget's disease of bone. J Clin Invest 89:46, 1992.

10. de Deuxchaisnes CN, Krane SM: Paget's disease of bone: clinical and metabolic observations. Medicine 43:233, 1964.

11. Kahn AJ: The viral etiology of Paget's disease of bone: a new perspective (editorial). Calcif Tissue Int 47:127, 1990.

12. Bataille R: Etiology of Paget's disease of bone: a new perspective (letter). Calcif Tissue Int 50:293, 1992.

13. Singer FR, Mills BG: Evidence for a viral etiology of Paget's disease of bone. Clin Orthop 178:245, 1983.

14. Ralston SH, Digiovine FS, Gallacher SJ, et al.: Failure to detect paramyxovirus sequences in Paget's disease of bone using the polymerase chain reaction. J Bone Miner Res 6:1243, 1991.

15. Collins DH: Paget's disease of bone: incidence and subclinical forms. Lancet 2:51, 1956.

16. Rosenkrantz JA, Wolfe J, Karcher JJ: Paget's disease (osteitis deformans). Arch Intern Med 90:610, 1952.

17. Frank WA, Bress NM, Singer FR, Krane SM: Rheumatic manifestations of Paget's disease of bone. Am J Med 56:592, 1974.

18. Barry HC: Paget's disease of Bone. Edinburgh: E & S Livingstone Ltd, 1969.

19. Hadjipavlou A, Lander P: Paget disease of the spine. J Bone Joint Surg 73A:1376, 1991.

20. Altman RD, Brown M, Gargano GA: Low back pain in Paget's disease of bone. Clin Orthop 217:152, 1987.

21. Weisz GM: Lumbar canal stenosis in Paget's diseases: the staging of the clinical syndrome, its diagnosis, and treatment. Clin Orthop 206:223, 1986.

22. Guyer PB: Paget's disease of bone: the anatomical distribution. Metab Bone Dis 4:239, 1981.

23. Dinneen SF, Buckley TF: Spinal nerve root compression due to monostotic Paget's disease of a lumber vertebra. Spine 12:948, 1987.

24. Hadjipavlou A, Shaffer N, Lander P, Srolovitz H: Pagetic spinal stenosis with extradural pagetoid ossification: A case report. Spine 13:128, 1988.

25. Nichjolson DA, Roberts T, Sanville PR: Spinal cord compression in Paget's disease due to extradural pagetic ossification. Br J Radiol 64:864, 1991.

26. Hepgul K, Nicoll JAR, Coakham HB: Spinal cord compression due to Pagetic spinal stenosis with involvement of extradural soft tissues: a case report. Surg Neurol 35:143, 1991.

27. Chines A, Villareal D, Pacifici R: Paget's disease of bone affecting a single vertebra: clinical, radiologic, and histopathologic correlations. Calcif Tissue Int 50:115, 1992.

28. Hanna JW, Ball MR, Lee KS, McWhorter JM: Spontaneous spinal epidural hematoma complicating Paget's disease of the spine. Spine 14:900, 1989.

29. Richter RL, Semble EL, Turner RA, Challa VR: An unusual manifestation of Paget's disease of bone: spinal epidural hematoma presenting as acute cauda equina syndrome. J Rheumatol 17:975, 1990.

30. Chen J, Rhee RSC, Wallach S, et al.: Neurologic disturbances in Paget diseases of bone: response to calcitonin. Neurology 29:448, 1979.

31. Schmidek HH: Neurologic and neurosurgical sequelae of Paget's disease of bone. Clin Orthop 127:70, 1977.

32. Schreiber MH, Richardson GA: Paget's disease confined to one lumbar vertebra. AJR 90:1271, 1963.

33. Lluberas-Acosta G, Hansell JR, Schumacher HR Jr: Paget's disease of bone in patients with gout. Arch Intern Med 146:2389, 1986.

34. Wick MR, Siegal GP, Unni KK, et al.: Sarcomas of bone complicating osteitis deformans (Paget's disease). Fifty years' experience. Am J Surg Pathol 5:47, 1981.

35. Schajowicz F, Velan O, Araujo ES, et al.: Metastases of carcinoma in the Pagetic bone. Clin Orthop 228:290, 1988.

36. Bannister P, Roberts M, Sheridan P: Recurrent hypercalcemia in a young man with mono-ostotic Paget's disease. Postgrad Med J 62:481, 1986.

37. Coulton LA, Preston CJ, Couch M, Kanis JA: An evaluation of serum osteocalcin in Paget's disease of bone and its response to diphosphonate treatment. Arthritis Rheum 31:1142, 1988.

38. Foldes J, Shamir S, Brautbar C, et al.: HLA-D antigens and Paget's disease of bone. Clin Orthop 266:301, 1991.

39. Dahlin DC, Unni KK: Bone Tumors: General Aspects and Data on 8,542 Cases, 4th ed. Springfield, Illinois: Charles C Thomas, 1986, pp 458–459.

40. Rosen MA, Matasar KW, Irwin RB, et al.: Osteolytic monostotic Paget's disease of the fifth lumbar vertebra: a case report. Clin Orthop 262:119, 1991.

41. Resnick D: Paget disease of bone: current status and a look back to 1943 and earlier. AJR 150:249, 1988.

42. Steinbach HL: Some roentgen features of Paget's disease. AJR 86:950, 1961.

43. Lewis RJ, Jacobs B, Marchisello PJ, Bullough PG: Monostatic Paget's disease of the spine. Clin Orthop 127:208, 1977.

44. Lander P, Hadjipavlou A: Intradiscal invasion of Paget's disease of the spine. Spine 16:26, 1991.

45. Waxman AD, Ducker S, McKee D, et al.: Evaluation of 99m Tc diphosphonate kinetics and bone scans in patients with Paget's disease before and after calcitonin treatment. Radiology 125:761, 1977.

46. Khairi MRA, Wellman HN, Robb JA, Johnston CC Jr: Paget's disease of bone (osteitis deformans). Symptomatic lesions and bone scan. Ann Intern Med 79:348, 1973.

47. Shih W, Riley C, Maggoun S, Ryo Y: Paget's disease mimicking skeletal metastases in a patient with coexistent prostatic carcinoma. Eur J Nucl Med 14:422, 1988.

48. Dunn EK, Vaquer, Strashun AM: Paget's disease: a cause of photopenic skeletal defect in indium-111 WBC scintigraphy. J Nucl Med 29:561, 1988.

49. Resnick D, Niwayama G: Paget's disease. In Resnick D, Niwayama G (eds): Diagnosis of Bone and Joint Disorders, 2nd ed. Philadelphia: WB Saunders Co, 1988, pp 2127–2170.

50. Zlatkin MB, Lander PH, Hadjipavlou AG, Levine JS: Paget's disease of the spine: CT with clinical correlation. Radiology 160:155, 1986.

51. Roberts MC, Kressel HY, Fallon MD, et al.: Paget disease: MR imaging findings. Radiology 173:341, 1989.

52. Lichtenstein L: Polyostotic fibrous dysplasia. Arch Surg 36:874, 1938.

53. Albright F, Butler AM, Hampton AO, Smith P: Syn-

drome characterized by osteitis fibrosa disseminata, areas of pigmentation and endocrine dysfunction with precocious puberty in females. N Engl J Med 216:727, 1937.

54. Mansfield FL: Case records of the Massachusetts general hospital. N Engl J Med 328:1836, 1993.

55. Schwindinger WF, Francomano CA, Levine MA: Identification of a mutation in the gene encoding the alpha subunit of the stimulatory G protein of adenylyl cyclase in McCune-Albright syndrome. Proc Natl Acad Sci 89:5152, 1992.

56. Mirra JM: Bone Tumors: Clinical, Radiologic, and Pathologic Correlations. Philadelphia: Lea & Febiger, 1989, pp 191–226.

57. Feldman F: Tuberous sclerosis, neurofibromatosis, and fibrous dysplasia. In Resnick D, Niwayama G (eds): Diagnosis of Bone and Joint Disorders, 2nd ed. Philadelphia: WB Saunders Co, 1988, pp 4057–4072.

58. Resnick D, Niwayama G: Diagnosis of Bone and Joint Disorders. Philadelphia: WB Saunders Co, 1981, pp 2949–2961.

59. Marks KE, Bauer TW: Fibrous tumors of bone. Orthop Clin North Am 20:377, 1989.

60. Kahn A, Rosenberg PS: Monostotic fibrous dysplasia of the lumbar spine. Spine 13:592, 1988.

61. Ehara S, Kattapuram SV, Rosenberg AE: Fibrous dysplasia of the spine. Spine 17:977, 1992.

62. Utz JA, Kranedorf MJ, Jelinek JS, et al.: MR appearance of fibrous dysplasia. J Comput Assist Tomogr 13:845, 1989.

63. Hosking DJ: Advances in the management of Paget's disease of bone. Drugs 40:829, 1990.

64. De Rose NJ, Singer FR, Avramides A, et al.: Response of Paget's disease to porcine and salmon calcitonins. Effects of long-term treatment. Am J Med 56:858, 1974.

65. Human calcitonin for Paget's disease. Med Lett Drugs Ther 29:47, 1987.

66. Altman RD, Collins-Yudiskas B: Synthetic human calcitonin in refractory Paget's disease of bone. Arch Intern Med 147:1305, 1987.

67. D'Agostino HR, Barnett CA, Zielinski XJ, Gordan GS: Intranasal salmon calcitonin treatment of Paget's disease of bone: results in nine patients. Clin Orthop 230:223, 1988.

68. Canfield R, Rosner W, Skinner J, et al.: Diphosphonate therapy of Paget's disease of bone. J Clin Endocrinol Metab 44:96, 1977.

69. Pamidronate. Med Lett Drugs Ther 34:1, 1992.

70. Fitton A, McTavish D: Pamidronate: a review of its pharmacological properties and therapeutic efficacy in resorptive bone disease. Drugs 41:289, 1991.

71. Mallette LE: Successful treatment of resistant Paget's disease of bone with pamidronate. Arch Intern Med 149:2765, 1989.

72. Harinck HIJ, Bijvoet OLM, Blanksma HJ, Dahlinghaus-Nienhuys PJ: Efficacious management with amino-bisphosphonate (APD) in Paget's disease of bone. Clin Orthop 217:79, 1987.

73. Altman RD: Long-term follow-up of therapy with intermittent etidronate disodium in Paget's disease of bone. Am J Med 79:583, 1985.

74. Ryan W, Schwartz TB, Perlia CP: Effects of mithramycin on Paget's disease of bone. Ann Intern Med 70:549, 1969.

75. Warrell RP Jr, Bosco B, Weinerman S, et al.: Gallium nitrate for advanced Paget disease of bone: effectiveness and dose-response analysis Ann Intern Med 113:847, 1990.

76. Reginster JY, Colson F, Morlock G, et al.: Evaluation of the efficacy and safety of oral tiludronate in Pag-

et's disease of bone: a double-blind, multiple-dosage, placebo-controlled study. Arthritis Rheum 35:967, 1992.

77. Gray RES, Yates AJP, Preston CJ, et al.: Duration of effect of oral diphosphonate therapy in Paget's disease of bone. Quart J Med 64:755, 1987.

78. Hosking DJ, Bijvoet OLM, van Aken J, Will EJ: Paget's bone disease treated with diphosphonate and calcitonin. Lancet 1:615, 1976.

79. Jawad ASM, Berry H: Spinal cord compression in Paget's disease of bone treated medically. J Roy Soc Med 80:319, 1987.

80. Ryan PJ, Gibson T, Fogelman I: Bone scintigraphy following intravenous pamidronate for Paget's disease of bone. J Nucl Med 33:1589, 1992.

81. Moore TE, King AR, Kathol MH, et al.: Sarcoma in Paget disease of bone: clinical, radiologic, and pathologic features in 22 cases. AJR 156:1199, 1991.

82. Healey JH, Buss D: Radiation and pagetic osteogenic sarcomas. Clin Orthop 270:128, 1991.

INFECTIVE ENDOCARDITIS

Capsule Summary

Frequency of back pain—rare

Location of back pain—lumbar spine

Quality of back pain—diffuse ache

Symptoms and signs—back pain an initial symptom in a minority, fever, weight loss

Laboratory and x-ray tests—anemia, leukocytosis, hematuria, rheumatoid factor, blood cultures

Treatment—antibiotics

PREVALENCE AND PATHOGENESIS

Infective endocarditis is a microbial infection of a heart valve or the mural endocardium. A similar disease occurs with intravascular infection of the endothelial surface of large arteries. Infections of these anatomic areas are not limited to bacteria alone, but can be caused by fungi, rickettsiae, and chlamydiae as well.

A variety of classification systems have been proposed for the definition of endocarditis.[1] Initial classification systems were based on the duration of illness before the demise of the patient. Acute bacterial endocarditis caused fatal disease in less than 6 week and was associated with infection of normal valves with virulent organisms, such as *Staphylococcus aureus* and *Streptococcus pneumonia.* Subacute and chronic endocarditis affected structurally abnormal valves with less virulent organisms, such as *Streptococcus viridans,* and would cause death between 3 months and 2 years of the onset of infection. This arbitrary system based on duration of illness has been supplanted in current medical literature for classification systems for infective endocarditis based on the type of valve (native, prosthetic), host infected (intravenous drug abuser), and infecting organism (*Streptococcus pyogenes*). Other systems have defined the infection as definite, probable, or possible depending on clinical and pathologic features.[1] Definite endocarditis is defined by histologic or bacteriologic evidence of infection of a valvular vegetation or peripheral embolus. Probable endocarditis is defined as persistently positive blood cultures in the setting of clinical evidence of infection including new heart murmur, fever, and embolic phenomena. Possible endocarditis has positive cultures and only one of the three clinical features.

The clinical manifestations of infective endocarditis include fever, cardiac murmurs, splenomegaly, and embolic events. When patients present with these signs, the diagnosis is an easy one to make. The difficulty arises when a patient presents with low back pain as the initial manifestation of the infection. The diagnosis of this potentially life-threatening infection is more difficult in those circumstances. The actual prevalence and incidence of this infection are not known. A number of studies from the 1960s and 1970s reported on large groups of patients with endocarditis, but the relative numbers of patients with this infection compared to groups of patients with other infectious diseases was not known.[2–4] The current incidence of infective endocarditis in the United States in the 1980s is 1.7 to 4 cases per 100,000 person years.[5–7] The overall proportion of men to women with infective endocarditis is 3:1.[8] The ratio may be as high as 8:1 in individuals more than 60 years of age.[9] The proportion of individuals who are 60 years or older with endocarditis has increased over recent decades. In Olmstead County, Minnesota, the comparison of individuals over 65 years old to those younger with endocarditis is 8.8:1.[6] The increased risk of the elderly to endocarditis is related to increased exposure to intravascular invasive procedures, genitourinary infections, and bowel lesions.[10]

Although the disease had been recognized at an earlier time, the disease complex that is associated with infective endocarditis was formulated by Sir William Osler. Osler, in the Gulstonian lecture in 1885, described the myriad of manifestations of malignant endocarditis, many of which are recognized during the present era.[11]

The pathogenesis of infective endocarditis seems to follow a regular sequence of events. Microbial proliferation occurs within a vegetation located within the circulatory system. These vegetations may occur in areas of endothelial damage (valvular heart diseases, prosthetic heart valves, indwelling catheters), hypercoagulable states, and cancer (marantic endocarditis). Once the organisms gain entry into the vegetation, they multiply within the interstices of the vegetation. Constant blood stream dissemination of microorganisms is a hallmark of this disease. Constant bacteremia occurs despite normal systemic host defense mechanisms, including antibodies and polymorphonuclear leukocytes. The process becomes a vicious circle as constant bacteremia reinfects the vascular vegetation. Over time, the host defense mechanism mounts an increasingly intensive antibody response, which leads to the formation of antigen-antibody immune complexes. As the vegetation increases in size, small pieces may loosen and embolize to any part of the body. In addition, if located on a heart valve, the increasing size of the vegetation may cause hemodynamic alterations in cardiac function. In its final stages, endocarditis can cause damage through local invasion of cardiac tissue, resulting in cardiac collapse. The problem in diagnosing this process is that the clinical symptoms associated with this disease are nonspecific and the possibility of the infection as a diagnosis is raised late in the course of the infection.[1, 12] The clinical manifestations of these pathogenic mechanisms are the damage to heart valves and the associated hemodynamic cardiac complications, septic or bland embolization to distant organs causing necrosis of tissues, metastatic infections, and circulating immune complexes causing disease similar to that associated with serum sickness.

The classic case of indolent, subacute endocarditis with multiple systemic complications in the young patient has decreased in frequency. The disease has evolved, in part, since the discovery and use of increasing numbers of antibiotics. The number of young individuals with heart lesions from rheumatic fever has diminished. Older individuals are the persons with degenerative valvular heart disease predisposed to infection. Other factors that have changed the spectrum of the illness has been the increased prevalence of prosthetic heart valves and vascular shunts, intravenous drug abuse, and hospital-acquired infections and antibiotic resistance.[13]

Back pain occurs in patients with infective endocarditis. While musculoskeletal symptoms of any sort have been reported in 40% of endocarditis patients, between 9% and 12% of patients have had back pain as an initial symptom or during the course of their disease.[14–17] The pathogenesis of back pain in endocarditis remains obscure. Proposed mechanisms have included septic foci in muscles, reactive arthritis, renal disease with kidney infarction, or circulating immune complexes. Of all these mechanisms, the presence of increased amounts of immune complexes is the most likely mechanism of pain production in the musculoskeletal system. Immune complexes are normally present in musculoskeletal structures.[18, 19] As a result of chronic antigenic stimulation and overriding of normal T lymphocyte suppression mechanisms, a hypergammaglobulinemic state is created. The bypassing of normal controls results in a polyclonal B lymphocyte proliferation and immunoglobulin secretion. Increased levels of antibodies activate the complement cascade, which helps kill bacteria but also contributes to the pathologic destruction of host tissues. The variable manifestations of the disease may correlate to the physicochemical nature of the immune complexes, their deposition in tissues, and their clearance by the reticuloendothelial system.[20] Musculoskeletal complaints develop later in the course of the illness. Also probably related is the fact that back pain resolves within 2 weeks of the initiation of antibiotic therapy. Arterial embolization also has been proposed as a possible mechanism.[21] Although an occasional patient has evidence of emboli, many individuals with endocarditis have symptoms of the disease without any evidence of embolization of vegetations.

CLINICAL HISTORY

The bacterial organisms that are the cause of the infection determine the clinical picture presented to the physician. A listing of these organisms and the relative frequency of each as a cause of endocarditis is presented in Table 18–2. Acute infective endocarditis develops over days or weeks and is associated with *S. aureus, S. pneumoniae, S. pyogenes,* or *Neisseria gonorrhoeae.* Patients with acute disease develop musculoskeletal symptoms about as half as often as patients with subacute infective endocarditis. Subacute endocarditis develops over weeks to months and is associated with low-virulence organisms such as the viridans streptococci including *S. mutans, S. sanguis, S. mitior,* and *S. salivarius.*

Patients with subacute infective endocarditis may present with generalized malaise, fever,

TABLE 18–2. MICROBIOLOGIC ETIOLOGY IN 2345 EPISODES OF INFECTIVE ENDOCARDITIS*

ORGANISM	TOTAL EPISODES	PERCENT OF TOTAL
Streptococci†	1,322	56.4
Enterococci‡	142	6.1
Pneumococci	71	3.0
Staphylococci	583	24.9
Coagulase-positive	447	19.1
Coagulase-negative	136	5.8
Gram-negative bacteria	135	5.7
Fungi	24	1.0
Other§	63	2.7
Culture-negative	218	9.3

Modified from Kaye D (ed): Infective Endocarditis, 2nd ed. New York: Raven Press, 1992, p 86.
*Representing cases from 1933–1987.
†Total includes viridans streptococci, enterococci, pneumococci, and other streptococcal species (e.g., *S. bovis*).
‡Now considered a separate genus.
§Includes *Erysipelothrix, Pharyngis sicca, Micrococcus, Spirillium, Bacillus, Corynebacterium, Clostridium perfringens, Lactobacillus, Listeria, Coxiella burnetti, Chlamydia,* and nonstreptococcal anaerobes.

fatigue, and weight loss. The onset of these symptoms is insidious. Back pain may be a presenting symptom in a minority. Other musculoskeletal complaints may include arthralgias, arthritis, or diffuse myalgias. The arthralgias and arthritis tend to involve proximal and lower extremity joints. Up to 44% of patients may have a musculoskeletal complaint during the course of their illness. Occasionally, a patient may develop vertebral osteomyelitis or septic arthritis as a result of endocarditis.[22, 23] While the usual organisms causing vertebral osteomyelitis are more closely associated with acute endocarditis, more indolent microorganisms associated with subacute endocarditis have also caused vertebral osteomyelitis.[24, 25] Patients with endocarditis may complain of radicular pain without muscle weakness on rare occasions.[26] A mechanical etiology may be suspected in these patients because they complain of increased pain with cough. However, no specific area of disc degeneration can be found in these patients. The source of their pain is undetermined.[15] Subacute bacterial endocarditis also has been reported to affect a patient with AS and aortic valvular disease.[27]

Other manifestations of subacute bacterial endocarditis include mental status changes, transient ischemic attacks, progressive heart failure, and skin rash.

PHYSICAL EXAMINATION

The duration of the infection before diagnosis plays a major role in determining the manifestations that will be apparent on physical examination. Since the diagnosis is considered earlier in the course of the disease than in the pre-antibiotic era, those manifestations which take a considerable time to develop (clubbing, splenomegaly, Osler and Janeway lesions, and glomerulonephritis) are less evident when the diagnosis is established.

Physical findings usually include fever and a heart murmur in 90% and 80% of patients, respectively. Splenomegaly occurs in a smaller proportion of patients. Skin rash is found in 20% to 40% of patients at the time of hospital admission.[4, 28]

Back examination may demonstrate spinal tenderness and decreased motion. Scoliosis and a list may be noted in patients with unilateral paraspinous muscle spasm. Muscle spasm may be the sole presenting symptom on occasion. Percussion tenderness without sacroiliitis on radiographs has been reported.[8]

Examination of the eyes may demonstrate a wide variety of lesions including petechiae, hemorrhages, cotton-wool exudates, Roth's spots, or endophthalmitis. Neurologic manifestations in 30% of patients may include hemiparesis, seizures, or transient ischemic attacks.

Patients with acute endocarditis develop high spiking fever, rigors, and chills. Petechiae may be very prominent if *S. aureus* is the cause of the infection. Meningitis along with signs of intravascular coagulation may be present. Septic emboli, which cause localized infections in various areas of the body, are characteristic. These manifestations may occur even in the absence of a heart murmur.

LABORATORY DATA

Screening blood tests are frequently positive but the findings are nondiagnostic. Anemia occurs in 90% and thrombocytopenia in 15%. The sedimentation rate is universally elevated. Gamma globulins, particularly rheumatoid factor, are present in patients with longer duration disease. Rheumatoid factor is detectable in patients with disease over 6 weeks in duration. Urinalysis may reveal proteinuria and microscopic hematuria. Elevated creatinine levels suggest renal failure secondary to immune complex glomerulonephritis. Hypocomplementemia is frequently present when endocarditis is complicated by glomerulonephritis.

The blood culture is the most important laboratory test in infective endocarditis. In patients with fulminant disease, three venous samples over a 1-hour period should be obtained. In patients with subacute disease, three to four venous samples drawn over a 24-hour period are adequate. Two more cultures should be drawn if the initial sets are negative for growth of an organism. Cultures should be incubated for 4 weeks to detect fastidious pathogens. The bacteremia of endocarditis is continuous so blood cultures may be obtained at any time and not exclusively at times of temperature spikes.

Infective endocarditis is usually caused by gram-positive cocci, with streptococci and staphylococci accounting for 80% to 90% of cases (see Table 18–2). *S. viridans* is the leading cause of streptococcal infection. Viridans streptococci normally inhabit the oral cavity. After dental manipulation, the organisms may enter the blood stream to infect abnormal heart valves. *S. bovis* is a group D streptococcus that inhabits the gastrointestinal tract. *S. bovis* bacteremia has occurred in patients with carcinoma of the colon and other lesions of the gastrointestinal tract. Gastrointestinal evaluation is appropriate in patients with *S. bovis* endocarditis.[29, 30]

Staphylococci cause 30% of cases, with *S. aureus* the most common organism of that group. *S. aureus* affects the elderly and drug abusers most often. *Staphylococcus epidermidis* has become an increasingly important cause of endocarditis, particularly in individuals with prosthetic heart valves.

Enterococci are normal inhabitants of the gastrointestinal tract, genital tract, and occasionally, the anterior urethra and mouth. They cause infections in older men after prostatectomy and young women after obstetric procedures.

Gram-negative organisms are infrequent causes of endocarditis except in intravenous drug abusers, recipients of prosthetic valves, persons with cirrhosis, and immunocompromised hosts. Among gram-negative organisms, *Pseudomonas aeruginosa* is the most common cause of endocarditis.

Fungal endocarditis is a problem for drug abusers and those who have been receiving prolonged parenteral antibiotic therapy. *Candida albicans* is the prime culprit in this group.

Approximately 5% of endocarditis is culture-negative. Reasons for the absence of growth may include use of antibiotics by patients and the presence of slow-growing fastidious organisms, anaerobic organisms, and obligate intracellular parasites as the infecting organisms.

Other laboratory measurements that may be obtained are complement, which is decreased, and immune complexes or cryoglobulins, which are increased. These tests help document the immune nature of the disease but are too nonspecific to help in the diagnosis. However, like the sedimentation rate and rheumatoid factor, these test results may normalize as the patient responds to therapy.

RADIOGRAPHIC EVALUATION

Radiographic evaluation of the back in patients with endocarditis is unrevealing. Any changes that may be present are more likely to be related to the patient's age than to the infection. Rarely, a hematogenous infection may involve the spine. These patients will have the radiographic changes associated with vertebral osteomyelitis or discitis.[25]

Great advances have occurred in the radiographic evaluation of endocarditis. Echocardiography is able to detect vegetations and intracardiac complications of endocarditis noninvasively. Transesophageal imaging has increased the sensitivity of detecting lesions compared to two-dimensional echocardiography. Doppler and color flow mapping has been a sensitive method for depicting the abnormal flow of blood in the heart.[1]

DIFFERENTIAL DIAGNOSIS

The diagnosis of infective endocarditis is considered in the patient with back pain who has associated constitutional symptoms. It may also be considered in the patient who is older and has "mechanical" back pain if there is no history of injury or previous episode of pain, and roentgenograms are normal or show minimal degenerative arthritis. The diagnosis may not be apparent initially, but persistent surveillance of patients should alert the clinician that he is dealing not with a mechanical problem but with one associated with a systemic illness. These are the patients who may be identified in the low back pain algorithm as the cohort of individuals with fever. They also might be identified as one of the group with persistent muscle pain. Laboratory evaluation of these patients would identify anemia, leukocytosis, elevated ESR, or CRP, which would alert the physician to the likelihood of a systemic illness.

TREATMENT

Once the cultures have been obtained and the diagnosis is established, antibiotic therapy is begun. The basic component of therapy is bactericidal drugs, administered parenterally, for a long enough period of time to eradicate the infection. The reasons for prolonged ther-

apy are that host defense mechanisms do not work well in vegetations and that older bacteria in vegetations are in a static state, less susceptible to the effects of antibiotics.

In subacute endocarditis, the usual therapy is penicillin G, 24 million units/day, along with an aminoglycoside. Bactericidal levels are measured routinely and antibiotic doses are given to maintain bactericidal levels. The course of therapy is 4 to 6 weeks, depending on the organism and its antibiotic sensitivity.[11, 12, 31]

Patients with acute endocarditis, which is usually secondary to staphylococci or gram-negative organisms, require parenteral oxcillin or nafcillin, 12 gm/day, and gentamicin or tobramycin, 3 to 5 mg/kg/day for a 6-week period. Alterations in dose, duration of therapy, or choice of antibiotic are determined by local environmental factors such as bacterial sensitivity to antibiotics.

The therapy for each form of endocarditis must be individualized. Antibiotic regimens change for specific organisms (streptococcal vs. enterococcal vs. staphylococcal disease), the sensitivity of the organism to antibiotics in that hospital at the time of the infection (i.e., hospital acquired), and the medical condition of the host. For example, the same species of bacteria in two different hospitals may have different antibiotic sensitivities. Current information from the hospital's bacteriology laboratory concerning antibiotic sensitivity should be reviewed in order to formulate the best therapeutic regimen.[20]

PROGNOSIS

The prognosis of patients with infective endocarditis is good if the diagnosis is recognized and prompt therapy given. Back pain resolves within 2 weeks of the start of antibiotic treatment if the pain is related to the infection.[14]

The overall survival rate for infective endocarditis is about 75%. The rate depends in large measure on the timeliness of initiation of therapy and the nature of the infecting organism. Survival is 90% with *S. viridans* and 50% with *S. aureus*. Endocarditis in the elderly is associated with a significantly higher mortality rate than in middle-aged and young patients (45.3%, 32.6%, and 9.1% respectively in one study).[10] Cardiac failure is a grave prognostic sign and is the most common cause of death. Valve replacement may be required not only in patients with acute endocarditis but also in patients with native-valve endocarditis with indolent organisms (coagulase-negative staphylococci), if recognition of the infection is delayed.[32] Patients with cardiac failure may require valve replacement, but they may not receive any benefit if their cardiac function has been too severely compromised.[20]

References

INFECTIVE ENDOCARDITIS

1. Kaye D (ed): Infective Endocarditis, 2nd ed. New York: Raven Press, 1992.
2. Cherubin CE, Neu HC: Infective endocarditis at the Presbyterian hospital in New York City from 1938–1967. Am J Med 51:83, 1971.
3. Lerner PI, Weinstein L: Infective endocarditis in the antibiotic era. N Engl J Med 274:199, 259, 353, 388, 1966.
4. Pelletier LL, Petersdorf RG: Infective endocarditis: a review of 125 cases from the University of Washington Hospitals, 1963–72. Medicine 56:287, 1977.
5. King JW, Nguyen VQ, Conrad SA: Results of a prospective statewide reporting system for infective endocarditis. Am J Med Sci 295:517, 1988.
6. Griffen MR, Wilson WR, Edward WD, et al.: Infective endocarditis. Olmstead County Minnesota, 1950 through 1981. JAMA 254:1199, 1985.
7. Hickey AJ, MacMahon SW, Wilcken DEL: Mitral valve prolapse and bacterial endocarditis: when is antibiotic prophylaxis necessary? Am Heart J 109:431, 1985.
8. Watanakunaknorn C: Changing epidemiology and newer aspects of infective endocarditis. Adv Intern Med 22:21, 1977.
9. Gladstone JL, Recco R: Host factors and infectious disease in the elderly. Med Clin North Am 60:1225, 1976.
10. Terpenning MS, Buggy BP, Kauffman CA: Infective endocarditis: clinical features in young and elderly. Am J Med 83:626, 1987.
11. Osler W: The Gulstonian lectures on malignant endocarditis. Br Med J 1:467, 522, 577, 1885.
12. Freedman LR: Infective Endocarditis and Other Intravascular Infections. New York: Plenum Medical Book Co, 1982.
13. Littler WA, Shanson DC: Infective endocarditis. In Shanson DC (ed): Septicemia and Endocarditis: Clinical and Microbiological Aspects. Oxford: Oxford University Press, 1989, pp 143–171.
14. Churchill MA Jr, Geraci J, Hunder GG: Musculoskeletal manifestations of bacterial endocarditis. Ann Intern Med 87:754, 1972.
15. Thomas P, Allal J, Bontoux D, et al.: Rheumatological manifestations of infective endocarditis. Ann Rheum Dis 43:716, 1984.
16. Meyers OL, Commerford PJ: Musucloskeletal manifestations of bacterial endocarditis. Ann Rheum Dis 36:527, 1977.
17. Harkonen M, Olin PE, Wenstrom J: Severe backache as a presenting sign of bacterial endocarditis. Acta Med Scand 210:329, 1981.
18. Myers AR, Schumacher HR Jr: Arthritis of subacute bacterial endocarditis (SBE). Arthritis Rheum 19:813, 1976.
19. Bayer AS, Theofilopoulous AN, Eisenberg R, et al.: Circulating immune complexes in infective endocarditis. N Engl J Med 295:1500, 1976.
20. Sande MA, Kaye D, Root RK (eds): Endocarditis. Edinburgh: Churchill Livingstone, 1984.
21. Irvin RG, Sade RM: Endocarditis and musculoskeletal manifestations. Ann Intern Med 88:578, 1978.
22. Kahn MF: Vertebral osteomyelitis and bacterial endocarditis. Arthritis Rheum 25:600, 1982.
23. Good AE, Hague JM, Kauffmann CA: Streptococcal endocarditis initially seen as septic arthritis. Arch Intern Med 138:805, 1978.
24. Allen SL, Salmon JE, Roberts RB: Streptococcus bovis endocarditis presenting as acute vertebral osteomyelitis. Arthritis Rheum 24:1211, 1981.
25. Ullman RF, Strampfer MJ, Cunha BA: Streptococcus mutans vertebral osteomyelitis. Heart Lung 17:319, 1988.
26. Holler JW, Pecora JS: Backache in bacterial endocarditis. NY State J Med 70:1903, 1970.
27. Hoppmann RA, Wise CM, Challa VR, Peacock JE: Subacute bacterial endocarditis in a patient with ankylosing spondylitis. Ann Rheum Dis 47:423, 1988.
28. Garvey GJ, Neu HC: Infective endocarditis—an evolving disease. Medicine 57:105, 1978.
29. Steinberg D, Naggar CZ: Streptococcus bovis endocarditis with carcinoma of the colon. N Engl J Med 297:1354, 1977.
30. Watanakunakorn C: Streptococcus bovis endocarditis associated with villous adenoma following colonoscopy. Am Heart J 116:1115, 1988.
31. Magilligan DJ Jr., Quinn EL (eds): Endocarditis: Medical and Surgical Management. New York: Marcel Dekker, Inc, 1986.
32. Caputo GM, Archer GL, Calderwood SB, et al.: Native valve endocarditis due to coagulase-negative staphylococci: clinical and microbiologic features. Am J Med 83:619, 1987.

VERTEBRAL SARCOIDOSIS

Capsule Summary

Frequency of back pain—rare
Location of back pain—lumbar spine
Quality of back pain—intermittent, dull or stabbing pain
Symptoms and signs—cough, dyspnea, vertebral percussion tenderness
Laboratory and x-ray tests—increased calcium, gamma globulins, mixed lytic-sclerotic lesions on plain roentgenograms
Treatment—corticosteroids, surgical decompression

PREVALENCE AND PATHOGENESIS

Sarcoidosis is a disease of unknown etiology that causes the formation of granulomas, a form of inflammation consisting of epithelioid cells surrounded by a border of mononuclear cells, in any organ in the body. It is most closely associated with granuloma formation in the lung and thoracic lymph nodes. A much smaller proportion of patients develop bony involvement, including vertebral bodies. The disease was first described by Hutchinson in 1877.[1]

The exact prevalence of sarcoidosis is unknown but may be as high as one case per 10,000 population. Autopsy studies suggest that the prevalence of sarcoidosis may be as high as 641 cases per 100,000 population in Scandinavian countries.[2] In the United States sarcoidosis is 14 times more common in blacks than whites.[3] The age of onset is between 20 and 40 years. The male to female ratio is 1:1. Vertebral sarcoidosis is a rare entity, with 12 reported cases.[4] Most patients with vertebral sarcoidosis are black males, with a mean age of 26 years.

The pathogenesis of sarcoidosis is unknown. The presence of granulomas in the lung and other tissues suggests an abnormality in immune function. Bronchoalveolar lavage has been used to sample immune cells from the lungs of sarcoid patients. Lavage fluid has a high proportion and absolute number of lymphocytes.[5] Normally, macrophages comprise 90% and lymphocytes 10% of lavage fluid. In sarcoidosis, the number of cells is increased several times the number from normal individuals, and the number of lymphocytes may be increased to 60% of total recovered cells.[6] T lymphocytes from patients with active sarcoidosis release substances that promote the formation of granulomas. T helper cells, as opposed to T suppressor cells, are found in increased numbers in the lung, while the ratio of helper to suppressor cells in the peripheral blood is decreased. In addition to increased numbers, T lymphocytes are in an activated state manifested by active proliferation, release of migration inhibiting factor, IL-2, and gamma interferon.[5] Macrophages are also activated to produce IL-1. In addition, T lymphocytes from patients with sarcoidosis cause B lymphocytes to produce immunoglobulin. These abnormalities in the number and function of immune cells correlate with the clinical findings of granuloma formation, anergy to delayed hypersensitivity reaction, and hypergammaglobulinemia.[7-9] The granuloma in an organ causes disorganization of normal tissue, and the process of healing results in the production of fibrosis in areas of granulomatous inflammation. Granuloma-associated fibrosis in the lungs, heart, kidney, eyes, and musculoskeletal system may be associated with dysfunction in all these organ systems and correlates with the wide range of clinical findings associated with this illness.

Osseous involvement in sarcoidosis has been estimated to be 15% to 20%. A proportion of sarcoid patients as high as 34% has been reported when consistent radiologic evaluation of patients is performed.[2] This proportion of patients with osseous involvement may be an underestimate because granulomas may be present in bone and not detected by radiographic techniques. Bone lesions are more common in patients with more persistent disease with chronic skin involvement.[10] The areas of involvement include the bones of the hands and feet, skull, pelvis, femurs, humeri, and ribs. The spine is rarely involved.

CLINICAL HISTORY

Osseous sarcoidosis almost invariably occurs when there is clinical or radiographic pulmonary involvement. Pulmonary symptoms include cough and shortness of breath. Osseous lesions may be asymptomatic or discovered by chance on radiographs, but this is rarely the case in vertebral sarcoidosis since it is usually painful. Patients complain of a dull or stabbing pain localized at the involved vertebrae. It may radiate from the back to the thighs and is relieved by rest and increased with activity. Patients with spinal cord compression complain of neurologic symptoms, including lower extremity weakness, loss of sensation, and abnormalities of bladder and bowel function.[11, 12] Symptoms related to a single nerve root infiltrated with sarcoid also have been reported.[13] Patients with generalized sarcoidosis may also give a history of anorexia, weight loss, and fever.

PHYSICAL EXAMINATION

Physical examination of patients with vertebral sarcoidosis demonstrates percussion tenderness over the involved area of the axial skeleton. Limitation of motion of the spine may be an accompanying finding. Those with neurologic involvement may demonstrate impaired sensation, weakness, and depressed or absent lower extremity reflexes. General physical examination may demonstrate other organ system involvement with sarcoidosis, including skin rash (erythema nodosum, macules or papules containing granulomas), abnormal breath sounds, splenomegaly, generalized lymphadenopathy, and eye inflammation (iridocyclitis, choroidoretinitis, conjunctivitis, enlarged lacrimal glands).

LABORATORY DATA

Several biochemical abnormalities have been described in sarcoidosis. These include hypercalcemia, increased serum alkaline phosphatase, and hypergammaglobulinemia. Serum angiotensin converting enzyme (ACE) is elevated in patients with sarcoidosis.[14] ACE is most active in lung lining cells. Granulomatous inflammation of the lung and lymph nodes may be the source of increased concentrations of ACE. ACE is elevated in 43% to 88% of patients with sarcoidosis.[15] This variability is in part due to differences in sensitivity of the test in different laboratories. The test also lacks specificity, since miliary tuberculosis, histoplasmosis, Gaucher's disease, and biliary cirrhosis are associated with increased ACE levels. Therefore, an elevated ACE level is supportive but not diagnostic of sarcoidosis. Cutaneous anergy (loss of delayed hypersensitivity), when tested with exposure to three antigens (PPD, *Candida,* and *Trichophyton*), occurs in a minority of patients.[16] Bronchoalveolar lavage has been used for determination of elevated proportions of helper T lymphocytes in sarcoid patients.[17] The results of bronchoalveolar lavage are not specific for sarcoidosis, and difficulty in obtaining fluid has limited its utility as a diagnostic test.

Pathologic specimens from patients with sarcoidosis demonstrate multiple noncaseating granulomas consisting of multinucleated giant cells. They are present in any organ involved with sarcoid, including the lung, skin, bone, and muscle. Nonsarcoid causes of granulomas (tuberculosis, berylliosis) must be considered before a diagnosis of sarcoidosis is entertained.

RADIOGRAPHIC EVALUATION

Radiographic abnormalities associated with vertebral sarcoidosis include bone lysis with marginal sclerosis that involves the vertebral body.[18] Occasionally the posterior elements of vertebra also may be affected (Fig. 18–9).[19] Contiguous vertebrae may be involved, some with narrowing of the intervertebral disc.[20] Other patients have noncontiguous vertebral body disease (Fig. 18–10).[21] The inflammatory process may progress to cause vertebral body collapse.[22] Paravertebral ossification with anterior bony bridges simulating AS has been reported.[4] It has been suggested that patients with sarcoidosis may develop sacroiliitis in addition to nonmarginal syndesmophytes and paravertebral ossification.[23] Occasionally, sarcoidosis may produce sclerotic lesions of bone that may be confused with metastatic disease to bone.[31]

Myelography may demonstrate defects compatible with soft tissue compression of spinal

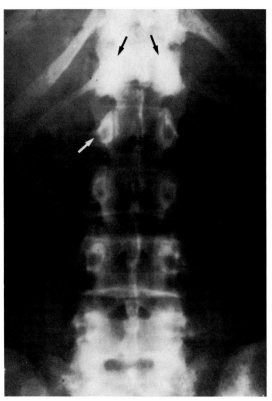

Figure 18–9. Sarcoidosis. AP view of the lumbar spine demonstrating sclerosis of the pedicles of T12 *(black arrows)* and the right pedicle of L1 *(white arrow)* and diffuse sclerosis of L5. (Courtesy of Anne Brower, M.D.)

cord elements.[18] Rarely, the spinal cord and cauda equina may be affected directly. Myelography may reveal intramedullary or intradural masses, arachnoiditis, or meningeal thickening.[24] The lower thoracic and upper lumbar vertebrae are the ones most frequently involved in vertebral sarcoidosis. CT and MR scans are particularly well suited to the evaluation of neurosarcoidosis. They are sensitive to detecting space occupying lesions in the spinal cord and other parts of the central nervous system.[25, 26]

DIFFERENTIAL DIAGNOSIS

The definitive diagnosis of vertebral sarcoidosis requires a biopsy of the lesion in patients with posterior element involvement or disc space narrowing. Diseases that may mimic sarcoid involvement of the spine include tuberculosis, pyogenic osteomyelitis, Hodgkin's disease, and metastatic carcinoma. These diseases also may cause posterior element destruction and/or disc space narrowing. Biopsy of the bone lesion may not be necessary in the pa-

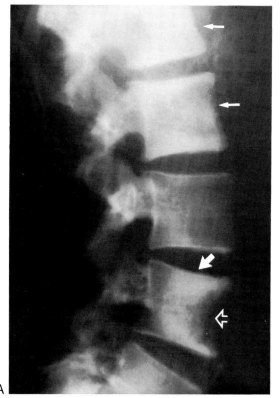
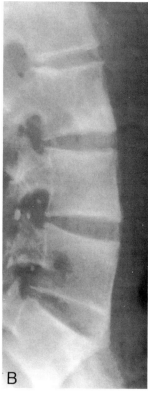

Figure 18–10. A 27-year-old black male with low back pain and sarcoidosis. *A,* Lateral view of the lumbar spine reveals sclerosis of L1 and L2 vertebral bodies *(small white arrows)* and mixed sclerosis *(white arrow)* and lysis *(open arrow)* of the L4 vertebral body. The radiograph was obtained in 1975. *B,* Lateral view of the lumbar spine taken in 1980 demonstrates continued sclerosis with paravertebral calcification. The patient developed hemoptysis secondary to an aspergilloma and expired in 1989. (Courtesy of Werner Barth, M.D.)

tient in whom previous biopsy has proved pulmonary and skin disease secondary to sarcoid. However, if an anterior lytic lesion of a vertebral body does not respond to therapy, further diagnostic tests, including biopsy, are indicated.

TREATMENT

Most patients with vertebral sarcoidosis require corticosteroids in the range of 15 to 80 mg/day to control the symptoms and the granulomatous inflammation.[4, 20, 22] Bone lysis and sclerosis may remain the same or lessen with therapy. In patients with persistent back pain or neurologic symptoms of cord compression, surgical decompression of the involved vertebrae is required.[4, 27] Surgical decompression may also be necessary to relieve radicular pain for nerve roots infiltrated with sarcoid granulomas.[13]

PROGNOSIS

The prognosis of patients with vertebral sarcoidosis has been generally good.[28] Surgical in-

tervention for biopsies of lesions is important in eliminating other causes of vertebral lysis and sclerosis and confirming the presence of noncaseating granuloma. Decompression and/or fusion of severely affected areas of the axial skeleton has helped prevent the progression of potentially life-threatening neurologic complications. In most circumstances, corticosteroids for sarcoidosis in general, and vertebral sarcoidosis in particular, have been effective in controlling the systemic inflammatory component of this illness. However, it should be remembered that patients with vertebral sarcoidosis have extrathoracic disease and patients with extensive systemic manifestations of sarcoidosis have a less favorable prognosis than those patients with exclusively intrathoracic disease.[29, 30]

References

VERTEBRAL SARCOIDOSIS

1. Hutchinson J: Illustrations of Clinical Surgery, Vol 1. London: Churchill, 1877, p 42.

2. Sharma OP: Sarcoidosis: Clinical Management. London: Butterworths, 1984.

3. Johns CJ, Scott PP, Schonfeld SA: Sarcoidosis. Annu Rev Med 40:353, 1989.

4. Perlman SG, Damergis J, Witrosch P, et al.: Vertebral sarcoidosis with paravertebral ossification. Arthritis Rheum 21:271, 1978.

5. Thomas PD, Hunninghake GW: Current concepts of the pathogenesis of sarcoidosis. Am Rev Resp Dis 135:747, 1987.

6. Soskel NT, Fox R: Sarcoidosis or something like it. South Med J 83:1190, 1990.

7. Hunninghake GW, Crystal RG: Mechanisms of hypergammaglobulinemia in pulmonary sarcoidosis: site of increased antibody production and role of T-lymphocytes. J Clin Invest 67:86, 1981.

8. Hunninghake GW, Crystal RG: Pulmonary sarcoidosis. A disorder mediated by excess helper T-lymphocyte activity at sites of disease activity. N Engl J Med 305:429, 1981.

9. Daniele RP, Dauber JH, Rossman MD: Immunologic abnormalities in sarcoidosis. Ann Intern Med 92:406, 1980.

10. Neville E, Carstairs LS, James DG: Sarcoidosis of bone. Q J Med 46:215, 1977.

11. Moldover A: Sarcoidosis of the spinal cord: report of a case with remission associated with cortisone therapy. Arch Intern Med 102:414, 1958.

12. Delaney P: Neurologic manifestations in sarcoidosis: review of literature and report of 23 cases. Ann Intern Med 87:336, 1977.

13. Baron B, Goldberg Al, Rothfus WE, Sherman RL: CT features of sarcoid infiltration of a lumbosacral nerve root. J Comput Assist Tomogr 13:364, 1989.

14. Lieberman S: The specificity and nature of serum angiotensin converting enzyme in sarcoidosis. Ann NY Acad Sci 278:488, 1976.

15. Fanburg BL: Angiotensin-1-converting enzyme. In Fanburg BL (ed): Sarcoidosis and Other Granulomatous Diseases of the Lung. New York: Marcel Dekker, 1983, pp 263–272.

16. Tannenbaum H, Rocklin RE, Schur PH, Sheffer AL: Immune function in sarcoidosis. Clin Exp Immunol 26:511, 1976.

17. Yeager J Jr, Williams MC, Beekman JF, et al.: Sarcoidosis: analysis of cells obtained by bronchoalveolar lavage. Am Rev Respir Dis 116:951, 1977.

18. Brodey PA, Pripstein S, Strange G, Kohout ND: Vertebral sarcoidosis: a case report and review of the literature. AJR 126:900, 1976.

19. Berk RN, Brower TD: Vertebral sarcoidosis. Radiology 82:660, 1964.

20. Baldwin DM, Roberts JG, Croff HE: Vertebral sarcoidosis: a case report. J Bone Joint Surg 56A:629, 1974.

21. Zener JC, Alpert M, Klainer LM: Vertebral sarcoidosis. Arch Intern Med 11:696, 1963.

22. Goobar JE, Gilmer S Jr, Carrol DS, Clark GM: Vertebral sarcoidosis. JAMA 178:162, 1961.

23. Curran JJ, Dennis GJ, Boling EP: Sarcoidosis and spondyloarthropathy. Arthritis Rheum 30:S42, 1986.

24. Bernstein J, Rival J: Sarcoidosis of the spinal cord as the presenting manifestation of the disease. South Med J 71:1571, 1978.

25. Chapelon C, Ziza JM, Piette JC, et al.: Neurosarcoidosis: signs, course and treatment in 35 confirmed cases. Medicine 69:261, 1990.

26. Sharma OP, Sharma AM: Sarcoidosis of the nervous system: a clinical approach. Arch Intern Med 151:1317, 1991.

27. Rodman R, Funderburk EE Jr, Myerson RM: Sarcoidosis with vertebral involvement. Ann Intern Med 50:213, 1959.

28. James DG, Neville E, Carstairs LS: Bone and joint sarcoidosis. Semin Arthritis Rheum 6:53, 1976.

29. Wurm K, Rosner R: Prognosis of chronic sarcoidosis. Ann NY Acad Sci 278:732, 1976.

30. James DG, Williams WJ: Sarcoidosis and Other Granulomatous Disorders. Philadelphia: W B Saunders Co, 1985.

31. Abdelwahab IF, Norman A: Osteosclerotic sarcoidosis. AJR 150:161, 1988.

RETROPERITONEAL FIBROSIS

Capsule Summary

Frequency of back pain—uncommon

Location of back pain—lower back and lower abdomen

Quality of back pain—dull

Symptoms and signs—weight loss, fever, decreased urine output, abdominal masses, peripheral edema

Laboratory and x-ray tests—impaired renal function, increased ESR; IVP—ureteral obstruction; MR—extent of fibrous plaque

Treatment—uterolysis, corticosteroids

PREVALENCE AND PATHOGENESIS

Retroperitoneal fibrosis is a disease of unknown etiology that causes fibrosis of the retroperitoneum and renal dysfunction secondary to ureteral obstruction. A grayish plaque of fibrosis envelops the retroperitoneum from the level of the renal arteries to the pelvic brim and laterally to the psoas margins. The structures enveloped in the fibrosis include the aorta, inferior vena cava, ureters, and spinal nerves.

The prevalence of retroperitoneal fibrosis is about 1 per 200,000 population.[1] Although the literature contains reports that review large numbers of patients with retroperitoneal fibrosis, it is an uncommon disorder with approximately 500 reported cases.[2, 3] Patients develop the disease between the fifth and sixth decades. The male to female ratio for retroperitoneal fibrosis is 3:1.

Albarran was the first to describe the disease, in 1905.[4] However, Ormond in 1948 described the disease so that it was recognized as a distinct clinical entity.[5] Retroperitoneal fibrosis has been associated with a variety of names including Ormond's diseases, nonspecific retroperitoneal inflammation, sclerosing retroperitonitis, retroperitoneal vasculitis, periureteritis fibrosa, and periaortitis.

The pathogenesis of retroperitoneal fibrosis is unknown. The association of vascular inflammation and panniculitis (Weber-Christian disease) has suggested an immunologic basis similar to that seen with other collagen vascular diseases. Patients with scleroderma, systemic lupus erythematosus, and retroperitoneal fibrosis have been reported.[6-9] Retroperitoneal fibrosis also has been described in patients with immune thrombocytopenia and those with polyserositis mimicking systemic lupus erythematosus.[10, 11] Another possible etiology is a disorder of uncontrolled fibrous proliferation.[12] Retroperitoneal fibrosis may occur in combination with other disorders, such as Dupuytren's contracture. Reidel's struma, or sclerosing cholangitis, which are associated with excessive fibrous proliferation in a number of organs.[13] Genetic factors may also play a role in light of a report of patients with HLA-B27 who developed retroperitoneal fibrosis.[14] However, retroperitoneal fibrosis has been reported in individuals with spondyloarthropathy who are HLA-B27 negative.[15, 16]

Retroperitoneal fibrosis occurs near areas of atherosclerotic disease affecting large, elastic arteries. One postulated theory for fibrosis is based on the hypothesis that fibrosis develops in response to the leakage of insoluble lipid, ceroid.[17, 18] Ceroid may be produced and deposited in atherosclerotic plaques by the oxidation of low density lipoproteins. Immunoglobulins, particularly IgG, are deposited with ceroid in vessel plaques. Characterization of the inflammatory cells in patients with ceroid deposits and fibrosis identifies a variety of activated immune cells including B and helper T lymphocytes. Retroperitneal fibrosis may be the result of an immune response to ceroid deposits. Fibrosis does occur in patients with abdominal aortic aneurysms.[19] However, this theory would not explain the presence of fibrosis in areas devoid of atherosclerotic disease.

Malignancy accounts for up to 10% of retroperitoneal cases.[2] In response to the presence of metastases, a desmoplastic response results in the production of fibrous tissue. A wide variety of tumors have been associated with fibrosis including breast, lung, thyroid, genitourinary including kidney, and cervix, and lymphomas.[20, 21]

A number of drugs have been associated with retroperitoneal fibrosis. Methysergide, an ergot derivative, accounted for 12% of cases when it was frequently prescribed for migraine headache.[2] Methysergide is a strong, competitive antagonist of serotonin and causes an increase in the amount of endogenous serotonin. Fibrosis is thought to occur secondary to increased concentrations of serotonin. Other medications including other ergot derivatives that may affect blood vessel function have been implicated as initiators of fibrosis.[22] Retroperitoneal fibrosis has also been reported subsequent to multiple celiac plexus anesthetic blocks.[23]

The largest group of patients with retroperitoneal fibrosis have idiopathic disease. Over two thirds of patients with this illness have no underlying explanation for the initiation of the fibrotic response in the retroperitoneum.

Approximately 44% of patients with retroperitoneal fibrosis have back pain as a presenting complaint. As the disease progresses, the back, flank, and abdominal lower quadrants become painful.[3]

CLINICAL HISTORY

The presenting symptom of patients with retroperitoneal fibrosis is pain located in the lower quadrants of the abdomen or the lumbosacral spine. The percentage of patients with flank pain and back pain is 42% and 32%, respectively.[24] Pain is insidious in onset, dull, and noncolicky. It may radiate, in the referred pain pattern of the ureter, from the flank to the periumbilical area and to the testes. Patients also may give a history of weight loss, anorexia, fever, and joint pain.[25] Symptoms of urologic compromise, hematuria or oliguria, occur in a later stage of the illness. Occasionally, patients may have spinal stiffness, muscle tenderness, and Raynaud's phenomenon as part of their symptom complex.

PHYSICAL EXAMINATION

The most common physical findings are masses found on abdominal and rectal examination. Compression of the inferior vena cava is associated with peripheral edema in the lower extremities. Patients may complain of pain with percussion over the lumbosacral spine. Hypertension may be noted in 68% of those with renal dysfunction. Testicular examination may reveal hydroceles, testicular atrophy, or scrotal edema. In rare circumstances, lower extremity weakness may be noted. If associated with sensory abnormalities, a lesion affecting the spinal cord or cauda equina should be suspected. A fibrotic epidural mass contiguous with the retroperitoneum may grow epidurally to compress neural elements.[26]

LABORATORY DATA

The most commonly abnormal laboratory finding associated with retroperitoneal fibrosis is an elevated ESR, which occurs in over 90% of patients.[3] Less often, but still in a majority of patients (67%), a decrease in hematocrit and an elevation in blood urea nitrogen are noted. Antithyroid, anti-smooth muscle, and Coomb's antibodies have been reported.[9, 27] Urinalysis may reveal a variety of abnormalities including proteinuria, microscopic hematuria, and pyuria. In two patients, elevated serum alkaline phosphatase was associated with active retroperitoneal fibrosis. The serum abnormality returned to normal with corticosteroid therapy of the fibrosis.[28]

On gross pathologic inspection, retroperitoneal fibrosis appears as a glistening, grayish-white, woody-hard, fibrous plaque that resembles a malignant retroperitoneal tumor.[3] The fibrosis envelops the retroperitoneal structures, including the aorta, vena cava, renal pedicle, ureters, and psoas muscle. The plaque usually is centered over the anterior surfaces of the fourth and fifth lumbar vertebrae. The tissue is adherent but does not invade the underlying structures. The process may involve the retroperitoneum and may spread as far as the mediastinum.[29]

Histologic specimens from biopsies of the retroperitoneum in patients with retroperitoneal fibrosis reveal dense fibrosis with distinct areas of chronic inflammation.[27, 30, 31] The chronic inflammation is centered on adipose tissue and blood vessels and is nonsuppurative. The inflammatory component includes lymphocytes, plasma cell, eosinophils, and polymorphonuclear leukocytes. Multinucleated giant cells and granulomas have been described. The inflammation has been associated with chronic inflammation of fibrofatty tissue, perivasculitis, vasculitis, necrotizing vasculitis, and fat necrosis.[3]

RADIOGRAPHIC EVALUATION

Radiographic techniques that demonstrate the location of retroperitoneal structures or obstruction of the genitourinary system help make the diagnosis. The classic triad of findings on intravenous pyelography (IVP) is bilateral ureteral narrowing at the level of the fifth lumbar vertebra, medial deviation of the ureters, and dilatation of the calyces, pelvis, and ureter (Fig. 18–11). Ureteral stenosis may be limited to the L4 and L5 vertebral body level in a majority of ureters evaluated by IVP.[32] Ret-

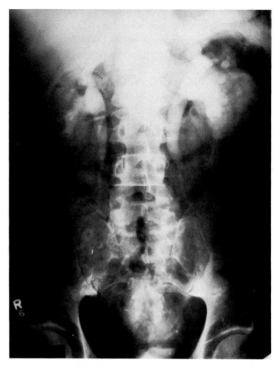

Figure 18–11. IVP of a 57-year-old man with acute onset of anuria with chronic, diffuse low back pain demonstrates dilatation of the calices, pelvis, and ureter of both kidneys. Obstruction of the ureters is greatest at the level of L4 and L5 vertebral bodies. (Courtesy of Arnold Kwart, M.D.)

rograde pyelography may show ureteral obstruction. The sonographic appearance of the retroperitoneum in retroperitoneal fibrosis is one of a smooth-bordered echo-free mass over the sacrum.[33] Lymphangiography is useful in distinguishing retroperitoneal fibrosis from lymphoma.[34] Gallium-67 imaging may be useful in measuring the state of inflammatory activity of fibrosis in the retroperitoneum. Gallium scan may identify an area of increased activity that would be an appropriate location for a diagnostic biopsy.[35]

In the past, CT was the most sensitive technique for evaluation of retroperitoneal fibrosis. CT scan is capable of detecting the presence and extent of the characteristic soft tissue mass as well as its relation to adjacent abdominal structures (Fig. 18–12).[36] However, CT scan is not able to identify the quality of soft tissue disease allowing the differentiation of the various causes of retroperitoneal fibrosis.[37] CT scan also may miss fibrosis that causes renal dysfunction in the form of obstructive uropathy but does not cause ureteral dilation.[38] In patients with renal failure, the use of contrast dye will worsen kidney dysfunction. Unenhanced scanning makes it difficult to distin-

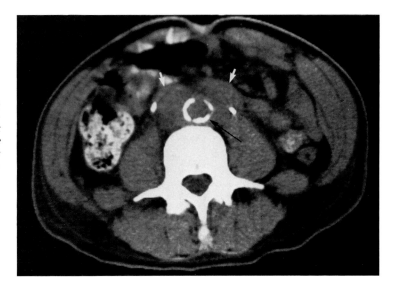

Figure 18–12. CT scan of the same patient in Figure 18–11 revealing encasement of the calcified aorta *(black arrow)* within a soft tissue mass *(white arrows)* that involves the ureters (white dots). (Courtesy of Arnold Kwart, M.D.)

guish the aortic lumen from surrounding tissues in some patients. Neoplastic tissues may not be differentiated from benign fibrosis. CT is limited to the axial plane.[39]

MR is the radiographic technique of choice to evaluate retroperitoneal fibrosis.[22, 40] T_1-weighted images of fibrotic plaque have low to medium signal. T_2-weighted images have high signal intensity. The presence of high signal intensity may be noted in patients with malignant fibrosis as well as those with an inflammatory stage of benign fibrosis because of high free-water content and hypercellularity.[41] The presence of low intensity signal on both T_1 and T_2 images suggests benign retroperitoneal fibrosis (Fig. 18–13).[42]

DIFFERENTIAL DIAGNOSIS

The diagnosis of retroperitoneal fibrosis can be suspected in a patient with back pain, con-stitutional symptoms, and evidence of genitourinary obstruction and is confirmed by biopsy of the retroperitoneum. There are many disease processes, including malignancy, trauma, infection, reactions to drugs, and connective tissue diseases, associated with retroperitoneal fibrosis (Table 18–3). Metastatic carcinoma from abdominal organs or breast may deposit in the retroperitoneum, causing ureteral obstruction and fibrosis.[43] Neoplastic diseases, such as Hodgkin's disease, non-Hodgkin's lymphoma, and sarcomas, may originate in the retroperitoneum and may produce extensive sclerotic reactions.[44] Rare tumors, such as teratomas, may present in adults and may mimic changes of retroperitoneal fibrosis.[45] Carcinoid tumors with increased production of serotonin have been associated with fibrosis.[46] Radiation therapy of the retroperitoneum given for the treatment of tumors may result in fibrosis.[47] The clinician must remember that retroperi-

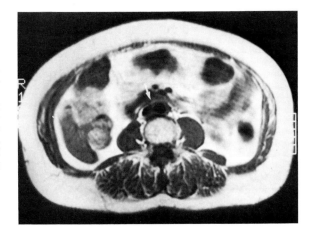

Figure 18–13. Retroperitoneal fibrosis. A 50-year-old woman with a history of lumbar laminectomy and fusion in 1983 who subsequently developed retroperitoneal fibrosis requiring right nephrectomy in 1988. In 4/92, MR scan was obtained to determine the extent and activity of her fibrosis. The T_2-weighted image demonstrated retroperitoneal fibrosis that had a slightly bright signal *(arrow)* suggesting mild activity of her disease. Her ESR was 85 mm/hr. She refused corticosteroid therapy. Over the following year, her ESR has fallen to 59 mm/hr and her renal function has been stable.

TABLE 18–3. CAUSES OF RETROPERITONEAL FIBROSIS

A. Malignancy
  Periureteral metastatic disease
  Primary retroperitoneal tumors
  Carcinoid
B. Retroperitoneal injury
  Bleed (anticoagulants, clotting factor deficiency)
  Trauma (blunt, operative)
  Ruptured diverticulum
  Appendicitis
  Urinary extravasation
  Radiation
C. Infection agents
  Genitourinary tract
  Histoplasmosis
D. Drugs
  Methysergide
  Amphetamines
E. Collagen vascular disease
  Vasculitis
  Weber-Christian panniculitis
  Mesenteric panniculitis
  Systemic lupus erythematosus
  Scleroderma
F. Miscellaneous
  Sclerosing fibrosis

Modified from Lepor H, Walsh PC: Idiopathic retroperitoneal fibrosis. J Urol 122:1, 1979.

toneal malignancy leaves subtle findings that are initially overlooked. Additional biopsies and close evaluation should elucidate those individuals with "idiopathic" retroperitoneal fibrosis who actually have fibrosis resulting from a malignant tumor.[48]

Trauma to the retroperitoneum may result in subsequent fibrosis. Examples of trauma include bleeding into the retroperitoneum secondary to a clotting factor deficiency or anticoagulant therapy.[49] Bleeding from Henoch-Schönlein purpura and abdominal aneurysm may also cause fibrosis. Trauma to the suprapubic area with hematoma formation may produce retroperitoneal fibrosis.[50] Inflammatory bowel disease that extends beyond the walls of the gut into the retroperitoneum may initiate fibrosis.[51]

Infections in the genitourinary tract may cause fibrosis. Infection may spread through the lymphatics from the bladder to the retroperitoneum and cause fibrosis in periureteral tissues.[52] Specific infections such as tuberculosis, syphilis, actinomycosis, and histoplasmosis have been implicated as causes of retroperitoneal fibrosis.[22]

Drugs are associated with the development of retroperitoneal fibrosis. Methysergide (Sansert), a drug used in the treatment of migraine headaches, has been implicated as a cause.[53]

Amphetamines have been blamed in a much smaller number of patients. Other drugs implicated for causing fibrosis include beta blockers, methyldopa, and hydralazine.[22]

Retroperitoneal fibrosis also may be caused by connective tissue diseases. Weber-Christian disease, a connective tissue disease associated with panniculitis (fat inflammation), causes fibrosis in the retroperitoneum and lymph gland inflammation in the abdomen.[54] Retroperitoneal fibrosis has been associated with vasculitis, including polyarteritis nodosa.[55]

TREATMENT

Treatment for retroperitoneal fibrosis may include surgery to remove ureteral obstruction and administration of corticosteroids (Fig. 18–14). Ureterolysis, freeing the ureters from the retroperitoneum and placing them laterally or intraperitoneally, is essential to relieve obstruction and preserve renal function.[27] Other surgical techniques, such as autorenal transplantation, or ureteral reimplantation are possible if ureterolysis is not successful.[56] These surgical procedures also may relieve back pain and normalize both the hematocrit and the sedimentation rate. Corticosteroids are useful in the early stages of the illness before dense fibrosis is encountered and for relapses of obstruction after initial ureterolysis (Fig. 18–15).[57] The optimum dose of corticosteroid to be employed has not been established. Most patients are treated with moderate doses of prednisone 60 to 80 mg/day. Pulse therapy also may be considered.[24] Most urologists are reluctant to use corticosteroids alone as the primary therapy for retroperitoneal fibrosis becasue of the risk of mismanaging a potentially malignant process. However, nonmalignant, early disease typically responds to corticosteroids in 7 to 10 days by relieving ureteral obstruction.[58] The use of MR should be helpful in identifying the benign nature of the fibrosis and the response to therapy. A preliminary report has suggested that immunosuppressive therapy, in the form of azathioprine over a 6-week course, may resolve ureteral obstruction.[59] A subsequent report has confirmed the utility of azathioprine therapy for retroperitoneal fibrosis.[60] Tamoxifen has been utilized successfully to reverse retroperitoneal fibrosis.[61]

PROGNOSIS

The prognosis and course of retroperitoneal fibrosis are variable. Cases of spontaneous re-

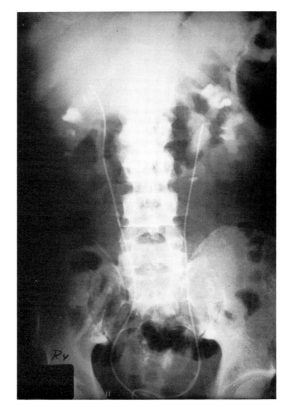

Figure 18–14. In the same patient as in Figure 18–11, ureteral catheters have been threaded up both ureters to relieve obstruction caused by retroperitoneal fibrosis. (Courtesy of Arnold Kwart, M.D.)

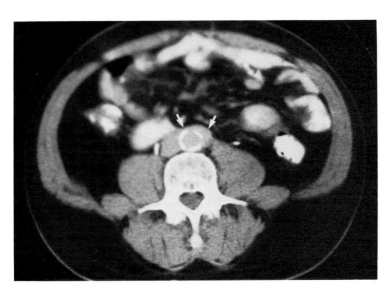

Figure 18–15. Repeat CT scan of patient in Figure 18–11 after ureterolysis and 12 months of corticosteroid therapy. Patient's back pain had resolved and soft tissue mass *(arrows)* encasing the aorta is diminished in size. (Courtesy of Arnold Kwart, M.D.)

missions have been reported.[62] Other patients have had resolution of the disease after surgical biopsy of the lesion.[6] An essential part of therapy is to relieve the obstruction of the ureters. Patients who are anemic at initial presentation have a poorer prognosis.[27] Patients who are older or who have more renal failure have a higher mortality.[24] Patients with early disease treated with surgery and corticosteroid therapy have the potential to achieve a complete remission of their illness.[63] The course of the illness and the resolution of inflammation and fibrosis may be followed by serial MR scans.[40, 64]

References

RETROPERITONEAL FIBROSIS

1. Debruyne FMJ, Bogman MJJT, Ypma AFGV. Retroperitoneal fibrosis in the scrotum. Eur Urol 8:45, 1982.
2. Koep L, Zuidema GD: The clinical significance of retroperitoneal fibrosis. Surgery 81:250, 1977.
3. Lepor H, Walsh PC: Idiopathic retroperitoneal fibrosis. J Urol 122:1, 1979.
4. Albarran J: Retention renale par petriureterite; liberation externe de l'uretere. Ass Fr Urol 9:511, 1905.
5. Ormond JK: Bilateral ureteral obstruction due to envelopment and compression by an inflammatory retroperitoneal process. J Urol 59:1072, 1948.
6. Hellstrom HR, Perez-Stable EC: Retroperitoneal fibrosis with disseminated vasculitis and intrahepatic sclerosing cholangitis. Amer J Med 40:184, 1966.
7. Ormond JK: Idiopathic retroperitoneal fibrosis: a discussion of the etiology. J Urol 94:385, 1965.
8. Mansell MA, Watts RWE: Retroperitoneal fibrosis and scleroderma. Postgrad Med J 56:730, 1980.
9. Lipman RL, Johnson B, Berg G, Shapiro AP: Idiopathic retroperitoneal fibrosis and probable systemic lupus erythematosus. JAMA 196:1022, 1966.
10. Wallach PM, Flannery MT, Adelman HM, et al.: Retroperitoneal fibrosis accompanying immune thrombocytopenia. Am J Hematol 37:204, 1991.
11. Morad N, Strongwater SL, Eypper S, Woda BA: Idiopathic retroperitneal and mediastinal fibrosis mimicking connective tissue disease. Am J Med 82:363, 1987.
12. Gleeson MH, Taylor S, Dowling RH: Multifocal fibrosclerosis. Proc Roy Soc Med 63:1309, 1970.
13. Hoffman WW, Trippel OH: Retroperitoneal fibrosis: etiologic considerations. J Urol 86:222, 1961.
14. Willscher MK, Novicki DE, Cwazka WF: Association of HLA-B27 antigen with retroperitoneal fibrosis. J Urol 120:631, 1978.
15. Golbach P, Mohsenifar Z, Salick AI: Familial mediastinal fibrosis associated with seronegative spondyloarthropathy. Arthritis Rheum 26:221, 1983.
16. Martinez FDLI, Gil JG, Veiga FG, et al.: The association of idiopathic retroperitoneal fibrosis and ankylosing spondylitis. J Rheumatol 19:1147, 1992.
17. Bullock N: Idiopathic retroperitoneal fibrosis (editorial). BMJ 297:240, 1988.
18. Parums D, Choudhury RP, Shields SA, Davies AH: Characterization of inflammatory cells associated with "idiopathic retroperitoneal fibrosis". Br J Urol 67:564, 1991.
19. Lindell OI, Sariola HV, Lehtonen TA: The occurrence of vasculitis in perianeurysmal fibrosis. J Urol 138:727, 1987.
20. Fromowitz FB, Miller F: Retroperitoneal fibrosis as host response to papillary renal cell carcinoma. Urology 38:259, 1991.
21. Rivlin ME, McGehee RP, Bakerower JD: Retroperitoneal fibrosis associated with carcinoma of the cervix: review of the literature. Gynecol Oncol 41:95, 1991.
22. Armis ES Jr: Retroperitoneal fibrosis. AJR 157:321, 1991.
23. Pateman J, Williams MP, Filshie J: Retroperitoneal fibrosis after multiple coeliac plexus blocks. Anesthesia 45:309, 1990.
24. Baker LR, Mallinson WJ, Gregory MC, et al.: Idiopathic retroperitoneal fibrosis: a retrospective analysis of 60 cases. Br J Urol 60:497, 1987.
25. Wicks IP, Robertson MR, Murnaghan GF, Bertouch JV: Idiopathic retroperitoneal fibrosis presenting with back pain. J Rheumatol 15:1572, 1988.
26. Sa JD, Pimentel J, Carvalho M, et al.: Spinal cord compression secondary to idiopathic retroperitoneal fibrosis. Neurosurgery 26:678, 1990.
27. Saxton HM, Kilpatrick FR, Kinder CH, et al.: Retroperitoneal fibrosis: a radiological and follow-up study of fourteen cases. Q J Med 38:159, 1969.
28. Barrison IG, Walker JG, Jones C, Snell ME: Idiopathic retroperitoneal fibrosis—is serum alkaline phosphatase a marker of disease activity? Postgraduate Med J: 64:239, 1988.
29. Utz DC, Henry JD: Retroperitoneal fibrosis. Med Clin North Am 50:1091, 1966.
30. Mitchinson MJ: The pathology of idiopathic retroperitoneal fibrosis. J Clin Pathol 23:681, 1970.
31. Webb AJ: Cytological studies in retroperitoneal fibrosis. Br J Surg 54:375, 1967.
32. Wagenknecht LV, Auvert J: Symptoms and diagnosis of retroperitoneal fibrosis. Analysis of 31 cases. Urol Int 26:185, 1971.
33. Sanders RC, Duffy T, McLoughlin MG, Walsh PC: Sonography in the diagnosis of retroperitoneal fibrosis. J Urol 118:944, 1977.
34. Bookstein JJ, Schroeder KF, Batsakis JG: Lymphangiography in the diagnosis of retroperitoneal fibrosis: case report. J Urol 95:99, 1966.
35. Jacobson AF: Gallium-67 imaging in retroperitoneal fibrosis: significance of a negative result. J Nucl Med 32:521, 1991.
36. Feinstein RS, Gatewood OMB, Goldman SM, et al.: Computerized tomography in the diagnosis of retroperitoneal fibrosis. J Urol 126:255, 1981.
37. Megibow AJ, Mitnick JS, Bosniack MA: The contribution of computed tomography to the evaluation of the obstructed ureter. Urol Radiol 4:95, 1982.
38. Spital A, Valvo JR, Segal AJ: Nondilated obstructive uropathy. Urology 31:478, 1988.
39. Mulligan SA, Holley HC, Koehler RE, et al.: CT and MR imaging in the evaluation of retroperitoneal fibrosis. J Comput Assist Tomogr 13:277, 1989.
40. Yuh WTC, Barloon TJ, Sickels WJ, et al.: Magnetic resonance imaging in the diagnosis and followup of idiopathic retroperitoneal fibrosis. J Urol 141:602, 1989.
41. Lee JKT, Glazer HS: Controversy in the MR imaging appearance of fibrosis. Radiology 177:21, 1990.
42. Arrive L, Hricak H, Tavares NJ, Miller TR: Malignant versus nonmalignant retroperitoneal fibrosis: differentiation with MR imaging. Radiology 172:139, 1989.
43. Usher SM, Brendler H, Ciavarra VA: Retroperitoneal fibrosis secondary to metastatic neoplasm. Urology 9:191, 1977.

44. Niz GL, Hewitt CB, Straffon RA, et al.: Retroperitoneal malignancy masquerading as benign retroperitoneal fibrosis. J Urol 103:46, 1970.

45. Bruneton JN, Diard F, Drouillard JP, et al.: Primary retroperitoneal teratoma in adults. Radiology 134:613, 1980.

46. Morin LJ, Zuerner RT: Retroperitoneal fibrosis and carcinoid tumor. JAMA 216:1647, 1971.

47. Moul JW: Retroperitoneal fibrosis following radiotherapy for stage I testicular seminoma. J Urol 147:124, 1992.

48. LeVine M, Schwartz S, Allen A, Narciso FV: Lymphosarcoma and periureteral fibrosis. Radiology 82:92, 1964.

49. Popham BK, Stevenson TD: Idiopathic retroperitoneal fibrosis associated with a coagulation defect (factor VII deficiency): report of a case and review of the literature. Ann Intern Med 52:894, 1960.

50. Webb AJ, Dawson-Edwards P: Malignant retroperitoneal fibrosis. Br J Surg 54:505, 1967.

51. Harlin HC, Hamm FC: Urologic disease resulting from nonspecific inflammatory conditions of the bowel. J Urol 68:383, 1952.

52. Mulvaney NP: Periureteritis obliterans: a retroperitoneal inflammatory disease. J Urol 79:410, 1958.

53. Utz DC, Rooke ED, Spittell JA Jr., Bartholomew IG: Retroperitoneal fibrosis in patients taking methysergide. JAMA 191:983, 1965.

54. Milner RDG, Mitchinson MJ: Systemic Weber-Christian disease. J Clin Pathol 18:150, 1965.

55. Hautekeete ML, Bakerabany G, Marcellin P, et al.: Retroperitoneal fibrosis after surgery for aortic aneurysm in a patient with periarteritis nodosa: successful treatment with corticosteroids. J Intern Med 228:533, 1990.

56. Mikkelsen D, Lepor H: Innovative surgical management of idiopathic retroperitoneal fibrosis. J Urol 141:1192, 1989.

57. Ochsner MG, Brannan W, Pond HS, Goodlet JS Jr: Medical therapy in idiopathic retroperitoneal fibrosis. J Urol 114:700, 1975.

58. Higgins PM, Bennett-Jones DN, Naish, Aber GM: Nonoperative management of retroperitoneal fibrosis. Br J Surg 75:573, 1988.

59. Cogan E, Fastrez R: Azathioprine: an alternative treatment for recurrent idiopathic retroperitoneal fibrosis. Arch Intern Med 145:753, 1985.

60. McDougal WS, MacDonell RC Jr: Treatment of idiopathic retroperitoneal fibrosis by immunosuppression. J Urol 145:112, 1991.

61. Clark CP, Vanderpool D, Preskitt JT: The response of retroperitoneal fibrosis to tamoxifen. Surgery 109:502, 1991.

62. Perlow S: Obstruction of the iliac artery caused by retroperitoneal fibrosis. Am J Surg 105:285, 1963.

63. Jones JH, Ross EJ, Matz LR, et al.: Retroperitoneal fibrosis. Am J Med 48:203, 1970.

64. Brooks AP, Reznek RH, Webb JAW: Magnetic resonance imaging in idiopathic retroperitoneal fibrosis: management of T1 relaxation time. Br J Radiol 63:842, 1990.

Section IV

THERAPY

Therapy of back pain has been based upon such diverse foundations as clinical experience, anecdotes, fads, and "scientific" articles in weekly magazines bought at grocery store checkout counters. For example, the following headline appears from time to time in one of the weekly tabloid papers: "Sex cures arthritis, prevents back pain and many killer diseases." The amount of scientific data that supports the use of sex as a treatment for back pain, as well as that for a wide range of other therapeutic interventions used in this disorder, is meager. Some physicians have used this fact to propose that therapies should be limited to those that have been proved effective in controlled clinical trials. Others take a more nonchalant attitude and use the patient's response "I feel better" as adequate evidence of efficacy. This difference of opinion should not preclude the use of therapies that have not been investigated in controlled trials but are believed to be safe and effective for back pain; on the other hand, one should not be satisfied with back pain therapy until it has been shown to be effective scientifically.

There is no single form of therapy that is effective for all forms of back pain. The various therapies that are effective treatment for specific disorders have been covered in the appropriate portions of Section III. This section gives a more detailed review of the components of therapy. The indications for specific therapies and the toxicities and complications associated with each are considered. Medical treatment in general and a specific therapeutic regimen that has been used successfully in the care of patients with uncomplicated back strain is presented in Chapter 19. Chapter 20 focuses on the indications for expected results from back surgery. The success of surgery depends on the careful selection of patients; the patient's physician can help the surgeon decide whether he is an appropriate operative candidate from a general medical and musculoskeletal standpoint. The epidemiology, impact, and cost of occupational low back pain are presented in Chapter 21. The treatment of patients with chronic low back pain is reviewed in Chapter 22.

The therapy of patients with back pain is arduous and taxing. It is easy for a physician to become frustrated and disillusioned with patients who do not improve. The following set of axioms will help a physician render appropriate care.

AXIOMS OF THERAPY

1. Most back pain is mechanical in origin.
2. Most mechanical back pain resolves over a 2 month period.
3. Common sense is the most important part of therapy. Both the patient and physician should use it during the course of treatment.
4. The goals of therapy must be the same for the patient and the physician.
5. The goals must be delineated at the start of therapy.
6. Do the patient no harm—limit the patient's exposure to addictive medications and operative procedures of questionable benefit.
7. Do not be too proud to accept the placebo response (an endogenous opiate effect) as an effective part of therapy.
8. Improved general physical condition is an important component of back therapy.
9. Consider improved physical function and increased self-reliance as good therapeutic outcomes.
10. Modify the therapeutic program in accordance with the changes (improvement or worsening) in the patient's condition.

In general, therapy of back pain is directed at controlling pain in the acute situation. In patients with mechanical causes of back pain, restoration of normal physiology (i.e., muscle length and strength) should commence as pain is relieved. Patients who are at risk for continuous "injuries" that result in back dysfunction should be instructed in appropriate body mechanics (good posture, appropriate work stance) to help prevent recurrent episodes of back pain. Patients who do not follow these recommendations may improve in any case or may develop chronic pain that can persist despite healing of the acute injury.

A number of components of therapy have been evaluated by scientific study. Controversies exist for most therapies utilized for low back pain patients. Conservative therapy limited to those components shown to be statistically significantly better than placebo would be limited to bed rest and back school.[1-4] Some physicians believe that most back pain is psychologic in origin and that controlling life stress or anxiety is the best way of treating back pain. The appropriate selection of patients for surgical intervention is debated in the literature. Intervertebral disc herniation may be treated effectively by nonoperative interventions.[5] Studies suggest that abnormal physical findings (positive straight leg raising test) correlate with anatomic abnormalities seen at surgery, but outcome is best related to the psychologic health of the patient.[6] If taken to an extreme, surgical intervention might be limited to the most severely affected individuals with marked neurologic compromise. Controversy exists in regard to the efficacy of surgical lumbar fusion in the treatment of patients requiring laminectomies or decompression procedures.[7] Increased morbidity and mortality are associated with older patients who undergo decompression procedures.[8] When is the risk associated with surgery outweighed by the benefit in quality of life associated with improved physical function? In this setting of conflicting studies and personal testimonials, thoughtful, unbiased clinical judgment must be the guide to the therapy of low back pain. In a time of increasing pressures on health care providers to deliver cost-effective care, thoughtful evaluation of the efficacy of the therapies we use for low back pain is appropriate. Our goal is to return the patient to full function. A variety of therapies may be needed to reach that goal. The choice for the physician is to pick those that are effective for that specific patient while exposing that individual to the least risk.

References

1. Fast A: Low back disorders: conservative management. Arch Phys Med Rehabil 69:880, 1988.
2. Spitzer WO, LeBlanc FE, Dupuis M, et al.: Scientific approach to the assessment and management of activity-related spinal disorders. Spine 12(Suppl):S22, 1987.
3. Deyo RA, Diehl AK, Rosenthal M: How many days of bed rest for acute low back pain? A randomized clinical trial. N Engl J Med 315:1064, 1986.
4. Hurri H: The Swedish back school in chronic low back pain: Part I. Benefits. Scand J Rehab Med 21:33, 1989.
5. Saal JA, Saal JS: Nonoperative treatment of herniated lumbar intervertebral disc with radiculopathy. Spine 14:431, 1989.
6. Spengler DM, Ouelette EA, Battie M, et al.: Elective discectomy for herniation of a lumbar disc: additional experience with an objective method. J Bone Joint Surg 72A:230, 1990.
7. Turner JA, Ersek M, Herron L, et al.: Patient outcomes after lumbar spinal fusions. JAMA 268:9087, 1992.
8. Deyo RA, Cherkin DC, Loeser JD, et al.: Morbidity and mortality in association with operations on the lumbar spine: the influence of age, diagnosis, and procedure. J Bone Joint Surg 74A:536, 1992.

Medical Therapy

CONTROLLED PHYSICAL ACTIVITY (BED REST)

Patients with acute low back pain have difficulty ambulating. Certain positions, particularly sitting and standing, exacerbate their pain. These patients spontaneously take to their bed to relieve their symptoms. The amount of scientific evidence to prove, in an objective manner, that bed rest works is relatively small. Also data on the appropriate duration of bed rest are limited. Despite this lack of scientific data, bed rest or controlled physical activity (a more honest term, since many patients find staying in bed for 10 to 14 days very boring and stand or sit during this period) is a mainstay of therapy.[1-3]

The biomechanical rationale for bed rest is that the lowest intradiscal pressures are recorded in the supine position.[4] The semi-Fowler position with the knees and hips flexed is even more helpful in reducing symptoms.[5] Whether the patient's symptoms are related to muscle strain or a herniated nucleus pulposus, controlled physical activity at bed rest will cause the least stress on the lumbosacral spine. The semi-Fowler position also may be comfortable for patients with apophyseal joint disease. These individuals experience less pain secondary to flattening of the lumbar lordosis by decreasing pressure on joint structures.

Patients with radicular pain are prescribed bed rest at home as long as family members or friends are available to aid them. The patient's position in bed is one of comfort. The patient lies on his back with hips and knees flexed to a moderate degree. Pillows behind the knees help to relieve pressure on the sciatic nerve (Fig. 19–1). Lying on either side with legs drawn up in the fetal position also affords comfort (Fig. 19–2). The only positions to be

avoided are lying prone (face down), which hyperextends the spine and can lead to additional disc extrusion in patients with a herniated disc, and sitting for prolonged periods, which increases intradiscal pressure.[5] Patients should be out of bed only to use a bedside commode, or if unavailable, the bathroom. Each patient is followed carefully and is not allowed complete mobility until objective signs of a list or paravertebral spasm disappear. As symptoms abate, patients are encouraged to take short walks, but to do as little sitting as possible. Increased physical activity is prescribed to increase mobility without incurring a return of symptoms.[6] Periods of bed rest longer than 2 weeks have a deleterious effect on the body in general. Patients with herniated discs will rarely stay at complete bed rest for longer than 2 weeks.

Scientific evidence demonstrating the efficacy of bed rest for low back pain unrelated to disc herniations is relatively meager.[3, 7-9] Garfin demonstrated some improvement for patients who used firm mattresses compared with softer mattresses, waterbeds, and foam on waterbeds. Lidstrom compared heat therapy with rest and traction, finding that the rest and traction group had greater improvement. Wiesel reported on an experience with military recruits who developed nonradiating back pain. Those who were ordered to bed rest had less pain and a faster return to full duty compared with those who remained ambulatory. The response to bed rest may be rapid, with improvement seen after 2 days, according to Deyo.[9] In a comparison of patients with nonradiating back pain who received 2 days and 7 days of bed rest, patients with 2 days of bed rest did as well as those assigned 7 days at 3-week and 3-month follow-up evaluations. The results of this study suggest that patients may be able to

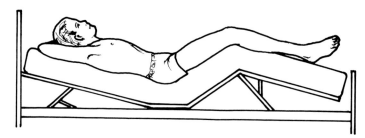

Figure 19–1. The preferred bed rest position for patients with low back pain. If a hospital bed is unavailable, pillows or wedges may be used to obtain the appropriate position for the patient. Pillows placed under the bed sheets remain more securely on the bed. The bed should be firm. A bed board (1 inch thick) may be inserted under the mattress to add support.

return to work more quickly, with a reduction in lost productivity. Other studies have reported improvement of muscle strain and herniated intervertebral discs with sciatica.[10, 11]

In realistic terms, busy patients rarely stay at bed rest for even a day unless their back pain is severe. Most patients will strictly limit their recreational activities and try to minimize time on their job. Explaining the importance of controlled physical activity as the cornerstone of conservative therapy cannot be overemphasized. It is essential for patients to understand the benefits of bed rest for pain relief. Those patients with acute low back pain who do limit their activities will have a faster return to normal function and are much less likely to experience recurrent, and eventually chronic, pain and limitation of function.

Recommendations regarding the balance between rest and activity must be based on good clinical judgment. During the acute phase of mechanical back pain, reduced physical activity is helpful. The recommendation should be to increase activity as tolerated. Too lengthy a time of bed rest can be detrimental. In one study, 60 of 171 (35%) patients had

prescriptions for bed rest that were too prolonged.[12] Extended bed rest has physiologic implications that are detrimental, particularly for geriatric patients. In the elderly, a number of organs including the cardiovascular, musculoskeletal, respiratory, gastrointestinal, and urinary systems are affected. Some of the abnormalities associated with prolonged bed rest include decreased cardiac output, orthostatic instability, atelectasis, muscle atrophy, decreased aerobic capacity, joint contracture, constipation, renal calculi, pressure sores, and impaired ambulation.[13]

On the other hand, chronic back pain patients should not be immobilized in bed.[14] Chronic low back pain patients should be encouraged to ambulate as much as possible. Activities can be selected that avoid specific tasks that increase the load on the spine without increasing pain. Increased activity may help bone and muscle strength, improve nutrition to intervertebral discs and cartilage, and increase endorphin levels and decrease sensitivity to pain. With these positive effects in mind, chronic back pain patients should be encouraged to be active.

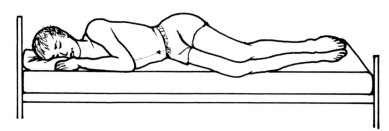

Figure 19–2. Lateral bed rest position with hips and knees flexed. This body orientation is the starting position for getting out of bed. Patients may use their arms to push themselves upright while maintaining a slightly flexed position of the lumbar spine. Patients should not flex the lumbar spine while coming to a straight sitting-up position with legs extended.

References

CONTROLLED PHYSICAL ACTIVITY (BED REST)

1. Rowe ML: Low back pain in industry: a position paper. J Occup Med 11:161, 1969.
2. Quinet RJ, Hadler NM: Diagnosis and treatment of backaches. Semin Arthritis Rheum 8:261, 1979.
3. Wiesel SW, Cuckler JM, DeLuca F, et al.: Acute low-back pain: an objective analysis of conservative therapy. Spine 5:324, 1980.
4. Nachemson A: The load on lumbar discs in different positions of the body. Clin Orthop 45:107, 1966.
5. Cailliet R: Low Back Pain Syndrome. Philadelphia: F A Davis Co, 1981, pp 80–81.
6. Wagner CJ: Williams's flexion regime in the treatment of low back pain. J Int Coll Surg 18:69, 1952.
7. Lidstrom A, Zachrisson M: Physical therapy on low back pain and sciatica. An attempt at evaluation. Scand J Rehabil Med 2:37, 1970.
8. Garfin SR, Pye SA: Bed design and its effect on chronic low back pain—a limited controlled trial. Pain 10:87, 1981.
9. Deyo RA, Diehl AK, Rosenthal M: How many days of bed rest for acute low back pain? A randomized clinical trial. N Engl J Med 315:1064, 1986.
10. Ellenberg M, Reina N, Ross M, et al.: Regression of herniated nucleus pulposus: two patients with lumbar radiculopathy. Arch Phys Med Rehabil 70:842, 1989.
11. Weinert AM Jr, Rizzo TD Jr: Nonoperative management of multilevel lumbar disk herniations in an adolescent athlete. Mayo Clin Proc 67:137, 1992.
12. Frazier LM, Carey TS, Lyles MF, et al.: Lengthy bed rest prescribed for acute low back pain: experience at three general medicine walk-in clinics. South Med J 84:603, 1991.
13. Harper CM, Lyles YM: Physiology and complications of bed rest. J Am Geriat Soc 36:1047, 1988.
14. Fast A: Low back disorders: Conservative management. Arch Phys Med Rehabil 69:880, 1988.

TRACTION

Traction is a nonstandardized conservative treatment modality for low back pain and sciatica that has been used over the centuries.[1] The basic premise of traction is that unloading the components of the spine by stretching muscles, ligaments, and functional spinal units will decrease intradiscal pressure, thereby relieving symptoms. When applied correctly, spinal traction can cause distraction or separation of vertebral bodies and facet joints, tensing of ligamentous spinous structures, widening of the intervertebral foramen, straightening of spinal curves, and stretching of spinal musculature.

There are many forms of spinal traction:

1. Continuous traction uses light weights applied for several hours at a time. This form of traction is not effective since patients cannot tolerate the amount of weight necessary to distract the spine for that length of time.

2. Sustained (static) traction uses a steady amount of weight for periods of up to 30 minutes. Heavier weights are tolerated for this shorter period of time. Force may be generated by hanging weights or a mechanical device that generates the pounds of traction force for the specified time. This form of traction is more effective if a split table is utilized, reducing friction.

3. Intermittent mechanical traction is frequently used in the United States and employs a mechanical device that applies and releases traction every few seconds.[2]

4. Manual traction is applied by a therapist who manually grasps the patient to generate the force. The traction can be in the form of a steady pull for a few seconds or a quick thrust.

5. Positional traction is applied by placing the patient in a variety of positions to obtain a longitudinal pull on spinal structures; this is usually used to stretch one side of the spine.

6. In autotraction a patient lies with flexed hips and knees and generates traction by pulling on a harness that is attached to an encircling belt. Sessions may last up to an hour.[3]

7. Gravity lumbar traction uses the force of gravity to stretch the spine in a patient who is suspended vertically by a harness or in an inverted position hanging by ankle boots.[4, 5]

The application of traction to the lumbar spine is used most often for patients with a herniated nucleus pulposus. The rationale for this therapy is that the stretching of the lumbar spine results in distraction of the vertebrae so that protruded discs return to a more normal anatomic position.

Friction hinders the transmission of force to the back. A force equal to 50% of body weight is required to move the body horizontally. The lower half of the body needs to be moved before any force is transmitted to the lumbar spine. Since 50% of the body weight lies beneath L3, 25% of applied force to the lumbar spine is lost overcoming friction. Therefore, a patient in a horizontal position in a conventional bed will receive effective traction only at weights equal to 25% to 50% of body weight. Weights over 50% of body weight will cause the patient to slide, while less than 25% will not overcome friction.

Another factor that must be overcome is the elasticity of muscles. A muscle pulled by a minimal force will behave as an elastic body, and as the force increases, the elongation of the muscle will be limited by a stretch reflex. Traction forces in the range of hundreds of pounds may be necessary to overcome this effect in the muscles that protect the lumbar spine. The application of pulley traction with conventional weights on a regular bed over a prolonged period is no more beneficial than bed rest since there is little distraction of the spine.[6] The efficacy of applying force to the lumbar spine is increased by the use of a split table, which eliminates lower body resistance. Traction on the spine will increase stature. Increased stature will occur when traction with ⅓ of body weight is placed on the lumbar spine. The increase in stature, measured in millimeters, was greatest within the first 15 minutes. This form of traction was more effective at increasing spine length than lying in a fetal position for a similar length of time. The clinical importance of this therapeutic intervention remains to be determined.[7]

Mathews used epidurography to study the effect of lumbar traction on returning protruded lumbar discs to their normal position.[8] Disc protrusion was reversed by the application of traction to the lumbar spine with vertebral distraction of 2 mm per disc. However, the amount of weight required to obtain this effect was 120 pounds and the duration of traction was between 30 and 38 minutes. The effect on the disc was of short duration with reappearance of disc prolapse within 14 minutes after the discontinuance of the traction forces. Gupta also demonstrated reduction of disc herniation with epidurography with associated clinical improvement in 9 of 12 patients given traction for 4 hours with 80 pounds for 10 to 15 days.[9]

Another rationale for the use of traction is reduction of intradiscal pressure. Nachemson and Elfstrom studied the reduction of intradural pressure in normal individuals placed in traction using a pelvic and thoracic harness, a split table, and 30 kg of tractive force for 3 seconds with 5 second intervals.[10] Intradiscal pressure was reduced by only 20% to 30%.

A number of therapeutic trials have been undertaken to study the efficacy of traction for the treatment of lumbar spine pain.[11–14] Many of the studies have design flaws that limit their scientific validity.[15] Weber undertook a controlled trial of effective weight traction (⅓ body weight) versus control weight traction (weight to tighten the harness) in patients with radiographically confirmed nerve root compression. Traction was given for 20 minute sessions. Clinical assessment of the two groups revealed no significant difference.[16] Mathews completed a study of patients with sciatica with dural tension signs, limited back movement, and pain who underwent lumbar traction with a minimum of 45 kg sustained for 30 minutes

compared with a control group of infrared heat treatments for 15 minutes.[17] Traction relieved pain but did not have a long-lasting effect. Traction was not thought to be more helpful than heat treatments except for women less than 45 years of age with sciatica.

Traction is not totally without benefit, however. In a later study, Weber found a positive psychologic effect in regard to the patient's expectations for recovery while in traction. However, the beneficial effect may have been more closely related to the enforcement of bed rest than to the tractive force on the spine.[18] Larsson found autotraction to be better than corsets for patients with low back pain.[3] The benefits of the autotraction system are that (1) the patient controls the amount of traction; (2) the device is portable and can be used at home; and (3) the device is relatively inexpensive. Autotraction is done for 15-minute periods, 2 to 5 times daily. This technique may be more beneficial for patients with muscle spasm as opposed to a herniated disc.[19] Andersson measured disc pressures in patients who underwent active (autotraction) and passive traction.[20] Patients using autotraction contracted their thoracic muscles and had increased intradiscal pressure in comparison with those who received passive traction with disc pressures that decreased, remained unchanged, or, occasionally, rose. Unilateral traction may be of benefit in patients with lumbar scoliosis associated with muscle spasm and unassociated with nerve root irritation. A constant, gentle pull on the muscles may relax the muscle, breaking the spasm cycle.[21]

Gravity techniques, which use the body's weight, have been proposed as a means of generating tractive forces. The Sister Kenney Institute Gravity Lumbar Reduction Program utilizes a harness placed under the ribs and a tilt bed to generate gravitational forces on the lumbar spine.[22] The patient needs to be hospitalized for a 10- to 14-day period. The program requires very close scrutiny by the health professional caring for the patient, making the program labor intensive.

Inversion therapy also uses gravity to provide traction. Inversion may be accomplished by using special boots clipped to an overhead bar or by kneeling over thigh platforms.[5, 23] Gianakopoulos and Waylonis evaluated a number of gravity techniques.[24] Patients experienced improvement in symptoms and distraction of the lumbar spine of 0.3 to 4.0 mm. However, side effects included elevated systolic and diastolic blood pressure, decreased heart rate, periorbital and pharyngeal petechiae, headache, blurred vision, nasal stuffiness, and conjunctival infection. Other potential complications are retinal detachment, bleeding from berry aneurysms, and gastrointestinal reflux. One other potential hazard is equipment failure. Unless therapy is done in the presence of another individual, the patient may fall on his head or cervical spine, sustaining spinal cord injury. The side effects of this therapy far outweigh its benefits.

In summary, the scientific proof for the efficacy of traction is sparse. The benefit of traction is most likely related to bed rest in patients with disc disease. Patients with muscle spasm may benefit from traction but it must be given in the setting of a comprehensive program for back pain. In a time of limited medical financial resources, the option of admitting a patient to the hospital for traction is gone. Traction, if used at all, is an outpatient therapeutic option.

References

TRACTION

1. Judovich B: Lumbar traction therapy. JAMA 159:549, 1955.
2. Hood L, Chrisman D: Intermittent pelvic traction in the treatment of the ruptured intervertebral disc. Phys Ther 48:21, 1968.
3. Larsson U, Choler U, Lidstrom A, et al.: Auto-traction for treatment of lumbago-sciatica. Acta Orthop Scand 51:791, 1980.
4. Swezey RL: The modern thrust of manipulation and traction therapy. Semin Arthritis Rheum 12:322, 1983.
5. Nosse L: Inverted spinal traction. Arch Phys Med Rehabil 59:367, 1978.
6. Youel MA: Effectiveness of pelvic traction. J Bone Joint Surg 49A:2051, 1967.
7. Bridger RS, Ossey S, Fourie G: Effect of lumbar traction on stature. Spine 15:522, 1987.
8. Mathews JA: Dynamic discography: a study of lumbar traction. Ann Phys Med 9:275, 1968.
9. Gupta R, Ramarao S: Epidurography in reduction of lumbar disc prolapse by traction. Arch Phys Med Rehabil 59:322, 1978.
10. Nachemson A, Elfstrom G: Intravital dynamic pressure measurements in lumbar discs: a study of common movements, maneuvers, and exercises. Scand J Rehabil Med (Suppl) 1:1, 1970.
11. Coxhead CE, Inskip H, Meade TW, et al.: Multicentre trial of physiotherapy in the management of sciatic symptoms. Lancet 1:1065, 1981.
12. Mathews JA, Hickling J: Lumbar traction: a double-blind controlled study for sciatica. Rheumatol Rehabil 14:222, 1975.
13. Jayson MIV, Sims-Williams H, Young S, et al.: Mobilization and manipulation for low back pain. Spine 6:409, 1981.
14. Lidstrom A, Zachrisson M: Physical therapy on low back pain and sciatica. An attempt at evaluation. Scand J Rehabil Med 2:37, 1970.
15. Deyo RA: Conservative therapy for low back pain: distinguishing useful from useless therapy. JAMA 250:1057, 1983.
16. Weber H: Traction therapy in sciatica due to disc prolapse: does traction treatment have any positive effect on patients suffering from sciatica caused by disc prolapse? J Oslo City Hosp 23:169, 1973.
17. Mathews JA, Mills SB, Jenkins VM, et al.: Back pain and sciatica: controlled trials of manipulation, traction, sclerosant and epidural injections. Br J Rheumatol 26:416, 1987.
18. Weber H: Lumbar disc herniation: a prospective study of prognostic factors including a controlled trial. Part 1. J Oslo City Hosp 28:36, 1978.
19. Lancort JE: Traction techniques for low back pain. J Musculoskel Med 3(4):44, 1986.
20. Andersson GBJ, Schultz HB, Nachemson AL: Intervertebral disc pressures during traction. Scand Rehab Med (Suppl)9:88, 1983.
21. Saunders H: Unilateral lumbar traction. Phys Ther 61:221, 1981.
22. Burton CV: The Sister Kenney Institute Gravity Lumbar Reduction Therapy Program. In Finneson BE (ed): Low Back Pain, 2nd ed. Philadelphia: J B Lippincott Co, 1981, pp 277–280.
23. Oudenhoven RC: Gravitational lumbar traction. Arch Phys Med Rehabil 59:510, 1978.
24. Gianakopoulos G, Waylonis GW, Grant PA, et al.: Inversion devices: their role in producing lumbar distraction. Arch Phys Med Rehab 66:100, 1985.

PHYSICAL MODALITIES

In addition to exercises, physical therapists may use various physical modalities to relieve patient symptoms. Treatment methods may include ice massage, hot packs, whirlpool, diathermy, ultrasound, transcutaneous electrical nerve stimulation (TENS), and high-voltage electrical stimulation. All of these counter-irritant modalities offer transient relief of symptoms but do not alter the underlying physical abnormality. Modalities may be used in conjunction with other therapies (e.g., exercises) that allow for greater motion and decreased postactivity symptoms.

Cold (Cryotherapy)

Patients with acute low back pain may experience analgesia with ice massage and cold packs. Therapeutic cold will reduce pain, swelling, and muscle spasm during the acute phase of an injury. Cold also reduces local metabolic activity, decreases muscle spindle activity, and slows nerve conduction.[1, 2] Initially, the patient experiences a burning sensation, which dissipates as the application is continued. The ice is applied in a stroking direction following the course of the muscle fibers. A cold pack is used first if a patient cannot tolerate ice massage. The cold pack may be placed in a wet towel to limit contact with the skin. Cold packs with silica gel can be refrozen and used again in patients who experience continued pain. A comparison of ice massage and cold packs reveals that ice massage cools the skin to a greater degree than the underlying muscle and may facilitate alpha motor neuron discharge.[3] Clinically, this explains the occasional patient who experiences increased muscle spasm with ice massage. Cold relieves pain and spasm longer than superficial heat. Cold therapy should not be used in patients with Raynaud's phenomenon or extreme sensitivity of the skin. Cryotherapy is also not indicated in patients with long-standing muscle contraction; in these patients, it will facilitate the return of shortened muscles to their contracted length after lengthening with stretching exercises. In evaluating forms of pain therapy in patients with chronic low back pain, Melzack found that over two thirds of affected individuals experienced a 33% reduction in pain following ice massage.[4]

Heat (Thermotherapy)

Heat is useful in easing pain and reducing muscle spasm. Heat cannot be used in patients with impaired mental status, diminished circulation, or decreased sensation because thermal damage to the skin can occur if heat is applied for an excessive period of time. Heat also is not indicated in patients with low back pain secondary to trauma where swelling may increase with heating. Heat causes vasodilatation with increased blood flow. It also increases the elastic properties of connective tissue. In addition, heat decreases gamma fiber activity, decreasing muscle spindle excitability and resting muscle tension. Heat to both skin and deeper structures will have the beneficial effects of decreasing pain through counterirritant mechanisms and by decreasing muscle ischemia associated with increased muscle spasm.

Superficial Heat. Superficial heat penetrates to the level of the subcutaneous tissues. Hydrocollator packs, heating pads, infrared heat, and whirlpools generate superficial heat. Hydrocollator packs (heated to 65°C) are wrapped in two towels and placed on the prone patient's back for 30 minutes.

Infrared Heating. Infrared heating allows the therapist to observe the area as it is treated. The amount of heat applied to the skin is determined by the size of the bulb generating the infrared radiation and its distance from the skin. Thirty minutes is the duration of therapy.

Whirlpool. Whirlpool therapy is difficult to use in patients with back pain. They may have difficulty getting in and out of the tub, and these movements may exacerbate their symptoms.

For all forms of superficial heat, the maximal safe exposure is 30 minutes at 45°C applied directly to the skin.

Deep Heat. Deep heat penetrates to structures below the subcutaneous tissues. Diathermy and ultrasound generate deeper heat.

Shortwave Diathermy. Shortwave diathermy penetrates the soft tissues and delivers heat to deeper structures, such as muscle, bone, and ligaments. Although diathermy has been shown to be effective in decreasing pain in trigger points including the low back, other heat modalities have been used in its place for deep heat therapy.[5] Microwave diathermy uses electromagnetic waves to transfer heat.

Ultrasound. Ultrasound delivers heat more deeply than diathermy. It is not used in the acute situation, where heat will cause additional swelling to the traumatized area. Ultrasound is used for 20-minute sessions 3 times a week for 2 to 3 weeks. Therapy is delivered to paraspinous structures but not over the spinal cord itself or gas-containing organs. It is contraindicated for patients with bleeding disorders.

Questions remain concerning the relative utility of heat and/or cold in the therapy of chronic back pain. Roberts studied the effects of cold packs and ice massage versus hot packs in 36 patients with chronic back pain 1 hour after therapy.[6] Ice massage gave the greatest amount of immediate post-treatment pain relief. At 1 hour after therapy, a significant difference remained between the ice massage patients and the other groups, although pain had increased for all groups in comparison to the immediate post-treatment period. Ice massage should be considered for chronic low back pain. Landon also reported his experience with temperature counter-irritant therapy in 117 patients with back pain. In acute conditions, patients treated with heat had shorter hospital stays than those treated with ice application. Cryotherapy was more effective than heat therapy in chronic conditions.[7]

References

PHYSICAL MODALITIES

1. Lehman JF, Delateur BJ: Diathermy and superficial heat, laser, and cold therapy. In Kottke FJ, Lehman

JF (eds): Kausen's Handbook of Physical Medicine and Rehabilitation, 4th ed. Philadelphia: WB Saunders Co, 1990, pp 283–367.

2. Ottoson D: The effects of temperature on the isolated muscle spindle. J Physiol 180:636, 1965.
3. Hartviksen K: Ice therapy in spasticity. Acta Neurologica Scand 38(Suppl 3):79, 1962.
4. Melzack R, Jeans ME, Straford JG, Monks RC: Ice massage and transcutaneous electrical stimulation: comparison of treatment of low back pain. Pain 9:209, 1980.
5. McCray RE, Patton NJ: Pain relief at trigger points: a comparison of moist heat and shortwave diathermy. J Orthop Sport Phys Ther 5:175, 1984.
6. Roberts DJ, Walls CM, Carlile JA, et al.: Relief of chronic low back pain: heat versus cold. In Aronoff GM (ed): Evaluation and Treatment of Chronic Pain. Baltimore: Urban & Schwarzenberg, 1985, pp 263–266.
7. Landon BR: Heat or cold for the relief of low back pain? Phys Ther 47:1126, 1967.

INJECTION THERAPY

Local and regional analgesia, either applied topically or injected locally or regionally, is part of the therapeutic regimen for patients with low back pain. The basic premise on which this therapy is based is that nociceptive input can be interrupted at its source by blocking the function of nociceptive sensory fibers in the peripheral nerve supplying the "injured" area as well as by interrupting the afferent limb of abnormal reflexes that increase muscle tension, which also contributes to pain. Depending on the type of agent used (topical cooling spray vs. short-acting analgesic vs. corticosteroid), the concentration of the medicine, and the site of application, the peripheral and central nervous systems can be affected in a number of ways. For example, low concentrations of local anesthetics can block the unmyelinated C and B fibers and small myelinated A-delta fibers without affecting A-alpha or motor fibers. If motor function must be blocked to decrease muscle spasm, this effect can be obtained through the use of an appropriate anesthetic at an increased concentration.

Bonica has suggested that blocks not only are therapeutic but also have diagnostic and prognostic indications (Table 19–1).[1] One must be careful in ascribing to much diagnostic importance to a response to an injection. The clinician should not confuse a response to an anesthetic with a definite diagnosis of the cause of back pain. Certainly, a response to an injection with relief of pain suggests that the area treated has been the source of nociceptive input, but referred pain may improve from

TABLE 19–1. INDICATIONS FOR NERVE BLOCKS WITH LOCAL ANESTHETICS*

Diagnostic Blocks
  Aid in the identification of the site(s) and cause(s) of pain.
  Identify nociceptive pathways (specific peripheral nerve).
  Determine mechanism of chronic pain syndromes.
  Determine patient's reaction to pain relief.
Prognostic Blocks
  Determine potential response to permanent blocks or neurosurgery.
  Allow patients to experience the sensation and side effects of permanent procedures on a temporary basis (decision concerning surgery).
Therapeutic Blocks
  Relieve acute postoperative pain and pain from self-limited diseases.
  Prolong pain relief by breaking reflex mechanisms.
  Provide temporary relief to allow the onset of action of other therapies with delayed effects.

*Modified from Bonica JJ: Local anesthesia and regional block. In Wall PD, Melzack R. (eds): Textbook of Pain. Edinburgh: Churchill Livingstone, 1984, p 541.

an injection as well. The physician must continue to observe the patient who receives a therapeutic injection. An initial beneficial response may wane if a more sinister problem than local muscle strain is the cause of the pain.

Soft Tissue Injections

A variety of topical and injectable anesthetics are available for use in patients with acute and chronic pain. All have advantages and disadvantages in specific circumstances. A brief review of their characteristics will help the clinician decide which agent is most appropriate for a given patient.

The local anesthetics produce their effects by blocking the depolarization of nerves inhibiting the flux of sodium ions across membranes. The local anesthetic blocks the mouth of the sodium channel and does this to a greater degree in nerves that are actively conducting impulses than in nerves that are inactive.[2] The sensitivity of nerves to local anesthetics relates to fiber size and myelination. Fibers that are thicker and myelinated transmit nerve impulses faster and are more resistant to local blockade than thin, unmyelinated fibers. The minimum amount of anesthetic that blocks impulse transmission (Cm) varies for each nerve and each agent. The Cm of A-alpha fibers (motor—greatest velocity) is approximately twice that of A-delta fibers (pain and temperature). B fibers (preganglionic autonomic nervous system) are the most sensitive of all fibers despite their thin myelination and have a Cm about one third that of unmyelinated C fibers (pain).[2] Agents also have different onsets of action correlated with diffusion capacity. Agents with greater lipophilic action (increased binding to tissue) have a slower onset of action. The characteristics of the most common local anesthetics are listed in Table 19–2.

Side effects of local anesthetic agents are uncommon but potentially serious. Systemic reactions occur when these agents are injected directly into the blood stream. Locally injected anesthetics slowly diffuse into the blood stream over time. Hypersensitive patients may develop systemic allergic reactions to locally injected medications. The neurologic toxicities range from slight dizziness to grand mal seizures, which occur when high concentrations of anesthetic reach the central nervous system. This complication can be prevented by using low doses of anesthetic, aspirating the area before injection, and injecting at a slow rate. Other toxicities include hypersensitivity reactions and cardiac toxicity in the form of conduction delays.[3, 4] Repeated injections of anesthetic into the same location may cause local irritation and muscle spasm.

Some patients with chronic pain obtain only short-term relief with short-acting anesthetics. These patients may benefit from injection with neurolytic agents, which destroy nerve fibers and produce prolonged, or sometimes permanent, nerve blockade. This procedure is reserved for patients with intractable pain who are not candidates for peripheral nerve section. The agents injected include 12% phenol in Renografin, 50% alcohol, 10% ammonium sulfate, and hypertonic saline.[5, 6] These agents may act on C pain fibers only or on the entire peripheral nerve. The choice of agent and its concentration will have variable effects on the degree of destruction of the peripheral nerve. These drugs are administered by an anesthesiologist.

Techniques of Injection

Identification of those patients who would benefit from injection is essential for a successful outcome. Patients who describe localized areas of muscle or ligamentous tenderness are candidates for local anesthetic therapy. These patients must be reliable; that is, they must be able to limit their activities to avoid increased tissue damage in areas with blocked reflex ac-

tion. If there is any doubt in our minds, we will not inject the patient.

The area of tenderness may be secondary to localized trauma or strain or may be a myofascial trigger point. Travell and Simons have popularized the theory of localized areas of muscle damage. The increased metabolism and decreased circulation in these areas cause accumulation of products that result in painful contracted muscles.[7] Active myofascial trigger points are those that are painful at rest, prevent full lengthening of muscles, weaken the muscle, refer pain on direct palpation, and cause a local twitch response in the muscle band containing the trigger point. Latent trigger points are those that are tender only on compression.[8]

In the lumbar spine, trigger points are located in the iliocostalis and longissimus muscles of the multifidus. Pain from these points may radiate down toward the buttock and then down the lateral thigh in the distribution of the tensor fasciae latae. The quadratus lumborum may also cause localized back pain. Trigger points are present in the muscle body that radiate pain to the sacroiliac joint area or the lateral thigh near the greater trochanter.[9, 10] Trigger points have also been described in the gluteal muscles with radiation down the leg below the knee. The injection sites that correlate with trigger areas (which also correspond to acupuncture points) include the sciatic outlet, deep in the gluteus maximus; the mid-belly of the gluteus medius between the greater trochanter and the iliac crest; and midway up the quadratus lumborum between the iliac crest and lower ribs.[11]

Whether undertaken to relieve pain associated with trigger points or, as some prefer to consider, local areas of muscle trauma, the use of local anesthetics is helpful in the treatment of low back pain. The procedure is started by identifying the area to be treated. Two cutaneous coolants are available: ethyl-chloride, which is flammable and very cold when applied, and fluorimethane, which is nonflammable and the preferred coolant. The spray is applied in sweeps in one direction only to match the pattern of referred pain. This procedure is used to stretch muscles that are foreshortened due to trigger points. The muscle is gradually stretched after the spray is applied.[7]

In many patients, local cooling with stretching is inadequate and injection of medication is needed to control local areas of pain. The skin must be cleansed with a suitable antiseptic and sterile technique must be utilized. Patients are questioned about any prior sensitivity to

TABLE 19–2. CLINICAL CHARACTERISTICS AND DOSAGE OF LOCAL ANESTHETICS*

	PROCAINE (NOVOCAIN)	2-CHLOROPROCAINE (NESACAINE)	LIDOCAINE (XYLOCAINE)	MEPIVACAINE (CARBOCAINE)	PRILOCAINE (CITANEST)	TETRACAINE (PONTOCAINE)	BUPIVACAINE (MARCAINE)	ETIDOCAINE (DURANEST)
Onset of action	Moderate	Fast	Fast	Moderate	Moderate	Very slow	Fast	Very fast
Dispersion	Moderate	Marked	Marked	Moderate	Moderate	Poor	Moderate	Moderate
Duration of action	Short	Very short	Moderate	Moderate	Moderate	Long	Long	Long
Optimal concentration (%)								
Local	0.5	0.5	0.25	0.25	0.25	0.05	0.05	0.1
Spinal nerve	1.5–2.0	1.0–2.0	0.5–1.0	0.5–1.0	0.5–1.0	0.1–0.2	0.25–0.5	0.5–1.0
Maximum safe dose (mg/kg)	12	15	6	6	6	2	2	2

*Modified from Bonica JJ: Local anesthesia and regional block. In Wall PD, Melzack R (eds): Textbook of Pain. Edinburgh: Churchill Livingstone, 1984, p 541.

injected anesthetics. Also, the possibility of vasovagal reaction is raised. If the patients have had vagal reactions in the past, they should be premedicated with atropine or placed in a supine position to limit potential hemodynamic effects. The choice of anesthetic depends on the desired effect (see Table 19–2).

Travell and Simons advocate the use of procaine for trigger-point injections since this agent has less systemic and local toxicity, in addition to its vasodilator effect.[7] Swezey has proposed the use of 2 to 5 ml of 1% lidocaine in combination with a depository form of corticosteroid.[12] Raj has used a mixture of 0.5% etidocaine and 0.375% bupivacaine for prolonged analgesia (the former for motor blockade, and the latter for sensory blockade).[13] Bonica has advocated using lower concentrations of anesthetics (0.25% lidocaine, 0.05% bupivacaine) since these concentrations are effective for local injections.[1]

The use of corticosteroids, in addition to anesthetics, is advisable for patients with soft tissue inflammation or with postinjection soreness, according to Travell and Simons.[7] Swezey has advocated the use of triamcinolone in conjunction with anesthetics.[12] Raj prefers 4 mg (1 ml) of soluble dexamethasone in 9 ml of local anesthetic. He reports no untoward effects other than a burning sensation in the area of the injection, which lasts 24 to 48 hours. We have used betamethasone sodium phosphate suspension (6 mg/ml) 1 ml/3 to 4 ml of anesthetic solution with good success.

After allowing the antiseptic to dry, the area to be injected is wiped clean with a sterile alcohol swab and anesthetized with coolant spray. The skin is entered and injection is started only after the area has been aspirated to assure that the tip of the needle is not in a blood vessel. Fingers are placed on the skin surface to try to localize the point of maximum tenderness. A small amount of solution is injected. If the appropriate area has been entered, the patient will experience an increase in pain before the analgesic effects of the injected solution commence. The tip of the needle is moved in a fanlike pattern to cover the entire painful area. During the injection, we test for tenderness over the injected area to be sure that the medication has been placed in the appropriate location. After removal of the needle, the patient is reminded of the potential for burning and redness over the area. Patients are instructed to call if symptoms persist or increase over the next 24 to 48 hours. It should be noted that dry needling or the injection of saline without anesthetic into trigger points also has been associated with decreased pain.[8]

After injection, patients may commence stretching exercises to maximize the length of contracted muscles. Additional modalities, including heat, massage, transcutaneous electrical nerve stimulation (TENS), or acupuncture, may be utilized to maximize normal activity in the muscle, allowing adequate blood flow and return of muscle strength.

If pain continues, repeat injections may be necessary. These may be done on a weekly basis for 3 to 4 additional sessions. If the pain still continues, other therapies are indicated since repeated injections cause local irritation and muscle spasm.

In regard to the efficacy of local injections, Garvey and coworkers reported the results of a double-blind, randomized study of trigger-point injection therapy for localized low back pain. A total of 63 patients with muscle strain with local, nonradiating pain, normal neurologic findings, and normal lumbar spine roentgenograms were treated with an injection of lidocaine, lidocaine with corticosteroids, acupuncture (dry needling), or vapocoolant spray with acupressure after 4 weeks of no response to conservative therapy. The percentage of improvement after therapy was 40% lidocaine alone, 45% lidocaine and corticosteroids, 61% acupuncture, and 67% acupressure and vapocoolant spray. The sole measure of outcome of this study was subjective patient response to improvement, a significant shortcoming of the study. Nevertheless, the benefit of injection may be related to pressure over the painful area similar to the mechanism implicated for counterirritant therapies including acupuncture.[14]

Sclerosant Injection

Ligamentous structures play a significant role in supporting the lumbar spine. Damage to these structures in the form of ligamentous strain is one mechanism of developing low back pain. Inflammation in these structures may result in pain and tenderness over the damaged area. The healing process may result in shortening of these ligamentous supporting structures resulting in stiffness and decreased motion. Attempts at increasing motion may result in recurrent reinjury and chronic inflammation. If this description of soft tissue injury is correct, optimal treatment of lumbar spine pain requires mobilization of stiffened structures while strengthening supporting connective tissue. This is the rationale for the use of sclerosant therapy. This therapy uses a chemical irritant to induce fibroblastic hyperplasia resulting in increased collagen formation.

In the 1930s, proliferant injection therapy was reported to be successful in decreasing back pain in 82% of treated low back pain patients.[15] The inadvertent injection of these agents (psyllium seed oil and zinc sulfate) into the subarachnoid space resulted in cases of paralysis and deaths, halting the enthusiasm for this form of therapy in the 1960s.[16, 17] A dextrose-glycerine-phenol solution used for varicose veins was substituted as a sclerosant solution. As part of sclerosant therapy, mobilization of the stiff joint to maximize motion was given prior to therapy, with flexion exercises encouraged after injection.

Sclerosant therapy was studied in a double-blind fashion in 81 patients with chronic low back pain. Injection therapy with dextrose-glycerine-phenol solution and flexion exercises resulted in a statistically significant decrease in disability compared with the 41 controls who received saline injections with exercises.[15] In another study by Mathews, sclerosant therapy was associated with decreased low back pain.[18] However, the number of patients was small and no specific conclusions could be drawn from the investigation. This form of therapy should be given only by physicians familiar with the appropriate sites for injection, the side effects of the injected sclerosants, and the necessary course of exercises needed to maximize return of physical function.

Epidural Corticosteroid Injection

The injection of epidural corticosteroids has been tried in patients in whom conservative therapy for lumbar nerve root compression has failed. The theory supporting the use of corticosteroids in the epidural space is the increased anti-inflammatory effect on the nerve root and its surrounding connective tissue in comparison with oral corticosteroids. Dilke's double-blind, controlled study of 100 patients demonstrated a significant difference in pain relief and resumption of usual activity at 3 months in patients receiving an extradural injection of 80 mg of methylprednisolone in 10 ml of saline versus an injection of 10 ml of saline into the interspinous ligaments as a control.[19] In contrast, White reported a study of patients who received epidural steroids that did little to alter the course of the disease.[20] Cuckler reported his experience with epidural

steroids, which showed no significant difference between the medicated and control groups.[21] In this double-blind study of 73 patients, epidural corticosteroids plus procaine were no better than epidural procaine alone in the reduction of symptoms secondary to acute herniated nucleus pulposus or spinal stenosis. A second injection was not associated with greater improvement. Power and coworkers described a study of 16 patients with sciatica who received epidural injection.[22] Patients were evaluated at 1 and 7 days after injection. Response was minimal and the 16 patients underwent surgical intervention for discectomy. Patients received only one injection. A retrospective study of 40 patients who received 1 to 4 epidural injections reported 50% of patients had temporary, acute relief of sciatic symptoms secondary to intervertebral disc herniation.[23] Long-term relief occurred in less than 25% of patients.

Other reports of epidural corticosteroid injections have appeared in the medical literature that have described beneficial effects from these injections. Ridley and coworkers completed a double-blind outpatients' injection study of 39 patients comparing epidural injection of 80 mg of methylprednisolone with an interspinous injection of 2 ml of saline.[24] Of the 35 patients who completed the study, 19 received active drug treatment. Seventeen of 19 (90%) patients had improvement in rest and walking pain during the blinded observation period of one month at the start of the study. Only 19% of the placebo group improved during this same time period. Fourteen patients in the placebo group were crossed over to the corticosteroid group. Approximately 38% of these patients were improved after steroid injection. At 6 months, only 11 of 17 patients who responded favorably to active injection maintained their improvement. The total group of patients who received pain relief from injection was 57%. Poor response was associated with previous sciatica and neurologic deficits. The benefits of injection are short term.

Bush and Hillier also completed a study of epidural injection in sciatica patients.[25] A total of 23 patients with radiculopathy were entered into a study without radiographic corroboration of nerve impingement. In this 1-year, double-blind, placebo-controlled trial, patients received 2 caudal injections of corticosteroids or saline at a 2-week interval. Patients were assessed at baseline, 4 weeks, and 1 year. At 4 weeks, the corticosteroid group demonstrated significant improvement in pain and motion.

At 1 year, both groups demonstrated improvement. Straight leg raising was the only objective measurement that improved to a greater degree in the steroid group at 1 year. In the discussion of this report, the authors suggest that previous studies which described little benefit of epidural injection assessed improvement too soon after injection.[21] Pain relief may occur 2 weeks or longer after injection. Mathews also reported greater improvement in patients who received epidural injections 3 months after injection compared to controls.[18] Hickey reviewed his experience of 250 patients with sciatica treated with epidural injections. He reported a better response in individuals who received epidural injection early in the course of sciatic pain.[26] Multiple injections improved the success rate of relieving pain.

The correct placement of the injection needle is another reason that epidural injections may not always be effective in reducing sciatic pain. Renfrew and coworkers reported that the placement of the epidural needle during a caudal injection was correct in 48% to 62% of procedures, depending on the experience of the physician.[27] In 9% of injections, the needle was placed intravenously. El-Khoury also reported the benefit of utilizing fluoroscopic control with a limited epidurogram to corroborate the location of the needle in the epidural space.[28] The blind placement of caudal epidural needles may be correct only 50% of the time. If an injection is unsuccessful, radiographic corroboration of needle placement may be required before assessing the lack of efficacy of the procedure.

The procedure is safe if meticulous technique is used.[29] However, complications include tuberculous meningitis, arachnoiditis, aseptic meningitis, and sclerosing spinal pachymeningitis,[30] and these risks must be considered in light of the 40% response rate to injection. One proposed mechanism explaining toxicities associated with epidural injection may be related, in part, to the presence of polyethylene glycol that gains access to the central nervous system causing a sterile meningitis.[31] In a study with epidural injection of depot corticosteroids in rabbits, there was no evidence of meningitis or inflammatory response in the meninges or nerve roots. This study concluded that steroids were not associated with detrimental effects on neural tissues.[32] Infection, in the form of epidural abscesses, is a rare but serious complication of epidural injection.[33] Until larger studies are conducted, epidurally administered steroid injections are an unproven therapy for lumbar

radiculopathy. In patients who have continued pain and are poor candidates for surgical intervention, epidural corticosteroid injections may be considered. The course of therapy includes 3 injections at variable intervals (days to weeks). After the initial round of injections is completed, patients do not usually receive a second course.

In the past, corticosteroids were injected directly into disc spaces,[34] but this technique has given way to the use of chymopapain or collagenase for radicular pain secondary to a herniated nucleus pulposus (see Chapter 20). The benefit of chymopapain injection for herniated disc is very limited. Chymopapain injection may have little effect on modifying the physical appearance of intervertebral disc herniations 3 months after injection when viewed by CT scan.[35] Although chymopapain injection may be associated with relief of sciatic pain in some patients, it is a form of injection therapy with potential toxicities that have limited its use as a therapeutic intervention to a very small, select group of patients. Most physicians recommend a small laminectomy, as opposed to a chymopapain injection, as the preferred procedure to remove herniated disc material.[36, 37]

In very rare circumstances, patients who are resistant to epidural injection may be considered for a short course (7 days or less) of oral corticosteroid therapy.[38] Dexamethasone (Medrol dosepak) is the form of corticosteroids most frequently used for this purpose. The highest dose administered is 40 to 60 mg for 1 or 2 days at most, and the drug is rapidly tapered over the next 5 to 6 days. Oral corticosteroids have been reported to be helpful in decreasing radicular pain.[39] The potential toxicity of the drug (hyperglycemia, fluid retention, hypertension, and infection) must be balanced against the potential benefit. In addition, the possibility of developing avascular necrosis of bone with 60 mg doses of dexamethasone must be considered.[40] If there is any doubt, the corticosteroid should not be given. Lower doses of corticosteroids (5 or 10 mg daily) may be considered for patients who are resistant to other therapies or who have experienced toxicities to other drugs. However, the patients must be fully informed of the benefits and risks of therapy and must be followed carefully for the development of any steroid-associated toxicities.

Facet Joint Injection

Patients with facet joint arthritis may develop pain that simulates radicular pain. If these patients do not respond to conservative therapy, they may benefit from facet joint anesthesia. Each facet joint receives sensory innervation from two spinal segment levels. Therefore, facets both at and above the level of the involved joint must be blocked or denervated in order to obtain adequate analgesia.

The procedure requires radiographic surveillance for placement of the spinal needle. Diagnostic block at the initial step employs 2 ml of 1% lidocaine at each level to confirm responsiveness. Patients then receive a solution of methylprednisolone (20 mg) in up to 4 ml of bupivacaine at each level to be blocked. If neurolytic therapy is being used, phenol in a contrast solution is given.[41] Repeat injections may be given every 2 to 4 weeks for three sessions.

The mechanism by which injections cause improvement (anti-inflammatory, neurolytic, or sclerosant action) is not apparent. Patients are told that symptoms will be aggravated before they improve.

Jackson and coworkers studied the effects of facet joint blocks in 454 patients.[42] The placement of the injecting needle was confirmed by facet joint arthrography. In this study, 30 (7.7%) patients had total pain relief after injection. Mean pain relief for all patients was 29%. No unique historic or physical examination characteristics would identify responsive patients. The characteristics of the patients who did respond included older age; history of back pain; normal gait; absence of leg pain, muscle spasm, and aggravation of pain with Valsalva maneuver. Many questions remained that were not answered by the Jackson study. The long-term benefit of the injections was not assessed. "Facet syndrome" patients were not exclusively studied. Some patients had discogenic disease that would not respond to joint injection.

Another large study using facet joint corticosteroid injections was completed by Carette and coworkers.[43] Patients who responded to local analgesic facet joint blocks were randomized to corticosteroid or placebo injections. At 1 month, there was no difference in 190 treatment and placebo patients. The steroid group had 42% of patients improved. The placebo group had 33% improved. At 6 months, the steroid group had greater pain relief, but the results of the study were clouded by the use of concurrent interventions. The use of facet joint blocks remains controversial in the treatment of patients with low back pain. Selection of patients for injection is essential for increasing the probability of success. Facet joint injections should be limited to patients with localized back pain that is exacerbated by extension of the spine, pain with ipsilateral bending, and who have had no response to other components of conservative management.

Facet joint denervation may be attempted with neurolytic techniques (chemical—phenol, heat—radiofrequency generator, cold—nitrous oxide cryoprobe). The major advantage of this procedure is that all afferent stimuli from the posterior elements of the vertebral segments are blocked. Success rates of up to 60% have been reported in patients receiving chemoneurolysis with phenol or corticosteroids.[44, 45]

Brechner reported on the effect of percutaneous cryolysis of facet joint nerves. She used the cryoprobe in patients who had pain for 6 months or longer, who were between 25 and 35 years old, and who had radiation of pain in a sciatic distribution but not below the knee. These patients had 75% relief of pain with local facet injection.[46]

The probe is placed with fluoroscopic guidance. A local anesthetic is injected for diagnostic purposes to locate the appropriate facet joint. The cryoprobe is placed near the facet joint until the patient's low back pain is elicited. If the probe is on the spinal nerve, radicular pain is produced and the needle is repositioned. One minute freeze-thaw cycles are performed 2 to 3 times at 2 or 3 levels. At 1 week follow-up, patients had 70% pain relief, but at 3 months, low back pain had recurred at its original level of intensity. Cryolysis must be considered a temporary measure for the control of facet pain.

Mehta reported his experience with a 1-year follow-up study of facet joint denervation associated with radiofrequency-induced heat lesions.[47] Approximately 50% of patients had an initial response to therapy. However, at 1-year follow-up, only 25% of the initial group of patients had continued relief of symptoms.

In light of these uncontrolled studies, denervation of the facet joint must also be considered an unproven therapy of short-term benefit. Additional studies are needed to investigate the therapeutic potential of these techniques. At this time, they can be offered to patients only after conservative methods have failed and with the recognition that there may be no long-term benefit.

Peripheral Nerve Blocks

The technique of differential nerve block is useful in the diagnosis of chronic pain and is discussed in Chapter 8. In addition to blockade of the conus medullaris and cauda equina, individual spinal nerves may be blocked. Not infrequently, patients with tumors may develop intractable pain if peripheral nerves are invaded. These patients may benefit from blockade of specific nerves such as the sciatic, femoral, obturator, or lateral femoral cutaneous nerve.[48] By accurately placing the needle with the aid of CT guidance before injection, paravertebral injection can be helpful in decreasing chronic peripheral nerve pain.[49] Injected medications may spread in an area beyond the local site of the injection. Radiographic guidance is warranted when longer lasting neurolytic injections are utilized for pain control.

Patients with radicular pain secondary to nerve root irritation of any cause and those with neurogenic pain of peripheral nerve origin may develop, in addition, a component of sympathetic nerve pain. "Causalgia" is the term used to describe this pain, which is of a burning, agonizing quality. The pain is constant and is not relieved by changing positions. The affected area also shows alteration in sweating and temperature function along with loss of motor power. Patients with sympathetic dystrophy also develop dysesthesias in the affected area so that the slightest touch causes unpleasant sensations. Reflex sympathetic dystrophies can occur in patients with postherpetic neuralgia; carcinomatous invasion of nerves; trauma, including nerve root damage, associated with subsequent scarring; and phantom limb pain. Sympathetic blockade is most often used for arterial disease of the lower extremities.

If patients do not respond to physical therapy and a course of oral medication, including nonsteroidal anti-inflammatory drugs and/or corticosteroids, paravertebral or regional sympathetic blockade with local anesthetics or other medications is indicated.[50–53] The procedure can be carried out on an outpatient basis. A series of 3 injections is usually given to obtain continued blockade. The efficacy of the blockade can be assessed by the rise in skin temperature of the toes within a few minutes of injection. Patients who have pain secondary to sympathetic nerve irritation will notice improvement within 12 to 24 hours of the injection. Increased physical activity is encouraged once pain relief starts. By increasing "normal activity" in the peripheral and central nervous system, the opportunity for "abnormal activity" to predominate in sensory pathways is diminished.

One additional area that may be benefited by local analgesic injection is the harvest site for bone for spinal fusion. These areas of bone where the periosteum has been removed may remain painful long after the operative site has healed. Neuromas also may form in these locations. If these sites remain painful, injection therapy can be helpful in decreasing pain. Longer-acting agents may be used if short-acting agents only provide temporary relief.

In summary, the role of injection therapy in the treatment of low back pain remains controversial. From the standpoint of scientific proof, a series of studies proving efficacy is lacking. Prime examples, in the setting of epidural injections, of studies that have shown no efficacy were poorly designed, measuring therapeutic effects of injections before the active agent had time to work or, at times, distant to the initial injection, when intervening events could alter responses. These studies cannot be used to prove or disprove the efficacy of this mode of therapy despite their presence in the medical literature. On the basis of pathophysiologic mechanisms, correctly placed injection therapy should have an effect on decreasing pain. In the patient who fails initial conservative management with controlled physical activity, physical modalities, and oral medications, injection therapy should be considered.

References

INJECTION THERAPY

1. Bonica JJ: Local anaesthesia and regional blocks. In Wall PD, Melzack R (eds): Textbook of Pain. Edinburgh: Churchill Livingstone, 1984, pp 541.
2. de Jong RH: Local anesthetics. In Raj PP (ed): Practical Management of Pain. Chicago: Year Book Medical Publishers, 1986, pp 539–556.
3. Incaudo G, Schatz M, Patterson R, et al.: Administration of local anesthetics to patients with a history of prior adverse reaction. J Allergy Clin Immunol 61:339, 1978.
4. de Jong RH, Ronfeld RA, DeRosa RA: Cardiovascular effects of amide local anesthetics. Anesth Analg 61:3, 1982.
5. Gregg RV, Constantini CH, Ford DJ, et al.: Electrophysiologic and histopathologic investigation of phenol in Renografin as a neurolytic agent. Anesthesiology 63:A239, 1985.
6. Raj PP, Denson DD: Neurolytic agents. In Raj PP (ed): Practical Management of Pain. Chicago: Year Book Medical Publishers, 1986, pp 557–565.
7. Travell JG, Simons DG: Myofascial Pain and Dysfunction: The Trigger Point Manual. Baltimore: Williams & Wilkins, 1983.
8. Simons DG, Travell JG: Myofascial pain syndromes. In Wall PD, Melzack R (eds): Textbook of Pain. Edinburgh: Churchill Livingstone, 1986, pp 263–276.
9. Reynolds MO: Myofascial trigger point syndromes in

the practice of rheumatology. Arch Phys Med Rehab 62:111, 1981.

10. Travell JG: The quadratus lumborum muscle: an overlooked cause of low back pain. Arch Phys Med Rehabil 57:566, 1976.

11. Melzack R, Stillwell DM, Fox EV: Trigger points and acupuncture points for pain: correlations and implications. Pain 3:3, 1977.

12. Swezey RL, Clements PJ: Conservative treatment of back pain. In Jayson MIV (ed): The Lumbar Spine and Back Pain, 3rd ed. Edinburgh: Churchill Livingstone, 1987, pp 299–314.

13. Raj PP: Myofascial trigger point injection. In Raj PP (ed): Practical Management of Pain. Chicago: Year Book Medical Publishers, 1986, pp 569–577.

14. Garvey TA, Marks MR, Wiesel SW: A prospective, randomized, double-blind evaluation of trigger-point injection therapy for low back pain. Spine 14:962, 1989.

15. Ongley MJ, Klein RG, Dorman TA, et al.: A new approach to the treatment of chronic low back pain. Lancet 2:143, 1987.

16. Hunt WE, Baird WC: Complications following injections of sclerosing agent to precipitate fibro-osseous proliferation. J Neurosurg 18:461, 1961.

17. Keplinger JE, Bucy PC: Paraplegia from treatment with sclerosing agents—report of a case. JAMA 73:13333, 1960.

18. Mathews JA, Mills SB, Jenkins VM, et al.: Back pain and sciatica: controlled trials of manipulation, traction, sclerosant and epidural injections. Br J Rheumatol 26:416, 1987.

19. Dilke TFW, Burry HC, Grahame R: Extradural corticosteroid injection management of lumbar nerve root compression. Br Med J 2:635, 1973.

20. White AH, Derby R, Wynne G: Epidural injections for the diagnosis and treatment of low-back pain. Spine 5:78, 1980.

21. Cuckler JM, Bernini PA, Wiesel SW, et al.: The use of epidural steroids in the treatment of lumbar radicular pain: a prospective, randomized double blind study. J Bone Joint Surg 67A:63, 1985.

22. Power RA, Taylor GJ, Fyfe IS: Lumbar epidural injection of steroid in acute prolapsed intervertebral discs. Spine 17:453, 1992.

23. Rosen CD, Kahanovitz N, Bernstein R, et al.: A retrospective analysis of the efficacy of epidural steroid injections. Clin Orthop 228:270, 1988.

24. Ridley MG, Kingsley GH, Gibson T, et al.: Outpatients lumbar epidural corticosteroid injection in the management of sciatica. Br J Rheumatol 27:295, 1988.

25. Bush K, Hillier S: A controlled study of caudal epidural injections of triamcinolone plus procaine for the management of intractable sciatica. Spine 16:572, 1991.

26. Hickey RF: Outpatient epidural steroid injections for low back pain and lumbosacral radiculopathy. N Z Med J 100:594, 1987.

27. Renfrew DL, Moore TE, Kathol MH, et al.: Correct placement of epidural steroid injections: fluoroscopic guidance and contrast administration. AJNR 12:1003, 1991.

28. El-Khoury G, Ehara S, Weinstein JN, et al.: Epidural steroid injection: a procedure ideally performed with fluoroscopic control. Radiology 168:554, 1988.

29. Barry PJC, Kendall PH: Corticosteroid infiltration of the extradural space. Ann Phys Med 6:267, 1962.

30. Dougherty JH Jr, Fraser RAR: Complications following intraspinal injection of steroids: report of two cases. J Neurosurg 48:1023, 1978.

31. Nelson DA: Dangers from methylprednisolone acetate therapy by intraspinal injection. Arch Neurol 45:804, 1988.

32. Cicala RS, Turner R, Moran E, et al.: Methylprednisolone acetate does not cause inflammatory changes in the epidural space. Anesthesiology 72:556, 1990.

33. Mamourian AC, Dickman CA, Drayer BP, et al.: Spinal epidural abscess: three cases following spinal epidural injection demonstrated with magnetic resonance imaging. Anesthesiology 78:204, 1993.

34. Feffer HL: Regional use of steroids in the management of lumbar intervertebral disc disease. Orthop Clin North Am 6:249, 1975.

35. Boumphrey FRS, Bell GR, Modic M, et al.: Computed tomography scanning after chymopapain injection for herniated nucleus pulposus: a prospective study. Clin Orthop 219:120, 1987.

36. Alexander AH, Burkus JK, Mitchell JB, et al.: Chymopapain versus surgical discectomy in a military population. Clin Orthop 244:158, 1989.

37. Nachemson Al, Rydevik B: Chemonucleolysis for sciatica: a critical review. Acta Orthop Scand 59:56, 1988.

38. Green LN: Dexamethasone in the management of symptoms due to herniated lumbar disc. J Neurol Neurosurg Psychiatry 38:1211, 1975.

39. Hakelius A: Prognosis in sciatica: a clinical follow-up of surgical and nonsurgical treatment. Acta Orthop Scand 129 (Suppl):1, 1970.

40. Fast A, Alon M, Weiss S, et al.: Avascular necrosis of bone following the short-term dexamethasone therapy for brain edema. J Neurosurg 61:983, 1984.

41. Boas RA: Facet joint injections. In Stanton-Hicks M, Boas R (eds): Chronic Low Back Pain. New York: Raven Press, 1982, pp 199–211.

42. Jackson RP, Jacobs RR, Montesano PX: Facet joint injection in low-back pain: a prospective statistical study. Spine 13:966, 1988.

43. Carette S, Marcoux S, Truchon R, et al.: A controlled trial of corticosteroid injections into facet joints for chronic low back pain. N Engl J Med 325:1002, 1991.

44. Hickey RFJ, Fregonning GD: Denervation of spinal facet joints for treatment of chronic low back pain. NZ Med J 85:96, 1977.

45. Mooney V, Robertson J: The facet syndrome. Clin Orthop 115:149, 1976.

46. Brechner T: Percutaneous cryogenic neurolysis of the articular nerve of Luschka. Reg Anaesth 6:18, 1981.

47. Mehta M, Sluijter MF: The treatment of chronic back pain. Anaesthesia 34:768, 1979.

48. Murphy TM, Raj PP, Stanton-Hicks M: Techniques of nerve blocks—spinal nerves. In Raj PP (ed): Practical Management of Pain. Chicago: Year Book Medical Publishers, 1986, pp 597–636.

49. Purcell-Jones G, Pither CE, Justins DM: Paravertebral somatic nerve block: a clinical, radiographic, and computed tomographic study in chronic pain patients. Anesth Analg 68:32, 1989.

50. Benzon HT, Chomka CM, Brunner EA: Treatment of reflex sympathetic dystrophy with regional intravenous reserpine. Anesth Analg 59:500, 1980.

51. Stanton-Hicks M, Abram SE, Nolte H: Sympathetic blocks. In Raj PP (ed): Practical Management of Pain. Chicago: Year Book Medical Publishers, 1986, pp 661–681.

52. Schutzer SF, Gossling HR: The treatment of reflex sympathetic dystrophy syndrome. J Bone Joint Surg 66A:625, 1984.

53. Hughes-Davies DF, Redman LR: Chemical lumbar sympathectomy. Anaesthesiology 31:1068, 1976.

CORSETS AND BRACES

The rationale for the use of external supports arises from the work of Bartelink, who proposed the theory that increased intra-abdominal pressure imparts force against the diaphragm and thoracic spine, decreasing the load on the lumbar spine.[1] Part of the load may be transmitted to transverse and oblique abdominal muscles. Nachemson has demonstrated a decrease of 25% in intradiscal pressure to a value intermediate between the supine and standing position by the use of an inflatable corset that increased intra-abdominal pressure and/or decreased the compressive force of the iliopsoas on the lumbar spine.[2]

In regard to decreasing movement of the spine, lumbar braces may actually increase lumbar motion during ambulation.[3, 4] The increase in motion is true for all standard braces, even those that stretch from the sacral area to the thoracolumbar junction.[5] The gross range of motion of the lumbar spine is decreased while individual segments have continued motion.[6]

According to a national survey, the use of corsets and braces by orthopedists is common, with only 1% never using the appliances in low back pain, despite a paucity of clinical controlled trials.[7-10] The rationales cited for use of braces included restriction of lumbosacral motion, abdominal support, and postural correction, although the previously cited studies challenge these concepts. In addition, the use of external supports may cause disuse atrophy of those muscles that specifically support the lumbar spine.[11]

The choice of a brace or corset is based on construction. The brace with its metal stays is built more sturdily, has less surface contact with the patient, and is therefore cooler. Otherwise there is no particular benefit of a brace over a corset. Corsets come in many forms. One that has been readily accepted by patients is an elastic cinch with a slot for a heat-molded rigid plastic lumbosacral insert that is custom fitted to the patient (Figs. 19–3 and 19–4).[12] Some patients prefer a narrow elastic band (sacroiliac trochanteric belt), which is prescribed more for a sense of security than for mechanical support.

External supports are indicated for only a short period in the average patient's recovery. Willner reported that patients who had pain relief when bent forward or in the supine position had pain relief with a rigid brace.[13] However, many patients with low back pain of un-

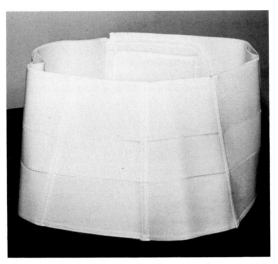

Figure 19–3. Flexible corset with pocket for removable plastic insert.

known etiology had no improvement with braces that decreased lumbar lordosis. A properly fitted corset will allow the patient to regain mobility faster. As recovery continues, the corset is abandoned in favor of an active exercise program. In those who are returning to heavy labor, a corset will keep the worker aware of his back and prevent him from applying maximum stress to the lumbosacral spine during work. After work is completed, the corset is removed. The patient who wears a corset at

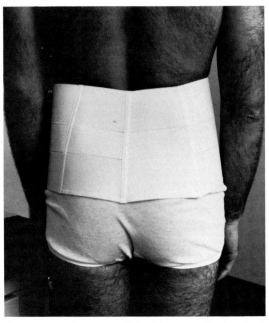

Figure 19–4. Placement of flexible corset for low back strain.

work is encouraged to perform strengthening exercises of the abdominal and paravertebral muscles. Once the patient feels confident, the corset can be removed while working. Patients may find leaving the corset off for the first half of the day and wearing it in the afternoon after fatigue sets in a way to wean themselves from the external support.

Excessively obese patients with weak abdominal muscles who have poor posture may benefit from long-term bracing. Realistically, these patients are very hard to fit in braces and may not be able to wear them for extended periods. Another group who may obtain greater benefit from bracing are elderly patients with multilevel degenerative disease who do not tolerate exercises and those with vertebral compression fractures. These patients may feel more comfortable and secure in a brace, although there is no scientific evidence to support its utility.

It should be remembered that bracing is a major part of therapy in idiopathic or genetic scoliosis. These patients benefit from Milwaukee braces or other similar appliances that slow the progression of scoliosis. Other individuals who may specifically benefit from a brace are those with spondylolisthesis. Also, a thermoplastic antilordotic low back brace along with muscle-strengthening exercises may be beneficial for individuals with spondylolisthesis.[14]

Alaranta and Hurri completed a study of 113 patients prescribed corsets for chronic low back pain.[15] In this compliance study, 37% of respondents described excellent or good results from wearing the brace. Only 60% had worn the brace during the preceding month. Men preferred the low, semirigid, elastic models, while women preferred the high semirigid corset. To improve compliance, a thorough explanation of the use and purpose of the corset is helpful.

References

CORSETS AND BRACES

1. Bartelink DL: Role of abdominal pressure in relieving pressure on lumbar intervertebral discs. J Bone Joint Surg 39B:718, 1957.
2. Nachemson A, Morris JM: In vivo measurement of intradiscal pressure: discometry, a method for the determination of pressure in the lower lumbar discs. J Bone Joint Surg 46A:1077, 1964.
3. Lumsden RM, Morris JM: An in vivo study of axial rotation and immobilization at the lumbosacral joint. J Bone Joint Surg 52A:1591, 1968.
4. Waters RL, Morris JM: Effect of spinal supports on the electrical activity of muscles of the trunk. J Bone Joint Surg 50A:51, 1970.
5. Norton PL, Brown T: The immobilizing efficiency of back braces. J Bone Joint Surg 39A:111, 1957.
6. Fidler MW, Plasmans CMT: The effect of four types of support on the segmental mobility of the lumbosacral spine. J Bone Joint Surg 65A:943, 1983.
7. Perry J: The use of external support in the treatment of low-back pain: report of the subcommittee on prosthetic orthotic education, National Academy of Sciences, National Research Council. J Bone Joint Surg 52A:1440, 1970.
8. Coxhead CE, Inskip H, Meade TW, et al.: Multicentre trial of physiotherapy in the management of sciatic symptoms. Lancet 1:1065, 1981.
9. Laisson U, Choler U, Lidstrom A, et al.: Auto-traction for treatment of lumbago-sciatica: a multicentre controlled investigation. Acta Orthop Scand 51:791, 1980.
10. Million R, Nilsen KH, Jayson MIV, Baker RD: Evaluation of low back pain and assessment of lumbar corsets with and without back supports. Ann Rheum Dis 4:449, 1981.
11. Hadler NM: Diagnosis and treatment of backache. In Hadler NM (ed): Medical Management of the Regional Musculoskeletal Diseases. Orlando: Grune & Stratton, 1984, pp 3–52.
12. Russek AS: Biomechanical and physiological basis for ambulatory treatment of low back pain. Orthop Rev 4:21, 1976.
13. Willner S: Effect of a rigid brace on back pain. Acta Orthop Scand 50:40, 1985.
14. Micheli LJ, Hall JE, Miller ME: Use of modified Boston brace for back injuries in athletes. Am J Sports Med 8:351, 1980.
15. Alaranta H, Hurri H: Compliance and subjective relief by corset treatment in chronic low back pain. Scand J Rehab Med 20:133, 1988.

MANIPULATION

Spinal manipulation—movement of parts of the axial skeleton through the use of external force—is controversial, since in the United States this therapy is associated with the practice of chiropractic. Spinal manipulation is based on the assumption that subluxation of the vertebra precipitates low back complaints and that these symptoms can be reduced with correction of the subluxation. In conflict with the basic premise of pain associated with malposition are studies of large groups of patients that have shown no relationship between vertebral malalignment and low back pain.[1, 2] Manipulation may also include massage or stretching techniques to relax muscles that are shortened and in spasm. Other explanations for benefits of manipulation include reduction of posterior disc herniations by tightening the posterior longitudinal ligament and freeing of adhesions around a prolapsed disc, mechanically stimulating large A-alpha fibers, and blocking nociceptive input.[3, 4] While Mathews and Yates demonstrated a reduction of small lumbar disc protrusions,[3] another study of 39 patients examined by myelography failed to demonstrate any persistent disc reduction after manipulation.[4, 5]

The terminology used by chiropractors must be defined. Mobilization is a less aggressive maneuver than manipulation. Mobilization starts where the active range of motion ends at the physiologic extreme of normal motion of the anatomic structure. Between the physiologic barrier and an anatomic barrier is the movement associated with manipulation. Chiropractors use the term adjustment for both maneuvers. Mobilization goes past the active range of a joint and stretches the elastic tissues in the joint capsule resulting in increased range of motion. With manipulation, a high velocity, short amplitude force is applied to stretch structures such as the capsule and ligaments. The cracking sound is caused by the negative pressure (vacuum) produced, resulting in the sudden production of joint nitrogen. Adjustments are directed at one specific joint with force applied in a specific direction.[6] A variety of concepts of pathophysiologic abnormalities have been proposed as explanations of the benefits of chiropractic intervention.[7] The Maitland concept suggests articular derangements of vertebral segments as the cause of pain. The Maigne concept suggests manipulation in the direction or opposite to the direction of limitation of motion depending on the abrupt limitation of movement with spinal palpation. The Sohier concept suggests abnormalities in articular structures and muscle tension.

Evaluation of patients considered for manipulation therapy involves measurement of active joint motion, passive joint motion, and accessory movements.[8] This is necessary in order to determine whether distraction, nonthrust, or thrust movements should be used. The manipulations may be given with varying force from different positions[8] but are always done in the direction that causes no pain for the patient. Manipulation does not require a forceful action to be effective. Patients are told to relax and are taken through a maximum range of passive motion. A gentle thrust at this point takes the joint or muscle to its maximum range of motion.

Manipulation has been recommended for uncomplicated acute and chronic low back pain, sciatica without neurologic deficit, sequestrated discs, facet syndrome, sacroiliac strain, piriformis syndrome, psoas syndrome, spondylolisthesis, and spinal stenosis.[9] The ideal patient for manipulative therapy is one with a degree of joint fixation or hypomobility. Absolute contraindications to mobilization include malignancy, osteomyelitis, osteoporosis, fracture, ruptured ligaments, acute arthritis, neurologic dysfunction, hypermobility, and pregnancy in the first trimester.

A number of studies have investigated the benefit of manipulation for low back pain.[4, 10–12] A recent review published by the Rand Corporation tabulated the benefits of spinal manipulation from 58 published articles including 25 controlled trials.[13] The majority of studies reported only a brief effect in relieving pain. The difficulty in determining the benefits of manipulation from these studies is the lack of definition of the specific therapies given in each study. Manipulation may mean a variety of therapies were given to a patient including modalities and exercises in addition to manipulation. It is difficult to determine the component of therapy that is effective when a number of therapies may be given as a part of a manipulative adjustment. Other methodologic problems included absence of placebo groups, inadequate blinding of patients, inadequate measurements of effects of therapy, small patient groups, and reasons for lack of response (patient drop-outs). In general, spinal manipulation is associated with transient benefit, lasting hours. Evaluation at periods of 3 months or longer does not show any significant difference among patients who have received manipulation and a variety of other therapeutic modalities. Patients who seem to benefit most are those who have a shorter history of pain. These findings may correlate with the spontaneous resolution of low back pain.[4] Many of the studies of manipulation are flawed by inappropriate control groups, indefinite entry criteria, and variable outcome measures.[14] In a recent study of 54 patients with low back pain, subjects were divided into those with pain less than 2 weeks and those with pain for 2 to 4 weeks. No benefit was noted by either group immediately after the treatment. However, by day 3, patients with pain for 2 to 4 weeks seemed to receive significant benefit from manipulation. The groups did not receive identical therapies. Those treated with manipulation seemed to have a more rapid response.[15]

Manipulation is not a benign procedure. Significant mechanical damage can result from physical force applied to the vertebral column. These complications include cauda equina compression, disc herniation, and vertebral pedicle fracture.[16, 17] The complications with chiropractic manipulation are rare compared with the number of treatments given, but the kinds of injuries are significant when they occur.[18–20]

In a study done in Utah, a comparison of physicians and chiropractors was undertaken to determine their effectiveness in the care of back pain patients.[21] Patients expressed confidence in both groups but were more satisfied with the therapy and explanations of the chiropractor. The chiropractors tended to spend more time talking to the patients and gave them emotional support. It seems that anyone "who is responsive to the emotional needs of the patient could achieve equal results in the vast majority of uncomplicated low back pain patients."[21] The essential beneficial factor in manipulation may not be the thrust but the conversation before and after the manipulation. Similar results were reported in a group of 467 patients with back pain of 2-weeks' duration who were treated by a family physician or a chiropractor. Overall satisfaction was three times greater with the chiropractors than with the physicians. Physicians were perceived as being less concerned about the patient's condition and pain. Physicians were also perceived as being less confident about the cause of the patient's pain. Patients who went to the chiropractor reported fewer days of limited activity associated with back pain.[22]

Another study reported the results of a 2-year study contrasting the results of private chiropractic therapy with hospital outpatient physical therapy.[23] Patients who received chiropractic therapy reported consistently greater benefit. However, the groups were not comparable, and the number of therapies were not equal. The recommendations of the authors included adding chiropractic treatment to the National Health Service in England.

Chiropractic therapy may also be cost effective when evaluating the total cost of a back injury. The Utah State Workmen's Compensation System calculated the total cost of medical therapy and days lost from work for low back pain patients treated by chiropractors and physicians. The total cost for chiropractic treatment was less than for physician's treatment for the same diagnostic codes.[24] All of these factors must be considered when considering the recommendation for treatment of a low back pain patient by a chiropractor. As with any other professional, some practitioners are excellent and have great experience; others do not. A relationship between a physician and another well-trained professional for appropriate referrals may be of benefit to a specific group of patients with acute low back pain and hypomobility.

Massage

Massage of back muscles provides mechanical stimulation of tissues that offers relaxation of contracted muscles along with increased circulation to the massaged areas. The exact mechanism of benefit is not known although the hypothesis of counter-irritant therapy and release of endorphins seems plausible.[7] The psychologic benefits of the therapy cannot be overlooked. Many patients mention the relaxation associated with massage as a significant component of this therapy. Demonstrating the benefit of massage therapy is difficult since it is used as part of placebo treatment in a variety of studies.[7] Therefore, although some patients state "they cannot get through the week without their massage," this form of therapy must be used in the setting of a total, conservative therapeutic program involving other forms of treatment.

References

MANIPULATION

1. LaRocca H, Macnab I: Value of pre-employment radiographic assessment of the lumbar spine. Can Med Assoc J 101:383, 1969.
2. Nachemson A: A long term follow-up study of non-treated scoliosis. Acta Orthop Scand 39:466, 1968.
3. Mathews JA, Yates DAH: Reduction of lumbar disc prolapse by manipulation. Br Med J 3:692, 1969.
4. Jayson MI, Sims-Williams H, Young S, et al.: Mobilization and manipulation for low back pain. Spine 6:409, 1981.
5. Chrisman OD, Mittnacht A, Snook GA: A study of the results following rotary manipulation in the lumbar intervertebral disc syndrome. J Bone Joint Surg 46A:517, 1964.
6. Raftis K, Warfield CA: Spinal manipulation for back pain. Hosp Prac 24:89, 1989.
7. Tan JC, Roux EB, Dunand J, et al.: Role of physical therapy in the management of common low back pain. Clin Rheumatol 6:629, 1992.
8. Paris SV: Spinal manipulative therapy. Clin Orthop 179:55, 1983.
9. Haldeman S: Spinal manipulative therapy in the management of low back pain. In Finneson BE (ed): Low Back Pain, 2nd ed. Philadelphia: J B Lippincott Co, 1981, pp 245–275.
10. Sims-Williams H, Jayson MI, Young SMS, et al.: Controlled trial of mobilization and manipulation for low back pain: hospital patients. Br Med J 2:1318, 1979.
11. Hoehler FK, Tobis JS, Buerger AA: Spinal manipulation for low back pain. JAMA 245:1835, 1981.
12. Hadler NM: Diagnosis and treatment of backache. In Hadler NM (ed): Medical Management of the Regional Musculoskeletal Diseases. Orlando: Grune & Stratton, 1984, pp 3–52.
13. Shekelle PG, Adams AH, Chassin MR, et al.: Spinal manipulation for low-back pain. Ann Intern Med 117:590, 1992.
14. Godfrey CM, Morgan PP, Schatzker J: A randomized

trial of manipulation of low-back pain in a medical setting. Spine 9:301, 1984.

15. Hadler NM, Curtis P, Gillings DB, et al.: A benefit of spinal manipulation as adjunctive therapy for acute low-back pain: a stratified controlled trial. Spine 12:703, 1987.

16. Dan NG, Saccasan PA: Serious complications of lumbar spinal manipulation. Med J Aust 2:672, 1983.

17. Gallinaro P, Cartesegna M: Three cases of lumbar disc rupture and one of cauda equina associated with spinal manipulation (chiroprosis). (Letter to the editor.) Lancet 1:411, 1983.

18. Slater RNS, Spencer JD: Central lumbar disc prolapse following chiropractic manipulation: a call for audit of "alternative practice." J Roy Soc Med 85:637, 1992.

19. Haldeman S, Rubinstein SM: Cauda equina syndrome in patients undergoing manipulation of the lumbar spine. Spine 17:1469, 1992.

20. Shvartzman P, Abelson A: Complications of chiropractic treatment for back pain. Postgrad Med 83:57, 1988.

21. Kane RL, Leymaster C, Olsen D, et al.: Manipulating the patient: a comparison of the effectiveness of physician and chiropractor care. Lancet 1:411, 1983.

22. Cherkin DC, MacCornack FA: Patient evaluations of low back pain care from family physicians and chiropractors. West J Med 150:351, 1989.

23. Meade TW, Dyer S, Browne W, et al.: Low back pain of mechanical origin: randomized comparison of chiropractic and hospital outpatient treatment. Br Med J 300:1431, 1990.

24. Jarvis KB, Phillips RB, Morris EK: Cost per case comparison of back injury claims of chiropractic versus medical management for conditions with identical diagnostic codes. J Occup Med 33:847, 1991.

PHYSICAL THERAPY AND EXERCISES

Physical therapy in conjunction with personal exercise regimens is recommended to many patients with low back pain. In the past, it was common practice to tear off an exercise instruction sheet (usually for flexion exercises) and give it to any patient with low back pain without further explanation. The therapeutic results of these exercises were varied: some patients had improvement; some had exacerbation of symptoms; some would follow the instructions incorrectly; and some would not do them at all. The results of this haphazard attempt at physical therapy exercises left some physicians skeptical of their benefit.

The goals of the exercise regimens vary greatly. Some strengthen lumbar spine extensors, while others strengthen abdominal muscles. Other exercises concentrate on lengthening contracted muscles. Physicians frequently choose a course of exercises for a patient based upon a general concept of strengthening muscles, whether paraspinous or abdominal, as the goal of exercise. They do not individualize the patient's regimen to the underlying disease or the associated abnormality in the musculoskeletal structures of the lumbosacral spine, and, consequently, the maximum benefit of therapy may not be achieved. For example, an ideal exercise program requires individualized therapy, which may include flexion or extension exercises that concentrate on strengthening and/or lengthening back muscles.

RATIONALE FOR PHYSICAL THERAPY

In a two part article, Jackson and Brown point out many of the fallacies and misconceptions associated with exercises and low back pain.[1, 2] The reasons for prescribing exercises for patients with low back pain are listed in Table 19–3.

Many theories have been proposed to explain how low back exercises result in pain relief. Williams postulated that back and leg pain resulted from compression of radicular nerves as they passed through the intervertebral foramen. Flexion exercises purportedly opened the foramen, relieving nerve root compression.[3, 4] In opposition to the flexion theory, McKenzie proposed that radicular pain was related to disc protrusion and that repeated extension exercises shifted extruded disc material anteriorly, relieving compression.[5] Flexion and extension exercises are not helpful in all patients with back pain. For example, neither of these exercise methods has been proved to be effective in relieving sciatic pain. Nerve compression is associated with numbness, not pain. It is the inflammation associated with chronic compression that causes pain. Neither flexion nor extension exercises relieve nerve inflammation or sciatic pain. Therefore, the potential for these exercises to

TABLE 19–3. REASONS FOR THE PRESCRIPTION OF EXERCISES FOR LOW BACK PAIN PATIENTS*

Decrease pain
Strengthen weak muscles†
Stretch contracted muscles
Decrease mechanical stress to spinal structures
Improve fitness to prevent injury†
Stabilize hypermobile segments
Improve posture
Improve mobility
As a last resort

*Modified from Jackson CP, Brown MD: Analysis of current approaches and a practical guide to prescription of exercise. Clin Orthop 176:46, 1983.
†Proven effective therapy.

significantly reduce radicular pain, acutely, is minimal. In regard to shifting disc material, both anterior and posterior compressive forces on the disc are associated with movement of nuclear material.[6] If pain is related to disc compression of nerve roots and exercises cause nuclear material to return to normal anatomic position, pain relief may gradually occur as the forces on the nerves are reduced.

Pain relief has been proposed as a beneficial component of aerobic exercise. Strenuous aerobic exercise is associated with increased endorphin levels, a sense of euphoria, and the potential for pain relief. Unfortunately, increases in levels of endorphins peripherally are not necessarily correlated with increased central nervous system levels.[7] Generalized pain relief cannot be obtained through generalized strenuous aerobic exercise and probably does not play a role in pain relief associated with exercises in back patients. In general, aggressive exercise programs are more successful in improving functional status, such as return to work, than in significantly relieving pain.[8] However, improved function may decrease the anxiety associated with fear of exacerbation of back pain. This decrease in anxiety may have beneficial psychologic effects. Early return to work after an aggressive exercise program is not associated with an increased rate of recurrence of low back pain.[9]

Strengthening of back muscles has been advocated as a beneficial aspect of exercise programs that are a part of a comprehensive program to control back pain.[10] Patients who have acute low back pain do not exhibit extensor muscle weakness.[11, 12] In contrast, those patients with chronic back pain of a month or longer do exhibit muscle weakness.[13] In these chronic pain patients, trunk extensors are weakened to a greater degree than flexors.[14, 15] This is in stark contrast to normal individuals without back pain who have stronger extensor muscles.[16, 17] In normal individuals, extensor strength is typically 30% greater than flexor strength.[18]

The paraspinous muscles are involved not only in job-related tasks but also in the maintenance of posture. The role of muscle weakness in the development of postural back pain was studied by De Vries.[19] Patients with back pain and bad posture had abnormalities on electromyographic (EMG) analysis of paraspinous muscles not elicited from normal controls without pain. He suggested that muscular deficiency was a cause of back pain and that this category of back pain was amenable to endurance exercises.

Posture also may play a role in causing pain in patients with occupations that require assuming one position for an extended period of time. The strength of the back muscles is important for completing certain tasks (lifting, carrying) but may not prevent the development of back pain in an individual who lacks the muscular endurance to maintain a certain posture.[20] Those workers who lack adequate strength or endurance relative to their work are at greater risk of developing back injury.[21] These findings suggest that abnormalities in strength or endurance of paraspinous muscles may act independently as sources of pain. Over time, back pain causes decreased muscle strength. In addition, the lack of muscle endurance may add to the perpetuation of back pain. A return of full muscle strength, joint movement, and endurance is necessary for a complete recovery of function. Back strength is more closely related to ability to work than to the degree of pain. Parnianpour and coworkers developed a device that can measure motor output (torque) and movement pattern (angular position and velocity profile) in three dimensions associated with work-related tasks that generated isoinertial forces. Isoinertial forces are generated by muscles contracting against a constant load. In a study, workers were asked to use maximum effort lifting a constant load.[22] With increasing fatigue, greater range of motion was noted in planes other than flexion and extension associated with the lifting task. The inability of the primary muscles to complete the task resulted in the recruitment of secondary muscle groups. The recruitment of these secondary muscles loaded the spine in a more injury-prone pattern. Fatigued muscles were less capable of compensating for any perturbation in the lifted load. The implication of this study is that endurance of back muscles related to a job task is a more useful predictor of the incidence of back pain than is the absolute strength of these muscles.

A number of studies have demonstrated the relationship between mechanical stress and low back pain.[23, 24] The relative benefit of flexion versus extension versus isotonic exercises in the relief of back pain remains controversial.[4, 25, 26] Whether specific exercises can be used to reduce mechanical loads on the spine and whether increased intradiscal stress on normal discs is necessarily associated with back pain remain to be determined.

Good general fitness is associated with decreased incidence of back injuries and decreased duration of incapacity with a back injury according to a prospective study of 1652 firefighters.[27] This study is strong evidence for improved fitness to prevent injuries but does not have relevance to those patients in poor physical condition with concurrent back pain.

Exercises directed at stabilizing a hyper- or hypomobile spinal segment by increasing muscle strength do not work. Paraspinous muscles lack the voluntary control to allow for specific segment strengthening. Patients must be evaluated for imbalances in muscle strength and length. Strengthening and lengthening the paraspinous, psoas, and hamstring muscles to achieve normal physiologic balance of the lumbosacral spine and its supporting structures give patients a greater chance of decreasing pain than does concentrating on strengthening an isolated area.[28]

Exercises to improve structural postural abnormalities are not effective. The degree of structural lordosis is unrelated to abdominal or back extensor muscle strength or to hip or trunk flexibility.[29] Flexion or isometric exercises that attempt to correct these postural abnormalities have been ineffective in altering nonpathologic structural back anatomy.[30, 31]

Although adequate mobility is necessary for normal function of the spine, the total range that has the greatest mechanical efficiency, tissue nutrition for discs and cartilage, and adequate facet joint motion has not been determined. Too little motion (less than 30°) may limit flexibility, while too much can excessively load the spine.[32] Exercises that attempt to increase spinal mobility beyond normal ranges of motion are not necessarily beneficial.

Exercise programs are occasionally prescribed for patients with chronic low back pain as a last resort after other therapies have failed. Exercise programs can have a beneficial effect even if the patient's physical condition is not dramatically altered. The active involvement of patients in their exercise program is an essential part of therapy. Exercise may decrease stress and foster better sleep habits and may also improve the patient's self-image and self-esteem.[33–35]

Exercise Programs

Therapeutic exercise can be defined as structural and controlled body movement to correct an impairment, improve musculoskeletal function, or maintain a state of well-being. Exercises can increase muscle strength, elasticity, range of motion, and endurance. A prescription for physical therapy must have a spec-

ified objective. The program of exercises may be modified as a patient's condition is altered and may include passive, active assisted, active, or active resistive exercises.

Passive exercise is produced entirely by an external force without any voluntary contraction of muscles by the patient. The exercises maintain range of motion and elasticity of soft tissue. Active assisted exercises, which require muscular contraction to move a portion of the body without an external force, maintain flexibility, and decrease potential for muscle atrophy. Isometric, isotonic, and isokinetic exercises are classified as active resistive. Isometric contraction is associated with increased muscle tension without change in muscle length. Strength is increased only at the length of muscle contraction; contraction at different muscle lengths is needed to increase generalized muscle strength. Isotonic exercise decreases fiber length without a change in muscle tension. Strengthening occurs through maximal effort of motion. Isokinetic exercises move body parts through ranges of motion at a constant speed. This kind of therapy is done with a Cybex machine.

Which is the best exercise program for patients with low back pain? Kendall and Jenkins studied three types of treatment: (1) mobility and strengthening exercises, (2) lumbar isometric flexion exercises, and (3) hyperextension exercises. At the end of the 3-month study, the isometric group had a statistically significant improvement in symptoms.[36] In contrast, Davies found that patients assessed at 4 weeks of treatment described greater improvement with extension exercises than with isometric exercises or heat. The period of time to return to work was shorter in the extension and control groups (2 weeks) than in the isometric group.[30] Data demonstrating the greater efficacy of one type of exercise over another are not available. The physician must decide whether flexion, extension, isometric, or general fitness exercises are best for specific problems their patients are experiencing.

FLEXION EXERCISES

Flexion exercises are used to open intervertebral foramina and facet joints, to stretch hip flexors and back extensors, to strengthen abdominal and gluteal muscles, and to mobilize the posterior fixation of the lumbosacral articulation.[3, 4] Williams' exercises have been modified over the years but basically consist of partial sit ups in the hook-lying position (feet on floor, knees flexed, head slightly raised) to strengthen abdominal muscles, pelvic tilts to flatten lumbar lordosis, knees to chest, and stretching hip flexors (Fig. 19–5).

These exercises are designed to increase intra-abdominal pressure to stabilize the spine. The muscles that actually generate abdominal pressure are the internal and external oblique muscles, which are involuntary muscles in the generation of abdominal pressure.[37] Voluntary efforts to increase pressure, such as contracting the rectus abdominis during a Valsalva maneuver, increase the load on the intervertebral discs and may be counterproductive. Exercises to increase strength in the oblique muscles without participation of the rectus abdominis include rotating the thorax on the pelvis, posterior pelvic tilt while standing, and hip roll.[38] The desired effect may also be obtained by lifting a shoulder during a modified sit-up in the hook-lying position.[39]

Other components of flexion exercises such as posterior pelvic tilts while supine, bilateral straight leg raising, and toe touches either have no benefit or increase intradiscal pressures.[2] In particular, flexion exercises are not indicated in patients with acute disc prolapse, immediately after periods of prolonged rest with hyperhydrated discs that are susceptible to injury, postural low back pain secondary to flexion, or lateral trunk list.[2]

EXTENSION EXERCISES

Extension exercises may be attempted with paraspinous extensors in a flexed or neutral position with the goal of improving motor strength and endurance, or attempted in the hyperextended position with the goal of improving mobility, strengthening the back extensors, or promoting a shift of nuclear material to a normal position (Fig. 19–6). People with strong paraspinous extensors have less postural fatigue and pain, greater capacity to lift weights and to withstand axial compression, and better overall physical fitness. Evidence exists demonstrating the effects of extension exercises on strengthening lumbar extensor muscles.[40] The primary functions of the paraspinous extensors are maintaining posture and controlling the descent of the trunk during flexion.[41, 42] Maximum trunk extensor movement occurs in 40° to 45° of flexion, and that is the range in which the muscles should be exercised. By positioning themselves at the edge of a table on their stomachs, patients can exercise the extensors by lifting and lowering their trunk without extending the lumbar spine. Electromyographic studies of

paraspinous muscles indicate that hyperextension exercises are the most effective for strengthening the extensor muscles.[43] Other components of a hyperextension exercise program include press ups in the prone position and strengthening and stretching of hip extensors (hamstrings and gluteal muscles)[44] (Fig. 19–6).

Low back pain patients often have tight hamstring muscles. Exercises to stretch and strengthen the hip extensors are an important component of an extension program. Stretching from a flexed, sitting posture may have limitations by hyperflexing the spine, increasing intradiscal pressure, and straining paraspinous muscles.[45] Unilateral hamstring stretches may be a safer alternative for improving hamstring muscle function without straining other lumbar structures.

Although extension exercises have been associated with relief of low back symptoms, not all patients benefit from them.[46] Patients who have an acute disc prolapse, have undergone multiple back operations, have limited flexion because of paraspinous scarring, or have facet joint disease (spinal stenosis) may have exacerbation of symptoms with extension exercises.[2]

ISOMETRIC FLEXION EXERCISES

Others propose isometric flexion exercises as the most appropriate for back patients.[26, 47] These exercises eliminate hyperextension and encourage contraction of trunk muscles and strengthening of abdominal muscles. The exercises are done in a supine position, although the same maneuvers may be attempted while sitting or standing. A sequence of active contractions involve the abdominal muscles; the gluteal muscles; the abdominal and gluteal muscles, resulting in a pelvic tilt; and finally, contraction of the hip adductors. The contractions are held for 5 to 15 seconds. The exercises are done frequently, for short periods, during the day. Progress is measured by increased duration and number of exercise completions. In a study comparing conventional physical therapy with mobilizing and strengthening exercises versus isometric flexion versus controls in 62 outpatients with sciatica, Lidstrom demonstrated significantly greater improvement in the isometric group than in the other two groups. Patients in the isometric group had decreased mobility.[48]

Elnaggar and coworkers studied the efficacy of flexion versus extension exercises in 56 patients with chronic mechanical low back pain

Text continued on page 622

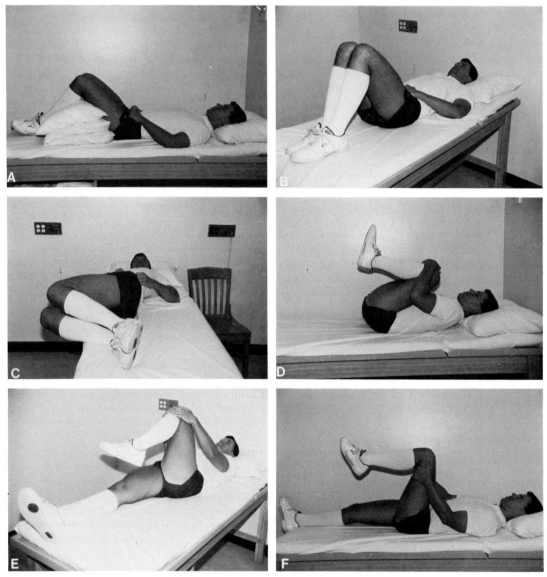

Figure 19–5. *See legend on opposite page.*

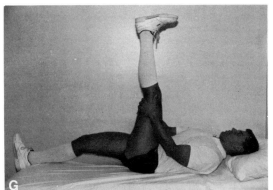

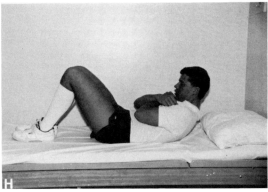

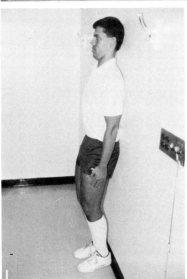

Figure 19–5. Flexion exercises. *A* to *C,* Acute (relaxation) phase. *A,* Resting position—hips flexed with pillows under knees. This flattens the lumbar spine. Duration: 15 minutes. *B,* Resting position without pillows. *C,* Back rotation—shoulders remain on the table while the pelvis is turned to one side to the patient's tolerance. This exercise stretches and strengthens the internal and external obliques. Duration: 1 minute. Patient alternates side to side. (These exercises promote relaxation of muscles.) *D* and *E,* Stretching phase. *D,* Knees to chest while raising the pelvis. This exercise stretches the paraspinous muscles. *E,* Crossover leg exercise—the heel is placed on the contralateral knee and the bent knee is pulled to tolerance toward the contralateral shoulder. Duration: The position is held to a count of 3, and the leg is rested in the neutral position for a count of 6. The legs are alternated with 10 repetitions. (These exercises stretch the paraspinous and hip abductor muscles.) *F* to *I,* Stretching and strengthening phase. *F,* Hamstring stretch with hip flexed, knee flexed. *G,* Hamstring stretch—fully extended knee. Duration: Hold for a count of 3, then count to 6 with the leg in the neutral position. *H,* Partial sit up—strengthens the abdominal muscles. Duration: Hold for a count of 3, then rest for a count of 6 for 25 repetitions. *I,* Pelvic tilt in standing position—back flattened against the wall, knees flexed. Duration: Count of 3, done hourly. (These exercises stretch and strengthen the paraspinous and hamstring muscles, and strengthen the abdominal muscles.) (Courtesy of Thomas Welsh.)

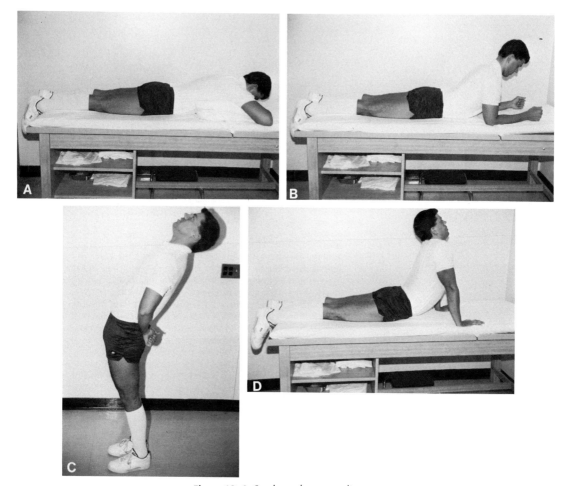

Figure 19–6. *See legend on opposite page.*

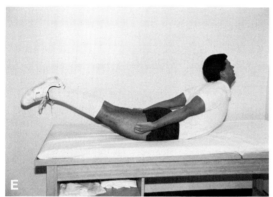
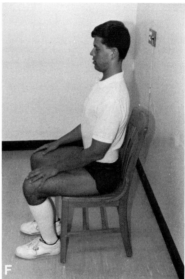

Figure 19–6. Extension exercises. *A,* Acute (relaxation) phase. Prone position resting on pillows. Additional pillows are used to patient's tolerance. Duration: 15 minutes. (This exercise promotes relaxation of paraspinous muscles.) *B* to *D,* Stretching phase. *B,* Patient is propped up on bent elbows. Duration: Hold to a count of 3, then rest for a count of 6. *C,* Extension of the lumbar spine in standing position. Duration: Hold for a count of 3, then rest for a count of 6. This exercise is done hourly. *D,* Full extension. Duration: Hold for a count of 10, with 10 repetitions. (These exercises stretch the paraspinous muscles.) *E* to *F,* Strengthening phase. *E,* Full extension with arms extended and legs lifted to tolerance. Duration: Hold for a count of 3, then rest for a count of 6. *F,* Extension—seated position. (Maintenance of lumbar lordosis.) (Courtesy of Thomas Welsh.)

TABLE 19–4. INDICATIONS FOR FLEXION EXERCISES

Pain relief on:
  Sitting
    and with:
  Repeated forward bending
  Increased lumbar lordosis
  Fixed lumbar lordosis with bending
Pain exacerbation on:
  Walking
  Standing
    and with:
  Sustained forward bending
  Repeated backward bending
  Sustained backward bending
  Extreme range of backward bending
Pain unchanged on:
  Stooping

for 3 months or longer.[49] Each patient received six therapist sessions and eight self-directed sessions over a 2-week period. Patients repeated the flexion or extension exercises 2 to 3 times over a 30-minute period. At the end of the 2-week exercise period, both groups experienced a significant decrease in low back pain. The flexion groups demonstrated increased sagittal motion compared with the extension group. This study points out the importance of exercise, in general, as a means to improve the function of low back pain patients.

AEROBIC EXERCISES

Jackson and Brown suggest a general aerobic program for back pain patients who have been medically screened for cardiovascular disease.[2] Exercise sessions, which involve large muscle groups, include a warm-up and cooldown period, last 30 to 40 minutes, and are completed 3 times a week. Temperature extremes should be avoided. Walking and swimming are probably the best aerobic exercises for the majority of back patients.

Just as there is no single therapy for all cases of back pain, there is no one physical therapy program for all patients with lumbosacral disease.[50] Some patients benefit from flexion, some from extension, and some from isometrics (Fig. 19–7); some do not improve at all. Listening carefully to the patient's symptoms and observing the movements that cause pain help the physician decide which physical therapy program has the greatest chance for success in an individual patient (Tables 19–4 and 19–5). It must be reiterated that the therapy program is not cast in stone. Communication among the patient, therapist, and physician is essential. As the patient improves, increasingly stressful tasks may be added to the exercise program in an attempt to increase endurance and strength in preparation for return to work. If symptoms increase, exercises may be discontinued or reduced, to be reinitiated once the patient's symptoms return to baseline. Individualizing exercise programs to patient symptoms leads to greater patient compliance and improved outcome.

The aggressiveness of the exercise program will have an effect on the degree of pain the patient experiences. Manniche and coworkers completed a study of 105 patients with low back pain dividied into three exercise groups.[51] One group received 30 sessions of intensive dynamic back extensor exercises over a 3-month period. Another group received six sessions of similar exercises over a 3-month period. The final group received massage and mild exercises. The treatment group that received the intensive exercise program had increased discomfort during the first month but felt better during the second and third months than did the individuals in the other study groups. Benefits from exercise can be long lasting. The physician should encourage the patient to continue with the exercise program even if there is some increase in discomfort initially. Most patients recognize the meaning of the saying "no pain, no gain." The full benefit of improved physical conditioning occurs after the initial phases of exercise that are more painful.[52]

Patients with nonmechanical back pain may also benefit from physical therapy and exercises. Patients with a spondyloarthropathy need to be involved in a regular home exercise program that includes chest expansion, range of motion, and strengthening exercises for the

TABLE 19–5. INDICATIONS FOR EXTENSION EXERCISES

Pain relief on:
  Lying
  Walking
    and with:
  Repeated backward bending
  Decreased lumbar lordosis
Pain exacerbation on:
  Sitting
  Driving
  Arising from chair
  Stooping
  Bending
    and with:
  Forward bending
  Repeated forward bending

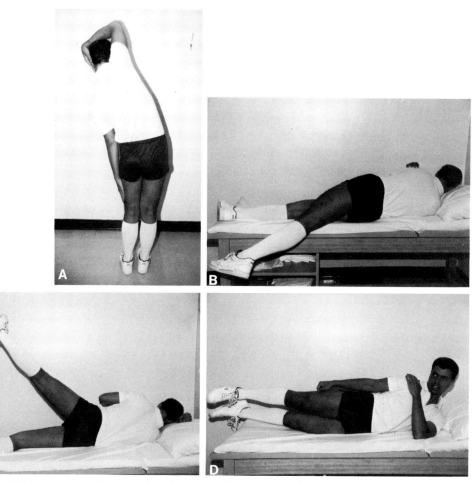

Figure 19–7. Two weeks after the start of flexion or extension exercises, the following set of exercises are initiated. *A,* Lateral bending in standing position. Duration: Hold for a count of 10; done hourly. (This exercise stretches the latissimus dorsi and the quadratus lumborum on the side with the list.) *B,* Hip abductor stretch. This exercise lengthens the side with the shortened iliotibial band. *C,* Hip abductor strengthening for the muscle opposite the shortened side. *D,* Oblique muscle strengthening and stretching. The oblique and latissimus dorsi muscles on the down side are lengthened, while the muscles on the up side are strengthened. (These exercises restore muscle balance to the patient with back list.) (Courtesy of Thomas Welsh.)

lumbosacral and cervical spine. Once again, the exercise program must be individualized, and this is best achieved under the direction of a physical therapist who communicates with both the patient and the physician.

References

PHYSICAL THERAPY AND EXERCISES

1. Jackson CP, Brown MD: Is there a role for exercise in the treatment of patients with low back pain? Clin Orthop 179:39, 1983.
2. Jackson CP, Brown MD: Analysis of current approaches and a practical guide to prescription of exercise. Clin Orthop 179:46, 1983.
3. Williams PC: Lesions of the lumbosacral spine, part I. J Bone Joint Surg 19:343, 1937.
4. Williams PC: Lesions of the lumbosacral spine, part II. J Bone Joint Surg 19:690, 1937.
5. McKenzie RA: The Lumbar Spine: Mechanical Diagnosis and Therapy. Waikanae, New Zealand: Spinal Publications, 1981.
6. Kramer J: Pressure dependent fluid shifts in the intervertebral disc. Orthop Clin North Am 8:211, 1977.
7. Fraioli F, Moretti C, Paolucci D, et al.: Physical exercise stimulates marked concomitant release of beta-endorphin and adrenocorticotropic hormone (ACTH) in peripheral blood in man. Experientia 36:987, 1980.
8. Mitchell RI, Carmen GM: Results of a multicenter trial using an intensive active exercise program for the treatment of acute soft tissue and back injuries. Spine 15:514, 1990.
9. Mayer TG, Gatchel RJ, Mayer H, et al.: A prospective two-year functional restoration in industrial low back pain injury. JAMA 258:1763, 1987.
10. Alston W, Carlson KE, Feldman DJ, et al.: A quantitative study of muscle fatigue in the chronic low back syndrome. Ann Surg 80:762, 1950.
11. Pedersen OF, Peterson R, Staffeldt ES: Back pain and isometric back muscle strength of workers in a Danish factory. Scand J Rehabil Med 7:125, 1975.
12. Beckson M, Schultz A, Nachemson AL, Andersson GBJ: Voluntary strengths of adults with acute low back syndrome. Clin Orthop 129:84, 1977.
13. Nachemson AL, Lindh M: Measurement of abdominal and back muscle strength with and without low back pain. Scand J Rehabil Med 1:60, 1969.
14. Addison R, Schultz A: Trunk strengths in patients seeking hospitalization for chronic low back disorders. Spine 5:539, 1980.
15. McNeill T, Warwick D, Andersson GBJ, Schultz A: Trunk strengths in attempted flexion, extension and lateral bending in healthy subjects and patients with low back disorders. Spine 6:529, 1980.
16. Davies G, Gould J: Trunk testing using a prototype Cybex II isokinetic dynamometer stabilization system. J Orthop Sports Phys Ther 3:164, 1982.
17. Schmidt GL, Amundson LR, Dostal WF: Muscle strength at the trunk. J Orthop Sports Phys Ther 1:665, 1980.
18. Beimborn DS, Morrissey MC: A review of the literature related to trunk muscle performance. Spine 13:655, 1988.
19. De Vries H: EMG fatigue nerve in postural muscles. A possible etiology for idiopathic low back pain. Am J Phys Med 47:175, 1968.
20. Magora A: Investigation of the relation between low back pain and occupation VI. Medical history and symptoms. Scand J Rehabil Med 6:81, 1974.
21. Poulsen E: Back muscle strength and weight limits in lifting. Spine 6:73, 1981.
22. Parnianpour M, Nordin MA, Kahanovitz N, Frankel V: The triaxial coupling of torque generation of trunk muscles during isometric exertions and the effect of fatiguing isoinertial movement on the motor output and movement. Spine 13:982, 1988.
23. Hirsch C: Studies on the pathology of low back pain. J Bone Joint Surg 41B:237, 1959.
24. Schultz A, Andersson GBJ: Analysis of loads on the lumbar spine. Spine 6:76, 1981.
25. Nachemson AL: The load on lumbar disc in different positions of the body. Clin Orthop 45:107, 1966.
26. Hadler NM: Diagnosis and Treatment of Backache. In Hadler NM: Medical Management of the Regional Musculoskeletal Diseases. Orlando: Grune & Stratton, 1984, pp 3–52.
27. Cady LD, Bischoff DP, O'Connell ER, et al.: Strength and fitness and subsequent back injuries in firefighters. J Occup Med 21:269, 1979.
28. Nachemson AL: The possible importance of the psoas muscle for stabilization of the lumbar spine. Acta Orthop Scand 39:47, 1968.
29. Flint MM: Lumbar posture: a study of roentgenographic measurement and the influence of flexibility and strength. Res Q 34:15, 1963.
30. Davies JE, Gibson R, Tester L: The value of exercises in the treatment of low back pain. Rheumatol Rehabil 18:243, 1979.
31. Fox MG: The relationship of abdominal strength to selected postural faults. Res Q 22:141, 1951.
32. Farfan HF: The biomechanical advantage of lordosis and hip extension for upright activity. Spine 3:336, 1978.
33. Collingwood TR: The effects of physical training upon behavior and self attitude. J Clin Psychol 28:583, 1972.
34. Morgan WP, Hortsman DH: Anxiety reduction following acute physical activity. Arch Phys Med 52:422, 1971.
35. Browman CP: Sleep following sustained exercise. Psychophysiology 17:577, 1980.
36. Kendall PH, Jenkins JS: Exercise for backache: a double-blind controlled trial. Physiotherapy 54:154, 1968.
37. Andersson GBJ, Ortengren R, Nachemson AL: Intradiscal pressure, intra-abdominal pressure and myoelectric back muscle activity related to posture and loading. Clin Orthop 129:156, 1977.
38. Partridge M: Participation of the abdominal muscles in various movements of the trunk in man. An EMG study. Phys Ther Rev 39:791, 1959.
39. Halpern A, Blech EE: Sit-up exercises: an EMG study. Clin Orthop 145:172, 1979.
40. Pollock ML, Leggett SH, Graves JE, et al.: Effect of resistance training on lumbar extension strength. Am J Sports Med 17:624, 1989.
41. Morris JM, Benner G, Lucas BD: An EMG study of the intrinsic muscles of the back in man. J Anat 96:509, 1962.
42. Floyd WF, Silver PHS: The function of the erector spinae muscles in certain movements and postures in man. J Physiol 129:184, 1955.
43. Pauley J: EMG analysis of certain movements and exercise: some deep muscles of the back. Anat Rec 155:223, 1966.
44. Farfan HF, Cassette JW, Robertson GH, et al.: The effect of torsion in the production of disc degeneration. J Bone Joint Surg 52A:468, 1970.

45. Liemohn W: Exercises and the back. Rheum Dis Clin North Am: 16:945, 1990.

46. Ponte DJ, Jensen GJ, Kent BE: A preliminary report on the use of the McKenzie protocol versus Williams protocol in the treatment of low back pain. J Orthop Sports Phys Ther 6:130, 1984.

47. Kendall PH, Jenkins JM: Lumbar isometric flexion exercises. Physiotherapy 54:158, 1968.

48. Lidstrom A, Zachrisson M: Physical therapy on low back pain and sciatica: an attempt at evaluation. Scand J Rehabil Med 2:37, 1970.

49. Elnaggar IM, Nordin M, Sheikhzadeh A, et al.: Effects of spinal flexion and extension exercises on low-back pain and spinal mobility in chronic mechanical low-back pain patients. Spine 16:967, 1991.

50. Sikorski JM: A rationalized approach to physiotherapy for low-back pain. Spine 10:571, 1985.

51. Manniche C, Hesselsoe G, Bentzen L, et al.: Clinical trial of intense muscle training for chronic low back pain. Lancet II:1473, 1988.

52. Balogun JA, Olokungbemi AA, Kuforji AR: Spinal mobility and muscular strength: effects of supine- and prone-lying back extension exercise training. Arch Phys Med Rehabil 73:745, 1992.

MEDICATIONS

A number of drugs have been advocated for the treatment of low back pain on a short- or long-term basis. The nonsteroidal anti-inflammatory drugs (NSAIDs) and analgesics, both non-narcotic and narcotic, have been used in the therapy of back pain. In general, the scientific evidence demonstrating efficacy of NSAIDs in back pain is small compared with the frequency of their use. Nevertheless, NSAIDs play a useful role in the control of pain in these patients.

A number of factors need to be considered when deciding whether to prescribe NSAIDs or analgesics for low back pain. The natural history of acute low back pain is one of resolution over a short period of time in 80% to 90% of patients. Patients may go through this period using physical measures (bed rest and physical therapy) alone. On the other hand, the pain the patients experience may be diminished through the use of NSAIDs or analgesics. In making the decision to use these drugs, the physician must remember not to exacerbate the condition or cause serious toxicities while the patient's back pain resolves. The clinical correlate of this prohibition is that NSAIDs and non-narcotic analgesics are appropriate agents in some patients with low back pain, but narcotic analgesics are reserved for only a very small group of patients with documented anatomic abnormalities for specified brief periods of time.

Nonsteroidal Anti-inflammatory Drugs (NSAIDs)

NSAIDs have analgesic properties when given in single doses and are anti-inflammatory and analgesic when given chronically in larger doses. Pure analgesics have no anti-inflammatory effect, while corticosteroids have anti-inflammatory but no analgesic effects except for those mediated through reduction of inflammation.

While narcotic analgesics act on the endorphin system in the central nervous system, NSAIDs act at the site of peripheral injury where peripheral nerves send nociceptive impulses to the cortex. Prostaglandins do not cause pain by themselves, but rather sensitize nociceptive nerve fibers to environmental chemical factors (bradykinin, histamine). In the presence of prostaglandins, small amounts of these chemical factors initiate nociceptive impulses. Cyclooxygenase inhibition by NSAIDs with decreased production of prostaglandins seems to play a role in the analgesic action of these agents. Other mechanisms must also act in the production of analgesia associated with these drugs since the potency of the NSAIDs as prostaglandin inhibitors does not necessarily correlate with their efficacy as analgesics. NSAIDs also have significant effects on other components of the inflammatory response including oxidative phosphorylation, superoxide production, and cellular activation.[1]

The pharmacokinetics and clinical pharmacology of these agents have little direct bearing on their time course of action; that is, the onset of analgesia does not parallel the peak plasma level. Agents that are rapidly absorbed do not necessarily have more rapid onset of analgesic effect. Determinations of peak plasma levels are not obtained clinically since they have little bearing in predicting qualitative or quantitative responses to a medication. Patient response to medications seems to be individualized and cannot be predicted by the pharmacokinetics of a drug.[2] The duration of anti-inflammatory effect of a medication may be different from that of the analgesic effect. An example given by Huskisson is that of piroxicam with a plasma half-life of 38 hours.[3] The anti-inflammatory effect of this drug lasts for 24 hours with a once-a-day dose, while the analgesic effect is only 6 hours in duration, similar to that of aspirin.

Although the NSAIDs are all weak organic acids, except nabumetone, a prodrug that is administered as a base, they belong to different chemical groups (Table 19–6). The drugs may be divided by their chemical grouping in

TABLE 19–6. NONSTEROIDAL ANTI-INFLAMMATORY DRUGS*

DRUG (CHEMICAL CLASS)	TRADE NAME	TABLET/CAPSULE SIZE (MG)	DOSE (MG/DAY)	FREQUENCY (TIMES/DAY)	ONSET (HOURS)	HALF-LIFE (HOURS)	METABOLISM
(Salicylates)							
Aspirin	Bayer	325	Up to 5200	4–6	1–2	4	Liver
Enteric coated	Ecotrin	325	5200	4–6	1–2	4	Liver
	Easprin	975	3900	4	1–2		Liver
Time release	Zorprin	800	3200	2	2	4	Liver
(Substituted Salicylates)							
Diflunisal	Dolobid	250,500	500–1500	2–3	1 (with loading dose)	11	Liver
Salsalate	Disalcid	500,750	3000	2	2	4	Liver
Choline magnesium trisalicylate	Trilisate	500,750, 1000, liquid (500 mg/5 ml)	3000	2	2	4	Liver
Choline salicylate	Arthropan	650 mg/ml	1950	4–6	1	4	Liver
Magnesium salicylate	Magan	545	3270	3–4	2	4	Liver
Sodium salicylate	Uracel	325	3900	3–6	1	4	Liver
Aspirin/antacids	Ascriptin	325	5200	4–6	2	4	Liver
(Propionic Acid Derivatives)							
Ibuprofen	Motrin	200	1200–3600	4–6	1–2	1–3	Liver
	Rufen	400					
	Advil	600					
	Medipren	800					
	Nuprin	200					
Naproxen	Naprosyn	250,375,500	500–1500	2–3	3	13	Liver
Sodium naproxen	Anaprox	275,550	550–1100	2	1–2	13	Liver
Fenoprofen calcium	Nalfon	200,300,600	600–3000	3–4	3	2–3	Liver
Ketoprofen	Orudis	25,50,75	150–300	3–4	2	3–4	Liver
	Oruvail	200					Liver
Flurbiprofen	Ansaid	50,100	300	2–3	1–2	6	Liver
Oxaprozin	Daypro	600	1800	1–2	3–5	25	Liver
(Pyrrole Acetic Acid Derivatives)							
Sulindac	Clinoril	150,200	300–450	2–3	2	18	Liver
Indomethacin	Indocin	25,50,75 SR, 50 suppositories	75–225	1–3	2	1–4	Liver
Tolmetin sodium	Tolectin	200,400	600–1600	4	1	1–4	Liver
(Benzeneacetic Acid Derivative)							
Diclofenac Sodium	Voltaren	25,50,75	75–225	2–3	2–3	2	Liver
Diclofenac Potassium	Cataflam	25,50	100–150	2–3	1	2	Liver
Oxicam							
Piroxicam	Feldene	10,20	20	1	5	38–45	Liver
Pyranocarboxylic Acid							
Etodolac	Lodine	200,300,400	800–1600	2–4	2	6	Liver
Fenemate							
Meclofenamate sodium	Meclomen	50,100	200–400	4	1	4	Liver
Mefenamic acid	Ponstel	250	1000	4	3	4	Liver
Pyrrolo-pyrrole							
Ketorolac tromethamine	Toradol	10	10–40	4	1	4–6	Liver
Naphthylalkanone							
Nabumetone	Relafen	500,750	1000–2000	1–2	4	26	Liver
Pyrazolones							
Phenylbutazone	Butazolidin, Azolid	100	400	4	2 (with loading)	72	Liver

*Modified from The Medical Letter 29:24, 1987.
†G = gastrointestinal; R = renal; CNS = central nervous system; BM = bone marrow; SR = slow-release

TABLE 19–6. NONSTEROIDAL ANTI-INFLAMMATORY DRUGS* *Continued*

DRUG (CHEMICAL CLASS)	EXCRETION	MAJOR TOXICITY†	COST ($/MONTH)	COMMENTS
(Salicylates)				
Aspirin	Kidney	G, R	16.00 (5200 mg)	Less expensive than other NSAIDS
Enteric coated	Kidney	G, R	16.39 (4000 mg)	Less G upset than aspirin
	Kidney	G, R	15.39 (3900 mg)	Less G upset than aspirin
Time release	Kidney	G, R	20.36 (3200 mg)	Less G upset than aspirin
(Substituted Salicylates)				
Diflunisal	Kidney	G, R	51.84 (1000 mg)	Loading dose for rapid onset of action; long half-life b.i.d. dosing
Salsalate	Kidney	G, R	43.24 (4000 mg)	Less G upset than aspirin
Choline magnesium trisalicylate	Kidney	G, R	43.72 (3000 mg)	Less G upset than aspirin
Choline salicylate	Kidney	G, R	27.30 (1950 mg)	Ease of swallowing
Magnesium salicylate	Kidney	G, R	34.31 (3270 mg)	Magnesium toxicity with impaired renal function
Sodium salicylate	Kidney	G, R	2.43–10.79 (5400 mg)	Simple analgesic, less effective than aspirin; increased sodium intake
Aspirin/Antacids	Kidney	G, R	21.58	Antacids do not buffer gastric acid adequately
(Propionic Acid Derivatives)				
Ibuprofen	Kidney	G, R	12.94–23.78 (generic–Motrin)	Need larger doses for anti-inflammatory effect (rheumatoid arthritis)
Naproxen	Kidney, stool	G, R	40.53 (1000 mg)	Effective in a number of musculoskeletal disorders
Sodium naproxen	Kidney, stool	G, R	40.40 (825 mg)	Onset of action more rapid than naproxen
Fenoprofen calcium	Kidney	G, R	28.69 (2400 mg) (generic)	Associated with renal toxicity more often than other nonsteroidals
Ketoprofen	Kidney, stool	G, R	65.36 (300 mg)	Newer nonsteroidal (extended release)
Flurbiprofen	Kidney	G, R	56.01 (200 mg)	More powerful form of ibuprofen
Oxaprozin	Kidney, stool	G, R	55.19 (1200 mg)	Convenient QD dosing
(Pyrrole Acetic Acid Derivatives)				
Sulindac	Kidney, stool	G	44.83 (400 mg) (generic)	Effective in a number of musculoskeletal disorders; less renal toxicity
Indomethacin	Kidney, stool	G, R, CNS, BM	15.80 (150 mg generic) 38.90 (150 mg SR)	Drug of choice for spondylitis; greatest CNS toxicity of all NSAIDs
Tolmetin sodium	Kidney	G, R	49.60 (1200 mg) (generic)	Cross reactivity with zomepirac sodium (Zomax)
(Benzeneacetic Acid Derivatives)				
Diclofenac Sodium	Kidney, stool	G, R	60.65 (150 mg)	Effective in a number of musculoskeletal conditions
Diclofene Potassium	Kidney, stool	G, R	72.27 (100 mg)	Potassium salt associated with more rapid onset of analgesia
Oxicam				
Piroxicam	Kidney	G, R	59.38 (20 mg) (generic)	Substantial G toxicity; long duration of action, which extends toxicity
Pyranocarboxylic Acid				
Etodolac	Kidney	G, R	57.75 (1200 mg)	Multiple dosage form allows for specific amounts for different disorders
Fenemate				
Meclofenamate sodium	Kidney, stool	G, R	43.34 (400 mg) (generic)	Diarrhea in 1/3 of patients
Mefenamic acid	Kidney, stool	G, R	42.34 (1000 mg) (generic)	Dysmenorrhea
Pyrrolo-pyrrole				
Ketorolac tromethamine	Kidney	G, R	77.96 (30 mg)	Effective, rapid onset analgesic
Naphthylalkanone				
Nabumetone	Kidney, stool	G, R	54.00 (1000 mg)	Only basic NSAID, less toxic to GI tract
Pyrazolones				
Phenylbutazone	Kidney, stool	G, R, BM	32.72 (300 mg) (generic)	Bone marrow toxicity limits utility in most back pain patients, limited availability

a variety of ways depending on the complexity of the classification.[4, 5] For example, aspirin may be considered a salicylate or a heterocarboxylic acid. These groups include the salicylates (heterocarboxylic acids), propionic acid derivatives (phenylacetic acid, naphthaleneacetic acid, oxazolepropionic acid, benzeneacetic acid), acetic acid derivatives (indoleacetic acid, pyrrole acetic acid), fenamates (anthranilic acids or heterocarboxylic acids), oxicams, naphthylalkanone derivatives, pyrrolo-pyrrole derivative, and pyrazolones (pyrazolidinediones). Within these groups are agents with a short half-life and rapid onset of action, and others with a longer half-life and slower onset of action. In general, the half-life of the drug plays a greater role in selection of a specific NSAIDs than the chemical grouping. However, when a NSAID is ineffective, the choice of the subsequent NSAID is usually one from a different chemical group with a similar half-life.

NSAIDs that are used as analgesics include aspirin, diflunisal, fenoprofen, ibuprofen, mefenamic acid, naproxen, naproxen sodium, piroxicam, ketoprofen, ketorolac tromethamine, etodolac, and diclofenac potassium. In general, the dosage needed for the production of the analgesic effect of these agents is lower than that required for anti-inflammatory effects. The doses required for analgesic effects might be 2600 mg aspirin, 1000 mg diflunisal, 1600 mg ibuprofen, 500 mg naproxen, 30 mg ketorolac tromethamine, 900 mg etodolac, or 100 mg diclofenac potassium.

Some of the NSAIDs have been studied in patients with acute and chronic low back pain. Indomethacin was found no better than a placebo in patients with sciatica.[6] Naproxen and diflunisal had greater efficacy than placebo in relieving chronic back pain according to patient opinion.[7] Diflunisal was also preferred to acetaminophen in another study of back pain.[8] Wiesel demonstrated a small preference for aspirin compared with acetaminophen and phenylbutazone that was not statistically significant in a study of acute back pain.[9] Mefenamic acid at high dose (500 mg) was better than low-dose mefenamic acid, low dose salicylate, and placebo in controlling chronic low back pain.[10] A double-blind study of piroxicam and indomethacin demonstrated efficacy of both NSAIDs in patients with back pain.[11]

Most of the NSAIDs, when used as analgesics, must be given every 4 to 6 hours. The exceptions are diflunisal, piroxicam, and naproxen sodium. The analgesic effect of diflunisal lasts up to 12 hours, so the drug should be given only twice a day. Although the analgesic effect of piroxicam lasts for 6 hours, the drug has a long half-life, which limits its use to once a day because of gastrointestinal intolerance. Therefore, piroxicam is not a first line agent for analgesia. Naproxen sodium should be given every 8 hours at a maximum.

It is important to remember that when the NSAIDs are used as anti-inflammatory agents, higher doses are necessary to obtain adequate anti-inflammatory effects. In addition, when the drugs are used for chronic diseases, the rapid onset of action is not as important as its eventual efficacy for that individual patient. Examples of the dosages of drugs that may be required for the therapy of the spondyloarthropathies or rheumatoid arthritis are aspirin 5300 mg, sulindac 400 mg, naproxen 1500 mg, ibuprofen 3600 mg, diclofenac sodium 225 mg, nabumetone 2000 mg, etodolac 1600 mg, and oxaprozin 1800 mg/day. For osteoarthritis lower doses of NSAIDs may be used to limit toxicity while decreasing pain and local synovial inflammation. Examples of therapy for osteoarthritis patients may include aspirin 2200 mg, sulindac 300 mg, naproxen 500 mg, ibuprofen 1600 mg, diclofenac sodium 100 mg, nabumetone 1000 mg, etodolac 800 mg, or oxaprozin 1200 mg/day. Although acetaminophen has been suggested as adequate therapy for osteoarthritis, no study has demonstrated the consistent benefit of this drug for patients with osteoarthritis of the spine.[12] In fact, many patients try acetaminophen for back pain before seeking medical attention. In many circumstances, they see a physician because acetaminophen was inadequate for decreasing their pain.

The toxicities of the NSAIDs are predominantly gastrointestinal and renal. Aspirin ingestion has been associated with acute gastrointestinal bleeding.[13] Other NSAIDs have also been associated with bleeding.[14, 15] The enteric coated salicylates and sulindac are less likely to cause acute gastric damage according to endoscopic studies in normal volunteers.[16] Approximately 10% of patients develop gastrointestinal toxicity, usually dyspepsia.[17] Nabumetone has been cited as being milder but not devoid of gastrointestinal tract toxicity.[18] Corticosteroids have a low risk of causing gastrointestinal bleeding because of gastrointestinal ulceration.[19] It is more likely that the illness for which the steroids are being given causes gastrointestinal injury (head trauma). However, the combination of NSAID and corticosteroids does increase the risk of injury.[20] Patients who receive both classes of drugs must be warned of the potential complications so that they can inform their physician of any alteration in gastrointestinal function.

Another major toxicity associated with NSAIDs is related to renal dysfunction.[21] A small group of patients develop an idiosyncratic reaction with interstitial nephritis. A larger group develop reversible renal failure secondary to diminished renal prostaglandins, which are directly associated with diminished renal blood flow. Sulindac, a drug with fewer active metabolites in the renal circulation, has less effect on renal blood flow and is rarely the cause of this form of renal toxicity.[21] Other forms of NSAID toxicity include neurologic, hematologic, and hepatic complications.[2] Dermatologic and hypersensitivity reactions also are associated with these drugs.[18]

The clinician should take into account the characteristics of both the patient and the drug in deciding on the best agent for a particular individual (Table 19–7). Of greatest importance is efficacy. When choosing an agent for acute back pain, one with rapid onset of action is preferred once its efficacy has been established. Most of the NSAIDs have similar safety profiles except for phenylbutazone, which is associated with rare but severe bone marrow toxicity. Most individuals tolerate the NSAIDs. Geriatric patients may require smaller doses because drug metabolism slows with age. If patients find an effective agent but develop gastric toxicity, alternative means of taking the medication may be tried (with meals, for example). Alterations in other habits (alcohol, coffee consumption, smoking) or adding antacids or antiulcer medications (H_2-receptor antagonists, cytoprotective agents, e.g., misoprostol) may be useful in increasing tolerability of an effective drug.[22] Misoprostol should be given in small doses (100 μg b.i.d.) initially. The drug must be given with meals to minimize the major complication of diarrhea. Eating allows the drug to remain in the stomach

and out of the small intestine where the prostaglandin will cause diarrhea. As the patient tolerates the agent, the frequency of administration should be increased to 3 to 4 times a day with meals. In general, agents that require ingestion of fewer tablets are associated with greater patient compliance. Flexibility in the amount of drug per tablet and of the total dose needed to attain and maintain efficacy is useful. Some patients will obtain adequate analgesia at low doses of a drug, while others require larger amounts to obtain pain relief. Some patients prefer aspirin because of its lower cost (Table 19–7).

In regard to patient characteristics, it is impossible to predict which chemical class will be effective in an individual patient. Patients with mechanical problems improve with the analgesic effects of NSAIDs, while those with spondyloarthropathies require the anti-inflammatory action of these drugs. Drug interactions may limit choices. Shorter half-life drugs may be safer in older patients who have a diminished capacity to metabolize drugs. The combination of all these factors should be considered before the physician chooses a NSAID for a particular patient.

Most patients obtain significant pain relief with a NSAID and are able to stop the drug when resolution of their back pain occurs. Occasionally after an initial recovery, a patient will experience intermittent recurrent attacks or complain of a chronic low backache. These patients benefit from a maintenance dose of a NSAID. Medication should be taken on a regular schedule. Delaying medication until pain is present is not an appropriate way to take a NSAID. The drugs work better before pain is maximum. Patients should take medicine for a set time until pain is resolved, and then discontinue the drug a few days later.

Analgesics

The analgesic medications are divided into non-narcotic (acetaminophen) and narcotic (codeine, oxycodone, meperidine) groups. Patients who are unable to tolerate the NSAIDs may benefit from a non-narcotic analgesic like acetaminophen. Acetaminophen, a paraphenol derivative, is a pure analgesic with antipyretic but without anti-inflammatory effects. Acetaminophen inhibits central nervous system prostaglandin production but not peripheral production; this corresponds to its activity as an analgesic and antipyretic and its lack of effect as an anti-inflammatory agent. The drug

TABLE 19–7. FACTORS AFFECTING CHOICE OF A NONSTEROIDAL ANTI-INFLAMMATORY DRUG

DRUG CHARACTERISTICS	PATIENT CHARACTERISTICS
Efficacy	Individual variations
Safety	Nature of the disease
Tolerance	Other drugs
Compliance potential	Age
Dose	Severity of disease
Formulation	Time factors
Cost	Pregnancy

is given in doses of 500 to 650 mg every 4 hours. The drug is probably a little less effective as an analgesic than aspirin but there is no gastrointestinal bleeding as there may be with acetylsalicylic acid. In addition, no cross tolerance exists between NSAIDs and acetaminophen. Added analgesic effects can be demonstrated in patients who take both agents simultaneously. The use of both agents occurs in the occasional patient who is on a NSAID and is prescribed Parafon Forte, a drug containing a muscle relaxant and acetaminophen. Acetaminophen should be considered as initial therapy for patients with osteoarthritis of the spine. For elderly patients, this drug has less toxicity than NSAIDs. However, many patients have tried acetaminophen before consulting a physician. In this circumstance, acetaminophen may be used in conjunction with a NSAID. The concomitant use of acetaminophen allows for a lower dose of NSAID to be effective for analgesia since both drugs have a synergistic effect for pain relief.

Patients who experience an acute herniated nucleus pulposus may develop severe low back and radicular pain that is not relieved by NSAIDs alone. These patients may obtain analgesia with the use of codeine 30 to 60 mg every 4 to 6 hours in combination with acetaminophen or aspirin. These medications are given in conjunction with a therapeutic program of home bed rest and temperature modalities.

If stronger analgesia is required, the patient should be admitted to the hospital for parenteral narcotics (meperidine, morphine). These drugs are given on a regular basis, in adequate doses to relieve pain, while the patient receives other therapies. The chance of developing addiction to narcotics during a short course of therapy is small. Therefore, physicians should prescribe sufficient doses of narcotics to provide adequate analgesia.[23] Ketorolac is an effective parenteral or oral analgesic with potency similar to some narcotics.[24] As pain decreases, non-narcotic analgesics are substituted for the more potent narcotic analgesics.

Narcotic analgesics, such as meperidine or oxycodone, should not be given on an outpatient basis, because potential for abuse of these drugs is very great. Patients become tolerant of the analgesic effects of the drugs, require higher and more frequent doses, and can eventually become addicted.[25] Also, patients may use narcotics to shortcut the period of bed rest, which is an essential part of therapy. Patients who attempt to use the drugs as a substitute for bed rest discover that pain re-

turns once the narcotics are discontinued. In unusual circumstances, patients require long-term narcotic therapy. These patients have metastatic cancer to the spine or osteoporotic vertebral compression fractures. In these patients, regular narcotic therapy, such as morphine sulfate in a controlled release form, may allow pain relief so that the patient is functional.[26] Patients who have a definite diagnosis associated with back pain are candidates for this therapy.

There is no role for narcotic analgesia in the therapy of chronic low back pain. Chronic pain patients who take narcotics experience the toxicities of the medications and none of the benefits. Many times these patients need to be detoxified before other therapies can be instituted to control their pain.

References

NONSTEROIDAL ANTI-INFLAMMATORY DRUGS/ANALGESICS

1. Abramson SB, Weissmann G: The mechanisms of action of nonsteroidal anti-inflammatory drugs. Arthritis Rheum 32:1, 1989.
2. Dahl SL: Nonsteroidal anti-inflammatory agents: clinical pharmacology/adverse effects/usage guidelines. In Willkens RF, Dahl SL (eds): Therapeutic Controversies in the Rheumatic Diseases. Orlando: Grune & Stratton, 1987, pp 27–68.
3. Huskisson EC: Non-narcotic analgesics. In: Wall PD, Melzack R (eds): Textbook of Pain. Edinburgh: Churchill Livingstone, 1984, pp 505–513.
4. Paulus HE, Bulpitt KJ: Nonsteroidal anti-inflammatory agents and corticosteroids. In Schumacker HR Jr (ed): Primer of the Rheumatic Diseases, 10th ed. Atlanta: Arthritis Foundation, 1993, pp 298–303.
5. Shaw J, Brooks PM, McNeil JJ, et al.: Therapeutic usage of the nonsteroidal anti-inflammatory drugs. Med J Aus 149:203, 1988.
6. Goldie I: A clinical trial with indomethacin (Indome) in low back pain and sciatica. Acta Orthop Scand 39:117, 1968.
7. Berry H, Bloom B, Hamilton EBD, Swinson DR: Naproxen sodium, diflunisal, and placebo in the treatment of chronic back pain. Ann Rheum Dis 41:129, 1982.
8. Hickey RFJ: Chronic low back pain: a comparison of diflunisal with paracetamol. NZ Med J 95:312, 1982.
9. Wiesel SW, Cuckler JM, DeLuca F, et al.: Acute low back pain: an objective analysis of conservative therapy. Spine 5:324, 1980.
10. Moore RA, McQuay HJ, Carroll O, et al.: Single and mutiple dose analgesic and kinetic studies of mefenamic acid in chronic back pain. Clin J Pain 2:39, 1986.
11. Videman T, Osterman K: Double-blind parallel study of piroxicam versus indomethacin in the treatment of low back pain. Ann Clin Res 16:156, 1984.
12. Brandt KD: Should osteoarthritis be treated with nonsteroidal anti-inflammatory drugs? Rheum Dis Clin North Am 19:697, 1993.
13. Levy M: Aspirin use in patients with major upper gastrointestinal bleeding and peptic ulcer disease. N Engl J Med 290:1158, 1974.

14. Hart FD: Naproxen and gastrointestinal hemorrhage. Br Med J 2:51, 1974.
15. Holdstock DJ: Gastrointestinal bleeding: a possible association with ibuprofen. Lancet 1:541, 1972.
16. Lanza FL: Endoscopic studies of gastric and duodenal injury after the use of ibuprofen, aspirin, and other nonsteroidal anti-inflammatory agents. Am J Med 77:19, 1984.
17. Simon LS, Mills JS: Drug therapy: nonsteroidal anti-inflammatory drugs. N Engl J Med 302:1179, 1237, 1980.
18. Borda IT, Koff RS: NSAIDS: A Profile of Adverse Effects. Philadelphia: Hanley & Belfus, 1992, p 240.
19. Carson JL, Strom BL, Schinnar R, et al.: The low risk of upper gastrointestinal bleeding in patients dispensed corticosteroids. Am J Med 91:223, 1991.
20. Piper JM, Ray WA, Daugherty JR, et al.: Corticosteroid use and peptic ulcer disease: role of nonsteroidal anti-inflammatory drugs. Ann Intern Med 114:735, 1991.
21. Clive DM, Stoff JS: Renal syndrome associated with nonsteroidal anti-inflammatory drugs. N Engl J Med 310:563, 1984.
22. Walt RP: Misoprostol for the treatment of peptic ulcer and anti-inflammatory drug-induced gastroduodenal ulceration. N Engl J Med 327:1575, 1992.
23. Stimmel B: Pain, analgesia, and addiction: an approach to the pharmacologic management of pain. Clin J Pain 1:14, 1985.
24. O'Hara DA, Fragen RJ, Kinzer M, et al.: Ketorolac tromethamine as compared with morphine sulfate for treatment of postoperative pain. Clin Pharmacol Ther 41:556, 1987.
25. Inturrisi CE: Narcotic drugs. Med Clin North Am 66:1061, 1982.
26. Hanks GW, et al.: Controlled-release morphine tablets: a double-blind trial in patients with advanced cancer. Anesthesia 42:840, 1987.

MUSCLE RELAXANTS

Although muscle relaxants have been employed in the treatment of low back pain for a number of years, their use has remained controversial. Not all physicians believe that these agents have a therapeutic role in the care of patients with back pain. There are a number of reasons why this is the case (Table 19–8). Muscle spasm in the low back may have a number of causes, including local pathology and referred mechanisms. No one therapy is effective in all forms of muscle spasm. Muscle relaxants do not relieve spasm in all patients with tonic muscle contraction. Some physicians believe muscle spasm to be a natural, protective mechanism by which the body heals itself; consequently, the dissipation of spasm should occur naturally as the underlying lesion heals and should not be speeded up with medications. Others do not believe that patients with back pain actually experience muscle spasm, since muscles are not damaged in this disorder. The anatomic abnormality is in the annular fibers of the disc. Therefore, muscle relaxants are not useful in improving the condition, since the medications have no effect on healing the disc disorder.

Other reasons for resistance to using muscle relaxants involve their site of action. Many of these drugs do not work on the muscles themselves, but instead act on the central nervous system to modify muscle tone. Differences of opinion exist in regard to the concentration of medication needed in the blood stream to achieve muscle relaxation. Some physicians believe that the concentration obtained in the blood is adequate to affect muscle spindle function. Others think that blood concentration is sufficient to cause sedation only by effects on the central nervous system. In other words these physicians view muscle relaxants as sedatives rather than relaxants and consider them to be ineffective in the therapy of this muscle disorder. In addition, some of these agents have serious potential toxicities including addiction (diazepam). The use of benzodiazepines causes depression, which compounds the difficulties of chronic low back pain patients who are already depressed from long-term pain and disability. Finally, the number of scientific studies that have investigated the role of these agents in the care of patients with low back pain, acute or chronic, is relatively small,[1-8] and the number of studies that actually demonstrate efficacy is even smaller.[9] Therefore, anecdotal evidence and clinical experience are often offered as proof of efficacy, but to some physicians that evidence is inadequate to justify the use of muscle relaxants.[10]

Some of these criticisms of muscle relaxants are valid. These agents are not indicated for all patients with low back pain. However, they do seem to relieve symptoms in carefully selected patients and should not be condemned outright.[2] In our experience, the combination of a muscle relaxant and a NSAID has been effective in decreasing symptoms and improving function, including return to work.[11] Patients with the combination of low back pain and involuntary, chronic muscle contraction

TABLE 19–8. REASONS CITED FOR RESISTANCE TO THE USE OF MUSCLE RELAXANTS IN LOW BACK PAIN

Multiple etiologies of low back spasm (posture, arthritis, referred pain from viscera)
Muscle spasm as ''natural protective mechanism''
Drug effect: central nervous system—sedation
Drug toxicity: addiction, depression (diazepam)
Few scientific studies demonstrating efficacy

benefit from a course of NSAID and muscle relaxant. In a study of patients with acute low back pain and tonic muscle contraction, the combination of naproxen and cyclobenzaprine was more effective than naproxen alone in decreasing pain.[12] A similar study using diflunisal and cyclobenzaprine also demonstrated a beneficial effect by day 4 of the combination therapy compared with placebo.[13]

Pathophysiology of Muscle Spasm

The interrelation of the sensory and motor systems is clearly recognized at the level of the spinal cord. This relationship involves the classic reflex arc in which stretching of a tendon (afferent-sensory input) results in a reflex contraction of the corresponding muscle (efferent-motor output). Adding to this simple arc are inputs from other levels of the spinal cord, the brain stem, and the cerebral cortex, which alter the threshold of the reflex arc. Increased muscle tension may occur as a consequence of intramuscular (trauma, fatigue), perimuscular (arthritis, bone fracture), or referred pain (kidney stone) processes.

Local trauma to muscles may cause reflex spasm. Tissue damage activates nociceptive (unmyelinated) nerve fibers that are distributed through tendons, fascial sheaths, and adventitial sheaths of intramuscular blood vessels. Increased muscle tension decreases muscle movement and allows for the damaged area to heal, usually in a contracted position. In addition to the nociceptive input derived from tissue damage, pain sensations may be generated through muscle fatigue associated with tonic contraction. Muscles that are chronically fatigued become locally painful and tender. This process may occur secondary to chronic contraction associated with trauma or to hyperactivity of muscles associated with poor posture and occupational or sports activities.[14] Muscle spasm may continue while the patient sleeps, as measured by nocturnal EMG recordings.[15] The pain associated with chronic fatigue may be related to the inadequate blood flow that accompanies muscle hyperactivity.[16] That component of muscle pain related to overuse may be relieved with rest and increased blood flow promoted by heat or massage.

Muscle spasm may also occur in response to disease processes in structures to which muscles and tendons attach. Inflammatory processes affecting joints in the axial skeleton can result in reflex muscle spasm, which limits mo-bility. Patients with spondyloarthropathies are prime examples of this mechanism. Patients with sacroiliitis may develop piriformis syndrome with contraction of that muscle and compression of the sciatic nerve. Therapy directed at decreasing joint inflammation, and thereby muscle spasm, decreases the symptoms of this syndrome. Patients who experience vertebral compression fractures develop severe spasm in paraspinous muscles. The muscles contract to splint the fractured bone, limiting painful motion. Once the fracture is diagnosed and pain relieved, muscle spasm diminishes. Continued spasm is not necessary for healing of the fracture. Relief of spasm while the patient limits his activities is appropriate and decreases pain.

Spasm that is secondary to sensory input from organs with common innervation results from the common connections of these nerve fibers in the spinal cord.[17] Abnormalities in the gastrointestinal, genitourinary, and vascular systems may cause reflex spasm in the lumbosacral spine. Therapy must be given to alleviate the primary disorder in order for muscle spasm to be relieved.

Action of Muscle Relaxants

The exact mechanism of action of the muscle relaxants is not known. Depression of polysynaptic, to a greater degree than monosynaptic, reflexes has been reported in animal studies.[18, 19] These effects are mediated through the central nervous system. The area of the central nervous system affected is the lateral reticular area of the brain stem, which monitors the facilitative and inhibitory nerve pathways that affect the activity of the muscle stretch reflexes.[20] The effects of these agents may be mediated through enhanced stimulation of gamma aminobutyric acid (GABA) neurons, which play a significant role in the inhibition of tonic facilitative input from supraspinal sources on motor neurons, both alpha and gamma. This effect on GABA receptors has been associated with the action of benzodiazepines (diazepam).[21] The oral doses of the muscle relaxants are below the levels needed in animal studies to achieve muscle relaxation. As mentioned, this fact has been used by some investigators to conclude that the beneficial effect of muscle relaxants is, in fact, sedation. Clinically, sedation is noted by most patients who ingest any of the members of this group of agents. It should be noted, however, that some patients obtain muscle relaxation without associated sedation.

The oral muscle relaxants have been shown to be better than placebo in acute muscle spasm. There are fewer studies demonstrating efficacy in chronic muscle spasm. Combinations of muscle relaxants and analgesics are more effective than their individual components in the control of muscle spasm.[22] The Drug Efficacy and Safety Implementation Program of the Food and Drug Administration has categorized all such combination products as possibly effective. The muscle relaxants alone do not provide analgesia.

The drugs included in the oral muscle relaxant group are cyclobenzaprine (Flexeril), chlorphenesin (Maolate), orphenadrine citrate (Norflex), chlorzoxazone (Paraflex, Parafon Forte DSC), methocarbamol (Robaxin), metaxalone (Skelaxin), carisoprodol (Soma), and diazepam (Valium). Combinations of these agents with analgesics include the drugs Norgesic, Parafon Forte, Robaxisal, Soma Compound, and Soma Compound with Codeine (Table 19–9).

Muscle relaxants have been studied and found to be better than placebo in both acute and chronic muscle spasm. Both carisoprodol and chlorphenesin were effective in acute but not chronic disorders.[23–26] In studies of acute pain, chlorzoxazone, metaxalone, and methocarbamol were also effective.[27–29] Cyclobenzaprine was compared with placebo in chronic disorders and was found to be superior.[3, 30, 31] Diazepam was not better than placebo in acute and chronic pain in hospitalized patients.[31] In unspecified musculoskeletal disorders, chlorphenesin, chlorzoxazone, and methocarbamol were found better than placebo, but diazepam was not.[6, 32, 33, 34]

Studies comparing muscle relaxants have been completed but the results do not demonstrate the clear superiority of any one agent.[22] Combination tablets appear to be more effective than single agents alone. However, no difference among the combination products was noted.[22]

The major side effect of these agents is drowsiness. Other central nervous system effects include headache, dizziness, and blurred vision. Cyclobenzaprine causes dry mouth. Nausea and vomiting occur rarely with all these agents. Orphenadrine may have a direct depressant and anticholinergic effect upon the heart, which may cause arrhythmias and cardiac arrest at lethal doses of 2 to 3 gm. Chronic use of carisoprodol may be associated with tolerance for the drug. Patients may ask for increasing doses of the medicine for the same muscle relaxing effect.

We have found muscle relaxants to be useful in patients who, on examination, have palpable evidence of muscle spasm or who have difficulty sleeping because of muscle pain. These patients may be experiencing spasm although their primary symptom is pain.[15] While superior efficacy has not been demonstrated for any one muscle relaxant, the chemical properties of cyclobenzaprine are very useful in the clinical setting. The drug is not combined with any analgesic, so it can be used with any of the nonsteroidals or analgesics. Its long half-life equates with once a day dosing in many patients. The medication is given 2 hours before sleep; this time interval allows the medicine to build up in the blood stream so that the patient is sleepy at the appropriate time. The patient awakens the next day feeling rested and not drowsy. If 10 mg causes drowsiness, the tablet may be cut in half; 5 mg is an adequate dose for many patients.

The sedation that occurs in some patients helps them to remain on bed rest, a key part of the therapeutic regimen of patients with acute pain. The sedation associated with the drug is not a toxicity but is a part of therapy. This sedative effect diminishes over time with continued use of the drug. The drug is continued for up to 2 weeks in patients with acute spasm. Patients are easily tapered off the medicine without any withdrawal symptoms. If there is no response to cyclobenzaprine, chlorzoxazone, orphenadrine, methocarbamol, or carisoprodol may be substituted (Table 19–9). Higher dosages and more frequent administration are necessary to achieve adequate levels of these other medications. These agents belong to different chemical groups, and as with the NSAIDs, a lack of response to one agent does not equate with inefficacy of the whole group of drugs. A series of agents may be tried before an efficacious and well-tolerated agent is found. The total dose of medication and frequency of administration must be individualized. Occasionally, combination tablets (Parafon Forte, Robaxisal) are used. These preparations are convenient because the muscle relaxant and analgesic are in the same tablet, but the amount of medicine is fixed, limiting the flexibility in dosage that some patients require.

Diazepam is a muscle relaxant that is not used in our back pain clinics. While the evidence for efficacy of this agent in back spasm is meager, its toxicities are real and troublesome. One cannot predict which patients with

TABLE 19–9. ORAL MUSCLE RELAXANTS

DRUG	BRAND NAME	TABLET/CAPSULE SIZE (mg)	DOSE (mg/day)	FREQUENCY (times/day)	ONSET (hours)	DURATION (hours)	HALF-LIFE	MAJOR TOXICITY	EXCRETION	COMMENTS
Cyclobenzaprine hydrochloride	Flexeril	10	20–60	3	1–2	12–24	1–3 days	Drowsiness, dry mouth, dizziness	Kidney, stool	10 mg 2 hours before sleep may be adequate dose with half-life; Caution: angle closure glaucoma, prostatic hypertrophy, myocardial infarction
Chlorphenesin carbamate	Maolate	400	1600–2400	3–4	3	4–6	5 hours	Drowsiness, dizziness	Kidney	
Orphenadrine citrate	Norflex	100	200	2	2	4–6	14 hours	Blurred vision, dry mouth, urinary retention	Kidney, stool	Intravenous form for therapy of acute spasm (Norgesic includes aspirin and caffeine)
	Norgesic	30 mg/dl								
Chlorzoxazone	Paraflex Parafon Forte DSC	250 500	1500–3000	3–4	1	3–4	1 hour	Drowsiness, dizziness	Kidney	Parafon Forte includes acetaminophen; Contraindicated—history of liver disease
Methocarbamol	Robaxin Robaxisal	500, 750 100 mg/dl	6000	4–6	1	3	2 hours	Dizziness, blurred vision	Kidney, stool	Intravenous form for acute spasm, tetanus (Robaxisal includes aspirin)
Metaxalone	Skelaxin	400	2400–3200	3–4	1	4–6	2–3 hours	Drowsiness	Kidney	Extreme weakness; Temporary loss of vision (rare); Mild withdrawal symptoms with abrupt cessation
Carisoprodol	Soma	350	1400	4	1	4–6	8 hours	Drowsiness	Kidney	Contraindicated—acute intermittent porphyria (Soma compound includes aspirin)
Diazepam	Valium	2, 5, 10 (5 mg/ml, 15 slow release)	4–40	4	1	8–12	24 hours	Drowsiness	Kidney	Withdrawal symptoms with abrupt cessation; Depression with prolonged use

acute low back pain will go on to develop chronic low back pain and depression. Diazepam will only worsen the depression and drug dependence of these patients. The drug is not indicated in this disorder.

It should be remembered that the use of muscle relaxants is not limited to traumatic muscle strain alone. Patients with arthritic conditions, particularly the spondyloarthropathies, may benefit from long-term use of a muscle relaxant. The following case is presented as an example of a patient with a spondyloarthropathy who had greater mobility because of the use of a muscle relaxant:

Case Study 19–1: J.A. is a 46-year-old white man admitted to the hospital because of neck, right buttock, left index finger, left great toe, and right heel pain that developed over a 3-week period after a fall from a 2-foot garden wall. The patient had marked limitation of cervical motion in all directions, associated with marked paravertebral muscle spasm. Swollen joints included the right knee, ankle, and heel and left great toe, and index finger. The diagnosis of incomplete Reiter's syndrome was made and the patient was started on indomethacin 50 mg t.i.d., which was increased to 75 mg slow-release t.i.d. The patient's lower and upper extremity arthritis improved, but severe muscle spasm of the cervical spine continued. Cyclobenzaprine 10 mg b.i.d. was added and the patient had gradual improvement in his neck motion. There was an exacerbation of symptoms after discharge from the hospital. Cyclobenzaprine was increased to 30 mg/day and prednisone 10 mg/day was added. Over the next 2 months, the patient's symptoms gradually resolved. One year after discharge, the patient was able to discontinue prednisone therapy. Attempts at reducing cyclobenzaprine were associated with decreased neck motion. The patient remains on indomethacin 75 mg b.i.d. and cyclobenzaprine 10 mg at night. He is active and is able to complete a full day's work without difficulty. He volunteers the fact that he believes that the muscle relaxant played a substantial role in his recovery.

An anecdotal case report does not prove efficacy scientifically. However, clinical observation is a reasonable means to study the effects of therapeutic interventions. Other patients with spondyloarthropathies have been placed on muscle relaxants and have noted decreased pain and improved motion with the addition of a muscle relaxant to the NSAID. Muscle relaxants are not indicated for all patients with back pain. In the carefully chosen patient, however, their use can relieve symptoms while the natural course of healing unfolds.

References

MUSCLE RELAXANTS

1. Baratta RR: A double-blind comparative study of carisoprodol, proxyphene, and placebo in the management of low back syndrome. Curr Ther Res 20:233, 1976.
2. Hindle TH: Comparison of carisoprodol, butabarbital, and placebo in treatment of the low back syndrome. Calif Med 117:7, 1972.
3. Brown BR, Womble J: Cyclobenzaprine in intractable pain syndromes with muscle spasm. JAMA 240:1151, 1978.
4. Hingorani K: Diazepam in backaches: a double-blind controlled trial. Ann Phys Med 8:303, 1966.
5. Gready DM: Parafon Forte versus Robaxisal in skeletal muscle disorders: a double-blind study. Curr Ther Res 20:666, 1976.
6. Valtonen EJ: A double-blind trial of methocarbamol versus placebo in painful muscle spasm. Curr Med Res Opin 3:382, 1975.
7. McGuinness BW: A double-blind comparison in general practice of a combination tablet containing orphenadrine citrate and paracetamol (Norgesic) with paracetamol alone. J Int Med Res 11:42, 1983.
8. Gordon EF: Carisoprodol in the treatment of musculoskeletal disorders of the back. Am J Orthop 5:106, 1963.
9. Deyo RA: Conservative therapy for low back pain: Distinguishing useful from useless therapy. JAMA 250:1057, 1983.
10. Hadler NM: Diagnosis and treatment of backache. In Hadler NM (ed): Medical Management of the Regional Musculoskeletal Diseases. Orlando: Grune & Stratton, 1984, pp 3–52.
11. Borenstein D, Feffer H, Wiesel S: Low back pain (LBP): an orthopedic and medical approach. Clin Res 33:757A, 1985.
12. Borenstein, DG, Lacks S, Wiesel SW: Cyclobenzaprine and naproxen versus naproxen alone in the treatment of acute low back pain and muscle spasm. Clin Ther 12;125, 1990.
13. Basmajian JV: Acute back pain and spasm: a controlled multicenter trial of combined analgesic and antispasm agents. Spine 14:438, 1989.
14. Simons DG: Muscle pain syndrome, Part II. Am J Phys Med 55:15, 1976.
15. Fischer AA, Chang CH: Electromyographic evidence of paraspinal muscle spasm during sleep in patients with low back pain. Clin J Pain 1:147, 1985.
16. Kuroda E, Klissouras V, Mulsum JH: Electrical and metabolic activities and fatigue in human isometric contraction. J Appl Physiol 29:358, 1970.
17. Kerr FWL: Neuroanatomical substrates of nociception in the spinal cord. Pain 1:325, 1975.
18. Smith CM: Relaxants of skeletal muscle. In Root WS, Hoffman FG (eds): Physiological Pharmacology, Vol II. New York: Academic Press, 1965, pp 1–96.
19. Roszkowski AP: A pharmacological comparison of therapeutically useful centrally-acting skeletal muscle relaxants. J Pharmacol Exp Ther 129:75, 1970.
20. Ginzel KH: The blockade of reticular and spinal facilitation of motor function by orphenadrine. J Pharmacol Exp Ther 154:128, 1966.
21. Study RE, Barker JL: Cellular mechanisms of benzodiazepine action. JAMA 247:2147, 1982.
22. Elenbaas JK: Centrally acting oral skeletal muscle relaxants. Am J Hosp Pharm 37:1313, 1980.
23. Cullen AP: Carisoprodol (Soma) in acute back conditions: a double-blind randomized, placebo-controlled study. Curr Ther Res Clin Exp 20:557, 1976.
24. Turner R, Rockwood CA: Chlorphenesin carbamate (Maolate) in the relief of muscle pain. Mil Med 132:371, 1967.
25. Jones AC: Role of carisoprodol in physical medicine. Ann NY Acad Sci 86:226, 1960.

26. Waltham-Weeks CD: The analgesic properties of chlorphenesin carbamate in the treatment of osteoarthrosis. Ann Phys Med 9:197, 1967–1968.
27. Ogden HD, Shackett L: Controlled studies of chlorzoxazone and chlorzoxazone-acetaminophen in treatment of myalgia associated with headache. South Med J 53:1415, 1960.
28. Dent RW, Ervin DK: A study of metaxalone (Skelaxin) vs placebo in acute musculoskeletal disorders: A cooperative study. Curr Ther Res Clin Exp 18:433, 1975.
29. Tisdale SA, Ervin DK: A controlled study of methocarbamol (Robaxin) in acute painful musculoskeletal conditions. Curr Ther Res Clin Exp 17:525, 1975.
30. Bercel NA: Cyclobenzaprine in the treatment of skeletal muscle spasm in osteoarthritis of the cervical and lumbar spine. Curr Ther Res Clin Exp 22:462, 1977.
31. Basmajian JV: Cyclobenzaprine hydrochloride effect on skeletal muscle in the lumbar region and neck: two double-blind controlled clinical and laboratory studies. Arch Phys Med Rehabil 59:58, 1978.
32. Kolodny AL: Controlled clinical evaluation of a new muscle relaxant—chlorphenesin carbamate. Psychosomatics 4:161, 1963.
33. Schiener JJ: Evaluation of combined muscle relaxant–analgesic as an effective therapy for painful skeletal muscle spasm. Curr Ther Res Clin Exp 14:168, 1972.
34. Payne RW, Xorenson EJ, Smalley TK, Brandt EN Jr: Diazepam, meprobamate, and placebo in musculoskeletal disorders. JAMA 188:229, 1964.

ANTIDEPRESSANTS

During the past 30 years, tricyclic antidepressants (TCAs) have been widely used for the treatment of chronic pain in patients with or without depression.[1, 2] The mechanism of action that results in pain relief remains unknown, although a number of theories have been proposed. In addition, the factors that might better predict a beneficial response to these drugs by chronic pain patients remain to be determined.[3]

Mechanism of Action

The basis for a response of pain to TCAs seems to be related to alterations in the central nervous system associated with chronic pain. Sternbach postulated that chronic pain results in depression, which is associated with depletion of serotonin in the brain. TCAs, which increase serotonin levels, might therefore be associated with pain relief.[4] This hypothesis was tested in a study using fenfluramine, a drug that causes a relatively selective release of serotonin, at a dose of 40 mg/day. This drug transiently reduced both chronic pain and depression in some patients, supporting this hypothesis.[5]

Another popular theory involves the activation of the endogenous opiate system in the central nervous system by TCAs. TCAs can exert analgesic effects either directly or indirectly on the endogenous opiate system.[6] TCAs can increase the low levels of endogenous opiates in patients with organic pain.[7]

As a neurotransmitter, serotonin may also play an important role as an inhibitor of pain. The pain inhibitory pathway descends from the raphe nuclei in the brainstem via the lateral columns of the dorsal spinal cord to the superficial laminae (substantia gelatinosa) of the dorsal horn.[8] Antinociceptive effects are generated by the application of serotonin and norepinephrine to the substantia gelatinosa in animal models.[9] From anatomic and neurophysiologic data, serotonergic pathways significantly modify transmission of nociceptive impulses.

Reduction of anxiety and relief of muscle tension may also decrease low back pain. Amitriptyline, a sedating antidepressant, has been associated with pain relief in individuals with chronic muscle tension.[10]

Pain relief by antidepressants also may be ascribed to therapy of masked depression. Pain may be a part of the symptom complex of the depressed patient. Although this may play a part in the resolution of symptoms, studies have demonstrated improvement in pain but not depression in depressed patients with chronic pain treated with TCAs.[11]

TCAs work by inhibiting the uptake of serotonin and/or norepinephrine by the nerve terminal that released them, thereby increasing the concentration of the neurotransmitter in the synapse. Increased neurotransmitter concentrations amplify the tone in corresponding neural pathways where these substances are neurotransmitters. TCAs that have been associated with potentiation of serotonin and related pain relief include imipramine, amitriptyline, doxepin, and desipramine.

A few clinical studies have investigated the use of TCAs in patients with chronic low back pain. Two double-blind studies comparing imipramine and placebo generated conflicting results. In a study using low-dose imipramine for a 4-week period, no difference was noted between imipramine and placebo.[12] In contrast, a study using higher doses for an 8-week period found statistically significant improvement with imipramine compared with placebo.[2] Doxepin has been found to be effective in reducing pain compared with placebo in clinical studies. Hameroff showed antidepressant doses of doxepin to be superior to placebo.[1]

TABLE 19–10. SELECTED ANTIDEPRESSANTS

CLASS	PAIN DOSE (mg)	DEPRESSION DOSE (mg)	SEDATION (Grade 1–4)
Tricyclic Tertiary Amines			
Imipramine (Tofranil)	10–75	200	3+
Amitriptyline (Elavil)	10–100	300	4+
Doxepin (Sinequan)	10–100	300	4+
Nortriptyline (Pamelor)	10–100	300	3+
Tricyclic Secondary Amines			
Desipramine (Norpramin)	10–100	300	1+

In Ward's study 60% of patients experienced pain reduction with doxepin and desipramine.[3] The findings supported the hypothesis of low serotonin concentrations being associated with chronic pain. Those patients who responded to fenfluramine were the same ones who were more likely to have pain relief with either antidepressant. Levels of endorphins, pain tolerance, and EMG findings were unaltered by the medications. Sedation was not a key factor in that the nonsedating drug (desipramine) was as effective as the sedating agent (doxepin). Patients, with or without depression, or with or without physical trauma, responded equally well. Doxepin has also been shown to be effective in patients with back pain who have failed other therapies.[13]

Amitriptyline, the agent with the greatest serotonergic activity, is also associated with pain relief in patients with chronic back pain. In a double-blind study, amitriptyline was associated with a significant decrease in the use of analgesics but no measurable change in activity level in patients with low back pain.[14]

The use of TCAs in the treatment of chronic back pain is not totally benign. In one study, 100% of patients taking TCAs developed side effects, however minor.[15] The toxicities of these agents are nicely summarized by Dudley Hart.[16]

[The TCAs] should be used with extreme caution in cardiovascular disease, liver disorders, epilepsy, patients with known suicidal tendencies, conditions where an anticholinergic agent would be undesirable, for example, glaucoma, urinary retention and pyloric stenosis, prostatic hypertrophy, pregnancy. Barbiturates alter the pharmacologic effects of tricyclic antidepressants, which can in turn alter the action of other drugs administered concurrently including other antidepressants (especially MAOIs); alcohol; some antihypertensives, for example methyldopa and guanethidine; anticholinergics and local anaesthetics with noradrenaline.

These toxicities are particularly troublesome in the elderly, who are more prone to the diseases and drug-related complications.[17]

In contrast to the use of TCAs in depression, the dose for analgesia should be kept low and raised slowly in light of the patient's clinical response.[18] Reaching antidepressant levels of 150 mg of amitriptyline has not been necessary in chronic pain patients. The drug is taken as a single dose, 2 hours before bedtime. Ten milligrams of amitriptyline is the initial dose, which may be increased to 25 mg within 2 to 3 weeks. Over the following 8 weeks, the dose may be increased to 75 to 100 mg. It is rare to use larger doses unless the patient is clinically depressed. The therapeutic ranges of the TCAs are listed in Table 19–10.

Newer antidepressants—fluoxetine, sertraline, and bupropion—are effective for treating depression, but their efficacy for pain relief similar to the tricyclic antidepressants has not been established. Studies in the future may demonstrate efficacy in low back pain patients making them a worthwhile addition to the drug therapy for chronic low back pain. The TCAs are relatively safe at the doses that are effective in patients with chronic pain. In patients with back pain who have failed other therapies, a trial of TCAs is indicated. The choice of agent is determined by the physician's familiarity with the individual TCAs and the need for sedation (amitriptyline). The trial should be continued for a number of weeks unless toxicity intervenes.

References

ANTIDEPRESSANTS

1. Hameroff SR, Crago BR, Cork RC, et al.: Doxepin effects on chronic pain, depression, and serum opioids. Anesth Analg 61:187, 1982.
2. Alcoff J, Jones E, Rust P, Newman R: Controlled trial of imipramine for chronic low back pain. J Fam Pract 14:841, 1982.
3. Ward NG: Tricyclic antidepressants for chronic low

back pain: mechanisms of action and predictors of response. Spine 11:661, 1986.

4. Sternbach RA: The need for an animal model of chronic pain. Pain 2:2, 1976.

5. Clineschmidt BV, Zacchei AG, Totaro JA, et al.: Fenfluramine and brain serotonin. Ann NY Acad Sci 305:222, 1978.

6. Spiegel K, Kalb R, Pasternak GW: Analgesic activity of tricyclic antidepressants. Ann Neurol 13:462, 1983.

7. Ward NG, Blood VL, Dworkin S, et al.: Psychobiological markers in coexisting pain and depression: toward a unified theory. J Clin Psychiatry 43:8(Sec 2)32, 1982.

8. Oliveras JL, Bourgoin S, Hery F, et al.: The topographical distribution of serotonergic terminals in the spinal cord of the cat. Biochemical mapping by the combined use of microdissection and microassay procedures. Brain Res 138:393, 1977.

9. Headley PM, Duggan AW, Griersmith BT: Selective reduction by noradrenaline and 5-hydroxytryptamine of nociceptive responses of cat dorsal horn neurons. Brain Res 145:185, 1978.

10. Lance JW, Curran DA: Treatment of chronic tension headache. Lancet 1:1236, 1964.

11. Watson CP, Evans RJ, Reed K, et al.: Amitriptyline versus placebo in post herpetic neuralgia. Neurology 32:671, 1982.

12. Jenkins DG, Ebbutt AF, Evans CD: Tofranil in the treatment of low back pain. J Int Med Res 4(Suppl 2):28, 1976.

13. Hameroff SR, Cork RC, Weiss JL, et al.: Doxepin effects on chronic pain and depression: a controlled study. Clin J Pain 1:171, 1985.

14. Pheasant H, Bursk A, Goldfarb J, et al.: Amitriptyline and chronic low-back pain: a randomized double-blind crossover study. Spine 8:552, 1983.

15. Pilowsky I, Hallett EC, Basset DL, et al.: A controlled study of amitriptyline in the treatment of chronic pain. Pain 14:169, 1982.

16. Hart FD: The use of psychotropic drugs in rheumatology. J Int Med Res 4(Suppl 2):15, 1976.

17. Shillcutt SD, Easterday JL, Anderson RJ: Geriatric pharmacology, part I: antidepressant medications. Hosp Formul 19:941, 1984.

18. Hollister LE: Treatment of depression with drugs. Ann Intern Med 88:78, 1978.

ELECTROTHERAPY

Transcutaneous Electrical Nerve Stimulation

Evidence has been reported suggesting that transcutaneous electrical nerve stimulation (TENS) therapy may alleviate chronic pain including back pain. The exact mechanism by which electrical current decreases pain is unknown, although there are a number of hypotheses. Most reports have assumed that TENS activates larger diameter afferent A-alpha nerve fibers. The input through these nerves presumably activates an intraneural network that pre- or post-synaptically inhibits ongoing transmission of nociceptive impulses supplied through the small C unmyelinated and alpha-D fibers or inhibits the C fibers directly.[1,2] TENS preferentially stimulates the low-threshold A-alpha fibers.[3] The effect of TENS on pain modulation does not seem to be directly related to endogenous opiates. Naloxone, an inhibitor of endogenous and exogenous opiates, failed to reverse the effect of high-frequency TENS in patients with acute and chronic pain.[4]

Electrical stimulation to the nerves may be accomplished by TENS using surface electrodes applied to the skin, subcutaneous implanted electrodes, or electrodes implanted directly on the nerve or dorsal column with stimulation applied directly to the spinal cord or through the dura. The transcutaneous stimulator is most frequently used.

The basic equipment for TENS therapy is an electrical pulse generator and transcutaneous electrodes. The pulses produced by the generator may be high-frequency, low-frequency, or variable-frequency. The pulse generator feeds its output to an amplifier that increases the signal to a level that delivers current to the electrodes. The wave forms most commonly used are rectangular and spike. The rectangular wave form can be adjusted for amplitude and pulse width, while the spike form can be modified by amplitude alone. TENS therapy uses alternating current to limit the flow of material on the surface of the skin (electrode gel) into subdermal structures resulting in irritation.

The electrodes receive the current and produce an electric field that excites the afferent fibers in the neighboring peripheral nerve. The current must be delivered without damaging the skin. The most widely used electrodes are silicone rubber impregnated with carbon particles. The electrodes are flexible and follow the contours of the body. An aquaphilic gel is needed to reduce skin resistance to facilitate current transmission and the electrodes must be taped appropriately to maintain a tight fit with the underlying skin; poor contact may result in sparking and damage to the skin. Disposable and reusable electrodes that have preapplied gel and adhesive are available, but they are more expensive and detach from the skin more easily, particularly when the patient perspires.

The choice of electrode placement depends on the location of the pain. The electrodes may be placed directly over the area, within the dermatome or myotome, or over a superficial peripheral nerve. The optimal site of stimulation is proximal to the painful area. The closer the electrodes are to the nerve, the lower the current required to stimulate the appropriate nerve fibers. Patients with back and radicular pain may benefit from electrodes placed on the leg in the distribution of the radiated pain in addition to electrodes placed over the lumbosacral area (Fig. 19–8) It is not possible to predict the most effective site for electrode placement, and different locations may need to be tested before the optimal site is identified. Some patients will need bilateral stimulation even in the circumstance of unilateral pain.[5]

Once the electrodes are placed, wave form parameters are altered to maximize pain relief. The parameters that can be modified are pulse rate, width, and amplitude. The rate regulates the number of electrical impulses delivered per second (pps). The range is from 2 to 200 pps, with 2 to 150 pps the most commonly used rates. The pulse width determines the duration of each impulse. A range of 50 to 250 μsec is commonly used. The amplitude of the signal is measured in milliamperes (mA).

Various combinations of rate, width, and amplitude will have a marked effect on the signal that reaches the stimulated area. The conventional mode of TENS therapy utilizes a high pulse rate (80 to 100 pps) and low pulse width (less than 100 μsec). The amplitude is increased until a tingling sensation is felt in the stimulated area. The aim is to activate large sensory myelinated fibers without producing muscle contraction or dysesthesias.

Other signal forms may be uncomfortable and are used only for short periods of time. High pulse width at low rates (2 to 4 pps) stimulates nerves at the superficial to deep levels and may cause muscle contraction. Like acupuncture, this form of TENS may stimulate endogenous opiate (endorphin) production.[6] Burst mode uses a low rate (4 pps) of a series of impulses (7 in number). The pulse width is wide and the amplitude high. In the burst mode, which is useful for chronic, deep pain,[7] rhythmic muscle contraction occurs. The subcutaneous and cutaneous nerves are stimulated with high rate, wide width, and high amplitude settings. Newer units allow the operator to alternate between modes that stimulate deep and superficial structures. This switching between modes may help prevent adaptation to TENS therapy.

The induction time for TENS to produce analgesia ranges from immediately to several hours, the average time being 20 minutes. The effect of TENS therapy may be cumulative in patients with chronic pain. Patients may not experience pain relief if duration of stimulation is limited to 30 minutes or less.[8] Therefore, TENS therapy should be used for a minimum of 30 minutes at a time. The pain relief from TENS may be present only during the stimulation or may last for an extended period of time.[9]

TENS therapy may be indicated for patients with acute or chronic pain. It has been used to decrease postoperative pain in patients who have undergone lumbar spine operations.[10] Patients with chronic pain from back conditions or neurogenic injuries have had pain relief with TENS therapy as well.[11, 12] Patients who have psychogenic pain not infrequently have increased discomfort with TENS therapy.[13]

Is TENS therapy better than placebo for the treatment of low back pain? Although TENS has been shown to be helpful in other pain conditions, a controlled trial has not been reported.[14] TENS, like other forms of pain therapy, has a significant placebo component.[15] In the early stages of therapy, it produces 60% to 80% relief of chronic pain. The placebo effect portion of the response quickly falls off while the therapeutic efficacy of TENS decreases more slowly, so that between 20% and 30% continue to experience pain relief at 1 year.[11] Patients with radicular symptoms and sciatic pain may benefit from TENS therapy.[16] This modality may also be helpful in patients with back pain without sciatica.

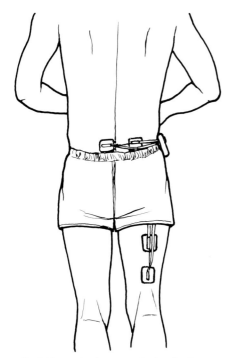

Figure 19–8. Electrode placement for low back pain radiating to the posterior aspect of the right thigh.

In an attempt to answer the concerns about the efficacy of TENS for treatment of low back pain, Deyo and coworkers designed a randomly assigned, controlled trial of TENS therapy for 145 patients divided into four groups: TENS alone, 36 subjects; TENS plus exercise, 37; sham TENS alone, 36; and sham TENS plus exercise, 36.[17] TENS therapy was employed over the maximum point of tenderness for 45 minutes, 3 times a day. The exercise program consisted of 13 exercises, including relaxation, stretching, and bending. Measurement of outcome included functional status, physical measures, and the use of medical services. Improvement was demonstrated in all four groups during the 4-week study but was diminished at the 3-month follow-up period. Exercise was the factor that was most closely associated with improvement. TENS was not a significant factor in improvement. Criticisms of this study have raised a number of issues including the improper placement of electrodes and improper machine settings. Jenkner suggests for optimal results, TENS must be set for monophasic pulses, using a frequency of 20 to 60 pulses per second, with unequal size electrodes on specific locations without modifications by the patient.[18] Other criticisms included inadequacy of blinding patients when physical therapies are involved. Deyo has responded to these criticisms suggesting that controls were appropriate for the TENS study.[19]

We offer TENS therapy applied by our physical therapists to patients with localized, chronic low back pain of traumatic origin. It is most useful in patients who experience limitations at work because of pain. The use of TENS therapy allows these patients to complete a usual day's work with much less discomfort. They can also use the units during recreational activities or activities of daily living. These patients use the units on an intermittent basis and have found this to be a way to sustain the beneficial effects of the therapy. Patients are always advised to rent, not buy, units initially. Only after a period of months of sustained pain relief should they buy their units. Whether through a placebo effect or direct effect on the nervous system, TENS therapy does help patients with back pain become more functional. However, in patients with chronic back pain who respond to TENS, the beneficial effect may not last. In a study of back pain using TENS therapy, a gradual reduction in efficacy occurred over a 2-month period.[18] TENS should be thought of as only a temporary therapy to be used while the patient tries to increase his physical status.

High-Voltage Stimulation

High-voltage stimulation is a form of TENS that utilizes high-voltage, monophasic pulses of short duration to stimulate soft tissue structures in the lumbosacral spine. High-voltage stimulation may be particularly helpful in eliminating persistent muscle spasm. Repeated electrical stimulation relaxes protective muscle spasm, thereby decreasing muscle fatigue. Patients may be able to exercise or stretch the muscle in spasm once electrical stimulation has been applied to the superficial area over the muscle. Electrical stimulation of muscles may maintain strength and endurance. In a 4-week controlled study, electrical muscle stimulation increased trunk endurance and strength in healthy women.[20] The ability of electrical muscle stimulation to increase strength of injured muscle requires additional study. This form of therapy may be considered only an adjunct to a therapy program, including active strengthening exercises.

Iontophoresis

Iontophoresis, also called common ion transfer, uses direct current, as opposed to the alternating current of TENS, to induce the transfer of an ion across a body surface. A variety of medications including corticosteroids, epinephrine, and local anesthetics may enter soft tissue without an injection. A study by Russo demonstrated that patients derived an equal amount of analgesia from an injection of lidocaine and lidocaine iontophoresis.[21] Harris reported on 50 patients with inflammatory musculoskeletal conditions; about 76% had marked relief of pain with iontophoresis of a solution composed of lidocaine and dexamethasone.[22] This technique may be of benefit to a patient with localized areas of pain that are irritated by injection. Pain may be diminished by iontophoresis with the instillation of a local anesthetic (lidocaine 4% solution) alone or in combination with a soluble corticosteroid. The effectiveness of iontophoresis continues to be studied. The beneficial effect of the therapy may not rely solely on the medication but also the effects of direct electrical current on tissues.[23]

Another proposed electrical therapy for low back pain is laser therapy. Lasers emit coherent photons that interact with biologic molecules to produce chemical reactions in the body. The use of laser in chronic back pain was no better than exercises alone in the treatment of pain.[24]

References

ELECTROTHERAPY

1. Woolf CJ: Transcutaneous and implanted nerve stimulation. In Wall PD, Melzack R (eds): Textbook of Pain. Edinburgh: Churchill Livingstone, 1986, pp 679–690.
2. Campbell JN, Taub A: Local analgesia from percutaneous electrical stimulation. Arch Neurol 28:347, 1973.
3. Bloedel J, McCreery D: Organization of peripheral and central pain pathways. Surg Neurol 4:65, 1975.
4. Abrams SE, Reynolds AC, Cusick JF: Failure of naloxone to reverse analgesia from transcutaneous electrical stimulation in patients with chronic pain. Anaesth Analg 60:81, 1981.
5. Picaza J, Cannon BW, Hunter SE, et al.: Pain suppression by peripheral nerve stimulation: Part 1. Observation with transcutaneous stimuli. Surg Neurol 4:105, 1975.
6. Sjolund B, Eriksson M: Endorphins and analgesia produced by peripheral conditioning stimulation. In Bonica JJ, Liebeskind JC, Albe-Fessard DG (eds): Advances in Pain Research and Therapy, Vol 3. New York: Raven Press, 1979, pp 587–591.
7. Eriksson MB, Sjolund BH, Nielzen S: Long term results of peripheral conditioning stimulation as an analgesia measure in chronic pain. Pain 6:335, 1979.
8. Wolf SL, Gersh MR, Rao VK: Examination of electrode placement and stimulating parameters in treating chronic pain with conventional transcutaneous electrical nerve stimulation (TENS). Pain 11:37, 1981.
9. Meyer GA, Fields HL: Causalgia treated by selective large fiber stimulation of peripheral nerves. Brain 95:163, 1972.
10. Solomon RA, Viernstein MC, Long DM: Reduction of postoperative pain and narcotic use by transcutaneous electrical nerve stimulation. Surgery 87:142, 1980.
11. Bates JAV, Nathan PW: Transcutaneous electrical nerve stimulation for chronic pain. Anaesthesia 35:817, 1980.
12. Cauthen JC, Renner EJ: Transcutaneous and peripheral nerve stimulation for chronic pain states. Surg Neurol 4:102, 1975.
13. Nielzen S, Sjolund BH, Eriksson MB: Psychiatric factors influencing the treatment of pain with peripheral conditioning stimulation. Pain 13:365, 1982.
14. Deyo RA: Conservative therapy for low back pain: distinguishing useful from useless therapy. JAMA 250:1057, 1983.
15. Thorsteinsson G, Stonnington HH, Stillwell GK, Elveback LR: The placebo effect of transcutaneous electrical stimulation. Pain 5:31, 1978.
16. Anderson SA: Pain control by sensory stimulation. In Bonica JJ, Liebeskind JC, Albe-Fessard DG: Advances in Pain Research and Therapy, Vol 3. New York: Raven Press, 1979, pp 569–585.
17. Deyo RA, Walsh NE, Martin DC, et al.: A controlled trial of transcutaneous electrical nerve stimulation (TENS) and exercise for chronic low back pain. N Engl J Med 322:1627, 1990.
18. Jenkner FL: TENS—an international perspective. Phys Ther 73:64, 1993.
19. Deyo RA, Walsh NE, Schoenfeld LS, et al.: Can trials of physical treatments be blinded? The example of transcutaneous electrical stimulation for chronic pain. Am J Phys Med Rehabil 69:6, 1990.
20. Kahanovitz N, Nordin M, Verderame R, et al.: Normal trunk muscle strength and endurance in women and the effect of exercises and electrical stimulation. Part 2: Comparative analysis of electrical stimulation and exercises to increase trunk muscle strength and endurance. Spine 12:112, 1987.
21. Russo J Jr, Lipman AG, Comstock TJ, et al.: Lidocaine anesthesia: comparison of iontophoresis, injection, and swabbing. Am J Hosp Pharm 37:843, 1980.
22. Harris PR: Iontophoresis: clinical research in musculoskeletal inflammatory conditions. J Orthop Sports Phys Ther 4:109, 1982.
23. Chantraine A, Ludy JP, Berger D: Is cortisone iontophoresis possible? Arch Phys Med Rehabil 67:38, 1986.
24. Klein RG, Eek BC: Low-energy laser treatment and exercise for chronic low back pain: double-blind controlled trial. Arch Phys Med Rehabil 71:34, 1990.

BACK SCHOOL

As part of the nonsurgical management of patients with back pain, back schools have been developed to educate patients to be better able to manage their own back problems. The modern back school was developed in 1969 in Sweden by Zachrisson-Forssell.[1] The basic concept behind the school was that if patients understand the anatomic, epidemiologic, and biomechanical factors that give rise to low back pain, they will be better able to control their back problems in activities of daily living. Education will help patients take responsibility for management of their spine problems. In patients with back pain, particularly those with chronic pain whose daily activities are curtailed, the encouragement to take responsibility for treatment of their back problems is an essential part of therapy.

Back schools may be used to prevent initial episodes of back pain or as part of a treatment program to prevent recurrent attacks; most schools deal primarily with prevention of recurrences. The goals of the back school in the short run are to reduce pain, encourage appropriate rest, and emphasize the good prognosis of most back pain problems. Teaching patients proper body mechanics, to develop coping skills for episodes of pain, to accept shared responsibility for their recovery, and to improve their general physical condition to help prevent recurrent back pain are the long-range goals.[2]

The methods used by back schools to teach patients may be cognitive (classroom instruction of basic facts), physical (demonstrations of appropriate exercises and work habits), and motivational (encouragement to be an active participant in their own care). A number of back schools have been developed that utilize a combination of these methods.

The Swedish Back School is designed as a general information program for patients with acute and chronic pain who can use knowledge about their back to be more active in their treatment program. The program also emphasizes the prevention of recurrences.[3] The school consists of four 45-minute lessons, given over a 2-week period. There are eight patients in a class, which is taught by a physiotherapist. The initial lesson, utilizing audiovisual materials, includes information on epidemiology, anatomy, function of the back, treatment modalities, and positions for resting. Subsequent lessons cover back strain associated with poor posture and work activities, ways to decrease physical strain, and general methods to improve physical conditioning.

The Canadian Back School is oriented toward the treatment of chronic low back pain through psychologic approaches to encourage patients to assume responsibility for their own health.[4] The faculty of the Canadian school includes an orthopedist, physiotherapist, psychiatrist, and psychologist who give 90-minute lectures on four successive weeks to 20 patients. The content of the initial 2 weeks of classes is similar to that of the Swedish school. During the third week, the psychiatrist explains emotional aspects of chronic pain and amplifies the interconnection among anxiety, muscle tension, and pain. The last class reviews physical therapy methods for relaxation and improved muscle strength.

The California Back School is directed primarily at the patient with acute low back pain.[1] The teachers are a physiotherapist and a consulting orthopedic surgeon. An essential component of the California program is an obstacle course that is used the first day to measure physical performance in an objective manner. The goals of the obstacle course are to identify postures or motions that produce pain that may alter the stated diagnosis of the patient; provide objective measurement of performance of standardized activities to be matched against a control population and as a baseline; demonstrate proper body mechanics; and correct specific job-related body mechanics problems.[6] The obstacle course consists of a number of motions and tasks that exert the lumbar spine. The course proper consists of three weekly 90-minute visits, with a fourth visit 1 month later with four patients in each class. The developers of the California school believe that the small classes foster group participation while allowing for individual instruction for specific mechanical problems. The first class includes the obstacle course and basic education on the natural history, anatomy, and physiology of back pain along with a review of activities to be avoided. The second class concentrates on training in the tasks included in the obstacle course, review of body mechanics, and a home exercise program. A retest on the obstacle course and a test on the information given during the course are given at the third class. At follow-up 1 month later, individual mechanical problems are discussed.

The back school programs are only as good as the educational materials (slides, tapes, pamphlets) used and, most importantly, the expertise and enthusiasm of the instructors. The ability to motivate course participants and answer their questions seems most closely associated with a good outcome for the patients.

Do back schools help patients decrease pain and prevent recurrences? Berquist-Ullman did a controlled prospective study of 217 Volvo employees with acute low back pain who were randomly assigned to physiotherapy, back school, and placebo.[7] The duration of symptoms was shorter for the physiotherapy and back school groups than for the placebo group. Back school patients were off work during the initial episode for a shorter period of time than the physiotherapy and placebo groups. The investigators concluded that back school was as effective as physiotherapy and was cost effective since one therapist treated a number of patients at the same time. The course of pain and the number of days lost from work during the first year due to recurrences were the same for each group.

Hall reported on 6418 participants in the Canadian program. Back pain improvement occurred in 64%, and 97% rated the program helpful.[4] The outcome was not adversely affected by previous back surgery or severity of pain, but use of a large number of consulting physicians and multiple physical therapy modalities prior to enrollment in the course had a negative prognostic value.

Mooney reported on his behavioral modification program at Rancho Los Amigos Hospital in Downey, California.[8] Approximately 75% of patients reported decreased pain and increased activity and 62% returned to work.

The California Back School has also reported similar success rates. A review of the first 300 patients with acute low back pain revealed 89% needed no further medical treatment, 95% resumed normal activities, and 64% had no change in lifestyle.[5]

How do back schools benefit patients? The goals of the various programs are to inculcate independence and self-reliance into their patients. This is accomplished through instruction by individuals who are considered authorities on back pain. Fisk proposes the notion that it is the influence of these authority figures and the promotion of self-sufficiency that account for the efficacy of back schools, rather than the actual educational or training procedures themselves.[9] Patients who have a close working relationship with a health care professional may be able to substitute that interaction for a formal school setting. What is important is the stress placed on self-reliance and better understanding of the way the back works and how to prevent recurrences. These methods can be helpful for the patient with acute or chronic back pain who is motivated to improve his condition. Back school is most effective when used as a part of a broader treatment program consisting of the modalities discussed in this section.

In summary, back school is an effective means of educating patients with acute and chronic low back pain. Back school has less impact when it is the sole therapy. It works best when it is one of a variety of therapies given for low back pain. Back school may be given after the patient's episode of pain has resolved or as a component of a multifaceted therapeutic program. The information given must be adapted to the needs of the participants. All the staff of the school must give consistent information to the patients. Patients with chronic low back pain will gain little from a program directed solely at acute problems.[10]

References

BACK SCHOOL

1. Zachrisson-Forssell M: The Swedish back school. Physiotherapy 66:112, 1980.
2. Andersson GBJ: Back schools. In Jayson MIV (ed): The Lumbar Spine and Back Pain, 3rd ed. Edinburgh: Churchill Livingstone, 1987, pp 315–320.
3. Zachrisson-Forssell M: The back school. Spine 6:104, 1981.
4. Hall H, Iceton JA: Back school. Clin Orthop 179:10, 1983.
5. Mattmiller AW: The California back school. Physiotherapy 66:118, 1980.
6. White AH: Back School and Other Conservative Approaches to Low Back Pain. St Louis: CV Mosby Co, 1983.
7. Berquist-Ullman M, Larsson U: Acute low back pain in industry. Acta Orthop Scand (suppl) 170:73, 1977.
8. Mooney V: Alternative approaches for the patient beyond the help of surgery. Orthop Clin North Am 6:331, 1975.
9. Fisk JR, DiMonte P, Courington SM: Back schools: past, present, and future. Clin Orthop 179:18, 1983.
10. Nordin M, Cedraschi C, Balague F, et al.: Back schools in prevention of chronicity. Clin Rheumatol 6:685, 1992.

WORK-RELATED EDUCATIONAL/EXERCISE PROGRAMS

Another component of patient education and physical therapy is job assessment, functional capacity evaluation, and work hardening.[1] These components of therapy are directed at returning the patient to the workplace. The prevention of back pain can be obtained when the ergonomics of a specific task are evaluated in relationship to the prevention of back pain. Some factors associated with occupational risk for back pain include heavy physical labor, sustained trunk posture, prolonged sitting, frequent twisting with lifting, and whole-body vibration. Modifications of the workplace to decrease exposure to these physical risks decrease the potential for back injuries. Education of workers in regard to proper body mechanics also can be helpful in decreasing injuries. After injury, workers may be evaluated in regard to their physical capabilities in relationship to the requirements of the work tasks. Exercises (work hardening) may be given to strengthen those physical characteristics that are inadequate to complete the work tasks. Vocational rehabilitation may be considered for those patients who have inadequate physical abilities to safely participate in their former employment. These individuals need to be retrained for jobs associated with less physically demanding work.

Reference

WORK-RELATED EDUCATIONAL/EXERCISE PROGRAMS

1. Halpern M: Prevention of low back pain: basic ergonomics in the workplace and the clinic. Clin Rheumatol 6:705, 1992.

MISCELLANEOUS THERAPY

Tryptophan

The rationale for using L-tryptophan in the treatment of chronic pain is related to the role of serotonin in the central nervous system (CNS). L-Tryptophan is a precursor to serotonin. Ingested tryptophan is absorbed in increased quantities by the CNS and is converted to serotonin. Increased serotonin heightens the tone in the serotonergic inhibitory nerve pathway. L-Tryptophan also potentiates opiate analgesia.[1]

Clinical studies of L-tryptophan have been completed in a small number of patients with chronic pain of maxillofacial origin.[2] Patients who received L-tryptophan in a double-blind study showed statistically greater reduction in pain than the placebo patients. Similar findings were reported by Brady, who measured pain relief in 10 patients with chronic pain, including two with back pain, who were treated with L-tryptophan.[3]

Therapy with L-tryptophan requires a high-carbohydrate, low-fat, low-protein diet in addition to oral administration of 4 gm of the drug. Dietary alterations are needed to favor CNS absorption of L-tryptophan over that of other neutral amino acids.[4] This therapy should be considered in patients with chronic pain who are willing to alter their diet as well as ingest 4 gm of the medication.

EOSINOPHILIA–MYALGIA SYNDROME

The use of tryptophan as a therapy for pain has been severely curtailed because of the association of the amino acid with eosinophilia–myalgia syndrome.[5] The source of tryptophan in the United States was a Japanese manufacturer. This tryptophan was thought to have a contaminant that caused the eosinophilia–myalgia syndrome.[6, 7] The abnormal metabolism of tryptophan resulted in eosinophil activation and release of eosinophil-derived toxic proteins into the extracellular space.[8] The disorder is characterized by peripheral eosinophilia, myalgias, rash, edema, dyspnea, neuropathies, and myopathies.[9] Patients with neurologic involvement have a poor prognosis.[10] Pathologic findings include inflammatory infiltrates in muscle, connective tissue, small blood vessels, nerves, and septa of subcutaneous adipose tissue.[11] The most effective method for controlling this disorder was the removal of tryptophan from the market, which has resulted in no additional cases. This amino acid is not available as a separate therapy for analgesia for low back pain patients.

Acupuncture

Acupuncture is based on the theory that the production of brief, moderate pain in specific locations will abolish severe, chronic pain. The same principle has been used in many forms over the years, including cupping, scarification, and cauterization. These counter-irritant therapies have been referred to by Melzack as "hyperstimulation analgesia."[1] Acupuncture points can be stimulated by heat, cold, pressure, electricity, ultrasound, or lasers. The most common method of stimulation is insertion of tiny needles into acupuncture points.[2]

The efficacy of acupuncture in diminishing pain is related to endorphin release and to stimulation of large myelinated fibers blocking nociceptive transmission from small unmyelinated C fibers. Stimulation of large fiber mechanoreceptors in a dermatome will inhibit the small fiber pain input in the ipsilateral or contralateral dermatome by "closing the gate" in the spinal cord that allows nociceptive impulses to reach the cerebral cortex.[3, 4] This mechanism would explain the lack of effect of acupuncture in disorders involving large fiber destruction, such as postherpetic neuralgia.[5] The importance of afferent transmission to achieve analgesia is also demonstrated by observations that the analgesic effect is blocked by procaine infiltration of acupuncture points. Acupuncture may also produce analgesia by stimulating a location distant to the site of pain. Acupuncture causes the release of endorphins, the endogenous opiates.[6] The effect of acupuncture analgesia can be partially abolished by injection of naloxone, an opiate antagonist.[7, 8] Opiate antagonists may prevent the beneficial effect on nociceptive reflexes when injected before acupuncture. The opiate antagonist fails to suppress the beneficial effect of acupuncture on nociceptive reflexes if given after the cessation of therapy. The hypothesis is that acupuncture causes the release of endorphins that set up a cascade effect that is not dependent on endorphins for sustained effect.[9] The long-term relief of pain associated with acupuncture may occur by two mechanisms: (1) normal physiologic activity may resume in a stimulated area with re-establishment of normal large fiber proprioceptive input, which blocks nociceptive input[10]; (2) pain, which may be a learned response or part of memory, is "forgotten" with brief intense stimulation.[1]

The response to acupuncture may result, in part, to the frequency of activation of the sensory system.[2] Low frequency electrical stimulation results in the secretion of enkephalins from the midbrain that inhibit primary afferent fibers via the dorsolateral funiculus to the spinal cord and endorphins from the hypothalamus that bind to opiate receptors that cause generalized analgesia. High frequency electrical activation enhances serotonin/norepinephrine descending inhibitory fibers that induce regional analgesia.

Acupuncture analgesia is obtained by stimulation of particular areas of the skin with fine needles (30-gauge steel, silver, or gold), which are slowly twisted after insertion. The specific areas to be stimulated follow specific meridians (14 in all) that have been plotted on charts.[11] The most effective acupuncture points are often located where nerves enter muscle.[12] The location of acupuncture points and the location for nerve blocks are similar.[13] Acupuncture points may have greater concentrations of pain fibers and vascular structures, which explains the enhanced sensitivity of these points. Most points are at or near the site of pain and a few are distant from it. The needles are left in place for 20 to 40 minutes. The needle insertion feels like a small prick, followed by an ache, numbness, and warmth in the area.[9] Electrical stimulation that directs current with a square or spike wave with variable frequency, pulse width, and voltage may be applied to the needles in situ. Low frequency electrical stimulation increases the efficacy of the acupuncture procedure.[14]

Patients who are overanxious or who have visceral pain should not receive acupuncture.[15] Potential complications of acupuncture include hemorrhage, pneumothorax, hepatitis and endocarditis.[15, 16, 17]

Acupuncture has been studied in the treatment of low back pain. In a placebo-controlled, double-blind, crossover study of low back pain, acupuncture was no better than placebo in relieving low back pain.[18] Meta-analysis of studies of acupuncture for the treatment of chronic pain have revealed contradictory results. The efficacy of acupuncture beyond placebo effect has not been demonstrated.[19]

How often should treatments be given? The first treatment may produce only a few hours of relief. Subsequent visits result in more lasting benefit. A chronic condition requires 5 to 7 treatments given weekly or biweekly. This regimen may result in 60% pain relief over a 6-month period.[15] The patient should be made aware that acupuncture also may increase pain.[20] Too strong a stimulus may result in tenderness that may last 48 hours or longer.

Auriculotherapy is acupuncture of the auricle. Nogier has proposed that an inverted homunculus is represented on the auricle.[21] In a double-blind study, Oleson was able to find abnormalities in other parts of the body by detecting areas of increased skin conductivity and tenderness over the ear.[22] Areas of the body that have been injured have altered conductivity of electrical current. Electrical current will follow the path of least resistance and will bypass injured areas. Diseased areas of the body may be located by measuring the electrical conductivity of the skin over suspicious areas, including the auricle, with an ohmmeter.[2] A hypothesis also has been proposed that visceral disorders may be discovered by identification of abnormal electroconductivity in specific meridians corresponding to individual organs. The explanation for this phenomenon is the viscero-skin-sympathetic nerve reflex. Abnormalities in the viscera are transmitted to the spinal cord and are reflected onto the skin via the efferent sympathetic nerves as longitudinal areas of electrical resistance. Electrostimulation of areas of the auricle has been demonstrated to increase cerebrospinal fluid endorphin levels.[23] Others have not been able to reproduce these results.[1] The efficacy of this therapy may be related to anatomic organization of the nervous system. Inputs from the ear project to central nervous system structures that play a role in referred sensation. Low frequency versus high frequency electroacupuncture may have a differential effect on the type of neurotransmitters (low frequency endogenous opioids, high frequency nonopioid neurotransmitters) resulting in analgesia.[24] Whether specific auricular stimulation or placebo stimulation alone accounts for analgesia with auriculotherapy remains to be determined. In their study, Katz and Melzack were unable to demonstrate any increased benefit of stimulating 'Nogier' points compared with placebo points in the auricle.[13] However, about a third of patients reported warmth and other sensations in distant parts of the body with ear stimulation. This suggests that referred sensations are generated by ear stimulation.[13] Acupuncture of the ear is associated with toxicities including auricular chondritis that is resistant to therapy.[25]

The same mechanism that results in analgesia with acupuncture also may cause the pain relief associated with TENS, ice massage, and needle effect (dry needling of trigger points). The counter-irritation of superficial structures may have analgesic effects of short, intermediate, or prolonged duration.[26, 27]

Acupuncture should be considered adjunctive therapy for patients with chronic low back pain. Patients should be considered candidates for this therapy even if they have not responded to TENS therapy. Acupuncture of the body and/or ear may be tried. Obviously, the availability of this therapy depends on the accessibility of an experienced acupuncturist. Electroacupuncture has been tested against paracetamol and was more effective for control of low back pain. A specialized unit that locates acupuncture points on the skin by virtue of properties of altered electrical resistance was helpful in identifying appropriate points of stimulation for patients.[24] Although this study of 40 patients is useful, additional studies will be needed to prove efficacy of this analgesic modalitiy in chronic back pain patients.

The amount of unconventional medicine utilized in the United States is significant.[28] Approximately 33% of people surveyed described visiting an acupuncturist or chiropractor for their medical problems. Unconventional therapy was used for chronic, nonlife-threatening conditions. Approximately 83% of individuals also sought advice from their medical doctor for the same condition, and of these, 72% did not tell their physician that they had seen another health care provider. Medical physicians should ask their patients about the use of unconventional therapy when they obtain a medical history.

Biofeedback

Chronic pain is associated with the development of a depressed or vegetative state. Pain, when associated with change in personality and mentation, may persist despite resolution of the physical trauma associated with the initial pain. In these circumstances, therapies directed only at relieving pain without attempting to modify the psychologic state of the patient may not be successful.

A number of techniques are available to alter the psychologic state of chronic pain patients. Biofeedback is a technique by which alterations in biologic processes are demonstrated by a proportional change in a sensory signal (visual or auditory). The biologic processes measured include muscle tension measured by electromyograms (EMG), skin temperature, pulse volumes, and waveforms on electroencephalograms. Biofeedback techniques are valuable in reducing anxiety and stress, emphasizing self-control, and manifesting the mind-body relationship. Biofeedback treatment is based on the premise that patients with low back pain have elevated levels of muscular tension, particularly in the paraspinal muscles.[1] EMG biofeedback

has been tried in chronic low back pain with mixed results. Nouwen reported increased paraspinal muscle EMG activity in patients with chronic pain.[2] A 3-week treatment period was associated with a decrease in EMG activity compared with controls but was not associated with decreased pain. Melzack reported decreased pain in patients using biofeedback who felt in greater control of their symptoms.[3] Kravitz was unable to demonstrate a correlation between paraspinal EMG reduction and pain reduction in chronic low back pain patients.[4]

Patients who may have the best outcomes from biofeedback were studied by Keefe. These individuals initially rated their pain as severe, were less likely to be receiving disability payments, had fewer years of continuous pain, and had fewer surgical procedures.[5]

The efficacy of biofeedback in low back pain remains to be determined. The reliance on control of a physiologic function ignores the complex psychologic, affective, and behavioral components of the pain experience. Biofeedback may work by allowing the patient to improve focused thinking resulting in increased relaxation.[6]

Biofeedback requires several weeks of training. It is indicated only in patients who have persistent chronic pain, and patient motivation must be high. In many circumstances, biofeedback is used in conjunction with relaxation training for control of pain.

Relaxation

The basic premise of this form of therapy is that elicitation of the relaxation response will result in an altered state of consciousness associated with a sense of well being and peace of mind and concomitant decrease in oxygen consumption, respiratory rate, and heart rate.[1] The proposed mechanisms include increased endorphin levels and presence of increased alpha waves on electroencephalography.[2] The scientific data to support these proposed mechanisms are inconclusive. The relaxation response leads to generalized decreased sympathetic nervous system activity. This response may be mediated by an area in the hypothalamus.[3] More than one relaxation technique is able to elicit the relaxation response.[4]

Relaxation may be induced by a simple technique as proposed by Beary and Benson.[5] The instructions are as follows:

1. Sit quietly with eyes closed.

2. Relax all your muscles starting with the feet and progressing to the head. Keep all muscles deeply relaxed.

3. Breathe through the nose. Say the word ''one'' silently after each breath. Continue for 20 minutes. Eyes are opened to check the time, but no alarm is used. After 20 minutes, rest with eyes closed, then opened.

4. Do not attempt within 2 hours of any meal.

This technique may be used alone or in conjunction with biofeedback or hypnosis to achieve the desired response.

Other relaxation techniques besides deep breathing also may be effective in achieving an appropriate relaxation response. Progressive muscle relaxation training will decrease muscular tension and pain. Mindfulness meditation uses imagery techniques to focus on distinguishing pain from other sensations.[6] Few studies have been completed comparing the efficacy of relaxation techniques with other therapies. Progressive muscle relaxation is effective and superior to placebo in the therapy of low back patients.[7] Relaxation techniques may not be proven better than placebo but are relatively cost-effective and lack lasting harmful side effects. Although the specific physiologic mechanisms resulting in pain relief are unproven, relaxation reduces muscle tension, decreases sympathetic nervous system tone, and provides a cognitive distraction from distress.

Hypnosis

Hypnosis is an altered state of awareness in which the patient experiences increased suggestibility. The hypnotic state narrows attention to exclude extraneous stimulation. Chronic pain is not purely a physical phenomenon. It is associated with emotions and thoughts that alter the patient's perceptions. Through its effects on emotions and thoughts, hypnosis can alter the perception of pain.

Hypnotic suggestion may decrease pain in a number of ways. Patients may attain a level of deep relaxation. The pain may be directly diminished by suggestion or by transfer to another part of the body. The quality of the pain may be altered to tingling or numbness. Patients may be distracted from the pain or told to think of a time prior to the onset of pain.[1] Hypnotic therapy is most useful if the patient can be taught self-hypnosis, eliminating the need for a hypnotherapist on a continuing basis.

References

TRYPTOPHAN

1. Ho Sobuchi Y, Lamb S, Bascom D: Tryptophan loading may reverse tolerance to opiate analgesia in humans: a preliminary report. Pain 9:161, 1980.
2. Seltzer S, Dewart D, Pollack RL, Jackson E: The effects of dietary tryptophan on chronic maxillofacial pain and experimental pain tolerance. J Psychiatr Res 17:181, 1982–1983.
3. Brady JP, Cheatle MD, Ball WA: A trial of L-tryptophan in chronic pain syndrome. Clin J Pain 3:39, 1987.
4. Fernstrom JD, Wurtman RJ: Brain serotonin content: physiological regulation by plasma neutral amino acids. Science 189:414, 1972.
5. Hertzman PA, Blevins W, Mayer J, et al.: Association of the eosinophilia–myalgia syndrome with the ingestion of L-tryptophan. N Engl J Med 322:864, 1990.
6. Silver RM, McKinley K, Smith EA, et al.: Tryptophan metabolism via the kynurenine pathway in patients with the eosinophilia–myalgia syndrome. Arhtritis Rheum 35:1097, 1992.
7. Henning KJ, Jean-Baptiste E, Singh T, et al.: Eosinophilia–myalgia syndrome in patients ingesting a single source of L-tryptophan. J Rheumatol 20:273, 1993.
8. Silver RM, Heyes MP, Maize JC, et al.: Scleroderma, fasciitis, and eosinophilia associated with the ingestion of tryptophan. N Engl J Med 322:874, 1990.
9. Swygert LA, Maes EF, Sewell LE, et al.: Eosinophilia–myalgia syndrome: results of national surveillance. JAMA 264:1698, 1990.
10. Krupp LB, Masur DM, Kaufman LD: Neurocognitive dysfunction in the eosinophilia–myalgia syndrome. Neurology 43:931, 1993.
11. Herrick MK, Chang Y, Horoupian DS, et al.: L-Tryptophan and the eosinophilia–myalgia syndrome: pathologic findings in eight patients. Hum Pathol 22:12, 1991.

ACUPUNCTURE

1. Melzack R. Folk medicine and the sensory modulation of pain. In Wall PD, Melzack R (eds): Textbook of Pain, 2nd ed. Edinburgh: Churchill Livingstone, 1989, pp 897–905.
2. Matsumoto T, Lyu BS: Anatomical comparison between acupuncture and nerve block. Am Surg 41:11, 1975.
3. Fitzgerald M: The contralateral input to the dorsal horn of the spinal cord in the decerebrate spinal rat. Brain Res 236:275, 1982.
4. Melzack R, Wall PD: Pain mechanisms: a new theory. Science 150:971, 1965.
5. Levine JD, Gormley J, Fields HL: Observations on the analgesic effects of needle puncture (acupuncture). Pain 2:149, 1976.
6. Pomerantz B, Chiu D: Naloxone blockade of acupuncture analgesia. Endorphin implicated. Life Sci 19:1757, 1976.
7. Mayer DJ, Price DD, Raffi A: Antagonism of acupuncture analgesia in man by the narcotic antagonist naloxone. Brain Res 121:368, 1977.
8. Chapman CR, Colpitts YM, Beneditti C, et al.: Evoked potential assessment of acupunctural analgesia: attempted reversal with naloxone. Pain 9:183, 1980.
9. McLean B, Fives HE: Stimulation-induced analgesia. In Warfied CA (ed): Principles and Practice of Pain Management. New York: McGraw-Hill, Inc, 1993, pp 413–425.

10. Melzack R: Prolonged relief of pain by brief, intense transcutaneous somatic stimulation. Pain 1:357, 1975.
11. Duke M: Acupuncture: The Meridians of Ch'i. New York: Pyramid House, 1972.
12. Gunn CC: Motor points and motor lines. J Acupunc 6:55, 1978.
13. Katz J, Melzack R: Referred sensations in chronic pain patients. Pain 28:51, 1987.
14. Omura Y: Electro-acupuncture: its electrophysiologic basis and criteria for effectiveness and safety. Part 1. Acupunct Electrother Res 1:157, 1975.
15. MacDonald AJR: Acupuncture analgesia and therapy. In Wall PD, Melzack R (eds): Textbook of Pain, 2nd ed. Edinburgh: Churchill Livingstone, 1989, pp 906–919.
16. Gilbert JG: Auricular complication of acupuncture. NZ Med J 100:142, 1987.
17. Evans D: Acupuncture. In Raj PP (ed): Practical Management of Pain, 2nd ed. St Louis: Mosby Year Book, 1992, pp 934–944.
18. Mendelson G, Selwood TS, Kranz H, et al.: Acupuncture treatment of chronic back pain: a double-blind, placebo-controlled trial. Am J Med 74:49, 1983.
19. Kent GP, Brondum J, Keenlyside RA, et al: A large outbreak of acupuncture-associated hepatitis B. Am J Epidemiol 127:591, 1988.
20. Scheel O, Sundsfjord A, Lunde P, Andersen BM: Endocarditis after acupuncture and injection—treatment by a natural healer. JAMA 267:56, 1992.
21. Nogier PFM: Treatise of auriculotherapy. Maisonneuve, France: Moulin-les-Metz, 1972.
22. Oleson TD, Kroening RJ, Bressler DE: An experimental evaluation of auricular diagnosis: the somatotopic mapping of musculoskeletal pain at ear puncture points. Pain 8:217, 1980.
23. Pert A, Dionne R, Ng L, et al.: Alterations in rat central nervous system endorphins following transauricular electroacupuncture. Brain Res 224:83, 1981.
24. Lee JH, Beitz AJ: Electroacupuncture modifies the expression of c-fos in the spinal cord induced by noxious stimulation. Brain Res 577:80, 1992.
25. Ter Riet G, Kleijnen J, Knipschild P: Acupuncture and chronic pain: a criteria-based meta-analysis. J Clin Epidemiol 43:1191, 1990.
26. Melzack R, Jeans ME, Stratford JG, Monks RC: Ice massage and transcutaneous electrical stimulation: comparison of treatment for low-back pain. Pain 9:20, 1980.
27. Lewit K: The needle effect in the relief of myofascial pain. Pain 6:83, 1979.
28. Hyodo M: Modern scientific acupuncture as practiced in Japan. In Lipton S, Miles J (eds): Persistent Pain: Modern Methods of Treatment. Orlando: Grune & Stratton, 1985, pp 129–156.

BIOFEEDBACK

1. Wallace RK: Physiological effects of transcendental meditation. Science 167:1751, 1970.
2. Nouwen A: EMG biofeedback used to reduce standing levels of paraspinal muscle tension in chronic low back pain. Pain 17:353, 1983.
3. Melzack R, Perry C: Self-regulation of pain: the use of alpha feedback and hypnotic training for the control of chronic pain. Exp Neurol 46:452, 1975.
4. Kravitz E, Moore ME, Glaros A: Paralumbar muscle activity in chronic low back pain. Arch Phys Med Rehab 62:172, 1981.
5. Benson H, Pomeranz B, Kutz I. The relaxation response and pain. In Wall PD, Melzack R (eds): Textbook of Pain. Edinburgh: Churchill Livingstone, 1984, pp 817–822.
6. Beary JF, Benson H: A simple psychophysiologic technique which elicits the hypometabolic changes of the relaxation response. Psychosomatic Med 36:115, 1974.

RELAXATION

1. Wallace RK: Physiological effects of transcendental-meditation. Science 167:1751, 1970.
2. Benson H, Pomeranz B, Kutz I. The relaxation response and pain. In Wall PD, Melzack R (eds): Textbook of Pain. Edinburgh: Churchill Livingstone, 1984, pp 817–822.
3. Benson H, Arns P, Hoffman J: The relaxation response and hypnosis. Int J Clin Exp Hypn 29:259, 1981.
4. Domar AD, Friedman R, Benson H: Behavioral therapy. In Warfield CA (ed): Principles and Practice of Pain Management. New York: McGraw-Hill, Inc, 1993, pp 437–444.
5. Beary JF, Benson H: A simple psychophysiologic technique which elicits the hypometabolic changes of the relaxation response. Psychosomatic Med 36:115, 1974.
6. Syrjala KL: Relaxation techniques. In Bonica JJ (ed): The Management of Pain, 2nd ed. Philadelphia: Lea & Febiger, 1990, pp 1742–1750.
7. McCauley JD, Thelen M, Frank R, et al.: Hypnosis compared to relaxation in the outpatient management of chronic low back pain. Arch Phys Med Rehabil 64:548, 1983.

HYPNOSIS

1. Pawlicki RE, Wester WC II: Hypnosis. In Raj PP (ed): Practical Management of Pain. Chicago: Year Book Medical Publishers, 1986, pp 829–833.

RECOMMENDED THERAPEUTIC REGIMEN

With so many different recommended forms of therapy, it is clear that there is no one therapeutic intervention that is effective for the universe of patients with back pain (Table 19–11). The physician faced with this myriad of therapeutic options should refer back to the axioms of treatment that introduced this section. These guidelines will help the physician decide on the forms of appropriate therapy for each specific patient with back pain.

Acute back pain of any cause is usually a self-limited illness. Educating the patient on this point is worth the effort. The time spent with the patient increases the confidence the patient places in the physician's recommendations and facilitates the therapeutic process. The patient is told that he will improve. Patients with acute pain of short duration can experience total relief of their pain and should expect to return to their usual activities. The physician will be right 80% to 90% of the time.

TABLE 19–11.   RECOMMENDED THERAPEUTIC REGIMEN

ACUTE LOW BACK PAIN
1. Controlled physical activity:
     Bed rest with bathroom privileges (minimum of 2 days)
2. Physical modalities:
     Cryotherapy—ice pack or
     Thermotherapy—hot towel in plastic bag
3. Nonsteroidal anti-inflammatory drugs
     Analgesic nonsteroidals
        Aspirin 650 mg q.i.d. *or* ketorolac 10 mg q.i.d. *or* diflunisal 500 mg b.i.d. (after loading with 1000 mg), *or*
           diclofenac potassium 50 mg b.i.d., *or* flurbiprofen 100 mg b.i.d., *or* naproxen sodium 550 mg b.i.d., *or* etodolac
           300 mg t.i.d. *or* ibuprofen 800 mg q.i.d.
     Muscle relaxants (palpable spasm or difficulty sleeping):
        Cyclobenzaprine 10 mg 2 hours before bedtime increased to 10 mg t.i.d. as needed and tolerated
        If ineffective, not tolerated:
        Orphenadrine citrate 100 mg b.i.d. *or* chlorzoxazone 500 mg q.d. to q.i.d. as tolerated
4. Injection therapy: anesthetic with/without corticosteroids
5. Optional therapy—prevent recurrence:
     Exercises or Back School

CHRONIC LOW BACK PAIN
1. Physical modalities:
     Cryotherapy or thermotherapy
2. Nonsteroidal anti-inflammatory drugs:
     Aspirin 650 mg q.i.d. *or* diclofenac sodium 75 mg t.i.d. *or* nabumetone 1000 mg b.i.d. *or* oxaprozin 1200 mg q.d. *or*
        sulindac 200 mg b.i.d. *or* naproxen 500 mg b.i.d. *or* etodolac 400 mg q.i.d. *or* piroxicam 20 mg q.d. *or* ketoprofen
        200 mg q.d.
     Other choices—ibuprofen, indomethacin, tolmetin (nonacetylated salicylates or coated preparations for patients
        with GI intolerance to the other NSAID)
3. Muscle relaxants (palpable spasm or difficulty sleeping):
     Cyclobenzaprine 10 mg q.d. increase to t.i.d. as tolerated
        If ineffective
     Amitriptyline 10 mg increasing to 100 mg q.h.s. *or* doxepin 10 mg increasing to 100 mg q.h.s. (less sedating)
4. Physical therapy:
   a. Exercises
        Flexion or Extension or Isometric
   b. Modalities
        Temperature (with exercise)
        TENS
        Electrical stimulation
   c. Corset
        Flexible with plastic molded insert (for return to work)
   d. Work hardening
        Determination of job capabilities

PERSISTENT CHRONIC LOW BACK PAIN
1. Pain clinic

During the initial period of injury, a short period of time with controlled physical activity is recommended to reduce pain and hasten return to work. Non-narcotic analgesics in the form of aspirin or other rapid-onset NSAIDs (diflunisal, naproxen sodium, ibuprofen, ketorolac, diclofenac potassium) should be added to decrease pain. If patients experience muscle spasm, which is noted on physical examination, or develop difficulty sleeping, muscle relaxants, which are nonaddictive, are indicated. Ketorolac may be used in the patient with acute pain, particularly when evaluated in the emergency room. An intramuscular injection is very effective for controlling pain without the need for narcotics. If anti-inflammatory therapy is needed, however, another NSAID should be chosen since ketorolac has a relatively mild anti-inflammatory effect compared with other NSAIDs. The sedating property of these agents will keep the patient in bed, which is the preferred location during the first few days of therapy. Instructing the patient to take the muscle relaxant 2 to 3 hours before bedtime decreases the likelihood of somnolence the following morning. Therapeutic modalities in the form of heat or cold may be applied to the painful area while the patient is at home.

With resolution of the back pain, the patient may resume his usual activities with or without additional education. A session in a back school or with a physical therapist is useful for those patients interested in learning to prevent recurrence of pain.

Patients who do not improve on this regimen are candidates for additional therapy, which may take the form of local injection of painful sites. A change in NSAIDs and/or muscle relaxant after a trial of 2 to 3 weeks may be warranted if pain continues. If the patient had a partial response to the NSAID without toxicity, the dose of the drug should be increased to the maximum.

Patients who have improved but who will resume strenuous physical activities are candidates for physical therapy and/or a corset. Exercises will improve their general physical condition and prepare them for increased strain on the lumbosacral spine. Patients should learn how to lift and carry objects. A corset makes the patient mindful of his back, limiting exposure to potentially damaging stresses encountered during work. The corset is only given with a course of strengthening exercises and the admonition for use only during working hours.

Patients who are concerned about returning to work may benefit from a functional capacity evaluation, quantifying their ability to complete tasks associated with their work in a controlled environment. If the patient is "weak" in comparison to the tasks required, a work-hardening program is worthwhile. In a work-hardening program, the patient "goes to work" at the work-hardening center. Over the 2 to 3 week period, the patient is given increasingly difficult physical tasks associated with work. By the end of the session, the patient has retrained for the work-associated tasks so that there is less risk of having a recurrence of injury when returning to work.

The therapy for chronic low back pain patients is more difficult. The goal of therapy for these patients is maximum physical function despite continued pain. The general internist or family practitioner may offer therapies which may diminish but not abolish discomfort. The patients must understand, from the outset, the goal for therapy and the likelihood of only partial pain relief. This understanding is an essential part of therapy. If these patients do not accept these goals and outcomes, they will be quickly disappointed and frustrated and will not improve.

Patients are instructed at the initial meeting with the physician that maximum function and return to work is the goal of therapy. Pain may continue and may be exacerbated at times but this is not necessarily indicative of past or present disease-associated damage. Patients can be functional despite pain. Patients with organic pain readily accept these goals. Malingerers are frequently disappointed with this regimen and miss appointments.

Patients with chronic back pain are treated with NSAIDs, muscle relaxants, and/or injection therapy when indicated. Other medications will be substituted for the initial agents if they prove to be ineffective. Tricyclic antidepressants will be used if patients have chronic pain and clinical symptoms of depression. Referral to a physical therapist is made for exercises to improve general conditioning as well as to correct any imbalance in the spine with stretching and strengthening exercises of the flexion, extension, or isometric variety.

Patients who continue to experience pain should try TENS therapy. Patients are fitted with the machine by the therapist, and those who find the unit useful can rent it for varying periods of time. Patients should buy units only if they obtain benefit from the TENS machine over a period of months.

Referral to a pain clinic should be considered for patients who continue to experience pain after receiving these therapies. Pain clinics offer a multidisciplinary approach to pain, employing neurosurgeons, anesthetists, psychiatrists, physical therapists, vocational rehabilitation counselors, and other professionals interested in the therapy of chronic pain. The number of people who require this type of therapy in comparison with those who present with low back pain is extremely small. However, the opportunity for this group of chronic pain patients to improve without this combined therapeutic approach is very small. Pain clinics are discussed further in Chapter 22.

20

Surgical Therapy

INDICATIONS FOR BACK SURGERY

Modern spinal surgery should produce very predictable and gratifying results. The indications are now clearly delineated and if one stays within accepted guidelines and is judicious in the selection of patients, surgery on the lumbar spine can be most rewarding for both the treating physician and the patient. In this day and age, there is no place for exploratory operations, which are associated with poor outcome and continued low back pain. Objective criteria for patient selection for back surgery exist; when these selection criteria are adhered to, good surgical outcomes can be expected.

Herniated Disc

A herniated disc can present clinically with varying degrees of severity, each with its corresponding indications for surgery. The most dramatic presentation of an acute disc herniation is the profound or progressive neurologic deficit referred to as a cauda equina compression (CEC) syndrome.[1] Affected patients may have loss of all neurologic function below the level of the lesion, including bowel and bladder control. It is a true surgical emergency. If bowel and bladder function are to be preserved, immediate surgical decompression of the cauda equina is imperative. The longer the delay, the less recovery can be expected; and in view of the complex interplay of compression, edema, and vascular insult to these delicate nerve roots, prediction of surgical results is difficult. These patients may fail to recover fully even with the most expeditious treatment.

The other indication for early surgical intervention is a progressive neurologic deficit. For example, a patient who was first seen with an absent Achilles reflex is then noted to be gradually losing muscle strength in the legs. Such patients must be kept under close observation because if the trend cannot be reversed, an operation may be the only way to prevent further progression. This presentation is unusual but must be kept in mind because of the serious risk of further neurologic impairment.

It is more common, however, for patients to present with an acute, stable neurologic deficit. If it is profound, such as complete paralysis of the quadriceps muscles of the thigh or the dorsal flexors of the foot, surgery is a viable option and in some centers is considered mandatory.[2] Some feel that the more prolonged the pressure on the spinal nerves and the more intense the compression, the less likely is return of function. It should be noted that there have been no controlled studies that have prospectively compared the return of nerve function with and without surgery. Anecdotes abound of "miraculous" return to full function after surgery was delayed or refused, so the final decision about surgical intervention is often predicated on the quality of the surgery available.

Uncertainty concerning the need for surgical intervention is even greater when motor weakness is less severe or when the situation is subacute. A stable neurologic deficit is not in and of itself an indication for surgery because an operation does not necessarily lead to a return of function. One should also keep in mind that the deficit may not have any temporal relevance; that is, it could very well be a residuum of a prior attack. A well-documented history can be a great help in these situations.

Weber, in an excellent prospective study, took a group of patients with stable neurologic deficits and operated on half of them.[3] After 3 years of follow-up, the neurologic residua were similar in both the surgically and conservatively treated groups. In a stable situation, the aim of surgery is to relieve pain, not to regain neurologic function. The stable deficit should not be used as an excuse for inadequate conservative management and premature intervention. Sensory loss and reflex change are helpful in terms of diagnosis, but they are not in themselves indications for surgical intervention. They have no prognostic value in terms of the ultimate outcome.

Sciatica

Occasionally an acute attack of sciatica will fail to respond to all forms of conservative treatment. The exact time when surgery should be recommended will vary from patient to patient according to pain tolerance, emotional stability, and socioeconomic factors. In general, the authors do not recommend consideration of surgery in acute sciatica until 4 to 6 weeks have elapsed. On the other end of the spectrum if there has been little or no improvement by 12 weeks, surgery should be done because further procrastination might adversely affect the end result.

After an initial successful course of conservative treatment, certain individuals will have recurrent sciatica that becomes incapacitating. Symptoms may be completely absent between episodes or what begins as low-grade pain may become increasingly severe. If the recurrent episodes are not too disabling and if the intensity of the symptoms is within the patient's tolerance, then continued conservative management is indicated. However, if the frequency and intensity of attacks are severe enough to interfere with the individual's ability to pursue gainful employment and enjoy the normal activities of daily living, then surgery should be seriously considered. In general, the authors would consider surgery after the third episode, but in this regard there is some difference of opinion.

In most instances, surgery is performed to relieve sciatic pain, and the effectiveness of the procedure will depend on the identification and relief of pressure upon the neural elements. Ideally, a mechanical nerve root compression will be found whenever an operation is done to relieve sciatica. Diagnosis of mechanical root compression requires (1) either a positive tension sign or a neurologic deficit and (2) radiologic confirmation by metrizamide myelography, CT scan, or MR. With the

availability of MR, which is noninvasive, it would be most unusual to undertake surgery without preoperative confirmation of the lesion. Surgery can be most efficacious when these guidelines are strictly adhered to. Certainly, with the advanced technology available, there is no excuse for relying on an "exploratory" operation to make the diagnosis. A variety of procedures for herniated discs exist and each will be briefly discussed.

Open (conventional) discectomy has proved to be safe and efficient in treating patients with herniated discs who have failed to respond to appropriate conservative therapy. With proper patient selection, conventional discectomy can be expected to initially provide good to excellent results in 90% to 95% of cases, but the long-term success rate in these patients may decrease to 70% over the subsequent decade due to recurrence or scarring.[4] It is estimated that conventional discectomy has a 0.03% mortality rate, with an incidence of neurologic complications of less than 0.5% and minor complications in 4.7% of cases.[5] Although acute lumbar disc herniation in the elderly is not a common problem, surgery yields a high rate of satisfactory results in selected patients over age 60.[6] With a high percentage of successful results and a low morbidity, this procedure has stood the test of time; other procedures must show definitive advantages before open discectomy can be abandoned in their favor.

Microsurgical discectomy involves the use of a small incision (2.5 to 3 cm), the operating microscope for high magnification, and intense illumination of the operative field. Its theoretical technical advantages are improved visualization of microanatomy, preservation of epidural fat, meticulous hemostasis, minimal nerve root trauma, and minimal dissection of paravertebral muscles.[7] An apparent economic advantage over conventional discectomy is the decreased hospital stay, although postoperative recovery time is similar.[8] At the extreme, ambulatory microsurgery for lumbar discs also has been reported.[9] However, retrospective studies have unfairly compared the length of hospitalization for microsurgical discectomies with that for open discectomies performed in the 1970s—a time when the average stay for all surgical procedures was much longer than it is today.

Most reports claim at least a 90% success rate for microsurgical discectomy at relieving leg pain and somewhat less success at relieving back pain.[10, 11] Concerns with this technique include the relatively high recurrence rate reported in some series[10] and an excessive number of dural tears.[12] A case of bowel perforation following microsurgical lumbar discectomy also has been reported.[13] In comparison with other techniques, the success rate of microsurgical discectomy appears to be superior to that of chemonucleolysis,[14, 15] and comparable to that of conventional discectomy.[12, 16, 17] It should be noted, however, that no prospective, randomized investigations with standardized monitoring of postoperative pain have been conducted.

Many surgeons, including the authors, are not convinced that the theoretical technical advantages and apparent cost savings with microsurgical discectomy are worth compromising surgical exposure.[18] The microsurgical technique does not facilitate adequate assessment or treatment of stenosis of the nerve root canal (which may coexist with disc protrusion), nor does it ensure visualization of disc fragments that may be forced above or below the disc level—two common reasons for reoperation. The authors agree that a technique that decreases hospital stay and lost work days is attractive; however, these advantages must definitively be proved in a prospective, randomized study with long-term follow-up.

Percutaneous discectomy is the newest technical method of removing a disc. By mechanically decompressing the disc, percutaneous lumbar discectomy may have the beneficial effects of chymopapain without the associated complications. Various posterolateral and lateral approaches have been reported, usually with manual removal of disc material with forceps after confirmation of location with fluoroscopy. The reported complications include leg dysesthesia and paraspinal muscle spasm. Early trials indicate that this treatment was effective in 65% to 75% of patients.[19, 20]

Onik and coworkers have described their experience with automated percutaneous discectomy.[21] The advantage of their technique is the introduction of a specially designed nucleotome through a narrow cannula (2.8 mm) to aspirate disc material without anterior perforation of the annulus. They reported an 86% success rate in 36 patients who met stringent clinical and radiographic criteria for surgery; those who had radiographic evidence of a free disc fragment or facet disease were excluded. When the procedure was performed under local anesthesia with fluoroscopic guidance, no neurologic complications occurred. As with chemonucleolysis, it is difficult to envision that removal of the nucleus pulposus will relieve pressure on neural elements caused by a large protrusion of disc material into the spinal canal. Regardless, these early results are promising and percutaneous discectomy may gain a place as a viable treatment option for some types of herniated discs pending larger studies with long-term follow-up.

Other percutaneous techniques are currently under investigation that attempt to remove the offending herniated disc fragment, rather than just center of the disc. These techniques use a larger working cannula often with endoscopic guidance and flexible instruments to retrieve contained posterolateral disc fragments.

Spinal Stenosis

Spinal stenosis is the narrowing of the spinal canal because of degeneration of the facet joints as well as the intervertebral disc spaces. If the narrowing is severe, constriction of the neural contents within the spinal canal will develop and cause symptoms, which may vary significantly from patient to patient and can be manifested by back pain, leg pain, or both. When pain constantly interferes with ambulation, surgery should be considered. Unlike the clinical syndrome associated with an acute disc herniation, there may be no objective clinical findings in canal stenosis; consequently, a carefully constructed history is particularly important and the patient's description of his discomfort should be carefully noted.

Routine roentgenograms are quite helpful in canal stenosis and show disc space narrowing as well as facet joint arthritis and decreased spinal canal diameter.[22] Similar findings also can be observed on a CT scan. Unfortunately, many asymptomatic patients will show these same radiologic findings, so a surgical decision cannot be based solely on these findings: the clinical and radiologic data must be compatible if a satisfactory operative result is to be expected. The patient must also be aware that the aim of surgery is to relieve leg pain; relief of back pain is less predictable.

Spondylolisthesis

Spondylolisthesis is the forward slipping of one vertebral body on another (horizontal translation). Routine roentgenograms are all that is necessary to make the diagnosis, but this is a relatively common condition that may be unrelated to the back pain in question and such an incidental radiologic finding can on occasion confuse the diagnostic process. Assuming that low back pain symptoms are due to the related instability, the spondylolisthesis can usually be treated successfully by limiting stressful activities, bracing, and exercises. Most people with spondylolisthesis do not require surgery.

In the majority of cases, once a patient becomes symptomatic, some form of job modification becomes necessary, since, regardless of treatment, heavy work will always be a problem. Surgery should be considered only after an adequate trial of conservative treatment has failed.[23] Most of these patients will complain of mechanical back pain with or without leg pain. It should be appreciated that surgery will relieve the pain but will not return these patients to unrestricted activity.

Spinal Fusion

The exact indications for spinal fusion are as yet unknown and will not be determined until the completion of long-term, prospective studies in which patients within specific diagnostic categories are treated in a controlled, randomized fashion. From what is known today, the authors feel that a spinal fusion should be considered only for the following indications:

1. The presence of surgical instability created during decompression with bilateral removal of the facet joints.

2. The presence of neural arch defects (spondylolysis or spondylolisthesis).

3. The presence of a symptomatic and radiographically demonstrable segmental instability that can be objectively identified by weight-bearing lateral flexion and extension roentgenograms. Instability can be assumed when there is more than a 3.5 mm horizontal translation, a reversal of the intervertebral angle at a specific interspace, or both.

TECHNIQUE OF LAMINECTOMY AND FUSION

The surgical excision of a herniated disc is straightforward. It is designed to minimize the postoperative recovery time yet effectively treat the source of nerve root compression.[24]

The operation may be performed with the patient under spinal or general anesthesia. The patient is placed in a kneeling position so that the abdomen is free and intra-abdominal pressure is reduced. A straight incision is made over the desired interspace and carried down to the lamina. The ligamentum is removed as well as bone from the adjacent lamina. The goal is to visualize the involved nerve root, which is retracted medially, and remove the disc. The procedure usually takes between 1 and 2 hours. There should be very little blood loss. Postoperatively, the patient may stand immediately and walk. Prolonged sitting is avoided for the first 6 weeks to decrease pressure on the involved disc space.

A lumbar fusion or arthrodesis of the spine is a more involved procedure. The anesthesia and position are the same. The object of the operation is to place bone between the transverse processes of the adjacent vertebrae to be fused. This is termed a bilateral lateral fusion. The fusion site has to first be decorticated and the bone harvested from one of the posterior iliac crests. There is significant blood loss, and two to four units need to be reserved for the patient.

Postoperatively the patients experience a great deal of pain. This is due to the decorticated surfaces of the fusion site and graft site. It may take as long as 12 months for fusion to occur, and some form of brace is usually prescribed.

Complications of Disc Surgery

Low back surgery is not without risks and should be undertaken only for the proper indications.[25] During the operation the most frequent problem is injury to the neural elements; this can involve just an isolated nerve root or the cauda equina itself. Another intra-operative complication is injury to the major vascular or visceral structures. This usually occurs during removal of the disc when an instrument violates the anterior longitudinal ligament.

Postoperative complications include wound infection, cauda equina syndrome, and urinary retention. These patients need to be watched very carefully for the first 48 hours. Due to the severity of the complications it should again be stressed that low back surgery should not be undertaken without due consideration and there is no place today for exploratory surgery.

Results of Surgery

If the expected pathology is found at surgery, the results of low back surgery are quite rewarding.[26] The average age of patients subjected to lumbar disc surgery is 40 years. In individuals with surgery on the L5-S1 disc space, 15% have persistent back pain postoperatively, 7% have persistent sciatica, and 14% have both back and leg pain. The results are essentially the same when the operation is done at the L4-5 interspace.

Preoperative physical findings such as muscle spasm, tenderness, limitation of motion, and positive straight leg raising test disappear in 90% of patients. Neurologic deficits clear less frequently. Reversal of preoperative motor and sensory deficits can be expected in 50% of patients, and lost reflexes will return to normal in only 25%.

In summary, if the appropriate indications for low back surgery are followed, one can expect 90% overall satisfaction with the operation. Although relief from leg pain is reasonably predictable, only 80% of patients achieve a satisfactory result as far as their back pain is concerned.

References

INDICATIONS FOR BACK SURGERY

1. Floman Y, Wiesel SW, Rothman RH: Cauda equina syndrome presenting as a herniated lumbar disc. Clin Orthop 147:234, 1980.
2. Spangfort EV: The lumbar disc herniation—a computerized analysis of 2,504 operations. Acta Orthop Scand(Suppl) 142:52, 1972.
3. Weber H: Lumbar disc herniation: a prospective study of prognostic factors including a controlled trial. J Oslo City Hosp 28:33, 1978.
4. Frymoyer JW: Back pain and sciatica. N Engl J Med 318:291, 1988.
5. Hill GM, Ellis EA: Chemonucleolysis as an alternative to laminectomy for the herniated lumbar disc: experience with patients in a private orthopedic practice. Clin Orthop 225:229, 1987.
6. Maistrelli GL, Vaughn PA, Evans DC, et al.: Lumbar disc herniation in the elderly. Spine 12:63, 1987.
7. Maroon JC, Abla A: Microlumbar discectomy. Clin Neurosurg 33:407, 1986.
8. Kahanovitz N, Viola K, Muculloch J: Limited surgical discectomy and microdiscectomy. A clinical comparison. Spine 14:79, 1989.
9. Cares HL, Steinberg RS, Robertson ET, et al.: Ambulatory microsurgery for ruptured lumbar discs: report of ten cases. Neurosurgery 22:523, 1988.
10. Mixter WJ, Barr JS: Rupture of the intervertebral disc with involvement of the spinal canal. N Engl J Med 211:210, 1934.
11. Thomas AM, Afshar F: The microsurgical treatment of lumbar disc protrusion. J Bone Joint Surg 69B:696, 1987.
12. Rogers LA: Experience with limited versus extensive disc removal in patients undergoing microsurgical operations for ruptured lumbar discs. Neurosurgery 22:82, 1988.
13. Schwartz AM, Brodkey JS: Bowel perforation following microsurgical lumbar discectomy. A case report. Spine 13:104, 1988.
14. Maroon JC, Abla A: Microdiscectomy versus chemonucleolysis. Neurosurgery 16:644, 1985.
15. Zieger HE: Comparison of chemonucleolysis and microsurgical discectomy for the treatment of herniated lumbar disc. Spine 12:796, 1987.
16. Nystrom B: Experience of microsurgical compared with conventional technique in lumbar disc operations. Acta Neurol Scand 76:129, 1987.
17. Sachdev VF: Microsurgical lumbar discectomy: a personal series of 300 patients with at least 1 year of follow-up. Microsurgery 7:55, 1986.
18. Fager CA: Lumbar microdiscectomy: a contrary opinion. Clin Neurosurg 33:419, 1986.
19. Davis GW, Onik G: Clinical experience with automated percutaneous lumbar discectomy. Clin Orthop 238:98, 1989.
20. Friedman WA: Percutaneous discectomy: an alternative to chemonucleolysis? Neurosurgery 13:542, 1983.
21. Onik G, Maroon J, Helms C, et al.: Automated percutaneous diskectomy: initial patient experience. Radiology 162:129, 1987.
22. Epstein BS, Epstein JA, Jones MD: Lumbar spinal stenosis. Radiol Clin North Am 15:227, 1977.
23. Henderson ED: Results of the surgical treatment of spondylolisthesis. J Bone Joint Surg 48A:619, 1966.
24. Wiesel SW, Bernini P, Rothman RH: The Aging Lumbar Spine. Philadelphia: W B Saunders Co, 1982.
25. Rothman RH, Simeone FA: The Spine, 2nd ed. Philadelphia: W B Saunders Co, 1982.
26. Hirsch C: Efficiency of surgery in low back disorder. J Bone Joint Surg 47A:991, 1965.

CHEMONUCLEOLYSIS

Chemonucleolysis is the injection of an enzyme (most commonly chymopapain) into a nucleus pulposus in order to dissolve the disc that is pressing on the neural elements (nerve root). Chymopapain is a proteolytic enzyme derived from the papaya plant that depolymerizes the chondromucoprotein of the nucleus pulposus, hastening the degradation of only the nuclear portion of the intervertebral disc. The improvement that results in a reduction in sciatic pain may be related to reduction in mechanical pressure on the nerve root or disruption of the vascular supply to the inflamed root, or both.

The strict selection of patients for this procedure is essential for a good outcome. Indications are the same as those for surgical intervention and include sciatic pain, paresthesias in a corresponding dermatome, positive sciatic tension signs, motor weakness, and positive myelogram for a posterolateral herniated disc with nerve root sheath swelling, deviation, or filling defect at the appropriate level. A CT or MR scan may be substituted for a myelogram if the scan is definitely positive. Patients should be excluded if they fail to meet diagnostic criteria for nerve root compression and have had an inadequate trial of conservative therapy including epidural blocks. Patients also are excluded if they have cauda equina syndrome, are pregnant, or experience anaphylaxis secondary to papaya. Relative contraindications are prior laminectomy, lateral stenosis in which back pain cannot be differentiated from disc pain, or a sequestrated disc fragment associated with a ruptured annulus fibrosus. Injected material may escape from the confines of the disc and then injure surrounding tissues, such as the arachnoid and arachnoid vessels.

Patients should be tested for papaya allergy with a monoclonal antibody screening test for IgE. This test identifies 99.8% of patients with allergy to chymopapain. The procedure itself requires histamine blockade (H_1-diphenhydramine, H_2-cimetidine), intravenous corticosteroids to decrease hypersensitivity reactions and back spasms, and local anesthetics. The level is confirmed by the use of saline, not dye, and first a test dose and then, after 20 to 30 minutes (the time during which anaphylactic reactions most commonly appear), a full dose of chymopapain are injected slowly to avoid extrusion of disc material. Patients are encouraged to walk within 24 hours and are discharged within 2 days.[1, 2]

In a review of 13,500 cases, Watts found a complication rate of 3%.[3] Back spasms are the most common complication, occurring in up to 40% of patients; they occur within hours of the injection and may be severe. Muscle relaxants may be given with analgesics to decrease the severity of spasms.

Other complications are rare but catastrophic. Anaphylaxis has been associated with deaths, usually in patients who have undergone general anesthesia. The use of local anesthesia has allowed for the early recognition of signs of anaphylaxis.[4] Acute transverse myelitis associated with chymopapain in the subarachnoid space can result in paraplegia.

In a double-blind, prospective study, 77% of 60 patients treated with chymopapain had moderate improvement at 2 years after injection compared with 45% of saline-injected controls. In the chymopapain group, 57% were pain free compared with 23% with saline injections.[5]

Macuinas reported on the Mayo Clinic experience with 268 patients treated with chymopapain at 10-year follow-up: 86% had less leg pain and 82% were employed in a job as strenuous as that held prior to the injection.[6] Chemonucleolysis did not prejudice the outcome of subsequent surgical treatment if it became necessary.

CT scan of patients after injection revealed a reduction in compression produced by a herniated disc in 71% of patients.[7] Diffuse disc swelling occurred after injection in 82%, suggesting that chemonucleolysis is not indicated when neural compression is due to annular bulging as opposed to a herniated nucleus pulposus.

Chymopapain appears to be better than placebo, but, in comparison with surgery, its effectiveness and safety are still unproved. The enthusiasm for the procedure has waned over the past few years. The company that originally sold the drug has stopped manufacturing it and has sold its interest in it to another company. As suggested in an editorial by Nordby, the procedure is only as good as the patient selection, meticulous technique, and follow-up care.[8] Whether intradiscal injection is better than surgery and is cost-saving remains to be determined. Until that time comes, when in doubt, surgical intervention is preferable.

References

CHEMONUCLEOLYSIS

1. Brown MD: Intradiscal Therapy. Chicago: Year Book Medical Publishers, 1983.
2. Brown JE, Nordby EJ, Smith L: Chemonucleolysis. Thorofare, NJ: Slack Incorporated, 1985.
3. Watts C: Complications of chemonucleolysis for lumbar disc disease. Neurosurgery 1:2, 1977.
4. Hall BB, McCulloch JA: Anaphylactic reactions following the intradiscal injection of chymopapain under local anesthesia. J Bone Joint Surg 65A:1215, 1983.
5. Fraser RD: Chymopapain for the treatment of intervertebral disc herniation. The final report of a double-blind study. Spine 9:815, 1984.
6. Macuinas RJ, Onofrio BM: The long-term results of chymopapain: ten-year follow-up of 268 patients after chemonucleolysis. Clin Orthop 206:37, 1986.
7. Konings TG, Williams FJB, Deutman R: The effects of chemonucleolysis as demonstrated by computerized tomography. J Bone Joint Surg 60B:417, 1984.
8. Nordby EJ: Editorial comments. Clin Orthop 206:2, 1986.

MULTIPLE OPERATIONS ON THE LUMBAR SPINE

Continued pain after low back surgery is a difficult problem. Fifteen percent of all patients who undergo an initial surgical procedure will have significant discomfort and disability.[1] The inherent complexity of these cases necessitates a method of problem solving that is precise and unambiguous.

The best possible solution for preventing recurrent symptoms is to avoid inappropriate initial surgery whenever possible.[2] Again, it must be stressed that proper surgical indications should be strictly adhered to for the first procedure. The idea of "exploring" the low back when the necessary objective criteria are not present is no longer acceptable. In fact, even when there are objective findings but the patient is psychologically unstable or there are compensation litigation factors, the outcome of low back surgery is uncertain. Thus, the initial decision to operate is the most important one. Once the situation of recurrent pain after surgery arises, the potential for a solution is limited at best.

The physician must differentiate the patient with symptoms secondary to a mechanical lesion from one with some other problem. Recurrent herniated disc, spinal instability, and spinal stenosis are the principal mechanical lesions and are amenable to surgical intervention. Scar tissue (arachnoiditis or perineural fibrosis), psychosocial instability, or a systemic medical disease is the nonmechanical problem commonly found in the patient who has undergone multiple low back operations; none of these entities can be relieved by additional surgery.

Successful treatment for these patients is dependent on obtaining an accurate diagnosis. This essential step is often omitted, and inappropriate care is rendered. The goals of this section are to review the major points in the evaluation of low back pain that continues after multiple back operations and to present an algorithm (flow chart) for obtaining a specific diagnosis.

Evaluation

The evaluation of the patient who has continuing low back pain following surgery can be quite confusing. The history, physical examination, and roentgenographic studies need to be assessed in a standardized fashion. With accurate information, a diagnosis usually can be obtained.

First, it should be determined if the patient's complaint is based on a medical cause such as pancreatitis or an abdominal aneurysm. Thus, a thorough general medical examination should be routinely performed. In addition, if there is any indication of psychosocial instability, evidenced by alcoholism, drug dependence, or depression, a thorough psychiatric evaluation is necessary. Persons with profound emotional disturbances do not derive any observable benefit from additional

surgery. In many cases, once a patient's underlying psychosocial problem has been treated successfully, his somatic back complaints and disability will disappear.

If the lumbar spine is the probable source of the patient's complaints, three specific historical points need clarification. The first is the number of previous lumbar spine operations the patient has undergone. It has been shown that with every subsequent operation, regardless of the diagnosis, the likelihood of a good result decreases. Statistically, the second operation has a 50% chance of success, and beyond two operations, patients are more likely to be made worse than better.

The next important historical point is determination of the pain-free interval following the patient's previous operation. If the patient awoke from surgery with pain still present, the nerve root may not have been properly decompressed or the wrong level may have been explored. If the pain-free interval was longer than 6 months, the patient's recent pain may be due to recurrent disc herniation at the same or a different level. If the pain-free interval was between 1 and 6 months, the diagnosis most often is arachnoiditis or infection.

Finally, the patient's pain pattern must be evaluated. If leg pain predominates, a herniated disc or spinal stenosis is most likely. If back pain is the main complaint, instability, tumor, infection, and arachnoiditis are the major considerations. If both back and leg pain are present, spinal stenosis and arachnoiditis are the possibilities.

Physical examination is the next major step in the evaluation of the patient in whom previous back surgery has failed to relieve pain. The neurologic findings and existence of a tension sign, such as a positive straight leg raising test or sitting root test, are noted. It is most important to have the results of a dependable previous examination so a comparison can be made between the preoperative and postoperative states. If the preoperative neurologic picture is unchanged and the tension sign is negative, mechanical compression is unlikely. If, however, there is a new neurologic deficit or the tension sign is positive, pressure on the neural elements is possible.

Roentgenographic studies are an important part of the patient's workup. Again, it is most helpful to have a previous set of plain roentgenograms, MRs, CT scans, and myelograms for comparison of the pre- and postoperative situations. The plain roentgenograms are evaluated for the extent and level of previous laminectomy(ies) and for evidence of spinal stenosis. Weight-bearing lateral flexion-extension films of the lumbar spine are examined to see if instability is present. An unstable spine may be the result of the patient's intrinsic disease or secondary to a previous surgical procedure.

Water-soluble myelography and CT play a limited role in evaluating the multiply operated lumbar spine. While these tests can identify extradural compressions, they cannot distinguish between disc material and epidural scar. The major use of these two tests in combination is for confirmation of arachnoiditis when the diagnosis is otherwise uncertain.

MR is perhaps the most valuable diagnostic test in these complicated patients. With the administration of an intravenous paramagnetic contrast material (gadolinium-diethylenetriaminepenta-acetic acid/dimeglutamine [Gd-DTPA]), a recurrent disc herniation may be distinguished from epidural scar. A herniated disc is avascular and will not enhance (light up) immediately after the injection of intravenous contrast material; scar tissue, on the other hand, is vascular and will enhance with contrast. MR is also extremely helpful in identifying inflammatory processes such as discitis, which demonstrates a decreased signal intensity on T_1-weighted images.

An Algorithm for Back Pain After Multiple Operations

A specific diagnosis is necessary if an additional operation on the spine is to succeed. Basically, the physician is trying to differentiate the patients whose symptoms have mechanical causes (e.g., recurrent herniated disc) from those who have pain secondary to scar tissue.

Each pathologic entity has associated specific symptoms, signs, and radiographic appearance. (Table 20–1), and this information can be reformatted into an algorithmic form (Fig. 20–1). Each of the pathologic problems that respond to surgery can be differentiated from scar tissue, which is not amenable to an invasive procedure. It must be stressed that the number of operative patients will always be much lower than that of nonoperative patients.

Three possibilities exist if the patient's pain is caused by a herniated disc. First, the disc that caused the original symptoms may not have been satisfactorily removed. This can happen if the wrong level was decompressed; the laminectomy performed was not adequate to free the neural elements; or a fragment of disc material was left behind. Such patients will continue to have pain because of mechanical pressure on and irritation of the same nerve root that caused their initial symptoms. They will complain predominantly of leg pain, and their neurologic findings, tension signs, and radiographic patterns will remain unchanged from the preoperative state. The distinguishing feature is that they will report no pain-free interval; they will have awakened from the operation complaining of the same preoperative pain. Patients in this group will be aided by a technically correct laminectomy.

A second possibility is that there is a recurrent herniated intervertebral disc at the previously decompressed level. These patients complain of sciatica and have unchanged neurologic findings, tension signs, and radiographic studies. The distinguishing characteristic here is a pain-free interval of greater than 6 months. Another operative procedure is indicated in these patients provided that an MR with gadolinium can demonstrate herniated disc material rather than just scar tissue.

Finally, a herniated disc can occur at a completely different level. Such patients generally will suffer sudden onset of recurrent pain after a pain-free interval of more than 6 months. Sciatica predominates and tension signs are positive. However, a neurologic deficit, if present, and the radiographic signs will be seen at a different level from that on the original studies. A repeat operation for these patients will be beneficial.

Lumbar instability is another condition causing pain on a mechanical basis in the multiply operated back patient. Instability is the abnormal or excessive movement of one vertebra on another causing pain. The etiology may be the patient's intrinsic back disease or an excessively wide bilateral laminectomy.[1, 2] Pseudoarthrosis resulting from a failed spinal fusion is included in this category, since the pain is caused by the instability created by the failed fusion.

Patients with instability will complain predominantly of back pain, and their physical examinations may be negative. Sometimes, the key to diagnosis of these patients is the weight-bearing lateral flexion-extension film; however, it is often difficult to precisely define the anatomic origin of back pain in the presence of radiographic instability. Relative flexion-sagittal plane translation of more than 8% of the anteroposterior diameter of the vertebral body or a relative flexion-sagittal plane rotation of more than 9° between segments is the most commonly cited guideline for instability of the lumbar spine.[3, 4] At the lumbosacral junction

TABLE 20–1. DIFFERENTIAL DIAGNOSIS FOR BACK PAIN AFTER MULTIPLE OPERATIONS

HISTORY/PHYSICAL FINDINGS	ORIGINAL DISC NOT REMOVED	RECURRENT DISC AT SAME LEVEL	RECURRENT DISC AT DIFFERENT LEVEL	SPINAL INSTABILITY	SPINAL STENOSIS	ARACHNOIDITIS	EPIDURAL SCAR TISSUE	DISCITIS
Previous operations						>1		
Pain-free interval	None	>6 months	>6 months			>1 month but <6 months	>1 month gradual onset	
Predominant pain (leg vs. back)	Leg pain	Leg pain	Leg pain	Back pain	Back and leg pain	Back and leg pain	Back and/or leg pain	Back pain
Tension sign	+	+	+					
Neurologic exam	+ same pattern	+ same pattern	+ different level		+ after stress	May be positive	May be positive	
Plain x-rays	+ if wrong level				+			±
Lateral motion x-rays				+				
Metrizamide myelogram	+ but unchanged	+ same level	+ different level		+	+	+	
CT scan	+	+	+		+		+	
MR	+	+	+		+		+	+

659

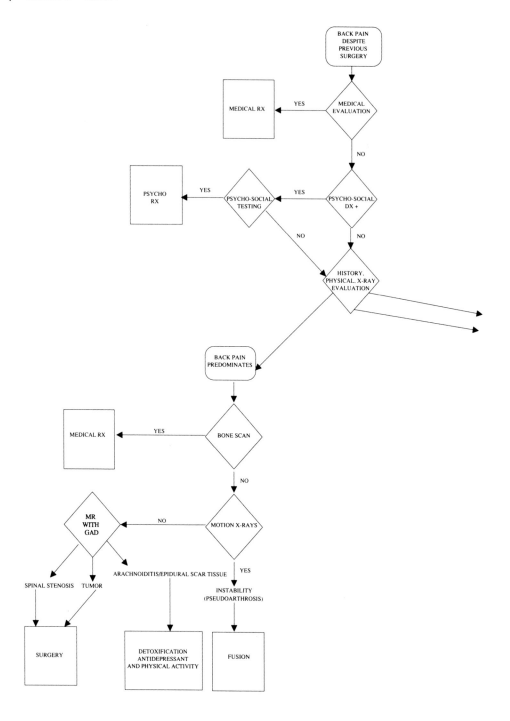

Figure 20–1. Algorithm for back pain after multiple operations.

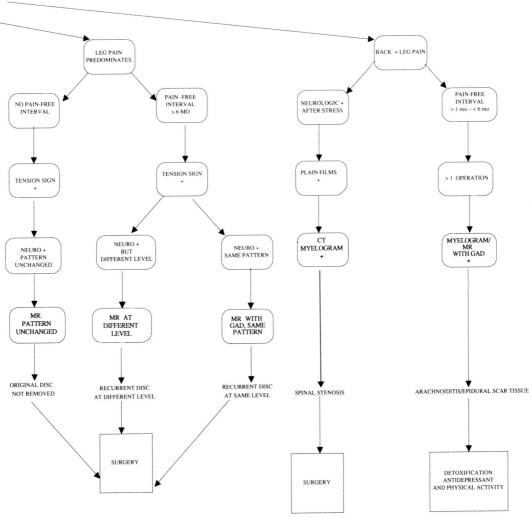

Figure 20–1. *Continued.*

the criteria are slightly different: relative translation of more than 6% or rotation of more than −1° is significant. These criteria are based on maximum displacements on a single flexion or extension view; however, calculation of relative dynamic translation and rotation from flexion to extension may prove to be a more reliable indication of true instability.[5]

Unfortunately, there is little information to explain why some patients with segmental instability develop back pain while others do not. If there is radiographic evidence of instability in symptomatic patients, spinal fusion (or repair of the pseudoarthrosis) may be considered.[6] Additional confirmatory evidence to determine the precise level of origin of the patient's symptoms may be gathered from facet injections and discography; however, these tests have a substantial rate of false-positive results.[7]

Spinal stenosis in the multiply operated back patient can mechanically produce both back and leg pain. The etiology may be secondary to progression of the patient's inherent degenerative spine disease, a previous inadequate decompression, or overgrowth of a previous posterior fusion. The physical examination is often inconclusive, although a neurologic deficit may occur following exercise; with reproduction of the patient's symptoms this phenomenon is termed a positive stress test.

The plain films can be suggestive and may display facet degeneration, decreased interpedicular distance, decreased sagittal canal diameter, or disc degeneration. A CT scan will demonstrate bony encroachment upon the neural elements; this is especially helpful in evaluating the lateral recesses and neural foramina. A myelogram or MR scan will show compression of the dural sac at the involved levels. It should be appreciated that spinal stenosis and scar tissue can co-exist.[8] Good results can be expected from surgery in at least 70% of properly selected cases, but if there has been a previous laminectomy and spinal fusion, surgery will be less successful. If there is definite evidence of bony compression, a laminectomy is indicated; however, if substantial scar tissue is present, the degree of pain relief the patient can anticipate is uncertain.

Scar tissue (arachnoiditis or epidural fibrosis) and discitis are nonmechanical causes of recurrent pain in the multiply operated back patient. While the etiologies and specific locations of these lesions are different, they are discussed in the same section because none of them will respond to another surgical procedure.

Postoperative scar tissue can be divided into two main types based on anatomic location. Scar tissue that occurs beneath the dura is commonly referred to as arachnoiditis. Scar tissue also can form extradurally, either directly on the cauda equina or around a nerve root.

Arachnoiditis is strictly defined as an inflammation of the piarachnoid membrane surrounding the spinal cord or cauda equina.[9] The condition may be present in varying degrees of severity, from mild thickening of the membranes to solid adhesions. The scarring may be severe enough to obliterate the subarachnoid space and block the flow of contrast agents.

This condition has been attributed to many factors: lumbar spine surgery and previous injections of intrathecal contrast material seem to be the most frequent precipitating factors.[10] This problem is much less common since the advent of water soluble contrast dyes. Postoperative infection also may play a role in the pathogenesis. The exact mechanism by which arachnoiditis develops from these events is not clear.

There is no uniform clinical presentation for arachnoiditis. Statistically, the history will reveal more than one previous operation and a pain-free interval of between 1 and 6 months. Often these patients will complain of back and leg pain. Physical examination is not conclusive; alterations in neurologic status may be due to a previous operation. As mentioned earlier, myelography, CT, and MR can be helpful in confirming the diagnosis.

At present there is no effective treatment for arachnoiditis. Surgical intervention has not proven effective in eliminating the scar tissue or significantly reducing the pain. Along with much needed encouragement, there are various nonoperative measures that can be employed. Epidural steroids, transcutaneous nerve stimulation, spinal cord stimulation, operant conditioning, bracing, and patient education have all been tried. None of these will lead to a complete cure, but when used judiciously they can provide symptomatic relief for varying periods of time. Patients should be detoxified from all narcotics, placed on amitriptyline (Elavil), and encouraged to do as much physical activity as possible. Treating these patients is a challenge, and the physician must be willing to devote time and patience to achieve optimal results.

Formation of scar tissue outside the dura on the cauda equina or directly on nerve roots is a relatively common occurrence.[11] This *epi-*

dural scar tissue acts as a constrictive force about the neural elements and frequently can cause postoperative pain. However, although most patients have some epidural scar tissue, only an unpredictable few become symptomatic.

Patients with epidural scarring may present with symptoms from several months to a year or two after surgery. They may complain of back pain or leg pain, or both. Commonly there are no new neurologic findings, but there may be a positive tension sign purely on the basis of scar formation around a nerve root. Epidural fibrosis is best differentiated from a recurrent herniated disc using gadolinium-enhanced MR.

As with arachnoiditis, there is no definitive treatment for epidural scar tissue. Prevention may be the best answer, and a free fat graft is sometimes used as an interposition membrane to minimize epidural scar tissue following laminectomy.[12] Use of too thick a fat graft may result in absorption of blood and swelling of the graft; there have been anecdotal reports of postoperative cauda equina syndrome associated with large fat grafts. Once scar has formed, surgery is not successful because scarring will often re-form in greater quantity. The treatment program should be similar to that already described for arachnoiditis.

Discitis is an uncommon but debilitating complication of lumbar disc surgery. Its pathogenesis is postulated to be direct inoculation of the avascular disc space but is not completely understood.[13] The onset of symptoms usually occurs about 1 month following surgery, and most patients will complain of severe back pain. Physical examination will sometimes reveal fever, a positive tension sign, and, occasionally, a superficial abscess.

If discitis is suspected from the history and physical examination, an ESR, blood cultures, and plain radiographs should be obtained. Plain films may not demonstrate the changes of disc space narrowing and end-plate erosion in the early stages. MR should confirm the diagnosis.

Effective treatment has been controversial.[13] The authors recommend placing the patient at bed rest acutely with immobilization of the lumbar spine using a brace or corset. If the patient experiences progressive pain after adequate immobilization or has constitutional symptoms, a needle aspiration biopsy should be performed. If a bacterial organism is identified, 6 weeks of intravenous antibiotics is indicated. There is no need for open disc space biopsy provided the patient responds to conservative therapy. With improvement of symptoms and laboratory findings the patient may ambulate as tolerated.

References

MULTIPLE OPERATIONS ON THE LUMBAR SPINE

1. Hopp E, Tsou PM: Postdecompression lumbar instability. Clin Orthop 227:143, 1988.
2. Johnsson KE, Willner S, Johnsson K: Postoperative instability after decompression for lumbar spinal stenosis. Spine 11:107, 1986.
3. Posner I, White AA, Edwards WT, et al.: A biochemical analysis of the clinical stability of the lumbar and lumbosacral spine. Spine 7:374, 1982.
4. White AA, Panjabi MM, Posner I, et al.: Spinal stability: Evaluation and treatment. American Academy of Orthopaedic Surgeons Instructional Course Lectures, Vol. XXX. St. Louis: CV Mosby, 1981, pp. 457–483.
5. Boden SD, Wiesel SW: Lumbosacral segmental motion in normal individuals. Spine 15:571, 1990.
6. Laasonen EM, Soini J: Low-back pain after lumbar fusion. Surgical and computed tomographic analysis. Spine 14:210, 1989.
7. Grubb SA, Lipscomb HJ, Gilford WB: The relative value of lumbar roentgenograms, metrizamide myelography, and discography in the assessment of patients with chronic low-back syndrome. Spine 12:282, 1987.
8. Epstein BS: The Spine. Philadelphia: Lea & Febiger, 1962.
9. Burton CV: Lumbosacral arachnoiditis. Spine 3:24, 1978.
10. Quiles M, Marchisello PJ, Tsairis P: Lumbar adhesive arachnoiditis: etiologic and pathologic aspects. Spine 3:45, 1978.
11. Rothman RH, Simeone FA: The Spine, 2nd ed. Philadelphia: W.B. Saunders, 1982.
12. Langenskydd A, Kiviluoto O: Prevention of epidural scar formation after operations on the lumbar spine by means of free fat transplants. Clin Orthop 115:92, 1976.
13. Dall BE, Rowe DE, Odette WG, et al.: Postoperative discitis: diagnosis and management. Clin Orthop 224:138, 1987.

21

Occupational Low Back Pain

Work-related low back pain has become the most common disabling musculoskeletal injury in the compensation setting. It has a large impact on society not only in terms of health care but also in terms of financial cost. The size of the economic impact has drawn the attention of business management and prompted efforts toward developing a comprehensive approach for prevention and treatment.

In this chapter, the epidemiology and impact of compensation with regard to the low back are outlined to establish a basis for the setting in which control strategies must function. Next, various approaches to the problem will be presented, including pre-employment variables, prevention, and treatment. Finally, permanent and partial impairment rating methods will be discussed.

PREVALENCE AND INCIDENCE

To accurately assess the significance of industrial low back pain, one must evaluate prevalence and incidence. Prevalence is the measure of how many individuals at some time in their lives have attacks of low back pain. Incidence, on the other hand, defines how many individuals have back pain during a specified time period.

The exact incidence and prevalence of low back pain in industry are unknown. It has been estimated that annually 2% of the United States workforce incur industrially related back injuries.[1] Several population studies in Sweden have demonstrated a prevalence of 60 to 80%.[2] Rowe reviewed data from a total of 237 employees at the Eastman Kodak Company just before their retirement and found that at some time during their career 56% had low

back pain severe enough to require medical care.[3]

The impact of low back pain in the workplace is formidable. Kelsey and Godlen reported that back symptoms were the most common chronic condition resulting in decreased work capacity and reduced leisure time activities for people below the age of 45 years.[4] In Sweden from 1960 to 1971, back pain was responsible for 12.5% of all sickness absence days; of all available workdays, 1% were lost each year because of back complaints (an average of 2.5 days for each working person yearly).[5] In Great Britain for 1969–1970, Benn and Wood found that 3.6% of all workdays were lost as a result of low back pain.[6] In 1974 Wood and Badley reported that 1011 days per 1000 working persons were lost each year for the same reason.[7]

In the United States, on the basis of estimates derived from the Bureau of Labor Statistics Annual Survey of Injuries and Illnesses, about 1 million workers suffered back injuries in 1980. Back injuries accounted for almost one out of every five injuries and illnesses in the workplace, although the frequency is variable, depending on the industry.[8] This 20% ratio is similar to that reported in Great Britain and Canada. Data from the National Health Survey indicate that in 1983 back impairment and intervertebral disc disorders were reported as chronic conditions by 8 million currently employed persons.[9] Only heart conditions and hypertension had a higher prevalence.

The most recent data from the Department of Labor Injury and Illness Survey demonstrate that back injuries made up 23% of all 1981 cases involving disability in the 18 states surveyed.[9] Most (87%) of these cases were sprains or strains, with 4% dislocations and 2% bruises or contusions. Although lumbosacral sprain is the most common diagnosis rendered in the compensation setting, herniated intervertebral discs, spinal stenosis, and spondylolisthesis also are seen. In addition, Rowe reported that inflammatory arthritis may be responsible for up to 20% of "nonspecific" low back pain.[3]

ECONOMIC IMPACT

The financial resources allocated to compensable low back pain are enormous. The most reliable estimate that could be obtained showed that $14 billion was spent in the United States in 1976 on treatment and compensation for low back injuries. This figure exceeded all other industrial injury payments combined.[10] By projecting these data into 1984 and using the consumer price index for all urban medical care, the costs would exceed $26 billion. In view of the fact that medical costs, technologic advancement, and utilization in this area probably are greater than the average for health care (because of widespread use of costly procedures such as CT scans and MR) and with the tremendous escalation of compensation costs, this dollar estimate is likely to be significantly lower than the actual current cost.

Another way to measure the economics of this situation is by looking at workers' compensation budgets, particularly in companies that are self-insured. A review of industrial compensation costs for several self-insured utility companies shows that such expenditures in 1983 were more than four times those in 1976. One would expect costs of low back injuries to have increased proportionally, if not more. The total projections from the two methods mentioned would put direct costs for back injuries between $26 and $56 billion—a staggering figure.

The cost distribution of this money has been carefully analyzed and is most interesting.[11] When disability lasted 9 months or less, the average total medical cost of back injury was no different from that associated with any other injury of the same duration. However, as more time elapsed, back injuries became more expensive. Of the total cost of low back pain, 45% was related to permanent disability payments, 22% to temporary disability payments, and 33% for physician fees and for hospital bills, including 7% for drugs, 5% for appliances, 9% for physical therapy and 12% for diagnostic tests.

Another interesting point is that a high percentage of these costs was concentrated in a small number of cases. For one insurance company, 25% of the low back cases accounted for 90% of their total costs. In a different group of patients (in 1971), the total average cost per case was $2197, but the median cost was $404. Although these dollar figures appear modest by today's standards, the relationship between the two figures is relevant. Only 22% of the cases had a total cost above the median. As might be expected, the high-cost cases were those that involved hospitalization, surgery, and compensation litigation.

RISK FACTORS FOR LOW BACK PAIN

It would be ideal if risk factors could be used to identify persons at high risk for low back pain or at risk for prolonged symptoms once injury occurs. Unfortunately the complex epidemiology of this problem makes early identification and screening somewhat difficult. Although as many as 65% of low back pain patients are unaware of any specific causative factor, several risk factors have been identified.

Low back pain typically begins in young adulthood, affecting the most productive years of life in an industrial worker. There is a rising prevalence with age until the fourth and fifth decades, after which there is a leveling off or decrease. Attacks of low back pain seem to be more common among those who have had previous back pain episodes. Buckle and colleagues found that of 68 patients, over 70% reported at least one previous episode.[13] Rowe similarly noted that 85% of low back pain patients had a history of intermittent episodes.[3]

Several studies have examined sex differences in relation to the risk of low back injury.[14] Women represent about 40% of the working population but develop only 20% of the industrial low back problems. This may be because women typically are employed in less physically demanding jobs. In a review of 31,000 employees from one manufacturer, Bigos and associates found that women had statistically fewer injuries than men but had an increased risk of making a high-cost injury claim.[11] Magora reported that in occupations demanding strenuous physical efforts, women had a higher incidence of low back pain than men.[15] Other investigators report equal prevalence of back pain in men and women.

Many investigators have examined the association between various radiographic abnormalities and the occurrence of back pain, usually concluding that no association exists.[16] Rowe reported that the prevalence of leg-length differences, increased lumbosacral angle, spondylolisthesis, transitional lumbosacral vertebrae, and spina bifida occulta among low back pain patients was not significantly different from that in a control group.[3] In a cohort study of 321 men, Frymoyer and Cats-Baril found no correlation of back pain with transitional vertebrae, Schmorl's nodes, or the disc vacuum sign.[12] However, when there were traction spurs or disc space narrowing between the fourth and fifth lumbar vertebrae, an increased incidence of severe low back pain was evident.

At least two studies have found low back pain to be more prevalent in cigarette smokers than in nonsmokers.[17] It is not clear whether this association is a result of increased intradiscal pressure from chronic coughing and straining or whether nicotine itself has a direct biochemical role in the pathophysiology of back injury.

Poor physical fitness may be a predisposing factor for back pain. Cady and associates, in a prospective study of firefighters, found that the least fit group of employees was 10 times more susceptible to develop back pain than the most fit group.[8]

One of the better-studied risk factors for industrial low back pain is job type; however, the data are inconsistent. The Bureau of Labor Statistics has identified construction and mining as the industries with the highest incidence of back injuries, followed closely by the trucking industry and the nursing profession.[9] Workers in government and finance are least likely to be affected. Accordingly, it has been hypothesized that the worker in heavy industry is most susceptible to a back injury. Sairanen and colleagues, however, found no significant difference between lumberjacks and controls doing light work with regard to low back pain occurrence.[18] Nachemson also has maintained that there is not a high incidence in heavy laborers.[19] In a retrospective study of 2000 workers, Rowe found that 35% of sedentary workers and 45% of heavy handlers had made visits to physicians for low back pain within a 10-year period.[3] Eastrand reported a survey of Swedish workers that suggested that the number of years spent doing heavy labor have a cumulative effect on predisposition to low back problems.[20]

Despite contradictory data, it does seem likely that certain tasks in the workplace are important in the development of low back pain. Snook and associates found that handling tasks were responsible for 70% of low back injuries, and Klein and associates later reported similar findings.[21, 22] The weight of the object lifted has been implicated in lifting injuries. In one study, more than half the injured workers had lifted objects weighing at least 60 pounds. The risk of low back pain is thought to be increased by prolonged sitting and exposure to vibration. Less physically stressful, but boring and repetitive jobs (assembly line work) also have been linked to increased incidence of back pain.

Magora reported that in workers who were not satisfied with their present occupation, place of employment, or social situation, there was a high incidence of low back pain.[15] This was also true of workers who felt that a high degree of responsibility and concentration was required of them. A correlation between back injuries and poor employee appraisal ratings by the supervisor has been demonstrated by Bigos.[11] Frymoyer and colleagues showed an association of diminished spinal motion with specific abnormalities on formal psychologic testing in back pain patients.[17] It is difficult, however, to determine whether any unusual psychologic characteristics in the low back patient are primary problems or secondary to medical illness. Certainly it is clear that many job and workplace factors other than mechanical loading of the spine play a role in the development of industrial low back pain.

PREVENTION OF LOW BACK PAIN

In view of the elusive nature of the etiology of industrial low back pain, it is not surprising that attempts at prevention in industry have not met with great success. Previous efforts have focused on careful selection of workers, training in proper lifting techniques, and designing the job to fit the worker.

The goal of careful worker selection is to screen job applicants in the hope of identifying and bypassing those potentially at increased risk for developing low back pain. The most commonly used screening tool is the pre-employment history and physical examination. Analysis of insurance company data from companies utilizing this method showed no significant difference in incidence of low back injuries compared with those that did not.[12] Another study estimated that 10% of workers who will have job-related, low back pain can be identified on a pre-employment medical examination.[23] The best predictor was a history of back trouble, especially if it occurred without a significant prior injury. While these observations are of interest, a more common one is that the person seeking employment may not be entirely candid with an examiner about past medical problems.

In summary, pre-employment history and physical examinations have not proven extremely helpful. However, before this time-honored, and apparently logical, procedure is abandoned, more facts are needed to determine if the incidence of back pain can be reduced when these assessments are made under carefully controlled conditions.

Radiographs as part of routine pre-employment assessment are in wide use. There have been a number of studies, however, that have shown conclusively that x-rays are of little value in identifying potential back problems.[16] The American Occupational Medical Association (AOMA) has recommended the following guidelines: "Lumbar spine x-ray examination should not be used as a routine screening procedure for back problems but rather as a spinal diagnostic procedure available to the physician secondary to appropriate indications."

In reviewing spinal x-rays of employees who have developed back pain, fewer than 1% of the films show any abnormality that would have been detected on pre-employment x-ray examination. This percentage of abnormal films is not different from radiographic findings of employees who have no back complaints. Individuals with a suspicious history or physical examination should be selected for x-ray evaluation, but routine use of pre-employment spinal films is neither medically justified nor cost-effective and involves unnecessary exposure to radiation. Techniques such as biplanar radiography and new dynamic measurements of flexion-extension views may prove to be more sensitive indicators of early spine dysfunction. Further investigation of these methods will determine their role in prediction of low back disorders.

One area that offers some promise is the attempt to match the physical characteristics of the job to the physical abilities of the prospective employee. It has been demonstrated that specific strength testing, using a battery of isometric strength measurements, is effective in screening potential employees to reduce the likelihood of back injuries.[24] A worker's susceptibility to back injury increases significantly when the lifting requirements of the job approach or exceed the individual's strength capacity as determined by the tests.

Pre-employment strength testing was not developed to exclude anyone from the work force, but there is concern that providing these kinds of guidelines for job placement will do just that. There is apprehension in some quarters that rather than being used to assist in determining the individual's capacity to do the job, the guidelines actually will be used to reject suitable candidates.

The application of such testing has been subjected to very close scrutiny by the legal profession. The possibility for discrimination, particularly against female applicants in the nontraditional workplace, must be carefully considered before any testing program is actually used. Women are now beginning to compete for physically demanding jobs that were traditionally held by men. Women have less experience in physically demanding activities than men and, given inherent biologic differences, the average female is not as physically strong as the average male. Thus, any strength testing program must be nondiscriminatory and designed to test only for the position under consideration.

The first step in designing a successful screening program is a thorough job analysis. The physical requirements of each task must be carefully delineated to determine just what is required from the worker. This includes a precise definition of the physical prerequisites.

After the analysis is completed, the next step is to design a battery of physical performance tests, which are linked to the job requirements. From these tests a predictive rating or score can be obtained so one applicant can be compared with another.

Each of these steps is time-consuming and expensive, but only after they have been taken can implementation of a program be considered. Even then, many industries are reluctant to start such programs because of the potential legal liability. Concerns include risk of injury during the testing process itself, legal requirements for access to the handicapped, and sex discrimination issues. In conclusion, even though pre-employment strength testing appears to offer a practical opportunity for job screening, the development of testing programs has been constrained by all of the above concerns as well as by high implementation costs.

Once a person is hired, the ideal situation would involve adjusting his job design and individual training to prevent the occurrence of low back pain. A great deal of research, time, and money have gone into this effort, but so far the results have been mixed.

Teaching employees the correct method of performing their jobs has been attempted in many industries. The most common instruction has been directed at proper lifting techniques. Safety departments have been cautioning workers to lift with their legs while keeping their back straight. This method has received wide acceptance by organizations such as the National Safety Council. Unfortunately, there have been many studies that cast serious doubt on the effectiveness of such training. It has been found that just as many back injuries occur among employees who have been through this type of safety training program as among those who have not. Also, general observation indicates that even though workers are instructed in appropriate lifting techniques and use them for a short period of time, they quickly revert to previous bad habits unless the training is updated and reinforced regularly.

Redesign of the job site has been under close scrutiny following several studies that showed relatively minor changes can significantly reduce the number of back injuries. The dynamics of changing a job site to reduce injuries is not within the scope of this chapter; however, while many of the changes appear simple and inexpensive, their implementation in the workplace, particularly when work patterns are long established, can be quite frustrating to both management and labor. What at first appears to be a minor environmental adjustment may be interpreted by employees, unions, or management as a rule change that requires a change in duty status, job reclassification, union approval, or pay adjustment. Thus, a change that appears to be a "cut and dried" issue can result in complex management negotiations.

Another problem relates to job equipment. Much of the machinery now in common use has been designed for larger, stronger males and is unsuited for smaller women with less strength. With the transition to more women in the workforce, accidents may occur more frequently. There is a natural reluctance on the part of management to replace equipment that has proved satisfactory in the past, particularly considering the high cost.

FACTORS AFFECTING THE DURATION OF WORK LOSS

Once a low back pain episode has occurred, efforts must be concentrated on returning the employee to work as soon as possible and iden-
tifying patients who may require a permanent adjustment of their work duties. Although 90% of patients return to work within 6 weeks of onset of the back pain, the importance of early return to employment cannot be overemphasized. Longer delays are clearly associated with a decreased likelihood of ever returning to the workforce. McGill reported that workers with back complaints who are away from work for over 6 months have only a 50% possibility of ever returning to productive employment.[25] If they are off work over 1 year this possibility drops to 25%, and if more than 2 years it is almost zero. Accordingly, Frymoyer and Cats-Baril have hypothesized that intensive rehabilitation early in the course of a low back disabling episode can prevent long-term disability and is cost effective.[12]

Although a multivariate model to predict disability from low back pain has not yet been developed, several factors have been shown to affect the duration of work absenteeism. First is the severity and type of injury. This may be difficult to evaluate because the history provided by the patient may be consciously or unconsciously biased. Patients who have a potential for seeking compensation will typically identify the onset of a problem as acute rather than chronic. Most injuries, however, produce few objective physical findings.

Because objective findings are usually absent, other factors must be considered. Gallagher and associates concluded that psychologic rather than physical factors predict return to work among patients with low back pain.[26] Waddell and colleagues estimated that objective physical impairment accounts for only one half the total disability that also is affected by psychologic reactions, such as emotional distress.[27] Similar conclusions were reached by Deyo and Tsio-Wu, who found that low educational level and low income are strong correlates with work absenteeism.[28]

The role that the secondary gain of compensation for low back pain plays in the length of disability is an issue that remains unresolved. Sander and Meyers found that patients injured on duty had a statistically significantly longer period of disability than those injured off duty.[29] Evaluation of the compensation patient may be complicated by malingering or conscious exaggeration, creation of symptoms, and subconscious amplification of the injury and symptoms. The conscious manipulator often arrives at the physician's office with extensive documentation and above-average command of the medical jargon pertinent to the injury. These patients take a persistently defensive attitude, may be hostile, and may selectively withhold vital information. In contrast, documentation is less important to the subconscious exaggerator, whose defensive attitude is more transient and who rarely and only briefly expresses anger; this individual will not knowingly withhold useful information.

Another factor affecting time off from work in industrial low back pain is financial compensation. The Federal Government and the individual states have developed their own regulations, and compensation payments can amount to as much as 100% of the worker's wage. Increased settlements for compensation claims and increased dollar value of compensation are highly associated with a subsequent increase in the number of claims made for alleged injury. Several investigations have concluded that a higher level of benefits prolonged the duration of back-related work loss.[30] The presence of compensation claims also is associated with a reduced rate of successful rehabilitation, as well as less successful surgical results.

Workers' compensation laws influence diagnostic evaluation, treatment, and recovery from injury. Beals suggested that, paradoxically, financial compensation may discourage return to work, the appeal process may increase disability, an open claim may inhibit return to work, and recovering patients may be unable to return to work.[6] Although one study concluded that personal injury litigants do not describe their pain as more severe than do nonlitigants, other studies have shown that if a lawyer becomes involved in the claim process, there is a greater probability of chronic pain and disability.

Health care providers also share responsibility for delaying return to work and escalating costs. Some physicians are less comfortable treating back pain and continue to see the injured worker at unnecessarily frequent intervals. Others take advantage of the third party fee-for-service payment system by liberally using their own x-ray and physical therapy facilities with questionable medical benefit to the patient. The result is a highly variable quality of health care and unnecessary expenditure of financial resources, both of which have served as the impetus for development of standardized approaches to the diagnosis and treatment of industrial low back pain.

STANDARDIZED APPROACH TO DIAGNOSIS AND TREATMENT OF INDUSTRIAL LOW BACK PAIN

The vast majority of low back injuries are not serious, and most employees can return to work in a short time. However, employees may return to work sooner and incur lower medical and compensation costs if an organized approach to evaluation, diagnosis, and treatment is made. There have been few standardized diagnostic or treatment protocols available to industry.

The authors recently evaluated the effect of such an organized approach in two industries. The study was prompted by a 1980 review of employee work loss at a public utility company, which revealed that 45% of all lost time was due to back injuries.[2] In addition, the number of back operations performed on these employees was much higher than in a noncompensation setting.

Under a newly developed program, the clinical approach to every patient was standardized by using an algorithm for low back pain diagnosis and treatment. The algorithm (see Fig. 20–1) was derived from information on previous patients with therapeutic successes as well as those who failed to respond. This protocol enabled the treating physician to make decisions based on well-delineated rules rather than intuition or emotion. The monitoring physicians were unbiased because they were not allowed to become involved in the patient's ongoing care. The algorithm has been modified to incorporate new data and technology since it was originally published.[31] We regard the use of a systematic and standardized approach as being the critical element, even as we expect the pathways of the algorithm to evolve.

Two employee populations were studied with monitoring programs of different intensity.[31] "Passive" surveillance was used to follow back pain patients from the U.S. Postal Service, which employs 14,000 people in the Washington, DC area. These patients were evaluated by one of the investigators (all orthopedic surgeons) after the initial episode of back pain. Computer forms were completed and, on the basis of diagnostic data and impressions, a prediction was made of when the patient should return to work. This estimate was based in part on previous averages for specific diagnostic entities. The patient was seen again only if return to work was not achieved within 5 days of the predicted date or if surgical intervention was subsequently proposed by the treating physician. The study was conducted for 1 year (1982–1983) and resulted in a 41% decrease in the number of low back pain patients, a 60% decrease in days lost from work, and a 55% decrease in compensation costs.

A second group of patients was "actively" followed. The Potomac Electric Power Company (PEPCO) employs 5380 workers, 75% of whom are blue collar. Under the "active" monitoring program, PEPCO patients with back pain were seen weekly or biweekly by one of the investigators until their return to work. If there was any disagreement in management according to the algorithm between the monitoring orthopedic surgeon and the treating physician, the latter was contacted for discussion. If an acceptable agreement could not be reached, a third physician was consulted for an independent medical opinion.

PEPCO patients were followed in this "active" fashion for 5 years (1981–1986). Using the standardized approach, there was an average decrease of 56% in the number of low back cases (from 98/year before the study to 42/year in the last study year). There was also a 54% average decrease in days lost (from 3640/year before the study to 2118/year in the last year). The cost savings were dramatic and nearly 2 million dollars were saved over the 5-year study (costs based on time lost from work, no direct medical cost savings were included). The number of surgical procedures decreased from nine in the year before the study to only nine over the next 4 years. Perhaps more significant is the fact that the surgical procedures performed under the algorithm criteria had a much higher success rate of patients returning to work.

Both the passive and active surveillance systems produced important savings and reductions in work disability. Although many of the reductions were greater in the active system, such a program is more expensive to employ. A cost-effectiveness study is needed to resolve this issue.

The etiology of these large reductions with the standardized approach remains speculative. Workers may have realized that they were being closely observed by low back experts and that they would not receive time off work without legitimate reasons. Light duty was made available to recovering patients, and although records prior to the study years were unavailable concerning light duty availability, this opportunity may have contributed to the savings. Finally, the acceptance of the fact that surgical procedures would never return workers to very heavy duty, and recognition that surgical indications were limited, helped decrease the number of surgical procedures.

The employee response to this program has been enthusiastic. Our experience to date with this standardized approach to the diagnosis and treatment of low back pain has certainly accomplished the goals required of any health care system in industry: (1) early return to normal activity, (2) avoidance of unnecessary surgery, (3) efficient and precise use of diagnostic studies, and (4) a treatment format with affordable costs to society.

This type of program has been tried in other industries with equally good results. It is a very attractive system because the program is automated and provides sophisticated medical guidance from the patient's first injury day. This greatly expands the productivity of company doctors and nurses by supplementing their medical training. Also, the program uses carefully designed forms to facilitate complete, accurate, and rapid data collection.

The date of the employee's return to work has been widely used to measure the rate of recovery from low back trauma in the industrial environment. This information often is quoted in support of the success or failure of various back programs, but there are a number of qualifying circumstances to be considered when using these figures.

Individual company policy concerning the availability of appropriate work for employees not yet fully recovered is an important limiting factor. The availability of a limited, light duty, or restricted work environment is frequently mentioned as one of the most significant factors in the encouragement of a rapid return to work. Although there is little published information to support this conclusion, a reduction in time lost due to back injuries has been apparent in work situations where job modification permits the employee to return to less than full regular duty status. When it is possible to assign the injured employee to a job in which he or she is temporarily protected from heavy lifting and repeated bending, the length of time the employee is out of work is markedly reduced. If nothing but heavy physical work is available, lost time is usually unnecessarily prolonged.

The amount of time away from work may, in itself, have a significant deleterious effect on the worker's capacity to ever return to productive employment. A report on a company's employees who were off work for 6 months showed only a 50% possibility of their eventually returning to productive employment. When employees were off work for more than a year, the possibility of their returning dropped to 25%, and if they were off more than 2 years, they rarely returned to work. Prolonged absenteeism appears to have a profound adverse psychologic effect on employees. It has been shown that employees off work for 3 or more months with back problems were more emotionally disturbed than those with injury to an extremity or those in a control group off work for a similar length of time.

The question of malingering or exaggeration of complaints often arises in conjunction with low back pain because subjective symptoms play such an important part in diagnosis. Authors of a careful study concluded that when the subjective complaints were out of proportion to objective physical findings, there was unconscious exaggeration of symptoms.[32] The study also showed that true malingering—the conscious effort by the individual to create symptoms not physiologically present—was a relatively rare occurrence. This is a subject that deserves much more careful investigation, because in some occupational environments, back pain without confirmatory objective findings is often construed by the employer to be malingering.

Another topic to consider is the effect of workers' compensation legislation on the low back pain patient and his return to work. The object of the original compensation laws was to provide workers with medical care and salary support for injuries that occurred on the job. Although each state and the Federal Government have developed their own unique sets of workers' compensation regulations, in most settings the employee who is hurt on the job has a free choice of physician or treatment facility, while his employer is responsible for payment of the costs involved. This financial obligation, however, is limited to some extent by the reasonableness and necessity of the care provided. The employee's reimbursement for lost time due to the accident varies widely in different jurisdictions. This usually is a percentage of his wages, most often 66 2/3% of the employee's current pay, with a designated maximum. Current maximum wage reimbursements range from $112/week in Mississippi to $966/week in Alaska. In addition, many companies provide supplemental reimbursement, which may increase the injured employee's salary to as much as 100% of his current wage, all of which is tax-free. These relatively large monetary payments have been targeted as the cause of unnecessary prolongation of complaints by employees.

Finally, there is no doubt that much of the unjustified lost time and expense in such cases is due to overutilization of services by certain health care providers. While most health care professionals are dedicated, conscientious individuals, a small minority have abused the workers' compensation system. The fee-for-service reimbursement of these providers has tended to encourage too frequent office visits, duplication of diagnostic tests, and prolonged use of a variety of unproven treatment modalities. It is hoped that an independent medical monitoring system, such as the algorithm system already discussed, will help limit this kind of abuse in the future.

LOW BACK IMPAIRMENT RATINGS

Despite successes in the diagnosis and management of low back problems with these standardized approaches, some patients are unable to return to their preinjury level of function. Any physical injury that occurs in the work-related setting must be quantitated, especially if the patient is unable to return to the previous level of employment. Such workers must be given a permanent partial impairment rating, a task that has enjoyed few satisfactory or accepted guidelines.

It is imperative to understand the distinction between physical impairment and physical disability. *Physical impairment* is an objective anatomic or pathologic dysfunction leading to loss of normal body ability. *Permanent impairment* is an objective assessment of functional abnormality or loss after the acute injury phase and after maximal medical rehabilitation. *Physical disability* is a measure of reduced capacity to engage in gainful everyday activity as a result of some impairment.

Assessment of physical impairment is solely a medical responsibility. However, the assignment of the more subjective disability rating should be made by someone independent of the treating physician. Disability rating is best calculated by administrative, vocational, or legal specialists from impairment ratings generated by the physician.

Guidelines for assigning a percentage impairment rating to a specific back injury are not available. In evaluating an extremity, the injured limb can be compared with the noninjured one, but, no such comparison can be made for back injuries. The American Medical Association's publication, *Guides to the Evaluation of Permanent Impairment,* is considered the best reference, but most experienced evaluators will not use it because it designates motion as the sole criterion of impairment and does not acknowledge pain as a factor in low back impairment except when associated with a peripheral nerve injury.[33] Chronic low back pain

TABLE 21–1. INDUSTRIAL BACK INJURY WORK RESTRICTION CLASSIFICATION

WORK CLASSIFICATION	WORK RESTRICTIONS	% PPI*	RELEVANT DIAGNOSES
Very Heavy Work	Occasional lifting in excess of 100 pounds Frequent lifting of 50 pounds or more	0	Recovered acute back pain Herniated nucleus pulposus treated conservatively with complete recovery
Heavy Work	Occasional lifting of 100 pounds Frequent lifting of up to 50 pounds	0	Healed acute traumatic spondylolisthesis Healed transverse process fracture
Medium Work	Occasional lifting of 50 pounds Frequent lifting of 25 pounds	<5%	Chronic back strain Degenerative lumbar intervertebral disc disease under reasonable control Herniated nucleus pulposus treated by surgical discectomy and completely recovered Spondylolysis/spondylolisthesis under reasonable control Healed compression fracture with 10% residual loss of vertebral height
Light Work	Occasional lifting of no more than 20 pounds Frequent lifting of up to 10 pounds	10%–15%	Degenerative lumbar intervertebral disc disease with chronic pain and restriction Herniated nucleus pulposus treated conservatively or operatively, but left with some discomfort, restriction, neurologic deficit Acute traumatic spondylolysis/spondylolisthesis, treated conservatively or operatively, but with residual discomfort and restriction Lumbar canal stenosis Moderately severe osteoarthritis accompanied by instability Healed compression fracture with 25% to 50% residual loss of vertebral height
Sedentary Work	Occasional lifting of 10 pounds Frequent lifting of no more than lightweight articles and dockets	20%–25%	Multiply operated back (failed back syndrome)

Modified from Social Security Rulings. Title 20—Employees' Benefits. 404.1567—Physical Exertion Requirements.
*PPI = Permanent partial impairment.

often exists with few or no objective clinical signs, and when there are clinical signs, they often are unrelated to the injury or disability in question. Also, measurement of spinal motion, even by the most experienced physician, is highly subjective.

The *AMA Guide* is useful in its "whole man" concept. Each part of the body is considered to represent only a section of the whole; the percentage each part contributes is based on the notion of function. Since the back is important to many functions, it contributes a maximum of 60% of the whole man. Therefore, once impairment of the back is estimated, the whole man impairment can be determined easily.

It must be realized that physical impairment ratings of spinal injuries are primarily "judgment calls" based on the history and physical findings. Inevitably, the rating system carries a heavy subjective component. Pain is the chief limiting factor in spinal disease, and there is enormous variation in individual response to pain. For example, a person with severe osteoarthritis of the spine undoubtedly has some discomfort every day. This is permanent and, in some cases, progressive. Should this individual sustain a superimposed back sprain and even be completely immobilized temporarily, the long-term prognosis for recovery from the sprain may be quite good. This assumes that he has not learned to enjoy inactivity during his immobilization period; if he has, his subjective complaints will not drop back to the previous baseline level.

A different approach to assignment of a permanent impairment rating is use of a specific diagnosis as the determining factor.[34] This was

TABLE 21–2. IMPAIRMENT RATING FOR COMPENSABLE LOW BACK PAIN

DIAGNOSIS	% PPI*	WORK PERMITTED
Acute back sprain—complete recovery	0	(Very) heavy work
Chronic back pain	5	Medium work
Degenerated disc—superimposed sprain		
Complete recovery	0	Heavy work
Acceptable level of discomfort and restriction	5	Medium work
Chronic pain and restriction	10–15	Light work
Herniated nucleus pulposus—conservative care		
Complete recovery	0	Heavy work
Acceptable level of discomfort	10	Light work
Herniated nucleus pulposus—surgical discectomy		
Complete recovery	5	Medium work
Acceptable level of discomfort	10	Light work
Pain and restriction without neurologic deficit	15	Light work
Pain and restriction with neurologic deficit		
Failed back syndrome	25	Sedentary work
Acute traumatic spondylolysis/spondylolisthesis		
Superimposed sprain		
Conservative care		
Complete recovery	0	Heavy work
Chronic pain	10	Light work
Recurrent pain	10	Light work
Pre-existing asymptomatic spondylolysis/		
spondylolisthesis		
Superimposed sprain		
Laminectomy and/or fusion		
Complete recovery	10	Light work
Chronic or recurrent pain	20	Sedentary work
Pre-existing lumbar canal stenosis		
Superimposed sprain		
Conservative care		
Status quo	0	Heavy work
Subjectively worse	10	Light work
Subjectively and objectively worse	15	Light work
Pre-existing lumbar canal stenosis		
Superimposed sprain		
Decompression with or without fusion		
Status quo	0	Medium work
Subjectively worse	10	Light work
Subjectively and objectively worse	20	Sedentary work
Pre-existing osteoarthritis		
Acute back sprain		
Conservative care		
Status quo	0	Heavy work
Subjectively worse	10	Light work
Subjectively and objectively worse	20	Sedentary work
Acute back sprain or herniated nucleus pulposus		
Conservative or surgical care		
No objective residuals		
Confirmed neurosis	5	Medium work
Compression fracture—healed with:		
10% compression	5	Medium work
25% compression	10	Light work
50% compression	20	Sedentary work
75% compression	20	Sedentary work
Transverse process fracture—healed with:		
No displacement	0	Heavy work
Malunited	0	Heavy work

From Wiesel SW, Feffer HI, Borenstein DG, Rothman RH: Industrial Low Back Pain: A Compenhensive Approach, 2nd ed. Charlottesville, VA: The Michie Company, 1989, pp 789–791.
*PPI = Permanent partial impairment.

attempted with a questionnaire circulated among 75 American members of the International Society for Study of the Lumbar Spine (ISSLS). The questionnaire included 41 specific clinical entities to be rated. Confirming the chaotic rating situation already described, the responses were anything but consistent, but with statistical analysis a medium range could be defined in most categories. Figures ranged from 0% for complete recovery from an acute low back sprain to 25% following failed back surgery. If a diagnosis was complicated by emotional problems or drug addiction, it was not unusual for the percentage to increase up to 50% (in actual practice one often finds even higher ratings in situations in which there is obvious bias).

An associated problem is assigning permanent work restrictions to a patient who has been given a permanent partial impairment rating. The best permanent work restriction classification system is defined by the Social Security Administration and can be modified to conform to the compensation setting:[35]

Very heavy work is that which involves lifting objects weighing more than 100 pounds at a time, with frequent lifting or carrying of objects weighing 50 pounds or more.

Heavy work involves lifting no more than 100 pounds at a time, with frequent lifting or carrying of objects weighing up to 50 pounds.

Medium work is defined as lifting of no more than 50 pounds at a time, with frequent lifting or carrying of objects weighing up to 25 pounds. Workers with 5% or less back-related permanent partial physical impairment can qualify in this category, but those with higher ratings cannot.

Light work is described as lifting of no more than 20 pounds at a time with frequent lifting or carrying of objects weighing up to 10 pounds. Applicants with between 10% and 15% permanent partial physical impairment because of a low back problem should be able to do this type of work.

Sedentary work is described as that involving no more than the lifting of 10 pounds at a time and occasional lifting or carrying of articles like docket files, ledgers, or small tools. Applicants with 20% or 25% permanent partial physical impairment should be capable of this type of work.

In practice one needs to have a practical approach to both permanent partial physical impairment and work restriction ratings. There are different ways to approach the problem. The authors use Tables 21–1 and 21–2 on a day-to-day basis with satisfactory results.

In conclusion, there is no good objective method for assigning physical impairment ratings to spine problems. Ratings based on a specific diagnosis appear to hold more promise of accuracy than those based solely on the patient's history and physical findings. There is much work to be done in this area. For now, physicians must strive to make their reports and evaluations reflect, to the highest possible degree, the true state of a patient's impairment, using methods that are organized and replicable.

References

1. Leavitt S, Johnston T, and Beyer R: The process of recovery: patterns in industrial back injury. Part 1. Cost and other quantitative measures of effort. Indust Med 40:7, 1971.
2. Bauer W: Scope of industrial low back pain. In Wiesel SW, Feffer H, Rothman R (eds): Industrial Low Back Pain. Charlottesville, VA: The Michie Co, 1985, pp 1–35.
3. Rowe ML: Low back disability in industry: updated position. J Occup Med 13:476, 1971.
4. Kelsey JL, Godlen AL: Occupational and workplace factors associated with low back pain. In Deyo RA (ed): Occupational Medicine: State of the Art Reviews, Vol. 3, No. 1. Philadelphia: Hanley & Belfus, 1988, pp 7–16.
5. Hansson T, Bigos S, Beecher P, Wortley M: The lumbar lordosis in acute and chronic low-back pain. Spine 10:154, 1985.
6. Benn RT, Wood PHN: Pain in the back. Rheumatol Rehabil 14:121, 1975.
7. Wood P, Badley M: Epidemiology of back pain. In Jeyson M (ed): The Lumbar Spine and Back Pain. London: Pitman, 1980, pp 29–33.
8. Cady L, Bischoff D, O'Connell E, et al.: Strength and fitness and subsequent back injuries in firefighters. J Occup Med 21:269, 1979.
9. Department of Labor, Bureau of Labor Statistics: Back Injuries Associated with Lifting. Bulletin 2144. August 1982.
10. Bergenudd H, Nilsson B: Back pain in middle age: occupational workload and psychologic factors: an epidemiologic survey. Spine 13:58, 1988.
11. Bigos SJ, Spengler DM, Martin NA, et al: Back injuries in industry: a retrospective study. II. Injury factors. Spine 11:246, 1986.
12. Frymoyer JW, Cats-Baril W: Predictors of low back pain disability. Clin Orthop 221:89, 1987.
13. Buckle P, Kember P, Wood A, et al.: Factors influencing occupational back pain in Bedfordshire. Spine 5:245, 1980.
14. Andersson GBJ: Low back pain in industry: epidemiological aspects. Scand J Rehabil Med 11:163, 1979.
15. Magora A: Investigation of the relation between low back pain and occupation. I. Age, sex, community, education and other factors. Indust Med Surg 39:465, 1970.
16. Gibson ES: The value of preplacement screening radiography of the low back. In Deyo RA (ed): Occupational Medicine: State of the Art Reviews, Vol. 3, No. 1. Philadelphia: Hanley & Belfus, 1988, pp 91–107.

17. Frymoyer JW, Pope MH, Clements JH, et al.: Risk factors in low-back pain. J Bone Joint Surg 65A:213, 1983.
18. Sairanen E, Brushaber L, Kaskinen M: Felling work, low back pain and osteoarthritis. Scand J Work Environ Health 7:18, 1981.
19. Nachemson A: Work for all—for those with low back pain as well. Clin Orthop 179:77, 1983.
20. Eastrand N: Medical, psychological, and social factors associated with back abnormalities and self-reported back pain: a cross sectional study of male employees in a Swedish pulp and paper industry. Br J Ind Med 44:327, 1987.
21. Snook SH, Campanelli RA, Hart JW: A study of three preventive approaches to low back injury. J Occup Med 20:478, 1978.
22. Klein BP, Jensen RC, Sanderson LM: Assessment of workers' compensation claims for back strains/sprains. J Occup Med 26:443, 1984.
23. Frymoyer JW, Newberg A, Pope MH, et al.: Spine radiographs in patients with low-back pain. J Bone Joint Surg 66A:1048, 1984.
24. Chaffin DB, Herin GD, Deyserling WM: Pre-employment strength testing: an updated position. J Occup Med 20:403, 1978.
25. McGill CM: Industrial back problems—a control program. J Occup Med 10:174, 1968.
26. Gallagher RM, Rauh V, Langeher R, et al.: Psychological, but not physical, factors predict return to work in low back pain. Psychosom Med 48:296, 1986.
27. Waddell G, Main CJ, Morris EW, et al.: Chronic low-back pain, psychologic distress, and illness behavior. Spine 9:209, 1984.
28. Deyo RA, and Tsio-Wu YJ: Functional disability due to back pain—a population-based study indicating the importance of socioeconomic factors. Arthritis Rheum 30:1247, 1987.
29. Sander RA, and Meyers JE: The relationship of disability to compensation status in railroad workers. Spine 11:141, 1986.
30. Walsh NE, and Dumitru D: The influence of compensation on recovery from low back pain. In Deyo RA (ed): Occupational Medicine: State of the Art Reviews, Vol. 3, No. 1. Philadelphia: Hanley & Belfus, 1988, pp 109–121.
31. Wiesel SW, Feffer HL, and Rothman RH: Industrial low-back pain—a prospective evaluation of a standardized diagnostic and treatment protocol. Spine 9:199, 1984.
32. Beals R, Heckman N: Industrial injuries of the back and extremities. J Bone Joint Surg 51A:1593, 1972.
33. American Medical Association: Guides to the Evaluation of Permanent Impairment, 2nd ed. Chicago: American Medical Association, 1984.
34. Wiesel SW, Feffer HL, Borenstein DG, Rothman RH: Industrial Low Back Pain: A Comprehensive Approach, 2nd ed. Charlottesville, VA: The Michie Company, 1989, pp 789–791.
35. Social Security Rulings. Title 20—Employees' Benefits. 404.1567—Physical Exertion Requirements.

22

Pain Clinics

MULTIDISCIPLINARY APPROACH TO CHRONIC PAIN

Although most patients with low back pain have resolution of their symptoms, a small percentage continue to experience pain. Even though the proportion of patients who continue with pain is small, the population at risk is so large (50 million people) that the number of patients with chronic pain is substantial. The monetary cost of chronic pain in general to the United States economy is 85 to 90 billion dollars each year.[1]

Chronic pain patients are taxing and frustrating to the general clinician. Attempts at improving the patient's condition have failed. Despite concern and clinical knowledge, the treating physician has patients who return with increasing pain, decreasing physical capacity, and debilitating psychologic difficulties and concomitant feelings of decreasing self-worth and insight, increasing depression, and inability to cope. It is impossible for the clinician to deal with all the physical, psychiatric, drug, and vocational concerns of these patients. When other therapies have failed, these patients can benefit from referral to a pain center.

Treatment Philosophy

In an attempt to identify those patients who might benefit from referral to a pain facility, Crue divides pain into six classes based upon a temporal classification:[2] (1) acute—days; (2) subacute—few months; (3) recurrent acute—continued new episodes—days; (4) ongoing acute—neoplastic disease—days; (5) chronic benign—6 months or longer; (6) chronic intractable benign pain syndrome (CIBPS)—

longer than 6 months. Patients with CIBPS have poor pain coping skills and pain is the focus of their existence. These are the patients who are most likely to benefit from a pain center. Patients in group 5 have chronic pain but are able to cope adequately and remain functional despite chronic pain; they usually do not require the multidisciplinary therapies of a pain facility.

Two schools of thought have promoted separate hypotheses to explain pain on a chronic basis. These theories play a role in the organization and staffing of pain facilities. The peripheral theory proposes a continuation of nociceptive input from the periphery related to the original location of tissue damage as the cause of chronic pain. The injury has not healed properly and the patient continues to experience pain. With time, psychologic abnormalities appear that add to the suffering associated with the peripheral nociceptive input.

The central hypothesis proposes that chronic pain is a central nervous system phenomenon that reverberates through the sensory networks connecting the spinal cord and cortex. The pain exists in the patient's mind even if the peripheral source of the nociceptive input has healed.

The differentiation of the two groups becomes important, since the therapy based on these hypotheses is different. Peripheralist therapy, used at the University of Washington Pain Center, is directed at control of nociceptive input and involves nerve blocks and other methods of anesthesia, while a smaller component of the regimen involves psychologic support therapies.[3] In centralist therapy control of pain through alterations of psychologic factors is the primary therapy, with drug and physical therapy as adjunctive modalities. This

676

type of treatment is employed at the New Hope Pain Center, Pasadena, California.[4] Other centers for chronic pain are located throughout the country, and include the Rehabilitation Institute of Chicago, the Boston Pain Unit, Johns Hopkins Pain Research and Treatment Program, Emory University Pain Center, University of Virginia Pain Clinic, Pain and Low Back Rehabilitation Program at the University of Miami School of Medicine, and University of North Carolina Pain Clinic. Outpatient therapy is offered at a pain clinic, while inpatient units are called pain centers. Other pain facilities work with patients with a specific problem (back pain, headache) or with a specific modality (acupuncture). The range of pain facilities is listed in Table 22–1. The Committee on Accreditation of Rehabilitation Facilities (CARF) has established guidelines for inpatient and outpatient programs. These guidelines set standards for physicians, allied health professionals, and facilities. The standards reflect the necessity of the interaction of a wide variety of health professionals for the management of chronic pain patients (Table 22–2).[5]

Pain Center Goals

The overall goals for therapy at pain centers or clinics are to help patients take more responsibility for their own lives and their health care and to help them become more functional. Additional goals are to improve patient

TABLE 22–1. PAIN FACILITIES

1. Unidisciplinary—physician or allied health professional from one specialty (i.e., neurosurgeon)
2. Interdisciplinary—a minimum of one physician interacting with allied health professionals as part of treatment team
3. Multidisciplinary—two or more physicians of different specialties working with allied health professionals
4. Pain clinic—outpatient facility organized as a pain treatment team
5. Pain unit—specialized inpatient program in a separate area for treatment of pain
6. Comprehensive pain center—offers inpatient and outpatient facilities for patients with a variety of chronic pain problems
7. Syndrome-oriented programs—a facility dedicated to patients with a specific pain problem (back pain, cancer)
8. Modality-oriented pain program—a specific form of therapy is offered for a variety of chronic pain problems (acupuncture, TENS)

Adapted from Aronoff GM: The role of pain clinics. In Warfield CA (ed): Principles and Practice of Pain Management. New York: McGraw-Hill, Inc, 1993, pg. 482.

TABLE 22–2. COMMISSION ON ACCREDITATION OF REHABILITATION FACILITIES STANDARDS FOR COMPREHENSIVE PAIN CENTERS

1. Multidisciplinary team led by a program director that manages chronic pain and is able to generate an interdisciplinary evaluation
2. Full-time professional staff offering adequate medical supervision
3. Medical, psychiatric and/or psychologic consulting services for patient evaluation along with appropriate allied therapies
4. Organized evaluative processes for screening and selection of patients
5. Adequate facilities to evaluate the cause and effect of chronic pain on the medical, psychologic, social, and environmental difficulties of patients
6. Expeditious synthesis of information to formulate a diagnostic opinion and management strategy involving multimodal treatment
7. Maintenance and review of medical records
8. Quantitative measure of dysfunction
9. Specific rehabilitation goals including detoxification, improved physical function, psychologic counseling, and stress management and pain control
10. Informed consent for treatment
11. Periodic review of treatment efficacy and patient progress
12. Vocational and avocational counseling for appropriate job placement

Modified from Ghia JN: Development and organization of pain centers. In Raj PP (ed): Practical Management of Pain, 2nd ed. St Louis: Mosby Year Book, 1992, pp 20–21.

comfort, diminish dependence on analgesic medication, and help patients feel more in control of their pain (Table 22–3). Patients who are referred to pain facilities most commonly have back (64%), neck (23%), or chest or limb pain (17%).[6] Similar types and percentages of patients have been treated at the Boston Pain Center.[7] A majority of the patients are on one or more medications including narcotics (codeine), antianxiety drugs (diazepam), or sedatives (pentobarbital, methaqualone).[8]

Pain Center Referrals

The tenor of the referral to pain center plays a role in the success of subsequent therapeutic interventions. Success is associated with a referral from a clinician who presents the combination of medical and psychologic therapies as a comprehensive approach to a complex process called chronic pain. This approach offers patients hope that the next phase of their therapy will be effective. In contrast, the referral of patients by a physician who no longer wants to deal with them and

TABLE 22–3. PAIN CENTER GOALS

I. Re-evaluate diagnosis—review medical records and consider necessity of additional diagnostic studies or invasive procedures to specify diagnosis
II. Improve pain control with physical therapy and modalities
   A. Improve comfort and physical activity resulting in a return to functional and productive life
   B. Promote pain-control modalities other than powerful drugs
   C. Reduce patient fear of reinjury with structured graduated exercise programs
   D. Teach proper body mechanics and postural awareness
   E. Evaluate limitations and restrictions
III. Improve psychologic functioning
   A. Define and address psychosocial issues affecting chronic pain syndrome
   B. Resolve drug dependency
   C. Treat depression and insomnia
   D. Determine secondary gain from pain
   E. Determine family dynamics
   F. Strengthen family and community support systems
IV. Vocational needs
   A. Access to occupational and vocational rehabilitation counselors
   B. Assess functional capacity and residual impairment
V. Communication with referring physician to establish mechanism for continued managment of patients
VI. Reduce inappropriate use of health-care system
VII. Decrease cost of medical care associated with chronic pain syndrome

Modified from Aronoff GM, McAlary PW: Pain centers: treatment for intractable suffering and disability resulting from chronic pain. In Aronoff GM (ed): Evaluation and Treatment of Chronic Pain. Baltimore: Williams & Wilkins, 1992, p 417.

sends them without explaining the role of the pain clinic has less chance of success. These patients are angry and will displace their frustration onto their new physicians.[9]

A patient who is an appropriate referral to a pain center meets the following criteria: (1) evaluated appropriately to eliminate active medical illnesses that had not been adequately treated, (2) failed conventional treatments, (3) developed psychosocial difficulties secondary to pain, (4) developed medication dependence or substance abuse, (5) has poor coping mechanisms, (6) motivated to change, and (7) unconcerned about secondary gains from family or work.

Treatment Plan

Four factors determine successful outcome of rehabilitation of chronic pain patients. In descending order of importance, they are motivation, social support system, chronicity, and degree of tissue pathology.[1] The patients must have the desire to improve their condition. If they do not, the therapeutic program will not be successful since one of its primary goals is to increase patient self-determination. Chronic pain has effects not only on the patient but also on his family and friends, and their understanding and support are important factors in recovery. Chronicity of pain shapes and maintains patients' pain behavior. In patients with chronic low back pain, it is the pain rather than the pathology that prevents them from leading a useful life or returning to work. The patients are helpless, depressed, anxious, demoralized, and dependent on others. They are under constant stress from being unemployed and financially insecure, with deteriorating home and marital lives, and increasing social isolation. In this setting, the extent of tissue damage is of some concern, but in most circumstances, the tissue damage has stabilized or healed and plays a small role in the patients' pain syndrome.

Patients who are addicted to narcotic medication, who require additional diagnostic evaluation, whose home environment is not conducive to regular visits, or whose psychologic impairment is such as to preclude active cooperation require inpatient therapy. Outpatient therapy is indicated for the other patients with chronic pain and has the advantage of keeping them in the home environment, thus allowing therapies to have a chance to be implemented in the family setting, limiting the stigma of being labeled "sick" because of being admitted to the hospital, and minimizing cost.

The goals of the treatment program (decreased drug dependence, increased physical fitness, improved coping skills, return to work) are reviewed with the patient and family at the outset. The treatment program includes pharmacologic, physical, psychologic, behavioral, and motivational/educational approaches aimed at restoring patients to functional lives. From a pharmacotherapeutic standpoint, patients must undergo narcotic detoxification. Analgesic medications are gradually withdrawn while antidepressants are added. Tricyclic antidepressants with sedative properties may be used if disturbed sleep is a major problem. Simple NSAIDs given on a regular basis may be substituted.

Physical modalities have a role in the treatment of chronic pain. A simple measure such as ice massage is safe and effective in partially or completely relieving pain for a variable length of time.[10] Depending on the school of thought (peripheralist or centralist), other pain modalities such as nerve block injections,

TENS, electroacupuncture, and high-voltage stimulation may be used.[11] The caveat in the use of physical modalities is that they should be used with a specific purpose of increasing function, not to reward pain behavior or to encourage passivity. Patients receive physical modalities so that they may participate in exercise programs or return to work, not because they have pain.

An important bridge between the physical and psychologic methods of pain control are relaxation techniques, which include biofeedback, hypnosis, and relaxation training. These methods reduce the intensity of the patient's emotional reaction to pain, and foster a feeling of greater mastery over the situation.

Although chronic pain is psychosomatic, the use of this term does not mean that the pain is imaginary or psychogenic. Chronic pain has an effect on the way patients think, interact with other people, and solve problems. These problems are best dealt with through individual or group therapy. The goals of counseling are to improve self-image, alter problem-solving techniques, and increase self-responsibility. Pain facilities are also organized to encourage appropriate behavior, rewarding evidence of increasing self-reliance (attaining stated goals of physical activity) while ignoring pain behavior (emergency appointments for increasing pain).[12]

Vocational rehabilitation is also an essential part of returning patients to full function. The secondary gain of symptoms must be ascertained in order to understand the potential for improvement. Patients may have limited resources, education, and familial support systems. For some, the pain facility offers a safe haven and security. Patients may fear relinquishing this security. Others may have an injury and resulting workmen's compensation from a job that they did not enjoy prior to their accident. Some individuals may also feel threatened by recovering too much. These patients must be offered the opportunity to become self-reliant. The vocational rehabilitation counselor, in conjunction with other health professionals, can assess physical capabilities along with educational and work skills. Return to the original place of employment is the ideal; however, this may not be possible, especially for jobs requiring heavy physical labor. A summary of the general principles in successful management of chronic pain patients is listed in Table 22–4.

The results seen at pain clinics have generally been good. Between 75% and 86% of patients completing a treatment program have

TABLE 22–4. PRINCIPLES FOR MANAGEMENT OF CHRONIC PAIN PATIENTS

1. Designate a definitive diagnosis early in the course of the disease
2. Communicate with and listen to patients
3. Develop a trustful doctor-patient relationship
4. Utilize a simple, constant, firm approach with patients
5. Avoid a dialogue of "organic versus psychologic" causes with the patient
6. Empower patients to be active in managing their problems
7. Treat concomitant medical disorders
8. Concentrate on function, not pain, as a goal of therapy
9. Avoid invasive diagnostic and therapeutic procedures, polypharmacy, addictive drugs
10. Schedule regular outpatient visits not contingent on the presence of symptoms
11. Continue support despite the failure of therapies
12. Promote physical activities of any variety including walking, swimming, and aerobic exercise
13. Treat depression, stress, and psychologic problems with the same vigor as physical problems
14. Refer complicated patients to comprehensive pain centers to facilitate the rehabilitation of chronic pain patients

Modified from Ghia JN: Development and organization of pain centers. In Raj PP (ed): Practical Management of Pain, 2nd ed. St Louis: Mosby Yearbook 1992, p 35.

returned to full activity and have been able to maintain this increased activity level for over a year.[13, 14] This group includes patients with work-related injuries. On admission to the Northwest Pain Center, 90% of patients were unemployed. At followup, 48% were employed.[13] Not all patients succeeded with the program with 20% returning to the use of narcotic medications. Those individuals who failed to maintain improvement continued to receive financial gain for pain. These individuals remained depressed and were passive in taking responsibility for their recovery. Little had changed in their social environment. Pain behavior continued to be rewarded.

In addition to the goals of reducing the dependence of patients on the health care system and the return of individuals to work is the goal of reducing the financial cost of treating the chronic pain patient. The use of outpatient facilities and the encouragement of patient responsibility for their own care result in cost savings.[15] Outpatient programs can achieve results comparable with inpatient facilities at a lower cost to both patient and community.

Clinicians should consider referral to a pain facility for chronic pain patients who have failed conservative therapy. Pain clinics may also be useful for surgical patients who continue to experience pain. As mentioned, the attitude of the referring physician is important to the ultimate success of this treatment program. The general goals of pain facilities and the opportunity they offer for patients to gain greater control over their lives should be emphasized.

References

1. Ng LKY: Perspective on chronic pain: treatment and research. In Ng LKY (ed): Research Monograph Series 36. Bethesda, MD: National Institute on Drug Abuse, 1981, pp 1–11.
2. Crue BL Jr: Multidisciplinary pain treatment programs: current status. Clin J Pain 1:31, 1985.
3. Bonica JJ, Black RG: The management of a pain clinic in relief of intractable pain. In Swerdlow M (ed): Monographs in Anesthesiology 1. New York: Excerpta Medica, 1974, pp 116–129.
4. Crue BL, Pinsky JJ: An approach to chronic pain of nonmalignant origin. Postgrad Med J 60:858, 1984.
5. Aronoff GM: The role of pain clinics. In Warfield CA (ed): Principles and Practice of Pain Management. New York: McGraw-Hill, Inc, 1993, pp 481–491.
6. Seres JL, Painter JR, Newman RI: Multidisciplinary treatment of chronic pain at the Northwest Pain Center. In Ng LKY (ed): Research Monograph Series 36. Bethesda, MD: National Institute on Drug Abuse, 1981, pp 41–65.
7. Aronoff GM, McAlary PW: Pain centers: treatment for intractable suffering and disability resulting from chronic pain. In Aronoff GM (ed): Evaluation and Treatment of Chronic Pain, 2nd ed. Baltimore: Williams & Wilkins, 1992, pp 416–429.
8. Gregg JM, Ghia JN: Comparative aspects of chronic pain in the head and neck versus trunk and appendages: experiences of the multidisciplinary University of North Carolina Pain Clinic. In Ng LKY (ed): Research Monograph Series 36. Bethesda, MD: National Institute on Drug Abuse, 1981, pp 112–121.
9. Aranoff GM: Pain Clinic 2: pain units provide an effective alternative technique in the management of chronic pain. Orthop Rev 11(7):95, 1982.
10. Grant AE: Massage with ice (cryokinetics) in the treatment of painful conditions of the musculoskeletal system. Arch Phys Med Rehabil 45:233, 1964.
11. Long DM: Electrical stimulation for the control of pain. Arch Surg 112:884, 1977.
12. Mechanic D: The concept of illness behavior. J Chronic Dis 15:189, 1962.
13. Painter JR, Seres JL, Newman RI: Assessing benefits of the pain center: why some patients regress. Pain 8:101, 1980.
14. Rosanoff HL, Green C, Silbret M, Steele R: Pain and low back rehabilitation program at the University of Miami School of Medicine. In Ng LKY (ed): Research Monograph Series 36. Bethesda, MD: National Institute of Drug Abuse, 1981, pp 92–111.
15. Simmons JW, Avant WS Jr, Demski J, Parisher D: Determining successful pain clinic treatment through validation of cost effectiveness. Spine 13:342, 1988.

Appendix

DISEASE ENTITY	BACK PAIN			ADDITIONAL HISTORY	PHYSICAL EXAMINATION
	Character	*Location*	*Radiation*		
Mechanical					
Cauda equina compression syndrome (deep somatic)	Sharp	Low back	Anteromedial thighs	Loss of bowel and/ or bladder control	Saddle anesthesia Decreased reflexes in legs Decreased rectal tone
Muscle strain (deep somatic)					
Mild	Sharp (acute) Ache (chronic)	Low back	Buttocks Posterior thigh	None	Point tenderness
Moderate	Sharp (acute) Ache (chronic)	Low back	Buttocks Posterior thigh	None	Point tenderness Spasm Decreased range of motion
Severe	Sharp	Low back	Buttocks Posterior thigh	None	Point tenderness Spasm Inability to walk Decreased range of motion
Herniated nucleus pulposus (radicular)					
L3-4 (L4 nerve root)	Sharp pain with numbness	Low back	Posterolateral aspect of thigh Across patella Along antero- medial aspect of leg	None	Weak knee extensor Quadriceps muscle atrophy Decreased patellar reflex
L4-5 (L5 nerve root)	Sharp pain with numbness	Low back	Anteromedial aspect of leg and foot	None	Weakness of great toe Dorsiflexion of foot Anterior tibial muscle atrophy Straight leg test + No reflex change
L5-S1 (S1 nerve root)	Sharp pain with numbness	Low back	Posterolateral aspect of leg	None	Weakness of plantar flexion of foot Calf atrophy Straight leg raising test + Decreased ankle reflex
Spinal stenosis (deep somatic, radicular)	Ache	Low back	Both legs with ambulation	Intermittent episodes of low back pain	May be normal Stress test + / −
Spondylolysis (deep somatic)	Ache	Low back	Legs	Trauma	Point tenderness
Spondylolisthesis (deep somatic)	Ache	Low back	Legs	Trauma	Increased lordosis Point tenderness
Adult scoliosis (deep somatic)	Ache	Low back	None	Deformity	Spinal deformity
Rheumatologic					
Ankylosing spondylitis	Sharp (acute) Ache (chronic)	Bilateral SI joint Midline	Posterior thigh	Male predominance Morning stiffness Pseudoclaudication	Decreased distance on Schober's test Decreased motion of LS spine in all planes Percussion tenderness
Reiter's syndrome (deep somatic)	Ache	Unilateral or bilateral SI joint Midline	Posterior thigh	Male predominance Morning stiffness Conjunctivitis Urethritis Skin lesions	Unilateral or bilateral SI joint tenderness Decreased motion of LS spine in all planes

LABORATORY ABNORMALITIES	RADIOGRAPHS	DIAGNOSIS	THERAPY	COMMENTS
Normal	Myelogram/MR	Clinical history Physical exam Myelogram/MR	Emergency surgery	Rapid surgical decompression necessary to prevent incontinence
Normal	Normal	Clinical history Physical exam	Controlled physical activity NSAIDs	Pain relief in 3–4 days
Normal	Normal	Clinical history Physical exam	Controlled physical activity NSAIDs	Pain relief in 7–10 days
Normal	Normal	Clinical history Physical exam	Controlled physical activity NSAIDs	Pain relief in 2 weeks
Normal	Plain radiographs − CT scan + Myelogram + MR +	Clinical history Physical exam Radiographs	Initial: rest, NSAIDs After 4–6 weeks with no response: epidural steroids Continued pain: surgery	70%–80% of patients with an HNP should respond to noninvasive therapy
Normal	Plain radiographs − CT scan + Myelogram + MR +	Clinical history Physical exam Radiographs	Initial: rest, NSAIDs After 4–6 weeks with no response: epidural steroids Continued pain: surgery	70%–80% of patients with an HNP should respond to noninvasive therapy
Normal	Plain radiographs − CT scan + Myelogram + MR +	Clinical history Physical exam Radiographs	Initial: rest, NSAIDs After 4–6 weeks with no response: epidural steroids Continued pain: surgery	70%–80% of patients with an HNP should respond to noninvasive therapy
Normal	Plain radiographs + CT scan + Myelogram +	Clinical history Radiographs	Controlled physical activity, NSAIDs, back support No response: epidural steroids No response: possible surgery	Majority of patients do well without surgery
Normal	Plain radiographs +	Plain radiographs	Controlled physical activity Back support	Few need surgery
Normal	Plain radiographs +	Plain radiographs	Surgery for Grades III and IV Controlled physical activity, back support for Grades I and II A few will need surgery	Surgery will not return people to full activity, just decreases pain
Normal	Plain radiographs	Plain radiographs	Bracing Progression or lack of response: surgery	Scoliosis in lumbar area usually asymptomatic— consider other diagnosis
Increased ESR HLA-B27 90%	Bilateral sacroiliitis Marginal syndesmophytes	Clinical history Plain radiographs (HLA)	Exercises NSAIDs Muscle relaxants	Pain improved with motion Iritis HLA confirmatory, not diagnostic
Increased ESR HLA-B27 80%	Unilateral or bilateral sacroiliitis Nonmarginal syndesmophytes Heel periostitis	History of clinical triad (HLA)	Exercises NSAIDs Antibiotics	Spondylitis may occur in absence of sacroiliitis

DISEASE ENTITY	BACK PAIN			ADDITIONAL HISTORY	PHYSICAL EXAMINATION
	Character	*Location*	*Radiation*		
Psoriatic spondylitis (deep somatic)	Ache	Unilateral or bilateral SI joint Midline	Posterior thigh	Morning stiffness Skin lesions	Psoriatic plaques Unilateral or bilateral SI joint tenderness Decreased motion of LS spine in all planes
Enteropathic arthritis (deep somatic, referred)	Ache	Bilateral SI joint Midline	Posterior thigh	Morning stiffness Abdominal pain Cramps	Abnormal abdominal examination Joint tenderness Decreased motion of LS spine in all planes
Behçet's syndrome (deep somatic)	Ache	Unilateral or bilateral SI joint	Posterior thigh	Morning stiffness Oral and genital ulcers Iritis Meningitis	Ulcerations Unilateral or bilateral SI joint tenderness
Whipple's disease (deep somatic)	Ache	Unilateral or bilateral SI joint	Posterior thigh	Gastrointestinal symptoms of malabsorption, fever, mental status changes	Hyperpigmentation Lymphadenopathy Percussion tenderness over SI joints Decreased motion of LS spine in all planes
Familial Mediterranean fever (deep somatic)	Ache	Unilateral or bilateral SI joint	Posterior thigh	Male predominance Episodic peritonitis	Normal between attacks
Hidradenitis suppurativa (deep somatic)	Ache	Unilateral or bilateral SI joint Midline	Posterior thigh	Skin disease precedes arthritis frequently	Axillary and inguinal disease Dissecting cellulitis Scalp lesions Acne conglobata
Rheumatoid arthritis (deep somatic)	Ache	Diffuse	Posterior thigh	Disease of long duration	Generalized involvement of hands and feet LS spine tenderness
Diffuse idiopathic skeletal hyperostosis (DISH) (deep somatic)	Mild ache	Midline	None	Dysphagia	Mild limitation of LS spine motion
Vertebral osteochondritis (deep somatic)	Ache	Midline	Hip Paravertebral muscles	Spinal angulation	Thoracic kyphosis Pain on palpation
Osteitis condensans ilii (deep somatic)	Dull ache	Bilateral or unilateral SI joint	Buttock	Pregnancy Postpartum	SI joint percussion tenderness
Polymyalgia rheumatica (deep somatic)	Muscle soreness	Shoulders Thighs	Arms Legs	Severe morning stiffness No muscle weakness	Muscle tenderness on palpation
Fibromyalgia (deep somatic)	Ache	Generalized	Tender points	Morning stiffness Fatigue Sleeplessness	Localized pain (tender points)
Infections Lumbosacral osteomyelitis (deep somatic) Bacterial	Sharp	Area infected	Paraspinous muscles	Extraosseous source of infection Fever	Percussion tenderness over involved bone Decreased motion
Tuberculous	Sharp	Area infected	Buttock	Low-grade fever Weight loss	Angular deformity Localized tenderness

LABORATORY ABNORMALITIES	RADIOGRAPHS	DIAGNOSIS	THERAPY	COMMENTS
Increased ESR HLA-B27 60%	Unilateral or bilateral sacroiliitis Nonmarginal syndesmophytes	Clinical history Skin rash Plain radiographs (HLA)	Exercises Topical skin care NSAIDs Methotrexate	Spondylitis may precede skin manifestations by many years Spondylitis may occur in absence of sacroiliitis
Increased ESR Blood in stool HLA-B27 50%	Bilateral sacroiliitis Marginal syndesmophytes	Clinical history Gastrointestinal x-ray, biopsy	Exercises NSAIDs	Activity of bowel and axial skeletal disease do not correlate
Increased ESR	Unilateral or bilateral sacroiliitis	Clinical history	Corticosteroids Thalidomide Colchicine	Ulcerations are painful
Decreased Hct Abnormal intestinal absorption studies	Unilateral or bilateral sacroiliitis	Small bowel biopsy	Procaine penicillin G Streptomycin Trimethoprim–sulfamethoxazole	Pathogenic organism—*Tropheryma whippleii*
Increased WBC Increased ESR with attacks	Unilateral or bilateral sacroiliitis	Clinical history	Colchicine	
Decreased Hct Increased ESR	Unilateral or bilateral sacroiliitis Asymmetric syndesmophytes	Skin rash Plain radiographs	Antibiotics Incision and drainage Corticosteroids Isotretinoin	Arthritis parallels activity of skin disease Sacroiliitis 80%
Decreased Hct Increased ESR Rheumatoid factor 80%	Sacroiliitis without sclerosis Lumbar spine malalignment	Clinical history Plain radiographs RA factor + Anemia	Exercises NSAIDs Antirheumatics Corticosteroids	
None	Flowing calcification on anterolateral aspect of 4 contiguous vertebral bodies	Plain radiographs	NSAIDs Exercises	
None	Vertebral body wedging Irregular endplates Limbus vertebrae	Radiographs	Exercises Bracing Surgery	Surgery for severe kyphosis, respiratory insufficiency
None	Triangular sclerosis on iliac side of SI joint	Radiographs	Exercises Firm mattress	SI joint changes confused with AS
Increased ESR Isolated increased alkaline phosphatase	None	Clinical history	Corticosteroids	Diagnosis by exclusion
None	None	Clinical history	Rest Graduated exercises NSAIDs Antidepressants	Diagnosis by exclusion
Elevated ESR Blood cultures (50%) Bone cultures (60%)	Subchondral bone loss Endplate loss Narrow disc space Contiguous endplate erosion	Positive culture Radiographs	Antibiotics Immobilization	Severe pain exacerbated by motion Hip pain Abdominal pain Meningeal signs
Bone biopsy: granulomas Cultures Positive PPD	Subchondral bone loss Endplate loss Narrow disc space Paravertebral soft tissue abscess	Positive culture Radiographs	Antibiotics Immobilization	X-ray changes occur less rapidly than with bacterial infection

DISEASE ENTITY	BACK PAIN			ADDITIONAL HISTORY	PHYSICAL EXAMINATION
	Character	*Location*	*Radiation*		
Fungal	Sharp	Area infected	Buttock	Low-grade fever	Localized tenderness
Spirochetal	Ache or none	Area infected	Buttock	Skin rash or ulcers	Localized tenderness
Parasitic	Ache or none	Area infected	Buttock	Geographic exposure	Localized tenderness
Discitis (deep somatic)	Severe, sharp	Disc infected	Flank Abdomen Lower extremity	Male predominance	Localized tenderness Marked limitation of motion
Pyogenic sacroiliitis (deep somatic)	Severe, sharp	SI joint	Buttock Thigh Calf	Male predominance Muscle spasm	Localized tenderness Patrick test + Soft tissue abscess Fever
Herpes zoster (superficial somatic, radicular)	Burning	Dermatomal	—	Fever Malaise	Vesicular dermatomal rash
Lyme disease (deep somatic, radicular)	Ache	Lumbar spine	Legs	Tick bite Erythema chronica migrans	Skin rash Radicular pain
Tumors and Infiltrative Disease *Benign* Osteoid osteoma (deep somatic)	Boring	Affected bone	Paravertebral muscles	Male predominance Young Nocturnal pain	Localized tenderness Scoliosis
Osteoblastoma (deep somatic)	Dull ache	Affected bone	Paravertebral muscles Posterior thigh	Male predominance Young	Localized tenderness and swelling scoliosis
Osteochondroma (deep somatic)	Mild ache	Affected bone	Paravertebral muscles	Male predominance Slowly progressive	Restricted spinal motion
Giant cell (deep somatic)	Intermittent ache	Affected bone		Female predominance Neurologic dysfunction	Localized bone tenderness and swelling Rectal mass with sacral involvement
Aneurysmal bone cyst (deep somatic)	Acute onset Increasing severity	Affected bone		Female predominance Young	Localized bone tenderness Skin erythema and warmth
Hemangioma (deep somatic)	Throbbing	Affected bone		Mid-life onset	Localized bone tenderness Limitation of motion with muscle spasm
Eosinophilic granuloma (deep somatic)	Persistent ache	Affected bone		Male predominance Young	Nontender swelling

LABORATORY ABNORMALITIES	RADIOGRAPHS	DIAGNOSIS	THERAPY	COMMENTS
Bone biopsy: granulomas Cultures	Anterior and posterior elements of vertebral body Spares disc	Positive culture Radiographs	Antibiotics Immobilization	Indolent course
Positive FTA	Localized lysis and sclerosis Marked dissolution	Serology Bone pathology	Antibiotics	Charcot spine Painless
—	Expansive osteolytic lesion containing trabeculae	Radiographs	Antihelminthics	
Increased ESR Increased WBC Blood culture Disc culture	Decreased disc height Reactive sclerosis adjoining vertebral bodies	Positive culture	Antibiotics Immobilization	Pain exacerbated with motion Severe muscle spasm Bone scan positive before plain radiograph MR positive before bone scan
Increased ESR Increased WBC Blood cultures (50%) Fluid culture	Blurred joint margins Erosions Sclerosis MR positive early	Positive synovial fluid culture	Antibiotics Surgical drainage if necessary	Unilateral involvement
Increased CSF WBC (33%)	Normal	Clinical history Physical examination	Analgesics Corticosteroids	Occult malignancy Often lymphoreticular
Elevated ESR Borrelia antibodies CSF pleocytosis	None	History Erythema chronica migrans	Antibiotics: early disease— oral; late disease—IV	Lyme antibodies are confirmatory, not diagnostic
Bone biopsy: nidus of osteoid, fibrous tissue, thickened cortical bone	Lytic area surrounded by sclerotic border Bone scan: hot spot	Bone biopsy	Excision Aspirin	Increased noctural pain Concave side scoliosis
Bone biopsy: osteoblasts, osteoid, giant cells	Posterior vertebral body expansile, well delineated, with periosteal new bone	Bone biopsy	Excision	Confused with osteosarcoma, but no cartilage or anaplastic cells in osteoblastoma
Bone biopsy: cartilage cap, woven bone with nests of cartilage	Posterior vertebral body well-demarcated sessile or pedunculated bone with cartilage cap	Radiographs Normal laboratory findings	Excision	Nerve impingement requires decompression Malignant degeneration with multiple osteochondromas
Bone biopsy: Osteoclastic giant cells, mononuclear stromal cells, thin-walled vessels	Anterior vetebral body expansile lesion Thin cortical margin No bony reaction	Radiographs Bone biopsy	En bloc excision	Recurrence common with partial excision Malignant transformation rare
Bone biopsy: cystic cavities lined with fibroblasts, osteoid, multinucleated giant cells	Posterior vertebral body osteolytic expansile lesion Thin dermarcated periosteal shell of bone	Radiographs	En bloc excision	Local recurrence with partial excision Pathologic fracture
Bone biopsy: increased capillary and venous vessels with sparse trabecular tissue	Anterior vertebral body prominent vertical striations with unchanged body configuration	Radiographs	Radiation therapy for symptomatic lesions	Most lesions asymptomatic Surgical excision for neural compression
Peripheral eosinophilia (10%) Increased ESR Bone biopsy: eosinophils, benign pleomorphic histiocytes	Osteolytic areas without sclerosis Vertebra plana Epidural extension on MR	Bone biopsy	Curettage	Bone biopsy findings confused with Hodgkin's disease

	BACK PAIN			ADDITIONAL HISTORY	PHYSICAL EXAMINATION
DISEASE ENTITY	*Character*	*Location*	*Radiation*		
Gaucher's disease (deep somatic)	Persistent ache	Affected bone		Abdominal distention Generalized fatigue Protracted course Intermittent exacerbations	Localized bone tenderness Abdominal organomegaly
Sacral lipoma (deep somatic)	Ache	Unilateral	Buttock Anterior thigh Lower extremity	Increased pain with compression (sleeping) Limited motion 40 years or older	Tender nodules over SI joints Flexion increases pain Obese
Malignant Multiple myeloma (deep somatic, radicular)	Mild ache (onset) Acute pain (fractures)	Affected bone	Radicular	Generalized bone pain Generalized fatigue Nausea, vomiting Mental status alterations Renal dysfunction (40 years or older)	Diffuse bone tenderness Fever Pallor
Chondrosarcoma (deep somatic, radicular)	Mild discomfort	Affected bone	Radicular	Male predominance (40–60 yr)	Painless swelling Rectal mass
Chordoma (deep somatic, radicular)	Dull or sharp Persistent	Sacral Lumbar	Hip Knee Groin	Male predominance (40–70 yr) Constipation Urinary dysfunction	Presacral mass on rectal examination Muscle flaccidity
Lymphoma (deep somatic, radicular)	Persistent ache	Affected bone	Radicular	Male predominance Pain increases with recumbency or alcohol ingestion	Localized tenderness and swelling
Skeletal metastases (deep somatic, radicular)	Gradual onset with increasing intensity	Affected bone	Radicular	Increased pain with recumbency, cough, motion Prior malignancy (over 50 years old)	Tenderness with palpation Limited motion Fever
Intraspinal neoplasms Extradural (deep somatic, radicular)	Increasing intensity Unrelenting	Affected bone	Radicular	Increased with recumbency or activity Unresponsive to mild analgesics	Tenderness with palpation Abnormal neurologic signs with compression
Intradural-extramedullary (deep somatic, radicular)	Slowly progressive	Back and leg	Radicular	Increased with recumbency, not by activity Neurofibromatosis	Gait disturbance Sensory changes Muscle atrophy Incontinence

LABORATORY ABNORMALITIES	RADIOGRAPHS	DIAGNOSIS	THERAPY	COMMENTS
Pancytopenia Increased nonprostatic acid phosphatase Decreased leukocyte glucocerebrosidase Bone marrow: Gaucher cells	Vertebral body radiolucency: accentuated vertical trabeculae Vertebra plana	Glucocerebrosidase Decreased leukocyte	Alglucerase	Accumulation of ceramide glucoside
Lipoma 1-5 cm, Fibrous capsule containing normal adipose tissue	None	Clinical history Physical exam	Local injection Surgical removal	Patients diagnosed with psychogenic rheumatism when lipoma unrecognized
Decreased Hct Increased WBC Decreased platelets Coombs' test + Increased ESR Increased calcium Increased uric acid Increased creatinine M-protein + Bence-Jones proteinuria	Diffuse vertebral body osteolysis without reactive sclerosis Spares posterior elements CT scan more sensitive	Abnormal plasma cells M-protein Electrophoresis	Chemotherapy Decompressing laminectomy and/or local radiotherapy for cord compression	Most common primary malignant tumor Bone scan does not identify bone lesion
Decreased Hct Increased ESR (late in course) Bone biopsy: verifying degree of malignant chondrocyte atypia with abnormal matrix production	Expansile, interior fluffy or lobular calcifications Thickened cortex CT scan: soft tissue extension	Bone biopsy	En bloc resection	Grade 1—slowly progressive Grade 3—more malignant, locally invasive
Decreased Hct Increased ESR (late in course) Bone biopsy: gelatinous tumor, physaliphorous cells interspersed in fibrous tissue	Osteolysis with calcific soft tissue mass Vertebral body without disc involvement initially	Bone biopsy	En bloc resection Radiotherapy for inaccessible tumors	Unpredictable clinical course, slow and indolent or rapid and destructive 10-year survival 10–40%
Decreased Hct Immunoglobulin abnormalities Disseminated disease	Osteolytic (75%) Sclerotic (15%) Mixed (5%) Periosteal (5%) Vertebral body compression fracture Spares disc space	Bone biopsy	Chemotherapy and/or radiotherapy	Potential for cure if diagnosed before extensive disease
Decreased Hct Increased ESR Urinalysis: RBC Increased alkaline phosphatase, prostatic acid phosphatase Bone biopsy: may or may not show characteristics of primary tumor	Osteolytic: lung, kidney, breast, thyroid Osteoblastic: prostate, breast, colon, bronchial carcinoid Spares disc Bone scan: 85% both symptomatic and asymptomatic areas Myelography: cord compression MR: most sensitive test	Bone biopsy if no primary neoplasm is identified	Palliative Radiotherapy Corticosteroids Decompressive laminectomy for spinal cord compression	Most common malignant lesion of the spine
Decreased Hct Increased ESR Bone biopsy: metastasis	Rapid bone destruction, body or posterior elements Myelogram: complete block, varying densities, displaces cord MR: contrast increases sensitivity	Lesional biopsy	Radiotherapy Corticosteroids Decompressive laminectomy	Metastatic lesions
Increased cerebrospinal fluid protein	Posterior scalloping of vertebral bodies Uniform dilatation of neural foramen Myelogram: sharp, smooth outline of lesion MR: contrast increases sensitivity	Radiographs	Surgical removal	Neurofibromas Meningiomas

DISEASE ENTITY	BACK PAIN			ADDITIONAL HISTORY	PHYSICAL EXAMINATION
	Character	*Location*	*Radiation*		
Intramedullary	Painless			Sensory deficits Weakness Incontinence	Abnormal pain and temperature sensation Hyperreflexia Spasticity
Endocrinologic and *Metabolic* Osteoporosis (deep somatic)	Acute (fractures) Dull (chronic)	Midline	Flank Posterior thigh Abdomen	Pain increases with motion Generalized bone pain Corticosteroids	Bone pain with spine percussion Paraspinous spasm Ileus
Osteomalacia (deep somatic)	Diffuse ache	Midline	Paravertebral muscles	Pain increases with activity and standing Muscle weakness and spasm	Bone pain with spine percussion Kyphoscoliosis Proximal muscle weakness
Parathyroid Hyperparathyroidism (deep somatic)	Diffuse ache Acute (fractures) Colic (stones)	Midline		Female predominance Gastrointestinal symptoms Genitourinary symptoms Mental status changes	Bone pain with spine percussion Kyphosis
Hypoparathyroidism (deep somatic)	Stiffness	Midline		Female predominance Muscle spasm Mental status changes	Tetany Decreased spine motion
Pituitary (deep somatic)	Ache	Midline	Lower leg	Headache Visual disturbances Muscle weakness Carpal tunnel syndrome 20–40 years old	Bone pain with spine percussion Normal range of motion Kyphosis Coarsened facial features
Microcrystalline Disease *(Deep somatic)* Gout	Acute (sharp) Chronic (ache)	SI joint Midline		Chronic peripheral gouty arthritis Male predominance	Straightening LS spine Tophi
Calcium pyrophosphate dihydrate disease	Acute (sharp) Chronic (ache)	SI joint Midline		Male predominance	Straightening LS spine Loss of motion
Ochronosis (deep somatic)	Ache	Midline		Peripheral joint arthritis Dark urine	LS spine Loss of motion Percussion tenderness Dark pigmentation of nose, ears, sclerae
Fluorosis (deep somatic)	Ache	Midline		Hand pain Weakness	Loss of motion in LS spine Generalized osteophytes Discolored teeth
Genetic Disorders Marfan syndrome (deep somatic)	Chronic ache	Diffuse low back	None	Family history Myopia Hypermobility	Arachnodactyly Scoliosis Aortic murmur

LABORATORY ABNORMALITIES	RADIOGRAPHS	DIAGNOSIS	THERAPY	COMMENTS
—	Myelogram: fusiform enlargement MR +	Lesional biopsy	Surgical removal	Ependymomas Gliomas
Primary: normal Secondary: decreased Hct, increased ESR Pyridinolines	Diffuse vertebral involvement Endplate "fish vertebrae" Compression fractures DEXA scan—decreased bone mineral	Clinical history Confirmed by bone biopsy	Calcium Vitamin D Estrogens Calcitonin Etidronate Fluoride—investigational	Women 65 years old 50% asymptomatic osteoporosis, 3% disabling Back pain with fracture may persist indefinitely
Decreased serum calcium, vitamin D, phosphate Increased alkaline phosphatase Decreased urinary calcium Increased parathyroid hormone Bone biopsy: increased osteoid, inadequate mineralization	"Cod-fish" vertebrae Scoliosis "Hot spots" on bone scan—Looser's zones	Clinical history confirmed by bone biopsy	Vitamin D Calcium Phosphate	
Increased serum calcium Decreased phosphate Increased chloride Increased alkaline phosphatase Increased serum parathormone	Resorption at symphysis pubis, SI joints Wedge vertebrae "Rugger-jersey" spine Schmorl's nodes	Surgical removal of abnormal parathyroid tissue	Surgery in symptomatic patients NSAIDs Braces	Clinical diagnosis: Hypercalcemia Secondary forms—renal osteodystrophy
Decreased serum calcium Increased serum phosphate Normal alkaline phosphatase	Osteosclerosis Calcification of longitudinal ligaments	Serum parathormone decreased	Vitamin D Calcium	
Increased growth hormone, somatomedin-C, phosphate, glucose, alkaline phosphatase	Anterior and lateral osteophytes Posteriorly scalloped vertebral bodies Increased disc space Disc calcification	Non-suppressible increased growth hormone concentrations	Ablation of pituitary tumor Bromocriptine Octreotide	Progressive degenerative back changes despite normalization of growth hormone concentrations
Monosodium urate monohydrate crystals Increased serum uric acid	SI joint erosions Marginal sclerosis	Monosodium urate monohydrate crystals	Colchicine NSAIDs Corticosteroids (acute) Uricosurics Xanthine oxidase inhibitors (chronic)	
Calcium pyrophosphate dihydrate crystals	Disc calcification and narrowing Osteophytes	Calcium pyrophosphate dihydrate crystals	NSAIDs Colchicine (33%)	Secondary forms: Hyperparathyroidism Hemochromatosis Hypothyroidism Wilson's disease Ochronosis
Dark alkalinized urine	Disc narrowing and calcification Osteophytes Bone scan—spinal whiskering	Homogentisic acid in urine	Rest NSAIDs Analgesics	Homogentisic acid oxidase deficiency Bony overgrowth Confused with ankylosing spondylitis
Increased urinary fluoride, serum alkaline phosphatase	Osteosclerosis Osteophytes Calcification of soft tissues, including entheses, ligaments	Urinary fluoride Radiographs Bone biopsy	Limit fluoride exposure and intake	Fluoride exposure: Drinking water Insecticides
None	Posterior scalloping Double curve scoliosis Spinal canal enlargement	Clinical criteria	Bracing Operative stabilization of scoliosis	Abnormal fibrillin gene chromosome 15

DISEASE ENTITY	BACK PAIN			ADDITIONAL HISTORY	PHYSICAL EXAMINATION
	Character	Location	Radiation		
Mucopolysaccharidoses Morquio's syndrome (deep somatic)	Chronic ache	Diffuse		Onset in childhood Decreased hearing Normal intelligence	Short stature Kyphoscoliosis Clouded corneas Ligamentous laxity Hepatomegaly
Hematologic Disorders Hemoglobinopathies (deep somatic)	Pressure ache	Midline	Flank	Black predominance Repeated episodes of bone pain Cholelithiasis Pulmonary infarcts Pneumonia	Bone tenderness increased with palpation Fever with crises
Myelofibrosis (deep somatic)	Severe sharp	Midline		Weakness Weight loss Abdominal pain or fullness 50 years old	Bone tenderness Splenomegaly
Mastocytosis (deep somatic)	Ache	Midline		Hyperpigmentation Urticaria Diarrhea Flushing	Bone tenderness Hepatosplenomegaly Skin pigmentation
Neurologic and Psychiatric Disorders Neuropathy (femoral, radicular)	Burning	Paraspinous	Thigh Knee	Episodes of lancinating pain, increased at night Pain not increased with cough	Pelvic girdle and thigh weakness Absent knee reflex
Psychogenic rheumatism Depression (psychogenic)	Dull ache	Low back		Listlessness Sleepiness Anorexia Constipation	Normal
Malingering (psychogenic)	Severe constant	Entire back	Nondermatomal	No relief with any therapy Job-related	Inconsistent abnormalities Nondermatomal sensory loss Pain with head compression
Referred Pain *Vascular (Visceral-referred)* Abdominal aortic aneurysm	Dull constant (chronic)	Left paraspinous	Hips Thighs	Caucasian men 60–70 years old Claudication Epigastric pain Hypertension Diabetes Smoking	Pulsatile abdominal mass Bruits Hypotension with rupture
Genitourinary (Visceral-referred) Kidney stone	Dull persistent and/or sharp cramping	Costovertebral	None *or* Genitalia	20–60 years old History of gout Acute severe pain Writhing with nausea and vomiting	Tender costovertebral angle Paraspinous spasm Acute scoliosis
Pyelonephritis	Dull persistent	Costovertebral angle (CVA)	None	Female 20–60 years old Diabetic UTI in childhood Foul-smelling urine Chills Neurogenic bladder	Tender CVA Fever
Ureteropelvic junction obstruction	Dull persistent Sharp	CVA	None	Flank pain with fluid intake or diuretics	Tender CVA

LABORATORY ABNORMALITIES	RADIOGRAPHS	DIAGNOSIS	THERAPY	COMMENTS
Increased urinary keratan sulfate	Platyspondyly Central beaking of vertebral bodies Increased kyphosis	Increased keratan sulfate	Bracing	Galactosamine-6-sulfate sulfatase deficiency Mild form of β-galactosidase deficiency
Decreased Hct Increased WBC Increased serum bilirubin	Coarsened trabeculae Osteoporosis "Fish-mouth" vertebrae Bone sclerosis	Hemoglobin Electrophoresis	Hydration Analgesics	Sickle cell anemia most common form
Decreased Hct Increased WBC Increased uric acid Bone marrow biopsy: fibrosis, hypocellularity	Osteosclerosis of inferior and superior endplates	Bone marrow biopsy	Transfusions Analgesics Radiotherapy Bone marrow transplant	Acute myelogenous leukemia (20%)
Decreased Hct Increased WBC Increased mast cells Bone marrow biopsy: fibrosis, bone matrix increased	Admixture of osteosclerosis and osteoporosis	Bone marrow biospy	Transfusions Analgesics H_2 blockers H_1 blockers Cromolyn	Mast cells mistaken for granulomas in bone marrow biopsy
Hyperglycemia Elevated CSF protein	Normal	Clinical examination Slowed nerve conduction	Analgesics Glucose control Mexiletene	Diabetes common cause
Normal	Normal	History	Antidepressants	
Normal	Normal	History Physical examination	Psychiatric	
Normal or decreased Hct	Cross-table lateral: curvilinear calcification CT scan or sonogram: vessel enlargement	Radiographic visualization	Surgical excision	Femoral nerve entrapment with retroperitoneal bleeding
Microscopic hematuria	KUB: stone IVP: confirms location, rules out obstruction	History Physical exam Urinalysis KUB IVP	Observation Extracorporeal shock wave lithotripsy Percutaneous removal	Open surgery has become less frequent
Pyuria WBC casts Culture +	IVP: renal swelling Sonogram: enlarged kidney Gallium scan +	History Urinalysis	Antibiotics	Obstruction Abscess must be ruled out
Normal urine	IVP: dilated renal pelvis, hydronephrosis Sonogram: same findings Renal scan: obstruction	History Radiologic studies	Surgical repair Observation Nephrectomy	Often asymptomatic and diagnosed incidentally Capsular distention

DISEASE ENTITY	BACK PAIN			ADDITIONAL HISTORY	PHYSICAL EXAMINATION
	Character	*Location*	*Radiation*		
Renal infarction	Acute sharp	CVA	None	Heart disease Atrial fibrillation Vascular disease Hypertension	Tender CVA Ileus
Renal cancer	None Dull Sharp	CVA	None	Gross hematuria	Abdominal mass Abdominal flank tenderness
Ureter Stone in upper ureter	Colicky Sharp	Flank Paraspinous	Genitalia Lower quadrant	20–60 years old Stone Gout Acute-onset nausea and vomiting	CVA tenderness Abdominal tenderness Paraspinous spasm Acute scoliosis
Stone in lower ureter	Colicky Sharp	Lower quadrant	Genitalia	Writhing with episode Frequency Urgency	
Vesicoureteral reflux	Dull	Flank, unilateral or bilateral	None	Female pyelonephritis Flank pain with voiding UTI childhood	Negative
Bladder Urinary retention	Dull	Sacral	None	Male over 60 Difficulty voiding Incontinence	Lower abdominal midline mass Prostatic enlargement
Urinary infection	Dull	Sacral	None	Sexually active women Frequency Urgency Afebrile	Tender lower abdomen Tender bladder on pelvic exam
Prostate Chronic prostatitis	Dull	Lumbosacral	None	Prior nongonococcal urethritis Discharge Urinary irritation Testicular perineal pain	Normal or lumpy, bumpy prostate
Carcinoma	Dull insidious Sharp focal	Vertebral bodies	Legs	Difficulty voiding Urinary frequency	Focal vertebral tenderness Rock-hard prostate
Testis Cancer	Dull	Lumbar	None	Testicular fullness Weight loss Gynecomastia	Testicular mass Abdominal mass Percussion tenderness along spine
Uterus Leiomyomas	Ache Pressure	Sacrum	Thigh	Abdominal heaviness +/− Abnormal menses	Palpable masses
Retroverted	Pressure	Sacrum	Thigh	Dysmenorrhea Dyspareunia	Retroverted uterus
Prolapsed	Pulling	Sacrum	—	—	Cervical descent to vulva

LABORATORY ABNORMALITIES	RADIOGRAPHS	DIAGNOSIS	THERAPY	COMMENTS
Normal urine	IVP: kidney not seen Sonogram: normal Renal scan: no flow Arteriogram: identifies location	History Radiologic studies	Surgical after <24 hours observation	Diagnosis often delayed, resulting in kidney loss
Hematuria	IVP: mass Sonogram: solid mass CT scan: solid mass, nodes, tumor, clot Arteriogram: mass, tumor, clot	History Radiologic studies	Radical nephrectomy	Incidentally found Commonly classic triad: flank pain, hematuria, abdominal mass
Microscopic hematuria	KUB: calcium stone IVP: stone site, obstruction	History Urinalysis Radiographs	Analgesics Antiemetics Extracorporeal shock wave lithotripsy Transurethral stone manipulation Percutaneous stone removal	Surgical removal infrequently indicated
Renal impairment in minority	Cystogram: reveals reflux IVP: dilated ureters, renal atrophy	History Cystogram	Ureteral reimplantation Observation Antibiotics	Ureteral reimplantation eliminates pyelonephritis
Renal impairment in minority	IVP: post-void residual, hydronephrosis Sonogram: bladder distention, hydronephrosis	Physical exam Radiographs	Catheterization Prostatectomy	Clinical presentation: slow progression
Hematuria Pyria Positive culture	None	History Physical exam	Antibiotics Bladder analgesics	Usually respond in 24 hours, otherwise complicating factors
Inflammation in prostatic secretion	None	History Prostatic secretion	Antibiotics Massage	Prostate is most frequently normal Secretion is obtained by massage Commonly overlooked cause of back pain
Elevated acid phosphatase Prostatic specific antigen	Bone scan: uptake in blastic lesions	Physical exam Radiographs	Hormonal therapy Observation	30–40% of prostatic cancer patients present with metastatic disease Acute paraplegia is rare complication
Elevated tumor markers: alpha-fetoprotein, beta-HCG	IVP: Deviated ureter CT scan: abdominal mass	Physical exam Radiographs	Orchiectomy Chemotherapy Surgery	Back pain is reflection of bulky retroperitoneal disease
Decreased Hct	Sonography: uterine masses	Sonography Physical exam	Surgery	
None	Sonography: posterior position	Physical exam	Surgery	
None	Sonography: prolapsed position	Physical exam	Surgery	

DISEASE ENTITY	BACK PAIN			ADDITIONAL HISTORY	PHYSICAL EXAMINATION
	Character	*Location*	*Radiation*		
Endometriosis	Cyclic cramping	Sacrum	Thigh	Dysmenorrhea	Beading of uterosacral ligaments
Pregnancy	Ache Pulling	SI joints Pubis	Thigh	Increases with duration of pregnancy	Hyperlordosis
Fallopian tube Pelvic inflammatory disease	Acute, sharp	Sacrum	Thigh	Fever Discharge	Pelvic tenderness on motion of cervix and adnexa
Ectopic pregnancy	Pressure Pain	Sacrum	Thigh	Missed menses	Adnexal tenderness, mass
Ovary Benign neoplasm	Pressure Ache	Sacrum	—		Adnexal masses
Malignant neoplasm	Ache	Paraspinous	Thigh	Weight loss Increased abdominal girth	Adnexal mass Ascites
Gastrointestinal (Visceral-Referred) *Pancreas* Pancreatitis Acute	Severe, sharp	Midline (L1)	From epigastrium	Alcoholism Gall stone Hypertriglyceridemia	Fever Tachycardia Hypotension Abdominal tenderness
Chronic	Boring, constant	Midline (L1)	From epigastrium	Anorexia Weight loss New-onset diabetes Greasy stools Jaundice Male predominance	Abdominal mass (pseudocyst)
Tumor	Dull or sharp Episodic or continuous	Midline	From epigastrium	Anorexia Weight loss Jaundice	Abdominal mass
Biliary Tree *Gallbladder* Acute cholecystitis	Severe Colicky	Right paraspinous	From right upper quadrant	Nausea Vomiting Female predominance 40 years old	Fever Abdominal guarding
Hollow Viscus *Stomach/Duodenum* Gastric ulcer Duodenal ulcer	Boring Burning	Midline (L1)	From epigastrium	Alcohol Caffeine Drugs Smoking	Epigastric tenderness
Colon Diverticulitis	Persistent cramp	Sacrum	From left lower quadrant	Change in bowel habits	Tender left lower quadrant Decreased bowel sounds Rectal or lower quadrant mass

LABORATORY ABNORMALITIES	RADIOGRAPHS	DIAGNOSIS	THERAPY	COMMENTS
None	Normal	Physical exam Laparoscopy	Hormonal supplementation Surgery	Rare episodes of sciatica
None	Normal	Physical exam Laparoscopy	Support Exercises Delivery	Relaxation of uterosacral ligaments, pain with increased load and strain
Gram stain Cultures	Normal	Culture	Antibodies	
Pregnancy test +	Sonography: adnexal enlargement	Laparoscopy	Surgery	
None	Sonography: mass	Physical exam Laparoscopy	Hormonal supplementation Surgery	
Decreased Hct CEA +	Sonography: mass	Physical exam Biopsy	Surgery Chemotherapy	Ovarian carcinoma with extension causes back pain
Increased trypsin, amylase, lipase	Pleural effusions Sentinel loop CT scan or sonogram: diffusely enlarged pancreas	Increased trypsin and amylase Compatible sonogram or CT scan	Hydration Nasogastric suction Treat complication: shock, renal or pulmonary insufficiency, abscesses	Pain lasts for days Increased in supine position, decreased in forward flexion Head—right of spine, tail—left of spine
Decreased Hct Decreased trypsinogen Increased alkaline phosphatase	CT scan or sonogram: pancreatic calcification, pseudocyst	Decreased trypsinogen Compatible CT scan or sonogram	Enzyme replacement Insulin Pseudocyst drainage	Common cause: Alcoholism Biliary tract disease
Decreased Hct Increased alkaline phosphatase Increased bilirubin	CT scan or sonography: pancreatic mass, liver metastases, enlarged intra-abdominal lymph glands	Needle biopsy or laparotomy	Pancreatectomy Diversion-bypass procedure	
Increased WBC Increased bilirubin Increased amylase	Scintiscan: non-visualization of gall bladder Sonography: stones	Scintiscan Sonography	Fluids Analgesics Antibiotics Nasogastric suction Surgery: perforation, abscess	Pain begins abruptly, subsides gradually Chronic cholecystitis and choledocholi-thiasis have similar clinical patterns Episodic pain
Decreased Hct Increased amylase	Posterior ulcer	Endoscopy	Histamine receptor antagonists Surface agents Antacids	Pancreatitis with duodenal penetration
Increased WBC Abnormal urinalysis	Localized diverticulosis Microperforations Obstructive gas pattern	Barium studies	Antibiotics Surgical drainage of abscesses	

DISEASE ENTITY	BACK PAIN			ADDITIONAL HISTORY	PHYSICAL EXAMINATION
	Character	*Location*	*Radiation*		
Cancer	Ache	Sacrum	Legs	Weight loss	Hard, nontender rectal or abdominal mass
Miscellaneous Disorders Paget's disease (deep somatic, radicular)	Deep, boring	Affected bone	Legs	40 years or older Pain with walking Increasing skull size Deafness	Decreased spine motion Percussion tenderness with bone fracture Scalp veins Angioid streaks
Endocarditis (deep somatic, radicular)	Diffuse ache	Low back	Legs	Fever Chills Anorexia Arthralgias Myalgias	Heart murmur Peripheral arthritis Skin rash
Vertebral sarcoidosis (deep somatic)	Intermittent stabbing Dull	Involved bone	Thighs	Black men Cough Dyspnea Anorexia Weight loss	Percussion tenderness Limitation of motion Skin rash Lymphadenopathy Abnormal breath sounds
Retroperitoneal fibrosis	Dull Insidious	Lumbar spine, flank	None	Over 40 years old Weight loss Decreased urine output Low-grade fever	Abdominal rectal exam Empty bladder Percussion tenderness over costovertebral angles and paravertebral areas

LABORATORY ABNORMALITIES	RADIOGRAPHS	DIAGNOSIS	THERAPY	COMMENTS
Decreased Hct Hemoccult positive stools Increased ESR	Abnormal barium enema	Colonoscopy Flexible sigmoidoscopy Biopsy	Surgery	
Increased alkaline phosphatase, urinary hydroxyproline Bone biopsy: increased osteoclastic activity with mosaic and woven bone osteoblastic response	Lytic and sclerotic areas in vertebrae "Picture frame" appearance Enlarged "ivory" vertebrae Scintiscan: increased bone activity	Laboratory abnormalities Biopsy rarely	NSAIDs Calcitonin Diphosphonates	Bone involvement Asymptomatic in many Cauda equina syndrome rare Slow virus infection
Decreased Hct Increased WBC Increased ESR Rheumatoid factor + after 6 weeks	Abnormal chest x-ray	Blood cultures New murmur	Antibiotics	Delay in diagnosis Worse prognosis in those with musculoskeletal symptoms Vertebral osteomyelitis, radicular "disc-like" symptoms in minority
Increased calcium Increased alkaline phosphatase Increased gamma globulins Increased angiotensin converting enzyme Increased ESR Cutaneous anergy Biopsy: noncaseating granuloma	Bone lysis with marginal sclerosis Vertebral body collapse Paravertebral ossification Disc space narrowing	Bone biopsy	Corticosteroids Surgical decompression	Patients with extrathoracic disease have worse prognosis
Impaired renal function No urine production Increased ESR	IVP: medial deviation of ureters Retrograde study: same CT scan: mass, ureteral and vascular encasement MR—extent and activity of fibrosis	Radiographs (biopsy)	Ureteral stents Ureterolysis Corticosteroids	Rare entity: may have idiopathic or neoplastic etiology

EVALUATION	BACK STRAIN	HERNIATED NUCLEUS PULPOSUS	SPINAL STENOSIS	SPONDYLOLISTHESIS/ INSTABILITY	SPONDYLO-ARTHROPATHY	INFECTION	TUMOR	METABOLIC	HEMA-TOLOGIC	VISCERAL
Predominant pain (back vs. leg)	Back	Leg (below knee)	Back/leg	Back	Back	Back	Back	Back	Back	Back (buttock, thigh)
Constitutional symptoms					+	+	+	+	+	+
Tension sign		+		+/−						
Neurologic exam		+/−	+/− after stress			+/−	+/−			
Plain x-rays			+	+	+	+/−	+/−	+	+	
Lateral motion x-rays				+						
CT/MR		+	+			+	+			+
Myelogram		+	+							
Bone scan					+	+	+	+	+	
ESR					+	+	+		+	+
Serum chemistries							+	+	+	+

+ / −, positive in only some patients with the condition

INDEX

Note: Page numbers in *italics* refer to illustrations; page numbers followed by (t) refer to tables.